GEORGE J. HILL, II, M.D.

Professor and Chairman,
Department of Surgery,
Marshall University School of Medicine,
Huntington, West Virginia

Outpatient Surgery

SECOND EDITION

1980
W. B. SAUNDERS COMPANY
Philadelphia • London • Toronto

W. B. Saunders Company: West Washington Square
                           Philadelphia, PA   19105

                           1 St. Anne's Road
                           Eastbourne, East Sussex BN21 3UN, England

                           1 Goldthorne Avenue
                           Toronto, Ontario M8Z 5T9, Canada

Outpatient Surgery   ISBN 0-7216-4676-X

Last digit is the print number: 9   8   7   6   5   4   3   2   1

To Lana, Sarah, Dave and Jim

Contributors

MENELAOS A. ALIAPOULIOS, M.D. Professor of Surgery, University of Massachusetts Medical School. Chief of Surgery, St. Vincent Hospital, Worcester, Massachusetts. Surgeon, Peter Bent Brigham Hospital, New England Baptist Hospital, and New England Deaconess Hospital, Boston, Massachusetts.

Metabolism and Endocrinology

MALCOLM DENNIS BARTON, M.D. Associate Professor of Anesthesiology (Clinical), University of Colorado School of Medicine, Denver, Colorado. Attending Anesthesiologist, Presbyterian Medical Centers, Aurora and Denver, Colorado.

Anesthesia for Outpatients; The Unconscious Patient

ROBERT W. BEART, JR., M.D. Consultant in Surgery, Mayo Medical School, Rochester, Minnesota. Attending Staff, Methodist Hospital and St. Mary's Hospital, Minneapolis, Minnesota.

Outpatient and Short Stay Fiberoptic Endoscopy

RICHARD A. BLATH, M.D. Attending Staff, St. Luke's Hospitals, DePaul Hospital, Christian Hospital Northeast, St. Louis, Missouri, and Christian Hospital Northwest, Florissant, Missouri.

Urology

PAUL W. BROWN, M.D. Clinical Professor of Surgery (Orthopaedics), Yale University School of Medicine, New Haven, Connecticut. Chairman, Department of Surgery, St. Vincent's Medical Center, Bridgeport, Connecticut. Consultant in Hand Surgery, Veterans' Administration Hospital, West Haven, Connecticut.

The Hand

JOHN D. BURRINGTON, M.S., M.D. Clinical Professor of Surgery, University of Colorado School of Medicine. Director of Surgical Education, Children's Hospital, Denver, Colorado.

Pediatric Surgery

JAMES R. CERASOLI, M.D. Associate Clinical Professor of Ophthalmology, University of Colorado School of Medicine. Attending Staff, Colorado General Hospital, Porter Memorial Hospital, Denver, Colorado, and Swedish Medical Center, Englewood, Colorado.

The Eye

BEN EISEMAN, M.D. Professor of Surgery, University of Colorado School of Medicine. Director of Surgery, Rose Medical Center; Attending Staff, Colorado General Hospital, Denver General Hospital, Fitzsimons Army Medical Center, and Veterans' Administration Hospital, Denver, Colorado.

> *Surgery and Medicine in the Field*

GERALD M. ENGLISH, M.D. Clinical Associate Professor of Otolaryngology, University of Colorado Medical Center. Attending Staff, Porter Memorial Hospital, Veterans' Administration Hospital, General Rose Memorial Hospital, National Jewish Hospital, St. Luke's Hospital, St. Anthony Hospital, Presbyterian Medical Center, Fitzsimons Army Medical Center, Denver, Colorado; Swedish Medical Center, Englewood, Colorado; and Lutheran Hospital, Wheat Ridge, Colorado.

> *Ear, Nose, Throat and Sinuses*

WILLIAM R. FAIR, M.D. Professor of Surgery and Chairman of Department of Urology, Washington University School of Medicine. Attending Staff, Barnes Hospital, St. Louis, Missouri.

> *Urology*

JOHN QUITER GALLAGHER, M.D. Associate Clinical Professor of Surgery, University of Colorado Medical Center. Attending Surgeon, Presbyterian Hospital and St. Joseph Hospital, Denver, Colorado.

> *The Breast*

JOHN D. HARRAH, M.D. Associate Professor of Surgery, Marshall University School of Medicine. Attending Thoracic and Cardiovascular Surgeon, St. Mary's Hospital, Cabell Huntington Hospital, and Veterans' Hospital, Huntington, West Virginia.

> *Organization and Functions of Emergency Department, Outpatient Clinic and Office Practice*

LELAND GREENE HAWKINS, M.D. Head of Medical Education Committee, St. Luke's Methodist Hospital and Mercy Hospital, Cedar Rapids, Iowa. Practicing Orthopedic Surgeon.

> *Musculoskeletal System: Fractures and Dislocations*

JOHN A. HIGGINS, M.D. Consultant in Gastroenterology, Mayo Clinic; Associate Professor in Internal Medicine, Mayo Medical School, Rochester, Minnesota. Attending Staff, Methodist Hospital and St. Mary's Hospital, Minneapolis, Minnesota.

> *Outpatient and Short Stay Fiberoptic Endoscopy*

GEORGE JAMES HILL, II, M.D. Professor and Chairman, Department of Surgery, Marshall University School of Medicine. Chief of Surgery, Family Care Outpatient Center; Staff Surgeon, Veterans' Administration Hospital; Active Surgical Staff, Cabell Huntington Hospital and St. Mary's Hospital; Consultant, Huntington (State) Hospital, Huntington, West Virginia. Courtesy Surgical Staff, Appalachian Regional Hospital; Honorary Surgical Staff, Raleigh General Hospital, Beckley, West Virginia.

> *Organization and Functions of Emergency Department, Outpatient Clinic and Office Practice; Metabolism and Endocrinology; The Abdomen and Gastrointestinal Tract; Cancer Chemotherapy*

PETER JOKL, M.D. Director of Athletic Medicine and Associate Professor of Surgery (Orthopaedic), Yale University School of Medicine, New Haven, Connecticut.

Orthopaedics

JAMES R. JONES, M.D. Professor and Chairman, Department of Obstetrics and Gynecology, College of Medicine and Dentistry of New Jersey, Rutgers Medical School, Piscataway, New Jersey. Senior Attending Staff, Middlesex General Hospital, New Brunswick, New Jersey.

Female Genitourinary Tract and Obstetrics

EKKEHARD KEMMANN, M.D. Assistant Professor, Department of Obstetrics and Gynecology, College of Medicine and Dentistry of New Jersey, Rutgers Medical School, Piscataway, New Jersey. Attending Staff, Middlesex General Hospital, New Brunswick, New Jersey.

Female Genitourinary Tract and Obstetrics

ROBERT R. LARSEN, M.D. Assistant Clinical Professor of Surgery, University of Colorado School of Medicine, Denver, Colorado. Chief of Surgery, Brighton Community Hospital, Brighton, Colorado.

Outpatient Surgery in Developing Countries

YEU-TSU N. (MARGARET) LEE, M.D. Associate Professor of Surgery, University of Southern California School of Medicine. Head Physician, Tumor Surgery Service, Los Angeles County–USC Medical Center, Los Angeles, California.

Tumors

MALCOLM A. LESAVOY, M.D. Assistant Professor of Surgery, Division of Plastic Surgery, UCLA School of Medicine, Los Angeles, California. Chief of Plastic and Reconstructive Surgery, Harbor General Hospital, Torrance, California.

The Integument

ANDREW M. MUNSTER, M.D., F.R.C.S. (Eng. and Ed.) Associate Professor of Surgery, The Johns Hopkins University School of Medicine. Director, Baltimore Regional Burn Center; Attending Surgeon, Johns Hopkins Hospital, Baltimore City Hospitals, and Loch Raven Veterans' Administration Hospital, Baltimore, Maryland.

Infections

MELVIN M. NEWMAN, M.D. Associate Professor, University of Colorado School of Medicine. Attending Staff, Colorado General Hospital, Denver, Colorado.

The Heart and Lungs — Thorax: Lungs and Esophagus

LAWRENCE W. NORTON, M.D. Professor of Surgery, University of Arizona College of Medicine. Associate Head, Department of Surgery, and Chief of General Surgery, University of Arizona Health Sciences Center, Tucson, Arizona.

Trauma

THOMAS R. O'DONOVAN, Ph.D. Administrator, Mount Carmel Mercy Hospital, Detroit, Michigan.

Recent Developments in Ambulatory Surgery

J. CUTHBERT OWENS, M.D. Professor of Surgery, University of Colorado School of Medicine. Attending Staff, Colorado General Hospital, General Rose Memorial Hospital, Denver General Hospital, and Veterans' Administration Hospital, Denver, Colorado.

Peripheral Blood Vessels

BRUCE C. PATON, M.R.C.P. (Ed.), F.R.C.S. (Ed.) Professor of Surgery, University of Colorado School of Medicine. Attending Staff, Colorado General Hospital, Denver General Hospital, Children's Hospital, Veterans' Administration Hospital, and Fitzsimons Army General Hospital, Denver, Colorado.

The Heart and Lungs — Heart and Great Vessels; Surgery and Medicine in the Field

ISRAEL PENN, M.D., F.R.C.S. (Eng.), F.R.C.S. (Can.) Professor of Surgery, University of Colorado Medical Center. Chief of Surgery, Veterans' Administration Hospital; Attending Surgeon, Colorado General Hospital, Children's Hospital, and Rose Medical Center, Denver, Colorado.

Transplantation

WILLIAM ROBERT ROSS, D.P.M. Chief of Podiatry Clinics, Denver General Hospital. Surgical Staff, Highland Medical Center; Consultant, Porter Memorial Hospital, Denver, Colorado, and Swedish Medical Center, Englewood, Colorado.

The Foot

ROBERT BARRY RUTHERFORD, M.D. Professor of Surgery, University of Colorado School of Medicine. Attending Staff, Colorado General Hospital, Veterans' Administration Hospital, and Denver General Hospital, Denver, Colorado.

Organization and Functions of Emergency Department, Outpatient Clinic and Office Practice; Peripheral Blood Vessels

JOHN EDWARD LAWSON SALES, M.A., M.Chir., F.R.C.S. (Eng.) Consultant Surgeon, Hillingdon Hospital, Oxbridge, and Mount Vernon Hospital, Northwood, Middlesex, England.

Anus and Rectum

NANCY S. SCHER, M.D. Assistant Professor of Medicine, Marshall University School of Medicine. Attending Staff, Veterans' Administration Medical Center; Associate Staff, St. Mary's Hospital and Cabell Huntington Hospital, Huntington, West Virginia.

Cancer Chemotherapy

ALEX M. STONE, M.D. Associate Professor of Clinical Surgery, State University of New York at Stony Brook, Health Sciences Center School of Medicine. Staff Surgeon, Long Island Jewish–Hillside Medical Center, New Hyde Park, New York.

The Abdomen and Gastrointestinal Tract

R. C. A. WEATHERLEY-WHITE, M.D. Associate Clinical Professor of Surgery (Plastic), University of Colorado School of Medicine, Denver, Colorado.

The Integument

PHILIP R. WEINSTEIN, M.D. Associate Professor, University of Arizona College of Medicine. Chief of Neurosurgery, Veterans' Administration Hospital; Attending Staff, University of Arizona Hospital, Tucson, Arizona.

The Skull and Nervous System

AUGUSTUS A. WHITE, III, M.D., D. Med. Sci. Professor of Orthopaedic Surgery, Harvard Medical School. Orthopaedic Surgeon-in-Chief, Beth Israel Hospital, Boston, Massachusetts.

Orthopaedics

CHARLES B. WILSON, M.D. Professor and Chairman, Department of Neurological Surgery, University of California (San Francisco) School of Medicine, San Francisco, California.

The Skull and Nervous System

LESLIE WISE, M.D. Professor of Surgery, State University of New York at Stony Brook, Health Sciences Center School of Medicine, Stony Brook, New York. Chairman, Department of Surgery, Long Island Jewish–Hillside Medical Center, New Hyde Park, New York.

The Abdomen and Gastrointestinal Tract

DAVID S. WOLF, D.P.M. Podiatric Medical Staff, Highland Medical Center, Denver, Colorado.

The Foot

Preface

The weary, frightened faces crowded together in the waiting rooms of large hospitals and busy offices are a constant reminder that our methods are imperfect and we must labor to improve them. This book was prepared to assist in the delivery of more effective, efficient care to all who appear at the doors of our medical facilities — to help surgeons and their assistants select, treat and release those patients who can be managed in the context of the Outpatient Department. Anyone who has heard the commotion, smelled the fear and anger, and seen the turmoil of the Outpatient Department will appreciate the need for better service in this area. It is to this end the authors have worked to prepare a guide for outpatient surgery.

GEORGE J. HILL
Huntington, West Virginia 25701

Acknowledgments

Preparation of this edition of *Outpatient Surgery* has been greatly helped by the many readers who have written to or spoken with us to offer suggestions and comments on the first edition and by those who reviewed the first edition for various journals.

I am especially grateful for comments offered by the students, surgical house staff and nurses at the University of Colorado, Washington University, and Marshall University and by the surgical staff of Colorado General Hospital, Barnes Hospital, St. Louis City Hospital, the Marshall University affiliated hospitals, and the Family Care Outpatient Center. The observations by scores of other surgeons, young and old, have helped us in the preparation of the present edition, including those in several U.S. Naval Hospitals and dispensaries, the University of Saigon's affiliated hospitals, and my colleagues in the Central Oncology Group and the Southeastern Cancer Study Group. I have been given courteous and helpful tours of many outpatient facilities and ambulatory surgical units during the past six years, too numerous to cite individually here, including many university hospitals, private hospitals and surgeons' offices. A substantial improvement in outpatient service is occurring, and I appreciate the opportunities I have been given to see the new facilities and new methods that are being used.

Encouragement to continue this work has come from my academic supervisors: Drs. William R. Waddell, Thomas E. Starzl, Walter F. Ballinger and Robert W. Coon. I was also encouraged by my family, including my patient wife, Lanie, my children—to whom this edition is dedicated—and my parents, who taught me to read and write well enough to have my work published. My father died as this edition was going to press, but he watched the work progress with a proud yet critical eye.

I am particularly indebted to the warm, enthusiastic and accurate advice I have received for nearly a decade from Mr. John Hanley, now Vice President and Publisher of the W. B. Saunders Company. Jack and I first became acquainted when he was assigned as an associate medical editor to the development of the first edition. His suggestions played a major role in every phase of development of

xiii

both editions, plus our foreign editions and the Spanish translation. Many others from the W. B. Saunders Company have helped with the second edition or both editions, particularly Janis Moore, Lorraine Battista, Herb Powell and Andrew J. Piernock, Jr. This group is Jack Hanley's team, and I am most grateful to him for bringing their efforts together for us. The work of Mrs. Dorothy Irwin, the artist for the first edition, continues to be the main body of illustration for the second edition, and we appreciate her ability to clarify our language with her brush and pen.

The burden of secretarial work in my office for this edition has been carried with care and accuracy by Mrs. Carole Mathi, Mrs. Barbara White and Ms. Catherine Tyson.

This work was supported in part by a Junior Faculty Fellowship from the American Cancer Society, NIH (NCI) grants 5R10 14241, 3 T12 08033, and 1 R25 17955, the Huntington Clinical Foundation, and a research award from the Veterans Administration.

Contents

Introduction to the Second Edition

Outpatient surgery has grown remarkably in scope and volume in the six years since publication of the first edition of this book. Various new terms have come into use to describe surgical treatment given in the office and in free-standing ambulatory surgical centers. These include phrases such as "short stay surgery," "ambulant surgery," "day care surgery," and "overnight surgery." This type of surgery is now being performed in major medical centers, utilizing the main operating rooms in some cases, with patients being sent home from the recovery room.

The major factor underlying all of these changes is the simplicity of outpatient surgery compared with the traditional inpatient approach. The simplicity of outpatient surgery allows lower cost and increased satisfaction for physicians and patients alike. A detailed cost analysis and a description of the present spectrum of procedures performed in ambulatory surgical centers is presented in our new Chapter 1. The movement toward outpatient surgery has been greatly helped by the participation of anesthesiologists, for most of the surgery performed in free-standing or hospital-based outpatient surgical centers is now done using light general anesthesia or heavy sedation. Safe observation and recovery have been assisted by anesthesiologists, who provide continuity in the units' operation, allowing the surgeons to arrive shortly before the procedure is scheduled to begin and to leave when the operation is over. Careful preparation of the patient and accompanying persons and a well-trained staff of nurses have made outpatient surgery safe and reliable. Cooperation by third party payers has helped facilitate the growth of outpatient surgery. The insurance carriers were slow initially to accept outpatient surgery because of pressure from hospitals and concern that unnecessary procedures would occur in the outpatient setting. These fears have not been substantiated, and the cost of operations for outpatients is actually far less than that for the same procedures performed on inpatients. The subject of the indications for outpatient surgery still remains an important one,[1] however. One of the features of the new accreditation system proposed for ambulatory health care facilities is a peer-review audit system, including a tissue committee, like those found in accredited hospitals.

As in the first edition, we have included in this book a description of surgical procedures and nonoperative aspects of surgical practice in the Outpatient Department, the Emergency Room and the surgeon's office. We have also included a description of some related topics, such as field medicine and surgery, when these topics are a part of the nonhospital practice of many surgeons and utilize procedures that are a part of standard outpatient practice. We have narrowed the scope of our definition of outpatient surgery to some extent, following the practice that has evolved in the past six years; we now define it as surgery that does not usually require hospitalization for more than 24 hours. Most of these procedures can be performed on patients who arrive and leave the office or outpatient surgical center on the same day. Some centers use overnight hospitalization preceding an early morning procedure, while in other cases an overnight period of postoperative rest and observation is considered to be desirable.

The rise in outpatient surgery has been reflected by a growth in the literature on this subject. Three or four articles appear monthly, and the National Library of Medicine's MEDLINE computer will provide the interested reader with a current list of articles on this subject. Topics range from the psychological and nursing aspects of ambulatory surgery to economic considerations, specific techniques and procedures, complications, and research topics. Several major publications on this subject have also appeared since our first edition was published, including the fifth edition of *Ferguson's Surgery of the Ambulatory Patient*,[2] the monthly commentaries published in *Same Day Surgery*,[3] two DHEW publications,[4,5] and a collection of important papers on this subject edited by O'Donovan.[6] Important legislation is also pending on the subject of ambulatory surgery.[7]

We hope the reader will find the present work to be as useful as the first edition of *Outpatient Surgery* and as helpful in practice as the eight editions of *Christopher's Minor Surgery* that preceded it.

REFERENCES

1. Hill, G. J.: Outpatient surgery—What are the indications for it? Surgery, 77:333–335, 1975.
2. Wolcott, M. W. (ed.): Ferguson's Surgery of the Ambulatory Patient, 5th ed. Philadelphia, J. B. Lippincott, 1974. Reviewed by G. J. Hill in Arch. Surg., 110:226–227, 1975.
3. "Same Day Surgery," a journal published monthly at 67 Peachtree Park Drive, Atlanta, GA 30309. Includes "Literature Review" by G. J. Hill in vol. 3, Jan.–Apr. 1979, pp. 16, 28, 40, and 52.
4. U.S. Government Printing Office: Surgical centers. Chapter 61 in Health Resources Statistics: Health Manpower and Health Facilities, 1978–79 ed. Washington, D.C., Dept. of Health, Education, and Welfare, 1979 (in press).

5. Orkand, D. S., Jagger, F. M., and Hurwitz, E.: Comparative evaluation of costs, quality, and system effects of ambulatory surgery performed in alternative settings. Executive summary, December 1977, by the Orkand Corporation for the Office of Policy Planning and Research, Health Care Financing Administration, U.S. Department of Health, Education and Welfare, 1977, 46 pp.

6. O'Donovan, T. R.: Ambulatory Surgical Centers: Development and Management. Germantown, MD., Aspen Systems Corp., 1976, 250 pp.

7. H. R. 5285, 95th Congress, May 17, 1978, Section 6: "Certain Surgical Procedures Performed on an Ambulatory Basis." This legislation would permit medicare reimbursement on the basis of an all-inclusive rate to free-standing ambulatory surgical centers and to physicians performing surgery in their offices for a listed group of surgical procedures.

Introduction to the First Edition

C'est par l'etude de La Petite Chirurgie que le chirurgien commence son apprentissage.

— MAISONNET

I think that there ought to be a book in the hands of the pupil to direct him in his studies . . . in which the lessons he has detailed to him at length by his teachers may be found more shortly expressed . . . to which, as a surgeon, he can turn for the detail of what is necessary to be done in preparing for an operation . . .

Every surgeon . . . ought to bring his judgment maturely to bear on all the points of the case; the objects to be attained; the dangers to be expected; the resources which he ought to have in readiness against probable mischance . . .

By anticipating he may avoid embarrassment, maintain his self-possession undisturbed, and save himself from the distraction of consultation and whispering.

SIR CHARLES BELL (1774–1842), *Professor of Surgery, University of Edinburgh ("Bell's palsy")*

This book was written to help young surgeons, interns and medical students in their work outside of the regular inpatient hospital wards. The major theme is the diagnosis and treatment of surgical patients in the Outpatient Clinic, Emergency Room and overnight ward.

We wish to encourage outpatient care whenever it can be done safely, for the economic burden is thereby reduced, the anxiety of the patient alleviated, and the danger of hospital-acquired sepsis is in part relieved.

Outpatient care is frequently delegated to junior house staff with relatively little supervision. A large patient load is thrust upon the young surgeon, and he has responsibility to make prompt and accurate decisions. The patient desires economy, speed, accuracy and sympathy. Since many outpatient procedures must be done under local anesthesia, awareness of the patient's pain and anxiety is essential for success.

Mixed in with routine or relatively minor problems, sudden emergencies may appear which require an entirely different magnitude of treatment. Usually these patients will soon be transferred to inpatient status, but responsibility for them is initially that of the outpatient surgeon. Guidelines for management of major surgical emergencies are therefore included as an integral part of this text.

Relatively minor complaints may be the hallmark of a serious impending crisis. The outpatient surgeon must be alert to these possibilities.

We have included descriptions of conditions and operations which can be treated by utilizing an overnight period of observation, because many hospitals have a small overnight ward adjacent to the outpatient-emergency facility under the control of the outpatient surgical team.[11] Patients may therefore be operated upon in the main operating room or undergo major diagnostic procedures such as angiography as part of their stay in the Outpatient Department, since they can be placed in a regular hospital bed to recover for up to 24 hours.[13] Many patients can be handled in this way only if they can return either to a good home or to an ambulatory care facility staffed with competent personnel. Procedures such as herniorrhaphy, saphenous vein surgery, lung biopsy, and cervical cone biopsy appear in this context.

All of the procedures described in this book have been performed as described by the authors. These are procedures which can technically be performed in an Outpatient Clinic and a well-outfitted Emergency Room which is equipped for brief major operations, and in which convalesence is speedy enough to permit release from the hospital within 24 hours. Nevertheless, we recommend that good judgment be used in selecting patients for outpatient surgery. It must be remembered that the patient should always be hospitalized if there is any question regarding the advisability of performing the procedure in the office or outpatient department, or as an overnight admission to the hospital.

Outpatient Surgery incorporates many of the ideas developed for American physicians by Frederick Christopher in *Minor Surgery* (1930), based on the previous textbooks by Wharton, Foote, Maisonnet and Hertzler, and the immensely popular *Manual of Minor Surgery* by Heath which appeared in 20 editions. Christopher's textbook was a classic which was published in six editions over an 18-year period and which was carried on in two additional editions by Drs. Alton Ochsner and Michael DeBakey. Members of the Department of Surgery at the University of Colorado began to work together on a description of their work in this field in 1967. The first publication of this team effort was the volume of Surgical Clinics of North America entitled "Improved Techniques in Everyday Surgery" (1969), edited by Dr. Ben Eiseman. *Outpatient Surgery* is a textbook which was designed to carry forward the work which was begun by Drs. Christopher, Ochsner, DeBakey and Eiseman.

The topics presented here cover subjects which comprise most of the entire field of surgery, which we define as the healing art which utilizes physical procedures such as incision, repair and other manipulations. Thus the specialties of gynecology and obstetrics, anesthesi-ology, podiatry, transplantation and oncology are represented, as well as the conventional categories of general surgery, trauma, cardiovascular and thoracic surgery, otolaryngology, urology, plastic surgery, pediatric surgery, orthopedics and proctology. Special chapters are presented regarding surgical considerations in areas far removed from teaching hospitals, such as developing countries and expeditions into remote areas. The latter topics are covered in this text because of the interest which many young surgeons have shown in extending their service into these very special outpatient situations. We also wish to acknowledge the fact that the procedures used in the outpatient department of American university hospitals are not necessarily the procedures which will or should be used in developing countries[8] or remote areas.

The authors have described the conditions and treatments which constitute the majority of their own outpatient practice. In some instances, the work is primarily diagnostic, whereas in other clinics it consists in large part of minor and major operations. In every case, each author has presented his personal experience as a guide for the young men and women who plan to work in the outpatient specialty clinics and offices.

The long-term follow-up of all patients will be emphasized, since the results of inpatient care must be measured by the surgeon in his office or outpatient clinic over an extended period of time.[2]

It is our hope that this text may serve as a useful reference for office practice as well as for the hospital Outpatient Department. The degree to which this will be possible will obviously vary greatly with the facilities, assistance, training and skill of the physician who uses this book.

REFERENCES

1. Bell, C.: A System of Operative Surgery Founded on the Basis of Anatomy. 1st

American ed. Hartford, Goodwin, 1816 (pp. iv–v).

2. Brook, R. H., Appel, F. A., Avery, C., Orman, M., and Stevenson, R. L.: Effectiveness of inpatient follow-up care. New Eng. J. Med., *285*:1509–1514, 1972.

3. Christopher, F.: Minor Surgery. 1st–6th eds. Philadelphia, W. B. Saunders Co., 1930–1948.

4. Eiseman, B. (ed.): Improved Techniques in Everyday Surgery. Surg. Clin. N. Amer., *49*(6):1199–1553, 1969.

5. Foote, E. M.: A Textbook of Minor Surgery. 1st–5th eds. New York, Appleton Century Crofts, 1908–1924.

6. Heath, C.: A Manual of Minor Surgery and Bandaging for the Use of House Surgeons, Dressers and Junior Practitioners. 1st–20th eds. Philadelphia, Blakiston and F. A. Davis Co., 1861–1930. Late editions by G. Williams.

7. Hertzler, A. E., and Chesky, V. E.: Minor Surgery. St. Louis, C. V. Mosby Co., 1927.

8. Ingelfinger, F. J.: Western medicine in tropical islands. New Eng. J. Med., *285*:1535–1536, 1972.

9. Maisonnet, P. J. F. R.: Petite Chirurgie. 1st–4th eds. Paris, G. Doin & Cie, 1928–1942.

10. Ochsner, A., and DeBakey, M. E. (eds.): Christopher's Minor Surgery. 7th–8th eds. Philadelphia, W. B. Saunders Co., 1955–1959.

11. Ruckley, C. V., MacLean, Mary, Smith, A. M., and Falconer, C. W. A.: Team approach to early discharge and outpatient surgery. Lancet, *1*:177–180, 1971.

12. Wharton, H. R.: Minor Surgery and Bandaging. 1st–6th eds. Philadelphia, Lea Bros., 1891–1905.

13. Zimmerman, C. E.: Techniques of Patient Care; A Manual of Bedside Procedures for Students, Interns and Residents. Boston, Little, Brown and Co., 1970.

1 Recent Developments in Ambulatory Surgery

THOMAS R. O'DONOVAN, Ph.D.

Major developments are taking place in efforts to improve the level of health care, reduce duplication of medical services and reduce or contain costs of health care delivery. One of the major innovations is ambulatory surgery,[1] which is being utilized increasingly in hospitals and independently operated facilities in the United States, Canada, Europe and Latin America.

This chapter is primarily concerned with formal, organized programs of elective ambulatory surgery, in which patients arrive and are discharged the same day. These patients are usually operated on under general anesthesia. The surgery is usually performed in hospitals, in hospital satellites, in buildings constructed near hospitals or in independently operated, freestanding facilities.

According to the American Hospital Association (AHA), "Many types of minor surgery do not require overnight hospitalization. Therefore, hospitals must plan and provide outpatient surgical facilities so that, whenever appropriate, surgery can be performed on an outpatient basis, thereby reducing costs to the patient, the hospital, and the community, and assuring optimum use of inpatient beds."[2]

The typical cases for ambulatory surgery are nonemergent, noninfected patients who are scheduled for elective operations. Performed under general anesthesia, these procedures usually take less than an hour and require less than a two hour stay in the recovery room (Table 1–1).

Ambulatory surgery reduces the average total cost per patient treated at a hospital. However, if hospitals establish a program of ambulatory surgery, and if this removes some of the inpa-

1

TABLE 1–1　Common Operative Procedures in Ambulatory Surgery*

Abscess, incision and drainage
Adenoidectomy and myringotomy
Adhesions of clitoris
Anesthesia—local, regional or spinal
Arch bars, removal or application
Arthrodesis (phalanges) (other joints)
Arthroplasty (phalanges) (other joints)
Arthroscopy
Arthrotomy, meniscectomy
Aspiration of aqueous
Augmentation mammoplasty (unilateral,
　bilateral)

Bartholin cystectomy
Basal cell cancer, excision
Benign intraoral lesions
Biopsy, conjunctiva or cornea
Biopsy, vulva
Blepharoplasty (upper, lower or combined)
Bone graft
Bone marrow biopsy
Bone reconstruction
Branchial arch appendages, excision
Branchial clefts
Breast implant, removal
Breast masses, excision
Bronchoscopy
Bunion operation
Bursae, removal of (olecranon)

Canthus excision
Capsulectomy
Carbuncle, excision
Cardioversion
Carpal tunnel decompression
Carpal tunnel ligament release
Cast change with manipulation
Cataract, by phakoemulsification
Caudal anesthesia
Cautery, vaginal cyst
Celiac (splanchnic) anesthetic block
Cervical amputation (Sturmdorf)
Cervical cone
Cervical node biopsy
Chalazion
Chemical face peel, limited
Circumcision
Cleft lip repair
Closed reduction (nose or zygoma)
Colonoscopy
Colostomy, revision
Colpotomy, diagnostic
Cryopexy for retinal tear
Cryoretinopexy
Cryotherapy, alone or with biopsy
Culdocentesis
Culdoscopy
Curettage or cauterization of corneal ulcer
Cystectomy—Skene's duct
Cyst excision
Cystoscopy

Débridement

Dermabrasion (partial or full)
Dermoid cyst of eyebrow, excision
Desiccation of condyloma
Dilation and curettage
Dislocated shoulder or elbow
Dorsal slit, preputial

Ear (prominent, correction)
Ectropion and entropion
Electroshock therapy
Enucleation
Episiotomy
Esophageal dilatation
Esophagoscopy
Ethmoidectomy
Examination under anesthesia
Excision, lesions, skin tags, cysts
Excision of parotid and submaxillary stones
Excisions of skin tumors (local vs. wide or
　radical—Wilz)
Excision of urethral caruncle
Exostosis, excision
Eye muscle operation—recession (unilateral)

Face lift, limited
Facial and neck lesions, removal
Facial wire, removal
Fasciectomy (finger, palm)
Fissure in ano
Fistula in ano
Fistulectomy
Flap revision
Foreign body excision
Foreign body excision with x-ray
Foreign body removal, ear
Foreign body, removal (with or without x-ray)
Fracture, closed reduction, uncomplicated
Fracture, closed reduction (with or without
　x-ray)
Frenulectomy, tongue—in children
Fulguration of bladder neck
Funduscopic exam in children
Fusion

Ganglionectomy
Gastroscopy
Gynecomastia, excision

Hair transplantations
Hammertoes with tenotomies and resection of
　bones
Hand fasciectomy for arthritis
Hand infections (minor and major)
Hardware, removal
Hardware, removal, hip
Hemangioma, removal, nostril
Hemangioma, removal
Hemorrhoidectomy
Hemorrhoid, thrombotic, evacuation
Herniorrhaphy, inguinal (infant or adult—
　unilateral or bilateral)
Herniorrhaphy, umbilical
Hordeolum

TABLE 1–1　Common Operative Procedures in Ambulatory Surgery (*Continued*)*

Hydrocelectomy
Hymenotomy
Hysteroscopy

Impacted wisdom teeth, removal of
Incision and drainage, dental
Inclusion cyst, excision
Inferior turbinate fracture
Inguinal/scrotal abscess, I and D
Intercostal anesthetic block
Intercostal neurectomy
Intervertebral disc injection
Intraoral biopsy
Iridectomy

Jaw, wiring of

Keratotomy
Kidney cannula, revision

Labia lesion, excision
Lacrimal duct probing or reconstruction
Laparoscopy
Laryngeal polypectomy
Laryngoscopy
Laryngoscopy with operative procedure
Lesion excision with graft
Limited rhinoplasty
Lipectomy
Lipoma, excision
Liver biopsy
Litholapaxy (Bladder stone crushing and
  removal)
Lymph node biopsy

Mammoplasty, augmentation or revision
Mandibular/maxillary cyst removal
Manipulation of joints (with or without x-ray)
Mass excision with scar revision
Mastoidectomy
Meatotomy
Medial ligament, knee, repair of
Meloplasty
Metatarsal heads, excision
Minor salivary gland surgery
Morton's neuroma
Mouth biopsy
Multiple teeth extractions
Muscle biopsy
Myotomy, recession or resection
Myringoplasty
Myringotomy with or without tubes

Nasal fractures
Nasal polyp, removal
Nerve repair
Neuroma (other)
Neurolysis (finger)
Nose, closed fracture reduction

Odontectomy, surgical
Odontectomy, uncomplicated
Olecranon bursa, excision
Olecranon spur, excision

Open and closed zygomatic fractures
Open reduction fracture, without x-ray
Oral biopsy
Oral surgery
Orchiectomy
Orchiopexy
Osteotomy
Otoplasty
Otoscopy
Otoscopy (with removal of foreign body)

Palate biopsy
Paracentesis
Pedicle flap, transfer
Pelvic endoscopy (Schirodkar)
Perineorrhaphy
Periodontal surgery
Periodontic surgery (full or partial)
Phalangectomy
Photocoagulation
Pilonidal cystectomy
Placement of dental arches
Plantar wart, excision
Polypectomy, cervical
Poly tubes, removal
Preauricular cyst excision
Preprosthesis surgery
Prostate biopsy
Pterygium

Rectal biopsy
Reduction of minor facial fractures
Reduction of nasal fractures
Removal of mandibular maxillary cyst
Renal biopsy
Resection, bilateral, unilateral
Rhytidectomy with blepharoplasty
Rhytidoplasty

Saline injection, intrauterine—therapeutic
Salivary gland surgery, minor
Scalene node biopsy
Scar revisions and relaxations
Septal reconstruction
Septo-rhinoplasty, limited
Sequestrectomy
Skin grafts, minor
Skin lesions, excision
Soft tissue tumor removal
Spinal tap
Splanchnic (celiac) block
Stapedectomy
Stellate ganglion anesthetic block
Strabotomy, pediatric
Sturmdorf repair of cervix
Subdural tap
Submucous resection
Synovectomy

Tarsorrhaphy
Tendon repair
Tenosynovectomy
Tenotomy, hand or foot

Table continued on the following page

TABLE 1-1 Common Operative Procedures in Ambulatory Surgery (*Continued*)*

Tension measurements in children	Urethral dilation—in children
Testes, excision	Urethroscopy—in children
Testicular biopsy	
Therapeutic abortion	Vaginal stenosis, release
Therapeutic retrobulbar injections	Vaginal tumor, excision
Thoracentesis, closed	Vaginal web, excision
Thyroglossal duct cyst	Vaginoplasty
Tongue biopsy	Varicocelectomy
Tongue surgery—glossectomy	Varicose vein ligation
Tonsillar tag excision	Varicotomy
Tonsillectomy, with or without adenoidectomy	Vasectomy
Torticollis, repair	Vasograms
Transvaginal ligation of tubes	Ventral femoral hernia
Trigger finger release	Vermillionectomy (both lips)
Tubal coagulation or ligation	Vermillionectomy (upper or lower lip)
Tympanoplasty	Vulva biopsy
Ulnar nerve transfer	Xanthoma, excision
Umbilical herniorrhaphy with bilateral inguinal herniorrhaphy	
	Z-plasty
Umbilical sinus, excision	Zygomatic arch procedures
Urethral catheter	Zygoma, reduction

*Adapted from O'Donovan, T. R.: Ambulatory Surgical Centers Development and Management. Germantown, Md., Aspen Systems Corp., pp. 203–207, 1976.

tient stays (without replacing them with new patients), ambulatory surgery can decrease occupancy and thus create an adverse financial impact on some hospitals. For this and other reasons, only 45 per cent of hospitals in the United States had programs of ambulatory surgery in 1977.

The question arises whether all hospitals should embark upon or enlarge a program of ambulatory surgery. Ambulatory surgery should be tailored to the needs of the community, which are often expressed by the degree of acceptance from patients and physicians. In most hospitals no ambulatory surgery program exists, yet in other hospitals over 20 per cent of all operative procedures are done on an ambulatory basis. Experts have indicated that nearly 30 per cent of all surgery performed in the U.S. could be performed on an ambulatory basis. However, if this actually occurred, and if there were no backlog to fill the gap, bed vacancies would result. This could place many fiscal challenges upon hospitals that are considering ambulatory surgery.

Nevertheless, our nation's health care system must seek reasonable ways to contain costs. Reducing the length of inpatient hospitalization is very important even when low occupancy exists. Ambulatory surgery should not be restricted solely to the hospitals with high occupancy.

Enormous savings in costs can result in the long run from the use of ambulatory surgery. When the length of stay for a large number of operative procedures decreases, the opportunity for cost reduction arises and fewer new beds need be provided. As our nation's population continues to expand, new inpatient beds will be needed in certain areas. A smaller number will be needed if more than 20 per cent of all future elective surgery is performed on a "same day" basis.

Much has been written about the financial importance of reducing a particular patient's hospitalization period for a hernia, for example, from six days to three days. Examples of the reductions in costs are shown in Table 1-2. It is likely that in the future Professional Standards

TABLE 1–2 Comparison of Costs of Procedures Performed in Ambulatory Surgical Center and in Hospital

CITY	PROCEDURE	INPATIENT SURGERY $	AMBULATORY SURGERY $
Wichita, KS	Dilatation and curettage	457.00	122.00
	Inguinal herniorrhaphy	751.00	165.00
Dallas, TX	Scar revision, tonsillectomy and adenoidectomy, dilatation and curettage, cysts, ganglions, ocular muscle procedure (average cost derived from 50 of each procedure)	349.00	246.00
Santa Barbara, CA	Therapeutic abortion	470.15	160.00
	Dilatation and curettage	467.95	160.00
	Local excision of shin	577.40	185.00
	Bilateral tubal ligation	464.00	185.00
	Laparoscopy	474.15	185.00
Phoenix, AZ	Carpal tunnel decompression	884.00	175.00
	Bronchoscopy	975.00	155.00
	Inguinal herniorrhaphy	897.00	175.00
	Dilatation and curettage	409.00	125.00
	Circumcision (adult)	1,209.00	155.00

Review Organizations (PSROs) will have a major impact on length of stay. This chapter will discuss the effect of reducing some procedures to zero days. In order to accomplish such a reduction, special programs for ambulatory surgery must be established. The patient who is discharged the day he arrives requires a wholly different system than does the patient who stays longer. Systems of patient charges must be different, as must physical facilities, planning, admitting, preop work-ups, postop care and discharge management. All these areas require fine points of distinction from inpatient management, simply because the patient arrives the day of surgery instead of one or more days before and is discharged the same day instead of at a future date.

Ambulatory surgery should be integrated within the community-wide plan for health services. Nonduplication of facilities must be documented in the planning process and a balance should be attained between excellent care and minimum cost. Ambulatory surgery can provide more hospital beds for seriously ill patients and reduce waiting time for elective surgery. This trend is occurring because of new techniques in anesthesia, in control of bleeding and other safeguards, as well as physician and patient acceptance.[3-6]

Ambulatory surgical patients often return to work sooner than if they had been hospitalized for the same procedure. An increasing number of hospital programs in ambulatory surgery are emerging, and the range of procedures is large.[7] Each case depends upon the judgment of the attending physician, as well as on the desires of the patient, the type of insurance coverage and access to short-stay surgical facilities.

EARLY AMBULATION

The general concept and theory of ambulatory surgery has been reviewed by Lahti.[8] His work relates to early ambulation of patients, which has an obvious application to ambulatory surgery. Lahti reported the effects of early ambulation and early discharge on 1000 consecutive patients. He has updated the original study reported in 1970, and now includes data on over 2000 patients. Lahti has observed that in the past 30 years the period of hospitalization necessary after surgery has decreased steadily.

Some of Lahti's observations and conclusions are (1) if a healthy person were put to bed for a week and given narcotics at various intervals, it would take several weeks for recovery from this experience; (2) it is now possible and desirable to discharge the majority of surgical patients on the first or second postoperative day; (3) the usual patient entering the hospital for major surgery is frightened of the unknown, and when he awakens from the anesthetic, his fears are brought to the surface so that any minor discomfort is magnified into real pain; and (4) narcotics only prolong the recovery, whereas the patient who knows that he will be up and about the afternoon of surgery and home the day after surgery is relaxed, not fearful, and requires much less postoperative medication. Infants and young children have not been conditioned to being ill following surgery and, as a result, they usually are not.

Some of the types of surgery noted in Lahti's report are unilateral and bilateral inguinal hernia, appendectomy, ligation and stripping of saphenous veins, hemorrhoidectomy, excision of breast tumor, simple and radical mastectomy, thyroidectomy and cholecystectomy. For an adult, one or two doses of 50 mg of meperidine (Demerol) is usually sufficient for relief of pain. If a patient is reluctant to go home, Lahti explains that as soon as the need for hospitalization ceases the patient is much better off at home. It is important that the patient know of the small but definite incidence of postoperative complications caused by being inactive and in a hospital. The patient is advised to bathe daily and to wash over the sutures with soap and water. Patients are advised that they may be up and about as much as they desire and may resume normal activities, including driving. Many patients return

to work before the sutures are removed.

In the data reported by Lahti, all patients were discharged by the seventh postoperative day, and 75 per cent of the first 1114 patients were discharged by the second day. According to Lahti, there are no valid reasons for keeping the usual patient in the hospital any longer than necessary to recover from the anesthetic. Patients' fears that something might go wrong if they go home can now be changed to the idea that something might go wrong if they stay in the hospital. Lahti's conclusion is that although it is difficult to overcome the traditions and habits of the past, the results are certainly worth the effort.

The lessons are clear: If patients spend a shorter time in the hospital, the result is more effective utilization of health care delivery resources. This, in turn, can help stem the tide of escalating hospital costs.

THE ADVANTAGES AND DISADVANTAGES OF AMBULATORY SURGERY

In the past few years the American experience with ambulatory surgery has increased dramatically. Much information can be drawn from this experience, but before definite conclusions are reached, we believe that more research should be conducted to properly document the major advantages and disadvantages.

For many years the reimbursement policies of insurance companies discouraged performance of ambulatory surgery in hospitals and in independently operated facilities. For example, there were many instances in which outpatient surgery was not reimbursed, forcing the patient to be hospitalized in order to receive coverage. This encouraged patients to request hospitalization rather than pay for their care as outpatients.

Advantages of Ambulatory Surgery

1. Reduced cost (by at least $200 per procedure). Less patient work-up is needed. For the same procedure, there are more lab tests given and pharmacy items prescribed for inpatients than for ambulatory surgical patients. There is a definite difference in the scope of medical management of inpatients and ambulatory surgical patients.
2. More effective use of physician's time. This tends to be a greater advantage in the independently operated facilities than in hospitals.
3. Reduced bed congestion in busy hospitals. This may make more room for seriously ill patients and reduce the need to provide new beds, or at least delay or reduce the number of new beds needed in a given community.
4. The patient may return to work a day or two earlier.
5. Reduction in the psychological stress associated with hospitalization, particularly in children with an easier and more agreeable recovery in the home.
6. Tailormade patient care to meet the needs of the "nonsick." Putting such patients in the hospital for one to three days forces them into the hospital's typical inpatient treatment pattern which, by necessity, requires some degree of aloneness and susceptibility to hospital-acquired infections.
7. Ambulatory surgical patients tend to receive less medication pre- and postoperatively than inpatients because they are under medical supervision for a shorter period of time.
8. When the hospital is able to attract "new business" by creating or expanding its ambulatory surgery program (from doctors' offices, from new doctors and so on), it can spread its fixed overall costs, to some extent, over a wider range of services.
9. Other advantages often occur when there is greater use of anesthesia and operating room services, such as attraction and retention of good anesthesiologists.

Problems and Possible Disadvantages of Ambulatory Surgery

Some of the problems that have come up in discussions of ambulatory surgery include the following:

1. Patient resistance, expressed in comments such as, "My friends always were hospitalized for a D and C, why shouldn't I be?" . . ., "My hospitalization insurance policy pays for inpatient care, and I want all that is coming to me." Or "It must be safer to be hospitalized because my doctor never uses the ambulatory surgery program of the hospital."
2. Physician resistance. This stems from force of habit, lack of general community acceptance and lack of immediate availability of care in case sudden complications occur. In addition, physicians are concerned about possible increased malpractice suits, a phenomenon that depends on area practice because court cases lean heavily on what is considered "common usage." In a community with little ambulatory surgery, a physician may tend to take a conservative view of "experimentation." Reduced physician income is seen by some, from loss of inpatient follow-up care.
3. Potentially reduced hospital income.

TYPES OF AMBULATORY SURGICAL CENTERS

Ambulatory surgery can take place in various settings. The most common setting is the hospital, but there are at least three different kinds of hospital controlled ambulatory surgical centers. In one very common model, the hospital creates a formal ambulatory surgical program by superimposing it upon its existing inpatient care system. In this way additional operating rooms are not constructed, and the ambulatory patients use the same preop, postop and admitting areas as inpatients do. Another hospital-type model is a specially created facility tailormade for ambulatory surgery on the grounds of the hospital. A third hospital model is the satellite, which is the creation of a separate ambulatory surgical facility located some distance from the hospital. The fourth model is the independently operated, free-standing ambulatory surgery center. The various advantages and disadvantages of each kind of center are detailed in this chapter.

With the decline in the nation's birthrate in recent years, a rather large number of obstetrical departments have closed. Some hospitals, such as Bethesda, Maryland's Suburban Hospital, have utilized a former obstetrical unit for ambulatory surgery. Sometimes ambulatory surgery is performed in emergency departments of hospitals. Phalen has noted that, when outpatient surgical services are provided within the emergency room, the same operating room that is used for minor emergency procedures also is used for minor elective procedures.[10] Constant staffing coverage and nonduplication of facilities are the primary advantages of this arrangement. A disadvantage is that the patient may not receive the individualized attention that he might otherwise expect. The tense emergency room environment, plus the unpredictable levels of activity and concomitant allocation of personnel resources, may result in a poorly functioning outpatient surgery facility.

THE FOUR BASIC MODELS OF AMBULATORY SURGERY CENTERS

I. Hospital Controlled: Using Existing Inpatient Operating Rooms and Admitting, Pre- and Postop Areas

There are also subvariations. For example, a hospital could use existing operating rooms but create a separate new admitting section.

Advantages

This model enables the hospital to establish a capability for ambulatory surgery, with limited capital investment. It is often possible to create this capability without adding admitting clerks or nurses, although in some cases some additional personnel may be needed, depending on how busy the unit is. Greater "economies of scale" are provided because the new subunit will be part of the overall system.

The capability can be established more quickly because the basic inpatient facilities already exist, eliminating construction time.

There is also great flexibility. If the medical staff, for whatever reason, does not utilize the ambulatory surgery program, there has been no great outlay in funds. If a complete new unit were constructed and not used sufficiently, serious financial problems would result.

This model allows the surgeon to perform more complex surgical procedures, which can result in greater utilization of the ambulatory surgical program. For example, if the pathology report on a breast biopsy shows cancer, more definitive surgery can be performed at that time rather than waiting until the patient is transferred to the hospital's inpatient area.

Disadvantages

Basically, the hospital is organized and established for inpatient care, and when ambulatory surgery or various other ambulatory programs are superimposed upon the existing inpatient system, many problems can result.[11-12] Hospital personnel often regard ambulatory surgery patients as second class citizens. This can lessen the dignity with which patients are treated. When these problems are not solved, utilization of the unit may not reach its full potential.

Longer waits may develop for admission for ambulatory surgery because the admission office may be busy with inpatients.

Some hospitals treat the ambulatory surgery patients who do not have Blue Cross or Medicare insurance differently from inpatients. For example, they may require full cash outlay in advance to pay for outpatient surgery if the patient has a commercial insurance policy, whereas that same patient might have had credit extended for his stay as an inpatient.

Higher charges may be billed than are necessary for ambulatory surgery, because of pricing structures modeled after the inpatient pricing system.

Outpatients scheduled for surgery may be displaced by emergency cases taken care of in the operating room. In addition, inpatient surgery often is awarded priority over ambulatory surgery.

Since the preop holding areas and recovery rooms are designed for inpatient surgery, ambulatory surgery patients must be accommodated in the same areas as inpatients who may be critically ill. This can result in unnecessary psychological stress. Often proper waiting room areas do not exist for ambulatory surgery patients. When families of inpatients and outpatients are mixed, a negative psychological impact can result on the families of outpatient surgery patients.

Since ambulatory surgery patients *awaken earlier* than inpatients, operating room personnel may not yet be familiar with the special needs of such ambulatory patients.

A greater incidence of nosocomial infections may occur, especially in comparison with the freestanding centers.

An excessive detailed medical record is needed, because of the comprehensive nature of inpatient care.

II. Hospital Controlled: Located on Hospital Grounds in a Specially Created, Newly Constructed or Remodeled Area, Tailormade for Ambulatory Surgery

Advantages

The biggest advantage of this program is that it relieves the disadvantages enumerated in Model I, although good management could also relieve many of those disadvantages.

A tailormade area is available for ambulatory surgery, to provide the best patient care from the point of view of the physical facilities. If the area is going to be remodeled rather than newly constructed, care should be taken that a suitable area is selected. For example, if a small space is chosen, it may be insufficient for a sound ambulatory surgery program.

There is greater satisfaction on the part of personnel, patients and physicians, because everything is "tailormade."

This type of community service may attract a large share of the market because it may appeal to physicians who are not currently members of the hospital's medical staff.[13]

Disadvantages

It can cost too much. A degree of flexibility is lost in this approach, because if the unit is not successful, it is not likely that the space can be utilized for other hospital services without additional capital investment.

Higher charges and problems with recovery from third party insurers may be seen with this model, as with Model I.

III. Hospital Controlled: The Satellite

Some hospitals have considered opening a satellite health care facility with ambulatory care as the central thrust, with or without ambulatory surgery. Ambulatory surgery, however, could be the main thrust of such a satellite system. Basically, a satellite ambulatory surgery facility is a freestanding facility in which the unit is located some distance from the hospital. It is created specifically for ambulatory purposes and is totally controlled by the hospital. Such satellites can be developed by joint hospital efforts as a "shared service."

Advantages are the same as those in Model II; in addition, the medical needs of a specific geographic area can be met on a tailormade basis.

Disadvantages are the same as those outlined in Model II, and those described in Model IV.

IV. Non-hospital Controlled: The Independently Operated Freestanding Surgery Center

Examples include the Phoenix Surgicenter® and the Minor Surgery Center® of Wichita.

Advantages

If a particular community has ambulatory surgery facilities, or if existing ambulatory surgery facilities are inadequate for whatever reason, the freestanding units fill a need by providing ambulatory surgery capability to the community.

Lower charges are usually seen in the freestanding independent units when compared to the hospital charge system.

There is a tendency for increased patient and physician satisfaction. There appears to be an excessive amount of bureaucratic red tape when patients have ambulatory surgery within the hospital setting. The freestanding units have capitalized on this and many perform admirably in terms of patient care and comfort.

Disadvantages

There is a possible increase in net community cost, under certain circumstances. This is an important issue and research is needed in this area.

There is also a greater distance from hospital emergency back-up facilities. The independent centers generally feel that such back-up is not needed for patient safety.

In *Business Week*, Dr. Herbert Notkin observed that, "Skimming off low-risk, no overhead surgery from hospitals will simply increase the cost of those operations that must be performed in hospital."[14] *Business Week* commented that one-day surgery could improve — or possibly destroy — the present health care system. Therefore, independently operated ambulatory surgical facilities can present a challenge to hospital delivery of such care.

MAJOR CONCLUSIONS REGARDING AMBULATORY SURGERY

Throughout the U.S. many patients who undergo surgery and are hospitalized from one to four days could be cared for on a "same day" basis. This concept of ambulatory surgery may be recommended by physicians to selected patients who are to undergo certain surgical procedures. From 20 per cent to 40 per cent of all surgery can now be performed without requiring an overnight stay in a hospital.

Acceptance by physicians of the concept of ambulatory surgery is increasing slowly but steadily in spite of the many pressures to avoid "come-and-go" surgery. Some of the factors that deter acceptance include conservatism, fear of malpractice suits and a general lack of facilities that help to create the appeal for short-stay surgery. A patient who develops bleeding may be less likely to sue if it happens during hospitalization than if it happens at home. We would be shocked at the economic cost of defensive medicine practiced by physicians as a result of court judgments in favor of the patient.

As hospitals enlarge or start a coordinated program of ambulatory surgery, they may experience reduced occupancy for the general acute hospital beds unless their surgical and medical patient waiting list is sufficient to cover the reduction. The net effect throughout the country will be a reduction in overall costs of health care delivery in the long run. Many hospitals should institute or expand such programs, based on need, existence of community facilities and their own individual capacities. It is interesting to note that if a hospital embarks successfully on a program of ambulatory surgery and has a high backlog, the internal medicine department may want an increased quota of beds, while surgery may want all the "bed savings" for themselves.

The federal government, through Professional Standards Review Organizations (PSROs) may require an increase in ambulatory or short-stay surgery within our nation's hospitals, although many hospitals are not sufficiently organized or philosophically prepared for this change at the present time.

Independently operated, private, come-and-go surgical facilities will be competing more and more with hospitals for patients. The new facilities often perform the services in a highly competent and well organized manner that provides a great deal of satisfaction to the patient. The net effect of such a trend in large urban centers with excess hospital beds could be to increase the cost of such delivery of health care to the community, because of the prevailing system of cost reimbursement.

There is no valid reason why a hospital should necessarily charge more for a surgical procedure on a come-and-go basis than an independently operated freestanding facility. Actually, a nonprofit hospital should be at an advantage, since the operating suites are already there, the lifesaving support equipment is available and the considerations of profit and property taxes necessary in an independent facility can be eliminated.

Unfortunately, the hospital can be placed at a disadvantage by the very agencies (government and Blue Cross) that should be most interested in allowing the existing facilities to be competitive and in the elimination of duplicated facilities, since such duplication can result only in increasing the total community cost of health care. This disadvantage results from the cost reimbursement mandated by some of the third-party payers, requiring allocation of costs for medical records, housekeeping, maintenance, depreciation and so forth. The allocation may be totally disproportionate to the realities of the added costs incurred, but the system often requires this allocation. The net result is that these so called "costs" force hospitals to charge more for procedures than freestanding facilities. The other side of the coin, and one that is never mentioned, is that by forcing hospitals to over-allocate costs to the ambulatory surgery program, the end result is really a reduction of allocated costs to other departments in the hospital. Hence, the end result well may be to reduce costs in roentgenography, the clinical laboratory, and other areas. This saving gets lost in the immense paperwork jungle of Blue Cross and Medicare, and the focus continues to be on why the hospitals cannot compete with freestanding facilities.

A policy statement adopted by the Board of Trustees of the AHA on May 9, 1973, cautioned that, "The overall impact of providing these services in a communitywide system of health care must be considered, rather than the unit cost per service in the individual facilities." If this factor could be truly and accurately measured, there is no way that any freestanding facility could compete with virtually any existing hospital. The necessary capital expenditures and operating costs at a freestanding facility almost by definition must exceed the *added* costs of a short-stay program in an existing hospital. The real problem is the inequitable distribution of overhead that appears to put the hospital at a cost disadvantage. Such overhead is not fully required to establish a hospital ambulatory surgical program.

As we approach the 1980s, over one-half of our nation's hospitals have no program of ambulatory surgery. If hospitals open or enlarge ambulatory surgery facilities, they can reduce their present number of inpatient admissions and reduce their percentage of occupancy. But if other strategies are developed, such as new programs, physician recruitment activities, outreach programs or development of satellites there can be an increase in inpatient stays. We should keep in mind that reducing inpatient stays is an important way of containing costs, even when low occupancy exists.

Quality care is vital. In short-stay surgery we are dealing with elective procedures on patients who are not sick. If death or any serious consequence occurs there is some doubt that the ambulatory surgery unit has a right to exist. Hospitals can do the job if such a priority objective is established. They have the facilities and personnel. All it takes is managerial expertise.

To date, the following views are held by various groups. The AHA tends to favor short-stay surgery to be performed in general acute hospitals rather than in independently operated surgical facilities. On the other hand, the American Medical Association has shown an interest in independently operated ambulatory surgical centers and tends to favor such programs over those controlled and operated within hospitals. To my knowledge, the AMA has issued no official policy statement on this subject.

Although the federal government has not made a clear policy statement, it favors a system that will generate the lowest costs. The strongest evidence of this is the high likelihood that PSROs will generate an increase in the number of ambulatory surgical procedures that will take place in the U.S. in the near future. Unfortunately, the Medicare program reimburses only hospitals for outpatient surgery, except for a few demonstration projects.

The Joint Commission on Accreditation of Hospitals (JCAH) has adopted guidelines that may soon become standards for ambulatory surgery. These guidelines hold that in order to minimize duplication of services, the objectives and plans of the ambulatory surgery center should be coordinated with those of other health service providers and planning agencies in the community. The main emphasis of JCAH is on quality care, in sharp contrast to the policy advocated by the federal government and certain other sources which tend to emphasize cost containment. Efficiently run units both in hospitals and in independently operated facilities can fully meet the future requirements of the JCAH. Those hospitals that have an established short-stay surgical unit have generally found it to be a useful service to the community, to patients and to physicians. Such units help the hospitals promote the establishment of a well rounded program of facilities for patient care. To the extent that existing surgical facilities can be utilized to handle short-stay surgery, this has the further effect of increasing the utilization of ancillary departments, and, as a result, fixed costs of many areas of the hospital are spread over a larger number of units. Therefore, fiscal advantages can accrue in many situations by having a solid program of ambulatory surgery.

Hospitals that do not at the present time have an ambulatory surgery program are, in some cases, thoroughly investigating the concept. As noted by Michigan Blue Cross, "Hospitals are not running over each other to set up ambulatory surgical units. Their big reason is that they create no *new* health dollars by doing so; they only reallocate existing dollars."[15] In such hospitals and in communities in general where a surplus of hospital beds exists, the advent of ambulatory surgery could create financial problems if supported on a large scale. It is estimated that Massachusetts has twice the number of hospital beds it needs. According to James Latham, provider reimbursement manager for Blue Cross of Massachusetts, guided by an estimate, said, "The real savings will be in closing hospitals that don't have to be there."

Many physicians support the concept of ambulatory surgery. It has been noted that "the future is almost unlimited; the surgical center can function successfully with greater savings to the patient while maintaining high standards of care, and such

centers will be a necessity under national health insurance; the patient who comes to the hospital for minor surgery is subsidizing the ones who have major surgery."[16] While many physicians believe that ambulatory surgery should be performed in the independently operated facilities, others fully support the program in hospitals. The real challenge among hospitals is to provide convenience to the physician and the patient in order to compete economically with the advent of independently operated ambulatory surgical facilities.

Blue Cross has a general concern regarding facilities for ambulatory surgery. The major conclusion of the organization is that such facilities should exist only when duplication is minimized. When a specific community has sufficient hospital facilities to provide care for meeting the needs of ambulatory surgery, independently operated facilities should be discouraged, since their creation would tend to increase the community cost of medical care. If hospital facilities are insufficient, then freestanding, independently operated programs could have a definite advantage for health care delivery within a specific community. Not all commercial insurance companies recognize outpatient surgery as a valid procedure for insurance coverage, hence, they encourage patients to be hospitalized rather than be discharged the same day.

The surgeon who is attempting to do come-and-go surgery must have his administration requirements adequately provided for, and he must be able to step immediately from the operating room, dictate the operating note, and move on to the next case. He also must be assisted in gathering whatever information is necessary for billing purposes. This makes his use of time efficient and convenient.

The concept of come-and-go surgery challenges health care leaders to maximize community utilization of such surgery. Traditional hospitals transfer short-stay surgical patients to a "recovery room." Since one "recovers" from "sickness" and the independently operated facilities do not regard ambulatory surgery patients as "sick," postoperative patients are transferred to a "wake-up area."

Hospitals are now receiving and will continue to receive many fiscal challenges as a result of new competition from non-hospital surgery centers. How well will administrators respond? My recommendation is that they concentrate on providing proper service to the community they serve and recognize that, under certain conditions, both approaches can coexist. This would leave us with only the cost issue to be researched and settled once and for all.

REFERENCES

1. O'Donovan, T. R.: Ambulatory Surgical Centers — Development and Management. Germantown, Md., Aspen Systems Corp., 1976.
2. Hospitals. JAHA, August 1, 1973, p. 132.
3. Cohen, D. D., and Dillon, J. B.: Anesthesia for outpatient surgery. *196*:11–14, 1966.
4. Doenicke, A., Kugler, J., and Laub, M.: Evaluation of recovery and 'street-fitness' by EEG and psychodiagnostic tests after anesthesia. Can. Anaesth. Soc. J., *14*:567, 1967.
5. Fahy, A., and Marshall, M.: Postanesthetic morbidity in outpatients. Br. J. Anaesth., *41*:433, 1969.
6. Janis, K. M.: Hospital-based outpatient anesthesia service: Organization and management. Hosp. Med. Staff, February 1973, pp. 12–16.
7. *The Wall Street Journal*, Vol. 54, No. 1, January 4, 1974, p. 15.
8. Lahti, P. T.: Early postoperative discharge of patients. Mich. Med., 69 (17):755–760, 1970.
9. Early postoperative discharge of patients from the hospital. Surgery, 63:410–415, 1968.
10. Phalen, J. F.: Planning a hospital-based outpatient surgery program. Hosp. Prog., 57(6): 65, 1976.
11. Kiser, J. M., and Kiser, R. L.: Gearing up for the ambulatory care crunch. Trustee, December 1975, p. 19.
12. MacStravic, R. E.: Hospital-based ambulatory care — the wave of the future. Hosp. Health Serv. Admin., Winter 1976, p. 60.
13. Phalen, op. cit. p. 65.
14. An answer to soaring hospital costs? *Business Week*, July 7, 1975, p. 63.
15. In and out surgery. Perspective, Blue Cross-Blue Shield of Michigan, Third Quarter, 1974, p. 3.
16. Ibid. p. 10.

2 Organization and Functions of Emergency Department, Outpatient Clinic and Office Practice

JOHN D. HARRAH, M.D.,
ROBERT B. RUTHERFORD, M.D.,
and GEORGE J. HILL, II, M.D.

b. Charge slip
c. Ledger card
d. Billing
e. Overdue accounts
6. Medical payments
    a. Fees and payments

b. Credit
c. Professional courtesy
7. Third party payments
    a. Insurance
    b. Medicare
    c. Workmen's compensation

CURRENT PROBLEMS IN EMERGENCY AND OUTPATIENT CARE

The patterns of utilization of Emergency Departments and Outpatient Clinics in U.S. hospitals have altered greatly in the last decade.[10, 18, 19, 24] Most of the changes were initiated if not brought about by the changing practices of patients, or "consumers." Indeed, a significant proportion of the operational problems currently plaguing our Emergency Departments and related outpatient facilities can be traced to our hospitals' failure to appreciate or to adjust adequately to changes in the public's attitude and approach to obtaining health care. We hope that most of these changes represent stopgap measures and quantitative adjustments rather than basic or qualitative changes in the system of health care delivery. However, physicians and hospital administrators are increasingly aware of the problems and the need for change.[9, 13, 20] Continuing public pressure will be felt, and federal and state governments and other "third parties" will play an increasing role as the patient's advocate in establishing standards for and exerting controls over the provision and cost of health care.[6] Already, these concerns have led to the development of the PSRO (Peer System Review Organization), utilization reviews, hospital service audits[23] and the regional Health Systems Agency (HSA) plan, which will control most new construction of health care facilities in the United States. Substantive and possibly even radical changes can be anticipated in the future. Concepts such as the health maintenance organization, the freestanding ambulatory surgical center, the "convenience clinic" or the neighborhood health center are no longer considered novel. And the Emergency Physician, the Emergency Department Nurse Practitioner and the Emergency Medical Technician are accepted as legitimate health professionals.

Most existing emergency rooms were originally designed, equipped, staffed and organized to deal with the acutely ill and injured.[2, 3] Outpatient Clinics, on the other hand, have generally been geared toward new or unsolved problems of a nonemergent nature. The emphasis of the Clinic has been on outpatient diagnostic evaluation as a basis for definitive therapeutic decisions, whether or not the decision involves admission or operation. In the past, any outpatient treatment or long-term follow-up of these problems was usually left to the patient's primary physician. This was the same physician who cared for the patient's acute self-limited illnesses and other "minor" medical problems and provided regular physical check-ups and the long-term care of chronic illnesses.

However, the balance that has governed patient-physician relations in the past decade was fundamentally altered by new developments. The increase in medical specialization, the decrease in number and availability of primary care physicians, the great mobility of American society and increased expectations of the patient and the physician for modern diagnostic and therapeutic equipment have caught most hospitals and Outpatient Clinics unprepared to meet the challenge of these fundamental changes. A further complication is the availability of third party medical payment plans, which sometimes tends to encourage patients to seek early medical attention for relatively minor or self-limited illnesses.

Most hospitals' Outpatient Clinics, particularly in the larger institutions, have not tried to accommodate this demand. To the contrary, many of them have followed, if not led the way in, the trend to increase specialization by emphasizing secondary or tertiary rather than primary medical care. In major hospitals today, the patient will find himself in a maze of clinics with labels such as "cleft palate," "cancer chemotherapy," "renal hypertension," "audiology," "epilepsy," "glaucoma," "hand," "orthopedics," "peripheral vascular," "speech," "adolescent psychiatry," "collagen vascular," "pediatric allergy" and others. An attempt to have even a simple complaint, such as "persistent headaches," evaluated and treated in such a setting frequently results in multiple visits to different specialty clinics interspersed with long delays, an unfortunate and common situation that has been labeled "outpatient Ping-Pong." Even if the cause of the patient's complaint is fairly evident, the decision about which clinic he should be sent to is not always clear to someone unfamiliar with the hospital's ground rules.

While these particular problems are more often encountered in major medical centers, the patient is likely to be confronted with a loosely coordinated organization of specialty clinics in any sizable hospital, each with limited hours of operation, restrictive admission policies and long waiting times. The cost, let alone the amount of time consumed (particularly for the working patient) in seeking medical care in the traditionally organized Outpatient Clinic, may be prohibitive. On the other hand, there stands the Emergency Department completely equipped, staffed in all specialties and open to the public night and day. The inevitable and predictable result, given these factors, has been called the "Emergency Room population explosion." The patient census of many hospital Emergency Departments has doubled and in some cases tripled in the last two decades, and only recently has this trend tapered off. Thus, while inpatient admissions increased by 8 per cent per capita in this country in the 1960s and outpatient visits increased by 18 per cent, Emergency Room visits increased by 79 per cent, and while the rate of increase in the outpatient census was four times greater than that of the inpatient between 1952 and 1962, in the following decade it was approximately eight times greater.

The problem is greater than statistics alone would indicate, because the same Emergency Departments that were designed, equipped and staffed to deal with emergent or at least urgent medical problems now find themselves obliged to provide services formerly rendered by office visits or house calls made by physicians practicing in the community.[11] Currently, these non-emergency patients constitute approximately two-thirds of the national Emergency Department census. Such patients indirectly interfere with the effective delivery of care to true or serious emergencies, although in general, once an acutely ill or injured person has reached a major medical facility, the emergency medical care he receives is excellent and continues to improve. Treatment priorities often dictate that patients with relatively minor or nonurgent problems must wait the longest time for the least treatment. Pressure on the Emergency Department staff to keep up with this flood of patients not only is responsible for treatment errors (mainly those of omission) but also often leads to hurried, impersonal care and long waiting times. Friction between the patients and the Emergency Department staff is almost inevitable under these circumstances and causes most of the unpleasant incidents that erupt there.

In general, the practice of treating nonemergent problems in an Emergency Department results in episodic, expensive and ineffective medical care. Patients pay twice for this convenience, since they are charged both a physician's fee for service and a facilities fee that is necessarily high because of the expensive equipment, drugs and other supplies kept on hand for the management of all kinds of emergencies. Furthermore, the attending physician tends to order more laboratory and x-ray studies on these patients than the patient's regular physician would, and often there is inadequate follow-up care or repetition by the several physicians who may treat these patients over the course of a year of episodic walk-in medical care. Thus, while it may be referred to as "supermarket medicine," the use of an Emergency Department to obtain nonemergent medical care provides only the convenience of availability and not the speed, efficiency or reasonably low cost one expects at the neighborhood supermarket.

It is clear, then, that major changes are still needed in our system (if it may be called that) of delivering ambulatory or outpatient care. To be successful, the changes not only must lead to better, more comprehensive medical care at a reasonable cost but will also have to do so in a way that is convenient, logical and attractive enough to gain public acceptance. Too much of the current public "abuse" of emergency care facilities has been blamed on lack of patient education. While this may be a problem, it must also be appreciated that the public will not use outpatient facilities in the intended way if they do not satisfy the patient's needs and expectations, regardless of how well patients are indoctrinated or how well the facilities are conceived and organized from the

point of view of the hospital and its medical staff.

GENERAL APPROACH TO DESIGN OF AMBULATORY CARE FACILITIES

The planning and building of an outpatient or emergency care facility involves several rather distinct phases:

1. The program planning phase, which includes determining the need for the facility and its role in the delivery of health care in the community at large and within the hospital complex itself. Planners must determine the intended scope of capabilities and the medical and surgical services the facility will offer, estimating its cost and its feasibility in terms of the availability of construction funds. A master plan and schematic drawings must be completed.

2. The physical planning phase, in which final architectural drawings are completed and construction documents are drawn up.

3. The actual construction phase.

4. The "moving-in" phase, in which painting, decorations and internal furnishings are completed and movable equipment is installed.

Bids for architectural and construction firms are let out between each of the first three phases, respectively, and the whole process usually requires three to five years from start to finish. Although it is recognized that most of the instructions from the medical staff must be given in the initial phase, the importance of involving the architects as early as possible is not generally appreciated. It is advantageous to include them during the conceptual period, long before the formal architectural work actually begins. One cannot expect architects to come up with good functional designs if they have not received adequate information from the hospital staff.

The individual characteristics of each hospital and its staff, the community in which it is located and the patient population which it serves vary so widely that no single design concept will prove universally satisfactory. Therefore, one should beware of prepackaged or "off the shelf" plans. Nothing less than a custom-tailored job will do, and nowhere is the advice that architectural "design must be based on function" more applicable. Careful prospective study of these variables offers the best prospect of success in planning for a new, expanded or renovated emergency or outpatient facility.

Before focusing on the actual design or internal features of the new facility, a series of basic preliminary steps must be taken. One must first establish the need for the new facility as well as the availability of construction funds before going very far. The next step is to establish clearly the type of care to be offered in this new facility. In doing this, differences must be resolved between the type of care the hospital can provide and the type of care the community needs and seeks. Considerations must be based on the desires and capabilities of the medical staff and the type of care offered by other facilities in the same area. The importance of these points and the need to have them settled at the outset cannot be overemphasized. It may seem that most hospitals let community needs determine the type of care they give and the manner in which it will be provided. However, this is rarely the sole determinant and sometimes not even the major one. Administratively, most hospitals exercise a number of constraints over outpatient as well as inpatient admissions. Such constraints frequently exist even when they are not formally set forth in the form of eligibility rules pertaining to residency, financial status, service-connected disability or other factors.

A subtler but equally powerful influence is the attitude of the medical staff toward patient care. For example, the faculty of a university hospital might feel that it should function as a referral center for problems of special interest or complexity and should not provide community health care in its broadest sense. Such an attitude might not be readily apparent to patients from the community who present themselves for care at that hospital, nor would it influence their choice. Those responsible for organizing outpatient and emergency care in such institutions will find themselves caught in the middle when this occurs.

The situation in community hospitals presents other difficulties. Established practitioners on the staffs of these hospitals understandably wish to center (and schedule) their own outpatient care activities in their offices. They may rarely use the hospital's Outpatient Clinics and may view the Emergency Department as a convenient place in which to meet their private patients to handle off-hour emergencies or to perform special procedures for which their offices are not adequately equipped. Many of these hospitals are encountering increasing difficulties in providing adequate coverage for their Emergency Departments and Outpatient Clinics from their own "volunteer" staff.

Obviously these two situations require entirely different approaches in the organization and planning of outpatient operations. It should be clear that the guiding philosophies behind each institution's outpatient activities need to be clarified formally at the highest administrative level and that the approval of the medical staff must be gained before proceeding very far with the actual design phase.

The patient population to be served by this outpatient facility should be analyzed and sufficient demographic data obtained to identify both the present patient population and the changing trends that will affect its future make-up. Finally, one must investigate all other existing or planned outpatient facilities in the community or region. More than one metropolitan medical center has found its outpatient facilities overwhelmed as one or more neighboring hospitals have joined in the flight to the suburbs. Nor is it unique for two neighboring hospitals to launch independent expansion programs almost simultaneously for their outpatient and emergency care facilities. This lack of interhospital cooperation, communication and coordination has been responsible for the emergence of regional and community health planning agencies.

The contemporary movement toward categorization of emergency medical facilities is a first step in regional medical planning. Standards have been drawn up by the AMA Commission on Emergency Medical Services for four distinct levels of capability in providing emergency medical services.[4] Professional staffing, facilities and equipment, supporting diagnostic services and intensive care units, and communications capabilities are evaluated in four categories: I (Comprehensive), II (Major), III (General), and IV (Basic Emergency Medical Services). It is anticipated that these or similar guidelines will be adopted, and it is hoped that categorization will be accomplished with the voluntary cooperation of the hospitals by survey questionnaire and site visit. It has been suggested that each hospital be allowed to achieve as high a category as it wishes, but then each should be expected to function effectively at its chosen level. This suggestion recognizes that not all hospitals have the capability or the desire to handle any and all emergencies but that all should have at least the facilities for resuscitation and referral.

It is also recognized that many hospitals will perceive an economic threat in any categorization plan if it appears to imply that they are not "first rate." This fear has impeded the implementation of such plans. It has been suggested that the capabilities of each hospital for handling different types of problems should be established, rather than attempting to assign each hospital to the appropriate category. Few hospitals fill *every* requirement for a given category. Most can provide higher levels of care

in some areas than in others. Thus, one hospital may have a burn center but not a cardiopulmonary bypass unit, while another has a thoracic surgeon but no neurosurgeon. A third hospital may have intensive care facilities for managing coronary occlusion and other cardiopulmonary emergencies but not the facilities or staff to handle poisonings, drug overdoses or multiple system traumas. An emergency care system that acknowledges rather than ignores these important differences and that can transport patients with specific problems to the hospital best equipped to handle them is not only more realistic but more logical.

A more efficient system of delivering emergency medical care should result from establishing the specific capabilities and desires of each hospital. Obviously the adopted standards must be kept in mind in building a new or enlarged facility, since such guidelines will probably serve as criteria for a successful application for federal funds to support the building program.

Other preliminary considerations include the determination of basic space needs, the choice between expansion and renovation versus rebuilding and the selection of the optimum building site. Space needs are difficult to estimate without the help of an experienced architect. There are no universally accepted factors for converting the patient load of an Outpatient or Emergency Department into square footage. Large facilities tend to be more efficient than small ones in minimizing poorly utilized or dead space.

Similarly, busy clinics that have staggered appointment systems and a predominance of multipurpose examining rooms, with a minimum of specialty examination or treatment areas, will function more efficiently and require less space for a given patient load. The average surgical patient can be seen in a twenty minute period, with a complete turnover time for the room of less than thirty minutes, which includes time allowances for the patient to dress and undress, for clinical personnel to change the linen and tidy the room and for the physician to complete the patient's records. Complicated or new cases will take approximately twice as long, while simple follow-up procedures and suture removals will take approximately half that time. One should not adhere too strictly to this observation in planning space, because a calculation of two patients an hour, eight hours a day, for each 100 square feet of examining room would be an underestimate of the overall space needed. Such an estimation does not account for the percentage utilization rate or for the additional space required for clinic support. Even the most efficient design will need an additional 50 per cent of space for waiting rooms, corridors and administrative and ancillary patient care areas. In clinic planning, provisions for future expansion and alteration should be considered carefully, since many busy clinics rarely achieve 50 per cent utilization initially. Thus, in practice, space needs for an Outpatient Clinic may run as high as 25 to 50 square feet per patient day.

One might think that an Emergency Department, open 24 rather than 8 hours daily, would utilize space more efficiently than an Outpatient Clinic. However, the Emergency Department must be designed to handle peak loads that may last for only a few hours a day, and its spacious and well-equipped trauma-resuscitation area may be used only 10 per cent of the time. Because of such essential but poorly utilized areas, the smaller Emergency Departments are usually less efficient in their use of space. There is no linear conversion factor, but a convenient figure to work from is 10,000 gross square feet for a daily patient load of 100 patients. This may seem high, but one must remember that there are few Emergency Departments in this country that are big enough to handle the clinical demands placed on them.

The choice between expansion and renovation as opposed to rebuilding is usually not difficult to make. The availability of construction funds and space in which to expand and the suitability of the arrangement of the present structure will ordinarily make the choice obvious. It should go without saying that the hospital's Emergency Department and its various outpatient components should be spatially related to each other in a functional manner and, to a lesser degree, to essential administrative and supporting services. Inappropriate external arrangements may seriously detract from an otherwise well-conceived Emergency Department plan.

For the internal design it is usually advisable to begin with a rough plan based on patient flow and services performed, and then to adjust the size of each area to meet expected peak demands. At this point the architect can complete the details after consultation with the personnel who will be involved in the daily operation of each area. Architects can only produce a satisfactory design if provided with proper and specified information such as the magnitude and type of patient load, the anticipated maximum rates of patient arrivals, the nature and frequency of services and procedures performed, the need for special diagnostic or therapeutic equipment and other considerations. For this reason it is often easier for experienced personnel to renovate and enlarge an existing facility than to build a new one, for they can see the shortcomings of the facility they now work in more clearly than those of one being created from architectural drawings.

The simplest ambulatory care facility will consist of a common receiving area for all outpatients that is served by a number of general examining rooms and one large multipurpose treatment area for special procedures and resuscitation. It should be located close to the hospital's x-ray and laboratory facilities. In larger hospitals, emergency and nonurgent outpatient care should be provided in separate (though preferably adjacent) areas. In most hospitals, a significant proportion of the outpatient traffic is of an unscheduled but non-emergent nature, so a screening clinic should be located immediately adjacent to the Outpatient Clinic's main entrance.

Some of these concepts can be better appreciated by a consideration of Figure 2–1, a schematic representation of the layout for an outpatient facility. The oversimplified arrangement depicted here does not indicate the vertical or horizontal access to important inpatient areas and supporting services, such as the operating room and blood bank. Important details of internal design are also deliberately omitted. This figure is not intended to recommend a specific plan but to illustrate the considerations involved in developing a functionally satisfactory layout. Note, for example, that the Emergency Department parking area is separate from that for general outpatient use. Each parking area should have well-marked, separate access ways to facilitate traffic control. The concept of separate but adjacent entrances is carried from the parking lot into the hospital so that the acutely ill and injured enter directly into the Emergency Department, whereas the ambulatory ill enter through the main outpatient entrance. The main outpatient entrance is flanked by a receiving and registration area on one side and a screening or triage clinic on the other. With this arrangement, the patient can receive proper directions as soon as he enters the outpatient area. He can be registered and his records sent for at the same station. The administrative core area is completed by the clinic cashier and outpatient administrative offices. After registration, the unscheduled patient is seen in the screening clinic and then either referred to the Emergency Department or to the appropriate Outpatient Clinic or given simple treatment on the spot. The diagnostic laboratory and the x-ray unit are positioned to serve both the Emergency Department and the Outpatient Clinics. There

is a general waiting area located on the outpatient side of the diagnostic facilities and this, in turn, is conveniently located across from a coffee shop or refreshment stand. Adjacent to it, at the exit from the Outpatient Clinic areas, is the pharmacy.

EMERGENCY DEPARTMENT

Design Planning

Many of the considerations mentioned in regard to the overall design of an ambulatory care complex apply individually to the design of an Emergency Department.[16, 21] Again, design should be based on function. However, few Emergency Departments function identically, so before proceeding with the actual design of a new, expanded or renovated Emergency Department, responsible members of the hospital staff must answer a number of practical questions pertaining to Emergency Department function.

For example:

Will the Emergency Department function as such in a strict sense, or will it also serve as an ambulance-admitting area or walk-in ambulatory care facility?

Will the surgical and orthopedic treatment areas be used for elective procedures such as minor surgery and cast changes?

Will there be an emergency observation ward, or will all patients be admitted to one of the inpatient services?

Will lacerations be sutured, casts applied and abscesses drained in special treatment areas or in examining cubicles in which portable equipment and sterile supplies are available?

Will patients with major trauma receive resuscitation and definitive diagnostic and therapeutic procedures in the Emergency Department, or will they be transferred immediately to either the operating room or intensive care areas?

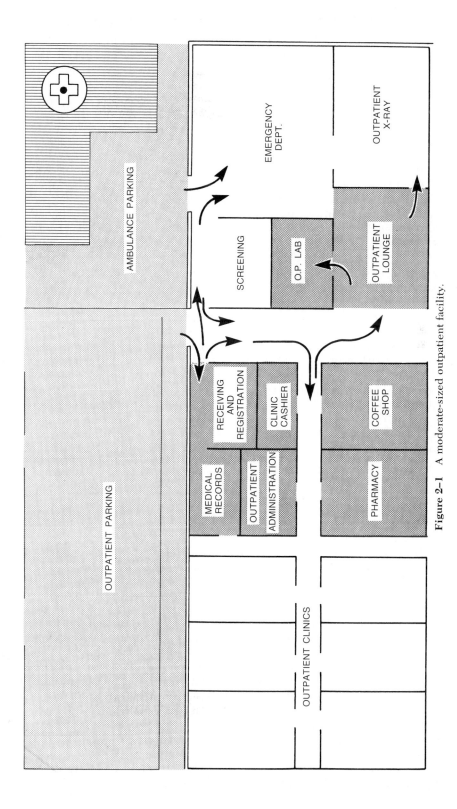

Figure 2–1 A moderate-sized outpatient facility.

Will pediatric, medical, surgical, obstetric and gynecological and psychiatric problems all be seen in a common suite of examining rooms, or will separate but adjacent facilities be required?

Will patient registration and financial arrangements be handled in the Emergency Department or elsewhere?

Will the Emergency Department serve as the outpatient complex's "front door," or will there be a separate receiving and screening clinic?

Will the Emergency Department serve as a focus for any of the institution's special treatment programs (for alcoholism, drug addiction, hemophilia or asthma, for example)?

Will clinical research be conducted in the Emergency Room?

Will a conference room be needed for educational programs conducted in the Emergency Department for physicians, medical students, nurses, emergency medical technicians or other allied health personnel?

Will basic diagnostic tests be performed in the Emergency Department, or will all specimens be sent to the main laboratory?

The answers to these and other basic questions about the functional requirements of the Emergency Department will place one in a better position to estimate the basic space requirements, as previously discussed, keeping in mind future growth, the need to plan for peak loading conditions and the fact that few Emergency Departments in this country (including many less than ten years old) are adequate for their current daily operations.[8]

Before turning to the details of internal design, the facilities and services that have external relationships important to the Emergency Department should be carefully considered: blood bank, x-ray department (if there is no x-ray unit in the Emergency Department), diagnostic laboratory, operating room, central receiving and admissions, screening clinic (if separate), other Outpatient Clinics, medical records, patient parking areas, pharmacy, central supply and the hospital's "front door." The spatial relationship of the Emergency Department to these other departments may be of great importance.

Attention must also be given to the following aspects of internal design: the need for controlled, orderly patient flow; separate access to the Emergency Department for ambulance and ambulatory patients and for Emergency Department personnel; adequate waiting areas for patients and the friends and relatives who accompany them; special and multipurpose treatment areas; lavatories; dressing rooms; lounges and sleeping quarters for physicians; nurses' lounges and conference rooms for in-service teaching programs; an area for extended observation and treatment (emergency observation ward); areas for storage and supplies, areas for clean and dirty linens and areas for x-ray and laboratory procedures.

As the details of the Emergency Department layout unfold, compromises will have to be made. For example, maximum visibility of the patients by Emergency Department staff is desirable, but on the other hand, an adequate degree of privacy is needed for special diagnostic or therapeutic procedures. Similarly, in this era of specialization there is a tendency to develop separate areas that are specifically designed and equipped for the management of certain emergencies. If this trend is followed to its inevitable conclusion, an Emergency Department might have a trauma receiving area, cardiac emergency area, laceration area, poison or overdose area, dirty or incision and drainage area, orthopedic area or cast room, eye, ear, nose and throat examining rooms, GYN or "pelvic" rooms and minor surgery areas. Only the largest Emergency Departments can justify this degree of specialization economically. In most medium-sized Emergency Departments, it is usually preferable to combine all of the special emergency equipment in one spacious trauma-resuscitation area. This equipment includes EKG monitoring, oscilloscope, defibrillator, respirator, Ambu bags, laryngoscopes, endotracheal tubes, emergency drugs, special procedure trays and catheterization equipment. To avoid unnecessary duplication, the multipurpose examining rooms should be equipped to be used not only for examination but also for minor treatments by bringing in portable equipment or special trays of instruments. A selection of equipment includes cast cart, IV cart, incision and drainage tray and suture tray. For this approach to be successful, the individual examining rooms must be larger than usual and must have good lighting, oxygen, suction and multiple electric outlets. They should be at least 9 by 12 feet in size, preferably 10 by 14 feet, and should be equipped with a good stretcher or mobile cart rather than a fixed examining table.

Following are some arbitrary recommendations regarding Emergency Department design and — indirectly — function. Of necessity, they reflect personal opinion and are not intended to represent the final solution. Since they are based on personal experience in specific Emergency Departments, they might be better appreciated by referring to Figure 2–2, a suggested layout for a moderate-sized Emergency Department that might comfortably accommodate about 25,000 visits a year. This plan is actually a stylized version of the layout of the Emergency Department at the Colorado General Hospital, with some of the undesirable features included to give a more functional design.

The Emergency Department entrance and parking area should be clearly marked and well lit, with the signs visible from a distance of 75 to 100 yards. Signs indicating the direction of the Emergency Department entrance should also be posted at other main hospital entrances and at major intersections leading to the hospital. The Emergency Department entrance should be partly covered for protection from the elements, and there should be room for at least two ambulances to pass and park easily. No extended parking privileges should be allowed at the ambulance entrance itself. If adjacent emergency parking is provided, it should be identifiably separate from ambulance parking, and approximately 12 parking spaces should be provided per 20,000 annual visits. Such emergency parking should be closely supervised or it will soon cease to serve the needs of the Emergency Department's patients. The ambulance unloading area should be visible from the front desk within the Emergency Department through clear glass windows or doors. The entrance doors themselves should be double-width, as should all the main corridors of the Emergency Department, easily accommodating a stretcher with people walking on both sides. There should be a double set of these doors, which open automatically as well as manually in case of power failure. This ambulance entrance should provide direct access to the Emergency Department's receiving area. Thus, the seriously ill and injured patients can pass directly into the trauma resuscitation area without going through the main waiting room. There should be a security station near this entrance as well as a "parking space" for additional stretchers and wheelchairs (2 for every 4,000 annual visits). Also near this entrance should be an "outside room" with direct and separate access from both outside and inside the Emergency Department. This room can serve as a decontamination station for patients contaminated with radionuclides, riot control gases or other noxious substances that would be undesirable if directly introduced into the internal environment of the Emergency Department. It can also be used for holding patients who are dead on arrival pending their transfer to the morgue or the medical examiner's office. In addition, it may be appropriate

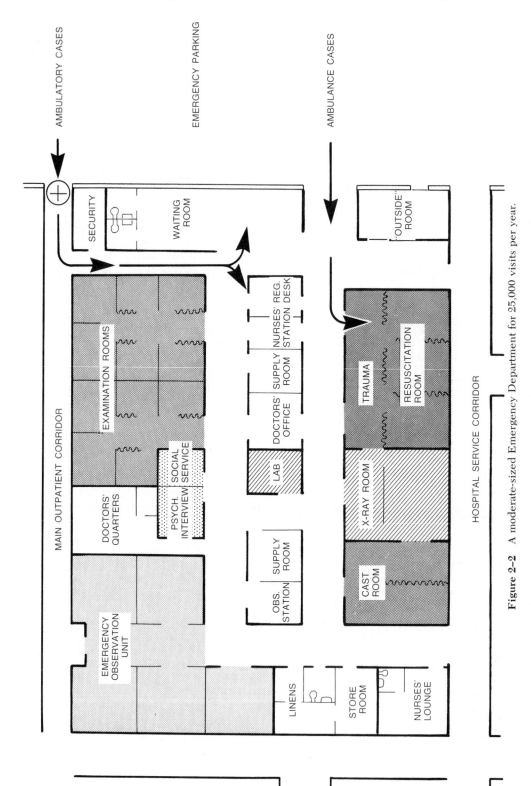

Figure 2-2 A moderate-sized Emergency Department for 25,000 visits per year.

to have an area with drop curtains, shower and hose immediately outside this room for large-scale decontamination procedures.

Clearly separate from the ambulance entrance should be an ambulatory entrance that allows patients to enter the Emergency Department waiting area from both the outside parking lot and a main hospital corridor. The waiting area of the Emergency Department should be large, with at least twice the number of seats as the average number of patients seen per hour. Waiting rooms are usually made too small because of the idealistic philosophy that patients shouldn't have to wait. However, the time and magnitude of peak patient arrivals are unpredictable, and allowance must also be made for friends and relatives accompanying the patient. The waiting area should be well furnished with television or background music, current reading material, beverage and candy vending machines, adjacent rest rooms and telephones. The reception desk should be open. It should face the Emergency Department entrances and the main waiting area. It is important to avoid having patients and their relatives or friends milling around the reception desk. Ordinarily, each new arriving patient, after stating his problem, should be given a number and asked to take a seat until registration can be completed. However, if the patient's condition is obviously an emergency requiring immediate evaluation and treatment on admission, he should be ushered promptly into a treatment room. The registration desk should be backed by a nurses' station from which the nurses can clearly see both registering and waiting patients and which will allow the nurses to be easily consulted by the clerks regarding problem patients. During overload periods when there is a backup of waiting patients, nurses should make an attempt to go out into the waiting room and interview each waiting patient at least briefly to assess the urgency of his problem and advise

him about the anticipated waiting time he will encounter. An operations control board placed across from the doctors' and nurses' office in the patient examining area has been found to be extremely helpful. The patient's name and time of admission to an examining room as well as the presenting problem is listed and initialed by the nurse at the time of admission. The physician initials the next column to indicate that he or she has accepted that patient. After examination and treatment, the physician lists the diagnostic studies and consultations ordered as well as any other items necessary for final disposition. A glance at this board as well as at the adjacent boxes of charts of patients not yet admitted enables the Emergency Department personnel to assess its operational status and to decide on appropriate action.

The supply room should be centrally located to minimize unnecessary movement. There should be a separate doctors' station where records can be completed, telephone calls received, consultations made and diagnostic studies reviewed. A small diagnostic laboratory should be provided, in which white blood cell counts, hematocrit readings and urinalysis can be performed and smears stained or cultured, even though most of the studies may be done in the main laboratory. Both the general examining rooms and special treatment areas should be readily accessible and within hearing — if not sight — of the doctors' or nurses' station. Ideally, an x-ray unit should be located inside or immediately adjacent to the Emergency Department, preferably between the orthopedic room and the trauma resuscitation area. The x-ray unit should have a multipurpose capability but, most important, it should have a rapid developer. The other features shown in Figure 2–2 are self-explanatory. More will be said about the emergency observation ward in the next section. The design in Figure 2–2 is adequate for a moderate-sized Emergency Department in the true sense of the words. A larger Emergency Department requires considerably more functional specialization, particularly when there is an admixture that includes nonurgent or ambulatory care problems. Figure 2–3 illustrates the basic layout of an Emergency Department designed to receive 100,000 or more emergency and nonemergent visits annually. It shows a degree of functional separation into specialty areas appropriate only in the largest of emergency departments.

Emergency Observation Unit

The emergency observation unit is a controversial feature of many large Emergency Departments and is more typical of a university, city or county hospital than of a private community hospital. Large Emergency Departments usually receive a higher proportion of "disposition cases." They are staffed by physicians on full-time duty and have a greater number of specialized, independent inpatient services. Observation units are sometimes denigrated on the theory that if a patient needs more than a few hours of observation or treatment he ought to be admitted as an inpatient. However, most large metropolitan hospitals find these units invaluable from a practical point of view. The situation is analogous to that of waiting rooms in Emergency Departments: ideally, there should be no need for a large waiting room, but it is a practical necessity in most Emergency Departments.

There are several valid reasons for the existence of these observation units. Their real *raison d'être* is to allow for continued, frequent observation of patients by the same physician over the course of several hours but for less than a day. The assumption is that the majority of these patients will be discharged from the hospital within 24 hours. Subsequent developments in some patients will clarify a need for continued hospitalization that was not apparent on admission. A typical example of this use of an observation unit is the patient with acute abdominal pain who may be developing a "surgical abdomen." Other examples are patients with a history of a significant blow to the head or frank concussion with no neurological signs of residual symptoms and patients with an acute psychiatric crisis, drug overdose or suicidal gesture for whom immediate admission to a psychiatric hospital would be a threat or stigma. Patients who have been involved in a serious automobile accident but who appear on initial evaluation to have escaped serious injury should be observed for several hours before discharge from the hospital. All of these patients deserve repeated evaluation or extended observation by the same physician. If these physicians are on full-time duty in a busy Emergency Department, their patients cannot readily be observed if they are scattered around the inpatient wards of the hospital. On the one hand, these patients do not need the degree of nursing care provided in an intensive care unit, but on the other, they need more observation than is usually provided overnight on a regular ward. Patients who present observation problems should be confined in one area, under the eye of a single nurse and conveniently close to the doctors who are responsible for their care. This plan not only is convenient and economical but promotes good patient care.

The real controversy usually arises when these observation units are used for other purposes, for instance, as a buffer against "undesirable," untimely or unrewarding admissions to inpatient services. These units are often used as overnight or weekend holding areas for other disposition cases until they can be sent to a more "appropriate" medical facility. Examples are their use as short-term admission areas for more complicated diagnostic procedures (arteriography, liver or spleen biopsy) and as places for the short-term treatment of selected "surgical infections" that

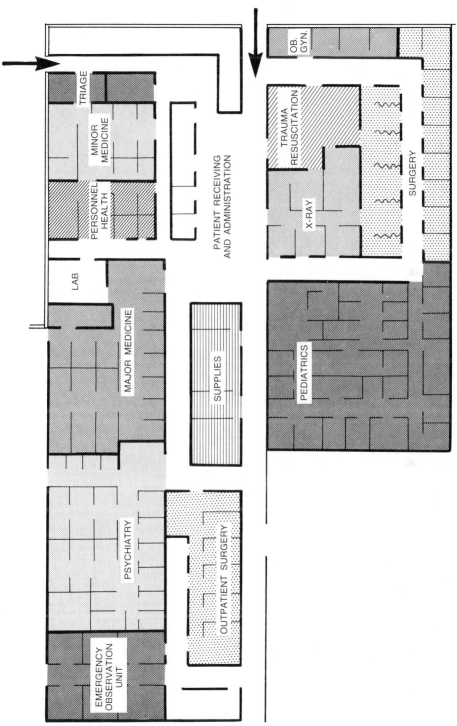

Figure 2–3   A large Emergency Department for 100,000 visits per year.

would benefit from a brief period of intensive antibiotic and topical therapy following drainage or débridement in the Emergency Department. The observation units are used for the treatment of selected hematological problems by the administration of whole blood, packed cells or other blood components and for short-term observation of "completed" abortions. Other uses are for short-term treatment of recurrent "medical" problems with established diagnosis for which prompt resolution under treatment can reasonably be expected (e.g. asthmatic crises, epileptic seizures, complications of ethanol intoxication and other problems). Therapeutic crises in cancer chemotherapy patients are sometimes managed in observation units to avoid unnecessary hospitalization. Depending on the particular circumstances in a given hospital, the indications just described for admission to an emergency observation unit may be considered acceptable. However, unless the allowable exceptions to the traditional indications for admission to the emergency observation unit are specifically set down in the Emergency Department's written procedures, this unit will tend to be used for the management of such conditions as acute pancreatitis, acute cholecystitis, spontaneous pneumothorax, acute pelvic inflammatory disease and other medical and surgical problems that usually cannot be controlled within 24 hours. As long as the use of emergency observation beds is carefully supervised, this area can have one of the best rates of bed utilization in a modern medical center. The minimum essentials of design for this unit include a central nursing station with good visibility of multiple semi-open patient cubicles, drug and linen supply areas and adequate toilet facilities. One or two of the units may be specially modified for the protective custody of patients with psychiatric problems or those under surveillance by a law enforcement agency. One observation bed per 75 inpatient beds usually suffices.

Equipment, Supplies and Drugs

It goes without saying that even the best trained professional staff cannot deliver emergency medical care without appropriate equipment, supplies and drugs. A discussion of specific choices is beyond the scope of this chapter. The following are offered as check lists and should not be considered complete or all-inclusive, since they were taken from the inventory of a single emergency department.

1. Equipment, Minor

alcohol lamp
bandage scissors
blood agar plates
blood sampling sets
blood sampling equipment
  (vacutainers, syringes, tubes)
catheters (intravenous, urinary, nasogastric, pediatric peritoneal
  dialysis, assorted thoracostomy, central venous)
counter pressure device (G-suit)
culture tubes, swabs
drains
esophageal balloon (Sengstaken)
flashlights, bulbs, batteries
hot water bottles
ice bags
incubator
instrument stands
ophthalmoscope
otoscope
selected special and extra instruments
  (in sterile pan)
selected suture material
soaking basins and tubs
sterile dressings
thermometers
tracheostomy tubes, multiple sizes
thioglycolate broth tubes

2. Equipment, Major

arm boards
cardiopulmonary resuscitation cart
defibrillator-monitor
irrigation stands

Kelly pads

operating or "laceration" tables

operating lights (overhead movable and portable)

orthopedic cart

portable oxygen tank (in addition to wall oxygen)

portable suction machine (in addition to wall suction)

refrigerator

splints (Thomas, universal, hand and other selected splints)

sphygmomanometers (wall mounted and portable)

trauma cart

trauma (x-ray) stretchers

ventilatory support equipment (oropharyngeal airways, padded tongue blades, laryngoscopes, endotracheal and nasotracheal tubes, McGill forceps, Ambu bags, mechanical ventilator)

3. Special Procedure Sets

burn dressing — major

central venous pressure catheterization tray

cutdown tray

D and C tray

lumbar puncture tray

ENT tray (including nasal packing)

gastric lavage tray

paracentesis tray

Kirschner wire set

minor dressing pack

minor pelvic tray

sigmoidoscopy tray

suture tray with plastic surgery instruments

thoracotomy tray (with vascular clamps)

tracheostomy tray

tube thoracostomy tray

COMMENT. The cardiopulmonary resuscitation cart includes all the equipment, drugs and supplies that might be needed in the event of a cardiopulmonary arrest. This would ordinarily be kept in the trauma-resuscitation area, particularly if one section of that area is specifically set aside for the management of cardiac and respiratory crises. In the same area, a defibrillator and electrocardiogram or cardiac monitor is kept. However, cardiac and respiratory arrests do not always occur where they are supposed to, so it is important that all this equipment be easily portable. On the other hand, except in the event of multiple injuries or minor disasters, most of the major trauma will be managed in the area designated for this purpose. It is wise to have a "trauma" cart separate from the cardiopulmonary resuscitation cart, on which is placed all the items that might ordinarily be requested by the physician or the nurse during the first ten minutes of arrival of a major trauma victim. These items should include, for example, lactated Ringer's solution, Plasmanate, infusion sets, venous pressure sets, Intracaths, Foley catheters, nasogastric tubes, blood sampling syringes and tubes, a variety of syringes and needles and a clipboard on which vital signs and other observations are recorded. The trauma cart or carts should also hold tourniquets, sterile gloves, oxygen nasal cannula and mask, organic iodide prep, antibiotic ointment, adhesive tape, sterile lubrication jelly, suction catheters, three-way stopcocks, alcohol sponges, large and small gauze dressings, arm boards, sand bags, lidocaine, epinephrine, calcium chloride and sodium bicarbonate. Since victims of serious multiple injuries are usually cared for by a team of physicians and nurses, we have found it appropriate to divide the materials among four smaller carts. The one placed near the patient's head includes all the equipment needed for airway control and the insertion of nasogastric tubes. A second one at the patient's side has all the equipment necessary for insertion of a central venous pressure catheter. A third cart on the patient's other side carries equipment for insertion of a peripheral intravenous catheter plus that needed for performing abdominal paracentesis. The fourth cart has everything needed for insertion of an indwelling urinary catheter. This allows each of the attending physicians to perform quickly those procedures that are almost routinely applied to serious trauma victims, without having to struggle to reach a common "crash" cart or having to bother the nurse. The nurse is in turn free either to monitor the patient's vital signs or to respond to special requests.

Although most orthopedic treatment can best be carried out in a specific area equipped with sinks having plaster traps, x-ray view boxes, splints, slings, traction equipment and so on, it is usually expedient (for simpler procedures) to take a plaster cart to the patient rather than to have the patient wait until this "cast room" is cleared of more complicated cases. This is just one example of the need for flexibility rather than commitment to one fixed procedure.

4. Drugs

Table 2–1 gives a partial list of drugs that might be maintained in an Emergency Department. Depending on the convenience and availabilty of the hospital or neighborhood pharmacy, it may be necessary for the Emergency Department to stock single days' supplies of important or commonly used drugs, such as antibiotics, as well as those listed here. In addition, the Emergency Department must stock crutches, canes, Ace bandages and other take-home supplies for the patients if they are not readily available elsewhere in the hospital on a 24-hour basis, including weekends.

5. Furniture

Each examining room should have a desk and two chairs and be stocked with changes of linen, examining gowns and commonly used supplies: cotton swabs, gloves, lubricants, adhesive tape, simple dressings, medical record forms, prescription pads, requi-

sition forms for laboratory and x-ray studies, disposable towels, Kleenex tissues, flashlight, reflex hammer, otoscope and ophthalmoscope, stethoscope, sphygmomanometer, and so on. The ideal patient cart or stretcher should have a radiolucent top that is flexible and adjustable so that the head can be elevated and the knees bent. It should be adjustable in height, have its own IV standard and be equipped with stirrups, safety straps, side rails and wheel brakes. Few models fit all these specifications.

Personnel Staffing and Duties

The staffing requirements of an Emergency Department have traditionally been broken down into categories for physicians, nurses and administrators. Unfortunately, this same separatism often carries over into the job descriptions of these personnel and into the lines of authority and responsibility. In the last few years, the clear lines of distinction between the roles of the doctor, the nurse and the clerk have been obscured by the appearance in the Emergency Department of emergency medical technicians, physician's associates, patient's ombudsmen, social workers and other allied health personnel. In addition, there has been a steady trend toward expanding and upgrading the duties of both nursing and administrative personnel in the Emergency Department. Thus, inflexibility regarding the roles of the various Emergency Department personnel is now being relaxed in the cause of efficiency and economy.

Efforts are being made to transfer many of the routine duties formerly performed by the physician and nurse to the nurse and clerk, respectively. The time and effort of each staff member are more efficiently spent performing the duties and using the skills for which he or she was trained. The objective is to allow the physicians to concentrate on those tasks that require

TABLE 2-1 Drugs Stocked in the Emergency Department

acetylsalicylic compound	hyperimmune globulin, tetanus
albumin, normal human serum	insulin
aminophylline	iodine and organic iodide solutions
ammonia, aromatic spirits	isoproterenol
amphetamine sulfate	isopropyl alcohol
antivenin, coral snake	kaolin with pectin mixture
antivenin, polyvalent snake	levarterenol bitartrate
antivenin, spider bite	lidocaine hydrochloride
apomorphine hydrochloride	magnesium sulfate
atropine sulfate	meperidine hydrochloride
bacitracin ointment	meprobamate
benzalkonium chloride solution	methylene blue
caffeine and sodium benzoate	morphine sulfate
calamine lotion	nalorphine hydrochloride
calcium chloride	neomycin sulfate ointment
calcium gluconate	neostigmine bromide
chloral hydrate	neostigmine methylsulfate
chlordiazepoxide hydrochloride	naloxone hydrochloride
chlorpromazine	norepinephrine
codeine	oxytocin
codeine terpin hydrate, dehydrocodeine cough	papaverine hydrochloride
mixture	paraldehyde
cortisone acetate	Peruvian balsam
dextran	phenobarbital
diazepam	phenol
digitoxin	phenylephrine hydrochloride
digoxin	phenytoin (Dilantin)
dehydroergotamine	physostigmine
diphenhydramine hydrochloride (Benadryl)	phytonadione
edathamil calcium–disodium	plasma protein fraction, human
ephedrine sulfate	potassium permanganate tablets
epinephrine	procainamide hydrochloride
ergonovine maleate	procaine hydrochloride
ethyl chloride spray	promethazine hydrochloride, NF
fibrinogen, human	protamine sulfate
fluorescein sodium	quinidine sulfate
glucose, 50% in sterile water	silver nitrate applicators
globulin, immune serum	sodium amytal
glycerine suppositories	sodium bicarbonate
glyceryl trinitrate	talc
heparin, sodium	tetanus antitoxin, bovine
hexachlorophene solution	tetanus toxoid
hydrocortisone acetate	tetracaine hydrochloride
hydrocortisone sodium sulfate	tincture of benzoin
hydrogen peroxide solution	zinc chloride

their skill and judgment. Then the nurse, technicians and other allied health personnel may carry out more of the routine procedures, such as gathering historical background, recording vital signs and making other simple physical observations, as well as performing some of the more common manipulative or therapeutic tasks. These include taking EKGs, starting IVs and drawing blood samples. These activities are carried out under the direction and supervision of the physicians rather than being performed by them personally.

Similarly, expanding the duties of the clerk in the Emergency Department will free the nurses of paperwork and allow them to concentrate on patient care. These upward shifts will gradually bring about changes in the relationships and ratios among the patient, physician, nurse and allied health personnel. Theoretically, since everyone will be working closer to the upper limits of his or her ability and skill, a greater degree of job satisfaction should result, and the entire operation should be more economical and efficient. The basic duties performed in an Emergency Department will not change, but there will be a gradual change in the personnel who perform them, with a broadening base of auxiliary staff. Even if new types of personnel, such as emergency medical technicians and physician's associates, are not introduced into an Emergency Department and the basic physician-nurse-clerk staffing pattern continues, the duties and responsibilities of each member of the team can be expected to shift upward.

To operate efficiently, the Emergency Department must have direction, and this can best be provided by interested and involved physicians, although it is not always feasible for every Emergency Department to have a full-time physician-director. While this may be a goal worth striving for in any large Emergency Department, practical considerations require that some compromise be made in smaller, less active Emergency Departments. Even though they usually have most of the appropriate leadership qualifications, few traditionally trained surgeons have the background or inclination to devote themselves full-time to this effort. The Emergency Department is an unpredictably busy, 168 hour per week operation that cannot be given full-time direction by any single physician, even if he or she works long hours. To achieve round-the-clock direction, a responsive system is necessary, with clear lines of authority that are followed in a responsible manner. Formalized, well-disseminated Emergency Department policies are essential. Standard procedures, lines of authority and delegated responsibility can provide this essential direction whether the director of the Emergency Department is immediately present or not.

Organizational Patterns

If an Emergency Department has a physician-director who devotes a significant proportion of time to this job, he or she will ordinarily work closely with the head nurse and either a unit manager or an administrative assistant, seeing that the operational policies of the Emergency Department, which they formulate together, are carried out on a daily basis. Another common organization pattern is the Emergency Department committee made up of staff physicians representing different clinical interests, one of whom acts as chairperson of the committee. Such a committee may provide overall policy direction, with day-to-day operation of the Emergency Department being left to the head nurse or manager who receives consultation as necessary with the head of the committee. Weekly "business" meetings of the Emergency Department committee, including appropriate nursing and administrative representatives, should be held. Current Emergency Department operational problems should be discussed, and operational statistics should be reviewed, including incidents, deaths and complications and overnight ward utilization.[22] In most Emergency Departments, the nurses and administrative staff are the only permanent professional personnel, since physician coverage of the Emergency Department tends to be temporary and fragmented.

Physician Coverage

Several basic patterns of Emergency Department physician coverage are commonly seen today: (1) a rotation of the entire attending staff of the hospital, (2) a rotation of interns and residents supervised by a small group of full-time staff members, (3) coverage provided by a large incorporated group from the hospital's own attending staff (Pontiac plan), (4) coverage by a group of full-time (contract) emergency physicians (Alexandria plan) and (5) various combinations of the above, including coverage by attending staff supplemented by "moonlighting" physicians who normally work in nearby university training programs or federal health care institutions.

There are advantages and disadvantages to each of these staffing plans. While no one plan will satisfy the needs of all Emergency Departments, one or a combination will prove more suitable than others for a given hospital.[7] The traditional approach in community hospitals has been a rotation of the entire "volunteer" attending staff, supplemented in some hospitals by house staff in training. The larger university-affiliated hospitals traditionally run the Emergency Department with a full complement of house staff. The interns serve as primary physicians. Specialty interests are covered by residents with varying degrees of experience, backed by faculty. The overall supervision is provided by one or more members of the full-time faculty. Both of these approaches have failed to stand up under the stresses of the previously described "Emergency Department population explosion."

In the community hospital, the heavier patient load has resulted in a need for greater staff coverage, which in turn has caused increasing conflicts with the private practices of the attending staff. This situation has been aggravated by the increasing competition of community hospitals with university-affiliated hospitals for qualified house staff. Furthermore, a larger proportion of the hospital's staff are specialists who find that Emergency Department problems frequently are outside their areas of special interest and clinical competence. As more and more of these specialists are excused from Emergency Department duty, a disproportionately greater load falls on the remaining "generalists." Frequently, Emergency

Department duty is neither financially nor professionally rewarding, particularly when a significant proportion of the case load is routine and when a large percentage of patients are either indigent or bad financial risks. Increasing medical-legal risks are also associated with Emergency Department practice. Therefore, many hospital staffs have abandoned traditional coverage in favor of other approaches. The Pontiac and Alexandria plans were developed from the necessity created by these circumstances.

THE PONTIAC PLAN. Emergency Department coverage by an incorporated group of the attending staff is typified by the Pontiac plan (named because of its origin at the Pontiac General Hospital in Pontiac, Michigan, in 1961).[1] This plan offers full-time Emergency Department coverage by a relatively large group of staff physicians who still retain their individual practices in the community but contractually agree to devote varying amounts of time on duty in the hospital's Emergency Department. When the group is large enough, part-time participation is more flexible and therefore can be varied to a degree compatible with the participant's private practice. Participating staff physicians retain their usual staff privileges and professional relationships at the hospital while participating in this plan. For this reason, they are more likely to work in harmony with the remainder of the medical staff in the community during the time they are covering the Emergency Department. This arrangement also provides the opportunity for the benefits of corporate practice, such as retirement plans, group insurance coverage and other benefits. Coverage by a larger group provides less of the consistency and continuity that a smaller group of full-time emergency physicians might provide. The heaviest contributors to this type of group coverage plan tend to be young physicians trying to get started in practice and older physicians wishing to withdraw from the rigors of an open private practice. Problems have occurred when some of the former have viewed the Emergency Department as a source of new private patients. In addition, some of these groups have had difficulty in attracting the participation and cooperation of the more established, successful practitioners in the community. In other groups, the income has been disappointing, partly because of the expense or inefficiency of the billing system and the high proportion of nonpaying patients. Some hospitals have solved these problems by letting the group use the hospital's billing system and by providing a guaranteed minimum income for services rendered to nonpaying patients.

THE ALEXANDRIA PLAN. The other major alternative to traditional Emergency Department coverage at a community hospital is called the Alexandria plan, after its city of origin (Alexandria, Virginia, 1961). This plan provides full-time coverage by physicians who have no outside practice, although they may serve more than one Emergency Department. These physicians, usually a minimum of four, may form a partnership or corporation. In general, an Emergency Department census of 18,000 to 20,000 visits a year is required to sustain a four-physician group without financial assistance from the hospital. As the Emergency Department census increases, an additional physician is usually added for every 7,000 to 10,000 patient visits a year. The advantage of this type of coverage is that clinical activities are performed by a few physicians who are accustomed to the problems presenting to an Emergency Department and who can see large numbers of patients efficiently. These physicians have no admission privileges and provide no follow-up care. Therefore, there is no concern about patient "stealing." Staff physicians may resent the fact that emergency physicians command relatively large incomes considering their negligible investment in setting up a practice,

limited hours of work and minimal responsibilities for on-going patient care. This resentment is usually offset by appreciation for relief from Emergency Department on-call responsibilities. A more lasting concern is whether this approach may perpetuate a system that provides ambulatory care on an episodic basis in Emergency Departments. This practice has also been criticized as being expensive and ineffective. There may also be grounds for challenging the validity of "emergency medicine" as a specialty and as a long-term solution to this aspect of health care delivery, even though it appears to be a *fait accompli* and certainly provides an attractive immediate solution to many of our current Emergency Department staffing problems. There is a potential conflict between the role of the emergency physician as he or she views it — the "compleat specialist" in emergency medical problems — and the practical role that he or she is usually asked to fill, namely, as someone to initiate resuscitation of the seriously ill or injured until the appropriate specialists can be summoned and to handle the increasing burden of general practice for minor medical problems that has fallen upon most Emergency Departments today.

TRAINING. The problems of who should train the emergency physician and what that education should consist of are also still unsettled. Two-year residencies in emergency medicine have been established in a few university hospitals. A vast majority of university medical centers favor the establishment of trauma or emergency medical care centers restricted to "true" emergencies, with the less urgent ambulatory care problems being handled in other outpatient facilities. Only time will tell whether either of these approaches will survive and flourish or whether some other approach — such as a modification of those used in certain European countries — will supervene.

University and university-affiliated

hospitals have usually seen an increase in trauma, and patients with emergency problems are turning to larger, better-equipped Emergency Departments. Nevertheless, the disproportionate part of the increase in patient census has come from nonemergent, general medical problems. Most of the trainees in university and university-affiliated hospitals are there for specialty training. Understandably, they and the heads of their departments or divisions resist their devoting an increasingly large proportion of their training period to this type of "service." Thus, an increasingly stronger effort is being made by many departments in university hospitals to restore and maintain a more favorable balance between "education" and "service."

OTHER CONSIDERATIONS. The other pressures forcing a reconsideration of the role of house staff in Emergency Departments are financial and ethical. Financially, university hospitals are losing the opportunity to collect significant sums in professional fees when most of the patient care is being provided by house staff. Ethically, a problem arises because a steadily increasing percentage of patients who present to university hospital emergency departments can no longer be considered indigent by any standards. The proportion of indigent to those who pay directly or are covered by some third party plan has been completely reversed. In addition, there is the recurring criticism that nowhere else in medicine are the most seriously ill left in the hands of the least experienced. Studies show that the emergency medical care of serious injuries provided by university hospitals is generally better than elsewhere in the community, but the pressure from this criticism persists. Triage systems have been developed in most large Emergency Departments, but these have simply moved the problem to other outpatient areas.

New approaches to emergency medicine will undoubtedly be developed, but at the moment an increasing number of university hospitals are abandoning their traditional coverage plan or at least significantly modifying it. Some have resorted to using salaried physicians to handle these service commitments, either in walk-in or evening clinics or in the Emergency Department itself. Others are superimposing faculty panels on top of house staff coverage to provide for better supervision and teaching as well as for the collection of fees for service to private patients.

Nursing and Administrative Staff

The problems with the nursing and administrative staffing in the Emergency Department are somewhat less complex but by no means simple. Fortunately, a number of traditional restraints are being overcome. Nurses are no longer considered to be simply physician's aides. They are being allowed to make many routine clinical decisions and to perform procedures such as withdrawing blood samples, starting intravenous therapy, taking and evaluating electrocardiograms, dressing wounds and other minor manipulative procedures. The parallel development of the emergency medical technician and physician's associate has served to break down resistance to upgrading the role of the nurse. In many institutions where nursing shortages are experienced, corpsmen returning from the armed forces, trained emergency medical technicians, licensed practical nurses and physician's associates are used to fill the professional ranks in the Emergency Department formerly held by nurses.

This effort to unburden the physician and nurse of "nonprofessional" responsibilities has resulted in an additional burden being placed on the nonprofessional administrative staff. Unfortunately, Emergency Department clerks usually have been saddled with these increasing responsibilities without adequate training or additional help. They are frequently underpaid as well as undertrained for their more important and sensitive duties. The clerks are asked to receive outside telephone calls regarding emergencies, to greet patients and to conduct registration and financial interviews. Rarely are they selected for their ability to maintain equanimity under pressure or for their natural respect for and sincere interest in patient welfare. In their position between the waiting patient and the physician and nurse, they hold one of the most important public relations positions in the hospital. For just as the Emergency Department is the hospital's "front door," so are these clerks the Emergency Department's front line, inasmuch as they hold a major responsibility for the impression patients receive of the Emergency Department.

Although staffing patterns are easier to work out for nursing and clerical personnel than for physicians, it is important to recognize that the traditional pattern of three shifts a day popularized by inpatient nursing services is frequently inappropriate when applied to an Emergency Department. One must recognize peak periods of clinical activity both by hour and by day and, in some instances, by season. Adequate coverage schedules for nursing and administrative personnel must be developed accordingly. Uneven and overlapping shifts may be required. In a smaller Emergency Department, a head nurse may handle the bulk of the administrative decisions and organizational tasks. In a larger Emergency Department, it is advisable to have both a head nurse and administrative assistant or manager. In addition, there should be an identifiable charge nurse or chief clerk, or both, for any period of the day when there is more than one nurse or clerk present. Contingency plans for backup personnel in all categories must be provided to meet every situation from natural disasters and civil disturbances to vacations and illnesses. In summary, one cannot overemphasize the importance of selection for proper attitude, careful orientation and training for specific duties, written policies and procedures, clear job descriptions and adequate salaries.

Patient Management and Records

The basic principles regarding the management of patients in the Emergency Department are generally accepted. Some of these are covered in the *Standards for Accreditation of Hospitals* of the American Medical Association.[23] Others have been included for the sake of completeness.

1. All patients presenting for treatment at the Emergency Department must be considered as having an emergent medical problem until proven otherwise.
2. From a practical point of view, the patient's definition of an emergency must be favored over the physician's.
3. All patients presenting to the Emergency Department should be seen (however briefly) by a physician, and the physician must bear the ultimate responsibility for that patient's treatment.
4. Within a short time of their arrival at the Emergency Department, all patients should be interviewed by a nurse, particularly if significant delays for evaluation and treatment are predictable.
5. The patient should be advised of potential treatment delays to be encountered in the Emergency Department.
6. The request of a patient or his private physician for transfer to another institution for evaluation and treatment should be honored as long as (and only if) the transfer is not expected to prove detrimental to the treatment of the patient.

7. Whenever possible, attempts should be made to contact the patient's private physician regarding treatment in the Emergency Department.
8. Financial considerations should have no bearing upon the emergency medical services provided by a particular Emergency Department.
9. A written record of each patient's Emergency Department visit should be kept and these records should be subject to periodic review.
10. There should be an up-to-date set of written policies and procedures covering every important aspect of Emergency Department operations, including policies regarding the management of specific conditions.

The patient's Emergency Department record should be written on a form specially designed for this purpose. There are almost as many emergency record forms as there are Emergency Departments. There obviously should be some uniformity, at least in terms of the minimum essential information. It is the authors' opinion that the more cluttered a form is with spaces reserved for specific aspects of the history and physical, the more impractical it is. Essential information should include patient's name, address, telephone number, means of arrival, name of personal or private physician and chief complaint. The time of arrival and departure should also be noted. The physician's note should include the time the patient is first seen, vital signs, history, results of physical, diagnostic impressions, diagnostic studies ordered, treatment administered, patient instructions and final disposition. The patient's instructions should be written legibly. An additional carbon copy tear-off sheet at the bottom of the record where disposition, treatment and instructions are written, along with the next clinic appointment and the doctor's signature, serves this purpose nicely. In addition, a carbon copy of the entire record is extremely useful in allowing for medical record audit on a daily basis without the need to hold up the permanent copy. In a teaching institution, a regular audit of the medical records of the Emergency Department is extremely valuable and brings to light a number of aspects of patient care that would otherwise go unnoticed.

OUTPATIENT CLINIC

Design Planning

The basic purpose of an Outpatient Clinic is to provide a convenient, pleasant area for the delivery of ambulatory surgical care. In choosing the area and designing the outpatient facility one must keep in mind the location and availability of the ancillary support services of the clinical laboratory and the radiology department. If utilization of the hospital laboratory and the radiology department is not feasible, then a satellite or free-standing laboratory and radiology section should be included. In its simplest form, an Outpatient Clinic unit combines a reception desk, a waiting area, a series of examination and treatment rooms and nurses' and doctors' stations equipped with some teaching facilities.

As in the case of the Emergency Department, there is the need for compromise between the desirable features of specialized rooms and the economic advantage of multiple purpose rooms. In the smaller hospital, one often finds a combination of general purpose and specialty examination and treatment rooms in a single Outpatient Clinic. Additionally, one finds in smaller hospitals specialty rooms shared by the Emergency Department and the Outpatient Clinics, such as those for otolaryngology and ophthalmology. Another room that may be shared in the smaller hospitals is the proctology room, or the room where proctoscopy and sigmoidoscopy is performed. In larger hospitals, one usually encounters a series of specialty clinics with unique equipment and supplies, such as those needed for ophthalmology and otolaryngology. It is desirable to have specialty rooms for proctology, and minor surgery. In other hospitals, well-designed rooms and specialty treatment carts allow the clinic to be used in an overlapping fashion by a wide variety of specialties. With minor adjustments, the treatment rooms can be used for applying casts, for surgical dressing changes and for sigmoidoscopy, with the judicious use of specialty treatment carts (such as dressing carts and cast carts). An Outpatient Clinic can thus be used for both medical and surgical subspecialties within the same day.

The most important aspect of the design of the outpatient clinic is the size and arrangement of the individual examination and treatment room. Figure 2–4 shows three variations on the same theme, each slightly different in size and detail. Each provides a patient interview area, dressing and undressing area and examination and treatment area (with portable treatment carts) within the same unit. This arrangement facilitates the process of the interview and the physical examination (with a relative or interpreter, if necessary). In this manner, examination and treatment can be given with a minimum of interruption, embarrassment or scene changing. The size of the room will vary between 9 by 12 and 10 by 14 feet. In most surgical clinics, these rooms include a sink and a modified dressing cart with a wash basin.

Equipment and Supplies

A surgical clinic has more complicated needs than the medical or pediatric clinic, but they are much simpler than those of an emergency room. Specific needs of specialized surgical clinics are beyond the scope of this chapter and are not included. The needs of surgical clinic facilities are determined by the scope and complexity of the outpatient practice and the procedures intended to be performed.

In most surgical clinics, adequately lighted rooms may be set aside for changing surgical dressings while other rooms are used for multiple purposes, including minor surgical procedures such as small superficial biopsies, débridement, aspiration of hematoma and incision and drainage of abscesses. Additional lighting must be available if minor surgical procedures are to be performed in the area, and ideally such rooms should have suction, oxygen and a small electrosurgical unit available.

Each of these rooms should have a surgical dressing cart, and either the room or the cart should be supplied with the necessary equipment and supplies needed for changing a minor surgical dressing, including:

band-aids, assorted
drains (Penrose and "cigarette")
sterile rubber bands
gauze packing (iodoform and plain),
　　gauze rolls and Kling or Kerlex
gauze squares (small, medium and
　　large)
gloves, nonsterile (rectal)
surgical lubricant (K-Y Jelly)
gloves, sterile
instruments: mosquito clamps, Crile
　　clamps, Adson forceps, Kelly clamps,
　　needle holder, sterile scissors, dissecting scissors, scalpel handle and
　　blades, probes and grooved directors
petrolatum gauze
prepping solutions: tincture of iodine,
　　tincture of merthiolate, organic iodide preparations, hexachlorophene
　　solutions, benzalkonium solutions,
　　merbromin solutions, ether, acetate,
　　70% alcohol and tape remover
tape (adhesive, Elastoplast or stretch
　　tape and nonallergic tape)
topical agents: Vaseline, zinc oxide, bacitracin ointment, Sulfamylon cream,
　　peroxide, balsam of Peru
tube gauze

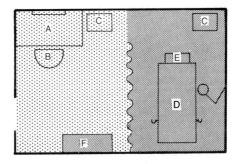

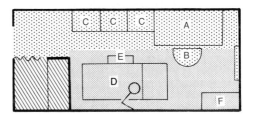

Figure 2–4 Example of treatment rooms
A – Physician's desk
B – Physician's chair
C – Chairs for patients and relatives, friends or interpreters
D – Examining table
E – Foot stool
F – Supply cabinet

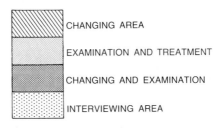

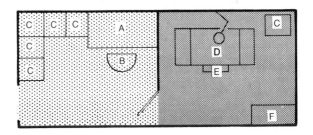

CHANGING AREA

EXAMINATION AND TREATMENT

CHANGING AND EXAMINATION

INTERVIEWING AREA

Each room of a surgical clinic should have a desk stocked with paper, medical examination sheets, progress sheets, clinic sheets, hospital admission order sheets, prescription pads and laboratory, x-ray and consultation request slips. The common instruments used in a physical examination should be included, such as: thermom-eter, sphygmomanometer, flashlight, pen, brush, tuning fork, reflex hammer, stethoscope, ophthalmoscope, oto-scope, sterile tongue depressors and Pap smear slides.

Both clean and sterile linens should be stocked in this room, particularly packs of sterile towels and drape sheets. If minor surgical procedures are to be performed frequently, individual packs for these procedures can be prepared and sterilized in central supply and stocked in this room. In a similar manner, suture removal instruments can be packaged by central supply. It is, of course, of utmost importance that the surgical dressing cart be used with scrupulous technique, using transfer forceps to take sterile dressings and instruments from the cart to a separate sterile field. One person should be responsible for assuring that the carts are restocked and that all items requiring sterilization are processed daily. It is not necessary to use a special surgical dressing room to see all postoperative patients and patients with simple wounds. A less well-equipped room could easily be utilized for common dressing needs. Its equipment should include gauze dressing, adhesive tape and suture removal packs as well as standard prepping solutions. For more complex procedures and specialty-equipped rooms for the clinic, refer to the preceding section on the Emergency Department.

A supply of less commonly used medications and equipment may be stocked in the supply or utility room of such a clinic to save space in the examining rooms while eliminating the need to request them from the pharmacy or central supply. These should include various suture materials, specimen cups and containers with formalin for biopsies. Other items may be stored in this area, such as additional instruments, biopsy forceps, biopsy needles, intravenous solutions, intravenous needles, ligation sheets, regular catheters, sterile catheters, urinary catheters, Ace bandages, Unna's paste boots and vaginal specula.

Regardless of how remote the possibility may seem, each major clinic should be equipped with an emergency cart for cardiopulmonary resuscitation. The cart should be used only for emergencies and its stock checked on a regular basis.

Staffing of the Surgical Outpatient Clinic

The staffing of the Outpatient Clinic is variable, depending on its type and organization and the volume of patients seen in the clinic. The simplest professional unit consists of a clerk, a nurse and a physician, while more complex clinics also involve dietitians, social service personnel, nursing aides, laboratory technicians and prosthetists. Aides and technicians may function as chaperones and assistants for the simplest of procedures, whereas nurses should be available if minor surgical procedures are being performed. Secretarial support may be provided by a centralized steno pool or may be supplied specifically to the clinic. The sharing of secretarial support by other outpatient and inpatient services increases the economy of the organization.

Convalescent care units and physical medicine and rehabilitation services are commonly involved because of disabilities associated with surgical operations and injuries and the special needs of some patients for provision of transportation and social service support.

In the consideration of staffing patterns, the organization and scheduling of patients and prompt attendance by physicians are extremely important. Infrequently, surgical clinics extend beyond an eight hour day, requiring additional time at the end of the day for personnel to clean instruments and prepare the facilities for the next day's operation. Therefore, the scheduling should be arranged so as to provide a one hour buffer period at the end of the day. If prolonged clinics are the usual case, rearrangement of the working period to ten hours a day, four days per week, may help solve the problems of staffing if the surgical clinic is too busy to be completed in an eight hour day. This will help correct many of the problems in staffing attitudes. Most of the problems in running a surgical clinic are not due to inadequate numbers or abilities of the ancillary staff but to the attitudes of the organization and the team.

Patient Management and Records

The key to a smooth, efficient clinic operation is timing of and preparation for the patient-doctor encounter. Patients should be given an appointment and instructed to arrive 10 to 15 minutes ahead of time. If laboratory or roentgenographic tests are needed prior to the visit, the patient should be scheduled for the ancillary tests earlier and the results should be available when the patient is seen by the physician.

Patients should be given staggered clinic appointments, the intervals being determined by the nature of the visit and the anticipated time for evaluation and treatment, for example, one hour for a complete evaluation, 30 minutes for a specialty consultation and 15 to 20 minutes for a follow-up visit.

The receptionist should greet the patient by name, log him in, prepare his old and new records and gather any other information not present in his file before introducing the patient to the nurse. New patients can complete the past history and review of systems with the help of a nurse or receptionist prior to the interview by the surgeon. The physician is then free to concentrate on the present illness and those aspects of the past history and the review of systems that relate to it. When patients are followed for certain conditions, such as anticoagulation therapy or cancer chemotherapy, they should arrive earlier than their appointment time so that the necessary lab work can be completed. When the patient's record is completed and reviewed, the nurse then ushers the patient to the examination room. At that time, specific instructions can be given regarding the patient's readiness for any examination needed. Reports

can be obtained while the patient is being prepared for the doctors arrival. The surgeon must arrive on time and must strive to move on to the next patient on schedule.

If the clinic receptionist or nurse is informed of the general nature of the patient's problem at the time the appointment is made, appropriate time can be allotted for the patient's visit. When a patient is scheduled for future clinic visits, a time is computed for examination and any special procedures that might be performed. The doctor's notes should be dictated or written immediately. A well-organized physician can dictate a patient's history while the patient undresses and the results of the physical examination while the patient dresses. If the receptionist and nurse obtain the pertinent past medical history and medical data, this will provide a more efficient operation. The physician should explain his or her instructions to the patient and, if feasible, write them legibly and give them to the patient along with any prescriptions and the future appointment date. Notes to referring physicians should be completed at this time.

In a larger, complex clinic, utilization of paramedical personnel such as the social worker and dietitian can augment total patient care and make it even more comprehensive.

Surgical clinic patients present no specific problems in record keeping; lack of prompt completion of the record is the main problem encountered.

In addition, cooperation with the medical records department is necessary to fill out disability affidavits and insurance forms. A note is frequently necessary for the patient's employer specifying the activities that the patient can perform and indicating when he will be able to return to work. Special forms may be necessary for subspecialty surgical clinics; for example, chemotherapy protocol dosage and laboratory data forms ("flow sheets"), vascular surgery follow-up forms and anticoagulation dosage sheets. It is helpful to use anatomical stamps to illustrate the results of physical examination, especially in the tumor clinic.

THE SURGEON'S OFFICE

Type of Surgical Practice and Office Desired

The type and size of a surgical office should be determined by the type of practice, the types of procedures to be performed and the desires of the surgeon or surgical group. From a financial standpoint, a surgical practice is primarily hospital-based rather than office-based. This is different from an internist's practice, which is predominantly an office-based one. Therefore, an elaborate surgical office that is utilized less than 50 per cent of the surgeon's working time may be a luxury and can become a financial burden. However, if the patient clientele is primarily of the "carriage trade," an attractive, well-appointed office would be essential. Many surgeons utilize their offices only for examinations, follow-up and business matters of the practice, while other surgeons use theirs to perform many small operative procedures as well as diagnostic tests. The surgical office is unique in that a large number of patients need to be seen in a pleasant and effective manner in a short period of time, which requires additional examining rooms for greater efficiency. This requirement must be met without becoming impersonal. Patients want to feel that they are being treated as individuals.

The patterns of office practice and the utilization of Emergency Departments and Outpatient Clinics have changed considerably over the past decade. Many of these changes have been brought about by the attitudes of patients and of the general public and as the result of social and economic forces. Some government agencies and third party carriers will reimburse hospitals and Outpatient Clinics for the use of surgical instruments and the services of nurses to set up and assist in certain procedures but will refuse to compensate physicians for instrument setups and the cost of personnel used if the procedures are done away from the hospital. This has forced many physicians to perform some procedures in Emergency and Outpatient Departments that could be done with less expense and more convenience in the office. Another factor is the increasing complexity of monitoring and defibrillator equipment. This equipment is felt to be desirable if outpatient surgery is to be performed in a physician's office. Therefore, before designing a surgical office, it is important to decide the type of practice, the anticipated patient volume, the number of physicians who will be utilizing the space and the types of procedures and laboratory studies to be performed.

Design of Office — General Approach and Planning

In planning an office practice, one must first determine its immediate short-range and long-range goals. A first consideration should be the location of the office relative to the hospital or hospitals and the traffic pattern in the area.

On first moving to a new area or upon opening a practice, one might consider renting or leasing an office for the first few years, if such space is available. In considering rental, before signing any agreements, one should be aware of (1) the adequacy of parking, (2) the physical appearance, both external and internal, of the building and (3) the understanding between the landlord and the renter regarding improvements and renovations, if necessary.

Before leasing, as with renting, there must be a well-defined agreement between the lessor and the lessee as to the terms of the lease and the responsibility of each for utilities, maintenance and renovations.

The planning phase for a surgical office practice includes determining the type of practice, the anticipated number of physicians and the proposed organization, both immediate and in a projected five-year period. This must include the intended scope of surgical services to be offered. Estimating the cost is important in determining the financial feasibility of the proposed project. The availability of construction funds and funds for equipping an office must be investigated early in the planning period, and the sources of these funds must be pursued. This will necessitate making a master plan, which must include the following items: the type of building, the internal layout, the location, the amount of parking available and the accessibility to the hospitals where inpatients and emergency cases will be served. The primary decision in any real estate venture is the location of the property.

Location

After the type of surgical practice is decided upon, the location of the office is the second critical feature. Factors to be considered are (1) proximity to the hospital that is to be used most often by the surgeon or surgeons' group —especially important if emergency duty for the hospital is taken by the practicing surgeon or group and not by hospital-based surgeons, (2) easy accessibility for patients with various types of infirmities, (3) convenient location in relationship to other practicing physicians or physician groups and especially to actual or potential referring physicians, (4) availability of office space, (5) safety of the area of the city or community, especially in larger cities, since office hours are frequently held in darkness during the winter months, and (6) availability of adequate parking.

Laboratory and other equipment needs should also be included in the master plan, as well as provision for patient records, patient record management, personnel working areas, examining areas, minor surgery rooms and laboratory facilities. A decision must be made about (1) minor surgical procedures to be performed in the office, (2) the need for office x-rays, (3) laboratory equipment needed and laboratory procedures to be performed and (4) other diagnostic procedures to be carried out in the office.

An ideal office location for the convenience of both physican and patients is one adjacent or in close proximity to the primary hospital that will be used. If this is not possible, convenience to the patient must still be kept in mind because often patients cannot go great distances from an office to a hospital or to another office for x-rays and then return. The inconvenience of the office to patients will ultimately be reflected in the nature and the volume of the surgical practice.

The other very important question to be decided is whether chemotherapy will be given in the surgical practice. Many patients receiving chemotherapy are quite ill and feeble and cannot tolerate the inconvenience and delay caused by having laboratory determinations made in one place and office visits and chemotherapy given in another. Influencing all of these decisions is the fact that time is the surgeon's most cherished and important asset. The success of the practice and the satisfaction of patients depend on the efficiency and availability of service provided by the surgeon's organization.

The availability and cost of real estate, the area's zoning codes and the permanency of the hospital are other significant determining factors. In recent years older hospitals have tended to move and build totally new structures rather than to build additions to existing structures. Additions and renovations may be false indications of permanency in a hospital.

Renovation or remodeling of existing office space may be more advantageous than constructing a new office. Every community, every surgeon and every surgical practice presents a different set of circumstances; therefore, only generalizations can be given here. In determining whether to rent or lease, the financial situation of the surgeon or group must be considered, without regard to the availability of financing, not only for building costs, but also for the cost of equipment to be placed in the office.

When these factors have been fully considered, the decision will have to be reached based on the current availability of office space and the possibility of renting or leasing space. Consideration should be given to both short- and long-term leases. Another option is to purchase an existing office or other structure and subsequently to modify it into a surgical office. Building a separate, free-standing surgical office is a very appealing idea; however, consideration should also be given to purchasing a unit in a developing medical office complex such as a medical office condominium or to purchasing stock and becoming involved in the development of a multioffice professional building.

Office Floor Plans and Rooms

Physical Planning

In the physical planning phase final architectural drawings are completed, construction documents are drawn up, bidding is opened and construction contracts are awarded. A surgeon should obtain professional help in designing the office and planning the construction. Financial advisors and lawyers are needed to point out minor loopholes that may create major headaches.

A decision should be made as to the number of square feet necessary and the expansibility of the unit to be built. Many new concepts have been developed in office design. One should decide whether a free-standing complex

with the potential to expand if the practice grows beyond its original inception would best suit his or her needs, or whether a condominium, self-owned office in a multi-office complex, or a closed leasing arrangement, in which a group of physicians forms a separate corporation to build an office complex to lease to their members, would be better.

The actual construction phase may take longer than anticipated and may be delayed by situations that surgeons are not usually accustomed to, such as the unavailability of construction materials, labor problems or problems in zoning.

Several months prior to the anticipated opening of the office, the surgeon should choose equipment for the waiting room, for records maintenance, for secretarial and steno activities and for the billing system.

In planning for a new office or for modification of an existing structure, consideration should be given to designing a good traffic pattern, where patients enter from one area and exit through another. Bottlenecks should be eliminated, and patients concluding an office visit should not feel so rushed that they can't say "goodbye" and should feel that they have been satisfied for the time and money spent.

The minimum size for a single surgical office is 900 to 1000 square feet. It is advisable for such an office to have approximately 1500 square feet if any special procedures or diagnostic tests will be performed. If two or more surgeons will be seeing patients simultaneously, a minimum of 1500 square feet is imperative, and 2000 square feet is recommended, especially if special diagnostic procedures, treatments and minor surgery will be included. For each additional surgeon who will be working at the same time in the office, another 500 square feet is necessary and 700 square feet is recommended. This provides 120 square feet for each of two examining rooms and the same amount for an office. The remaining 140 square feet in each 500 square foot multiple addition can be utilized for additional waiting area and additional offices for staff functions. One means of saving space in a group surgical practice is to stagger the times at which the surgeons see patients in the office. In this manner, the surgeons can work at different times of the day and on different days without conflict.

The rooms in an office floor plan are (1) an entry area, (2) a reception room or reception area, (3) a waiting room, (4) a doctor's office, (5) two to three examining rooms per surgeon, (6) a minor surgery room, (7) a special examination and treatment room, (8) a laboratory, (9) a room for storage, equipment, preparation and supplies, (10) a secretarial office or offices and (11) a library and interview room.

An entry area should be provided, and two doors are recommended to avoid heat loss from the office. A coat and hat rack or a closet should be available.

The reception room and the waiting room are the first areas of the office that are seen at length, and therefore they establish impressions about the surgeon and the practice in the minds of patients and their families. The waiting room should be bright, neat and clean and have a cheerful atmosphere. It should be large and have adequate, comfortable seating that is serviceable and easily kept clean and that will maintain a good appearance. Two sets of neatly arranged, recent magazines should be provided. Smoking should be discouraged, but if permitted, ashtrays should be provided. If the surgical practice includes children, children's books and toys that are quiet, safe and easily kept clean should be provided. The waiting area should be ample for the size of the practice. Additional space should be provided to handle unforeseen delays. This is especially important when the surgeons are late because emergencies or unexpected events prevent them from arriving at their offices on time. Some form of music system should be provided, such as commercial piped-in music, tapes or primary radio receivers with speakers placed in the waiting area and treatment rooms and with a central control system at the reception desk and a speaker switch in each of the treatment rooms.

Examination Rooms

The examination rooms should be at least 9 by 12 feet in size and should contain cabinets for supplies, a sink, a small desk or writing platform and stool and an intercom system communicating with the front desk, reception area or control desk. This should be placed so that communications cannot be heard in the waiting room. The examining tables that are needed should be determined by the type of surgical practice and should be of good quality. A spotlight should be provided. If minor surgical procedures are to be performed, wall-mounted lights that provide illumination and do not occupy floor space are recommended. A dressing area with draw curtain or door is essential. For best utilization of space, a triangular or corner dressing cubicle is adequate. The number of examining rooms will be determined by the specific type of practice, but there should be at least two examining rooms for each surgeon who is in the office at one time. If brief office visits are the rule in a practice, a third room will be necessary. The economics of an office practice is related to the efficiency and productivity of the surgeon and is augmented by nurses and paramedical personnel. Therefore, the office rooms must be as efficient as possible.

Doctor's Office

One type of floor plan places the doctor's office between two examining rooms so that in the period between examinations, while one room is being vacated and another patient is coming in, the surgeon may complete charts, order appropriate tests and finish any paperwork before seeing the next patient. If this plan is not possible or desired, a second idea is to place a dictating booth between examining rooms. These booths must be soundproof and the privacy of the dictation is mandatory.

A dictating system is recommended rather than handwritten notes, since dictation is less time consuming and easier to use for later office visit reviews. The physician's productivity may be increased because less time is spent in dictating than in writing. The doctor's office will vary with the specific tastes and desires of each surgeon, but in most situations it will contain a desk, a desk chair, a bookcase and one or two soft chairs.

Minor Surgery

If minor surgical procedures are to be performed, a larger room, at least 12 by 12 feet, is needed. This should be arranged to facilitate access to the patient from all directions, with the table in the center of the room and a light mounted overhead. This room should be designed as a dual purpose room, for examinations as well as minor surgery. It should be fully stocked with dressings, sutures, tape, minor surgical supplies and solutions in addition to examination equipment.

Depending on the specialty of the practice and the type of procedures to be performed in the office, a room with a table designed for proctoscopies and related procedures may be necessary. This type of table provides as pleasant and atraumatic an area as possible for carrying out endoscopy and minor anal and rectal surgery.

If the office practice involves pacemaker follow-up, a room for electrocardiograms and other pacemaker evaluation functions will be needed. If the room is to be used for diagnostic vascular procedures, it must be of sufficient size and be equipped with Doppler flowmeters and pulse volume recorders.

Laboratory

If the office is to perform laboratory procedures, a room with a refrigerator should be provided. An autoclave may be installed in this room or in the storage and equipment room. A decision about the type of laboratory procedures to be performed depends not only on available space but also on the cost-benefit ratio for personnel. A very important additional factor is the patient's convenience and comfort, since many surgical patients are elderly and sick. As previously noted, if chemotherapy is given, the patient may find it inconvenient to drive to the hospital to have laboratory tests made and then to return to the physician's office. Many tests can be performed right in the office. However, if the volume of patients does not justify the continuous performance of high-quality laboratory work, a laboratory should not be included in the office. As with the other specialty rooms, specific needs for a laboratory depend upon the type of surgical practice involved.

A room for storage, equipment and supplies, for preparing and cleaning instruments, and for preparing suture and minor surgery packs is needed. The best provision of linens and surgical drapes as well as gowns and caps depends upon the type of practice, the availability of a linen service and the consideration for disposable drapes. Some offices may find it advantageous to have washers and dryers in this room to provide for the office's linen needs.

Secretarial and Insurance Offices

The number of office personnel is determined by the magnitude of the practice. A central control desk or a reception room control area is necessary for patient record files, card indexes and central billing information. If possible, a separate room or area away from the reception room should be provided for the insurance secretary or clerk so that the financial aspects of the practice may be kept separate and the noise of the adding machine removed from the hearing of patients. This type of noise is somewhat distracting to patients and gives them a feeling that the orientation of the office is to money rather than to providing medical care for the patient's needs. An interview room is helpful if there is a large volume of new patients.

Library

A central library may double as an interview room and may also be utilized as a secretarial office or as a luncheon area for office personnel.

Office Organization, Scheduling, Appointments, Procedures and Policies

The key reason for scheduling is to produce an organized office operation. An effort should be made to run the office in a systematic fashion, with patients being seen on certain days or during certain periods of certain days. Some days should be reserved for operations and hospital work, and scheduling procedures in the office at specific periods of the day or on specific days should relate to the tests being performed, to patient comfort and to the efficient use of the physician's time.

In setting the appointment schedule, an estimated period of time should be established for new patients, follow-up patients and short-term follow-up patients so that arrivals can be spaced to produce a reasonable semblance of order. Scheduling should be arranged to correspond with the type of surgical patients being seen and to the length of time that a specific physician needs for each type of patient. These needs

should be established prior to instituting the office schedule.

Data needed on new patients being referred include (1) the patient's name, (2) his address, (3) his age and family status, (4) his occupation, (5) the problem or need causing him to seek medical help, (6) the name of the person who referred him to the doctor and (7) the method of payment and type of insurance coverage he will use.

A list of procedures that will be performed in the office should be established and an estimate should be made as to the time required per procedure for each surgeon. Some surgeons work faster than others and require different periods of time for each procedure. Schedule interruptions may be transitory or prolonged, particularly when caused by important phone calls or by emergencies in the office or those requiring the physician to go to the hospital. Depending on the type of practice, other surgeons in the group may take over that surgeon's patients, or the patients may be informed that there will be some delay and given the opportunity either to wait or to be rescheduled. In every office, walk-ins will occur even though great effort is made to schedule specific appointments. Some time should be scheduled daily for the surgeon to see additional patients or walk-in patients as necessary.

Patients with emergencies such as bleeding, dyspnea and pain should be taken directly to a treatment room or minor emergency area if one is available and should not be asked to stay in the waiting room in a routine fashion. Most patients with routine appointments understand this. A phone listing for ambulance service, fire department, police department, coroner or medical examiner, poison control centers and adjacent physicians should be maintained and readily accessible in case of emergencies.

Some offices arrange for a rest break to give the surgeons time to regroup their thoughts before continuing with the busy office load. Frequently, however, scheduled rest breaks are filled by unscheduled patients and recurring chores.

Patients who do not arrive for appointments should be sent a very pleasant request for rescheduling. A form letter can be devised for this purpose. An example is:

Dear (Blank):

Yesterday you were scheduled to see Dr. (Blank) and failed to appear for your appointment. We assume some unexpected situation arose so that you were unable to keep this appointment. If you will call this office or correspond with the above address, a return appointment will be scheduled. In the future, if you would be kind enough to notify us of any cancellations, we would be very appreciative.

Sincerely,

(Blank)
Secretary to Dr. (Blank)

Operating Policies and Rules

When establishing an office or hiring new employees, certain items should be clarified as soon as possible, and a procedures, rules and policies manual should be written. Specifically mentioned should be the orientation and philosophy of the office. The ultimate purpose of all employees of a medical office has been amply described by Conomikes Associates.[15] The organization, philosophy and implementation of a surgical office should be designed to increase the efficiency of the surgeon, because the physician's time is the most valuable asset of the medical practice. At times this can be overlooked, and it becomes a question of who is running the office and for whom the office is actually being managed. A properly managed office is oriented to the patients and their needs and to facilitate a good patient-physician relationship in as pleasant an environment

as possible. The confidence a patient develops in his physician is not uncommonly initiated by the patient's communication with the secretary-receptionist, who should be cheerful, neat, tactful and cooperative.

The working hours, office hours, requirements for occasional extra time, the doctor's schedule and sick leave, holidays, vacations and other fringe benefits should be discussed as well as the salary at the time of interviewing and employing office personnel. It must be emphasized to employees that all the information in a physician's office is confidential and that this confidence is not to be violated. It should also be emphasized that office personnel should not give advice to patients on personal or medical matters without consulting with the physician.

If house calls or nursing home visits are part of the surgical practice, this should be filled into the doctor's daily schedule.

Personnel

Office Staff — Supporting Personnel

In its simplest form, the surgical office may consist of one physician and one assistant. The other extreme may be a very complex multi-specialty group or a large surgical practice with many employees. Depending on the office arrangements and type of practice, various numbers and types of employees will be necessary; however, certain generalizations may be made. In structuring an office, a specific job description should be drawn up for each position, with a clarification of the previous education and experience needed for the job. The duties of the job should be clearly stated to eliminate any confusion, and the person to whom each employee is responsible for specific facets of his or her work should be identified.

For example, in a one-physician, one-assistant office, the assistant will be responsible for making appointments, keeping the books, sending out bills, preparing the examining rooms for patients, preparing the patients for examination, sterilizing of instruments, and many other tasks. If the surgeon is male and the assistant is female, she can serve as chaperone for female patients. Billing and bookkeeping in small operations are sometimes handled by outside services or part-time employees.[15]

At the other extreme, in very large practices, specific and well-defined tasks are assigned. The job description should be a workable understanding and never serve as an excuse for an employee to say, "That's not my responsibility." All employees should be willing to help and cross-cover for staff illness and periods of peak patient load. In a two-employee office, one person should be designated as the office manager or nurse-in-charge and one person made responsible for the reception desk and for providing patients with admission slips or receipts for paid office visits. Depending on the type of surgical practice, a nurse, nurse's aide or medical assistant may be utilized. In a predominantly gynecological practice, a greater number of female employees will be necessary to function as chaperones, if the surgical staff is largely male. Some of the female nurses or assistants may be utilized for this. The secretary and insurance clerk may function in a full-time capacity; however, in a smaller office practice the secretary may function as a receptionist during office visits and as secretary and insurance clerk when the surgeon has only a half day each day or alternates full days with days when he or she is not in the office. For this reason, it is especially important to have an office manager or a nurse-in-charge to whom all personnel report. Regardless of the size of the practice, it is important to have an odd number of employees so that one half of the office staff will not

be competing with the other half, or else a split in personnel may develop. In a medium-sized office with either two or three surgeons, the following staffing pattern is an example.

Nurse

This position may be filled by a registered nurse or a practical nurse, depending on the complexity of the practice and of the treatment program with regard to medication and blood-drawing. If the practice is not of adequate size to need an office manager, the nurse may serve in this capacity with an overall idea of the needs of the physician in practice.

The nurse would be responsible for assisting the doctor directly in the treatment of patients by providing patient care. The nurse can take vital signs, prepare patients for examinations, take medical history information, measure height and weight, draw blood if there is no laboratory technician, administer medication, give injections and administer other tests and treatments, such as EKG and pulmonary function tests. If a limited laboratory is provided without a medical technician, the nurse may perform simple laboratory tests. Nurses may be taught to perform routine tests, for example, complete blood counts, differential blood counts, platelet counts, hematocrit and hemoglobin readings and urinalysis, if chemotherapy is to be given. Blood can also be drawn and separated for multiple types of analysis and sent to a commercial lab or hospital. The nurse can also take responsibility for ordering supplies, sterilizing instruments and maintaining the medical equipment.

Secretary or Office Assistant

The secretary or office assistant will answer the telephone, greet patients and other callers, handle correspondence, make appointments for patients, keep track of the doctor's daily schedule, type insurance reports and medical histories, open the mail, receive payment from patients, maintain patients' financial records and send out bills.[15]

Receptionist or Secretary

The receptionist or secretary should have a pleasant smile and friendly greeting. The words "May I help you," spoken frequently by the receptionist, may expeditiously and pleasantly inquire about the needs of the patient and the reasons for his visit to the office. The receptionist should engage in conversation with the patients to make them feel relaxed and at ease; however, time does not permit lengthy conversations with each patient.

Medical Technologist

If the size of the office justifies it, a medical technologist would administer blood tests, electrograms, radiographs and other tests, perform laboratory work, obtain the results of those laboratory tests referred to other hospitals or laboratories and file the laboratory reports in the patient's records after review by the physician. The results of laboratory tests should be reviewed before they are noted on the patient's chart. If the practice is not large enough to warrant a medical technologist, most of these duties can be handled by a nurse.

Other Personnel

In large offices, an office manager with the help of a bookkeeper can maintain records of charges, receipts and expenditures, follow up on delinquent accounts and handle other money matters. In small offices, part-time bookkeepers can service several physicians.

Part-time personnel may be hired to augment the full-time office staff. Part-time registered nurses, licensed practical nurses or aides may assist during office hours, and part-time stenographers may be utilized for typing patient records, billing and other tasks. One thing to keep in mind is that if part-time employees work in several different offices, loyalty of personnel may become a problem. This is usually nòt significant if the part-time employee does not work elsewhere.

Communications and Telephones

Proper communications with patients and referring physicians are the lifeline of an office practice. First impressions are often lasting, and in most situations the first impression is a telephone call for an appointment or a request for the doctor's services. In answering the telephone, the secretary or receptionist should be polite, organized and pleasant, saying, for example, "Dr. (blank)'s office. May I help you?" or "Mountain State Surgical Group. May I help you?"

It should be established which calls will be put through immediately to the physicians, which calls are to be handled by office personnel and by whom, and which calls will be returned later by the physician. Frequent interruptions of the physician's schedule are not only disturbing to patients but also interfere with the efficiency of the practice. Calls that are often put through directly to physicians are (1) calls from another physician, (2) true medical emergencies and (3) prescription refills, especially if called in from another city. Calls that can be held to be returned later by the physician include (1) general calls to the physician, (2) most requests for medication refills and (3) calls for clarification of an appointment. In recording messages from telephone callers, the secretary should obtain (1) the name of the person calling, (2) his telephone number, (3) the time the call was received, (4) the nature of the call and (5) the anticipated time when the call may be returned. The office staff should not give medical advice over the telephone unless directed by the physician, and information about patients that might violate confidentiality or the patient's privacy should not be given. Telephone call prescriptions and treatment should be noted in the patient's record in case this information is needed at a later time.

In determining the number of telephones that an office should have, the size and complexity of the practice must be taken into consideration. An adequate number of telephone lines and extensions should be available so that the lines are not occupied the majority of the time. A private line is beneficial to permit access to the surgeon by other doctors, to provide a line for dictation of admission, history and physical examination information to the hospital steno pool at the time the patient is seen in the office, and to permit readily available communication with the hospital about patient care. An additional phone listed under insurance billing is beneficial if the surgical practice is large enough to justify it.

Medical Records

Medical records are among the most important aspects of the office filing system. In addition to being the source of information about the patient's past and present medical problems, medical records have an important legal significance. If a lawsuit were to arise regarding the patient's health care, a doctor's records may be summoned or may be needed for the defense. Medical records are also used in legal matters regarding injury claims by treated patients. Therefore, these records should be well maintained, clean, neat, complete and without erasures. If changes are made, the original notation should be marked through and the correction written above it.

Organization

Proper organization of the medical records is extremely important to provide the maximum information to the physician with a minimum of time needed to find it. Therefore, each chart should contain a summary sheet of all diagnoses, hospital admissions and medications. Each chart should then be organized chronologically to contain information about the patient's past history, present history, physical examinations, diagnoses and treatment programs. As with hospital records, the patient's family and social histories are very important features of the initial medical record. Allergies should be noted in a prominent place in the record. The summary sheet containing current and past diagnoses, allergies to medications and medication currently being taken should be placed in the front of the chart.

Separate areas should be provided for the recording of ongoing laboratory data, and these data should be filed by either taping or stapling them together in a chronological order with both the date and the results readily available to the physician. A "shingling" technique is frequently helpful. Radiographs and financial records are maintained in other folders; x-ray reports, however, are recorded in the primary medical chart.

Certain points need to be reemphasized, particulary that (1) medical records are always the property of the doctor, (2) office personnel should not permit the patient to read his chart unless directed by the physician and (3) records should never be released to any other source nor copies made without the written authorization of the patient and the direction of the physician. A filing system that is designed for the physician's own practice and office arrangement should be maintained. Filing methods include the alphabetical system, number system and color coding system. A numerical method using the Acme record system can be utilized, or a filing system using alphabetical order, last name first, may be more appropriate. Files should be kept where they may be easily retrieved and refiled, as quickly and efficiently as possible. Separate patient files should be maintained rather than grouping files by cases or by families. Inactive files may be stored in a safe, fire-protected place that does not interfere with the operation of the present patient care area. When a portion of the chart is removed, a filler or note that tells where the information has been filed should be added, or if the chart has been completely removed, where the chart can be located. All information should be recorded in the patient's medical record, including telephone transactions, discussions with the patient, prescription renewals, hospitalization and any communication with attorneys.

Medical History

A complete medical history may be obtained by a physician's assistant, nurse or office assistant to facilitate acquisition of data and prevent unnecessary expenditure of the physician's time. This history should be obtained in complete privacy, in the absence of accompanying family; additional information may be obtained later from the family. The history should be taken in a comfortable, quiet area, with the answers recorded precisely. The patient should be observed for any unusual actions, comments or facial expressions. Several standard history forms are available from commercial sources, or the physician may wish to design his or her own and have them prepared by a printing company. Included on the form should be: present occupation, past occupation, past medical history, social history and family history, as well as the current problem and a review of systems. Questionable information should be clarified by the assistant before the patient sees the physician.

If a new patient appears at the office to make an appointment to see the physician at a later date, a "release of information" form for the patient's former physician should be signed at that time. The information should be requested promptly so that it will be available at the time of the initial office visit to the new physician. Information to be collected on the first visit includes:

1. Patient's full name
2. Date of birth
3. Social Security number
4. Marital status
5. Number of dependents
6. Current address
7. Past address, for the preceding two years
8. Telephone numbers for both residence and work
9. Name and relationship of person(s) legally responsible for payment
10. Patient's and spouse's occupations and names and addresses of employers
11. Name, address and telephone number of person to be notified in case of emergency
12. Name of neighbor or friend in the area and phone number if no immediate family is available.
13. Referring doctor or other referring person
14. Health insurance information and numbers[12]

To obtain information from other physicians, a letter should be written, for example:

Dear Dr. (blank):

I am to see a former patient of yours, Mr. (Ms.) Blank (or I have seen a former patient of yours, Mr. [Ms.] Blank). I would very much appreciate your forwarding to me any medical history on the patient or other information that you think would be helpful in his (her) care. Enclosed is a consent form signed by the patient.

Sincerely yours,

(Blank), M.D.

An example of the consent form follows:

AUTHORIZATION FOR RELEASE
OF MEDICAL INFORMATION

I, _____, do
hereby authorize _____
to release any and all medical information
to _____ _____.
(Name)

_____
(Address)

_____
Signed

_____
Date

_____
Witness

There are many types of medical history forms and medical record forms available from commercial vendors. Forms can also be custom-made to the specific wishes of a physician.

Office Procedures — Examinations and Treatments

Most important for each office procedure is that the office assistant or nurse makes the most effective use of the doctor's time, with a minimum delay between patients. The best designed pattern of traffic flow in the office may be ineffective if personnel do not realize the necessity of placing patients promptly in examining rooms or treatment areas. The examining room should be checked, cleaned and refurnished, if necessary, before the patient enters it. After the patient is shown to the room and before the examination, all charts and laboratory information should be made available to the surgeon. The nurse or assistant can prepare the patient and take basic vital sign data to save time. Appropriate gowns for the area to be examined or treated should be provided, and the nurse should obtain the specific historical information requested by the physician. Assisting in the examination is a very important task and may range from aiding in treatment and taking notes on the examination to serving as chaperone in the examination of female patients for male physicians. The nurse or office assistant should be sure that the patient has all necessary information, prescriptions and dressings before leaving the room.

Depending on the type of practice, the forms of treatment and the diagnostic tests performed, the procedures of each office will vary considerably. Specific procedures, physician requests and instruments to be used should be established for each of the treatments given. If minor surgery is performed, the instrument packs, local anesthetics and dressings should be prepared beforehand. If local anesthetics are administered, injections given or minor surgery performed in the office, it is recommended that an emergency box, an Ambu bag, airways, endotracheal tubes, a laryngoscope and an oxygen tank be available, as well as the emergency medications listed earlier in this chapter. A strict record should be kept of all medications given from the office, and a log should be maintained if narcotics or sedatives are utilized. At the end of the day, all instruments should be cleaned and sterilized in preparation for the following day. An ample number of instrument packs and suture removal packs should be available so that cleansing and sterilizing will not be necessary during office visits, unless personnel are specifically designated for that function. A procedure should be established in the office for instrument sterilization, either by autoclave or cold sterilization.

Business and Business Records

Bookkeeping

A professional accountant, an accounting firm or a business manager should be involved in setting up the bookkeeping operation and in supervising and regulating it. Business records must be easily understood, kept in a regular, up-to-date manner and be neat, legible and accurate. Since physicians are primarily deliverers of health care and not primarily businesspersons, this part of the practice usually should be overseen by an accountant, business manager or accounting firm.

The bookkeeping system begins with the *charge slip* provided by the physician, which lists the specific charges or specific services rendered. This is then entered in the *daily log*, which is a detailed record of all patients' charges and payments. Entries from the daily log are then recorded in each *patient's ledger* on a daily basis and include additional charges, payments or payments from third party carriers received in that 24-hour period. The information from the daily log is then recorded in a *combined journal*, a chronological record of all business transactions of the medical practice listing the grand totals on a daily basis. The combined journal shows the cash flow in and out of the medical practice and gives a running account of the current financial situation. Information from the combined journal is then recorded by the business manager, accountant or accounting firm into the *general ledger*, which is a final listing of income, expenses, value of property and equipment owned and amounts owed. The business operation must be maintained on a daily basis.

The ledger cards, when they are completed daily, include (1) charges for medical services, (2) payment for the services of the day and (3) payment of previous charges. The patient's ledger cards and all business records should be maintained in a safe area protected from theft and fire and away from the general office staff and patients.

PETTY CASH. Petty cash must be maintained for such items as postage due and other small expenses requiring a petty cash fund. This fund, however, should not utilize collected sources of revenue but should be maintained with a petty cash ledger or book and be drawn upon by check from the office account.

BANKING. A total discussion of banking and medical business is beyond the scope of this book. The following points, however, are important: A bank account should be established and a specific person identified to whom the office personnel, accountants or physicians may communicate regarding the banking interests of the medical practice. All checks received from patients should be immediately endorsed for bank deposit. The safest type is called a restrictive endorsement because it eliminates the possibility of the check being cashed in any other way. An example would be, "Pay to the Order of First National Bank For Deposit Only in the Account of Surgical Associates, Inc." The total of bank deposit tickets and cash deposited should equal the column totals in the *combined journal* daily. If cash receipts cannot be deposited during regular working hours, use of a night depository is recommended. Deposit slips preprinted with name and account number should be utilized.

DISBURSEMENTS. All bills and salaries should be paid by check in order to keep complete and accurate records. Before checks are written, all bills should be checked for authenticity and for accuracy of arithmetic and all equipment should be received and verified.

Employees should be paid on a regular basis, and this should be supervised by the accountant or business manager, who will make sure that the checks are properly written and will also take care of federal, state and local tax deductions, Social Security (FICA) and other payroll deductions.

Insurance

MALPRACTICE INSURANCE. Malpractice insurance and other forms of insurance are essential in the practice of medicine. The nature of malpractice insurance, the specific carriers and the limits and requirements of a policy should be fully understood. When the possibility of a malpractice claim arises, the malpractice insurance carrier should be notified. Other forms of insurance are necessary to protect the office building against fire, vandalism, flooding and public liability. If office space is rented, insurance is necessary to protect the equipment against theft and damage.

HEALTH INSURANCE. The physician and his or her family and employees may have a group policy under the office practice if so arranged.

UNEMPLOYMENT INSURANCE AND WORKMEN'S COMPENSATION INSURANCE. Unemployment insurance and workmen's compensation insurance are necessary for any business operation.

Licensing Requirements

A log or record should be kept of relicensing requirements: (1) a practice license granted by the state licensing board requires periodic reregistration, either annually or biannually, (2) the narcotics license or BNDD number requires an annual reregistration and (3) a business privilege license requires renewal annually.

Stationery, Records and Office Forms

The following items are needed or should be considered (optional):

1. Appointment stationery
2. Scheduling book
3. Telephone message book
4. Telephone prescription book or pad
5. Telephone conversation book or pad, if information is not dictated into patient's chart
6. Professional cards
7. Appointment cards
8. Letterhead paper and envelopes, in two sizes: $8^{1}/_{2} \times 11$ and $5^{1}/_{2} \times 8^{1}/_{2}$
9. Billhead statements and envelopes.
10. Announcement cards, for example: "is announcing the opening of a practice," "... the relocation of an office" or "... the addition of a new associate"
11. Treatment or prescription blanks (Some physicians duplicate treatment blanks for office records, others prefer single blanks and some prefer multidrug or treatment blanks.)
12. Memorandum slips (optional)
13. Ledger cards
14. Receipt book (Some physicians use specific receipt books, e.g., one specifically for Medicare, that list diagnosis, service, supplies and date.)
15. Charge slips or patient transaction slips
16. Recall notification letters (change of appointment letters)
17. Missed appointment letters
18. Direct insurance payment order forms
19. Operative consent forms for minor surgery to be performed
20. Referral forms
21. Specific instruction forms (for patients preparing to have laboratory tests recommended after specific treatments)
22. Surgical and hospital estimated cost forms (optional)
23. Return to work forms
24. Disability forms
25. Collection and overdue bill reminder forms
26. Health insurance claim forms
27. Medicare and Medicaid forms
28. Surgery scheduling book
29. Patient information forms
30. Patient medical questionnaires or medical history forms and medical history and physical examination forms, depending upon the type of practice and

the desires of the individual physician

31. Laboratory procedure and x-ray report forms as appropriate to the type of practice and procedure performed
32. Petty cash vouchers
33. Drug record book—absolutely necessary if DEA-controlled drugs are maintained in the office and of value if any types of drugs are kept there
34. Compensation forms
35. Report to referring physician forms (if a letter is not sent)
36. Pegboard (e.g., PEGMaster[R])[17]
37. Daily transaction control book

Patient Charges, Billing, and Other Records

An accurate record system is mandatory in the medical office because it assures constantly updated information about the physician's financial condition, fulfills the doctor's obligation to the Internal Revenue Service and assures prompt and fair dealing with patients regarding their charges and payment of their bills. Record keeping should be in three forms: (1) daily master records, (2) charge slips and (3) a charges and receipts book.

DAILY MASTER RECORD. The daily master record summarizes patient charges, records the names of patients, briefly describes the service performed, states the amount of charge and records cash payments made. These transactions are listed in the order in which they occur. The information is recorded and summarized daily. It is then entered in the charges and receipts book so that there is an ongoing record of all charges and receipts for all patients and sources in the book. This provides a means of checking on other financial records and gives up-to-date information about the current financial status of the practice.

Procedures performed outside the hospital, hospital operating charges, hospital inpatient care charges and nursing home charges should be recorded on the daily master record in whatever system is most effective for the practice. Some offices record the charges on the day of surgery; others record the charges on the day of discharge. The essential factor is that some regular system be established.

CHARGE SLIP. The charge slip is a piece of paper on which the doctor records items for which the patient should be charged. This provides for the listing of laboratory, x-ray and other data, medications and suture trays, as well as the physician's fee. Information from the charge slip is recorded onto the daily master record when the patient brings the slip to the checkout desk. This gives the patient a breakdown of the charges incurred for that visit. A pegboard system (Histacount)[17] is used in many offices.

LEDGER CARDS. A separate ledger card is maintained on a daily basis for each patient or possibly for each family, depending on the office situation. All entries from the daily master record sheet are transferred to the patient ledger card. The ledger cards should be completed in their entirety, with an adequate explanation of the service performed and of identifying codes (CPT, or current procedural terminology, codes).[14]

BILLING. The ledger card becomes the source for billing of patients and recording of payments. A system should be arranged so that each patient statement is sent out on a specific day of the month and so that these bills can be prepared several days in advance. Many systems may be utilized, and the one that is most compatible with the practice should be chosen; for example, a ledger card that is photocopied and sent each month to the patient is one effective method.

One way to keep track of patients is to provide a daily patient list to the physician or physicians and to re-issue a new list at the end of each day. Physicians then can add to this list all admissions, emergency visits, house calls and consultations.

A large portion of the physician's income arrives at the end of each billing period, either monthly or bimonthly, depending on the practice. Three factors can influence the effectiveness of billing and the amount collected: (1) the completeness of the bill, itemized to eliminate confusion and misunderstanding, (2) the neat appearance of the bill, which impresses patients with the financial organization of the office and appears to give a more favorable overall image of the doctor and the office and (3) the promptness with which the bill is sent. The patient's awareness of a doctor's services and willingness to pay decrease as time elapses after his visit.

OVERDUE ACCOUNTS. Many people do not pay their medical bills promptly, which causes a great deal of extra work and expense for the office practice. Even in the face of this frustrating situation, such patients must be treated courteously and in a manner that will not interfere with the doctor-patient relationship. A system recommended by Conomikes Associates[15] is: first month: a bill is sent explaining the services and methods of payment; second month: the words *Second Statement* are typed on the bill and underlined; third month: the bill is marked *Final Statement*; fourth month: a collection letter is sent; and fifth month: a stronger collection letter is sent. Some offices utilize an inquiry or call at either the third month or the second month. This should be made in a very courteous and efficient manner.

At some point, an uncollected bill will be sent to either a collection agency or a bad debt bureau or will be written off. When this is done, a memorandum recording the name and address of the patient, the services performed and the reason for nonpayment is written. This is stapled inside the patient's financial record and filed with other noncollectable accounts. Financial records are generally kept separate from patients' charts; however, uncollected bills and written-off charges may be noted in the medical records.

Medical Payments

FEES AND PAYMENTS. An establishment for any business or professional activity depends upon payment from customers, patients, or clients for its livelihood. In medical schools and in residency training, the business aspect of medical practice is frequently omitted. The focus in medical education in this country is to help the physician understand his or her responsibility to the sick rather than any monetary consideration. The lack of instruction in medical economics in formal education programs has caused many physicians opening a practice to be very naive in the business world.

Setting fees is a personal matter, and amounts are quite varied among different sections of the country and even among sections of a state. It may be easier to establish a fee schedule in surgical practice than in medical practice, since medical services vary from patient to patient and from day to day. Infrequently in a surgical practice, patients have not prepared themselves to pay for surgical procedures necessitated by an accident or complicated illness, as they might if planning to purchase a new automobile or garment. A realistically structured fee schedule should be developed for the more common operative procedures to help eliminate the myths that (1) physicians do not have a rational basis for their fees and (2) charges are made based on what the physician believes the individual is able or willing to pay. In setting a fee program, however, allowances for more complex procedures and those requiring more time in recurring medical care must be built into the system. One system that has worked very well in determining fees is the relative value scale, for example, the California Relative Value Scale.[5] This is a printed index of hundreds of medical procedures, which assigns values to each on a numerical scale. These have been compiled by several state medical associations and are based upon the practices of a large number of physicians. Numerical units are multiplied by a charge factor that is based upon the physician's experience, the training experience and the locality. Some physicians utilize relative value scale on a regular basis and others use them only for procedures not commonly performed.

One of the primary problems that arises in the fee-based medical practice is misunderstanding between the patient and the physician. Open discussion of fees with the patient by the physician or the physician's medical designee, i.e., secretary, medical assistant or other person, can eliminate confusion and lead to a better understanding. In certain facets of surgical practice third party carriers do not provide for payment, for example, in some plastic surgical procedures. In this situation the patient may ask for a medical cost estimate. If the surgical practice will make estimates, a form should be provided that includes all charges for medical care, including operations, hospitalization, surgeon's, surgical assistant's and anesthesiologist's fees, and other fees for professional services.

Insurance companies have frequently misled their policyholders by propagating the myth that physicians will always accept the fees they are paid. In the practice of surgery, one should remember that fees are established for the medical and surgical services rendered and are not set arbitrarily by an insurance company's board of directors. The problem arises when patients do not realize that the insurance company has not paid the full fee, and they receive a secondary bill from the doctor's office. The agreement between an insurance company and a patient, purely an individual contract between a corporation and a person or persons purchasing a policy, does not determine medical fee structure.

CREDIT. Credit is a necessary part of business; however, even if everyone paid his credit obligations on time, credit would be expensive because of the paperwork involved and the postage and personnel time required. Many patients prefer to pay for their medical services immediately following an office visit or at the time of follow-up after a surgical procedure. This system eliminates additional paperwork, personnel time and postage.

A patient who has not been seen previously in the office should complete an information form at the time of the follow-up visit. Also at this time the patient can be requested to sign all third party insurance carrier forms.

Cooperation between hospitals and physicians' offices helps both the hospital and the practitioner to complete insurance information and collect due bills more efficiently and effectively. Many hospitals provide the physician with a copy of the admission data, including insurance information and current address, when the patient is admitted to the hospital. Many physicians provide similar information to the hospitals when a patient is scheduled for admission.

Many patients are unable to pay large medical bills in a lump sum but are willing to make installment payments on a regular and well-defined basis. Patients frequently are proud and unwilling to ask for this opportunity. The physician's office should mention this possibility to the patient in the event that bills are unpaid. A standard form containing this information should be prepared by the office to be sent out with delinquent bills.

PROFESSIONAL COURTESY. Physicians often provide their services free of charge or at reduced rates to other physicians and to certain other professional groups. In establishing the office the guidelines for professional courtesy should be clarified and the way this will be carried out should be decided. A list of the groups who will receive professional courtesy should be made, and the per cent reduction of the normal fee for each category should be established.

Third Party Payments

With the appearance of third party insurers to pay medical fees, medical care is no longer considered a privilege but a right. The different forms of third party payment are insurance, Medicare, Medicaid, workmen's compensation and group health maintenance organization (HMO) prepayment plans, such as those of the UMW and C & O Employees Association. In some prepaid plans, the physician must apply for and be considered a participant in the program, and this should be accomplished before seeing patients who are members of these plans.

INSURANCE. Relationships with third party carriers, especially of health insurance, are now a way of life in medical practice. These plans make it easier for most patients to handle unforeseen medical expenses; however, they are somewhat misleading to patients, and the system is poorly represented and poorly understood. Medical insurance is a contract between a potential patient and an insurance company and is not a contract between a physician and an insurance company. Insurance creates a lot of paperwork for medical office personnel. The approach to insurance claims should be a very complete, prompt and accurate processing by the office staff, with quick filing of forms. Accuracy and completeness will decrease the frequency of returned claims.

Many systems are used in surgical offices, one of which is to list, on the day either of the patient's discharge or operation, the patient's name, date of admission, date of discharge, admission diagnosis, discharge diagnosis, and operative procedure performed. This can either be written by the physi-

cian or called in to the office. This facilitates completion of the insurance forms prior to completion of the discharge summary, which may be delayed in the hospital's clerical department.

Blue Cross, one of the best known forms of medical insurance, pays part or all of the hospital costs in participating hospitals. Blue Shield, similarly, pays for physician's services or other medical services. There are many different kinds of medical insurance plans and many different types of plans within individual insurance companies, such as Blue Cross and Blue Shield. Many insurance plans pay the patient directly. To eliminate confusion, when a patient is likely to receive payment directly from the insurance company, a *form assignment of insurance benefits* may be signed by the patient authorizing the insurance company to make payment to the physician rather than to the insured patient. A combined form on which the patient permits the release of information about his medical diagnoses to the insurance company as well as assignment of benefits may be utilized (Fig. 2–5).[15]

The insurance forms, if not completed rapidly and effectively, may create havoc in office finances. Conomikes Associates recommends keeping an *"insurance claim log"*[15] in which the patient's name and insurance company, the date the form was received and the date the form was mailed are recorded. Some insurance companies require a policyholder to file a preliminary notice with the company within 20 days of an accident or illness, and they subsequently forward a claims form to the patient. Many insurance companies have a number of different forms of varying degrees of complexity. If the forms appear to be too complicated or difficult, one may utilize a standard Health Insurance Council form, known as CONB-1(10–67), and staple this to the insurance forms. If adequate space is not provided on the insurance form for the necessary information, attach

```
RELEASE OF MEDICAL INFORMATION

ASSIGNMENT OF INSURANCE BENEFITS


                             Date_____

Patient_____

Employer_____

Date of Injury or Illness_____

Insurance Carrier_____

Group_____
In consideration of Medical Services rendered to

_____
           (patient's name)
I hereby authorize and direct_____
                             (insurance carrier)
to pay directly to Dr._____
any benefits that may accrue to me under the above indi-
cated insurance and/or disability benefits plan.  I
agree to pay Dr._____ for all ser-
vices incidental to the said treatment not paid for by
the Medical Insurance Plan named above.

I hereby authorize Dr._____
to release to said Insurance Company any information re-
garding my illness and/or injury including laboratory re-
ports, X-rays and diagnosis which is needed by said
Insurance Company to process the claim.

Witness_____

          Signature of Subscriber_____
```

_____ ConomikesAssociates _____

Figure 2–5 Combined form for release of medical information and assignment of insurance benefits. (From: Guidebook for the Medical Office Staff. Greenwich, Connecticut, Conomikes Associates, Inc., 64 Greenwich Avenue, Greenwich, 06830, 1973.)

such information to it to avoid having the form returned. Remember that promptness and completeness will facilitate rapid claims, keep patients happy and create a better financial situation for the office.

MEDICARE. The federal government insurance program called Medicare covers patients over 65 years of age. A person covered by this program will carry a Medicare identification card that say "Health Insurance Social Security Act." There are two types of Medicare insurance. *Part A*, which is hospitalization insurance, is financed by the contributions of working individuals through the Social Security system and by employers' matching contributions. *Part A* on the identification card states that the person "is entitled

to hospital insurance." *Part B* is medical insurance coverage. Patients must apply for and pay a monthly premium for Part B. If a person is entitled to Part B Medicare, the card is labeled "entitled to medical insurance." As with other forms of insurance, the patient must be aware that the program does not pay all of his or her medical costs but only a portion. A physician may approach Medicare in one of several ways: (1) The Medicare form may be filed with the insurance carrier for the 80 per cent of the fee that Medicare will pay. However, in this situation the physician must sign the fee assignment line of the Medicare form. With this method, the surgeon must acknowledge to the insurance carrier that the 80 per cent reimbursement is based on an average fee and will not necessarily be 80 per cent of the usual fee and is frequently based on a period of time earlier than the present year of billing. A surgeon accepting fee assignment may bill the patient for the remaining 20 per cent of the charges. (2) A bill may be sent directly to the patient for the entire amount. After receipt of payment, the physician may issue a receipt with the necessary medical information (diagnosis and operation) for the patient to submit directly to Medicare for reimbursement. (3) A promissory note can be signed by the patient for the full amount of the fee. With this the patient receives a receipt for the bill, which can be sent to the insurance carrier for reimbursement. The patient is responsible for payment of the entire amount.[15]

WORKMEN'S COMPENSATION. Workmen's compensation is a compulsory insurance program in which an employer pays the premium for medical care and loss of wages resulting from illness or accident sustained on the job. This is required by state law. Each state has individual requirements, and the surgeon or office manager should contact the workmen's compensation commission in his or her state for the regulations. Some insurance companies retain their own doctors and refer patients to them; however, most states give the worker the right to choose his or her own physician.

If a surgical practice has a large volume of workmen's compensation claims, a workmen's compensation form log should be maintained as well as an insurance log, since workmen's compensation frequently requires a report from the physician to (1) the employer of the patient, (2) the workmen's compensation board and (3) the insurance carrier at the time of initial medical treatment. Frequently, progress reports are required after two weeks, and subsequent progress reports are required at monthly intervals or as otherwise specified, along with a final report listing any permanent dis-

ability. These reports should be maintained in a separate folder or a separate filing system.

REFERENCES

1. Abbott, V. C.: Emergency department staffing: Five-year experience with the Pontiac plan, Bulletin of the American College of Surgeons, January-February 1966, pp. 1–2.
2. Accidental Death and Disability: The Neglected Disease of Modern Society. Washington, D.C., National Academy of Sciences, National Research Council, September 1966. (Printing and Publishing Office, National Academy of Sciences, 2101 Constitution Avenue, Washington, D.C., 20418)
3. Accidental Death and Injury Statistics. Washington, D.C., U.S. Department of Health, Education and Welfare, Public Health Service Publication Number 1111, October 1963. (U.S. Government Printing Office, 20401)
4. Categorization of Hospital Emergency Capabilities. Chicago, American Medical Association, 535 North Dearborn Street, 60610, 1971.
5. Committee on Relative Value Studies, California Medical Association. Report. San Francisco, Sutter Publications, Inc., 731 Market Street, 1974. (Revision of 1969 *California Relative Value Studies.*)
6. Developing Emergency Medical Services: Guidelines for Community Councils. Chicago, American Medical Association, 1976. (Order Department OP-386, American Medical Association, 535 North Dearborn Street, Chicago, Illinois, 60610)
7. Emergency Department: A Handbook for the Medical Staff. Chicago, American Medical Association, Department of Hospitals and Medical Facilities, 1966.
8. The Emergency Department in the Hospital: A Guide to Organization and Management. Chicago, American Hospital Association, 840 North Lake Shore Drive, 1962. (publication no. M47)
9. Emergency Medical Services: Proceedings of the Airlie Conference on Emergency Medical Services. Airlie House, Warrenton, Virginia, May 5–6, 1969. (American College of Surgeons, 55 East Erie Street, Chicago, Illinois, 60611)
10. The emergency room and the outpatient clinics. Resident and Staff Physician, January 1970, pp. 94–106.
11. Facts and Trends on Hospital Outpatient Services. Washington, D.C., Division of Hospital and Medical Facilities, Public Health Service, U.S. Department of

Health, Education and Welfare, 20201, 1964. (Public Health Service Publication Number 930-C-6)

12. Frederick, P. M., and Kinn, M. E.: The Medical Office Assistant, 4th ed. Philadelphia, W. B. Saunders Co., 1974.

13. Frey, C. F.: University Association for Emergency Medical Services. Charter meeting. J. Trauma, *11*:541–559, 1971.

14. Gordon, B. L. (ed.), et al.: Current Procedural Terminology, 3rd ed. Chicago, American Medical Association, 1973.

15. Guidebook for the Medical Office Staff. Greenwich, Conn., Conomikes Associates, Inc., 64 Greenwich Avenue, 06830, 1973.

16. Guidelines for Design and Function of a Hospital Emergency Department. Chicago, Committee on Trauma, American College of Surgeons, 55 E. Erie Street, 60611, 1970.

17. Histacount Corporation, subsidiary of SEM Corp., Melville, Long Island, New York, 11746 (Summer 1978 catalog).

18. Hospital Emergency Room Utilization Study: A Report on Emergency Room Visits in 22 Michigan Hospitals. Detroit, Michigan Blue Cross, 441 E. Jefferson Avenue, 48226.

19. Hospital Outpatient Emergency Activities. Rockville, Md., U.S. Department of Health, Education and Welfare, Public Health Service, Health Services and Mental Health Administration, Health Care Facilities Service, 20852, 1977. (Publication number 930-H-1)

20. Mills, J. D.: Emergency department management. South. Med. Bull., December 1971, pp. 18–22.

21. A Model of a Hospital Emergency Department by the Committee on Trauma, American College of Surgeons. Chicago, American College of Surgeons, 55 E. Erie Street, 60611.

22. Owens, J. C.: Auditing daily emergency department care. J. Trauma, *11*:359–362, 1971.

23. Standards for Accreditation of Hospitals, 1979. (Distributed by: American Medical Association, Joint Commission on Accreditation of Hospitals, 645 N. Michigan Avenue, Chicago, Illinois 60611)

24. What's wrong with emergency rooms. Resident and Staff Physician, August 1971, pp. 96–102.

3 Anesthesia for Outpatients

DENNIS BARTON, M.D.

There are many procedures that require anesthesia but do not require overnight hospitalization. This chapter will examine anesthetic techniques and point out methods that have been found useful for outpatients.

In-hospital charges for patients in the United States are rapidly approaching two hundred dollars per day. With such inflationary pressure an overnight stay in the hospital can no longer be a part of a minor surgical procedure. Outpatient surgery programs have been organized in which patients come to the outpatient facility, are examined for their fitness for surgery, undergo necessary preoperative laboratory examinations and are then given written instructions to prepare them for the day of surgery.[1] Patients may then return at a later date for surgery or proceed directly to the operating room.[2]

Freestanding surgical facilities, separated from hospitals, have also been organized.[3] These surgical clinics offer the advantage of better cost control, but they may require an initial capital investment of some magnitude. If patients are preselected for fitness, transfer of patients with unexpected complications to hospitals is rare.[4] Both hospital and freestanding surgical clinics expect to admit outpatients, perform elective surgery and discharge patients to responsible companions for return home on the same day. There are many patients who arrive at hospitals seeking emergency surgical care. Some of these patients can be treated and sent home also.

There are many patients and proce-

65

TABLE 3-1   Pharmacology of Local Anesthetic Agents*

Drug (Trade Name)	Supplied	Maximum Permitted Dose	Onset of Action	Duration	Toxicity
Cocaine Not for injection	As powder made up in 1–4% solution	100 mgm total Some authors use up to 6.6 mgm/kg	Rapid — topical	1 hr	Convulsions, coma, respiratory arrest
Dyclonine (Dyclone) Not for injection	Solution, 0.5% concentration	200 mgm in adult	Rapid — topical	20–30 mins	Very rarely reported
Procaine (Novocain)	1–2% solution	10–15 mgm/kg	Rapid	30 mins to 1 hr	Tinnitus, nausea, convulsions rare
Chlorprocaine (Nesacaine)	1–2% solution	10–20 mgm/kg	Very rapid	1 hr	Less toxic than Procaine
Tetracaine (Pontocaine) Topical	1–3% solution Also ingredient of Cetacaine (see text)	1.5 mgm/kg (not to exceed 150 mgm)	Moderate speed (*Topical use*) Sometimes combined with other agents (see text)	2 hrs	Drowsiness→coma Convulsions rare
Lidocaine (Xylocaine)	0.5–2% solution	4 mgm/kg	5–30 minutes	2 hrs	Drowsiness→coma Convulsions also seen
(Lignocaine)	2–4% solution	4 mgm/kg	Rapid (*Topical use*)	1 hr	Drowsiness→coma Convulsions also seen
Mepivacaine (Carbocaine)	1.0–2.0% solutions	7 mgm/kg (do not exceed 1000 mgm/ 24 hrs)	5–30 minutes	2–3 hrs	Drowsiness→coma Convulsions
Xylocaine with 1:200,000 Epinephrine	0.5–2.0% solution	7 mgm/kg	5–30 minutes	2–3 hrs	Drowsiness→coma Convulsions. Do not use more than 50 cc 1:200,000 epinephrine solution
Prilocaine (Citanest)	1.0–3.0% solutions	Dose not to exceed 700 mgm in adult	5–30 minutes	2–3 hrs	Drowsiness→coma or convulsions. Methemoglobinemia with overdose (see text)
Bupivacaine (Marcaine)	0.25–0.75% solution with and without epinephrine	Max. dose 175 mgm in adult or 225 mgm with epinephrine solutions	7–30 minutes	12 hrs on peripheral nerves	Tremor, shivering, nausea. Rare convulsions
Etidocaine (Duranest)	0.5% to 1.5% with and without epinephrine	400 mgm in adult	7–10 minutes	12 hrs on peripheral nerves with epinephrine, 10 hrs without epinephrine	Slurred speech, circumoral numbness, lightheadedness.

*1% solutions of drugs listed have 10 mgm drug per 1 cc; 2% solutions have 20 mgm per cc, etc.

dures not suitable for outpatient anesthesia. The procedure itself may be relatively minor, but the patients may be poor anesthetic risks because of severe systemic disease. Some patients have no one to look after them at home. One series found that 5.4 per cent of patients previously selected for outpatient surgery were unable to follow their normal occupation on the day after anesthesia.[5] This incidence alone warrants the precept that no patient should be returned to an isolated home environment. Elderly and mentally retarded patients, unable to follow written instructions, must also be hospitalized.

Emergency patients with head injuries or stupor resulting from alcohol or drug abuse cannot be sent out but must be kept for observation. Patients undergoing surgical procedures with a high incidence of postoperative blood loss or other complications must also be kept in the hospital: mammoplasty, extensive varicose vein stripping and perhaps tonsillectomy fall into this category.

This chapter will consider regional and general anesthetic techniques. The pharmacology of local anesthetics will be presented first, followed by presentations of useful regional anesthetic techniques. The regional anesthetic techniques in this chapter have wide application to various surgical disciplines. Those techniques peculiar to a particular surgical specialty are found elsewhere in the appropriate chapter. The last section of this chapter will consider pertinent facts relating to drugs for premedication and general anesthetic agents.

Table 3–1 summarizes the pharmacology of the well-known local anesthetic agents. The maximum permitted doses in a typical adult are shown in Table 3–2.

The physician desires local anesthetic drugs of rapid onset, low toxicity and prolonged duration. Unfortunately, local anesthetics of rapid onset tend

TABLE 3–2　Maximum Volume of Solution of Local Anesthetics for a 70 Kgm Adult*

ANESTHETIC	MAXIMUM VOLUME
Procaine (Novocain) 1%	70–105 cc
Chlorprocaine (Nesacaine) 1%	70–140 cc
Lidocaine (Xylocaine, Lignocaine) 1%	28 cc
Lidocaine with epinephrine 1%	50 cc
Mepivacaine (Carbocaine) 1%	50 cc
Prilocaine (Citanest) 1%	70 cc
Bupivacaine 0.25%	70 cc
Bupivacaine 0.25% with epinephrine	100 cc
Etidocaine 0.5%	80 cc

*Calculations based on maximum doses specified in Table 3–1.

to be of short duration, and one must choose a drug compatible with the length of the proposed procedure. Long-acting local anesthetics are available, indeed peripheral nerve blocks with bupivacaine may last longer than 12 hours.

One will occasionally encounter allergy to local anesthetic agents. This is usually manifested as a rash, urticaria or even wheezing.[6] One must distinguish between allergy to the anesthetic drug and allergy to the preservative in the drug vial (methylparaben).[7] If a patient has a history of allergy to a drug in the para-aminobenzoic acid-ester series (procaine, chlorprocaine, tetracaine), skin testing may reveal no allergy to anesthetics in the amide-linked series (lidocaine, mepivacaine, or bupivacaine). Anaphylactic shock reaction to minute amounts of local anesthetic drug is extremely rare.

Most histories of allergy to local anesthetics are actually histories of inadvertent intravascular injection, especially with epinephrine-containing solutions. Fright at the sight of an injection needle is probably the most common cause of "allergy to local anesthetics." One still encounters cases where the well-publicized dose limits of various anesthetic drugs have been exceeded by physicians somehow ignorant of the deadly potency of local anesthetic agents.

Close verbal contact is kept between the physician and the patient undergoing local block so that early signs of toxicity can be detected. The patient may become nauseated or drowsy, or complain of tinnitus or generalized numbness and tingling. High blood levels of local anesthetic resulting from either intravascular injection or too great a total dose, may cause excitatory central nervous system effects. These reactions may be transient or absent, and toxicity will be manifest as drowsiness merging into unconsciousness and respiratory arrest.

The management of such an emergency is treated elsewhere in this book (see Chapter 26). Major blocks should not be attempted unless resuscitative gear is at hand. An intravenous line should be set up in cases in which drug doses near the permitted maximum are planned.

Blocks may fail or may need renewal. As a general rule, the maximum permitted dose should never be exceeded at one sitting. Many of the blocks described in this chapter will require the maximum permitted dose and should not be renewed until several hours have passed. Less extensive blocks that fail can be attempted several times, provided a drug with a high maximum dose is chosen. Tachyphylaxis to local anesthetic agents is often encountered with repeated injection of a certain drug. The block can be re-established with a different local anesthetic drug.

TOPICAL ANESTHESIA — COCAINE, CETACAINE, TETRACAINE, DYCLONINE

Cocaine, dyclonine (Dyclone), and Cetacaine, a local anesthetic mixture, are used exclusively as surface analgesics. Lidocaine (Xylocaine) in viscous form, or as a 4 per cent solution, as well as tetracaine (Pontocaine) are also available as topical agents. Cocaine is the only agent in the series that has vasoconstrictive properties, and this may be the reason why the drug still enjoys popularity. Great care must be exercised in its use — a measured amount of the drug in a 1.0 to 2.0 per cent solution is placed in a medicine cup (totaling 50–100 mgm) and this dose is never exceeded. (However, one author has used up to 6.6 mgm per kg cocaine and has never encountered a toxic reaction.)[8] The cocaine is applied with a swab; a spray is inefficient. Overdose with cocaine is manifested by hyperirritability leading to convulsions, coma and respiratory arrest.

Tetracaine (Pontocaine, Amethocaine) can be employed as a topical anesthetic either alone or in combination with other topical anesthetic agents.

If tetracaine alone is chosen, a 1.0 to 2.0 per cent solution is used. The limit of the dose for tetracaine is 1.5 mgm per kg. Overdose usually results in drowsiness, progressing to shallow respirations and coma. Convulsions are rarely encountered. The use of other topical agents with tetracaine gives the physician a faster onset of anesthesia. Cetacaine, a combination of tetracaine with ethylamino and butylamino benzoate, is used frequently at our hospitals. The latter two chemicals are poorly soluble in water, a property which causes these drugs to be absorbed slowly into the body, and they provide only surface anesthesia. Cetacaine is not helpful in diagnostic work. The drug leaves a yellowish deposit that obscures oral and pharyngeal mucosa.

Dyclonine (Dyclone) is an excellent topical anesthetic,[9] differing in its structural formula from other anesthetic agents. It is confined to topical use because it is rather irritative to tissue when injected locally. The topical effect lasts around 20 minutes. In dose ranges used clinically (4–20 cc of 0.5 per cent solution) no toxic reactions have been reported; indeed doses of 200–500 mgm IV in man have been without toxic effects.

LOCAL AND REGIONAL DRUGS

Procaine (Novocain)

Procaine has a wide margin of safety, and up to 15 mgm per kg total dose of the drug can be used. The onset of action is extremely rapid, seven minutes for nerve blocks, but it cannot be expected to last for more than an hour. Convulsions occur with overdose, but extremely large and unrealistic doses are necessary to achieve these symptoms.

Chlorprocaine (Nesacaine)

This drug is said to be even less toxic than procaine.[10] Twenty mgm per kg of this drug have been used without toxic effects. Again the onset of action is extremely rapid, but the drug cannot be used for prolonged surgery. Both procaine and chlorprocaine are deactivated via hydrolysis by the pseudocholinesterase system in the blood. This fact may have practical importance, for there are certain rare patients that are hereditarily deficient in this enzyme system.

Lidocaine (Xylocaine)

Lidocaine offers fairly prolonged anesthesia (one to two hours). The addition of epinephrine 1:200,000 prolongs the action to two to three hours. The volume of 1:200,000 epinephrine solution should not exceed 50 cc to avoid side effects from the epinephrine. The onset of action varies from 5 to 30 minutes. The most common cause of block failure with this drug is impatience. A patient who has spent days getting ready for surgery can afford to wait 20 to 30 minutes more for the onset of solid anesthesia.

The maximum doses of lidocaine are listed in Table 3–1. Solutions of 0.5 to 1.0 per cent are used for sensory anesthesia, while 1.5 to 2.0 per cent concentrations are more suitable for motor nerve block, or blocks where a longer duration is required. Minor lacerations can easily be handled with 0.5 per cent solutions. Solutions with epinephrine should never be used on the finger, the toes, or the penis, since the resultant ischemia may cause necrosis. Toxicity is usually manifested by drowsiness deepening into coma and cardiorespiratory collapse. Convulsions are rare.

Mepivacaine (Carbocaine)

This is roughly equivalent to xylocaine with epinephrine in both duration of anesthesia and maximum permitted dose (see Table 3–1). Addition of epinephrine to mepivacaine will prolong the action of the drug only slightly.[11] Mepivacaine accumulates in the body with repeated blocks, and it has been recommended that no more than 1000 mgm of mepivacaine be used in a 24-hour period.[12] Toxicity is manifested by stupor and coma, or rarely by convulsions.

Prilocaine (Citanest)

Prilocaine was felt to be an advance in local anesthetics because the maximum permitted dose was stated to be 10 mgm per kg. Unfortunately, methemoglobinemia occurs with this drug, owing to the accumulation of a metabolite of prilocaine in the red cells of the patient. Methemoglobinemia is seen as 5 per cent of total hemoglobin at doses of 600 mgm prilocaine.[13] The methemoglobinemia can be reversed with 1–2 mgm per kg IV methylene blue. Nevertheless, the early enthusiasm for the drug has been dimmed by this side effect. As with mepivacaine, the addition of epinephrine will not greatly prolong the action of the drug. Overdose is manifested by tremor, shivering, nausea and vomiting.

Bupivacaine (Marcaine)

This drug has an extremely long duration of action in peripheral nerve blocks.[11] Its onset of action is moderately long. It is marketed both with and without epinephrine. Epinephrine serves to delay the uptake of the drug by the body, thus improving the margin of safety, but it has no effect on the duration of the drug's action. The drug should not be used when rapid sensory and motor return is desired. Its prolonged action is especially useful in therapeutic nerve blocks such as intercostal blocks for the pain of fractured ribs, or sympathetic blocks done for vascular insufficiency or causalgic pain. Solutions of 0.25 per cent strength are used for local infiltration and peripheral sensory and sympathetic nerve blocks. The 0.5 per cent strength solution also gives additional motor blockade. The 0.75 per cent solutions are used in epidural anesthesia.

Etidocaine (Duranest)

Etidocaine also has a prolonged duration of action, but somewhat shorter than bupivacaine. Addition of epinephrine will prolong its action. The 0.5 per cent solution is roughly equivalent to 0.25 per cent bupivacaine. As etidocaine wears off, sensation may return before motor power has been reestablished. Toxicity is manifested by convulsions, but more commonly by drowsiness deepening into coma and respiratory arrest.[14]

REGIONAL ANESTHETIC TECHNIQUES

All these techniques will be more satisfactory if premedication with tranquilizers, somnifacients or analgesics is used. For outpatients these drugs are best given IV to allow rapid recovery after the procedure. (See the section on premedication later in this chapter.)

Intravenous Regional Anesthesia

This method was first established by Bier in 1908, but owes its current revival to Holmes, who reintroduced the technique in 1963.[15] The technique is especially useful in emergencies or other procedures in which a tourniquet time of an hour or less is foreseen. The technique is illustrated in Figure 3–1. A scalp vein needle is inserted into a vein near the proposed site of operation, and a double cuffed tourniquet is fitted about the upper arm. The hand and arm below the tourniquet are exsanguinated either with an Esmarch bandage, or by gravity drainage in the case of fracture or trauma. The upper (proximal) cuff of the tourniquet is then inflated, and a local anesthetic is injected (see below for dosage) into the scalp vein needle. Analgesia suitable for operation will appear in 10 to 15 minutes in the arm below the tourniquet. (Cuts on fingers that prevent venous spread of the drug may not allow analgesia distal to the cut.) The injected drug spreads through the venous system in the arm and then diffuses through the tissues.[16] Once analgesia is established, the lower (distal) tourniquet is inflated and the upper (proximal) tourniquet is deflated. The inflated tourniquet is now over an analgesic area, and the occurrence of tourniquet pain is reduced. Tourniquet pain can still be a problem with this method, especially if the procedure is prolonged over an hour. Tourniquet time limits analgesia. When the tourniquet is released, sen-

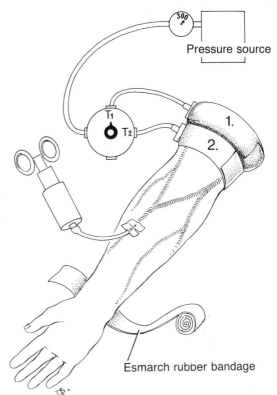

Pressure source

300

T₁

T₂

1.

2.

Figure 3–1 Intravenous regional analgesia. A double cuffed tourniquet permits inflation of an occlusive tourniquet over a previously anesthetized area. Such tourniquets are commercially available.

Esmarch rubber bandage

sation is quickly restored. Intravenous bupivacaine evidently allows the physician 20 minutes of analgesia after tourniquet release,[17] but this drug is not yet available commercially in the United States.

DOSAGE. Three mgm per kg of 0.5 per cent lidocaine is used for intravenous regional analgesia (42 cc in a 70 kgm adult). There will be no motor nerve block with this concentration. The physician should not use the drug made up with preservative or with epinephrine. If flaccidity is desired, 1 mgm d-tubocurarine per 40 pounds of body weight can be added to the injection. This small dose will be harmlessly redistributed when the tourniquet is released.

Axillary Block

This block is easily learned, and has been found suitable for emergency and elective surgery of the forearm and hand.[18] The technique is quite useful in children. Needle placement for the block is illustrated in Figure 3–2. The brachial artery is invested with a perivascular fascial sheath. The sheath holds not only the artery but also the median, radial and ulnar nerves.

The patient lies supine, with the arm to be blocked placed so that the hand rests above or near the top of the head. A Penrose drain is tightened circumferentially about the arm distal to the injection site. This aids in spreading the anesthetic solution cephalad, and increases the chances of a successful nerve block. A 23 gauge needle is inserted close to the brachial artery near the lateral border of the pectoralis major muscle. A paresthesia is sought, indicating needle contact with one of the nerves in the perivascular sheath. (The sheath is fairly superficial in the axilla, and the physician will err in

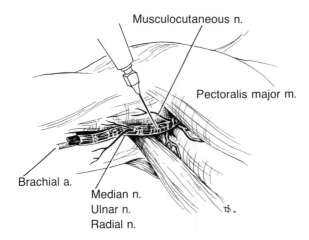

Musculocutaneous n.

Pectoralis major m.

Brachial a.

Median n.
Ulnar n.
Radial n.

Figure 3–2 The axillary block. Note that the musculocutaneous nerve is often missed with this block. The anesthetic solution is held in place by the perivascular sheath that encases both the artery and the nerves. A Penrose drain is tightened circumferentially about the arm distal to the injection site while the injection is made. This increases the spread of the anesthetic solution in a cephalad direction.

going too deep.) The radial nerve lies behind the artery, so the median nerve (above) or the ulnar nerve (below) is usually encountered with the needle. The patient will experience tingling or an electric shock sensation down the forearm into the hand. The patient should be instructed to say "Now" when the paresthesia is elicited. The entire anesthetic solution can be deposited at the site of the paresthesia. An alternate technique is to deposit half the anesthetic solution at each of two separately elicited paresthesiae, usually the median and ulnar nerves. (See later for dosage.) The anesthetic solution will spread within the perivascular sheath and surround all three nerves. Some patients find this block an unpleasant experience and premedication is required. The physician will also encounter patients who will not experience a paresthesia. In this instance the 23 gauge needle is inserted directly into the brachial artery and its position is checked by aspiration of blood. The needle is then withdrawn to a point just outside the artery where blood can no longer be aspirated. The tip of the needle is presumed to be in the perivascular space, and again the entire amount of anesthetic solution is deposited. The circumferential Penrose drain is removed and replaced by a standard pressurized tourniquet.

The injection site may not give anes-thesia to the musculocutaneous nerve. A sensory branch of this nerve, the lateral antebrachial cutaneous nerve, has a variable distribution in the radial border of the forearm and down into the thenar eminence. The physician will occasionally encounter patients who will experience some sensation if surgical dissection is carried into these areas. The problem is usually solved by local infiltration at the surgical site.

Tourniquet pain is sometimes experienced with this block, owing to tourniquet pressure on the intercostobrachial nerve that innervates a portion of the upper medial aspect of the arm. A line of subcutaneous infiltration of local anesthetic across the axilla above the tourniquet will solve this problem.

DOSAGE. Lidocaine with epinephrine will give around three hours of anesthesia with this block. Dosage of lidocaine with epinephrine 1:200,000 should be limited to 7–8 mgm per kg. A sufficient volume (¼ cc per pound in the adult) to fill the axillary sheath must be used. In children 7–8 mgm per kg of 1 per cent lidocaine with epinephrine will supply sufficient volume. As an example, in a young, fit, 80 kg man, one would use 30 cc of 1.5 per cent lidocaine with epinephrine plus 10 cc of 1.0 per cent lidocaine with epinephrine. This is a volume of 40 cc with a total dosage of 550 mgm. The maximum allowable dose in this man would be 560–640 mgm. Mepivacaine 1 per cent, also 7–8 mgm per kg can be used. Bupivacaine (Marcaine) 0.25 to 0.5 per cent will give a prolonged block of up to 12 hours' duration. Forty ml of 0.25 per cent solution (100 mgm) bupivacaine is below the maximum permitted dose in a 70 kg patient (175 mgm). The 0.5 per cent solution can be used if motor block is desired.

In all blocks with near the maximum allowed dose, an IV drip should be placed in the patient. Resuscitation gear should be at hand wherever blocks are done.

Interscalene Block

This block has been developed and promulgated by Dr. Alon P. Winnie.[19] Because of its site of injection it provides immobility at the shoulder joint and anesthesia of the musculocutaneous nerves, features missing with an axillary block. As the intercostobrachial nerve is still intact with the block, subcutaneous axillary infiltra-

tion is required if a tourniquet is used on the arm. The approach to the block is different from that used for the classic supraclavicular approach to the brachial plexus. The supraclavicular approach entails a risk of pneumothorax (0.5 to 4 per cent incidence),[20] while the interscalene approach avoids this complication. Rarely, injection into the subarachnoid space with the interscalene technique has been reported. Such an injection will result in high spinal anesthesia.

The approach to the block is illustrated in Figure 3–3. The anatomy of the patient's neck is brought into relief by tilting the head backward and sharply away from the arm to be blocked. The patient is then asked to stretch the arm as if reaching for his knee, and the muscles are brought further into relief by asking the patient to raise his head. The anterior scalene muscle can be felt just lateral to the sternocleidomastoid muscle. The interscalene groove is palpated lateral to the anterior scalene. A line perpendicular to the interscalene groove is drawn on the skin of the neck from the

Figure 3–3 The interscalene block. The needle is inserted into the interscalene groove at the level of the cricoid cartilage. The needle points inwardly and slightly caudal.

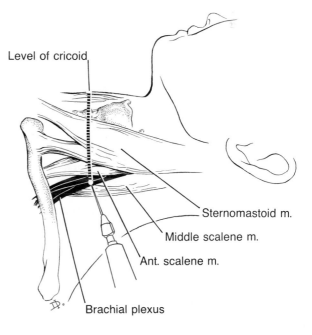

Level of cricoid

Sternomastoid m.

Middle scalene m.

Ant. scalene m.

Brachial plexus

cricoid cartilage and a 21 gauge needle is inserted at the junction of the interscalene groove with this perpendicular cricoid line. The needle is advanced inwardly and slightly caudad and is kept in an imaginary plane that is perpendicular to the neck at the interscalene groove. Three or four attempts may be needed to elicit a paresthesia, which is mandatory before injection of a drug. The patient will feel the paresthesia down into the hand. No injection is made if the patient has paresthesia in the posterior shoulder, as the block will not succeed. The physician may feel a distinct "pop" as the fibrous tissue investing the brachial plexus is penetrated.

DOSAGE. Adequate volume is necessary for this block. In adults, Winnie suggests the formula $\dfrac{\text{Height (Inches)}}{2} =$ Volume (ml) as a starting point. One to one and a half per cent lidocaine with epinephrine, mepivacaine, 0.5 per cent etidocaine or 0.25 per cent bupivacaine can be used, provided the maximum allowed dose of these drugs is not exceeded. Low volumes usually result in incomplete block of the ulnar nerve. Larger volumes (40 ml in the adult) will result in block of the supraclavicular nerves as well. Care must be taken not to exceed the maximum allowed mgm per kg dose.

Sciatic-Femoral Block

Sciatic-femoral block was perfected in the United States by the pioneer anesthesiologist Gaston Labat.[21] It is technically more difficult to perform than the other blocks listed in this chapter, but it is included here because of its usefulness in outpatient and emergency surgery. Surgical incision or manipulation can be performed from 2 cm below the patella. The block will also cover closed manipulation of the knee and the lower portion of the femur. The tourniquet cannot be applied with this block without the addi-

tional block of the lateral femoral cutaneous nerve.[20]

The anatomy for the sciatic-femoral block is illustrated in Figures 3–4 and 3–5. The patient lies laterally with the leg to be blocked uppermost and drawn up (Sims' position). A line is drawn from the posterosuperior spine of the ilium to the greater trochanter. The midpoint of the line is located and a perpendicular bisecting line is drawn at this point down the leg. The injection site is 3–5 cm down this bisecting line. A 22 gauge spinal needle is inserted perpendicular to the skin at this point, a depth of 6–8 or even 10 cm being necessary to locate the sciatic nerve. Paresthesia is manifested by tingling or an electric shock sensation down the back of the leg. The patient should be instructed to say "Now" when this paresthesia is obtained.

Bone may be encountered while advancing the needle at this site. This is the rim around the greater sciatic notch. The nerve is usually close to

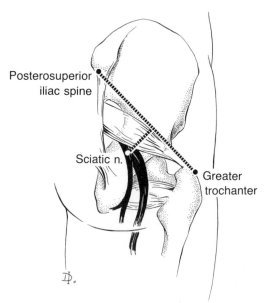

Figure 3–4 Sciatic femoral block. Block of the sciatic nerve. If the needle encounters bone, the operator is at the correct depth, but the needle must be redirected until a paresthesia is elicited.

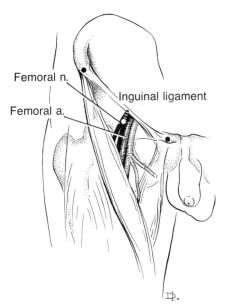

Figure 3–5 Sciatic femoral block. Block of the femoral nerve. No paresthesia is required for this block. The success rate is quite high.

this depth, so the needle need not be advanced much farther.

If no paresthesia is obtained, the needle is redirected either upward or downward in a plane in the body perpendicular to the original bisecting line drawn on the skin surface.

The femoral nerve block is performed with the patient lying supine. The femoral nerve lies lateral at the same depth as the femoral artery. The nerve is best approached from a point 1 cm below the inguinal ligament and just lateral to the artery. The anesthetic solution should be injected in an imaginary triangle. The apex of the triangle is the injection site, while the base is on a plane passing slightly below the femoral artery and nerve (3–3.5 cm). The line of the base is parallel to a line 1 cm below and parallel to the inguinal ligament. The injection is carried from the artery laterally at least 1 inch. Usually no paresthesia is elicited.

DOSAGE. Lidocaine (1.0 to 1.25 per cent) with 1:200,000 epinephrine is used. The volume injected at the sciatic nerve varies from 20 to 30 cc. The

femoral nerve is injected with 10–15 cc with epinephrine at the femoral nerve. The total dose would then be 450 mgm, while the maximum permitted dose in a 70 kg man is between 490 and 560 mgm.

Anesthesia for Inguinal Hernia[6, 21]

Although many surgeons have never used regional anesthesia for this operation, it is a commendable technique. Routine herniorrhaphy is followed by early mobilization and lack of hospitalization. Obviously, complicated hernia repair should not be attempted on an outpatient basis, but, in experienced hands, the routine herniorrhaphy is of short duration. As will be seen by the description below, the volume of drug injected is fairly large; thus procaine, chlorprocaine or 0.5 per cent xylocaine with epinephrine might be considered the drugs of choice for this surgery. Bupivacaine, 0.25 per cent with epinephrine, will give a longer block. Reference is made in this description to Figure 3–6. Step 1 (Fig. 3–6 A and B): The operator starts at point X, located on the line from the anterior superior iliac spine to the umbilicus. Here 10 cc of anesthetic solution is deposited along the inside shelf of the iliac bone. Step 2 (Fig. 3–6 C): The needle is again inserted at point X and a fan-shaped infiltration in the anterior abdominal musculature is made in a plane perpendicular to the line drawn in A. Fifteen to twenty cc of solution are used. Multiple redirections are necessary to block the hypogastric and ilioinguinal nerve as well as thoracic nerves T11 and T12. Step 3 (Fig. 3–6 D): Here the needle is directed subcutaneously on the line drawn in Step 1 (Fig. 3–6 A). Twenty-five cc of solution is deposited along this line to block thoracic nerves coming down into the operative area. Step 4 (Fig. 3–6 E): Subcutaneous infiltration is carried out ½ inch below the inguinal ligament from the anterior superior iliac spine to

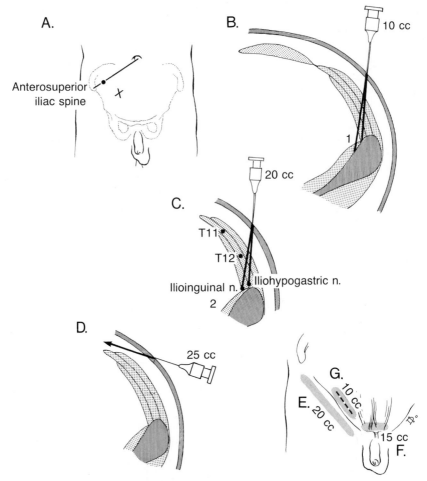

Figure 3–6   Herniorrhaphy. *A.* Point X is roughly 1 inch from the anterior superior iliac spine along the line from this spine to the umbilicus. *B.* Here anesthetic solution is deposited along the inside shelf of the iliac bone. The needle insertion is made at point X. *C.* Muscles lying below the line drawn in *A* are infiltrated in order to block the hypogastric, ilioinguinal and thoracic nerves. *D.* A subcutaneous line of infiltration is carried out on the line drawn in *A. E.* Branches of the gluteal and femoral nerves are blocked by a subcutaneous infiltration ½ inch below the inguinal ligament. *F.* Attachments of the rectus abdominis are infiltrated at the pubic bone. *G.* A subcutaneous line of anesthesia is infiltrated where the incision is to be made.

the groin. This blocks branches of the gluteal and femoral nerves that may go to the operative area. Step 5 (Fig. 3–6 *E*): A deep injection of 15 cc is made along the superior ramus of the pubic bone into the attachment of the rectus abdominis muscle, and into the space between the bladder and pubic bone. Steps 6 and 7 (Fig. 3–6 *E*): Ten cc is injected along the incision line. Tissue in the spermatic cord at the external

ring must be blocked when it is exposed, as must the genitofemoral nerve at the internal ring. This should be done by the surgeon after the operation has begun. Attempts at transcutaneous blocking of these structures may result in hematoma formation.

DOSAGE.   One hundred cc of either 1 per cent procaine, 1 per cent chlorprocaine or 100 cc of 0.5 per cent xylocaine with 0.25 cc of 1:1000 epinephrine. (Epinephrine concentrations in local anesthetics must not exceed 0.25 cc of 1:1000 total dose.)[20]

Epidural and Subarachnoid Anesthesia[20, 22]

These techniques are infrequently used in an outpatient setting for surgery. Spinal anesthesia can be followed by postpuncture headache, a condition caused by the slow leak of cerebrospinal fluid through the puncture hole in the arachnoid membrane. Treatment usually requires bed rest, as the symptoms of this headache are exacerbated by an erect posture. Spinal anesthesia may also result in urinary retention that continues for many hours after sensory nerve block has worn off. This phenomenon is thought to be the result of residual autonomic nerve blockade.[22]

Epidural anesthesia avoids the possibility of postpuncture headache, provided that the epidural needle does not penetrate the arachnoid membrane. This difficulty can occur even in experienced hands, and postpuncture headache may follow. Urinary retention can also follow epidural anesthesia.

Sympathetic Nerve Blocks

Diagnostic or therapeutic blocks of the sympathetic portion of the autonomic nervous system are useful in outpatient work.

Sympathetic nerve blocks can be attempted to improve blood flow to an ischemic limb. Examples include arteriosclerotic disease, arterial embolism, frostbite, arterial dysfunction as seen in Raynaud's disease and unhealed cutaneous ulcers.

Trauma to sensory nerves can result in the well known syndrome of causalgia. The pain of causalgia can be relieved by sympathetic nerve blocks.

PARAVERTEBRAL LUMBAR SYMPATHETIC BLOCK (Figure 3–7). This block is used to interrupt temporarily the sympathetic innervation of the leg. The block is done with the patient in a prone position. A pillow is placed under the patient to flatten the lumbar curvature of the vertebral spine. The tips of the lumbar spines of the second, third and fourth lumbar vertebrae are located and marked on the patient's skin with a pen. The points are connected, and a line parallel to the midline is drawn 4 to 5 cm from this midline on the desired side. Lines drawn

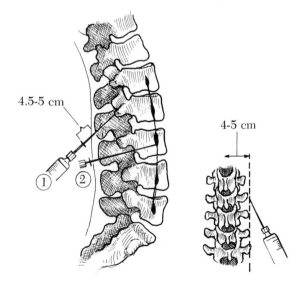

Figure 3–7 Lumbar paravertebral sympathetic nerve block. A 4-inch, 22 gauge block needle is used and is inserted first as is needle "1" to determine the depth of the transverse process, 4 to 5 cm lateral to the midline (see insert). A 4.5 to 5 cm distance is noted on the needle shaft above the skin. The needle is reinserted at the same point on the skin. The needle passes between the transverse processes to the vertebral body, which is 4.5 to 5 cm below the processes. This position is marked in the figure as needle "2". For the sake of clarity two different needles are shown in the lateral figure.

Local anesthetic infiltration at the skin and along the point of needle insertion is required.

4.5-5 cm

4-5 cm

from the tips of spinous processes perpendicular to this lateral line locate the points of needle insertions.

The operator wishes to pass the needle between the transverse processes of the lumbar vertebrae to a point just lateral to the vertebral body. This point lies 4.5 to 5 cm deep to the transverse process. To find this point, the depth and location of the transverse process must first be determined. The needle is inserted at a 45 to 60 degree angle to the skin, directing the needle cephalad. The transverse process depth is noted when the needle strikes it. The depth to the transverse process is noted and the needle is withdrawn and reinserted the extra 4.5 to 5 cm length at an 80 to 90 degree angle to the skin, thus passing between the transverse processes to the lateral edge of the vertebral body. Somatic sensory paresthesias may be encountered, as the needle must pass close to the lumbar nerves as it is advanced. The author increases the chance of success by blocking the nerves at the second, third and fourth lumbar sympathetic ganglia with 10 ml each of anesthetic solution.

Bupivacaine, 0.25 per cent, or 0.5 per cent lidocaine with epinephrine, is used for therapeutic sympathetic nerve block. A series of blocks can be used to relieve causalgic pain. Sometimes dramatic, long lasting results can be achieved after a single block for causalgic pain. Vascular insufficiency that responds to sympathetic block should be treated with surgical sympathectomy.

STELLATE GANGLION BLOCK (Figure 3–8). This block is done to interrupt temporarily the sympathetic innervation of the arm. The patient is placed in a supine position with the head fully extended to stabilize the soft tissue structures of the neck. The stellate ganglion is located 1/8 of an inch anterior to the transverse process of the seventh cervical vertebra.

The operator locates the transverse

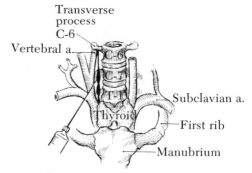

Figure 3–8 Stellate ganglion block. The needle is inserted at a point 1¼ inches above and 1¼ inches lateral to the midpoint of the manubrium. The reader can appreciate the necessity of retracting the carotid artery laterally to perform this block. The tip of the needle may lie within the vertebral artery, and must be readjusted if it does. The stellate ganglion lies 1/8 inch anterior to the transverse process of the seventh cervical vertebra, and is separated from the transverse process by the longus colli muscle. Blocks placed directly on the transverse process may fail if this anatomy is neglected.

process by marking a point 1¼ inches above and 1¼ inches lateral to the midpoint of the upper edge of the manubrium. A clinical rule, "two fingers up, two fingers over," may be used. The location can be checked by finding the sixth transverse process of the cervical vertebrae, which is lateral to the cricoid cartilage. The seventh process, which is the one desired, is ½ inch below the sixth transverse process.

The needle is inserted at the correct point over the seventh cervical transverse process, perpendicular to the skin. The operator pulls the sternocleidomastoid muscle laterally, and the carotid artery pulsation must be felt lateral to the needle. After the transverse process is felt at the needle tip, the needle is withdrawn 1/8 of an inch. A test dose of 1 ml of anesthetic is slowly injected. This is necessary, for despite aspiration with the syringe, the tip of the needle may rest in the vertebral artery. If no untoward reaction is seen, a total dose of 10 ml of anesthetic solution is injected. Bupivacaine, 0.25 per cent, is most frequently used. Horner's syndrome (ptosis, constricted pupil and enopthalmos) results with a successful block. The anatomical location of the stellate ganglion results in anesthetic spread into the brachial plexus or the recurrent laryngeal nerve upon occasion. Subarachnoid injection can occur on rare occasions.

INTRAMUSCULAR AND INTRAVENOUS DRUGS FOR OUTPATIENT SURGERY

Premedication

Premedicant or sedative drugs should be kept to a minimum for outpatient surgery. Regional block, however, is more successful with sedation. Thus if sedative drugs are to be administered, they should be of short duration and noncumulative, an ideal difficult to achieve. The drugs are best given in fractional intravenous doses as required.

Cholinergic blocking agents are used to prevent excessive salivation during general anesthesia and to reduce parasympathetic effects on the heart. Their use results in a decrease in the incidence of bradycardia. Patient discomfort (dry mouth) is increased unnecessarily if these drugs are used with regional blocks. Their use with modern anesthetics is felt to be optional. Atropine, IM 0.1 mgm per 15 lb body weight, can be used to a total dose of 0.4 to 0.5 mgm. Glycopyrrolate (Robinul), 0.3 to 0.5 mgm in the adult, acts for a longer duration than atropine.

Scopolamine is a superior drying agent and has the effect of amnesia and sedation. Patients will sometimes become delirious with scopolamine, especially in the presence of pain, and therefore the use of it alone in outpatient surgery is not advised.

Narcotics

This group of drugs is useful when preoperative pain is present or postoperative pain is anticipated. The author is best able to gauge the dose by repeated intravenous administration of small doses of narcotics. As a general rule, 2.5 mgm morphine sulfate IV, 20 mgm meperidine (Demerol) IV or 0.025 mgm fentanyl (Sublimaze) IV give about the same degree of pain relief. The doses can be repeated as required. The frequency of nausea is the same with all these drugs.[23] The effect of morphine will last somewhat longer than that of meperidine (one to two hours). Fentanyl, given IV, has a duration of action of only 15 to 30 minutes. Combination of fentanyl with an intravenous barbiturate, the short-acting muscle relaxant succinyldicholine and inhalational nitrous oxide has been very successful in outpatient surgery. Overdose with fentanyl, and indeed with all narcotic drugs, is manifested primarily by respiratory depression.

Overdose with narcotic drugs can be combatted with the narcotic antagonist naloxone (Narcan), 0.2 to 0.4 mgm IV. A "pure" narcotic antagonist, naloxone has no narcotic depressing properties. Naloxone has a short duration of action, and narcotic depression caused by morphine or Demerol may reappear after the antagonist effect wears off. The short duration of action is related to the drug's rapid appearance and disappearance from the brain after injection.[24]

Pentazocine (Talwin) was originally investigated as a narcotic antagonist but is now used as an analgesic. Thirty mgm doses of Talwin can be roughly equated with 10 mgm morphine.[25] The drug was formerly believed to have no addictive effects, but reports of addiction have appeared.[26] The drug also has a "ceiling effect": doses above a certain point — usually 60 mgm — produce no additional analgesia. Nausea and vomiting can be seen with pentazocine.

Most postoperative pain following outpatient surgery can be treated with aspirin or codeine.

Diazepam (Valium)

This well known benzodiazepine can be given IV in 2.5 mgm increments. The author gives this drug slowly in an intravenous drip because the drug is irritating to the vein. It offers the advantage of sedation without altering cardiovascular stability. Large doses may cause respiratory depression, especially noticeable when the drug is used with narcotics. Diazepam enhances alcoholic intoxication. Curiously, chlordiazepoxide (Librium), another benzodiazepine, antagonizes the depressant effects of alcohol.[27]

Diazepam has a slower onset of action than intravenous barbiturates. The onset of sedation is delayed by 30 to 120 seconds. Only intravenous use brings out the amnestic properties of diazepam. Another benzodiazepine, lorazepam, is stated to be an even more effective amnesic drug than diazepam.[28] The long term effects of lorazepam in outpatient surgery have not been studied.

Outpatient dentistry utilizing local anesthesia and diazepam has been studied several times.[29] These reports show that diazepam is a valuable adjunct in outpatient surgery, provided that it is not used to produce deep sedation, and that the patient is taken home by a responsible party. There is evidence that pharmacologically active metabolites may reappear in the blood stream some hours after the drug has appeared to have worn off.[30] This phenomenon may be related to the ingestion of food.[31] Patients receiving diazepam, or any intravenous sedative, are cautioned against alcoholic ingestion on their return home.

Short-Acting Barbiturates

Thiopental (Pentothal) and methohexital (Brevital) are mainstays in an outpatient surgical practice. Administration of these drugs may result in respiratory obstruction, hiccups, laryngospasm (usually caused by surgical stimulation and too little drug), apnea (caused by overdose), vomiting with consequent aspiration, and cardiovascular depression. Intravenous short-acting barbiturates should not be given to a patient with a full stomach without the prior or subsequent rapid insertion of a cuffed endotracheal tube. The pain of injury will slow gastric motility, and a patient who ate shortly before injury may have food in the stomach *24 hours* after injury. The physician should not use these drugs unless he is prepared to handle the unfortunate consequences that sometimes result.

Thiopental was originally investigated clinically by Lundy at the Mayo Clinic in the early 1930's.[32] The drug is given intravenously in 2.5 per cent concentrations. A test dose of 50 mgm (2 cc) is first administered, followed by gradual injection of the drug to the point where the eyes are fixed and the eyelids no longer contract when the lashes are stroked (blink reflex). The 50 mgm dose alone will occasionally produce anesthesia in the infirm or cause hypotension. Small doses of thiopental can be used with success to mask the transient pain caused by placing nerve blocks, especially in plastic surgery. The total dose required will vary from 100 mgm to 1 gm in the adult, and give three to ten minutes of anesthesia.

The patient rapidly recovers consciousness from thiopental because of the redistribution of the drug in the body, but drowsiness persists for hours. Longer procedures should not be attempted with thiopental, as the cumulative effects of the drug will produce unnecessary cardiovascular and respiratory depression.[29]

Methohexital (Brevital) is an adequate substitute for thiopental. It is approximately 3.3 times as potent as thiopental. The drug is administered in a 1.0 per cent solution. Some patients complain of transient pain with injection at the IV site. Hiccups are common if the drug is given too rapidly. Many authors feel that methohexital has a shorter recovery period with less residual drowsiness than other intravenous barbiturates.[33,34,35] Methohexital is also a respiratory and cardiovascular depressant and should not be used in repetitive doses to prolong anesthesia.

KETAMINE (KETALAR, KETAJECT). This drug marks a new departure in anesthesia and has proved useful in outpatient anesthesia. Miyasaka and Domino[36] have offered evidence that ketamine acts to block or dissociate sensory input from nonspecific thalamic nuclei to the cortex of the brain. Ketamine anesthesia is sometimes termed a "dissociative state." Careful induction leaves respiration unimpaired. The patient appears to be in a deep sleep, with oropharyngeal reflexes intact. Roving eye movements and random muscle movements are seen. Usually the airway is maintained, but sometimes the head must be fully extended or a nasopharyngeal airway used to keep the breathing unobstructed. Preoperative atropine or glycopyrrolate is required to dry secretions in the mouth. The cardiovascular system is stable, and indeed there is an increase in blood pressure. The drug is contraindicated in hypertensive patients. Ketamine is contraindicated in operations that cause blood or irrigating solutions to enter the mouth or nose. Laryngospasm may be precipitated by these fluids under ketamine anesthesia, for the laryngeal reflexes are not suppressed.

Ketamine for outpatient anesthesia is best given intravenously, for the intramuscular route requires larger doses and results in a more prolonged recovery. The doses recommended when the drug first appeared on the market are too large. The author uses 0.4 to 0.8 mgm per kg IV ketamine to produce a short amnesic analgesic state. Brief, painful procedures can be accomplished while the drug is effective. Recovery will begin in 2 to 3 minutes, with a longer disruption in reasoning ability observed.[37,38] The propensity of ketamine to cause postoperative hallucinations is well known. The incidence of these hallucinations is reduced with the lower dose recommended here, and with the concomitant use of intravenous thiopental or diazepam. The incidence will also be decreased if the patient is left to recover quietly without external stimulation.

The drug has a wide application in pediatric surgery, since children either do not experience or are not bothered by hallucinations. The reason for this difference is not known. Prolonged procedures are possible utilizing ketamine alone, but the recovery period is too long and the hallucinations too frequent to recommend ketamine as the sole anesthetic agent in longer outpatient surgery.

PROPANIDID (EPONTAL). This intravenous anesthetic drug is useful in outpatient surgery because of its transient action and the rapid recovery that follows its use.[38] The rapid recovery is caused by the drug's metabolism by serum cholinesterase as well as by drug redistribution. Following its administration, first hyperventilation, then hypoventilation and apnea can occur. Administration of larger doses can also cause hypotension and its use appears contraindicated in patients with cardiovascular disease. Propanidid also has an unfortunately high incidence of nausea. The drug can be considered equipotent with thiopental for induction, but with a faster recovery time. Dose ranges are generally accepted as 5 to 10 mgm per kg for surgical procedures. The drug is not yet available in the United States.

ALPHADIONE (ALTHESIN). This is a viscid liquid that is a mixture of two steroid molecules. Each milliliter of liquid contains 9 mgm of alphaxalone and 3 mgm of alphadolone acetate. Doses are recorded in μL per kg. Sixty

μL per kg appears equipotent with 4.0 mgm per kg thiopental or 1.2 mgm per kg of methohexital. Only a small volume is required for induction and a clear headed recovery usually follows. The drug is not available in the United States.[40]

Both propanidid and alphadione offer more rapid recovery than intravenous barbiturates.[41] However, hypersensitivity to propanidid and alphadione has been reported with some frequency. Hypersensitivity to intravenous barbiturates is rare.[42]

Neurolept-Analgesia

This method of anesthesia is available to the American physician by the use of Innovar, a combination of the ultrashort-acting narcotic fentanyl (Sublimaze) (see earlier discussion), and droperidol (Inapsine), a long-acting tranquilizing agent of the butyrophenone group. Other combinations of drugs, of similar pharmacological properties, are available in other parts of the world. Neurolept-analgesia would appear best reserved for inpatient anesthesia because of the long action (6 to 12 hours) of droperidol (Inapsine).[43]

AGENTS FOR INHALATIONAL ANALGESIA AND ANESTHESIA

Outpatient anesthesia in ambulatory surgical clinics in the United States is mainly a matter of general anesthesia at the present time, administered under the supervision of anesthesiologists. This section describes the agents in common use.

The ideal agent for outpatient anesthesia (as yet undiscovered) should offer rapid onset, rapid recovery, no side effects of nausea, vomiting or hallucination, no cardiovascular or respiratory depression and no need to maintain an airway artificially. Some of the inhalational agents approach this ideal as closely as the drugs previously discussed. Analgesia with inhalational agents may be defined as a state in which peripheral sensation is markedly diminished, but the patient retains consciousness, responds to commands and still maintains his own airway.

Analgesia with inhalational methoxyflurane (Penthrane) or with nitrous oxide fulfills many of the requirements for an analgesic agent in outpatient anesthesia. The analgesia produced by these agents is usually insufficient to mask completely the pain of surgical procedures. Intelligent patients will tolerate dental extractions, sprain and fracture manipulations, joint injections, abscess incision and other similar procedures with inhalational analgesia.[44]

Methoxyflurane can be self administered by various commercially available hand held inhalers. Penthrane is used in a Cyprane or Duke inhaler with the setting in a "Full-on" position. General anesthesia can result if too high a concentration is used. This is to the physician's disadvantage as the patient will loose protective cough and gag reflexes, and possibly aspirate stomach contents. Inhalational anesthetic agents should not be used except by those physicians with the proper facilities and training to handle any consequence of the administration of these drugs.

General Anesthetic Agents

General anesthetic agents in common use are summarized in Table 3–3. Explosive anesthetic agents are no longer in common use and are omitted from the table. General anesthesia can never be given in an emergency unless the patient's airway is fully protected by a cuffed endotracheal tube. Equipotent minimum alveolar concentrations (MAC) are listed to give the reader an idea of the potency of various agents.

TABLE 3-3 Pharmacology of Inhalational Anesthetic Agents

AGENT	ADMINISTERED	MAC IN O_2	AD_{95}	BLOOD GAS SOLUBILITY COEFFICIENT	PROBLEMS
Nitrous Oxide	Gas machine	101%		0.468	Inadequate for most procedures
Halothane (Fluothane)	Gas machine	0.76%	0.9%	2.3	Emergence shivering, little muscle relaxation, rare incidence of hepatitis
Methoxyflurane (Penthrane)	Gas machine Hand-held vaporizer	0.16%	0.22%	13.0	Renal damage seen. Prolonged emergence
Enflurane (Ethrane)	Gas machine	1.68%	1.88%	1.91	Emergence shivering, coughing with induction, seizure patterns on electroencephalogram
Isoflurane (Forane)	Gas machine	1.15%	1.63%	1.41	Expensive. Not available in U.S.

The MAC of an anesthetic gas is defined as that concentration required to prevent muscular movement in 50 per cent of subjects in response to a painful stimulus.[45]

The anesthetizing concentration of an anesthetic is higher than the minimum alveolar concentration. Ninety-five per cent of patients will be anesthetized at the AD_{95} concentration, listed for some agents in Table 3–3.[46]

Agents that have a low blood gas solubility or low tissue solubility will have a shorter induction and emergence time. The concentration of anesthetic agents in the brain rapidly approaches the concentration of the anesthetic agent in the alveoli when the blood gas solubility is low. When an agent with high blood gas solubility is used, the brain will take longer to receive a sufficient concentration of the agent to induce anesthesia. Emergence time will be delayed by its high blood and tissue solubility. Thus after a methoxyflurane anesthetic, the patient tends to remain somnolent and has diminished postoperative pain for many hours. This may be a distinct advantage with inpatient surgery, but not for the patient who is expected to return home. Agents with a high incidence of postoperative nausea, vomiting, emergence delirium and hallucinations are less acceptable than those agents with a low incidence of these undesirable side effects. These side effects can be controlled with sedatives and antiemetic agents, but such drugs, in turn, will impair the patient when he leaves the hospital.

Halothane (Fluothane)

This drug has a low incidence of postoperative nausea and vomiting; it is nonexplosive and it has a relatively low blood gas solubility coefficient. One can predict a brief emergence following short outpatient procedures. Halothane does have a high body fat solubility, and emergence from a longer operation will be prolonged unless the inspired concentration of the agent is gradually reduced during the course of the operation.

Halothane is metabolized in the body, and a small portion of the gas will be broken down rather than exhaled. One of the products of halothane metabolism, the bromide ion, has been held responsible for prolonged emergence and postoperative sedation in lengthy halothane anesthesia.[41]

Halothane anesthesia can be used alone in outpatients or with atropine premedication. Lack of heavier preoperative sedation may result in postoperative headache.[48] Other preoperative medication will prolong emergence. Even thiopental induction of anesthesia will result in a longer time to complete recovery.[49]

It is highly probable that in rare instances halothane will cause postanesthetic hepatitis.[50, 52] This statement is made against the background of the National Halothane Study, which concluded that halothane was as safe as, if not safer than, the other anesthetic agents available at that time.[51] It is not known why halothane causes postanesthetic hepatitis, but authors have argued that the agent should not be used in any patient with liver disease, sepsis or a recent history of flulike symptoms. A history of previous administration of halothane followed by unexplained fever or jaundice is also an indication to avoid further halothane anesthetics.[48]

Methoxyflurane (Penthrane)

Methoxyflurane was considered an alternative to halothane in the sixties. However, metabolism of methoxyflurane in the body yields a serum level of inorganic fluoride ion that can cause nephrotoxicity. This is not a problem when the drug is used as an analgesic agent, but has curtailed its use in general anesthesia.[53]

Enflurane (Ethrane)

This drug was introduced into anesthetic practice in the early 1970s. It is a nonexplosive, halogenated ether with a low incidence of postoperative nausea. The drug has a low blood gas solubility coefficient and its uptake and washout compare favorably with halothane (Table 3–3).[54] The agent can be used in outpatients without atropine premedication. As with halothane, gas induction of pediatric patients can easily be accomplished. Enflurane has muscle relaxing properties not seen with halothane, and the intraoperative use of muscle relaxants can be reduced. There is a higher threshold for epinephrine-induced cardiac arrhythmia with enflurane than with halothane, thus offering the surgeon an advantage if epinephrine is used for hemostasis during surgery.[56]

The metabolism of enflurane results in the production of fluoride ion, but in contrast to methoxyflurane, the blood level of the ion appears insufficient to cause nephrotoxicity.[55] As a halogenated molecule enflurane has been suspected to be a cause of postoperative jaundice. Evidence for such causality has not yet appeared. The electroencephalogram of patients under enflurane anesthesia exhibits a seizure pattern. This phenomenon appears to be of no clinical consequence.[56]

Endotracheal General Anesthesia

Endotracheal intubation is a necessary adjunct for many types of outpatient anesthesia. Adding intubation to an anesthetic will increase the morbidity of the procedure. Mild sore throat is by far the most commonly seen complication. An incidence of 46 per cent has been reported.[57] Low pressure cuff endotracheal tubes have a higher incidence of sore throat after intubation than other varieties of endotracheal tubes.[58]

Succinyldicholine (Anectine)

Intubation can be facilitated with the use of succinyldicholine, a short-acting muscle relaxant. Its use is mandatory for rapid emergency intubation to gain control of the airway (see Chapter 26). Use of this drug will also increase postanesthetic morbidity, as any dose greater than 10 mgm is associated with varying degrees of muscle ache in patients. The aching, especially in the back of the neck and chest, occurs 18 to 72 hours postoperatively. The incidence can be reduced but not eliminated by small doses of d-tubocurarine or gallamine IV preceding succinyldicholine injection.[59] Succinyldicholine administration can also increase intraocular pressure,[60] although here the phenomenon can be blocked by 3 or 6 mgm d-tubocurarine IV. Caution is urged when succinyldicholine is planned for any patient with glaucoma.

Succinyldicholine is metabolized by plasma pseudocholinesterase. Thus apnea following succinyldicholine injection normally lasts only three to five minutes. There are patients who have a hereditary deficiency of this enzyme. The incidence of heterozygous deficiency is about 1 in every 25 patients. Heterozygous patients show a slight prolongation of the drug's action that is not clinically significant. Apnea prolonged up to several hours follows in homozygotes, the incidence being roughly one in every 2500 patients.[61] The deficiency is usually discovered after the injection, as there is no widespread screening procedure for this condition. There is no antidote for succinyldicholine, but some antagonism of succinyldicholine overdose has been reported with the use of neostigmine.[62] Apneic patients must be ventilated until the drug wears off.

Despite these drawbacks, succinyldicholine is quite useful in outpatient surgery. The profound but brief relaxation is useful for intubation, reducing fractures and dislocations or to facilitate abdominal examination under anesthesia. The drug can be given by an intravenous drip or by intermittent injection for periods of muscle relaxation longer than one to three minutes. This drug should be used only by physicians well trained on an anesthesiology service.

Summary

This chapter has attempted to cover enough separate anesthetic techniques to allow the reader to intelligently select from among them while dealing with outpatient surgical patients. This chapter is not encyclopedic; many useful variations of the techniques described can be found by consulting the appropriate references listed at the end of the chapter.

Anesthetic drugs do not cure disease; their use constitutes a certain risk to every patient who receives them. Intelligent administration of these drugs requires training in a separate branch of medicine, and no physician should attempt these techniques without previous training in anesthesiology.

REFERENCES

1. Barton, M. D.: Outpatient surgery and anesthesia. Primary Care, 4:183–197, 1977.
2. Steward, D. J.: Outpatient pediatric anesthesia. Anesthesiology, 43:268–276, 1975.
3. Reed, W. A., Crouch, B. L., and Ford, J. L.: Anesthesia and operations on outpatients. *In* Public Health Aspects of Critical Care Medicine and Anesthesiology, Vol. X. Philadelphia: F. A. Davis & Co., 1974.
4. Outpatient Anesthesia. K. F. Schmidt (ed.). International Anesthesiology Clinics, Vol. 14. Boston: Little Brown & Co., 1976.
5. Fahy, A., and Marshall, M.: Postanesthetic morbidity in outpatients. Brit. J. Anaesth., 41:433–438, 1969.
6. deJong, R.: Physiology and Pharmacology of Local Anesthetics. Springfield: Charles C Thomas, 1970.
7. Aldrete, J. A., and Johnson, D. A.: Allergy to local anesthetics. J.A.M.A., 207:356–357, 1969.
8. Proctor, D. F.: Anesthesia for peroral endo-scopy and bronchography. Anesthesiology, 29:1025–1036, 1968.
9. Harris, L. C., Parry, J. C., and Greifenstein, F. E.: Dyclonine — a new local anesthetic agent: Clinical evaluation. Anesthesiology, 17:648–652, 1956.
10. Foldes, F. F., Molloy, R., McNall, P. G., and Koukol, L. R.: Comparison of toxicity of intravenously given anesthetic agents in Man. J.A.M.A., 172:1493–1498, 1960.
11. Scott, D. B. (ed.): Proceedings of a symposium on local anesthetics. Brit. J. Anaesth., 47(Suppl. Ed.): 1975.
12. Moore, D. C., Bridenbaugh, L. D., Bagdi, P. A., and Bridenbaugh, P. O.: Accumulation of mepivacaine hydrochloride during caudal block. Anesthesiology, 29:585–588, 1968.
13. Lofstrom, B.: Aspects of the pharmacology of local anesthetic agents. Brit. J. Anaesth., 42:194–206, 1970.
14. Lofstrom, B.: Clinical experience with long acting local anesthetics. Acta Anesth. Scand., Suppl. 60, 1975.
15. Holmes, C. McK.: Intravenous regional analgesia: A useful method of producing analgesia of the limbs. Lancet 1:245–247, February, 1963.
16. Adams, J. P., Kenmore, P. I., Russell, P. H., and Haas, S. S.: Regional anesthesia in the upper limb. Curr. Pract. Orthop. Surg., 4:238–261, 1969.
17. Watson, R. L., Brown, P. W., and Reich, M. P.: Venous and arterial bupivacaine concentrations after intravenous regional anesthesia. Anesth. Analg. (Cleveland), 49:300–304, 1970.
18. DeJong, R. H.: Axillary block of the brachial plexus. Anesthesiology, 22:215–225, 1961.
19. Winnie, A. P.: Interscalene brachial plexus block. Anesth. Analg. (Cleveland), 49:455–466, 1970.
20. Moore, D. C.: Regional Block. 4th ed. Springfield: Charles C Thomas, 1965.
21. Adriani, J. (ed.): Labat's Regional Anesthesia. Philadelphia: W. B. Saunders Co., 1967.
22. Greene, N. M.: Physiology of Spinal Anesthesia. Baltimore: Williams and Wilkins Co., 1969.
23. Ordy, J. M., Kretchmer, H. E., Gorry, T. H., and Hershberger, T. J.: Comparison of effects of morphine, meperidine, fentanyl, and fentanyl-droperidol. Clin. Pharmacol. Ther., 11:488–495, 1970.
24. Ngai, S. H., Berkowitz, B. A., and Yang, J. C.: Pharmacokinetics of naloxone in rats and man. Anesthesiology, 44:398–401, 1976.
25. Potter, D. R., and Payne, J. P.: Newer analgesics: With special reference to pentazocine. Br. J. Anaesth., 42:186–193, 1970.
26. Weber, W. F., and Rome, H. P.: Addiction to

pentazocine: Report of two cases. J.A.M.A., *212*:1708, 1970.

27. Greenblatt, D. J., and Shader, R. I.: Benzodiazepines in Clinical Practice. N. Y.: Raven Press, 1974.

28. Pandit, S. K., Heisterkamp, D. V., and Cohen, R. J.: Further studies of the anti-recall effect of lorazepam. Anesthesiology, *45*:495–500, 1976.

29. Dundee, J. W., and Haslett, W. H. K.: The benzodiazepines. A review of their actions and uses relative to anaesthetic practice. Br. J. Anaesth., *42*:217–234, 1970.

30. Kortilla, K., Mattila, M. J., and Linnoila, M.: Prolonged recovery after diazepam sedation. Brit. J. Anaesth., *48*:333–340, 1976.

31. Ghonein, M. M., Mewaldt, S. P., and Ambre, J.: Plasma levels of diazepam and mood ratings. Anesth. Analg. Curr. Res., *54*:173–177, 1975.

32. Dundee, J. S.: Intravenous anesthesia: Preliminary report of the use of two new thiobarbiturates. Proc. Staff Meet. Mayo Clin., *10*:536–543, 1935.

33. Clarke, R. S. J., Dundee, J. W., Barron, D. W., and McArdle, L.: Clinical studies of induction agents. XXVI: The relative potencies of thiopentone, methohexitone and propanidid. Br. J. Anaesth., *40*:593–601, 1968.

34. Whitwam, J. G.: Methohexitone. Brit. J. Anaesth., *48*:617–619, 1976.

35. Breimer, D. D.: Pharmacokinetics of methohexitone following intravenous infusion in humans. Brit. J. Anaesth., *48*:643–649, 1976.

36. Miyasaka, M., and Domino, E. F.: Neuronal mechanisms of ketamine-induced anesthesia. Int. J. Neuropharmacol., *7*:557–573, 1968.

37. Harris, J. A., Biersner, R. J., Edwards, D., and Bailey, L. W.: Attention, learning, and personality during ketamine emergence. Anesth. Analg. Curr. Res., *54*:169–172, 1975.

38. Liang, H. S., and Liang, H. G.: Minimizing emergence phenomena: Subdissociative dosage of ketamine in balanced surgical anesthesia. Anesth. Analg. Curr. Res., *54*:312–316, 1975.

39. Clarke, R. S. J.: The eugenols. *In* Intravenous Anaesthesia. J. W. Dundee and G. M. Wyant (eds.). London and Edinburgh, Longman, 1974, pp. 162–192.

40. Clarke: Steroids. *In* Intravenous Anesthesia.

41. Kortila, K., Linnoila, M., et al.: Recovery and stimulated driving after intravenous anesthesia with thiopental, methohexital, propanidid, and alphadione. Anesthesiology, *43*:291–299, 1975.

42. Watkins, J., Udnoon, S., Appleyard, T. N., and Thornton, J. A.: Identification and quantitation of hypersensitivity reactions to intravenous anesthetics. Brit. J. Anaesth., *48*:457–461, 1976.

43. Edmonds-Seal, J., and Prys-Roberts, C.: Pharmacology of drugs used in neuroleptanalgesia. Br. J. Anaesth., *42*:207–216, 1970.

44. Packer, K. J., and Titel, J. H.: Methoxyflurane analgesia for burns dressings: experience with the analgizer. Br. J. Anaesth., *41*:1080–1085, 1969.

45. Eger, E. I.: Anesthetic Uptake and Action. Baltimore: Williams & Wilkins Co., 1975.

46. deJong, R. H., and Eger, E. I.: MAC expanded: AD_{50} and AD_{95} values of common inhalation anesthetics in man. Anesthesiology, *42*:384–389, 1975.

47. Tinker, J. H., Gandolfi, A. J., and Van Dyke, R. A.: Elevation of plasma bromide levels in patients following halothane anesthesia. Anesthesiology, *44*:194–201, 1976.

48. Zohairy, A. F. M.: Postoperative headache after nitrous oxide-oxygen-halothane anesthesia. Br. J. Anaesth., *41*:972–976, 1969.

49. Doenicke, A.: Street fitness after anesthesia in outpatients. Acta. Anaesthesiol. Scand. Suppl., *17*:95–97, 1965.

50. Trey, C., Lipworth, I., and Davidson, C. J.: The clinical syndrome of halothane hepatitis. Anesth. Anal. (Cleveland), *48*:1033–1040, 1969.

51. Summary of the national halothane study: Possible association between halothane anesthesia and post-operative hepatic necrosis. J.A.M.A., *197*:775–788, 1966.

52. Lomanto, C., and Howland, W. S.: Problems in diagnosing halothane hepatitis. J.A.M.A., *214*:1257–1261, 1970.

53. Mazze, R. I., Trudell, J. R., and Cousins, M. J.: Methoxyflurane metabolism and renal dysfunction. Anesthesiology, *35*:247–255, 1971.

54. Rolly, G. (ed.): Symposium on enflurane. Acta Anesth. Belgica, *25*: 1974.

55. Greenstein, L. R., Hitt, B. A., and Mazze, R. I.: Metabolism *in vitro* of enflurane, isoflurane, and methoxyflurane. Anesthesiology, *42*:420–424, 1975.

56. Reisner, L. S., and Lippman, M.: Ventricular arrhythmias after epinephrine injection in enflurane and halothane anesthesia. Anesth. Analg. Curr. Res., *54*:468–470, 1975.

57. Lewis, R. N., and Swerdlow, M.: Hazards of endotracheal anesthesia. Br. J. Anesth., *36*:504–515, 1964.

58. Loeser, E. A., Orr, D. L., Bennett, O. M., and Stanley, T. H.: Endotracheal tube design and postoperative sore throat. Anesthesiology, *45*:684–687, 1976.

59. Virtue, R. W.: Comparison of gallamine with d-tubocurarine: Effects on fasciculation after succinylcholine. Anesth. Analg. Curr. Res., *54*:81–82, 1975.

60. Miller, R. D., Way, W. I., and Hickey, R. F.: Inhibition of succinylcholine-induced increased intraocular pressure by nondepolarizing muscle relaxants. Anesthesiology. 29:123–126, 1968.

61. Lehmann, H., and Liddell, J.: Human cholinesterase (pseudocholinesterase): genetic variants and their recognition. Br. J. Anaesth., 41:235–244, 1969.

62. Miller, R. D.: Antagonism of neuromuscular blockade. Anesthesiology, 44:318–329, 1976.

4 Trauma

LAWRENCE W. NORTON, M.D.

I. INTRODUCTION

II. MASS CASUALTIES
A. *Overall plan and communication*
B. *Triage*
C. *Preoperative care*
D. *Ambulatory care*
E. *Tear gas*
F. *Radioactive contamination*

III. MAJOR TRAUMA—PRINCIPLES AND PROCEDURES
A. *Immediate reaction of the outpatient surgeon and his team*
B. *Examination*
   1. Respiration and circulation
   2. Head and spine
   3. Lungs and heart
   4. Abdomen and extremities
   5. Blood vessels
C. *Priorities and treatment*
   1. Airway and ventilation
   2. Cardiac and pulmonary resuscitation
   3. External bleeding
   4. Treatment of shock
   5. Burns
D. *Superior vena cava catheterization*
   1. General discussion
      a. Advantages
      b. Complications
   2. Subclavian vein puncture
      a. Infraclavicular approach
      b. Supraclavicular approach
   3. Internal jugular vein puncture
      a. Lateral to sternocleidomastoid muscle
      b. Through sternocleidomastoid muscle
   4. External jugular vein puncture
E. *Venesection*
   1. Advantages and disadvantages
   2. Sites available
   3. Saphenous vein "cutdown" at ankle
F. *Diagnostic procedures*
   1. X-rays
   2. Bladder catheterization
   3. Nasogastric intubation
   4. Paracentesis
      a. Four-quadrant tap
      b. Peritoneal lavage
      c. Laboratory examination
      d. Complications
   5. Sinography of stab wounds

IV. SPECIFIC INJURIES
A. *Closed wounds*
   1. Contusions, bruises, hematomas and blebs
   2. Nonsurgical treatment; ice pack; aspiration
B. *Open wounds*
   1. Principles
   2. Abrasions
   3. Debris
   4. Healing: scabs and dressings
C. *Puncture wounds*
   1. Nail wounds of the foot
   2. Lesser puncture wounds
   3. Specific problems; draining sinuses; fish hook
   4. Superficial stab wounds
   5. Deep stab wounds
   6. Gunshot wounds
   7. Legal aspects of gunshot wounds
   8. Shotgun wounds
D. *Lacerations*
   1. Principles
   2. Anesthesia
   3. Débridement and irrigation
E. *Bites*
   1. Animal and human bites
   2. Snakebite
   3. Insect bites
      a. Brown recluse spider
      b. Black widow spider
      c. Scorpion
      d. Bee sting

V. SUTURES AND DRESSINGS
A. *Suture repair*
   1. Principles
   2. Types of sutures
   3. Placement of sutures
   4. Knot-tying
      a. Two-hand knot
      b. One-hand knot
      c. Instrument tie
B. *Wound dressing*
   1. Closed wound dressing
   2. Open wound dressing
   3. Pressure dressing
   4. Bandaging

INTRODUCTION

The outpatient surgeon must be capable of managing injured patients. The scope of trauma encountered may range from minor injury of an individual to major injuries in mass casualties. While treating the former definitively, the outpatient surgeon initiates for the latter a sequence of treatment involving many hospital services. Common to both functions is the role as first surgeon to receive the injured.

About 60 million persons are injured each year in the United States.[11] One-third of accidents occur in the home. In 1975, 102,500 accidental deaths were recorded, a decrease of 2 per cent from the previous year. Motor vehicle-related deaths, which account for 45 per cent of the total, decreased only 1 per cent. The estimated national cost of accidents in 1975 was $47.1 billion.

More than one-third of hospital Emergency Department visits are necessitated by trauma. Most injuries are minor and manageable on an outpatient basis. Injuries make up about 17.5 per cent of all acute conditions that require medical attention or restrict usual daily activity.[14] The incidence of injury per 100 persons per year has risen from 29 in 1968 to 34 in 1975. No other acute medical problem, with the exception of influenza, is increasing in incidence as rapidly as trauma.

Important principles of treatment pertain to all forms of trauma. First, the patient must be quickly attended whether his injury is major or minor. Treatment of minor wounds may be delayed in favor of more pressing problems provided that prompt initial appraisal of the patient is made. Second, care when given must be competent and complete. Complications of injury result from failure to treat as well as incorrect therapy. Third, disposition home or to other care must avoid unnecessary delay. Instructions for

further care should be written in precise, clear language.

The outpatient management of trauma will be described in terms of mass casualties from a community disaster, major injuries in an individual patient who will require hospitalization and minor injury in a person who can return home after treatment.

MASS CASUALTIES

Overall Plan and Communications

An active hospital emergency service can seldom receive more than 15 to 25 seriously injured patients at one time without immediately expanding staff, supplies and treatment space. A community disaster in which more than this number of casualties are brought to a single hospital should activate a well-rehearsed Disaster Plan. Such a plan assumes that the hospital facility remains intact and that all personnel are capable of reporting for duty. Problems involving radioactivity and toxic gases require separate protocols to protect the hospital staff from contamination. The aim of a Disaster Plan is to give definitive care to all patients within 24 hours of admission. No patient is considered hopelessly injured and the most severely injured are treated first.

The success of an individual hospital's Disaster Plan depends upon community resources for reporting the disaster, triaging victims at the site, transporting patients to local hospitals and maintaining communications among civil authorities, hospital personnel and nonprofessional volunteers. This integration is best accomplished at a municipal or regional level. All agencies to be involved in disaster response should meet under the aegis of a local authority, often the Director of Civil Defense. Police are given responsibility for notifying medical agencies that a disaster has occurred. Word is first given to the hospital that is to supply a field triage team. Such a team consists of at least three doctors and an equal number of clerks or assistants. A communications support person accompanies the team.

The field triage team should be the first medical personnel to reach the disaster scene. Their job is to sort casualties for immediate removal to nearby hospitals. As a doctor assesses the degree of injury, the accompanying clerk tags the patient with information giving number, condition and hospital assignment. The latter is determined arbitrarily by the triage doctor on the basis of known capabilities of local hospitals. Resuscitation is limited to insertion of oral airways in unconscious patients, pressure control of severe external bleeding and splinting of obvious fractures.

As victims are removed from the disaster site, the communications support person contacts a community radio control center, indicating the number of casualties, the proportion severely injured and the number of patients being sent to each local hospital. Central radio control personnel then advise hospitals of similar information and coordinate the assignment of victims among community health facilities if the primary receiving hospitals become overtaxed.

Word of a disaster usually reaches each receiving hospital through a telephone operator. Details of site, type of disaster, estimated number of casualties and the identity and location of the caller are relayed to the designated Director of Disaster Planning, who is empowered to activate the Disaster Plan. The Director may be a hospital administrator or chief of a clinical service. Essential personnel in all departments of the hospital are then notified in the order of their importance. The hospital is thereby prepared to receive the injured before existing facilities and personnel are overwhelmed.

Triage

An outpatient surgeon may be designated Triage Officer with responsibility to evaluate arriving casualties, assign priorities of treatment, initiate lifesaving procedures and insure rapid disposition for definitive care. Triage Officers are the key to the success of disaster planning. They should be mature and experienced, for while receiving casualties, they must often deal with irrational relatives of patients, demanding newsmen and confused assistants. Unless they maintain rigid authority and awareness of their duties, organization collapses and previous planning becomes valueless.

The first duty of Triage Officers is to sort casualties in preparation for treatment. They must not neglect this duty by involvement in individual patient care. Upon activation of the Disaster Plan, the Officer moves to the triage area, usually a large open space with access to emergency vehicle portals, and is stationed at a point from which it is possible to inspect arriving casualties and supervise assistants. Each victim is judged dead-on-arrival (DOA), preoperative or ambulatory. Clerks tag each patient with brief descriptions of number, time of arrival, condition and treatment given. The most seriously injured are selected for priority treatment and identified by special markers such as red ribbons. Ambulatory injured are immediately sent to an Ambulatory Care Area from which they may be hospitalized or treated and discharged. After sorting and tagging, the Triage Officer assigns medical personnel to individual patients as numbers allow to begin emergency treatment. Care in the triage area is limited to maintenance of airway by means of oral airway insertion or endotracheal intubation, ventilation by mouth-to-mouth or resuscitator techniques, control of hemorrhage by pressure dressing, restoration of blood volume by intravenous fluid administration and stabilization of fractures by splinting. A permanently stocked kit containing oral airways, resuscitator bags and masks, laryngoscopes, endotracheal tubes, elastic bandages, splints, intravenous needles and tubing, liter bottles of intravenous crystalloid solution and fresh ampuls of bicarbonate, epinephrine, isoproterenol and morphine should be stored near the triage area. Diagnostic procedures such as thoracentesis or paracentesis are deferred until the patient is admitted to the Preoperative Care Area, although emergency procedures such as pericardiocentesis may be required during triage.

With the opening of a Preoperative Care (Shock) Area, the Triage Officer orders the removal of the most seriously injured (red-tagged) patients from the triage area. It is essential to clear the triage space as rapidly as possible, recognizing strict rules of priority treatment.

Preoperative Care

Critically injured victims are triaged to the Preoperative Care Area whether or not surgery is urgently indicated. Intensive care of the patient begins here and is directed toward reversal of shock and preoperative preparation. Diagnostic procedures including x-ray are now possible and further resuscitative measures such as tube thoracostomy, tracheostomy and mechanical ventilation can be performed.

Ambulatory Care

Outpatient physicians not involved in triage may be assigned to evaluate, treat and arrange disposition of walking wounded. Some of these patients will have no significant injury, while others may be emotionally distraught and still others may be ambulatory despite serious injury that requires surgery or plaster immobilization of an extremity. Treatment of lacerations should be as thorough as time and assistance permit, with attention to cleaning, débridement, early wound closure, proper dressing, tetanus prophylaxis and follow-up appointment. Sheer numbers may limit individual patient care. In this case closure of wounds by adhesive strips or dressings should replace suture techniques. To all patients with minor injuries, instructions are given to return to the hospital the next day for wound inspection and thorough physical reexamination.

While casualties are being received and treated, the Director of Disaster Planning insures a flow of supplies and personnel to the triage and treatment areas. The security of the hospital and especially the triage area is maintained by locking all but essential doors and by posting security guards at entrances and exits. Access for hospital personnel and volunteer staff requires identity cards. Control must extend to ambulance areas and nearby streets to maintain open access for emergency vehicles. Relatives, newsmen and curious visitors should be barred from the triage and treatment sites and sequestered in adjacent facilities where information regarding victim identity and condition can be disseminated by hospital administrators.

Tear Gas

Lacrimotor agents (tear-producing substances) are used both by law enforcement agents and by private citizens for riot control, dislodging barricaded persons and personal protection. The most commonly used agents are CN (L-chloroacetophenone) and CS (chlorobenzalmalononitrile).[6] CR (dibenzoxazepine), a newer, more potent skin and mucosal irritant, currently is being tested in the United States, while DM (diphenylaminearsine chloride) is available only to military personnel.

CN and CS are crystalline powders dispersed as aerosol clouds of finely divided particles. Dispersal is by blowers, bursting grenades or burning with a fuel. CN (Chemical Mace) produces a blue-white cloud on release and has an apple blossom odor. Its primary effect is to produce conjunctival irritation and heavy lacrimation, a burning sensation of the nose, increased salivation and a burning sensation of the skin with blistering at high concentrations. Allergic contact dermatitis has been reported after repeated exposure.

CS produces a white cloud and has a pepperlike odor. The mean incapacitating dose of CS is slightly lower than that for CN and its clinical effects are more pronounced. CS produces immediate irritation that persists for five to ten minutes after the victim is removed to fresh air. In addition to skin and mucosal irritation, it may cause nasal discharge, coughing, tightness in the chest with a sense of suffocation, malaise and a panic reaction. The dose of CS required for such severe effects is only 10 to 20 milligrams per cubic meter of air. Thus even limited exposure results in incapacitation. Death or serious complications resulting from CS contamination are very rare.

Decontamination of the tear gas victim varies with the type of lacrimotor agent used. Because of its high volatility, CN can be removed from clothes by aeration and vacuuming. If necessary, skin decontamination can be achieved by using a 5 per cent sodium bicarbonate solution to decompose CN. Decontamination of CS is more difficult because of its lower volatility. Shaking out clothes may recirculate CS, contaminating ambient air and producing recurrence of symptoms in the original victim and induction of symptoms in others. Flushing with large amounts of water will relieve symptoms, and solutions of 5 to 10 per cent sodium bicarbonate specifically decompose CS. A solution of 6.7 per cent $NaHCO_3$, 3.3 per cent Na_2CO_3 and 0.1 per cent ben-zalkonium chloride in water is an effective skin decontaminant in small amounts. Aqueous solutions of 10 per cent monoethanolamine and 0.3 per cent of a nonionic detergent, such as Triton X-100, dissolve and decontaminate CS on clothes in about two minutes. The decontaminant is then washed off with water.

Management of victims with tear gas exposure should be in a treatment area located within the emergency department but having a separate outside entrance. Under no circumstances should contaminated patients be brought into a patient care area without advance notice. Ideal facilities for decontamination include overhead shower, floor drain and adequate ventilation independent of common ventilator ducts.

Hospital personnel treating contaminated patients should wear surgical gowns, caps, gloves, boots and masks. After the patients are disrobed, they are washed thoroughly with soap and water and dressed in clean clothes. All contaminated clothes and linen are placed in plastic bags or buckets of soapy water. After transfer of the patients to an uncontaminated treatment area, attendants should remove their own clothing to soak in soapy water and shower before dressing in fresh clothing.

Radioactive Contamination

Nuclear explosion or industrial contamination with radioactive materials can cause radiation injuries in mass casualties.[13] In the case of explosions, trauma and thermal burns are initially more important problems than radiation injury. Contamination can exist without serious radiation damage. Symptoms are dependent upon total dose of irradiation. In general, if a patient has not vomited within 24 hours after injury, he has not been seriously injured by radiation.

If fallout particles, grossly contaminated with radioactive substances, whether due to military explosion or industrial accident, are not visible during fall or after settling on surfaces, they are likely to have no acute effects. Fallout loses about 90 per cent of its radioactivity within the first seven hours and is virtually inactive after 48 hours. Early fallout carries a high irradiation dose. As radiation accumulates over several days, however, an increasing dose may result in symptoms. It is important to establish for each victim his distance from the irradiation source and his degree of shielding.

Monitoring for radioactivity should be conducted outside of the triage area. Counters for this purpose are often available from Civil Defense agencies. If counts of radioactivity are high, either on the clothing or the body, decontamination procedures begin before moving the patient inside the hospital. Ambulatory patients should remove all clothing, avoiding contact of outside clothing with unexposed parts of the body. Bathing with soap and water is best accomplished under a shower. Face, hands, fingernails and hair are scrubbed with a brush. Contaminated clothing is placed in tightly covered receptacles until disposed of by trained personnel. Before decontaminated victims are allowed to enter the triage area, they are remonitored for residual radioactivity.

Seriously traumatized and contaminated patients who cannot walk must be undressed and washed. A tub or tank is useful for this purpose. If a tub is unavailable, water may be poured over the skin, concentrating on exposed areas. Open wounds can be sealed with plastic film or tape during bathing. Later they are decontaminated by irrigation with large amounts of water and débridement. Clipping of hair is preferable to shaving, which enhances skin absorption. Alkaline soaps, abrasives and organic solvents also increase skin permeability and penetration of radioactive particles. Wash water used in decontamination is potentially hazardous and should be disposed of without contaminating water supplies. When no water is available for decontamination, wiping or brushing the skin is of some benefit.

Whole body radiation delivered over a relatively short period of time causes (1) central nervous system symptoms at higher doses, (2) gastrointestinal symptoms at intermediate doses and (3) hematopoietic symptoms at lower doses. The greater the dose, the sooner the onset of symptoms.

Very high doses of irradiation (3000 rads or more) quickly result in tremor, convulsions, ataxia, lethargy and, within two days, death. Nothing can be done for such lethal radiation injury. Exposure to 500 to 1000 rads, causing early nausea, vomiting and diarrhea, results in death within four weeks. Later onset of symptoms is associated with a better prognosis, but diarrhea and subsequent dehydration and electrolyte imbalance may complicate accompanying wounds.

Radiation in the range of 200 to 500 rads depresses bone marrow. Patients with this degree of injury may be free of symptoms for two to four weeks before developing leukopenia, anemia and purpura. Presumably protection during this interval is due to relatively radio-resistant circulating cells. B-cell lymphocytes are more radiosensitive than T-cell lymphocytes or macrophages. Circulating gamma globulins will remain after radiation, but no new circulating antibodies will be produced until new B cells appear.

The most important treatment category is the lower exposure (200 to 500 rads) group. These patients will probably constitute the maximum casualty load and provide the best opportunity for effective treatment. Survival in this group is in the range of 50 per cent to 75 per cent, the variation being due to differences in individual response to radiation. The LD_{50} of radiation-injured man at six weeks is about 350 rads of uniform whole body irradiation, which is equivalent to an exposure of 425 roentgens "free in air." Within a few hours of exposure, these patients experience nausea, vomiting and malaise. Recovery thereafter depends upon the severity of hematologic complications. Initially, patients are supported with antiemetics to control nausea and vomiting. Whole blood or antibiotics are helpful later when bleeding diatheses and infection due to leukopenia occur.

Persons receiving under 200 rads of irradiation have had light exposure and rarely die. Transient nausea and vomiting may occur but should disappear within 72 hours. After monitoring and decontamination, these persons may be discharged.

MAJOR TRAUMA – PRINCIPLES AND PROCEDURES

Immediate Reaction of the Outpatient Surgeon and Team

Initial care of a critically injured patient is the responsibility of the outpatient surgeon. Competent early management is often the key to later recovery. Conversely, initial mistakes cause subsequent morbidity or mortality.

In active hospital emergency rooms a team of doctors, nurses and technicians is available at all times for resuscitation of the severely injured patient. The role of the outpatient surgeon is to command this team by recognizing treatment priorities, assigning individual duties, avoiding confusion and assessing progress. As team leader the surgeon should be certain that personnel are trained, rehearsed and ready and that facilities are organized, adequate and available. After the emergency event, the team is reviewed to confirm successful management and to correct errors.

The outpatient surgeon who does not have such a team and facilities is responsible for using what is available in the best possible way. The surgeon acts alone to preserve the patient's life. Diagnostic and therapeutic measures are limited to the most urgent needs. If help is not imminent and if local facilities are inadequate, the patient must be prepared for referral to a larger treatment center.

Both the team surgeon and the solo outpatient surgeon are confronted by the critically injured patient in terms of immediate life-threatening problems. A detailed accident history is rarely available and time does not permit extensive questioning before treatment begins. When acute needs have been met, medical history relevant to the patient's present condition can be sought.

Examination

In the absence of history and immediate laboratory values, the outpatient surgeon treats the injured patient on the basis of physical findings. Examination is first directed toward respiration and circulation. When these vital functions are assured, overall evaluation of systems may begin. Vital signs are recorded several times within the first quarter hour. If formal records are initially unavailable, state of consciousness and values of blood pressure, pulse and respiration with the time of observation may be written on the linen of the Emergency Room cart.

The state of consciousness must be determined. Pupil size and reaction are recorded. Spinal fluid drainage from the nose or ears, indicating basal skull fracture, should be looked for, though it may easily be missed in the presence of adjacent bleeding wounds. Skull fractures may be palpable. Similarly, injuries of the cervical spine are often associated with deformity and tenderness. The anterior neck is palpated to detect tracheal displacement or injury.

The chest is thoroughly inspected for evidence of paradoxical movement, sucking wounds or abrasions resulting from blunt injury. Auscultation may reveal diminished or absent breath sounds. The quality of heart sounds is rated while auscultating the chest. Fractures may be felt by gently compressing the ribs.

Penetrating abdominal wounds, with or without protruding viscera, are covered with sterile moist dressings while examination is made for abdominal muscle spasm, tenderness and peristalsis. Extremities are rapidly surveyed by requesting active motion in a conscious patient. If the patient cannot comply, extremities are moved passively in a slow, gentle way and are palpated for dislocations or fractures. With thighs in abduction the perineum can be inspected, giving special attention to the perianal area where lacerations related to "blow-out" injuries of the pelvis may be seen. The pelvis should be tested for fracture by manual compression of the iliac crests and by pressure on the pubic symphysis.

An important aspect of the examination is palpation of peripheral pulses. Skin color, temperature and muscle activity are affected by major arterial occlusion in the legs.

Priorities and Treatment

The first priority in caring for an injured patient is to assure an open airway and ventilation. Audible or sensible expiration is the most reliable confirmation of an adequate airway and spontaneous breathing. Moving of the chest as respiratory effort does not insure adequate ventilation.

Airway obstruction by the tongue can be relieved by hyperextending the head on the shoulders and advancing the mandible. Foreign bodies obstructing the airway are eliminated by suctioning or cleaning the mouth with a finger. With an open airway, ventilation is possible by means of mouth-to-mouth or mouth-to-nose respiration. These techniques require no apparatus and should be used before attempting endotracheal intubation (see Chapter 26).

Cardiac and pulmonary resuscitation is essentially one activity but adequate ventilation must be achieved before cardiac resuscitation will succeed. The diagnosis of cardiac arrest or inadequate cardiac effort is made when pulsation in a large vessel such as the femoral or carotid artery cannot be felt. Pupillary dilation confirms arrest except in patients with head injury. Electrocardiography is seldom of immediate help unless the equipment is already in place. A normal ECG pattern can exist in the presence of inadequate cardiac output.

Closed cardiac massage begins and ventilation is established as soon as the diagnosis of cardiac arrest is made. Delay of eight to ten minutes is fatal. As the interval is shortened, the chances of complete resuscitation improve. The purpose of massage is to maintain circulation to vital organs until the heart resumes normal pumping. This may require one hour or longer. Successful massage depends upon restoration of blood volume, correction of acidosis and return of myocardial contractile force. The technique of closed massage is described in Chapter 26.

Severe external bleeding can be controlled in most cases by applying finger pressure over the wound. This technique is fast and effective and can be used during cardiorespiratory resuscitation. Later, a pressure dressing replaces the finger. A mound of gauze pads compressed by an elastic bandage makes a satisfactory pressure dressing. The bandage is wrapped tightly enough to tamponade the bleeders but not to occlude intact major vessels. Tourniquet compression of the artery proximal to the wound is very rarely necessary. Tourniquets often increase bleeding by obstructing venous return. They can cause ischemic injury in extremities unless released for several minutes every quarter hour.

Blindly clamping bleeding vessels in a deep wound is unwise. Tissue damage rather than hemostasis usually results. Lacerated major arteries are best controlled by pressure until adequate exposure is possible in the operating room. Ligation of large arteries is seldom justified in the Emergency Room, especially when the risk of subsequent limb ischemia is great. Profuse bleeding is alarming and diverts attention away from more important needs such as restoration of airway and ventilation. Experience and discipline are required to focus on these priorities in the face of dramatic hemorrhage.

After adequate ventilation, effective cardiac function and control of external bleeding have been assured, the outpatient surgeon is responsible for estimating the degree of shock. Shock is peripheral circulatory failure to maintain tissue perfusion. Such failure is caused by hemorrhage in most traumatized patients. Hypovolemic shock may also result from decreased blood volume due to loss of plasma or body water and electrolytes. Other types of shock — cardiogenic, neurogenic and septic — may be encountered in the injured patient. Each results in insufficient microcirculatory flow and yet requires different treatment.

Monitoring the patient with shock involves recording pulse and blood pressure at frequent intervals, observing temperature and color of skin, measuring urine output on an hourly basis and assessing cardiac output and oxygen transport. Arterial blood gases (Pao_2, $Paco_2$ and pH) are indispensable therapeutic guides during restoration of oxygenation and tissue perfusion. Using a nomogram, base deficit can be calculated and corrected with appropriate amounts of bicarbonate solution. Arterial oxygen tension below 60 mm Hg indicates marginal respiratory reserve and requires increased concentrations of oxygen in inspired air. A $Paco_2$ over 45 mm Hg suggests serious hypoventilation or, in the presence of adequate ventilation, severe pulmonary insufficiency. Arterial pH values reflect the efficacy of resuscitation. As perfusion improves, metabolic acidosis should diminish. Serum lactate levels may be useful as prognostic guides. Levels of 2 mM/liter (normal 0.44 to 1.8 mM/liter) have been found to be associated with a mortality rate of 15 per cent, and levels of 10 mM/liter or greater are associated with a mortality rate of 95 per cent.

Central venous pressure (CVP) is a guide to vascular volume replacement, especially when colloids are given. Since colloids remain in the vascular system, CVP rather accurately reflects volume restoration and prevents overtreatment. Pulmonary artery pressure, a more reliable guide to blood volume, especially during administration of crystalloid solutions, can be measured by passing a balloon catheter (Swan-Ganz) from a peripheral vein through the right heart into the pulmonary artery.

The object of treatment of hypovolemic shock is to restore blood volume. Two types of fluid are used: crystalloids and colloids. Crystalloids such as normal saline or lactated Ringer's solution restore vascular volume for short periods. They lower blood viscosity and improve microcirculation. Time is thereby gained for definitive typing and cross-matching of blood. It is nearly impossible to dilute blood sufficiently to prevent adequate tissue oxygenation. As salt and water are lost from the circulation, however, both pulmonary and tissue edema may result. Ideally, then, initial volume replacement with crystalloid should be followed by the administration of blood. Only cross-matched or type-specific blood should be transfused. Minor mismatch often results from emergency transfusion of type O Rh-negative blood and may, after repeated transfusion, cause serious morbidity.

Colloids other than blood which are useful in hypovolemic shock are plasma, serum albumin and plasma substitutes such as Dextran. Solutions containing albumin should be avoided during resuscitation of profound hypovolemic shock, since they may later contribute to prolonged interstitial edema.

A venous channel is urgently required to administer either crystalloid or colloid solutions and to monitor fluid replacement. Large bore catheters can be placed in peripheral veins such as the basilic vein in the antecubital space. A short catheter is preferred when fluid is to be infused under pressure. A long catheter can occasionally be placed in the superior vena cava for measurement of CVP. When peripheral veins are collapsed or inaccessible, superior vena cava catheterization or a peripheral vein "cutdown" (venesection) is indicated.

Burns

Initial evaluation and treatment of a major burn victim often begins at the site of injury. The burn source must be removed by smothering flames, applying wet towels or immersing in water. Chemical burns should be flushed with large volumes of water. The patient must be moved immediately from an area where dangerous fumes are present. Fires commonly generate carbon monoxide, cyanide and phosgene, especially when plastics are burned.

Concern for airway and ventilation is as great after a burn as after any other severe injury. Inhalation burn is suspected in the presence of facial burn, noxious fumes or signs such as wheezing, coughing, hoarseness, tachypnea and cyanosis. Measurements of arterial blood gases confirm such injury. Treatment is endotracheal intubation and positive-pressure ventilation. Methylprednisolone sodium succinate, 40 mg per kg body weight, is given intravenously every 24 hours for two days.

With an airway assured, a large-bore catheter is inserted in a peripheral vein for administration of a balanced electrolyte solution such as Ringer's lactate. Most patients with a major burn will require a central venous line for measurement of pressure and, possibly, infusion of fluid. At the time an intravenous line is inserted, blood samples are drawn for baseline determinations of blood count, hemoglobin, hematocrit, blood urea nitrogen, serum electrolytes, blood glucose, total protein and albumin-globulin ratio. Fluids are given according to an appropriate formula (see Chapter 9), but after the first few hours fluid administration is correlated with urine output, central venous pressure and other estimates of blood volume.

A nasogastric tube is passed to empty the stomach. The tube is connected to intermittent suction to prevent gastric dilation, aspiration and ileus. An indwelling catheter is placed into the bladder to permit measurement of hourly urine output, which should be 35 to 75 ml per hour if fluid replacement is adequate.

At this point a brief history documenting the type of burn, the place of injury, associated injuries and the emergency treatment given previously can be obtained. Physical examination gives the extent of burn but not, with accuracy, the depth. Using the rule of nines (Chapter 9), the total body surface area burned is calculated. It is important to remember that in children under age ten the proportion of surface area on the head and neck is greater than in adults. Circumferential burns of extremities, chest or neck may cause constriction and require surgical escharotomy. The Doppler flowmeter is valuable in monitoring circumferential vascular compression.

Vital signs are recorded every 15 minutes during the early hours of a major burn. Evidence of hypovolemia should be detected from decreasing urine output before change occurs in blood pressure. Pain is relieved by intravenous narcotics, usually morphine, 8 to 10 mg every four hours. Intramuscular narcotics are contraindicated because of their slow absorption during resuscitation. Tetanus toxoid, 0.5 ml, or tetanus immune globulin (human) (Hyper-Tet) should be given intramuscularly. Antibiotics such as penicillin or a cephalosporin are sometimes given to prevent infections by *Streptococcus* and *Staphylococcus aureus*, which can be associated with sepsis and pneumonia. Others prefer to withhold antibiotics unless later evidence of gram-negative invasion requires their use.

Superior Vena Cava Catheterization

General Discussion

Placement of an indwelling catheter in the superior vena cava for measurement of central venous pressure and administration of fluids is a widely accepted technique in the management of a critically injured patient. Advantages of the technique are (1) rapid procurement of a large caliber intravenous line in a patient with inaccessible peripheral veins, (2) long-term maintenance with relatively few complications and (3) accurate placement of a catheter tip near the right heart.

Several techniques are available for catheter placement. All are subject to hazards and complications.[10] Common to each is the risk of perforating the vein, causing extraluminal catheter placement with possible hematoma, hemothorax or mediastinal infiltration. A misdirected needle can puncture lung, artery, lymphatic duct or brachial plexus. Properly positioned catheters are capable of displacement, thrombus formation and infection.

Observing certain principles of technique in catheterizing the superior vena cava, even under emergency circumstances, will minimize the risk of serious complications. The patient should be flat or, preferably, in Trendelenburg position to increase venous filling and to decrease the chance of air embolism. A firm board placed beneath the head and thorax and a rolled sheet placed behind the vertebral column tend to reflect the shoulders dorsally, improving the angle of venipuncture.

Skin preparation should be as thorough as conditions allow to minimize infection of both catheter tip and skin puncture site. The anterior chest should be shaved if necessary. Skin is scrubbed with an iodine-containing solution for seven to ten minutes over an area extending at least 15 centimeters from the puncture site. An iodophor paint is applied after scrubbing and before placement of sterile drapes. The surgeon wears sterile gloves, a mask and a hat and works from a sterile instrument tray.

Subclavian Vein Puncture

The subclavian vein can be cannulated by means of a supraclavicular or an infraclavicular approach. While the former entails less risk of pneumothorax,[16] the latter is technically easier and more commonly used.

Infraclavicular subclavian vein puncture is illustrated in Figure 4–1. Landmarks are the sternal notch and the anterior scalene muscle, which inserts on the first rib between the subclavian vein (anterior) and the brachial plexus and subclavian artery (posterior). Using these landmarks the operator can visualize the target area of the vein. An anesthetic solution, such as 1 per cent lidocaine, is infiltrated in the skin at the puncture site, which is just medial to or at the midpoint of the clavicle. With skin held taut, a 2¾ inch

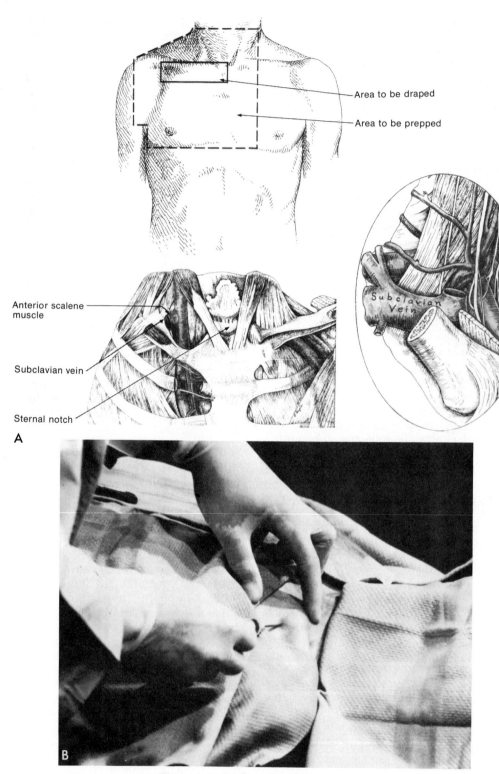

Figure 4–1 *See legend on the opposite page.*

long 14 gauge needle connected to a 5 ml syringe is inserted through the skin wheal. The angle of approach is determined by placing one finger in the sternal notch and another over the anterior scalene muscle, lowering the barrel of the syringe toward the patient's shoulder and slowly advancing in a frontal plane to the target. Slight negative pressure is maintained in the syringe as the needle is advanced. The patient is instructed to "look away" from the operator, press his shoulders to the bed, "reach for his feet" and hold his breath at the end of expiration.

When a free flow of venous blood is obtained, the needle is advanced a few millimeters to ensure that the entire bevel is within the lumen of the vein. The needle is steadied with a clamp while the syringe is removed and a 12 inch long 16 gauge radiopaque catheter is inserted using forceps and no-touch technique. The needle is then withdrawn, a guard is placed on the needle and the syringe is attached to the catheter. If backflow of blood is not satisfactory the catheter is withdrawn to a point that yields adequate flow. If this maneuver is unsuccessful, the catheter is replaced.

With proper backflow confirmed, the catheter is connected to an intravenous administration set. The catheter may be fixed to skin at the puncture site by fine nonabsorbable sutures. An iodine-containing antiseptic rather than an antibiotic ointment is applied to the catheter exit site and an occlusive dressing

is fashioned with sterile gauze pads, tincture of benzoin and nonporous tape to seal the wound. The dressing also secures catheter and tubing.

Chest x-ray is obtained soon afterward to exclude the possibilities of pneumothorax or catheter displacement. Catheter aftercare requires dressing changes under aseptic conditions three times a week. Evidence of catheter sepsis or occlusion by clot generally demands immediate replacement.

Supraclavicular subclavian puncture entails less risk of pneumothorax than the infraclavicular approach, especially in patients with emphysema. In these patients the subclavian vein, normally overlying the pleural dome, rises to a higher position. Ideal for supraclavicular puncture are patients with a horizontal clavicle and a wide costoclavicular space or obese patients in whom the needle may not reach the subclavian vein when inserted below the clavicle. In this approach the operator stands at the head of the supine patient and presses his index finger, pointing toward the feet, behind the clavicular head of the sternocleidomastoid muscle on the side of the puncture to feel the anterior scalenus tubercle on the first rib. The subclavian artery lies lateral to this tubercle. A needle is inserted in a horizontal plane above and parallel to the anterior scalenus muscle, medial to the subclavian artery. The needle is withdrawn with constant aspiration until a free flow of blood is obtained. The

Figure 4–1 *Superior Vena Cava Catheterization. A.* The infraclavicular approach to the subclavian vein is based on relationships of the vein to the anterior scalene muscle, the clavicle and the first rib. Visualizing these structures establishes the "target" area of the subclavian vein.

B. The angle of approach for infraclavicular subclavian vein puncture is determined by placing one finger in the sternal notch and another over the anterior scalene muscle. The needle is introduced near the midpoint of the clavicle and advanced to the "target" area. If the vein is missed and the needle is parallel to the clavicle, the target is probably more cephalad and not deep toward the cupula of the lung.

syringe is then lowered toward the shoulder and rotated 180° to place the needle along the axis of the vein with the bevel facing the superior vena cava. Catheter insertion and fixation are performed as described above.

Internal Jugular Vein Puncture

Perhaps the safest technique for placement of a superior vena cava catheter is percutaneous puncture of the internal jugular vein. The incidence of pneumothorax and hemothorax with this technique is negligible. Air embolism, thromboembolism, septicemia and mediastinal infusion of fluid may occur.[9] The internal jugular vein occupies an almost constant anatomic position deep to the sternocleidomastoid muscle and, during a Valsalva maneuver, will be distended to a diameter of at least 2 centimeters in an adult.

With the patient in Trendelenburg position and the head rotated to the opposite side, a needle is introduced at a site along the outer border of the sternocleidomastoid muscle two fingerbreadths above the clavicle. The needle tip is advanced toward the suprasternal notch while suction is maintained. When venous blood returns, a catheter is advanced and secured as described in subclavian puncture.

An alternative technique for internal jugular puncture is to introduce the needle at the apex of the triangle formed by the dividing sternal and clavicular heads of the sternocleidomastoid and the clavicle. The center of this triangle is directly over the internal jugular vein. The needle is advanced from the apex while maintaining back pressure on the plunger of the syringe, toward the center of the triangle at a 30° angle with the skin. Inadvertent puncture of the carotid artery is seldom dangerous if the needle is withdrawn and direct pressure is applied for several minutes.

External Jugular Vein Puncture

Central venous catheterization via the external jugular vein using a J-wire virtually eliminates the possibility of pneumothorax and other complications that may result from subclavian or internal jugular vein puncture.[3] The technique utilizes a flexible stainless steel "J" tip spring guide to place a catheter in the central venous system. The "J" tip is especially helpful in traversing tortuous vessels, which are commonly found with the external jugular vein. Once the wire guide is placed, insertion of the catheter is easily accomplished. Utility of the technique in a severely injured patient depends upon sufficient filling of the external jugular veins to permit venipuncture.

Venesection

Percutaneous superior vena cava catheterization has largely replaced venesection as a means of securing a reliable intravenous route in severely traumatized patients. The technique of subclavian or internal jugular puncture is easier and faster than cannulating the saphenous or cephalic veins in the extremities. Nevertheless, the cutdown technique of intravenous infusion occasionally is useful and is essential when superior vena cava catheterization fails and peripheral veins cannot be punctured. It remains a common procedure in pediatric patients in whom percutaneous puncture is technically difficult. Venesection avoids pulmonary or mediastinal complications due to needle puncture or catheter displacement. Problems of thromboembolism and sepsis are not avoided and, in fact, catheters are less well tolerated for prolonged periods in peripheral veins than in larger vessels.

The greater saphenous vein is easily exposed and cannulated at the level of the medial malleolus. Contraindications for venesection at this site are previous excision or thrombosis of the vein, contamination of overlying skin and local injury. Alternate sites are the cephalic vein in the anatomical snuffbox at the wrist, cephalic or basilic veins proximal to the antecubital space and tributaries of the long saphenous vein in the upper thigh. Cannulation of the basilic vein at the antecubital fossa can be performed through a horizontal or longitudinal cutdown incision. Upper extremity routes are preferred for patients with injuries of the liver or vena cava.

The technique of venesection ("cutdown") at the ankle is illustrated in Figure 4–2. A tourniquet is applied about the calf to distend the greater

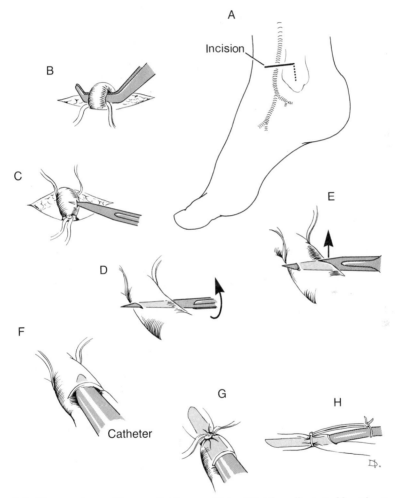

Figure 4–2 *Venesection — Greater Saphenous Vein "Cutdown" at Ankle.* The technique of greater saphenous venesection at the ankle is illustrated. *A.* A 2 cm incision is made anterior and cephalad to the medial malleolus. *B.* The subcutaneous saphenous vein is freed from fascia and the accompanying saphenous nerve. *C.* After tying the vein distally and passing a silk ligature proximally, venotomy begins. *D.* The tip of a #11 scalpel blade is inserted horizontally through the middle of the vein. *E.* As the blade is rotated vertically the venotomy is completed. *F.* Polyethylene tubing is advanced proximally through the venotomy and (*G*) secured with the silk ligature. *H.* The ligature is passed around the catheter and tied securely to prevent accidental withdrawal.

saphenous vein. Skin over the medial aspect of the ankle is prepared with application of an iodophor (organic iodine) paint and draped with sterile towels. The saphenous vein is often visible just anterior to the medial malleolus. One centimeter above and 1 centimeter anterior to the malleolus a 2-centimeter transverse incision is made in the skin over the vein and carried through the scant subcutaneous tissue. By blunt dissection, using the tips of a hemostat, the vein is separated from adjacent tissues, particularly the saphenous nerve, and exposed over a distance of 2 centimeters. Two silk ligatures are passed around the vein. The distal ligature is tied and placed on traction. The untied proximal ligature is retracted upward while a venotomy is made with scissors or pointed scalpel blade midway between ligatures. A polyethylene catheter, 12 or 14 gauge in adults, is beveled slightly at its tip and inserted through the venotomy. As the proximal ligature is relaxed, the tubing is advanced into the vein so that at least 10 centimeters of the catheter lie above the venotomy. The proximal ligature is tied about the vein and tubing in order to secure but not occlude the catheter.

Skin is closed with two or three vertical mattress sutures of silk, one of which is used to encircle the tubing. Antibiotic ointment is applied around the catheter site before a dressing is placed over the wound. Adhesive secures the dressing and further retains the catheter as it lies on the skin of the ankle.

Diagnostic Procedures

Detection of obscure injury, especially after severe blunt trauma, depends upon repeated physical examination of the patient and specific diagnostic procedures performed in the Emergency Room.

X-rays

Head injuries can be studied by skull x-rays, ultra-sound encephalography, carotid arteriography and computed axial tomography (CAT) (Chapter 8). Neck pain or tenderness demands that cross-table lateral cervical x-rays be obtained with portable equipment before the patient is moved to avoid spinal cord injury from fractured or dislocated cervical vertebrae. An unconscious, motionless patient should be assumed to have a fractured neck until proved otherwise, especially if found to have a skull fracture. Chest x-ray documents rib fracture, pneumothorax, hemothorax, atelectasis, mediastinal widening or displacement and changes in the cardiac silhouette. X-rays of extremities and the pelvis can, of course, demonstrate fractures or dislocations and peripheral arteriography can show major vessel patency or perforation.

Abdominal injuries are not often detected by routine x-ray. Free peritoneal air on upright chest x-ray is usually apparent after "blow-out" injuries of the stomach or bowel. Retroperitoneal or subserosal air may be seen in some patients with retroperitoneal rupture of the duodenum or colon. Laceration of organs with bleeding must usually be diagnosed by means other than x-ray, although obliteration of the psoas shadow may be a clue to the presence of retroperitoneal hematoma.

Angiographic techniques may be helpful in diagnosing injury to liver, spleen, pancreas and kidney. Ultrasound occasionally detects rupture of spleen and pancreas. Radio nuclide scanning of the spleen may also detect rupture.

Bladder Catheterization

An indwelling bladder catheter assures precise measurement of urine output which helps in monitoring shock and fluid therapy. Inability to pass a catheter suggests urethral injury and requires percutaneous bladder catheterization or cystostomy. Gross or microscopic hematuria is a sign of urinary tract trauma and is an indication for intravenous pyelography (Chapter 19).

Nasogastric Intubation

A nasogastric tube of 18F size or larger should be passed in every severely injured patient to reduce gastric content, thereby lessening the risk of aspiration during surgery, and to detect the presence of blood in the stomach. Significant amounts of bright blood returned from the stomach usually indicate gastric or esophageal injury. Stress ulcer bleeding and most types of hemobilia are not seen immediately. Small bowel injuries including duodenal perforation seldom present with blood in the stomach. If gastric perforation is suspected, intermittent suction should be applied to the nasogastric tube. Irrigation is allowed only to maintain tube patency. Sterile saline in small amounts is used for this purpose.

Paracentesis

Paracentesis or peritoneal tap with lavage is a means of detecting injury of abdominal viscera after trauma. It is especially useful in patients unconscious after blunt trauma, in whom physical signs of intraperitoneal injury are often unimpressive. When the tap is positive for blood, laparotomy is usually indicated. When the tap is negative, however, the possibility of intraabdominal injury cannot be excluded and continued observation with repeated abdominal examination is mandatory.

The four-quadrant needle puncture technique of paracentesis, while simple and rapid, is often falsely negative in cases of slight to moderate hemoperitoneum. It is useful, however, for immediate confirmation of massive intraperitoneal bleeding. A 10 centimeter 18 or 20 gauge spinal needle attached to a sterile syringe is used to puncture the anterior abdominal wall in the middle of each abdominal quadrant. Skin preparation is limited to a single application of tincture of iodine or iodophor antiseptic. Local anesthetic is seldom required. The needle can be felt to perforate the peritoneum by the sudden release of a temporary resistance. Thereafter, the needle is slowly advanced perpendicular to the skin while negative pressure is maintained until blood is obtained or the hub is reached. Very often blood returns as the needle is being withdrawn. Injury to the bowel or other viscera rarely occurs with this technique. Ordinarily the needle tip displaces normal intestine. Perforation of distended or adherent bowel, however, can result in leakage and peritonitis, which require laparotomy. Similar peritoneal inflammation has been caused by perforation of an intraabdominal abscess.[8] Troublesome bleeding from epigastric vessels in the rectus muscle can occur after needle paracentesis. Hematoma is usually prevented by exerting pressure over the puncture site for several minutes.

Peritoneal lavage is currently used in preference to four-quadrant paracentesis. The accuracy of peritoneal lavage in establishing the diagnosis of hemoperitoneum is reported to be as high as 96 per cent. False negatives (3 per cent) were more common than false positives (1 per cent) in a series of 304 patients.[12] The test consists of introducing a catheter into the peritoneal cavity and aspirating for gross blood. If no blood is obtained, the abdominal cavity is irrigated with a balanced salt solution and returning fluid is examined for blood.

The abdomen may be punctured with a trocar, a dialysis catheter or a large bore needle (Fig. 4–3). The needle is preferred because it causes fewer false positive taps due to abdominal

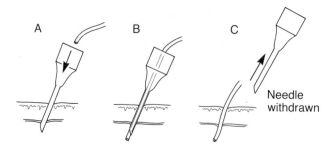

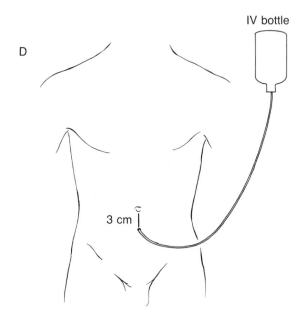

Figure 4–3 *Paracentesis and Peritoneal Lavage. A–C.* After inserting a two inch 14 gauge needle with stylus through the linea alba 3 cm below the umbilicus, a 16 gauge polyethylene catheter is passed into the abdominal cavity and the needle is withdrawn. *D.* If gross blood is not obtained, peritoneal lavage is performed by introducing one liter of normal saline solution rapidly into the abdomen and allowing it to freely drain back through the catheter onto a clean white gauze pad.

wall vessel perforation. A 2 inch 14 gauge needle with a 16 gauge intraluminal catheter, identical to that used for subclavian puncture, is recommended. After painting the skin of the midabdomen with an antiseptic, a skin wheal is raised with local anesthetic in the midline 3 cm below the umbilicus. The needle is advanced perpendicularly through the abdominal wall to its hub. If aspiration yields gross blood, the procedure is terminated and the patient prepared for laparotomy. If not, the catheter is advanced into the peritoneal cavity and the needle entirely withdrawn. One liter of normal saline solution is introduced rapidly into the abdomen of adults. In children only 500 ml is used. The fluid is then removed by allowing free drainage through the catheter onto a clean white gauze pad. Evidence of even pink-tinged fluid is considered a positive tap.

Examining returned fluid microscopically for erythrocytes and leukocytes has been recommended. Although the exact number of red cells constituting a positive test has not been determined, it appears that 100,000 erythrocytes per cubic millimeter of lavage fluid can be considered significant.

Complications of peritoneal lavage,

although unusual, include perforation of bowel, injury of mesentery, transection and loss of the catheter into the abdomen, extra-peritoneal infusion and bleeding from abdominal wall vessels. Peritonitis secondary to lavage has not been reported.

Sinography

Puncture wounds of the abdomen may be superficial or they may penetrate the peritoneum. Surgical exploration is sometimes required in the latter to repair intraperitoneal injury. The outpatient surgeon may wish to determine whether or not the peritoneum has been penetrated by performing stab wound sinography.[4] Shock, peritonitis, a protruding viscus or any other indication for immediate operation obviate the use of sinography. The technique is principally useful to avoid unnecessary exploration when physical findings are inconclusive. Sinography becomes less frequent when a policy

of selective rather than mandatory exploration is followed.

Skin about the stab wound is prepared and draped sterilely and wound edges are infiltrated with local anesthetic solution. A 12–18 French rubber catheter is inserted into the wound for a distance of 2 centimeters. The catheter is not pushed more deeply into the wound tract. A purse-string suture of heavy silk is secured in the skin around the catheter to occlude the tract opening. At least 50 cc of meglumine diatrizoate (Renografin 60 per cent) is injected into the catheter by sufficient hand force to evert the skin closed around the tract. The catheter is then clamped and anteroposterior, lateral and oblique roentgenograms of the abdomen promptly taken. Sinography may also be performed under fluoroscopy, following which x-rays are taken (Fig. 4–4).

In penetrating wounds of the peritoneum, contrast medium outlines intraabdominal structures. In superficial wounds, the medium tends to diffuse

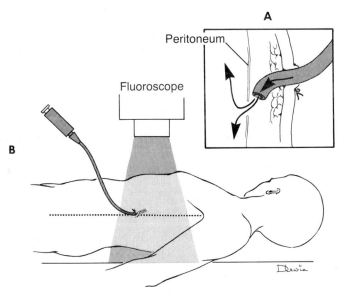

Figure 4–4 *Abdominal Sinography.* A. A 12–18 French rubber catheter is inserted into a flank stab wound and secured by a purse string suture of heavy silk which occludes the open wound. Contrast media is injected under some pressure just before anteroposterior, lateral and oblique roentgenograms of the abdomen are taken. B. Contrast media passes into the peritoneal cavity and surrounds visceral structures if the peritoneum has been penetrated.

along extraperitoneal soft tissue planes. If the chest has been entered, intrathoracic structures may be outlined.

With multiple stab wounds, each tract should be individually injected and x-rayed to eliminate superimposition of contrast media.

Falsely negative results may occur in as many as 10 per cent of examinations. Insufficient volume of contrast medium in multiple stab wounds or simultaneous chest and abdominal tracts contribute to this error. It is important to perform sinography before diagnostic peritoneal lavage to avoid dilution of radiopaque material within the abdominal cavity.

Complications of sinography include hypersensitivity reactions to the contrast medium and moderate transient pain with injection. The incidence of wound infections, however, is not increased.[4]

SPECIFIC INJURIES

Most trauma encountered by the outpatient surgeon will consist of minor injuries in patients who return home after treatment. Such injuries include contusions, abrasions, lacerations, bites and burns. The essence of treatment in each case is proper wound care. This requires an understanding of tissue injury, inflammation, infection, débridement, repair and healing. Local and constitutional factors influencing these events are discussed elsewhere (Chapters 5 and 7). The practical management of simple wounds, based on knowledge of tissue damage and repair, will be discussed here.

Closed Wounds

Contusions and bruises are nonpenetrating wounds caused by blunt trauma in which subepithelial blood vessels rupture. When blood or pigments disseminate throughout intercellular spaces without forming a collection of blood, an ecchymosis results. This is identified by an initial blue-black color in subcutaneous tissues which later fades to a brown-green discoloration. If extravasated blood collects in subcutaneous tissue or muscle, a hematoma is formed. Blebs or blisters caused by minor burns or blunt force are another form of closed wound. Because of its thin, easily ruptured wall, however, a bleb is often treated as an open wound.

The important injury in most minor closed wounds is the rupture of capillaries. Other structures are seldom seriously damaged. Inflammatory reaction to the extravasation of blood is generally moderate and, in simple contusions, subsides within a few days. Absorption of blood or serum is rapid unless a hematoma has been formed in large tissue spaces. Then inflammation persists while a capsule of connective tissue encircles the fluid and destroyed cellular elements. Blood in a hematoma ordinarily clots, organizing itself by ingrowing capillaries and connective tissue. Aspiration at this stage is impossible and slow resolution is inevitable.

Treatment of contusions is nonsurgical. Local cold such as an icepack, used early, tends to limit swelling as with any inflammatory process. Later, heat reduces pain and accelerates resolution. Occasionally, a large, early hematoma that is well-defined in subcutaneous tissue and is fluctuant on palpation may require needle aspiration to relieve pain and to hasten healing. The danger here is infecting the evacuated space with microorganisms introduced with the needle. Aseptic technique in aspirating blood is essential. Overlying skin is painted with tincture of iodine or an iodophor compound. A skin wheal is raised with local anesthetic solution directly over the fluctuant mass. An 18 gauge needle with attached syringe is inserted into the cavity and the syringe advanced and withdrawn or rotated gently until all unclotted blood and serum are aspirated. A sterile gauze dressing is loosely bunched over the site and secured under slight pressure with elastic adhesive to obliterate the empty space and to prevent hematoma recurrence. If drainage is unsatisfactory or if the evacuated space becomes secondarily infected, incision with open drainage is indicated. Rest, elevation, sedation and mild analgesics control pain after such a procedure.

Wringer injury of the arm is an example of a severe closed wound. Patients with such trauma should always be hospitalized and observed for evidence of muscle ischemia that might require fasciotomy. Initial treatment is elevation and ice packs to reduce edema. Muscle function and pulses in the involved extremity are monitored for early detection of ischemia.

Open Wounds

Certain principles apply to the care of all open wounds regardless of cause, size or location. Inspection must be done aseptically using sterile gloves and a face mask to avoid secondary contamination. No further injury should be caused by unnecessary manipulation during examination, dressing or diagnostic procedures such as x-ray. The whole patient must be evaluated by obtaining an accurate history and performing a physical examination. When multiple injuries have occurred, priority of care is determined so that immediate treatment is given to the most serious problem while no minor injury is neglected.

Abrasions are superficial open injuries in which epithelium of skin or mucous membrane is lost. The wound area may be extensive. Wound depth usually is uneven but no greater than the level of accessory skin structures in the dermis. If all epithelial elements are lost, the lesion is termed "wound with loss of substance." Since nerve endings are exposed, abrasions are painful and may limit the mobility of underlying joints.

Blood, serum and inflammatory cells exuding from abrasions dry to form a crust or scab. Beneath the crust new exudate is formed by inflammation. This either escapes from beneath the crust edge or dries to thicken the eschar. Eventually, mesodermal elements grow from midwound sites and epithelium grows from wound margins to cover the surface. The scab thins and separates to expose an epithelized surface within about ten days.

Dirt and other foreign material may be incorporated into the eschar or imbedded in dermal layers. If inorganic particles remain, a "tattoo" effect is evident after healing. It is important to remove all dirt particles imbedded in abrasions within the limits of pain and new tissue damage. Vigorous washing or scrubbing with sterile water or saline may be required to remove this debris. A sterile toothbrush can be used to clean abrasions. Occasionally only the firm bristles of a surgical scrub brush can dislodge debris. If all such techniques fail, excision of tissue or dermabrasion should be considered. Foreign particles should not be allowed to remain in facial wounds.

Mild antiseptics, such as Betadine and hexachlorophene may reduce the number of bacteria in the wound. Stronger antiseptics are not indicated, as they cause pain and compound tissue injury. It is unlikely that even potent antiseptics kill all contaminating microorganisms in abrasions, since solutions cannot reach deeper tissue spaces.

Scabs serve to protect abrasions from further trauma and bacterial invasion, so they should be preserved during healing. External dressing is optional and dependent upon susceptibility to further trauma. When infection is developing beneath an eschar, however, the scab must be removed and the wound treated with nonadherent dressings, saline irrigation and wound support. Infected abrasions may become full thickness defects if dermal remnants are destroyed. Dressings then involve "wet-to-dry" fine mesh gauze applications.

Fine mesh gauze is moistened with saline and wrung out to leave the dressing moist but not dripping wet. The gauze is then applied to the wound surface for a four hour period, during which time it will dry and become partially adherent to the underlying coagulum of leukocytes and fibrin. The dry gauze is gently removed, debriding the surface, and replaced with a new damp gauze. The cycle of dressing changes every four hours is continued until the wound has healed or until a suitable clean granulating surface has developed, to be covered with a skin graft.

Puncture Wounds

Long, sharp objects may penetrate visceral cavities or injure deep structures in the head, neck and extremities. Evaluation and treatment of such injuries generally require hospitalization. The most frequent puncture injury treated by the outpatient surgeon is nail wound of the foot. Because of the potential for clostridial infection in deep, virtually closed wounds of this type, treatment of nail punctures should be aggressive.

Skin surrounding the puncture site of a nail wound is excised to allow wound irrigation and drainage. After infiltration of skin edges with local anesthetic solution, approximately 3 millimeters of skin is debrided with scissors or knife around the wound margin. Saline irrigation of deeper tissue planes is facilitated by using a syringe and large bore needle. The wound is not closed but dressed lightly for protection if on a weight-bearing surface. Antibiotics in addition to tetanus prophylaxis are indicated.

Lesser puncture wounds caused by needles, wooden splinters or glass may require no treatment except administration of tetanus toxoid. Imbedded foreign bodies need not be removed unless symptomatic, unsightly, infected or the cause of undue patient alarm. Wooden splinters usually produce more pain than metal objects. Often they can be pulled out by grasping a protruding end. A common circumstance is a splinter under the fingernail. Removing a V-shaped segment of the nail edge, with the apex overlying the end of the splinter, allows the operator to grasp the splinter. With gentleness the procedure can be carried out painlessly. If necessary, digital nerve block can be used for anesthesia (Fig. 4–5).

While metal objects are readily identified in tissue by x-ray examination, wood and many glass foreign bodies are not. Glass containing lead may be faintly radiopaque. Retained glass is difficult to find by x-ray unless a "no screen" soft tissue technique is used. Glass in a wound is rarely identified visually and more often is recognized by a grating sensation when touched by an instrument.

All foreign bodies associated with draining wounds must be removed. If extensive search in deeper tissue spaces is planned or if mechanical aids such as magnets are needed, the procedure is better done in a well-equipped operating room than in an outpatient clinic. It is distressing for both patient and surgeon to hunt unsuccessfully for a possible foreign body under inadequate conditions of light, anesthesia, asepsis and assistance.

An imbedded fish hook is a unique form of puncture wound. The barb must be forced through a wound of exit so that it can be cut off with a wire shears. The remainder of the hook is then withdrawn through the site of entry (Fig. 4–6). An alternative approach for removing a fish hook is described in Chapter 28.

Simple stab wounds and gunshot wounds that do not penetrate the neck or thoracic or peritoneal cavities and

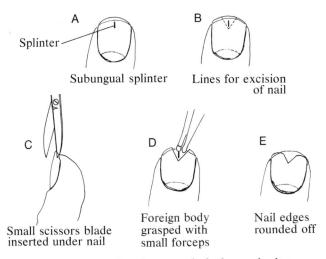

Figure 4–5 Procedure for removal of subungual splinter.

do not involve deep structures such as vessels, nerves, tendons or bones can usually be treated on an outpatient basis.

Stab wound tracks seldom require excision or débridement. The cardinal point in care is to keep open the wound of entry, allowing free drainage of the wound track until complete healing has occurred. An effective means of accomplishing this is to excise from ½ to 1 centimeter of full thickness skin circumferentially at the site of entrance. If the depth of the wound is more than 2 to 3 centimeters, packing with iodine-impregnated gauze keeps

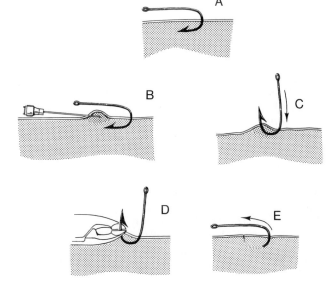

Figure 4–6 *A.* The barb of a fish hook is embedded subcutaneously. *B.* A skin wheal is raised with anesthetic solution at the proposed site of exit. *C.* The shaft of the hook is angled to force the barb through the skin wheal. *D.* The barb is cut off with a wire shears. *E.* The remainder of the hook is then withdrawn through the site of entry.

skin edges separated and prevents a closed space infection. Packing is replaced during each wound dressing until the deep portion of the tract is healed as determined by gently probing with a sterile applicator stick. At the time of dressing, saline or dilute hydrogen peroxide is used to irrigate the wound tract. If infection develops deeply, the track must be opened widely or excised to allow adequate drainage. Stab wounds of the neck may be associated with injury to the carotid artery, jugular vein, esophagus and various mediastinal structures. Probing wounds to ascertain such damage is unrewarding. Most stab wounds of the neck merit exploration in the operating room to exclude deep injuries. This is especially true of supraclavicular stab wounds, in which the potential for mediastinal penetration is great.

Abdominal stab wounds penetrate the peritoneum in only one half of patients. One fourth of these have life-threatening injury. Because of this relatively low risk, many surgeons prefer to observe patients with abdominal stab wounds for evidence of intraperitoneal injury rather than to perform immediate laparotomy. Exceptions are patients in shock or those with obvious signs of peritoneal perforation such as protruding viscera. During the period of observation, the care of an abdominal stab wound consists largely of cleaning and covering.

Gunshot wounds present a special problem in wound care. The degree of tissue damage sustained is related to the tissue velocity and mass of the missile. Entry and exit wound size cannot be related to tissue injury along the bullet track. Missiles fired from low velocity weapons such as the .22 caliber rifle cause relatively little tissue damage. In superficial wounds of this type, entry and exit wounds should be debrided, but the track need not be explored unless heavily contaminated with clothing or other foreign material.

High velocity missile tracks are as-sociated with considerable tissue necrosis.[12] Wounds caused by such missiles should be opened along the entire track and obviously nonviable tissue debrided. It is unwise to close such wounds primarily. They may be packed loosely, dressed and allowed to heal secondarily. The most common outpatient surgical errors in managing gunshot wounds are failing to recognize injury of deep structures and incompletely debriding high velocity missile wound tracks. If any question exists concerning the adequacy of outpatient débridement, the patient should be hospitalized.

Occasionally the outpatient surgeon will be asked to remove a subcutaneous bullet or missile fragment. It is important that he mark the removed bullet in such a way as to be able to identify it later in court. All bullets removed from patients must be given to police authorities, and gunshot wounds should be reported to the police.

Shotgun wounds carry a greater threat of subsequent infection than do most penetrating gunshot wounds. The reason is contamination of wadding materials used in shotgun shells. Home-packed shells may contain wadding composed of felt, hair or beeswax. Commercial wadding is less often contaminated but is still capable of inciting infection. Pellet wounds must therefore be inspected carefully. Wadding, clothing and the pellet itself are removed when identified. Individual wounds may require débridement and extensive cleaning before dressing. Such wounds are never closed.

Lacerations

Open wounds caused by objects that incise or tear full thickness skin are termed lacerations. If deeper tissue damage is slight, as in injury caused by a sharp knife, the lesion is called an "incised wound." Most lacerations are irregular, although skin edges remain well-defined. The tendency to gape is due to gravity, contraction of underlying muscle and retraction of tissue fibers lying perpendicular to the laceration. The mechanism of wound healing in lacerations is discussed in Chapter 9.

Minor lacerations are easily managed in the Emergency Room, office and clinic so long as facilities allow adequate anesthesia, débridement and suturing. When deep structures such as nerves, vessels, tendons or bone are involved, repair is best accomplished in the operating room. Since all accidental open wounds are considered contaminated with microorganisms, the surgeon must decide whether or not to attempt primary closure. Wounds of the body and extremities over six hours old are likely to be infected in the sense that contaminating bacteria have invaded tissue. Such wounds are better treated open — anticipating healing by secondary intention. An exception to this principle is wounds of the head and neck which, because of abundant blood supply, can be closed primarily within 12 hours of injury without undue risk of infection. Extensive débridement that removes dead tissue as well as bacteria imbedded in adjacent viable tissue can, of course, transform a potentially infected wound into a relatively clean, moderately contaminated lesion.

Infiltration of anesthetic solution into wound edges is usually sufficient to permit cleansing, débridement and suture repair. Nerve block techniques (Chapter 3) are sometimes more effective and avoid excessive wound manipulation. Minor lacerations are gently irrigated with sterile saline or washed with surgical soap before infiltration of anesthetic solution. More thorough cleansing follows anesthesia. Under aseptic conditions using sterile gloves, mask and wound drapes, lidocaine 1 per cent or 0.5 per cent is injected subcutaneously by means of a 22 or 25 gauge needle around the circumference of the wound. Edges are not grasped with forceps until anesthesia is obtained. The proper plane of injection is the corium which contains nerve endings. Injection into subcutaneous fat is unnecessary.

The addition of epinephrine to the anesthetic solution decreases bleeding from wound edges. Because of its vasoconstrictive effects, epinephrine solutions should not be used for infiltration of fingers, toes, ears or genitalia. Wounds infiltrated with epinephrine should be inspected within 24 hours for evidence of hematoma.

The most important factor in managing lacerations is adequate débridement. Surface dirt and foreign matter can be removed by vigorous irrigation with saline solution. Several liters may be required in large, heavily contaminated wounds. A pressure irrigation device is seldom indicated. Surgical soap should not be used in deeper lacerations where muscle, tendon, nerves and blood vessels might be chemically irritated. Soap is useful, however, for cleansing surrounding skin. Iodophor antiseptic solutions usually are applied to skin edges only, although their use in the wound is increasingly common.

Dead or ischemic tissue should be sharply debrided. Devitalized fat or muscle is especially apt to cause wound infection. In sharply incised wounds, the skin border may require no débridement, whereas in avulsion or crush injuries large areas of skin may need excision. Débridement of skin edges is easily accomplished with forceps and scalpel or scissors, and excision is extended to normal-appearing, normal-bleeding tissue. Bleeders seldom require ties or ligatures, but if they do, an absorbable suture material is used.

It is essential to persist in irrigation and débridement until all devitalized and contaminated tissue is removed. The incidence of wound infection is inversely related to the amount of débridement done at the time of injury.

The technique of débridement is further described in Chapter 9.

Bites

Animal and Human Bites

These bites produce a combination of puncture and laceration wounds. Common sites of injury are the ankle, forearm and hand. Dog bites of the face, especially in children, are fairly common. Because of the penetrating nature of the bite injury, infection is a prime concern. Of particular importance in human bites is infection with anaerobic microorganisms, notably *Bacteroides* and *Fusobacteria*. The bite of a dog or cat is often contaminated with *Pasteurella multocida*, a facultative anaerobe that is usually sensitive to penicillin and ampicillin. The virulence of *Pasteurella multocida* wound infection is such that osteomyelitis of underlying joints or inflammation of adjacent tendons is a common complication. Since any bite may be contaminated with *Clostridium tetani*, tetanus prophylaxis is mandatory.

Treatment of animal and human bites can be summarized as débridement and drainage to prevent deep wound infection. Débridement of human bites over metacarpal phalangeal joints, a common injury of fist fighting, must include the full thickness of skin and subcutaneous tissues, with inspection of tendons and, possibly, exposure of periosteum, since a tooth can easily penetrate a metacarpal head. Such débridement is done best in the operating room. All human bites are left open after débridement. Preferred treatment of significant wounds is hospitalization, elevation of the affected part, moist dressings, antibiotics and frequent inspection of the wound for evidence of inadequate débridement or infection. Delayed closure or coverage may be required.

Dog or cat bites also require deep, and sometimes extensive, débridement. With the single exception of a face bite, these animal wounds are not closed. Treatment seldom requires hospitalization but includes elevation, soaks, dressing and antibiotics. An argument can be made for primary closing of dog bites on the face or on other exposed areas, since only 10 to 15 per cent of such closed wounds become infected. The cosmetic advantages of closing a large skin injury on the face of a child are obvious. Before such closure can be undertaken, painstaking débridement of devitalized tissue must be done. Skin closure should be somewhat loose, in contrast to usual plastic techniques of skin repair. After repair, warm, moist soaks are applied at home or in the hospital and antibiotics are prescribed. If the wound is not dressed it can be inspected readily and evidence of infection detected early.

Bites of field animals, such as the fox, bat, raccoon and squirrel, are managed similarly to those of dogs and cats. In all animal bites the question of rabies is raised. If the offending animal cannot be observed, initiation of rabies prophylaxis should be considered[15] (Table 4-1). Further description of the treatment of bites is in Chapters 5, 9, 14 and 28.

Snakebite

Four types of venomous snakes are found in the United States. Three are pit vipers (Crotalidae): the rattlesnake, the cottonmouth moccasin and the copperhead. The fourth, the coral snake, differs from pit vipers in that it has a venom similar to the Indian cobra. Snake venom causes local tissue necrosis by means of proteolytic enzymes and other substances. Secondary edema may compound local ischemia, endangering viability of an extremity. In addition to local effects, venom may cause neurotoxic or hemotoxic reactions. Among the latter are decreased levels of fibrinogen and platelets and hemolysis of red cells.

TABLE 4–1 A Guide to Prophylaxis Against Rabies in Exposed Persons*

A. GENERAL CONSIDERATIONS
1. Rabies occurs in many wild animals, bats and domestic animals such as dogs, cats and cattle, but rarely, if ever, in rodents.
2. A dog or cat that remains healthy for 10 days after a bite does not have rabies, and prophylaxis for a person bitten by that animal is not indicated.
3. A negative fluorescent antibody (FA) examination of an animal brain in an experienced laboratory is reliable evidence that the animal did not have rabies.
4. Saliva of a rabid animal on an open wound (usually a bite) or mucous membrane constitutes exposure to rabies.
5. A decision to initiate postexposure prophylaxis is based upon balancing two probabilities: (1) that rabies virus was introduced into an exposed person and (2) that a serious reaction to prophylaxis material might occur.
6. The Center for Disease Control's approach to rabies postexposure prophylaxis is summarized in the figure below. The guidelines illustrated constitute an algorithmic interpretation of the U.S. Public Health Service's official treatment recommendations.

B. POSTEXPOSURE RABIES PROPHYLAXIS ALGORITHM

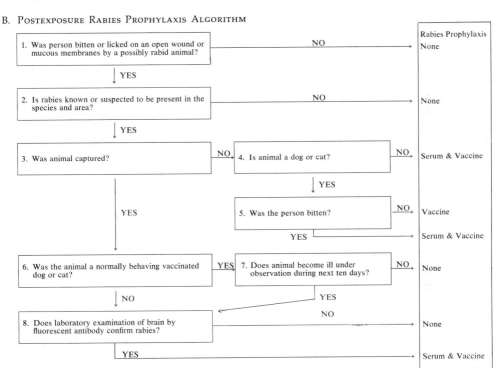

C. PRINCIPLES OF POSTEXPOSURE PROPHYLAXIS
1. Local wound treatment—very important. Thoroughly scrub the wound with soap and water.
2. Indications for immunization, dosages, injection sites and adverse reactions (see algorithm):
   a. For all bite exposures, unless rabies can be excluded, and for all nonbite exposures if animal is proven to have or is strongly suspected of having rabies, provide both passive and active immunization.

Human Rabies Immune Globulin (RIG): Give 20 international units per kg of body weight.

or

Equine Antirabies Serum (ARS): Give 40 international units per kg of body weight.

With either RIG or ARS, infiltrate the wound with up to 50 per cent of the material and give the remainder intramuscularly in the buttocks. RIG eliminates the hazards of sensitivity to horse serum. RIG or ARS is administered only one time, at the initiation of antirabies therapy.

and

Table continued on the following page

TABLE 4-1   A Guide to Prophylaxis Against Rabies in Exposed Persons* *Continued*

Rabies Vaccine (V): Give a total of 23 doses, one dose daily for 21 days (or two doses daily for seven days and then one dose daily for seven days). Then for either schedule, give an additional dose 10 and 20 days after the primary series. Give vaccine subcutaneously in abdomen or thigh, rotating sites of injection.

    b. For nonbite exposures from escaped dogs or cats in a rabies endemic area (this is the only indication for using vaccine prophylaxis alone):

        Rabies vaccine: Give a daily dose for 14 days subcutaneously in abdomen or thigh, rotating sites of injection.

ADVERSE REACTION

Human rabies immune globulin (RIG) or Hyperab® is the "biological of choice" for passive immunization of persons exposed to rabies. Local pain and slight febrile response may occur following the administration of RIG. Although not reported after RIG, angioneurotic edema, nephrotic syndrome and anaphylaxis have been reported very rarely after injection of ordinary human immune serum globulin.

*Based on recommendations of the Committee on Trauma, American College of Surgeons. Bulletin of American College of Surgeons, October 1978, pp 16–17.

Secondary bleeding into tissue may exacerbate local pressure effects.

Of American snakes, the Mojave rattlesnake may possess the most lethal venom. While the coral snake's venom is nearly as deadly, it is injected in smaller amounts and kills less often. Next in order of danger are the eastern diamondback rattler, the western diamondback rattler, the cottonmouth and the copperhead.

Treatment of venomous snakebite varies widely in this country. Techniques popular in one area are sometimes ignored in another. Reasons for such variation are regional differences in venom potency and the fact that envenomation occurs in only 50 to 70 per cent of bites. Thus each wound is a singular challenge in terms of both treatment and prognosis.

First aid in the field for the victim of a poisonous snake bite is immobilization. Walking should be minimized. Evacuation by any other means is preferred. If the bite is on an extremity a flat tourniquet should be placed proximally to occlude lymphatic but not arterial flow. The purpose of tourniquet compression is to retard venom absorption. Once applied, the tourniquet should not be removed until definitive care is available. If distal swelling develops, the tourniquet can be loosened.

After applying a tourniquet, a linear full thickness skin incision is made through puncture wounds. It is often possible to connect fang sites. A linear incision is preferred to cross-hatching. The benefit of applying suction to the wound by mouth or bulb syringe has not been proven. When the patient has reached a treatment facility, deep excision of the wound site is advisable. The tourniquet is removed when the wound is excised. An ellipse is made in skin surrounding puncture wounds and carried through underlying tissue to deep fascia. Venom, loculated in deep subcutaneous tissue, can be removed with the specimen. The extremity is then kept in an elevated position.

Use of antivenin either in the field or in the Emergency Room is controversial. Known allergy to the horse serum in antivenin precludes administration until a physician can effect desensitization. When antivenin is indicated a polyvalent preparation (Wyeth) is used. One vial in 100 milliliters of saline is given intravenously over 15 to 20 minutes. With evidence of generalized envenomation such as muscle fibrillation, unresponsiveness, and a bleeding tendency the same dosage should be repeated. Additional administration of antivenin is of questionable benefit. Antivenin for patients bitten by coral snakes differs from Crotalidae antivenin. Separate antivenin is required after bites of the North American coral snake and coral snakes found in Arizona and New Mexico.

Steroids may be given during the acute treatment of snakebite. A bolus of methylprednisolone (1 gm) given intravenously is recommended. Tetanus prophylaxis and antibiotics are also given.

In the absence of generalized life-threatening envenomation, local and regional tissue injury is the target of therapy after first aid. The value of injecting antivenin locally around the bite is debated. Certainly antivenin should not be injected into a closed tissue space such as a finger. The question of fasciotomy in an extremity that is rapidly swelling is best answered by a surgeon, although primary care physicians must occasionally confront this issue. Disappearance of palpable distal pulsation with signs of tissue ischemia are signs that fasciotomy may already be too late to save the extremity. Mechnical devices such as the

Doppler ultrasound make determination of peripheral pulses more accurate, despite soft tissue swelling and ecchymosis that may obscure an underlying normal artery.

With evidence of envenomation, coagulation defects should be assessed and treated with fresh blood or plasma. Renal function requires monitoring to detect acute tubular necrosis due to hemolysis.

Insect Bites

BROWN RECLUSE SPIDER (Fig. 4–7). While insect bites are potentially dangerous in terms of hypersensitivity reactions, they seldom result in lesions requiring surgical treatment. A notable exception is the bite of the brown recluse spider (*Loxosceles reclusa*), which can cause severe local reaction with tissue loss, intravascular hemolysis and death.[1]

The brown recluse spider thrives in dark corners of outbuildings, attics and storehouses. It is prevalent in southern

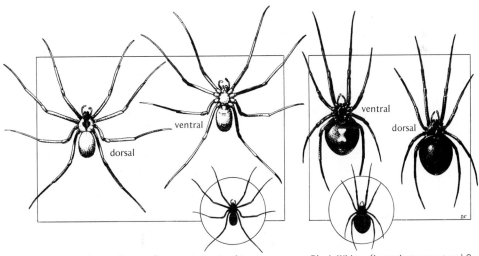

Brown Recluse (*Loxosceles reclusa*) ♀   Black Widow (*Latrodectus mactans*) ♀

Figure 4–7   (Left) The brown recluse spider (*Loxosceles reclusa*) is light brown in color with a darker violin-shaped marking on the back.

(Right) The black widow spider is shiny black with a ventral marking that resembles a red hourglass.

Comparative sizes of two spiders (females) are shown in the insets.

and southwestern United States but ranges from the Midwest to the Gulf of Mexico and from the Rocky Mountains to the Atlantic coast. The spider's body, 10 to 15 millimeters long, is brown in color with a darker, violin-shaped marking on the back that extends caudally from three pairs of eyes. Other spiders of the genus *Loxosceles* resemble the brown recluse in having the same fiddle marking on the carapace and in having the capacity to produce loxoscelism.

The venom of the brown recluse spider is primarily cytotoxic. The initial injury is endothelial damage to arterioles and venules, which become occluded with thrombi. Capillary stasis with tissue infarction and necrosis follow. A spreading zone of hemorrhage, stasis and thrombi occurs with focal abscesses in the superficial fascia.

The diagnosis of loxoscelism is often made in retrospect. The bite may be inconspicuous. Two to eight hours later the area becomes painful when a transient erythema develops at the site. A pale, mottled, cyanotic ischemic center becomes apparent with formation of a bleb. On the third or fourth day the center turns dark red or violet in color and, within another day or two, sloughs to form an ulcer that is often several centimeters in diameter. Surrounding tissue becomes gangrenous in some cases and underlying joints may be destroyed. Healing is slow, as the ulcer remains indolent for several weeks.

Systemic manifestations of loxoscelism result from intravascular hemolysis of blood and can include hemolytic anemia, thrombocytopenia and hemoglobinuria. Transient fever, malaise, nausea, vomiting, joint pain and a petechial skin eruption may occur within 48 hours. Crampy abdominal pain, jaundice, convulsions and phlebitis have been reported. Diffuse intravascular coagulation, probably secondary to hemolysis, may cause multiple hemorrhages. Such complications are

more severe in children. Death follows renal failure, hemorrhage into a vital structure or sepsis. Surprisingly, systemic symptoms are not proportional to the severity of skin lesions.

Treatment of the brown recluse spider bite varies with the degree of local and systemic reaction. Small areas of mild cutaneous involvement may regress without treatment. Local pain and swelling are reduced by cold compresses, immobilization and elevation. Ulcers measuring 1 cm or larger usually require excision with simultaneous removal of underlying tissue, including toxin-bearing superficial fascia. If gangrene surrounds the ulcer, excision of all diseased tissue is necessary.[2] This is especially true when the ulcer overlies a finger joint and the danger of secondary osteomyelitis with joint destruction exists. Established ulcers heal slowly over several weeks. Skin grafting may accelerate wound closure.

Systemic disease requires early, vigorous treatment. Steroid therapy is recommended in decreasing doses over ten days. Antihistamines are often used but with unproven benefit. Heparin is indicated if there is evidence of diffuse intravascular clotting. Renal function should be monitored closely, since renal failure is the most common cause of death. Antibiotics are prescribed for secondary infection.

BLACK WIDOW SPIDER (Fig. 4–7). The black widow, in contrast to the brown recluse, causes little local tissue damage but kills by direct toxicity. It is found typically in rocks, debris, basements and privies in the South, Ohio Valley and West Coast but may be seen in any state except Alaska. The spider is shiny black and shaped like a shoe-button. On the ventral surface is a red hourglass marking shared by no other arachnida. The female black widow is 10 mm in length and 7 mm wide.

The black widow's bite may cause no more than a pinprick sensation. Dull pain at the site occurs later when the fang marks are surrounded by redness and edema. Abdominal pain often is associated with a bite on the lower extremity, while pain in the chest, back or shoulders may follow a bite on the arm. Patients may groan persistently and grunt with expiration. Restlessness, fever and hypertension are seen later.

Treatment of the black widow spider bite is local cleansing, an ice pack and antivenin (Antivenin, Lyovac). Skin testing is essential because the antivenin is in horse serum. Desensitization material is usually available with the antivenin. The usual dosage is 2.5 milliliters of restored serum given intramuscularly. If pain recurs, one or more additional doses may be given. In the absence of antivenin, pain may be treated with a muscle relaxant or with 10 per cent calcium gluconate given intravenously.

SCORPION. This arachnid can be found in the Southwest and is occasionally transported elsewhere in packages or products from infested areas. It resides under rocks, in debris and in dark places in the home. Its activity is nocturnal. Scorpions vary in length from ½ to 8 inches and are black or yellow in color. Their appearance is crablike with a segmented tail terminating in the stinger.

The scorpion's sting brings sharp pain followed by paresthesia. There is no local swelling or discoloration. Untreated patients develop itching of nose, mouth and throat, speech impairment, restlessness, muscular spasm, pain, vomiting and convulsions. Symptoms last 24 to 48 hours. If the bite is not fatal within three hours, the prognosis is good.

Initial treatment is to place ice packs around the sting site and to apply a tourniquet proximally if the sting is on an extremity. The victim is immobilized to delay spread of venom. Species-specific antivenin is indicated but is difficult to obtain. A foreign source is Laboratories MYN, S. A., in Mexico.

Multiple scorpion stings can be rapidly fatal. A sting on the face, back of neck or genitalia is especially dangerous.

BEE STING. Stinging insects (Hymenoptera) include bees, bumblebees, wasps, yellow jackets, hornets and ants. Identifying features of these insects are commonly appreciated. The venom of bees and wasps contains histamine, amino acids, hyaluronidase and acetylcholine. Antigenic proteins in venom are species-specific, allowing cross-reactivity between insects. Reaction to stinging depends upon the amount of venom injected, the site, the number of stings and the presence or absence of sensitivity. Local reaction to a single sting begins as a small red area at the site surrounded by a flare of erythema and a ring of pallor. A wheal forms and subsides within a few hours followed by itching and heat.

Treatment for local reaction is symptomatic. The site is cleansed and ice packs are applied. Elevation of an extremity is helpful. Oral antihistamines may reduce urticaria. The stinging apparatus often is seen to be anchored at the site by two barbed lancets. Pulling out this apparatus may release more venom. An exuded poison sac can be removed, however, by scraping with a fingernail or knife blade.

The danger of hymenoptera stings is severe systemic and anaphylactic reaction.[7] General reactions range from urticaria, itching and malaise through generalized edema, wheezing and vomiting to dyspnea, dysphagia and confusion. A severe shock state with cyanosis, hypotension and coma may supervene. Treatment for these complications is adapted to the nature and severity of symptoms, for example, barbiturates for extreme restlessness, IV fluids for repeated vomiting and diarrhea.

Emergency treatment for anaphylactic reaction is to inject 0.2 to 0.5 milliliter of epinephrine (1:1000) subcutaneously and repeat smaller doses as often as every 15 minutes if needed.

An antihistamine such as diphenhydramine, 20 to 50 mg, should be given intravenously. Steroids, methylprednisolone 0.5 to 1.0 g, should be added to an IV solution. If the sting is on an extremity, a tourniquet is tied proximally and loosened every 15 minutes. Oxygen is administered by nasal prongs or endotracheal tube if the patient is cyanotic.

SUTURES AND DRESSINGS

Suture Repair

Principles

The technique of suturing, as used by the outpatient surgeon in closing wounds, is intended to provide precise coaptation of skin edges and obliteration of subcutaneous spaces. Suturing is a skill resulting from both instruction and experience and it requires that no further tissue damage follow its use. All elements of the procedure must be kept sterile to guard against infection. To minimize trauma, the smallest possible diameter of suture consistent with adequate strength is used. The suture must be easily manipulated, easily tied and, once tied, securely knotted. Occasionally superficial lacerations may be closed securely without sutures, using the "butterfly" adhesive strip shown in Figure 4–8 or individually packaged adhesive strips of ⅛ or ¼ inch widths (Steri-Strip). Such strips can also be used to support a wound following suture removal. The choice of a nonsuture technique in primary wound closure requires easy skin coaptation, sufficient surface for tape adhesion and patient acceptance of possibly less than ideal cosmesis.

Types of Sutures

There are two types of suture material, absorbable and nonabsorbable. Absorbable sutures are made of animal

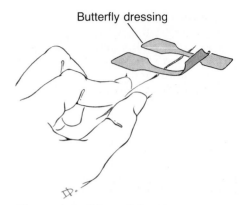

Figure 4–8 *"Butterfly" Adhesive Wound Closure*. Simple, rapid closure of clean superficial lacerations can be accomplished without sutures by applying "butterfly" adhesive strips to coapt skin edges.

tissue and are proteolytically dissolved by the host. Plain catgut, made from the submucosa of sheep small intestine, dissolves in human tissue within a week. Impregnating catgut with chromic oxide (chromic catgut) extends resistance to proteolysis for 10 to 40 days, depending upon the degree of impregnation. Polyglycolic acid suture has greater tensile strength than catgut, handles more easily, but is absorbed between 7 and 30 days. The absorbable suture materials are used for closing of subcutaneous tissues and for ligation of small blood vessels. Their disadvantages are the stimulation of greater local tissue reaction than nonabsorbable materials and the absorption of water which, by causing swelling, loosens knots. Since they are readily absorbed, these substances do not cause chronically draining suture sinuses as do silk sutures.

Nonabsorbable sutures are useful for skin closure and for ligation of larger blood vessels. Silk is a commonly used nonabsorbable suture material. It consists of the protein fibroin extruded by the silkworm. Its advantages are good tensile strength, little tissue reaction, pliability and secure knots. Cotton shares many of these advantages. Other nonabsorbable materials are mono-filamentous synthetic polymers, such as Dacron or nylon, and stainless steel. These substances elicit less trauma reaction than silk but involve either more difficult tying or less knot security. Polypropylene suture (Prolene) currently is popular for use in skin closure.

The size of suture selected for any purpose is determined by its diameter and knot-pull tensile strength. The material used need not be stronger than the tissue it will hold together. Thus catgut used in subcutaneous tissues can be size 3–0. Silk or synthetic suture for approximating the skin is usually size 4–0. Sutures used on the face are often smaller than this and those suitable for injuries of the eye are not larger than size 6–0.

Individually wrapped, sterile sutures are now available in plastic envelopes which open easily by cutting or tearing off the end of the envelope. Material for ties, either absorbable or nonabsorbable, can be unraveled and stored in or under a towel with only the tip of each piece protruding. Thus, each length can be readily grasped. Spools of tie material are not needed in the outpatient repair of most lacerations.

Both absorbable and nonabsorbable suture materials are usually swaged into suitable needles. This arrangement minimizes tissue trauma and the surgeon's effort. Having separate suture material and needle requires that the surgeon place the suture in the needle and hold it there. To do this rapidly the empty needle is best held in the needle holder as it will later be used, the middle of the curve squarely placed about 2 millimeters from the tip of the instrument. While the needle is immobilized in the needle holder, the suture is advanced through the eye for at least one quarter of its length. It is unnecessary to lock the ends through the holder tips. French-eye needles, which allow the use of heavy sutures on relatively small needles, are threaded by first passing the suture around the tip of the holder and then with tension slipping the material through the notch in the needle eye. Tapered or "round" point needles are used to suture subcutaneous structures. Cutting edge needles which more easily puncture tissue are used to suture skin.

Placement of Sutures

Most minor lacerations require only closure of the skin. If a significant subcutaneous defect exists, the surgeon should suspect injury to deeper structures. When this cannot be confirmed, the subcutaneous tissues are approximated by absorbable sutures placed in Scarpa's fascia. Few sutures are needed to accomplish this closure in most wounds. Subcutaneous sutures provide support for skin closure and are the principal source of wound strength during the first week or two following removal of skin sutures. Since tissue apposition without necrosis from tight sutures is the goal, skin is closed with simple interrupted nonabsorbable sutures. The depth of the suture bite in terms of distance from the skin edge should equal the distance between bites (Fig. 4–9). The skin edge can be manipulated by the use of fine-tooth tissue forceps placed on subcuticular structures. This avoids pressure necrosis of epithelial edges. If

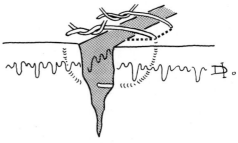

Figure 4–9 *Simple Interrupted Suture.* In simple interrupted suture technique, the distance from the skin edge should equal the distance apart to avoid tissue ischemia. Bites are taken well through the full thickness of skin.

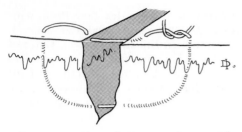

Figure 4–10 *Vertical Mattress Suture.* The vertical mattress suture, which includes bites at the skin edges, coapts layers precisely to enhance appearance and healing.

coaptation of edges is difficult, especially in the center of the wound, vertical mattress sutures can be used (Fig. 4–10).

Arterial bleeders in the depths of a lacerated wound can be securely controlled by means of a suture ligature, as illustrated in Figure 4–11. The ligature is useful when the vessel cannot be grasped with a hemostat. An alternate technique is to pass the needle through the vessel wall and to tie the suture on both sides.

Knot-tying

The outpatient surgeon ties knots to achieve wound hemostasis and closure. Since sutures usually are placed superficially in nonvital tissues, techniques of knot-tying receive little attention. Actually it is just as essential to tie surgical knots well in repairing a laceration as it is in performing other surgery, since the complications of poorly tied knots may be significant. Complications of poor knot-tying include the release of bleeders, skin necrosis and wound separation.

Tension ties are to be avoided but occasionally are needed to approximate wound edges. Simple overhand knots will loosen by the time the rest of the knot is completed unless strands are kept taut throughout.

TWO-HAND KNOT (Fig. 4–12). This is the most reliable way to tie a square knot. Although slower than the one-hand technique, it insures a more dependable knot, especially under tension. For this reason many surgeons prefer the two-hand tie. It is important to lay the first half of the knot "flat." Unless strands have been crossed initially, this requires crossing the hands between the first and second halves. Two-hand knots tied without crossing the hands at the end of either the first or second half do not lie flat and may become untied.

ONE-HAND KNOT (Fig. 4–13). This tie is executed rapidly and allows the surgeon to retain a needle holder in the opposite hand along with one strand of suture. Again, hands must cross to lay the knot flat and to insure stability.

INSTRUMENT TIE (Fig. 4–14). Another technique of tying a surgical knot while retaining a needle holder is the instrument tie. Here the instrument acts as a hand in forming loops. The tie is useful only when tension is not required. It is of value when one end of the suture is short and cannot be held.

Wound Dressing

Dressings are used primarily to protect wounds from trauma and contamination. In some instances, they contribute to healing by controlling bleeding, obliterating dead space, supporting structures or relieving pain by immobilizing the wound area. Clean wounds treated early and closed primarily seldom require a protective dressing for more than 24 hours. Wound infection rates in dressed and undressed surgical wounds are not significantly different. Open, draining or otherwise complicated wounds, however, benefit from dressings which protect regenerating epithelium, debride developing granulation tissue and absorb exuded fluid. (See "wet-to-dry" dressings, page 110.)

Surgical dressing is less formalized
Text continued on page 128

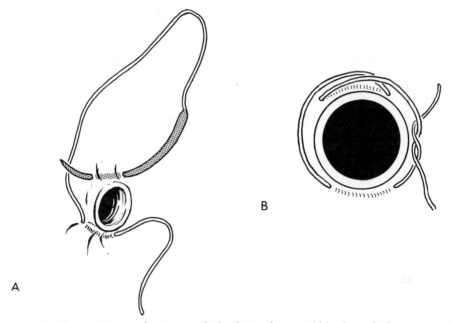

Figure 4–11 *Suture Ligature for Retracted Blood Vessel.* Arterial bleeders which retract into the wound and cannot be clamped and tied adequately are controlled by means of a suture ligature, usually of fine silk, which circumferentially compresses the vessel.

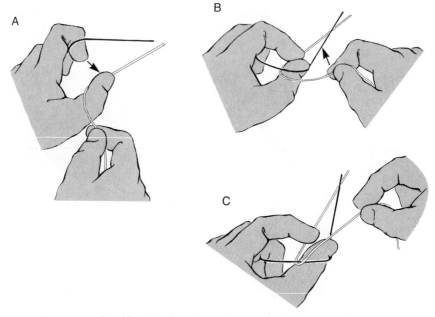

Figure 4–12 The *two-hand knot* is illustrated. Suture ends are uncrossed as Step A begins. Hands must cross at the end of the first loop tie (Step F) *(opposite page)* to produce a flat knot. Hands are not crossed at the end of the second loop tie (Step J) *(opposite page)*.

Illustration continued on opposite page.

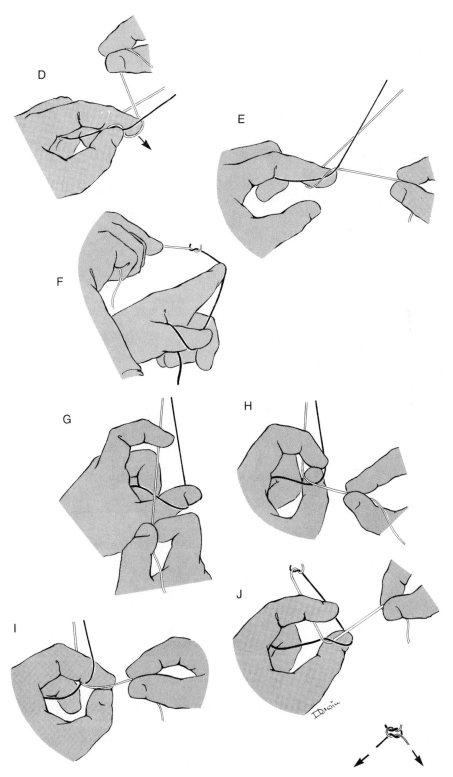

Figure 4–12 *Continued.*

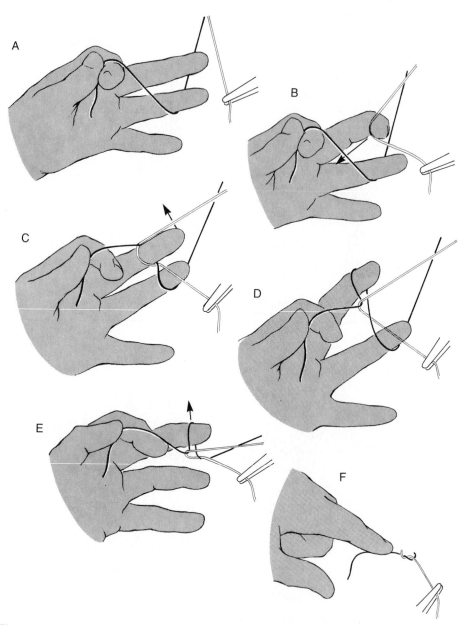

Figure 4–13 The *one-hand knot* is illustrated with one end of the suture grasped by an instrument. In Step A the light colored suture end is crossed over the dark colored suture before beginning the tie. Hands are uncrossed at the end of the first loop tie (Step F) but must be crossed after the second loop tie to produce a flat square knot.

Illustration continued on opposite page.

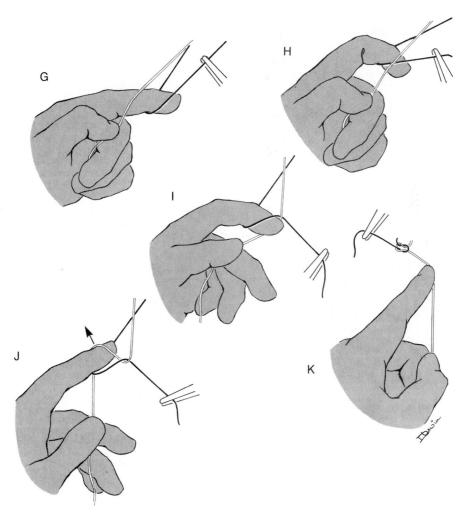

Figure 4–13 *Continued.*

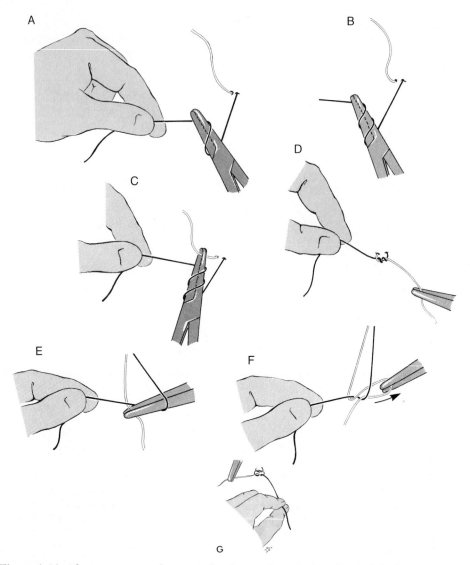

Figure 4–14 The *instrument tie* begins with either single or double (illustrated) looping of the long end of the suture about the needle holder. The first loop is laid flat without crossing hands. Hands must be crossed after the second loop tie (Step G) to produce a flat square knot.

today than previously. Newer materials allow less bulky dressing and are easily applied and reliably secured. Nevertheless, dressing techniques are important. Certain principles will be discussed here while specific techniques are illustrated in chapters appropriate to the body region.

Closed Wound Dressing

Most closed wounds, such as contusion and hematoma, require no dressing. Recently sutured lacerations may be protected by covering with wide-mesh gauze secured by adhesive. Squares of gauze, individually wrapped and sterile, are readily available to the outpatient surgeon. After suture repair, the skin is gently washed with sterile water or saline. Sterile gauze pads, two to three layers thick, are placed over the wound when the skin is dry. Antiseptic paint is not required on the suture line. Two or three strips of adhesive secure the gauze without preventing ventilation through the dressing.

Shaving skin hair and applying tincture of benzoin increases the adhesiveness of tape strips. Cloth-backed adhesive, while strong and moderately waterproof, occasionally causes skin irritation that may result in blisters. It is frequently painful to remove from hairy parts of the skin. Tape backed by a nonwoven viscose rayon largely avoids these disadvantages while remaining strongly adherent. It is easily cross-torn by the hands or by a dispenser and is considerably lighter than conventional adhesive. If occlusive or waterproof dressings are required, tape backed with polyethylene plastic may be used. This material contains no sensitizing ingredients and is transparent. Its elasticity makes tearing difficult. Commercially prepared adhesive strips with central gauze squares (e.g., Band-Aid) are ideal for protecting small wounds.

Another method of protecting sutured wounds or holding dressings in place is the use of collodion or plastic aerosol sprays. No additional benefit has been shown to result from combining the spray with an antibiotic. When the spray dries, a tough, thick, clear film protects the wound and allows continuing observation. Wounds of the face and neck where dressing is difficult are well treated with this technique.

Open Wound Dressing

Open wounds exude serum which dries to form a surface eschar. Porous dressings such as gauze become incorporated into the eschar and are sealed to the wound. This can be both helpful and harmful in terms of wound healing. Removing adherent gauze from infected granulations removes tissue debris, thereby debriding the wound. Delicate new epithelium growing across the wound, on the other hand, may be lost by dressing with adherent gauze. Nonporous materials lack debriding benefits but protect regenerating epithelium. The type of open wound thus dictates the type of dressing needed.

Adherent, porous dressings are ideal for granulating wounds which are heavily contaminated or infected. Fine mesh gauze is used because only small tufts of granulations become fixed in mesh pores and are debrided by dressing removal. The resulting surface is cleaner and more even. Soaking facilitates dressing change and débridement. When a healthy granulating surface is obtained and re-epithelization is likely, nonporous dressings may be used.

Initially, clean superficial open wounds, such as abrasions, are dressed with a nonadherent material such as Telfa. This is a cellophane-like substance with many fine perforations too small to allow tissue ingrowth but large enough to permit circulation of air. Wax or petrolatum-impregnated gauze is another nonadherent dressing. Its disadvantage is skin maceration due to lack of ventilation and drying. Both adherent and nonadherent dressings are backed with gauze and secured by adhesive, plastic spray or bandaging.

Draining wounds present a special problem. Sufficient gauze should cover the wound to absorb all drainage and to keep the skin dry. Dressings of open wounds should be inspected daily and changed if saturated with drainage. Larger amounts of absorbent gauze may be needed to avoid rapid resaturation. Change of dressing is an aseptic procedure requiring sterile gloves, instruments and face mask.

Dressings impregnated with antibacterial agents are helpful in treating minor burns and superficial wounds. In general, however, topical antibiotics are of limited value and may in some cases interfere with tissue regeneration. Deep lacerations that cannot be closed primarily are packed loosely with sterile gauze to keep skin edges apart until secondary healing obliterates the open base.

Pressure Dressing

In order to tamponade superficial wound bleeders or to obliterate tissue spaces, flat or fluffed gauze is heaped over the wound site and maintained under pressure by circumferential bandaging or noncircumferential elastic adhesive. The latter is particularly useful in applying local pressure. Since this type of bandage tends to unroll at the ends or sides, it is surrounded by narrower strips of adhesive plaster.

Bandaging

Bandage materials, once limited to gauze, muslin or flannel, now include a variety of elastic cottons and adhesives. Elastic cotton is commonly available in rolls 2 to 6 inches wide. It

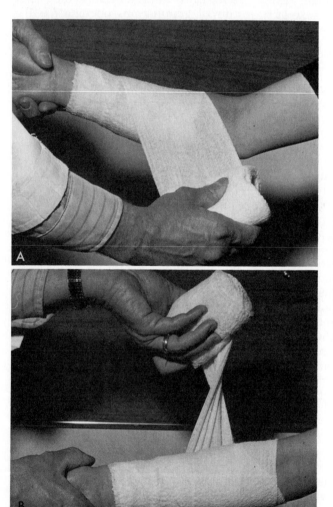

Figure 4–15 *Forearm Bandage Technique. A.* Elastic cotton is ideal material for bandaging an extremity. To secure a forearm dressing, three inch bandage is wrapped twice around the arm distally and advanced proximally with circular, overlapping turns. *B.* Snugness of the bandage is increased by rotating the bandage roll 180° after each circular turn to effect a reverse spiral.

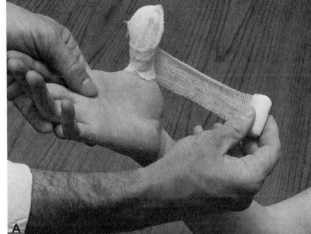

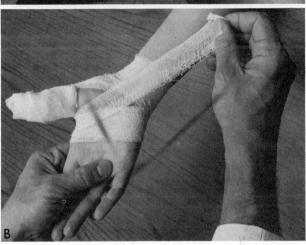

Figure 4–16 *Stump Dressing Technique. A.* Bandaging a finger with elastic cotton narrowed to one inch in width begins by passing the bandage lengthwise over the digit to effect coverage and locking it in place by circular turns. *B.* The bandage is secured by passing the roll above the palm and wrist and taping the end.

can be rapidly, snugly and neatly applied regardless of previous experience. The elastic qualities of the bandage allow it to conform closely to body contours. While a moderate degree of pressure can be exerted by circular wrapping, occlusion of major arteries is quite unlikely. The material is washable, allowing reuse. This is of some advantage to the outpatient who may be responsible for changing his dressing.

Elastic cotton (Kerlix) is well-suited for use on extremities where circular bandaging is required to stabilize dressings. Figure 4–15 illustrates the application of such a dressing on the forearm. After covering the wound with gauze squares, sterile elastic cotton bandage, 3 inches wide, is wrapped twice around the arm distal to the wound to fix the bandage. The material is unrolled by advancing proximally with circular, overlapping turns. The end of the bandage is secured to the material by adhesive. This dressing may be made more snug by rotating the roll 180 degrees after each circular turn to effect a reverse spiral.

In bandaging any distal area such as an amputation stump or finger, elastic cotton is again useful. Strips of the bandage are rolled lengthwise over the stump and locked in place by circular turns (Fig. 4–16). An alternative technique is to use tubes of elastic cotton

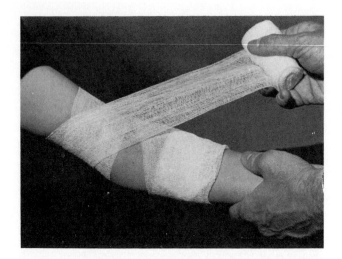

Figure 4–17 *Figure of Eight Bandage Technique.* To bandage joints, elastic cotton is anchored proximally by taking several turns and then unrolled obliquely across the joint and anchored below by a complete turn. The process is repeated until dressings are securely covered.

(Tubex) and special applicator frames. Elastic cotton bandaging of joints allows mobility while maintaining dressings in place. When elastic materials are unavailable, a figure-of-eight bandage of gauze or muslin may be used to bandage joints. The technique is shown in Figure 4–17. Several turns are taken distal to the joint to anchor the bandage. The material is then unrolled obliquely across the joint and anchored above by a complete turn. Again the bandage is brought obliquely across the joint space and anchored below by a complete turn. The process is repeated until dressings are securely covered.

The use of elastic adhesive bandages as part of pressure dressings has been described. These materials are also of value in fixing dressings to the chest, abdomen or pelvis. Elastic adhesive allows the chest to expand and contract without dislodging the bandage, and it can be maintained in areas where other bandages fail to hold. Because of a tendency to unroll at both ends and sides, elastic adhesive should be bordered by ordinary adhesive plaster.

Plaster splints are sometimes incorporated into bandages to reduce mobility and thus to promote healing. These splints are most commonly used on the volar aspect of the forearm, wrist and hand, on the extensor surface of the elbow and on the posterior aspects of the lower leg and the sole of the foot. Plaster is particularly useful if a skin graft has been applied.

The primary purpose of bandaging is to secure and protect underlying wound dressings. The appearance of the bandage is important, however, in that patients may judge the excellence of their treatment by the neatness of their bandage. While aesthetic considerations are not crucial, they contribute to the technique of bandaging. A trim bandage usually indicates that care has been taken to avoid wrinkles that might create undue pressure and loose turns that might shorten the effective life of the dressing.

REFERENCES

1. Arnold, R. E.: Brown recluse spider bites: Five cases with a review of the literature. J. Am. Coll. Emerg. Phys., 5:262–264, 1976.
2. Aver, A. I. and Hershey, F. B.: Surgery for necrotic bites of the brown spider. Arch. Surg., 108:612–618, 1974.
3. Blitt, C. D., Wright, W. A., Petty, W. C. and Webster, T. A.: Central venous catheterization via the external jugular vein: A technique employing the J-wire. J.A.M.A., 229:817–818, 1974.
4. Cornell, W. P., Ebert, P. A., Greenfield, L. F. and Zuidema, G. D.: A new nonoperative technique for the diagnosis of

penetrating injuries to the abdomen. J. Trauma, 7:307–314, 1967.

5. Demuth, W. E., Jr.: Bullet velocity as applied to military rifle wounding capacity. J. Trauma, 9:27–38, 1969.

6. Fine, K. S., Bassin, R. H. and Stewart, M. M.: Emergency care for tear gas victims. J. Am. Coll. Emerg. Phys., 6:144–146, 1977.

7. Frazier, C. A.: Those deadly insects. R. N., 4:49–55, 1971.

8. Hickman, T. C.: Abdominal paracentesis. Surg. Clin. North Am., 49:1409–1412, 1969.

9. Jernigan, W. R., Gardner, W. C., Majr, M. M. and Milburn, J. L: Use of the internal jugular vein for placement of central venous catheter. Surg. Gynecol. Obstet., 130:520–524, 1970.

10. Mitty, W. F., and Nealon, T. F.: Complications of subclavian sticks. J. Am. Coll. Emerg. Phys., 4:24–28, 1975.

11. National Safety Council: Accident Facts. Chicago, 1976, p. 3.

12. Perry, J. F., McMeules, J. E. and Root, H. D.: Diagnostic peritoneal lavage in blunt abdominal trauma. Surg. Gynecol. Obstet., 131:742–744, 1970.

13. Radiation Injury. *In* McCarroll and Skudder (Eds.): The treatment of mass civilian casualties in a national emergency. Washington, Medical Education for National Defense, 1967.

14. U. S. Department of Health, Education and Welfare: Acute conditions: Incidence and associated disability. Rockville, Maryland, 1977, pp. 1–3.

15. U.S.P.H.S.: Recommendations of Advisory Committee on immunization practices. Washington, 1976.

16. Yoffa, D.: Supraclavicular subclavian venipuncture and catheterization. Lancet, 2:614–617, 1964.

Infections 5

ANDREW M. MUNSTER, M.D.

"If thou examinest a man having a diseased wound in his breast: while the two lips of that wound are ruddy, and that man continues to be feverish, his flesh cannot receive a bandage. I will make cool applications for drawing out the inflammation, applications for drying up the wound, and poultices."

(Anon., 3000 B.C. *In* Breastead, H. H. (Ed.): The Edwin Smith Surgical Papyrus. Chicago, University of Chicago Press, 1930, Case 41, pp. 371–391.)

INTRODUCTION

The prevention and treatment of infections in an outpatient setting represent a substantial amount of effort and time for the surgeon. At the Baltimore City Hospital Emergency Room and walk-in clinic, of 64,000 patients seen in 1976, 18.8 per cent presented some infectious problem, and in 4.8 per cent the problem was deemed surgical. This represents 3072 visits per year, or 8.4 each day. The scope of the problem is therefore considerable.

There are two distinct aspects to the surgical infection — that of prevention and that of treatment. In prevention,

the outpatient surgeon should adhere to sound principles of asepsis in preparing patients for elective minor surgery, and in the cleansing and débridement of traumatic injuries. The surgeon should also be thoroughly familiar with the indications for the use of prophylactic antibiotics and tetanus prevention. In treatment, the primary task is the recognition of infection, followed by the exercise of considerable judgment in when to intervene surgically in the natural history of an infection. Other considerations include the technique of drainage of abscesses and the selection of appropriate antibiotics when indicated. The goal of treatment

134

at all times should be the early restoration of intact function and the prevention of morbidity and mortality.

Infections involving some areas demand special expertise and, since they are fully discussed elsewhere in this book, will not be considered in this chapter. These include infections of the eye, ear, nose and throat, the gastrointestinal tract, bones and joints, teeth and venereal disease.

PREVENTION OF INFECTION IN THE OUTPATIENT DEPARTMENT

The Environment

Surgeons sometimes assume that because most procedures performed in the outpatient setting are "minor," aseptic principles in the performance of these procedures can be relaxed. Nothing could be further from the truth. Admittedly, the full degree of asepsis aimed at in the hospital operating room is almost impossible to achieve, but one must remember that infection is a quantitative, not qualitative, event. Just because a wound is already contaminated we are not at liberty to contaminate it further by neglect of aseptic principles, since there is, in most situations, a "critical mass" of bacteria beyond which host defenses are overwhelmed and infection occurs.

The basic design of the Emergency Room/outpatient clinic area is important. One may rarely get the opportunity to contribute to the design of such an area in the blueprint stage, but existing facilities can often be utilized so as to substantially diminish the risk of cross contamination. Each outpatient clinic should have three basically distinct areas. The first is for the treatment of major emergencies; this must be well lit and roomy. Contamination by clothing, soil, attendants and so on is almost unavoidable here and this must be taken into consideration in planning. The second area is for "clean" elective minor surgery, such as the removal of sebaceous cysts, moles and the repair of small, clean lacerations. This area should have all the amenities of an operating room, including its own supply cabinet, scrub sink, gowns, masks, caps and gloves, a proper operating room table complete with appropriate armboards, and a good light with spotlights. Instruments prepackaged in a central supply area should be stored here for use only in this area. Traffic should be restricted to the patient and his immediate attendants. The borrowing of equipment and instruments from other areas of the outpatient clinic should be minimized. The third basic area is the "dirty" room, where abscesses may be drained and procedures that do not require asepsis, for example, the application of plaster casts, may be carried out.

Outside these three basic areas there must be a triage area where a decision is made on where to send each patient and from which a patient may be transported into one of the three basic areas without crossing another. These principles are illustrated in Figure 5–1.

Attention to environmental surveillance and handwashing techniques is part of the responsibility of the outpatient surgeon. The outpatient clinic is an integral part of the hospital, and regular bacteriological sampling of floors, walls, equipment and personnel

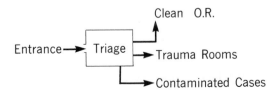
Clean O.R.

Entrance → Triage → Trauma Rooms → Contaminated Cases

Figure 5–1 Organization of clinic facilities to reduce contamination: receiving rooms for trauma near entrance, and inner rooms for "dirty" and "clean" cases.

should be carried out in coordination with the hospital infection control committee, much in the same way it is for the intensive care unit or any other critical care area. The housekeeping service must establish regular cleaning procedures for floors and other surfaces, using modern techniques such as wet-vacuum pickup and a germicide that is acceptable to the hospital infection control committee. Materials that harbor bacteria and are difficult to clean, such as cloth isolation curtains, should be replaced by pretreated or plastic materials. Handwashing is particularly important for the outpatient surgeon and staff, since the chance of contamination by hand carriage is so great in the outpatient department. The iodophors, which are water-soluble complexes of iodine with organic compounds, reduce hand bacterial counts most efficiently. If drying or cracking of the hands occurs after prolonged use, a hexachlorophene preparation may be used.[1] With either preparation, gloves should be worn when handling any wound, clean or otherwise.

Preparation and Draping for Surgery

Preparation and draping should be carried out as carefully as for any elective surgical procedure. In the management of traumatic wounds, hair in the vicinity of the wound must be shaved, care being taken not to allow the shaved hair to fall into the wound. If this is not done, hair may be turned into the sutured wound and act as a foreign body. On the scalp, it is advisable to clip the hair around a wound with a clean pair of scissors first, followed by shaving. The area for repair is then prepped in the usual fashion, the antiseptic of choice again being the iodophor group.

In the case of repair or débridement of contaminated wounds, copious irrigation with saline and removal of gross

obvious contaminants such as clothing or tar particles should be carried out prior to prepping and draping. Tincture of iodine, removed rapidly by alcohol, is a satisfactory substitute for the iodophors as a prepping agent, but the tincture is more irritating. Both iodine and the iodophors are irritating to the eyes and should not be used around the face, where benzalkonium chloride (Zephiran, a quaternary ammonium compound) is more advisable. Benzalkonium is an inferior antiseptic agent when compared with the iodophors because it is inactivated by protein, cellulose fibers and other organic material; it is also relatively ineffective against *Pseudomonas aeruginosa*.[1] However, the face is so vascular that infection of surgical wounds is comparatively rare here and the safety of benzalkonium chloride for the conjunctiva makes it a more acceptable agent. Tinted tinctures of benzalkonium are available and outline the prepped area conveniently. For clean and elective procedures, the technique for prepping is centrifugal, as illustrated in Figure 5–2. For massively contaminated wounds — abscesses

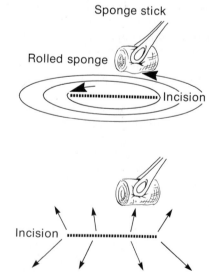

Figure 5–2 Skin preparation: Two acceptable techniques of centrifugal scrubbing and application of disinfectant.

and so on — prepping should be centripetal, that is, it should begin at the periphery of the area to be prepped and work carefully toward the center.

In draping, the outpatient surgeon should remember that the patient is often in pain or afraid and is usually under local anesthesia; therefore, he is likely to move on the operating table. The use of "area sheets" — drapes with small pre-cut holes allowing exposure of the surgical area only — is unsuitable in most instances, since the "hole" tends to move around, forcing the surgeon to drag and pull at the drapes in the middle of the procedure. This is inconvenient and leads to contamination. It is far better to prep a large area (for example, the entire face in the case of a facial laceration) and fix the drapes firmly at the periphery of the prepped surface, exposing a large prepared area.

Principles of Débridement

The prevention of infection in traumatic wounds is one of the most important duties of the surgeon working with outpatients. Despite the advent of powerful new antibiotics over the last few decades and despite our increased understanding of the mechanisms of infection and resistance, there is still no substitute for compulsive care of the wound. The technical principles involved in this care may be summarized as gentle handling of tissues, effective removal of foreign material and devitalized tissue, adequate hemostasis and elimination of dead space. Large, crushing instruments should not be used. Hemostats that inevitably crush tissue must not be applied to skin edges. Fine, nonirritating suture material such as nylon is preferable to silk for skin closure. The decision to excise devitalized tissue requires a great deal of judgment; skin should always be saved if possible, especially on the face. If there is a question about the viability of tissue it

is wise to leave the wound open and inspect it again the following day, at which time the viability of deep tissue is usually more obvious.

The search for a foreign body should begin with the finger and continue with gentle probing with an instrument. X-rays may be of help, in case the foreign body is radiopaque; x-rays should always be taken in at least three planes to aid localization. Glass may or may not be radiopaque, and if a fragment is available from the glass that caused the injury, the piece should be placed on the x-ray plate near the injured part so that its radiolucency may be defined with the identical exposure technique. If the presence of a foreign body is demonstrated or strongly suspected but not readily found, the operation should be approached without haste, using extreme care and excellent anesthesia. The removal of metallic foreign bodies, especially needles, which are deeply embedded may exceed the facilities available in the outpatient department, in which case admission of the patient and operative extraction under full anesthesia and a tourniquet may be wise.

Hemostasis should be obtained with equal care. There is no place for the hurried placement of blind sutures, or groping with hemostats in the depths of poorly illuminated wounds. Bleeding can almost always be slowed considerably with simple pressure, and the gradual release of pressure from one part of the wound, then another, will help identify the bleeding site so that it can be secured with certainty. The use of fine ligatures tied gently is recommended. If the bleeding point cannot be visualized with accuracy, figure-of-eight or horizontal mattress sutures of fine catgut may be tied around the suspected bleeding point. In the scalp, which usually bleeds profusely, temporary hemostasis can be obtained by placing hemostats on the galea aponeurotica and turning the hemostats back to lie on the scalp. The wound can be approximated with through-and-through interrupted simple sutures, which will encompass the retracted bleeding vessels and secure hemostasis.

A difficult decision is whether the method of closure should be primary or delayed. If the wound is recent (under 12 hours), if contamination is minimal, dead space can be eliminated, débridement has been satisfactory and the wound edges can be closed without tension, then the wound should be closed primarily. If the wound is old, contamination is massive, tissue damage extensive or if there is doubt whether débridement has effectively removed all dead soft tissue and foreign body, it is better to pack the wound lightly with gauze and plan for delayed primary closure after two to three days, or to allow the wound to granulate and heal spontaneously without sutures. This last-named method is termed "healing by secondary intention." In either case, the injured part should be gently immobilized with a splint, a sling or both, in a position of function; rest is important in the prevention of infection. Antibiotic therapy should be considered in the presence of massive contamination.

The introduction of quantitative microbiology has provided some new information on the indications for primary closure. In one recent study of 59 hand injuries,[2] the presence of 10^5 or more microorganisms was considered a contraindication to primary closure; three of four wounds that were closed with higher counts became infected. Of the total of 18 infections, only eight grew out pure cultures. The remainder grew out a mixed growth of several organisms, attesting to the difficulty in predicting proper antibiotic therapy for these injuries.

The rate of infection following traumatic injuries is difficult to ascertain, but has been reported as high as 23 per cent.[3] Obviously, every effort must be made in the individual patient to reduce this potentially high incidence.

DOCUMENTATION AND FOLLOW-UP

Proper documentation and adequate follow-up of outpatients with wounds or infections is imperative. In the case of a wound, documentation should include the location and extent of the injury, the degree of contamination, the time elapsed since injury when first seen, vascular and neurological findings distal to the injury, the results of exploration and the technique of repair. If the wound was closed primarily, it should be reinspected the next day. If it was left open, it should be inspected and repacked every day until a decision regarding delayed primary closure has been made. The patient must be warned to look for possible signs of infection such as increasing pain, or fever, and instructed to return if these symptoms appear. If an abscess was drained, the sending of material for culture should be documented and arrangements should be made for the resulting information to reach the surgeon as soon as possible, since a change in antibiotic therapy may be indicated. A sketch in the chart depicting the injury or abscess is entirely appropriate and often illustrates the problem better than a written description.

LABORATORY STUDIES

In the diagnosis and treatment of suspected or proven surgical infections in the Outpatient Department, a few basic laboratory studies are helpful. X-rays for the detection of foreign bodies have already been mentioned; radiology may also be valuable in the detection of soft tissue masses, osteomyelitis or air in the tissues (see Fig. 5–5). A hemoglobin or hematocrit and white blood count determination with differential count may be helpful, as well as an analysis of the urine and determination of the blood sugar for the detection of occult diabetes. More important, microbiological tests must be readily accessible in the outpatient department. As a minimum standard, facilities for the Gram-staining of specimens, a centrifuge for examining urinary sediments and a microscope to examine smears and stains must be available in the outpatient area. Optimally, an incubator in which bacteriological samples can be stored overnight in appropriate media and culture plates on which specimens can be immediately smeared should also be located in the area. The surgeon should, in addition, be familiar with the techniques of aspiration with saline to obtain bacteriological samples, transportation and storage techniques for anaerobic organisms, biopsy for culture, particularly for fungi, and scraping of lesions for fungi.

The simplest and quickest technique for obtaining information is the Gram stain. The steps are as follows:[4]

(1) Place specimen on a clear slide and make a thin film.

(2) Air dry, then heat gently. Do not overheat.

(3) Flood slide with crystal violet for 10 seconds, rinse with tap water.

(4) Decolorize with 95 per cent ethanol until practically colorless and rinse with tap water.

(5) Flood with safranin for 10 seconds. Wash off with tap water and dry. The specimen is now ready for microscopic examination. The reader is referred to Gardner and Provine[4] for various other techniques of staining and illustrations of typical organisms under the microscope.

Anaerobic cultures may be important, since unless they are cultured immediately after opening an abscess, anaerobic organisms are killed by contact with oxygen and become unrecoverable on the surface, although still causing continued infection in the deeper tissue planes. In gathering anaerobic cultures, pus or fluid should be obtained instead of a swab if at all possible, and the specimen placed in a special anaerobic transport medium for the laboratory. Several satisfactory anaerobic transport media are available commercially. Some rely on a vacumsealed transport tube; the specimen must be injected through a rubber stopper into the oxygen free environment. Others utilize tubes filled with an inert gas heavier than air, into which the specimen may be placed. It is important to understand the requirements for each type of medium; in case of doubt, the hospital clinical laboratory should be consulted.

Biopsy of the edge of hard-to-diagnose lesions may be required to recover an organism. The biopsy may be performed under local anesthesia. The specimen should be placed on a sterile piece of gauze, and sectioned into two pieces. One should be placed in 10 per cent formalin for pathological examination, the other placed sterile into transport medium for the microbiology laboratory. This technique is particularly useful for chronic, indolent lesions when a low grade fungal infection is suspected (for example, *Aspergillus* and *Actinomyces*).

For surface scrapings in suspected fungal skin lesions, the following technique is recommended:[5]

(1) Clean skin surface with ethanol.

(2) Scrape scales and epidermis with a number ten blade, place on a clean slide and cover with coverslip.

(3) Apply 1 to 2 drops of 10 per cent potassium hydroxide to the edge of the coverslip, allowing the peroxide to seep under the coverslip. Heat gently on a bunsen burner and cool. The slide is now ready for examination.

DIAGNOSIS OF INFECTION

Infection in the normal host causes local inflammation; therefore, the classic signs of heat, redness, swelling, pain and loss of function will be pres-

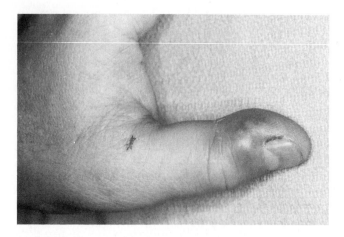

Figure 5–3 This 30 year old housewife pricked the nail-fold of her left thumb with a diaper pin while changing the baby. Within three days, throbbing pain and swelling developed, her temperature was 101° F, and she was feeling ill.

Diagnosis: Paronychia, acute. Controlled promptly by antibiotic therapy, incision and drainage. The pus grew out a pure culture of *Escherichia coli*, which is unusual in cases of paronychia but understandable in view of the history.

ent to a greater or lesser degree, perhaps accompanied by fever, malaise and an elevated white cell count with a "shift to the left" in the differential. That these symptoms and signs are present in the *normal host* is emphasized, because they are altered in many patients. Moreover, these are features only of an acute pyogenic infection: infection by many other organisms does not produce these manifestations. A deep seated abscess, such as an ischiorectal abscess, is usually manifested by fever and malaise and vague perineal pain, but on physical examination only some induration may be found in the perianal area, with no obvious redness or edema. A chronic in-

fection by staphylococci of low virulence is sometimes present on the dorsal aspect of a finger; the symptoms consist of discomfort and swelling; and physical findings will reveal slight brawny induration and flaking of the epidermis of the skin, but little more. Such relatively low grade findings usually accompany the inflammatory process in immunosuppressed patients, and in these patients the clinician must have a high index of suspicion that an infection is present, even if the classic signs of inflammation appear in a subdued form. These patients include diabetics, individuals receiving corticosteroids or anti-inflammatory agents (aspirin, aceta-

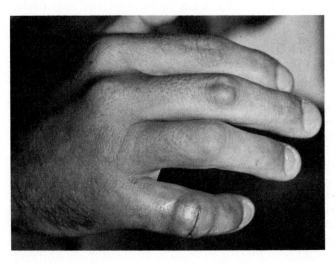

Figure 5–4 A 24 year old man cut the back of his right little finger with a knife. Within 12 hours he was feeling unwell and the finger began to swell slightly. By 24 hours he had a fever of 103° F, marked erythema and tenderness around the cut, with red streaks visible along the forearm and tenderness in the axilla.

Diagnosis: Acute streptococcal cellulitis by Group A β-hemolytic *Streptococcus*. Prompt response to penicillin. Since there was no suppuration, surgical intervention was unnecessary.

minophen), cancer chemotherapy or radiation therapy, and individuals with some uncommon congenital immunodeficiency syndromes. Some surgical infections are illustrated in Figures 5–3 to 5–10, which show the wide variety of problems that may be encountered in an outpatient department.

A few infections have characteristics that enable the clinician to make an immediate diagnosis or at least strongly suspect it. A partial list follows.

Bright red, rapidly spreading (hours), poorly localized infection; fever; little or no pus; Group A, β-hemolytic Streptococcus

Abscess with creamy yellow odorless pus: *Staphylococcus aureus*

Brownish foul pus, especially in immunosuppressed patients: *Bacteroides spp.*

Tissue crepitation: Clostridial gas gangrene (especially if foul odor is present) or nonclostridial, possibly polymicrobic, anaerobic infection

Persistent suppuration in relation to an air sinus or orbit, commonly seen in a diabetic: Mucormycosis

Chronic skin infections with considerable induration and inflammation but little pus: Blastomycosis (especially of the scrotum), histoplasmosis, actinomycosis

Relatively painless infection of fingers and toes, especially with ulceration: pyogenic infection secondary to neuropathy; look for diabetes, leprosy, neurological disease

Chronic suppuration or "cold" abscess with little fever, erythema or pain in a cervical lymph node-bearing area: Tuberculosis

Abscesses and sinuses in the face and neck area discharging "sulfur granules": Actinomycosis

Reddish-purple subacute infection on the hands of humans who work with fish, swine and cattle: *Erysipelothrix rhusiopathiae*

Painless ulcer of genitalia, lips or perianal area: Syphilis

Chronic paronychia: Atypical myco-

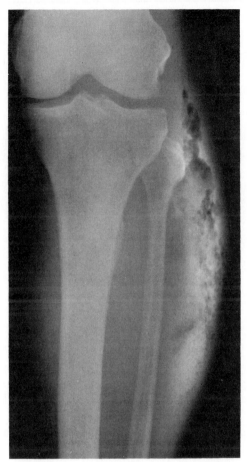

Figure 5–5 A 54 year old laborer was seen in the Emergency Room after a blunt injury to the calf. No break in the skin was noted and the patient was treated with rest, heat and analgesics. Eighteen days later he returned with fever, marked toxicity and considerable local pain. This x-ray was taken, showing gas in the soft tissues.

Diagnosis: An unusual case of gangrene. The leg was saved by prompt surgery and extensive débridement of dead muscle. Cultures grew *Clostridium welchii*.

bacterium (tropical fish fancier) or fungus

Chronic suppuration and sinus formation of the feet in certain tropical areas of the world: Fungus, especially Maduromycosis

Recurrent boils, especially in hospital personnel: *Staphylococcus aureus* (penicillinase producing)

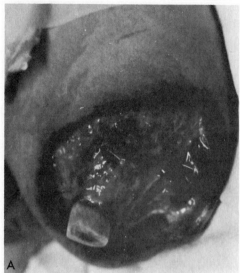

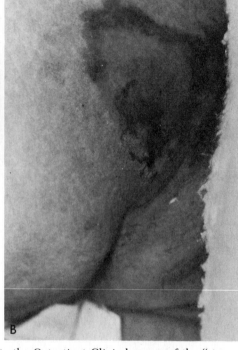

Figure 5–6 Two lesions characteristic of infection by *Pseudomonas aeruginosa*. A. The thigh of an above-knee amputee recently discharged from the hospital with a healed stump. He fell, injured the stump and did not report for several days, at which time the above picture was taken.

B. An elderly nursing home resident brought to the Outpatient Clinic because of the "strange appearance" of a pressure sore on the sacrum. Note the circumferential discoloration around both lesions, which *in vivo* was purplish-black. The lesion is due to vasculitis by an advancing margin of *Pseudomonas* infection. Both patients required surgical débridement.

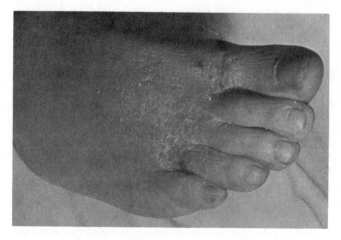

Figure 5–7 The dangers of topical corticosteroids. This patient had an itchy lesion on the dorsum of the foot, and the skin had been broken in several places by scratching. The diagnosis of dermatitis was made and he was given a steroid ointment to rub into the foot. Within three days he presented with pain, swelling, redness and fever. Saline aspiration of the subcutaneous tissues grew out a pure culture of *Staphylococcus aureus*. He responded slowly to discontinuation of steroid therapy, bed rest with elevation of the foot, local heat and antibiotics.

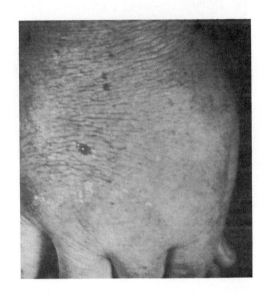

Figure 5–8 A dangerous occult lesion. This 250-pound diabetic sustained a second-degree burn and in the course of therapy received intravenous therapy through a scalp-vein needle inserted into a hand vein. Although the needle was removed after just a few hours, he presented five days later with high fever, delirium and a red, edematous hand. Pressure above the old venipuncture site produced the drop of pus illustrated in the picture. Culture of the pus and blood culture grew out *Staphylococcus aureus.* Case of suppurative thrombophlebitis. This patient required surgical exploration of the back of the hand, resection of a length of vein filled with purulent thrombus and intensive antibiotic therapy.

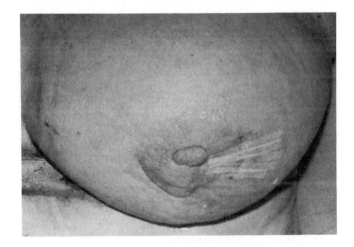

Figure 5–9 This 53 year old patient presented with the history of an injury to the breast three weeks previously, followed by the development of marked swelling and pain in the breast. Physical examination showed acute tenderness, induration and edema of the breast with tender axillary nodes. She had a fever of 101.4° F. A small incision placed over the maximal point of induration, as shown, revealed only solid tissue.

An example of a condition that often masquerades as an infection. The preoperative diagnosis was breast abscess. The frozen section showed tumor. Case of mastitis carcinosa.

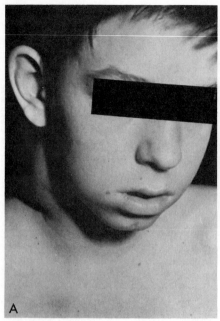
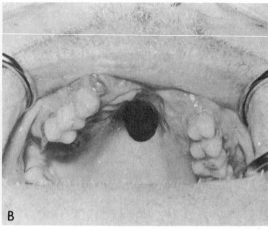

Figure 5–10 Two classic surgical lesions that are still seen occasionally. *A*, A young boy with a soft, painless, fluctuant swelling in the neck. No tenderness, redness or heat is present. Case of scrofula, or cold abscess: tuberculous lymphadenitis of the cervical lymph node with abscess formation. *B*, The palate of a 74 year old man who had never sought medical help for a speech defect of several years' duration. Case of a syphilitic gumma.

Purulent, painful urethral or vaginal discharge: *Gonococcus*

Axillary or groin abscess: Cat-scratch fever, lymphoma, bubonic plague

Chronic fever and weight loss associated with formation of small abscesses: Tularemia, brucellosis

Drug addicts with fever and local abscesses at injection site: Malaria, tetanus, suppurative thrombophlebitis and its complications — septicemia, endocarditis, pulmonary embolism

Each community and state has specific requirements for reporting infections, but, in general, a call to the County Health Department regarding any bizarre infection is wise; in addition, the hospital Infection Control Committee should be notified.

TREATMENT OF INFECTIONS

Once the diagnosis of a surgical infection is made, treatment must be commenced. The modality of treatment has to be decided upon, and it will generally fall into one or a combination of three methods: local nonsurgical, surgical or chemotherapy. The choice of therapy and particularly its timing can tax the judgment of the most experienced surgeon, yet it is of crucial importance because the wrong choice may lead to much increased morbidity or even mortality. The main questions that usually arise are these: Can the progression of the infection be aborted by local treatment and, if so, should antibiotics be used or not? When is surgical intervention such as incision and drainage necessary? Should antibiotics be used in addition to surgical intervention? We will attempt to consider each of these problems.

Local Therapy

The mainstays of local nonsurgical therapy are rest, heat and elevation of the affected part. Rest relieves pain and restricts the spread of infection by allowing the host defense mechanism such as inflammation to localize the offending microorganisms. Heat causes vasodilation and allows the increased exudation of antibodies, opsonins, and neutrophil leukocytes to the site, again increasing the capability of the host to deal with the infection. Heat may be applied by towels wet with warm water wrapped around an extremity or, more conveniently, by simply wrapping the area with wet towels and enclosing it in a plastic bag, allowing the body to generate its own heat. In the case of a finger or toe, soaking for twenty minutes in warm water three to four times a day will achieve the same effect. If the infected area is open, edema may be reduced by adding an osmotic agent such as Epsom salts to the soak. Elevation reduces edema and helps to increase lymphatic flow, which increases comfort. It is important that the patient be given precise rather than vague directions. Elevation should be carried out by means of a sling, and the patient taught how to put it on. At night, or in the case of the lower limb, the extremity should be elevated on two or three soft pillows. Two heaped tablespoonfuls of Epsom salts dissolved in half a pint of warm water provide a simple hyperosmotic solution for soaks.

The indications for this type of therapy are diffuse, nonfluctuant infections that are poorly localized, such as a mild paronychia or minor cellulitis consequent upon a small laceration. Topical antiseptics such as Mercurochrome may be helpful; in the case of open wounds with signs of mild infection, the use of a topical antibiotic such as bacitracin or polymyxin may be employed, but the possibility of patient sensitization must be borne in mind. These simple principles are illustrated in Figure 5–11.

In infections that appear to be more severe and accompanied by fever, malaise or other systemic symptoms, yet are not well enough localized for drainage, the surgeon may choose to add antibiotics to this regimen. It is often preferable, however, to avoid antibiotics unless the patient is either really ill or the affected part is of vital functional importance, such as one of the fascial spaces of the hand. If antibiotics are not used, the infection may

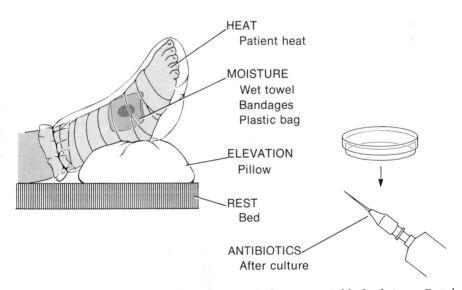

HEAT
Patient heat

MOISTURE
Wet towel
Bandages
Plastic bag

ELEVATION
Pillow

REST
Bed

ANTIBIOTICS
After culture

Figure 5–11 Nonsurgical treatment for infections which are not suitable for drainage. Rest, heat, moisture, elevation, and antibiotics if infection is serious. Watch for lymphangitis, which should be treated with antibiotics.

resolve or proceed to suppuration, in which case it may be drained surgically. If antibiotics are used the infection may also resolve; on the other hand, it may become a lingering chronic infection harboring resistant organisms and may not either resolve or suppurate. These are among the most difficult to deal with.

Surgical Intervention

Surgical intervention is clearly indicated if a foreign body is suspected within an area of infection, dead or devitalized tissue is present, the infection is thought to be anaerobic (crepitus) or when fluctuation becomes apparent in an area of infection. Foreign bodies may consist of sutures in a repaired wound, which must be removed if they are causing infection, or other embedded foreign matter in an infected area of traumatic injury which must likewise be removed. Devitalized and necrotic tissue should be debrided by sharp dissection.

Incision and drainage (I and D) is probably the most common intervention practiced in the case of surgical infections, and good results demand close attention to technique. To perform I and D in the outpatient department, one must first be certain that it can be done adequately without hospitalization and general anesthesia. The latter is often preferable with children and in the case of deep seated abscesses (for example, most perirectal abscesses). When in doubt, the error should be made in the direction of admission and anesthesia, for inadequate drainage will inevitably lead to recurrence and prolongation of morbidity. For most abscesses, simple infiltration of the line of incision with local anesthesia is adequate. Anesthetic techniques for special areas such as fingers are described in specific chapters related to regional anatomy.

Ethyl chloride spray was formerly used as a topical anesthetic for I and D of superficial abscesses, but its use should be abandoned. Ethyl chloride anesthetizes by temporarily freezing the skin as it vaporizes. It does not produce good anesthesia in most cases, and there is also the risk of frostbite or damage to other structures, such as the eyes of the patient or of the physician. Furthermore, ethyl chloride vapor is highly inflammable and can easily be ignited with a spark or electrocautery.

The technique of I and D is illustrated in Figure 5–12 (I). Immediately upon entering the abscess cavity, aerobic and anaerobic cultures should be taken. Following spreading, if the incision is large enough, a gloved finger should be introduced gently into the abscess cavity and loculations broken down. After evacuation of the pus, the cavity must heal by granulation from the bottom up; therefore the skin incision must be kept open until the cavity is obliterated. To facilitate this process, to provide further drainage by capillary action and to help débridement, it is customary to lightly pack the abscess cavity with plain or iodoform ribbon gauze, or 4 × 4 inch gauze. If more than one piece of foreign material is introduced into the cavity, the pieces should be tied together because it is easy to lose one otherwise. Packing should be removed and reintroduced daily.

Some abscesses that are extremely superficial and nearly ready to rupture may be treated simply by aspiration with a needle and syringe. A dry sterile dressing is then applied, and the patient soaks the area intermittently in warm water for a few days until healing is complete. A culture may be made from the aspirated pus if an unusual organism is suspected.

When the abscess is deep to an area of necrotic skin or fat, simple I and D may not be sufficient and the abscess may need to be "de-roofed," with actual removal of the necrotic cover. Examples are carbuncles and deep perirec-

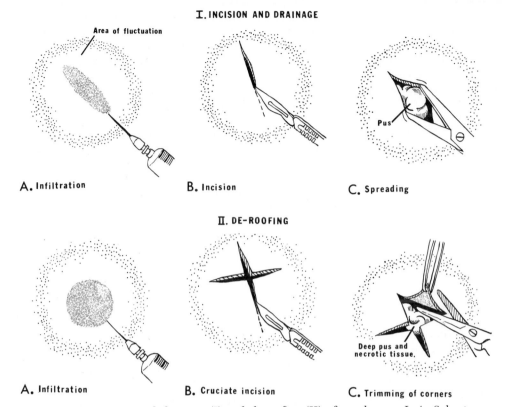

I. INCISION AND DRAINAGE

Area of fluctuation

A. Infiltration

B. Incision

Pus

C. Spreading

II. DE-ROOFING

A. Infiltration

B. Cruciate incision

Deep pus and necrotic tissue.

C. Trimming of corners

Figure 5–12 Incision and drainage (I) and de-roofing (II) of an abscess. I. *A.* Subcutaneous infiltration of local anesthetic over the fluctuant area. *B.* Incision carried over the entire extent of fluctuation. *C.* Widening or spreading to allow the escape of pus.
II. *A.* Infiltration of a circular area over the abscess. *B.* Cruciate incision over the area of induration. *C.* Conversion of cruciate incision to a diamond-shaped defect with actual removal of tissue of the abscess roof to allow for free drainage of pus and necrotic material.

tal abscesses. The author's technique is illustrated in Figure 5–12 (II).

Without question, the most crucial aspect of the I and D is its timing. An area of inflammation or induration in which central fluctuation is beginning is usually not ready for incision, since more pus is likely to form. Such an area should be treated conservatively, with or without antibiotics, for a few days and watched closely until the area of fluctuation is maximal and surrounding inflammation has begun to subside. If an abscess ruptures spontaneously, the surgeon must not assume that drainage is adequate. The opening usually needs to be enlarged surgically, and the cavity explored as described above.

Chemotherapy

Chemotherapy, in addition to the other measures described above, is indicated when the infection is in a functionally crucial area such as the hand, or if the patient shows signs of systemic toxicity such as fever, malaise or leukocytosis. Even if these are present, one may elect to withhold chemotherapy if the abscess is considered ready for drainage, particularly if there is doubt about the nature of the causative organism.

Principles of Antimicrobial Therapy

The principles of antimicrobial therapy are simple, yet it is surprising how often they are totally neglected. The patient pays the price of inappropriate therapy by increased morbidity from the infection, development of resistant organisms and side effects from the drug. These principles, as they apply to the outpatient surgeon, may be stated as follows.

(1) Antimicrobial therapy is *never* a substitute for adequate drainage, débridement and removal of foreign material from the wound.

(2) Antimicrobial therapy should be based, wherever possible, on adequate microbiological information.

(3) One antibiotic is usually preferable to two, unless sound bacteriological evidence indicates the need for multiple drugs.

(4) A change in the drug used should always be based on adequate bacteriological information, follow an adequate trial of the first drug and be justified by clear cut evidence of clinical failure of therapy by the first drug.

(5) A penicillin is usually preferable to a broad-spectrum antibiotic unless there is either bacteriological evidence or strong clinical suspicion that the causative organism is resistant.

In electing to use prophylactic antimicrobial therapy, experience must show that infection is highly likely to supervene in the absence of such therapy; furthermore, the antimicrobial agent must be thought capable of penetrating to the site of potential infection. Once the decision is made to give antibiotics, administration must be prompt. Optimal wound levels may be obtained by simultaneous IV and IM therapy to begin with.[6] On occasion, the surgeon is confronted with situations in which antimicrobial therapy must be used empirically, that is, without evidence of the nature of the pathogen. In such cases, it is useful to know what the normal flora of the area of the body involved is, so that a rea-

sonable guess can be made about the possible pathogen. A list of normal potential pathogenic flora in various parts of the body is presented in Table 5–1.

There are many antibiotics available in today's market, and the resemblance among various trade names is confusing. Table 5–2 lists the generic and commercial names of some of the most commonly used antibiotics and the recommended adult doses. Some of these antibiotics will now be considered in more detail.

ANTIBIOTICS AND OTHER ANTIMICROBIAL AGENTS

In general, antibacterial chemotherapy should be reserved for treatment of specific established infections, rather than in prophylaxis of infection. The use of antibiotics should be instituted advisedly, considering the possibility of drug reaction. The patient and his family should be told the nature of possible drug reactions, so that therapy may be changed immediately if a reaction is noted.

Penicillin

The natural and semisynthetic penicillins are bacteriostatic and bactericidal for multiplying bacteria at low concentrations. The penicillins act by inhibition of cell wall synthesis in bacteria. Relatively high concentrations of penicillin are well tolerated in most individuals. The major problems observed are the emergence of drug-resistant strains of bacteria — especially penicillinase-producing staphylococci — and drug sensitivity. A prior history of allergy to penicillin is, in general, a contraindication to the use of any of the penicillins in outpatient therapy.

PENICILLIN G. Useful against a wide variety of gram-positive organisms, Neisseria and spirochetes. Many streptococci and staphylococci and all

**TABLE 5-1   Empirical Antibiotic Therapy: Guide to Decision Making
Based on Common Habitat of Pathogenic Organisms***

Site	Normal Flora, Potentially Pathogenic	Other Common Pathogens	Antibiotics Most Likely to be Effective
Skin	*S. epidermidis*	*S. aureus* Streptomyces Group A	Nafcillin[1] Cephalosporins[2]
Naso-pharynx	*S. epidermidis* *S. aureus* Streptomyces Group A *Diplococcus pneumoniae* *H. influenzae* Anaerobic streptococcus (Peptostreptococcus)	Candida Fusobacterium Bacteroides	Penicillin Nafcillin Erythromycin Cephalosporins
Lower GI tract	*Bacteroides fragilis* *E. Coli* Enterococcus (Strep. Group D. or *S. faecalis*) *Proteus sp.*[3] Enterobacter sp.[4]	*S. aureus*	Clindamycin *or* chloramphenicol, both with Gentamicin alone *or* with gentamicin and penicillin (Enterococcus)
Soil (wounds)	Clostridia *Proteus vulgaris*[3] *Ps. aeruginosa*[5]		Penicillin Nafcillin Cephalosporins

*For further details, the reader is referred to Hoeprich, P. D. (Ed.): Infectious Disease. Hagerstown, Maryland, Harper & Row, 1972; and Gardner P., and Provine, H. T.: Manual of Acute Bacterial Infections. Boston, Little, Brown & Co., 1976.

[1]A penicillinase-resistant penicillin is advisable because of the increasing incidence of penicillinase-producing staphylococci in the community. The precise choice of drug depends on whether primarily oral or parenteral therapy is being considered (see Table 5–2).

[2]The cephalosporins are here considered as a group. In moderately serious infections, an initial systemic dose with simultaneous commencement of oral therapy (e.g., cephazolin plus cephalexin) should be considered.

[3]Indole-positive strains of proteus (e.g., vulgaris) should be treated with parenteral aminoglycosides. Indole-negative strains (e.g., mirabilis) usually respond to ampicillin. Obviously, a decision here must be based on culture results.

[4]The Enterobacter spp. are a mixed group of bacteria of which the antibiotic sensitivity is unpredictable — hence no recommendations are made.

[5]*Ps. aeruginosa* is of low pathogenicity except in the immunosuppressed host. Normally, no antibiotic prophylaxis is recommended against this organism.

pneumococci, actinomyces, clostridia and treponema are sensitive to penicillin. Resistance has appeared in staphylococci, many strains of which produce penicillinase, and in increasing numbers of gonococci. Emergence of resistance to penicillin G has not yet become a serious problem with other previously sensitive organisms. Because it is poorly absorbed by mouth, penicillin G is usually administered intramuscularly (see Table 5–2). Adequate blood levels are difficult to maintain on an outpatient basis except for organisms highly susceptible to penicillin. A syndrome similar to serum sickness is a rare but serious side effect of penicillin therapy.

PENICILLIN V. Has a spectrum of activity and resistance similar to that of penicillin G. It is well absorbed by mouth and causes little gastrointestinal toxicity. For outpatient therapy of sensitive organisms, one week of ther-

TABLE 5–2   Trade Names and Dosages of Commonly Used Antibiotics (Adults)*

Generic Name	Trade Names	Oral Dose	Parenteral Dose
Ampicillin	Penbritin, Polycillin, Omnipen, Principen, Totacillin, Pensyn, Amcill	0.5–1.0 G q6h	1.0 G q6h
Carbenicillin	Geopen, Pyopen, Geocillin	2 tablets (382 mg/tab) q6h	20–30 G/day (follow package insert)
Cephalexin	Keflex	0.5 G q6h	—
Cephalothin	Keflin	—	1–2 G q6h
Cephazolin	Kefzol, Ancef	—	0.5–1.0 G q6h
Dicloxacillin	Dynapen, Pathocil, Veracillin	0.5 G q6h	—
Erythromycin	Erythrocin, Ilotycin, Pediamycin, Robimycin	0.5 G q6h	0.5 G q6h
Gentamicin	Garamycin	—	3–5 mg/kg/day in 3 divided doses; follow renal function
Methicillin	Celbenin, Staphcillin	—	1–3 G q6h
Nafcillin	Unipen	0.5 G q6h	0.5–1.0 G q6h
Oxacillin	Prostaphlin, Bactocill	0.5–1.0 G	0.5–1.0 G q6h
Penicillin G	Many names	400,000 U (250 mg)– 800,000 U (500 mg) q6h (before meals)	Procaine penicillin 1.2 mill. U. q12h
Penicillin V	Many names	250–500 mg q6h	—
Tetracycline	Achromycin, Mysteclin, Panmycin, Sumycin, Tetracyn, Tetrex	0.5 G q6h	0.25–0.5 G q6h

*Commercial combinations of antibiotics are not recommended.

apy with 250 to 500 mg p.o. every six hours is generally advisable. It should be given on an empty stomach since food interferes with its absorption. Increasing numbers of relapses of gonorrhea following a course of penicillin have been observed during the past few years. Diligent follow-up information is therefore required to demonstrate cure in these patients. Long-term therapy is needed for actinomycosis, but outpatient treatment of this condition can be effective as long as the necessary surgical therapy has also been performed.

AMPICILLIN. A broad-spectrum penicillin with activity against gram-positive cocci and also against gram-negative bacteria such as salmonella, shigella, *Escherichia coli, Hemophilus influenzae, Neisseria gonorrhoeae* and indole-negative strains of proteus spp. It is useful in the treatment of infections of the urinary tract, ear, nose, throat, and lower respiratory tract, for typhoid carriers and other gastrointestinal infections. It should not be used in outpatient therapy of patients with a prior history of allergy to penicillin. It is not resistant to penicillinase and should not be used for staphylococci resistant to penicillin.

Although ampicillin may be started empirically, a culture and sensitivity test is indicated to guide further therapy. Ampicillin is available in oral and parenteral forms. Superinfections with Pseudomonas, Enterobacter or fungi may emerge during ampicillin treatment.

CLOXACILLIN. This, along with dicloxacillin and oxacillin, is an oral semisynthetic penicillin that is especially useful in the outpatient treatment of penicillinase-producing staphylococci. Methicillin and nafcillin are related drugs that must be given parenterally to achieve satisfactory blood levels, and they are therefore rarely used in outpatient therapy. Cloxacillin is well absorbed and well tolerated by mouth. It has a good spectrum of activity against pneumococci and streptococci, but it is not the best drug for these organisms — penicillin G or V would be preferable. Cloxacillin is indicated as the initial drug in staphylococcal infections, especially if the infection was acquired in the hospital. Fortunately, most strains of staphylococci in the U.S. are still sensitive to cloxacillin and the other semisynthetic, penicillinase-resistant penicillins.

CARBENICILLIN. A benzyl penicillin derivative, particularly useful in treatment of gram-negative bacilli, especially pseudomonas, proteus and some of the rare organisms such as Herellea and Serratia. Pseudomonas frequently develops resistance rapidly, and Klebsiella is usually resistant. Like the other penicillins, it is relatively free of renal toxicity, though blood levels increase rapidly in the presence of poor renal function. Carbenicillin is also effective against gram-positive cocci, but it is not resistant to penicillinase. Parenteral outpatient therapy utilizes 1 to 2 gm IM every six hours. It is mainly used for urinary tract infections in this dosage.

Cephalothin

Cephalothin, cephalexin and cephaloridine are broad-spectrum antibiotics structurally related to penicillin, derived from cephalosporin C. These antibiotics are produced by the fungus *Cephalosporium*. They are powerful bacteriostatic and bactericidal drugs, but multiple daily doses of the parenteral forms required are usually not practical for outpatients. The oral form (cephalexin) is now available and, when used in large doses, it has reportedly been useful in treatment of respiratory and urinary tract infections. Patients with penicillin allergies should receive these drugs with caution, because of crossover allergy due to a structural similarity to penicillin. Nevertheless, a history of penicillin allergy is currently a major indication for the use of cephalosporin derivatives in inpatients. Pseudomonas is notably resistant to cephalosporin derivatives and superinfection with pseudomonas is common in patients treated with cephalosporins. Troublesome proteus or *E. coli* urinary tract infections may be treated with the cephalosporins in cooperative outpatients if sensitivity studies indicate that the organisms are sensitive.

Tetracycline, Chloramphenicol and Erythromycin

These are potent antibacterial agents that act by inhibition of protein synthesis.

TETRACYCLINE. Tetracycline and the tetracycline derivatives are bacteriostatic antibiotics that are mainly useful in treatment of gram-negative infections. Minor infections with gram-positive cocci also occasionally respond to these antibiotics. Tetracycline is relatively less dangerous for short-term outpatient therapy than other broad-spectrum antibiotics. It is particularly useful for treatment of bacterial infections of the biliary, respiratory or urinary tracts. It is also used in treatment of syphilis in patients who are allergic to penicillin. Many problems have been associated with chronic or intensive therapy, including staphylococcal enterocolitis, candidiasis, hepatic failure, deposition of tetracycline in bones and teeth and abnormalities of skin, kidneys and blood. The drug is contraindicated in pregnancy. The most common problem is nausea or diarrhea from mild gastrointestinal toxicity, which subsides when therapy is discontinued. It should be emphasized that tetracycline resistance is common in staphylococci and emerges rapidly during treatment.

CHLORAMPHENICOL. This drug is highly effective in the treatment of a broad spectrum of gram-negative infections, but hematological toxicity generally precludes its use in outpatient surgical infections. Hematological toxicity may occur as an idiosyncratic fatal aplasia, but fortunately this is rare. It is more common to see a dose related and time related leukopenia occur gradually, subsiding when treatmen is stopped. If chloramphenicol is believed to be indicated because of in vitro and in vivo studies, the manufacturer's brochure should be studied carefully and blood counts monitored frequently during therapy.

ERYTHROMYCIN. This is a broad-spectrum macrolide type of antibiotic that is active against multiplying bacteria. Erythromycin is bacteriostatic at low concentrations and bactericidal at high concentrations. It is relatively ineffective against gram-negative infections, except *Corynebacterium diphtheriae*, but it is a very useful alternative to penicillin in many infections with gram-positive cocci. It is well absorbed and well tolerated by mouth. Troublesome side reactions are very rare and ordinarily all side effects disappear when therapy is discontinued. Erythromycin is particularly useful in treatment of β-streptococcal infections, and for other penicillin-sensitive bacteria in patients who are allergic to penicillin.

Streptomycin

Streptomycin is an antibiotic produced by *Streptomyces griseus*. It is useful against a broad spectrum of organisms not affected by penicillin. It is bactericidal in its effects on the cell wall, on nucleic acid formation and on protein synthesis. It is effective against salmonella, Klebsiella and many other gram-negative organisms, but resistance may appear within 24 hours. The rapid emergence of resistant populations and toxicity for the eighth cranial (auditory) nerve have been major problems limiting the usefulness of streptomycin. The discovery of other broad-spectrum antibiotics has essentially reduced the use of streptomycin to short courses, in combination with penicillin G, in mixed infections caused by unknown organisms and in tuberculosis. It is given with careful sequential studies of auditory and vestibular nerve function. The usual course for nontubercular infections is five days.

Kanamycin

Kanamycin (Kantrex) is an antibiotic, derived from streptomyces, with activity against a very broad spectrum of bacteria, including gram-positive and gram-negative cocci and many gram-negative rods. Most strains of Enterobacter and *E. coli* and most strains of proteus are sensitive to kanamycin. It is also effective against salmonella, shigella and *E. histolytica*. Systemic therapy requires parenteral administration, and it is therefore difficult to use kanamycin in outpatients. It also produces renal and eighth nerve toxicity, so careful monitoring is required. Oral therapy is used for preoperative sterilization of the bowel and treatment of sensitive gastrointestinal infections, since kanamycin is not absorbed from the GI tract. Clostridium, bacteroides and yeast overgrowth may occur and should be watched for in patients receiving kanamycin by mouth. Parenteral therapy may be given with doses of 0.5 gm IM every 12 hours and should be limited to five days. Oral therapy for preoperative bowel preparation is given with 1.0 gm per hour for four hours, followed by 1.0 gm every six hours for 36 to 72 hours.

Neomycin

Neomycin is an aminoglycoside antibiotic obtained from *Streptomyces fradiae.* It is bacteridical against a wide variety of gram-positive and gram-negative bacteria, including Proteus. It is useful as an oral, nonabsorbable antibiotic for preoperative preparation of the colon, and for other conditions requiring suppression of intestinal bacteria. It is also used in topical ointments and solutions for treatment of localized, accessible infections. Side effects occurring after oral administration include mild diarrhea, yeast or staphylococcal overgrowth and renal toxicity if ulcerative lesions or large burns are present, permitting absorption into the blood stream. It is a potent intestinal antiseptic and should not be used for more than 36 hours. If symptoms suggesting enterocolitis appear, the patient should be hospitalized promptly. If staphylococcal enterocolitis is demonstrated, treatment may require methicillin and restoration of normal flora with oral lactobacillus (Lactinex) or fecal enemas. Neomycin is given by mouth in doses of 1.0 gm per hour for four hours, then 1.0 gm every four hours for 24 to 36 hours. Topical neomycin is available in ointments, alone and in combination with polymyxin B and bacitracin (Neosporin).

Colistin

Colistin (Coly-mycin) is a polypeptide antibiotic that is bactericidal by absorption into specific receptor sites in gram-negative organisms. It also prevents chromosomal recombination. Since its mechanism of action is different from other antibiotics, its spectrum of action is also different. It is effective against *Pseudomonas aeruginosa,* and also against a wide variety of other gram-negative bacilli. Unfortunately, it is not absorbed from the GI tract and requires parenteral therapy (2.5 mg per kg per day in two to four divided doses, deep IM). Neurotoxicity should be watched for, but outpatient therapy is possible. The patient should receive one dose daily in the clinic and subsequent doses can be given at home by a trained member of the family or by a visiting nurse.

Polymyxin B

Polymyxin B (Aerosporin) is a bactericidal antibiotic derived from *Bacillus polymyxa.* It is effective against most of the troublesome gram-negative bacilli, except proteus. It can be used effectively against Pseudomonas, Klebsiella, Aerobacter and *E. coli,* but systemic use or absorption may produce significant renal toxicity. It must be given parenterally in systemic therapy and frequent checks of renal function are required during therapy, which requires restriction of its systemic use to inpatients. Polymyxin B is a useful and relatively safe topical antibiotic used in treatment of accessible localized infections. It is available in combination with bacitracin (Polysporin) and bacitracin and neomycin (Neosporin).

Gentamicin

Gentamicin (Garamycin) is an aminoglycoside antibiotic with a broad spectrum of activity against gram-negative and gram-positive organisms. Cross-resistance is rare. It has drawbacks similar to the other parenteral antibiotics, and is used infrequently in outpatient therapy.

Bacitracin

Bacitracin is a bactericidal polypeptide antibiotic derived from *B. subtilis*. It is highly effective against grampositive organisms, but because of renal toxicity its use is restricted to topical chemotherapy, usually in ointments, in combination with polymyxin (Polysporin) and polymyxin and neomycin (Neosporin).

Amphotericin B

Amphotericin B (Fungizone) is a potent polyene antifungal antibiotic derived from a streptomyces species. It is supplied as a solubilized desoxycholate salt, and it may be applied topically, administered by mouth or — for systemic administration — given parenterally. It has significant renal toxicity and is usually administered intravenously only to inpatients. However, long-term therapy may be performed intermittently in the outpatient clinic for disease such as meningitis or draining abscesses due to coccidioidomycosis, blastomycosis, cryptococcosis and other systemic fungi. Amphotericin B can also be instilled into spinal fluid or bladder for localized fungal infections.

Mycostatin

Mycostatin (Nystatin) is a nonabsorbable antifungal agent used predominantly in treatment of oral and intestinal or vaginal candidiasis.

Sulfa Drugs

Sulfisoxazole (Gantrisin) is one of several derivatives of sulfanilamide which are useful in systemic antibacterial therapy. The "sulfa" compounds act by competitive inhibition with the essential metabolite p-amino benzoic acid, which is necessary for synthesis of folic (pteroylglutamic) acid. Folic acid is a coenzyme required in synthesis of many nucleic and amino acids. Sulfisoxazole is useful in outpatient treatment of Group A β-hemolytic streptococcus, *E. coli,* Nocardia and lymphogranuloma venereum infections. It is rarely used in acute streptococcal infections, but is well tolerated, inexpensive and relatively potent in acute urinary tract infections such as cystitis and prostatitis. In these cases, symptomatic relief can be accelerated wtih phenazopyridine (Pyridium), a topical mucosal analgesic excreted through the urinary tract. Phenazopyridine is given by mouth in tablets of 200 mg three times daily. Sulfisoxazole is also useful in suppression of chronic urinary tract infections. The effectiveness of sulfisoxazole may be more apparent clinically than in vitro. Sulfisoxazole is effective in long-term therapy with 500 mg four times daily, although acute infections should be treated with twice this dosage for the first few days.

Sulfathalidine and Sulfasuxidine are nonabsorbable sulfadiazine derivatives used for intestinal antisepsis, especially in preparation for surgery of the colon. They appear to be less effective but are also less dangerous than kanamycin and neomycin. Azulfidine is a well tolerated, nonabsorbable sulfa derivative that is commonly used in chronic therapy of ulcerative colitis. Allergy to sulfonamides is relatively common and must be guarded against.

Nitrofurans

Nitrofurans are synthetic antimicrobial compounds that interfere with anaerobic and aerobic carbohydrate metabolism in bacterial cells. A broad spectrum of activity is seen, and resistance rarely appears. Topical nitrofurazone (Furacin) is a highly effective antibacterial agent, useful in secondarily infected excoriations. Most patients tolerate it well, though approximately 1 per cent develop atopic allergic reactions. Nitrofurantoin (Macrodantin, Furadantin) is excreted rapidly in the urine and is a highly effective antibacterial agent for many gram-negative bacillary infections. Its use is limited partially by nausea, and it is also considerably more expensive than sulfisoxazole. The adult dose is 50 to 100 mg four times daily. The drug is satisfactorily absorbed and better tolerated when given with milk. Furazolidone (Furoxone) is used in the treatment of a variety of gastrointestinal infections, including giardiasis. The nitrofurans may cause anemia in patients with glucose 6-phosphate dehydrogenase deficiency, so black patients and patients of eastern Mediterranean ancestry should be observed closely for hemolytic reactions. Monoamine oxidase inhibition has also been reported in association with furazolidone, so sympathomimetic amines and foods containing tyramine should not be given in conjunction with this drug. Chronic pulmonary fibrosis has been demonstrated in some patients treated with nitrofurantoin. The nitrofurans are no longer recommended for the outpatient treatment of burns.

Metronidazole

Metronidazole (Flagyl) is a potent systemic trichomonacide, effective against these organisms in the vagina, in extravaginal sites and in the genitourinary tract. It is given by mouth in doses of 250 mg two to three times daily. Metronidazole has also recently been described as an effective agent in amebic abscesses due to *E. histolytica.* It is currently being used in doses of 1 to 2 gm per day for seven to ten days as an amebicide. The potential of metronidazole against *Bacteroides fragilis* is currently under investigation.

Adverse Interactions

Some antimicrobial agents interact adversely with other pharmaceutical agents or other antibiotics.[7, 8] Some of the more important include the following.

AMINOGLYCOSIDES. Combination with cephaloridine, cephalothin, ethacrynic acid and the polymyxins may lead to increased toxicity. Combination with digoxin may lead to decreased digoxin effect. Simultaneous administration of curariform agents leads to increased neuromuscular blockade.

CEPHALOTHIN AND CEPHALORIDINE. Combination with aminoglycosides, ethacrynic acid, or furosemide may lead to increased nephrotoxicity.

CHLORAMPHENICOL. Combination with oral anticoagulants may lead to increased anticoagulant effect. Combination with oral hypoglycemic agents may increase hypoglycemia.

TETRACYCLINES. Combination with oral antacids, barbiturates and iron may lead to decreased tetracycline effect.

PROBENECID. (BENEMID). Interferes with renal excretion of penicillin, causing elevation of penicillin blood levels.

For further details, the reader is referred to The Medical Letter[7] and Hansten.[8]

SOME SPECIFIC INFECTIONS

A number of surgical infections or clinical situations which may lead to infection are serious enough to warrant specific discussion.

Tetanus

The incidence of tetanus in the U.S. has declined from 300 cases in 1965 to 101 in 1974[9], a tribute to the success of active immunization. The mortality rate still remains approximately 40 per cent[9], so efforts at immunization in prophylaxis and therapy in established cases must remain intense. Tetanus should be suspected in any patient who, following an injury or operation — no matter how minor — and after an incubation period of between a few days to three weeks, complains of muscle spasm, particularly in the muscles of mastication (trismus). All such patients must be hospitalized immediately. The prognosis of tetanus depends on the length of incubation (the shorter the incubation the worse the prognosis) and the rate of progression of symptoms from stiffness around the mouth to full opisthotonos. A progression of a few hours heralds a poor prognosis; several days suggests a more favorable prognosis. Tetanus is more likely to occur, although by no means exclusively, in the presence of massive con-

TABLE 5–3   Guidelines for Tetanus Prophylaxis

Type of Wound	Patient Not Immunized or Partially Immunized	Patient Completely Immunized: Time Since Last Booster Dose		
		1* to 5 Years	5 to 10 Years	10 Years
Clean minor	Begin or complete immunization per schedule; tetanus toxoid, 0.5 cc	None	Tetanus 0.5 cc	Tetanus toxoid 0.5 cc
Clean major or tetanus prone	In one arm: **Human tetanus immune globulin 250 mg. In other arm: **Tetanus toxoid 0.5 cc., complete immunization per schedule	Tetanus 0.5 cc.	Tetanus 0.5 cc	In one arm: **Tetanus toxoid 0.5 cc. In other arm: **Human tetanus immune globulin 250 mg
Tetanus prone	In one arm: **Human tetanus immune globulin 500 mg. In other arm: **Tetanus toxoid 0.5 cc., complete immunization per schedule thereafter. Antibiotic therapy	Tetanus toxoid 0.5 cc	Tetanus toxoid 0.5 cc amd antibiotic therapy	In one arm: **Tetanus toxoid 0.5 cc In other arm: **Human tetanus immune globulin 500 mg and antibiotic therapy

*No prophylactic immunization is required if patient has had a booster within the previous year.
**Use different syringes, needles and sites.
Note: With different preparations of toxoid, the volume of a single booster dose should be modified as stated on the package label.

tamination with soil or animal excreta.

When a patient presents with an open cut or injury, evidence of prior immunization should be obtained. Satisfactory immunization can be presumed in school children who have completed a course of DPT (diphtheria, pertussis, tetanus) vaccination, and in members of the armed forces who have completed the basic course of three immunizing injections. In all cases, however, documentation should be sought; in the absence of satisfactory documentation, the patient must be presumed to be nonimmune. The length of protection after an initial course of immunization is currently debated by authorities[10] and is probably between five and ten years. A great deal depends on the nutritional status of the patient: the length and degree of protection after primary immunization is shorter in patients with less than adequate nutritional status. Table 5–3 shows the current recommendation of the Committee on Trauma, American College of Surgeons.[11]

Rabies

While the incidence of human rabies in the U.S. is now restricted to one to two cases a year, the wild and domestic animal reservoir has remained constant over the last 15 years in the range of 4000 cases a year;[9] therefore, the risk of human disease is ever present. The disease is almost uniformly fatal in man, so reliance must be placed on immunoprophylaxis of clinical disease by immunizing all patients who have been bitten by unimmunized or wild animals, particularly if the animal has exhibited strange behavior. The following points summarize current recommendations of the World Health Organization.

(1) If the animal is unvaccinated and captured, it should be quarantined for a ten day period of observation. If the bite is slight, duck embryo vaccine (DEV) should be given to the patient in doses of 1.0 ml daily for 14 days using different subcutaneous sites.

(2) If the animal is known to be rabid, develops rabies during the period of quarantine, or if the bites are severe, deep, multiple or affecting the head and neck or arm, then in addition to DEV, rabies antiserum should be given.

(3) Under some circumstances this regimen may be modified. If the suspect animal has been quarantined but shows no signs of rabies by day five, and if the wound is minor, immunization of the patient may be suspended after five injections and resumed only if the animal is subsequently proven rabid. Individuals at high risk, for example, veterinarians, should be vaccinated prophylactically and boosted every one to two years.

As this book goes to press, the Food and Drug Administration is considering for approval a new rabies vaccine prepared from human diploid cell lines. If approved, a full course of vaccination will require only four injections of the new vaccine, and it will improve the length and the height of immunity provided by the duck embryo vaccine. Readers would be well advised to be aware of this new development and, when approved and released for general use, consider the new vaccine for use in their emergency rooms.

Human and Animal Bites

These injuries are in general so heavily contaminated that, as a general rule, primary suture should not be done, but the wound should be debrided, irrigated and the patient treated with systemic penicillin. Tooth lacerations on a knuckle such as may follow an altercation should be treated as a bite (Fig. 5–13). An exception to this

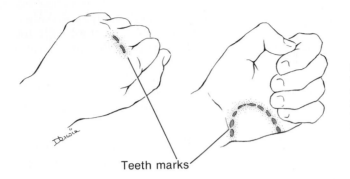

Teeth marks

Figure 5–13 Human bites are particularly dangerous wounds because of the high incidence of sepsis. Should be irrigated, debrided and treated with systemic antibiotics. Do not close with sutures.

rule is an injury where healing by secondary intention would produce unsightly scarring, such as a dog bite on a child's face or lip. In such a circumstance it is permissible to debride devitalized tissue carefully and to perform closure, using fine monofilament nylon skin sutures. The comments made about rabies prophylaxis in the preceding section apply. Prophylactic antibiotics are frequently used in cases where primary closure is performed for an extensive dog bite.

Gas Gangrene

Gas gangrene may be recognized by the history of a highly contaminated injury, followed by local pain, induration and the presence of air in the tissues as evidenced by crepitation or gas on an x-ray film in the soft tissues. Gas gangrene may be caused by Clostridia or by a symbiotic infection with aerobic and anaerobic nonclostridial organisms. Treatment must be immediate, with wide opening of the wound to allow access of oxygen to all injured parts, débridement of necrotic tissue and foreign material, Gram stain of the exudate and penicillin therapy. Hospitalization and supportive therapy for possible systemic effects are mandatory. The administration of antigas gangrene sera is currently not recommended, since most authorities feel that the anaphylactic reactions caused by these sera outweigh their potential benefit.[11] Although some authorities

espouse the use of hyperbaric oxygen for treatment of gas gangrene, adequate and — if necessary — repeated surgical débridement is the essential aspect of therapy.

ALLERGIC REACTIONS TO CHEMOTHERAPEUTIC AGENTS

Most untoward reactions can be avoided by taking a careful history. Patients who have had antibiotics in the past without side effects but who have a positive history of other allergic reactions such as urticarial eruptions, asthma or food intolerance should be considered potentially allergic. Epinephrine 1:1000 and aminophylline 1.0 gm ampoules should be available for injection in all outpatient departments in case of a reaction. In suspected allergic patients, skin or conjunctival tests should be performed as described in manufacturers' brochures. Adverse reactions to drugs in an outpatient setting were found in 17.5 per cent of patients in one study.[12]

SUMMARY

In the treatment of outpatient infections, the emphasis is on correct diagnosis, appropriate timing of surgical intervention, adequate débridement when necessary and close adherence to the principles of antibacterial therapy. This includes the bacteriological investigation of exudates by Gram stain and culture, selection of appropriate antibiotic agents and careful follow-up of all patients until they are fully healed.

REFERENCES

1. Center for Disease Control: National Nosocomial Infections Study, Quarterly Report. U.S. Department of Health, Education and Welfare, Public Health Service, March 1974.
2. Marshall, K. A., Edgerton, M. T., Rodeheaver, G. T., et al.: Quantitative microbiology: Its application to hand injuries. Amer. J. Surg., *131*:730, 1976.
3. Day, T. K.: Controlled trial of prophylactic antibiotics in minor wounds requiring suture. Lancet, *II*:1174, 1975.
4. Gardner, P., and Provine, H. T.: Manual of Acute Bacterial Infections. Boston, Little, Brown & Co., 1975.
5. Hall-Smith, P., Cairns, R. J., and Beare, R. L. B.: Dermatology. 2nd Edition. New York Grune & Stratton Publishers, 1973.
6. Alexander, J. W., and Alexander, N. S.: The influence of route of administration of wound fluid concentration of prophylactic antibiotics. J. Trauma, *16*:488, 1976.
7. The Medical Letter: Vol. 19, No. 2, The Medical Letter Inc., Publishers, 1977, p. 5.
8. Hansten, P. D.: Drug Interactions. 3rd Edition. Philadelphia, Lea & Febiger 1975.
9. Center for Disease Control: Morbidity and Mortality Report. Vol. 23, No. 53. U.S. Department of Health, Education and Welfare, Public Health Service, March, 1974.
10. Furste, W.: The fourth international conference on tetanus. J. Trauma, *16*:755, 1976.
11. American College of Surgeons, Committee on Trauma: Early Care of the Injured Patient. Philadelphia, W. B. Saunders Co., 1972.
12. Steward, R. B., and Cluff, L. E.: Studies on the epidemiology of adverse drug reactions. Hopkins Med. J., *129*:319, 1971.

Tumors 6

YEU-TSU N. (MARGARET) LEE, M.D.

INTRODUCTION

When a patient presents with a new growth or tumor anywhere in the body, the most important information the physician needs to have is whether the lesion is benign or malignant. For benign lesions, the principles of treatment are fairly straightforward. For malignant lesions, delayed diagnosis or inadequate initial treatment jeopardizes the patient's chance of long-term control. Although a good history, physical examination and proper interpretation of laboratory studies may pro-

vide strong clues regarding the diagnosis, in many cases it is impossible to determine benignity or malignancy of a particular lesion until a biopsy is taken.

Once the definitive histological diagnosis is made, recommendations for further treatment will depend on type, extent of the lesion (stage) and condition of the host. After a general discussion of the initial management of patients with external tumors, subsequent sections in this chapter will deal specifically with tumors of the skin, soft tissue, and oral cavity; and

160

the work-up of a patient presenting with a neck mass or lymphadenopathy.

After proper treatment of the malignant tumor, the patient should be followed at regular intervals in the tumor clinic. This emphasizes the uniqueness of surgical oncology, because long-term follow-up care is essential for detecting recurrence or progression of disease, discovering second primary lesions and dealing with the effects of disease and treatment. Postoperative adjuvant chemotherapy has recently been found to be of value in certain cancers and this has been incorporated in outpatient tumor practice.

BIOPSY

Indications

DEFINITIVE TREATMENT. There are clinical situations in which a histological diagnosis is not mandatory before proceeding with definitive therapy. An example is a small lesion of the skin that can be excised and closed primarily without leaving a significant cosmetic defect (Fig. 6–1).

DIAGNOSIS AND PROGNOSIS. A le-

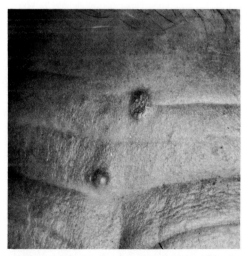

Figure 6–1 Example of lesion suitable for excisional biopsy in the Outpatient Department: basal cell carcinoma of forehead.

sion large enough to require cosmetic reconstruction after excision presents another problem. To properly advise the patient, a histological diagnosis is frequently necessary. A basal cell carcinoma of the skin is much more curable than squamous cell carcinoma. Also, a malignant melanoma involving upper papillary dermis has a much better prognosis than another lesion invading the subcutaneous fat.

STAGING WORK-UP. In patients with known malignant solid tumors, the appearance of distant suspicious lesions, either before or after treatment of the primary cancers, necessitates biopsy to define the extent of involvement and to document recurrent or metastatic spread. For instance, metastasis in a supraclavicular lymph node indicates that the primary breast or lung lesion is surgically incurable. The presence of cervical and inguinal lymphadenopathy in Hodgkin's disease would place the patient in stage III.

Prebiopsy Record of Information

Accurate information is important in making management decisions on patients, and better records may make these decisions easier. The first step in a biopsy is the accurate recording in the chart of a description of the lesion. The exact location, outline, consistency, color, mobility and dimensions (measured with a millimeter ruler) are described. In some tumors, the auscultatory findings may also be important. The use of drawings or anatomical stamps with the lesion diagrammed is enthusiastically endorsed (Fig. 6–2 A and B).

Types of Biopsy

It is impossible to illustrate biopsy techniques in a manner that will apply to every clinical condition. However, guidelines applicable in most situa-

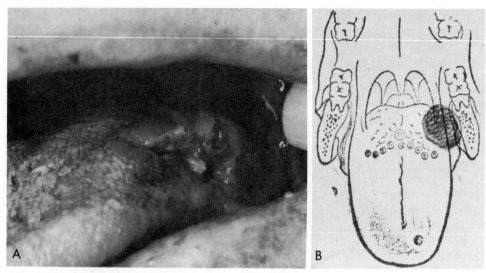

Figure 6–2 Use of anatomical diagram to record size and location of tumor. Squamous carcinoma of the tongue (A), Stage T_1; N_0; M_0 (B). Biopsy performed in OPD. Patient refused definitive surgery; he received Co^{60} therapy, but induration persisted, and neck node developed. He underwent resection ("Commando") and was free of tumor five years later.

tions are suggested here and modifications can be made as needed. There are several types of biopsies; the particular clinical setting usually determines the selected type.

EXCISIONAL BIOPSY. An excisional biopsy (Fig. 6–3) is the complete removal of the lesion for a histological diagnosis. Excisional biopsy provides the advantage of definitive one-stage treatment in many instances while the diagnosis is being made. If the lesion is benign, no further procedure is necessary. If the lesion is malignant, and if the margin of normal tissue removed is adequate for the type of malignancy,

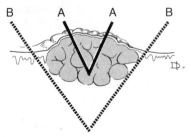

Figure 6–3 Incisional (A) and excisional (B) biopsy.

the excisional biopsy is all that is necessary.

For epidermoid carcinoma of the skin, a margin of 1 cm in width and depth of grossly normal tissue should be excised.[34] For basal cell cancers, a margin of 5 mm is adequate, but for most malignant melanomas, the optimal margin is around 5 cm.[11] Thus, skin lesions 2 cm or more in size usually should have incisional biopsies before treatment.

INCISIONAL BIOPSY. An incisional biopsy (Fig. 6–3) is the removal of part of a large lesion for histological examination, leaving the remainder to be controlled by subsequent therapy. Whenever possible, a section of normal tissue adjacent to the tumor should be included in the specimen. A cup or alligator jaw biopsy forceps can also be used for incisional biopsy, and hemostasis can be achieved with pressure or silver nitrate sticks.

There is a possible objection to incisional biopsy in a potentially curable tumor because of the theoretical chance of spreading tumor by the biopsy. Although this objection may be valid, the danger has been exaggerated; the value of an exact diagnosis before planning specific treatment has significant benefits. The danger of spreading tumor cells is minimal if definitive care is carried out within a few weeks of the biopsy.

Donegan[25] showed that patients with stage A breast carcinoma treated with radical mastectomy without biopsy did not have a better five-year survival rate than those with biopsy. Also, there was no difference in survival rate, whether the biopsy was incisional or excisional. Soft tissue sarcoma tends to spread by infiltration of the surrounding muscle and connective tissues, and wide excision of the lesions, except small ones, may require excision of entire muscle bundles. Without a prior biopsy, lesions resected with limited margins had a much higher local recurrence rate (78 per cent as contrasted with 17 per cent for those with biopsy).[47]

For malignant melanoma a tissue diagnosis is mandatory, since only 2 per cent of black lesions of the skin are malignant melanomas.[27] The survival rates of patients who have initial biopsies or incomplete excision followed by definitive surgery are similar to those who have immediate definitive surgery. In fact, at ten years, those patients who have biopsies survive better than those without (83.5 versus 66.5 per cent). Knutson and colleagues[41] also found that the survival curves are similar among those who had previous biopsies, whether incisional or excisional, and those who did not. In melanoma of the trunk, Sugarbaker and McBride[70] found that previous biopsy, whether excisional or incisional, did not correlate with treatment failure.

OTHER METHODS OF BIOPSY. *Punch or needle biopsies* have advantages for both the patient and the physician when they can be used. These are simple techniques to master and require minimal anesthesia, equipment and postbiopsy care. However, the specimens obtained often are distorted by crushing or squeezing. One needs the cooperation of a pathologist who has enough experience and is willing to make a diagnosis from a small segment of tissue. Two types of needles are commonly used: the Vim-Silverman needle (Fig. 6–4) and the disposable biopsy needle (Fig. 15–5). A core of tissue is removed and submitted in formalin, fixed and stained, as are other incisional biopsies.

Recently, fine needle aspiration biopsies, using 18 to 22 gauge needles in which cells are drawn into the syringe, have gained popularity. Aspiration specimens are smeared on glass slides, air-dried and placed in 95 per cent alcohol. They are then examined for cytological findings in a manner similar to the cervical "Pap smear." With the cooperation and experience of the cytopathologist, aspiration biopsies can have an overall accuracy rate of about 90 per cent. This technique has been used in diagnosing lesions of the breast, lymph node, subcutaneous nodules, lung, pancreas, prostate and so on.[40]

Curettage or scraping biopsies are infrequently used in the general surgery outpatient area but are applicable more often in gynecological and orthopedic procedures. Biliary tract tumors are often diagnosed by curettaged specimens. The *needle aspiration of fluid* for cytological examination is used most frequently in patients with ascites, pleural effusions or cystic fluids. Usually a positive cytological finding still requires confirmation of malignancy by tissue biopsy, except in patients who previously had cancer documented by histological examination or in patients who had x-ray and physical findings typical of advanced cancer.

Anesthesia and Incisions

Prior to inducing anesthesia, the area designated for biopsy and its immediate surroundings should be prepared

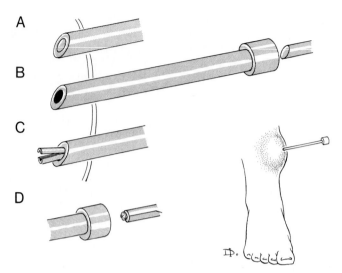

Figure 6–4 Vim-Silverman needle biopsy technique. *A.* Skin is punctured with a No. 11 blade and needle is inserted with obturator in place. *B.* Obturator is removed. *C.* Biopsy forceps introduced through the hollow needle. While holding the inner forceps stable, outer needle is advanced to the tip of forceps with a continuous twisting motion, shearing off the entrapped tissue. *D.* Forceps, containing a core tissue, are then removed. Often it is preferable to remove the inner forceps and outer needle together.

and draped as a sterile field. Disposable plastic sheets with self-adhering edges, such as those used for eye surgery, are ideal for minor excisional procedures.

Prior to administering any local anesthetic a history for possible allergic reaction must be obtained. Also, gentle aspiration should be performed prior to any injection, to guard against intravascular injection. Topical sprays can be used occasionally, but the best anesthesia is achieved with local injection of 0.5 or 1 per cent lidocaine without epinephrine. A 25 gauge needle is used to raise a skin wheal next to the biopsy site, followed by infiltration of the deeper tissues using a 21 to 23 gauge needle. It is preferable to use field block technique and avoid direct injection into the tumor.

Whenever possible the surgical scar should be parallel with the lines of skin tension (Langer's lines). For incisional biopsy, the direction of the scar should be placed so that it can be readily and widely removed at the time of definitive surgery. Occasionally, a pa-

tient may have had unusual reactions to a particular type of suture. Such information would be helpful to avoid wound healing problems. The traditional silk or nylon nonabsorbable sutures have been replaced by newer synthetic materials that can be absorbed and yet last for over two weeks.

Preparation of Specimen

Once the specimen has been obtained it must be handled with tender loving care. No specimen should be allowed to dry out, nor should it be crushed. As a general rule, frozen section diagnosis of outpatient biopsies is not performed. However, a frozen section may be requested to ensure that a diagnosis can be made from the tissue submitted, allowing further specimens to be taken if necessary without requiring a second procedure. Quick knowledge of the diagnosis also expedites treatment decisions.

For routine pathological examinations, solid tissues should be placed in 10 per cent formalin for fixation. However, surgeons must remember that there are occasions when fresh specimens are essential for special studies:

(1) In difficult cases, such as soft tissue sarcomas, a piece of the fresh tissue should be prepared for electron microscopic study.

(2) For patients with breast masses suspicious of carcinoma or for patients with lesions suggestive of recurrent breast carcinoma, about 1 gm of the tumor tissue should be kept aside for estrogen receptor (ER) study. If the frozen section report shows the lesion to be that of breast carcinoma, the fresh specimen should be quickly frozen in dry ice to avoid disintegration of the ER receptor protein.

(3) For patients with lymphadenopathy suspicious of malignant lymphoma, part of the fresh specimen may be used for special study of T and B lymphocytes,[50] and bacterial cultures taken to rule out infectious processes.

The importance of proper labeling of all specimens must be stressed. The responsibility belongs to the surgeon and to no one else. Diagrams on the pathology requisition and special markings on the specimen can help the pathologist to orient the specimen. Each questionable part of the excised tissue must be identified with a stitch.

When an excisional biopsy is carried out, it is important to know that there is an adequate margin of normal tissue present. To help the pathologist identify the true margin of resection and to avoid artifacts produced during sectioning of the fatty tissues, the excised specimen can be coated with India ink before it is fixed in formalin.[34] The margins of excision are thus permanently marked, and, if the ink is observed at the microscopical margins of the cancer, the lesion is inadequately excised (Fig. 6–5).

The transportation to the pathologist of the properly labeled specimen in

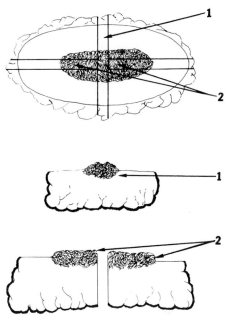

Figure 6–5 Technique of cutting specimen to determine adequacy of excision. India ink coating applied to surface of specimen prior to processing in order to mark the margin of resection. (Courtesy of Dr. Carlos M. Perez-Mesa.)

the correct solution is usually done by the outpatient administrative staff. However, a wise surgeon may wish to carry the specimen to the pathologist personally and to consult him or her directly.

Operative Note and Rebiopsy

After completing the procedure and sending the properly labeled specimen to the Pathology Department one more recordkeeping task remains to complete the job: the operative note. This information is very important and should be accurate and complete. When several physicians rotate through Tumor Clinics, accurate records assume even greater importance. A complete operative note should contain:

Date and time of operation
Surgeon's name
Anesthesia used

Preoperative diagnosis
Postoperative diagnosis
Operation (including diagram of the location, shape, dimensions of lesions and normal margins removed)
Special studies requested
Sutures and drains
Postoperative condition
Follow-up plans

In situations in which small samples or an incisional biopsy is taken, when the pathologist's report is benign, non-diagnostic or undiagnostic, and if the clinical picture of the patient warrants it, the surgeon should repeat the biopsy. I have seen a patient whose third breast biopsy showed carcinoma while two previous biopsies within two months were benign. Remembering that both the surgeon and the pathologist can have sampling errors, one should include rebiopsy as part of the diagnostic armamentarium.

Postbiopsy Care

All patients who undergo local excision of tumors should be instructed on aftercare of their wounds. Incisions should be kept clean and dry, allowing routine showers or bathing after the third day. Limitations in activity, if any, should be explained. Most incisions around the face and neck do not limit activities as do those crossing a joint or located on the sole of the foot.

Provisions for postoperative discomfort must be made. The patient should always have the name and telephone number of the surgeon in case he develops unexpected problems. If only absorbable sutures were used, there is no need to remove them. Otherwise, the time to remove skin sutures depends on the location of the wound and the type of closure.

Sutures can be removed from the face and neck in five days, from the scalp and trunk in seven days and from the extremities in ten days. If subcutaneous sutures are used the skin sutures

can come out two days earlier than if they are not used. The early removal of sutures is important in decreasing visible scar formation on the skin. One additional postoperative visit after the sutures are removed is all that is usually required in benign conditions, and this can be scheduled for four weeks after the operation. Malignant conditions require arrangements for further therapy and long-term follow-up care.

SKIN CANCERS

General Comments

Both benign and malignant lesions of the skin and its appendages have common clinical presentations and are approached similarly. The three most frequent types of cutaneous cancer, accounting for the great majority of all primary malignant tumors of the skin, are basal cell carcinoma, squamous cell carcinoma and malignant melanoma. Overall, about 68 per cent are basal cell, 29 per cent squamous cell and 3 per cent of other histological types.

Other less frequent, but nonetheless important, cancers that may arise primarily on the skin include Bowen's disease (squamous cell carcinoma in situ), as well as tumors of the cutaneous adnexal structures (sweat gland adenocarcinomas); vascular system (Kaposi's sarcoma, lymphangiosarcomas), connective and muscular tissues (dermatofibrosarcoma protuberans, leiomyosarcoma); reticuloendothelial system (malignant lymphoma) and others. The skin may also be a site for cutaneous metastases, particularly from melanoma and cancers of the lung, large intestine, breast and ovary.[13]

A great deal is known about the causes of skin cancer. It may result from exposure to electromagnetic radiation (sunlight, x-ray), chemical carcinogens (arsenic, coal tar derivatives etc.), genetic predisposition (nevoid basal cell carcinoma syndrome, xeroderma pigmentosum), thermal burns and so on.[35] Thus, skin cancer is more common where sunlight is most intense and on those areas of the body that receive the most sunlight. Caucasians are most susceptible, particularly those who have light eyes, light hair, fair complexions, sunburn easily and spend more hours outdoors than the general population.

Presenting Complaints

In general, basal cell carcinomas are most frequently found around the nose, eyelids and cheeks, but they can occur anywhere on the skin. Approximately 75 per cent of the squamous cell carcinomas are found on the skin of the head (face, cheeks, ears, nose, lips), 15 per cent on the hands and 10 per cent elsewhere. This tumor can metastasize to the regional lymph nodes and, therefore, shows a higher mortality rate than basal cell carcinoma.

Both basal and squamous cell carcinomas may be multicentric and commonly appear as a "growth" or a "sore" (ulceration). Basal cell carcinoma usually is plaquelike with a raised margin of "pearly" or waxy border, while squamous cell carcinoma varies from a scaly lesion or a nodular mass to a large ulcerated or fungating tumor.

Malignant melanoma is a much more lethal cancer, because it tends to spread not only through local extension and regional lymphatics but also through the blood stream. Etiologically, melanomas often appear to be related to previous pigmented nevi or birthmarks. There are certain signals suggestive of malignant transformation of pre-existing nevi. These are (1) change in color or shades of color, including spreading of pigmentation at the periphery; (2) sudden growth of the lesion either at its margins or in elevation above the surface; (3) change in surface characteristics, such as when it becomes scaly, crusted, ul-

cerated or bleeds; (4) appearance of new symptoms such as itching, tenderness or pain; and (5) signs of redness or swelling of surrounding skin or appearance of satellite nodules or regional lymphadenopathy.[35] In adults nevi located in areas subjected to chronic irritation, such as the palm, sole, waist, hair-bearing scalp, neck or bra areas, should be excised prophylactically.

Principles of Management

All benign tumors and almost all of the early malignant tumors require only adequate local excision for treatment. Accurate histological diagnosis of all skin cancers is essential. Electrodesiccation of skin lesions without pathological examination is hazardous. When a lesion is suspected of being malignant melanoma, punch, shave or curettage biopsy is not enough to define the depth of invasion. Clark and Breslow and associates[10, 11, 20] have shown that the depth or thickness of invasion of primary melanoma has important prognostic value, and that it does influence the decision of how wide a margin is necessary when excising the primary and whether or not to perform a regional lymph node dissection as part of the initial therapy (Fig. 6–6, Tables 6–1 and 6–2). Thus, total excisional biopsy is preferred in suspected melanoma.[44] Exceptions include lesions that are so large or so anatomically situated that total removal would involve a disfiguring procedure, or one in which closure could not be accomplished by more than a simple primary suture technique. In such instances an incisional biopsy is indicated.

When excising carcinomas of the skin, a margin of 1 cm in width and depth of grossly normal tissue should be included with epidermoid cancers and 5 mm with basal cell cancers. If the defect is too large to be closed primarily, split thickness or full thickness skin should be used to cover the de-

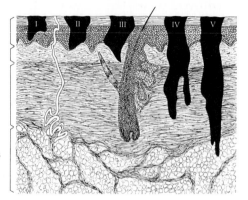

Epidermis

Papillary
dermis

Reticular
dermis

Subcutaneous
fat

Figure 6–6 Clark's levels of depth of invasion of melanoma. Level I: Tumor does not penetrate deep to basement membrane. Level II: Tumor extends into papillary dermis. Level III: Tumor extends to and impinges on interface between papillary dermis and reticular dermis. (Some level III lesions may be deeper than other level IV melanomas because papillary dermis extends around hair follicles.) Level IV: Tumor extends into reticular dermis. Level V: Tumor extends into subcutaneous fat.

fect. Undermining of skin edges or the use of pedicles for covering excisional defects should *not* be done, because cancers that recur under flaps are often far advanced when they are detected. When a sufficiently wide excision would produce disfiguration, radiotherapy is indicated. Radiotherapy is also the preferred treatment for all but the smallest lesions of the eyelid, nasal ala and inner canthus.

For basal cell carcinoma, an "inadequately" excised lesion has a local recurrence rate of 33 per cent, while only 1.2 per cent of "adequately" excised lesions recurred.[57] For epidermoid cancers, 66 per cent of those lesions that were inadequately excised in depth recurred, and 33 per cent of those that were inadequate in width recurred.[34] Thus, skin cancers that are excised with inadequate margins should have immediate wide reexcision or curative radiotherapy, unless conscientious postoperative follow-up is maintained.

ORAL CAVITY LESIONS

The mouth can be involved in a large number of benign and malignant growths. Seventy-five per cent of all head and neck cancers begin in the

TABLE 6–1 Incidence of Occult Regional Nodal Metastasis at Time of Prophylactic Nodal Dissection of Patients With Stage 1 Malignant Melanoma

REFERENCE	YEAR	CASES	PRIMARY SITE	CLARK'S LEVEL (%)				
				II	III	IV	V	SUB-TOTAL
Wanebo, et al.	1975	159	Extremity	4	7	25	70	18
Fortner, et al.	1977	162	Trunk and extremity	0	14	31	33	20
Holmes, et al.	1976	60	All	—	16	45	—	27
Holmes, et al.	1977	160	All	—	18	27	33	22
Cohen, et al.	1977	61	All	15	14	35	33	21
Goldman, et al.	1978	42	All	—	4	← 26 →		14
Kapelanski, et al.	1979	26	All	0	18	← 17 →		15
TOTAL		670						
Minimum (%)				0	4	17	17	14
Maximum (%)				15	18	45	70	27
Median (%)				4	14	27	33	20

Detailed references available on request.

TABLE 6–2   Five-Year Survival Rates of Patients With Stage 1 Malignant Melanoma According to Clark's Pathological Classification

REFERENCE	YEAR	CASES	PRIMARY SITE	CLINICAL STAGES[a]	CLARK'S LEVEL (%)				
					II	III	IV	V	SUB-TOTAL
Donnellan, et al.	1972	104	Head and Neck	I	95	75	70	55	—
Mehnert and Heard	1973	75	All	I	85	← 43 →		11	59
Wanebo, et al.	1975	151	Extremity	I	100	88	65	15	79
Veronesi, et al.	1977	249	Extremity	I	—	79	64	—	71
Hansen and McCarten	1974	141	All	I, II	100	70	50	40	—
Breslow	1975	138	All	I, II	96	67	38	22	67
Das Gupta	1977	150	All	I, II	100	95	50	37	76
Cohen, et al.	1977	118	All	I, II	80	53	58	45	—
Balch, et al.	1978	205	All	I, II	94	71	43	27	68
Kapelanski, et al.	1979	104	All	I, II	85	63	38	23	55
McGovern	1970	183	All	I–III	84	65	49	29	62
Cady, et al.	1975	176	All	I–III	86	67	67	11	67
Elias, et al.	1977	248	All	I–III	62	46	30	10	—
TOTAL		2042							
Minimum (%)					62	46	30	10	55
Maximum (%)					100	95	70	55	79
Median (%)					90	68	50	28	67

Detailed references available on request.
[a]Clinical stages: I = Localized primary melanoma.
II = Clinical metastases to regional lymph nodes.
III = Disseminated melanoma.

oral cavity. With the possible exception of malignant tumors of the skin, no human cancers are more accessible or easier to diagnose. Thus, every physician and dentist should be familiar with the methods of examining the oral cavity and with the appearance of benign and malignant tumors.

Technique of Routine Examination

A complete examination of the mouth requires a tongue blade, a finger cot and a light. The finger cot is not essential but it is certainly more esthetic and safer for the examiner. A systematic approach is desirable to avoid omissions. Dentures and false teeth should be removed. Note any asymmetry or recent changes such as erosion, leukoplakia, mass or swelling.

With the mouth open wide and the tongue in its normal anatomical position the lips are examined, followed by inspection of the buccal mucosa bilaterally, the upper and lower gingiva, the soft and hard palates, the tonsillar fossa and the oropharyngeal wall posteriorly. The tongue blade is then used to hold the tongue aside while the floor of the mouth and the inner aspect of the gingiva on each side are explored. Next, wrap a piece of gauze around the tip of the tongue and pull the tongue gently forward and to one side. The junction of the posterior aspect of the middle third of the tongue with the anterior tonsillar pillar (faucial arch) should always be checked, as this is the most common site of cancer of the tongue (Fig. 6–2).

The lips, floor of the mouth and tongue should routinely be palpated, in addition to any suspicious areas in other sites. Mirrors and topical anesthesia are needed to examine the oropharynx, nasopharynx and larynx. Both sides of the neck, from mandible to the clavicle, should be carefully palpated for lymphadenopathy. Small submental or submandibular lymph nodes can only be felt by bimanual examination: one gloved finger inside the mouth pushing against the other hand under the chin.

Presenting Complaints

The majority of oral cancers cause no symptoms in their early stages. Sometimes the patient complains of a mucosal sore that does not heal, pain or bleeding, Rarely, the first symptom is a lump in the neck indicating metastatic spread to a cervical lymph node.

MUCOSAL SORE. Since the oral cavity is generously endowed with sensory nerves in addition to the tongue, which can roam almost everywhere anterior to the faucial arch, early recognition of even a small tumor or mucosal irregularity by the patient is ensured. Often a persistent nonhealing ulcer, frequently attributed to defective teeth or ill-fitting dentures, brings the patient to seek medical care.

PAIN OR BLEEDING. Small, painful ulcerated lesions are often viral in origin (herpetic ulcers), and occasionally benign vascular tumors such as hemangiomas will present with blood-tinged sputum. But neither pain nor bleeding is the early symptom of an oral lesion. When bleeding occurs with a cancer, it is almost always associated with an ulcerated advanced tumor. When pain occurs, it is often due to secondary infection of the tumor or to invasion of adjacent structures. Referred pain to the ear may occur in cancers situated more posteriorly in the oral cavity or in the pharynx, such as the tonsillar region, base of the tongue or hypopharynx. Occasionally, a patient with oral cancer will complain of difficulty in chewing, swallowing or speaking.

Squamous cell carcinomas of the mouth are seen most often in males over the age of 40. The use of tobacco predisposes to the development of oral cancer; this includes not only smoking of cigarettes, pipes and cigars, but also the use of chewing tobacco or snuff. Cancers of the posterior tongue and hypopharynx are frequently associated with a history of heavy drinking. Risk increases with poor oral hygiene and lack of dental care.

Types of Lesions and Diagnosis

Inflammatory ulcerations are the most frequently encountered benign oral conditions. Foreign body or inclusion cyst with secondary infection and induration can be confused with tumors. The more common benign and malignant oral conditions are listed below:

Benign
  (1) Inflammatory ulceration
  (2) Epulis
  (3) Hemangioma
  (4) Granuloma
  (5) Cheilosis
  (6) Leukoplakia
  (7) Mucocele
  (8) Papilloma

Malignant
  (1) Squamous cell carcinoma
  (2) Adenocarcinoma
  (3) Sarcoma
  (4) Lymphoma

The most common sites of oral cancer are shaped like a horseshoe: the lower lip, sides of the mobile tongue, floor of the mouth and tonsillar arches. Often large tumors involve contiguous structures and it may be impossible to determine the exact site of origin.

About 90 per cent of malignant oral lesions arise from the mucosa and are epidermoid carcinomas. Adenocarcinomas of the minor salivary glands, usually occurring near the junction of hard and soft palate, are uncommon, accounting for 1 to 2 per cent of the malignancies. Sarcomas from the submucosa of the tongue and soft palate are extremely rare.

Either incisional or excisional biopsies are acceptable for diagnosis of most oral lesions. The clinical setting will determine which type to use. In patients whose neoplastic lesion may be masked by diffuse leukoplakia or dysplasia, the areas of invasive carcinoma or carcinoma in situ may be better delineated after staining with toluidine blue solutions.[36, 62]

A few oral lesions can be removed locally as excisional biopsies. The major requirement is that enough normal tissue be present around the lesion to permit approximation by sutures without tension (Fig. 6–7). It is rare to expose bone with biopsy procedures, but if this occurs the bone must be covered with soft tissue to prevent osteomyelitis.

Lip Shave and V-Excision

Solar keratosis and in situ carcinomas of the lower lip are found with some frequency in men who spend a great deal of time outdoors. In these patients, removal of the involved tissue can be accomplished with a lip shave, achieving an excellent cosmetic result (Fig. 6–8). In patients with invasive epidermoid carcinoma of the lower lip, the malignant lesion can be treated with a V-excision and the adjacent areas of keratosis or in situ carcinoma removed with a lip shave.

The procedure can be done under local or general anesthesia. One per cent lidocaine without epinephrine (1 to 2 cc) is used to anesthetize the submental nerves bilaterally at the foramen between the apices of the bicuspid teeth.[51] Supplemental injections of 2 to 3 cc at the lateral commissures insure complete anesthesia for the entire lower lip.

After appropriate preparation, drapes are applied to isolate the lower lip, leaving the nose uncovered to allow easier breathing. Every maneuver should be explained to the patient before it is done. One or two 4 inch by 4 inch gauze sponges are placed in the back of the mouth to prevent blood from trickling into the pharynx. A total lip shave will be described, but it is emphasized that less than the total can be done if only a part of the lip is involved by a lesion.

The initial incision is made along the entire vermillion border from com-

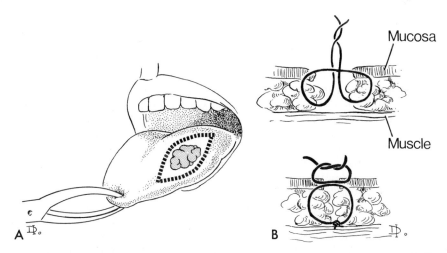

Figure 6–7 Tongue lesion suitable for excisional biopsy in Outpatient Department. *A.* Exposure and elliptical lines of excision. *B.* Two-layer closure of tongue with buried 3–0 chromic in muscle and 3–0 chromic catgut in mucosa.

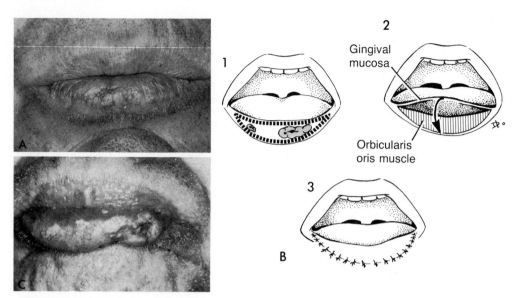

Figure 6–8   Lip carcinomas treated in Outpatient Department under local anesthesia. *A. In situ* carcinoma with adjacent leukoplakia, treated with lip shave. *B.* Lip shave technique. Submental nerves are blocked bilaterally with 2 to 3 cc of 1 per cent plain lidocaine. Similar injections are given at commissures of the mouth. (1) Lines of excison. (2) Buccal mucosa is undermined to prepare a flap for advancement. (3) Closure of defect with 5–0 nylon sutures. *C.* Invasive carcinoma and adjacent leukoplakia, treated with V-excision and lip shave.

missure to commissure. The incision is carried down to the orbicularis oris muscle. Small dissecting scissors are then used to undermine the mucosa in the plane above the orbicularis muscle posteriorly toward the gingival sulcus. The extent of the undermining depends on the posterior extent of the lesion, because the normal mucosa must be freed enough to allow it to be advanced anteriorly to meet the skin. The lesion should not be resected until all the undermining has been accomplished. Once this is done, the involved lip mucosa is resected.

Bleeding may or may not be a problem, depending on whether or not the labial artery or vein is entered during the undermining maneuver. A large amount of hemorrhaging must be controlled by clamp and ligation, but small oozing is best ignored, as it will stop when the mucosa is advanced and sutured. Four-0 or 5-0 nonabsorbable simple sutures are used to approximate the mucosa to the skin of the lower lip.

There will be some inversion of the lip, but this is minimal after complete healing. No drains are needed.

For V-excision of lower lip cancers, special right angle lip clamps can be applied to compress the tissue. After excision of the lesion from skin side to the oral mucosal side with about a 5 mm margin, the defect can be approximated in three layers: oral mucosa and middle muscular layers with absorbable sutures and external layer with nonabsorbable sutures. The first external stitch should be placed in such a way that the vermillion border is lined up perfectly.

Antibacterial ointment is applied to the suture line and the tube is sent home with the patient to be applied three times a day. Xylocaine ointment, analgesics or both can be used every four hours for pain. A cold wet washcloth can be applied for 15 minutes every two hours to reduce swelling and give comfort. The patient is instructed to eat whatever he wishes, but initially jello, soups and other soft foods are preferred. When the patient returns for his postoperative visit, the pathology report must be available and should be explained to the patient. Further plans can then be made for follow-up or discharge from care, depending on the report.

TUMOR MASS IN THE NECK

Differential Diagnosis

Tumor mass in the neck is a common complaint and offers challenging diagnostic problems. Of 3027 patients with neck masses, which represented about 1 to 2 per cent of surgical admissions, 1411 had thyroid masses.[64] The differential diagnosis of neck masses among the remaining 1616 patients is presented in Table 6–3. It must be emphasized that 85 per cent were of neoplastic origin. In general, the average age of patients with neoplastic disease was about 60 years; with inflammatory,

16 years; with congenital lesions, 8 years. Inflammatory tumors existed for approximately seven days, neoplasms for seven months, and tumors of embryonic origin were present for seven years before causing trouble.

For tumor surgeons, any mass present in the neck region is presumed to contain metastatic cancer until proven otherwise. The cervical lymphatic system has a wide potential for filtering out metastatic cancer cells from both infraclavicular and supraclavicular sources. The correct evaluation of a patient who presents himself with a mass in the lateral neck is not difficult if certain points are kept in mind and proper diagnostic maneuvers are performed.

History and Physical Findings

The length of time the mass has been present is helpful in the differential diagnosis. If it has been present several months or even years and has remained the same size, it is very apt

TABLE 6–3 Distribution of Nonthyroid Neck Masses
Among 1616 Surgical Admissions*

Histological Type		No. of Cases		Percent
Neoplastic		1370		85
Benign		309		23
Salivary gland	165			
Others	144			
Malignant		1061		77
Primary	161			
Metastatic	900			
Inflammatory		52		3
Acute infections		50		96
Chronic infections		2		4
Others		194		12
Congenital masses		113		58
Thyroglossal cyst	82			
Bronchogenic	26			
Cystic hygroma	5			
Salivary duct stenosis		54		28
Miscellaneous		27		14
Totals		1616		100

*Adapted from Skandalakis et al.[64]

to be a benign process. An enlarging mass of recent origin is a strong indication of cancer. Associated complaints referable to the head and neck area are important, especially hoarseness, sore throat, dysphagia or a painful sore in the mouth. However, often the mass itself is the only complaint.

The patient should be asked if he has a history of heavy smoking or drinking. The former habit predisposes to lung cancer, which can present as cervical lymph node enlargement. Smoking and excessive use of alcohol are commonly associated with cancer of the upper alimentary and respiratory passages.

The location of the mass is an important clue to its origin as well as to the location of the primary tumor in the case of a metastatic lymph node. Oral, pharyngeal and hypopharyngeal cancers metastasize to cervical lymph nodes as a natural course of the disease (Fig. 6–9).

The consistency of the tumor may also be helpful in the diagnosis. A rock-hard mass is very likely to be cancer, especially if it is fixed to the adjacent tissue, whereas a soft mass may be a cyst or a lipoma. Metastatic lymph nodes adherent to carotid sheath, if still movable, can only be moved from side to side but not up and down, while benign lumps can be moved in all directions.

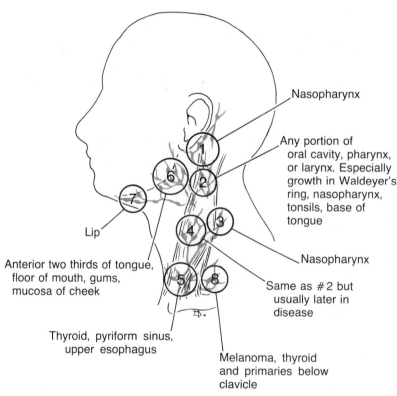

Nasopharynx

Any portion of oral cavity, pharynx, or larynx. Especially growth in Waldeyer's ring, nasopharynx, tonsils, base of tongue

Nasopharynx

Same as #2 but usually later in disease

Melanoma, thyroid and primaries below clavicle

Lip

Anterior two thirds of tongue, floor of mouth, gums, mucosa of cheek

Thyroid, pyriform sinus, upper esophagus

Figure 6–9   Lymph nodes of the neck and most likely sites of primary tumor. (1) Nasopharynx. (2) Oral cavity, Waldeyer's ring (nasopharynx, tonsil, base of tongue), pharynx, larynx. (3) Nasopharynx. (4) Same as (2), but usually later in disease. (5) Thyroid, pyriform sinus, upper esophagus. (6) Tongue (anterior two-thirds), floor of mouth, gums, buccal mucosa. (7) Lip. (8) Melanoma, thyroid and primaries below clavicle.

Work-up

In addition to a meticulous history and a complete physical examination, the head and neck should be investigated very carefully before removing any mass in the neck. If the mass is metastatic from primary cancer of the head and neck, open biopsy may compromise the possibility of cure from subsequent therapy.

The scalp, skin of the head and neck, mouth, base of the tongue, nasopharynx, oropharynx, hypopharynx and larynx must be examined closely. Examinations should be repeated if necessary on more than one occasion. No biopsy specimen should be taken until head and neck x-ray studies have been completed.

All patients should have a chest film and soft tissue x-rays of frontal and lateral views of the neck. Calcification of the mass implies a benign process. The air column on lateral x-rays of the neck can outline the nasopharynx, base of the tongue, hypopharynx and larynx to good advantage. Tomograms of the nasopharynx or larynx and contrast studies of the upper alimentary and respiratory passages can be useful, but they yield little as a screening procedure. Sinus films give little information in the asymptomatic patient because silent cancers in the paranasal sinuses almost never present as a cervical mass. Intravenous pyelogram, upper gastrointestinal series, barium enema and endoscopic studies may be ordered when the clinical symptoms suggest difficulty in the gastrointestinal or genitourinary tract.

If a neck mass appears to be metastatic cancer, and a primary site is not readily apparent, blind biopsies should be performed of the base of the tongue, nasopharynx and tonsil, along with a direct laryngoscopy. If these are negative, needle biopsy of the neck mass, wherever applicable, is the initial diagnostic step, because the subsequent operative field is not violated. If the needle aspiration biopsy specimen is nondiagnostic, open biopsy of the neck mass is then in order.

Management Guidelines

In patients with a solitary metastatic node in the supraclavicular region, or if the biopsy shows the lesion to be adenocarcinoma — which accounts for less than 10 per cent of the cervical metastasis — the primary malignancy is more likely to be below the clavicle.[7, 46] For both left and right supraclavicular metastases, the site of primary cancer is most likely to be lung, breast, stomach, prostate or ovary.[55] For all adenocarcinoma of unknown origin, 40 per cent of patients have pancreatic carcinoma and another 40 per cent have cancer of the colon, stomach, liver or biliary system.[53]

Despite intensive and extensive pre- and paraoperative work-ups, large series have shown that the primary lesion was found subsequently only in about one third of the patients with metastatic lesions in the neck,[42] and about 15 to 25 per cent of the patients could survive five years if the lesions were treated aggressively.[7] Thus, it is justifiable to treat the cervical metastasis for cure.

When open biopsy of a neck mass is necessary, it should be done under general anesthesia, with plans for immediate radical neck dissection if the lesion is resectable and especially if it is metastatic epidermoid cancer. Although surgical resection or radiotherapy is equally effective in controlling the disease in the more favorable clinical stages, a radical neck dissection is preferred in these patients because of the potential morbidity of radiation.[58] Postoperative radiotherapy can improve the local control rate, and radiation therapy is highly effective in preventing the development of subsequent contralateral metastatic nodes and in treating a primary cancer in the nasopharynx, oropharynx or hypopharynx. Advanced unresectable metastatic lesions in the neck should have radiotherapy after a tissue diagnosis is obtained.

PERIPHERAL LYMPHADENOPATHY

Other than cervical metastasis as described above, metastatic lesions can appear in axillary or inguinal nodes before primary cancer is discovered. Among 254 patients with metastatic carcinoma from occult primary tumors, 33 (13 per cent) presented with enlarged nodes in the axilla or groin.[24] In another series of 617 patients, 57 had involvement of cervical lymph nodes, 5 had axillary, 6 had inguinal and 39 had general lymphatic involvement.[37] In addition, malignant lymphoma (Hodgkin's disease and non-Hodgkin's lymphoma) can originate in lymph nodes. All such cases need outpatient biopsy of peripheral lymphadenopathy for diagnosis.

Axillary Node

To biopsy axillary lymph nodes, the conventional approach is to have the patient lying supine, with the ipsilateral upper extremity abducted 90 degrees and supported on an armboard. An improved technique is this: The forearm is suspended anterior to the chest in an adducted position to an overhead anesthesia screen.[56] This way, the pectoralis major muscle is displaced medially and the apical axillary lymph nodes are moved closer to the hair-bearing area of the skin (Fig. 6–10).

Among patients needing axillary biopsy for diagnosis, one third had unilateral adenopathy. About 70 per cent of such lesions were of nonspecific changes; malignant lymphoma occurred in 14 per cent, 10 per cent had metastatic adenocarcinomas and 7 per cent had granuloma.[59] In approximately one third of the patients with axillary metastasis the primary tumor was in the breast. Excluding patients with breast lesions, 24 of 42 died with site of origin still undetermined, and nine survived two to ten years after resection with no evidence of disease.[21] Nine (21 per cent) subsequently were found to have malignant lesions in the stomach, lung, pharynx and sarcoma.

Excluding cancers of the lung, skin or melanoma of the arm or trunk, carcinoma of the breast is the most common hidden primary in female patients with a metastasis in the axilla. Thus, mammography should be performed before biopsy of an axillary node in a woman.

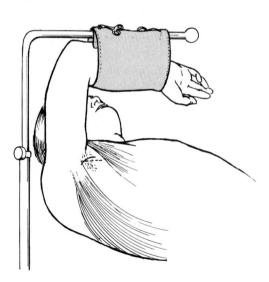

Figure 6–10 Method of securing arm for biopsy of axillary nodes. Solid and broken lines indicate usual orientation of incisions. Note that incisions are limited to hair-bearing (stippled) area. (Adapted from: Arch. Surg., *112*:1124, 1977. Copyright 1977, American Medical Association. Used with permission of the authors and the AMA.)

In 1951, before mammography was generally available, Weinberger[75] reported five cases of axillary metastases in which radical mastectomy revealed a small primary tumor of the breast. In three patients, despite extensive metastatic involvement of one lymph node, no other axillary nodes were involved. Ashikari and colleagues[4] reported a series of 42 patients who presented with an axillary mass without significant clinical findings in the breast. Twenty-two of 25 cases had negative mammograms, and three were suspicious for carcinoma. Suprisingly, the survival rate after radical mastectomy in such patients was better than in those who presented with a palpable breast mass and axillary metastasis.

Inguinal Node

In the female, metastases to inguinal lymph nodes when the primary is not apparent are usually due to cancer of one of the pelvic organs, such as the cervix, uterus or ovary. Special diagnostic studies include dilation and curettage of the uterus, conization of the cervix and cul-de-sac punctures. In a series of patients with ovarian tumors found on pelvic examination, histological diagnosis of carcinoma could be made in 45 per cent by cul-de-sac puncture and routine inguinal node biopsy on the affected side.[42] Inguinal node metastases also occur from carcinomas of the vulva, vagina and urethra. The primary tumors in these patients can usually be seen or palpated on physical examination.

In the male, the prostate should be carefully examined. A transrectal prostate biopsy should be considered when the serum acid phosphatase is elevated, even if the rectal examination is normal.

In both sexes the anus and rectum should be meticulously investigated. The possibility of mucosal or cutaneous melanomas must be kept in mind. Proctoscopy and barium enema should be routine; pelvic lymphangiography may also be helpful. Inguinal node enlargement may occur as the first sign of lymphoma in patients of either sex.

Nodal Biopsy For Malignant Lymphoma

The most frequent surgical procedure essential to the histological diagnosis of malignant lymphoma is a biopsy of the peripheral lymph nodes. This procedure established the diagnosis in 94 per cent of the patients with Hodgkin's disease and in 77 per cent of the patients with non-Hodgkin's lymphoma. About 15 per cent of the diagnoses were made by biopsy of the axillary nodes and 10 per cent by biopsy of the inguinal nodes.[45]

In general, for diagnosis of both Hodgkin's disease and non-Hodgkin's lymphomas, 23 per cent of the patients required more than one lymph node biopsy, and the average number of biopsies per patient was 1.4. These figures not only reflected the intrinsic difficulty of diagnosing such lesions by the pathologists, but also emphasized the need for special care by the surgeons who performed the node biopsy.

(1) When more than one anatomical area is involved, the site of biopsy should be carefully selected. It is better to remove a lower cervical node and to avoid the submandibular and inguinal nodes, since the latter often exhibit chronic inflammatory changes. It is better not to biopsy axillary lymph nodes because this is sometimes followed by troublesome hematoma formation.

(2) If there are multiple nodes present in one region, my preference is to remove the firmest node and, wherever possible, two or three lymph nodes should be removed. Some authors recommend removal of the largest node; others feel the largest node often becomes necrotic, and in certain instances, the critical nodes

might be the fresh, smaller nodes about the periphery of the conglomerate mass.

(3) It is important that the entire node be removed in one piece and with the capsule intact, since changes typical of benign hyperplastic lymph nodes are evaluated much more easily in the intact node than in segments of a fragmented node. If a question arises between histiocytic lymphoma (reticulum cell sarcoma) or metastatic poorly differentiated carcinoma, the presence of carcinoma in the subcapsular sinusoid will make the latter diagnosis obvious.

(4) When the pathologist cannot make a definite diagnosis from a biopsy specimen, the physician's thought should not be to "let time be the best therapy," but "when and what to biopsy the second time." When rebiopsy is necessary it is better not to take nodes at or near the previous incision, since chronic inflammation and suture granulomatous reactions will make the histological interpretation difficult.

SOFT TISSUE MASS

General Comments

Small soft tissue tumors rarely cause diagnostic problems, as they are readily accessible to local excisional biopsy and histological diagnosis. Lipomas, fibromas, hemangiomas and so on are representative of this group. The problems arise when a patient presents with a large mass, often very firm. If it is soft tissue sarcoma, wide excision requires removal of the entire muscle bundle or even amputation. Local excision of a large benign tumor can be a major undertaking.

Soft tissue sarcomas represent about 1 per cent of all malignant tumors. Among soft tissue sarcomas, the most common types are liposarcoma, fibrosarcoma, rhabdomyosarcoma and synovial sarcoma. Each accounted for about 15 to 20 per cent of the cases in large series.[16] The clinical characteristics of these sarcomas are summarized in Table 6–4. Some of the tumors that used to be called fibrosarcomas are now classified as malignant fibrous histiocytomas because it has been shown that the fibroblastic elements actually are derived from histiocytes.[30]

Presenting Complaints

Painless swelling is the most common complaint. The fact that pain is absent lulls many patients into a false sense of security and they ignore the mass until it becomes very large. This lack of concern is reflected in an average delay of six to twelve months from onset of symptoms to diagnosis.

Pain can be a complaint, but not often. It is likely to occur in retroperitoneal tumors, which can achieve a large size without detection because of their inaccessible location. Occasionally a soft tissue mass can achieve a size large enough to interfere with function. Motion of the knee can be compromised by a popliteal mass, for example, or a retroperitoneal tumor can produce obstruction of the inferior vena cava.

Physical Examination

It is rarely possible to make a definitive diagnosis from a physical examination, since the consistency, mobility and size of the tumor are not reliable tests of benignity or malignancy.

The exact anatomical location should be diagrammed and the dimensions recorded. Is the tumor located in the subcutaneous tissue, within a muscle or in a deep fascial plane? If the tumor is within a muscle, the exact muscle involved should be determined, as well as adjacent ones that may be involved. The proximity of important structures, such as vessels, nerves, tendon sheaths

TABLE 6-4　Summarized Characteristics of Common Varieties of Soft Tissue Sarcoma*

	LIPOSARCOMA	FIBROSARCOMA	RHABDOMYOSARCOMA	SYNOVIAL SARCOMA
Origin of Tissue	Adipose tissue	Connective tissue	Striated muscle	Synovium
Sex Preponderance	None	None	Slightly more often male	M:F = 3:2
Mean Age	All ages	50 yrs.	All ages	32 yrs.
Common Locations	Gluteal region, thighs and popliteal and retroperitoneal regions	Extremities and trunk	Popliteal, inguinal, gluteal and interscapular regions	About tendon sheaths and immediate vicinity of knee and ankle joints

*Adapted from Ackerman and del Regato's Cancer—Diagnosis, Treatment and Prognosis.[23]

and joint space often determines the extent of major ablative procedures.

Work-up and Management

It is not practical to order an extensive work-up for metastatic disease before the histologic findings of the tumor are known. However, all patients with large soft tissue tumors suggestive of malignant lesions should have (1) roentgenogram of the tumor; (2) chest film; (3) electromyogram and nerve conduction tests if there is a suggestion that major nerves may be involved; and (4) angiographic studies if there is a suggestion that major arteries or veins are affected. Patterns of vascularity may help differentiate between benign and malignant lesions. The angiograms can be useful in delineating the anatomical extent of lesions and in planning the appropriate boundaries for resection.

When the tumor is small enough for an excisional biopsy this is the procedure of choice. In large tumors, needle aspiration biopsy may be tried if the pathologist can make a definitive diagnosis. However, a good tissue sample is difficult to obtain from large soft tissue tumors, because of central necrosis and hemorrhage. Furthermore, major resection or amputation of an extremity should rarely be performed on the basis of aspiration biopsy alone. Thus, incisional biopsy of a generous wedge of tumor should be obtained. The wound should be closed without dead space. It is better not to use a drain to avoid growth of tumor along the sinus tract. Whenever possible, frozen section should be performed prior to closure of the wound to make sure that a representative tissue has been taken.

In most instances, a permanent section that gives precise information of histogenesis and degree of anaplasia of the sarcoma is needed before one can plan definitive therapy. If the tumor turns out to be malignant, tomogram of the lung and laparotomy should be done to rule out distant metastases be-

fore radical amputation such as hemipelvectomy is carried out.

It can not be overemphasized that inadequate excision increases the incidence of local recurrence. Occasionally a locally recurrent sarcoma is more aggressive than the primary tumor. Although radiotherapy has been shown to be of benefit to control the local lesion,[71] and chemotherapy can treat the subclinical systemic metastasis,[8] the best opportunity for cure is obtained with a carefully planned multimodality approach combining accurate diagnosis, adequate resection, optimal radiotherapy and adjuvant chemotherapy.

TUMOR CLINIC

The functions of a tumor clinic are several:
(1) Detection and early diagnosis. Physicians should screen asymptomatic patients for cancer and examine patients with complaints suggestive of cancer.
(2) Pre-therapy staging work-up. This includes biopsy procedures and laboratory and radiographic tests that can be done in the outpatient department.
(3) Postoperative care including adjuvant therapy. Early use of systemic chemotherapy or immunotherapy has been shown to be effective in treating subclinical micrometastases in certain cancers.
(4) Long-term follow-up care. Patients who had surgical treatment for cancer should be followed for problems relating to therapy, recurrent disease or new malignancies.

Detection and Early Diagnosis

It is well known that treatment at early stages improves functional results and long-term survival for nearly all forms of human cancer. However, high cost, lack of medical manpower and facilities and low yield have dampened the enthusiasm for mass screening. In the tumor clinics, however, one should not overlook the possibility of new or additional primary malignancies among patients of the high risk groups or patients with symptoms suggestive of cancers.

For some of the common human cancers, the high risk groups are listed in Table 6–5. The occurrence of multiple primary cancers in the same individual, whether simultaneous, nonsimultaneous or cumulative, is a common phenomenon. Cancer incidence increases with age. It has been calculated that about 10 per cent of all persons living to the age of 60 years would develop one cancer, 1 per cent would develop two and 0.1 per cent would develop three separate cancers.[68] By age 90, the corresponding figures are 52 per cent, 18 per cent and 6 per cent. Statistically, certain primary cancers are more likely to be associated with malignancies of another site, for example, larynx — lung; lip — skin; oral cavity — pharynx —

TABLE 6–5 High Risk Factors for Leading Human Cancers

Site	Estimated New Cases for 1978 Male	Female	High Risk Factors
Skin			
Melanoma	4600	5000	Radiation overexposure
Others	200,000*	100,000*	
Colorectum	49,000	53,000	1. Adenomatous polyps 2. Familial polyposis 3. Previous cancer of colorectum 4. Ulcerative colitis
Lung	79,000	23,000	Cigarette smoking caused at least 80% of lung cancer
Breast	700	90,000	1. Previous cancer of breast 2. Family history of breast cancer
Prostate	57,000	—	Uncommon in Asia, Africa and Latin America.
Female genital organs			
Uterine cervix	—	20,000	Sexual promiscuity
Endometrium	—	28,000	Prolonged use of estrogens
Ovary	—	17,000	Family history of ovarian cancer
Urinary organs			
Bladder	22,000	8000	Chemical/industrial workers
Kidney, etc.	9400	5700	
Oral cavity and pharynx	17,400	7000	Tobacco and alcohol overusages
Stomach	14,000	9000	1. Country of origin (i.e., Chile, Iceland, Finland), Orientals 2. Family history of gastric cancer
Pancreas	12,000	9900	Etiological factor obscure, but twofold increased risk noted for cigarette smokers and diabetic patients
All sites	352,000*	348,000*	

*Skin cancers of 300,000 are not included in the total.

esophagus; breast—ovary—endometrium, breast—colorectum.

For the general public, the American Cancer Society has publicized seven warning signals, using the acronym CAUTION:

(1) Change in bowel or bladder habits;
(2) A sore that does not heal;
(3) Unusual bleeding or discharge;
(4) Thickening or lump in the breast or elsewhere;
(5) Indigestion or difficulty in swallowing;
(6) Obvious change in size or color of a wart or mole; and
(7) Nagging cough or hoarseness.

It is estimated that about 80 per cent of the most common cancers can be found early by a simple thorough physical examination. In addition to asking relevant questions, one should have a systematic plan to examine organs most frequently involved with malignant disease. Annual check-up examinations should include:

(1) complete inspection of the entire skin area;
(2) inspection and palpation of the oral cavity;
(3) indirect laryngoscopy;
(4) careful palpation of the mammary glands;
(5) examination of all peripheral lymph node areas: neck, axilla and groins;
(6) pelvic examination including Pap smear for females; and
(7) rectal examination and testing stool for occult blood.

Other examinations, such as endoscopic procedures and special radiological or laboratory tests, should be done as indicated for each patient. For example, women who are older than 50 years of age or those with a family history of breast cancer should have a mammogram as a screening procedure. The benefit of mammography in finding early cancers appears to outweigh the very small increased risk of radiation carcinogenesis several decades later. Proctosigmoidoscopy has been advocated as an annual examination for patients older than 40 years. However, the yield of cancer is so low (less than 1 per cent) that it probably should be used only in patients with symptoms of rectal bleeding, unexplained anemia or abdominal pain.[72] The feasibility of using fecal occult blood testing to detect early colorectal neoplasia is presently being actively studied.[76]

Staging Work-up

Clinical staging of malignant disease, in general, reflects the extent of involvement based on physical findings supplemented by standard diagnostic procedures. Histological diagnosis and pathological information also are essential in the meaningful evaluation of the tumor patient. The objectives of clinical and pathological staging are: (1) aiding the clinician in planning treatment; (2) aiding the clinician in estimating the prognosis; (3) assisting in the evaluation of results of treatment; (4) facilitating the exchange of information among treatment centers; and (5) assisting in the continuing investigation of human cancer.

The American Joint Committee for Cancer Staging and End-Result Reporting has recently published a "Manual for Staging of Cancer" based on the TNM system.[52] The classification is applicable to all solid tumors and is based on the life history of such cancers. As the primary tumor (T) increases in size, at some point local invasion occurs, followed by spread to the regional lymph nodes (N) draining the area of the tumor. Later, distant spread or metastasis (M) becomes evident.

This new staging system can classify the extent of disease at different sites and at different time periods, for instance, (1) clinical-diagnostic staging (cTNM) before any treatment is carried out, (2) surgical-evaluation staging (sTNM) for cases that had surgical exploration, biopsy or both (3) post-surgical-pathological staging (pTNM) following the complete examination of the resected specimen and (4) retreatment staging (rTNM) for cases in which treatment has failed and additional therapy is needed. Well-designed forms for initial and follow-up examinations can facilitate data collection and avoid omission of important information (Figs. 6–11 and 6–12).

It is well known that the treatment of all human solid cancers depends on the stage of disease. If the lesion is localized to one area, local treatment offers hope of cure. If, however, the tumor has

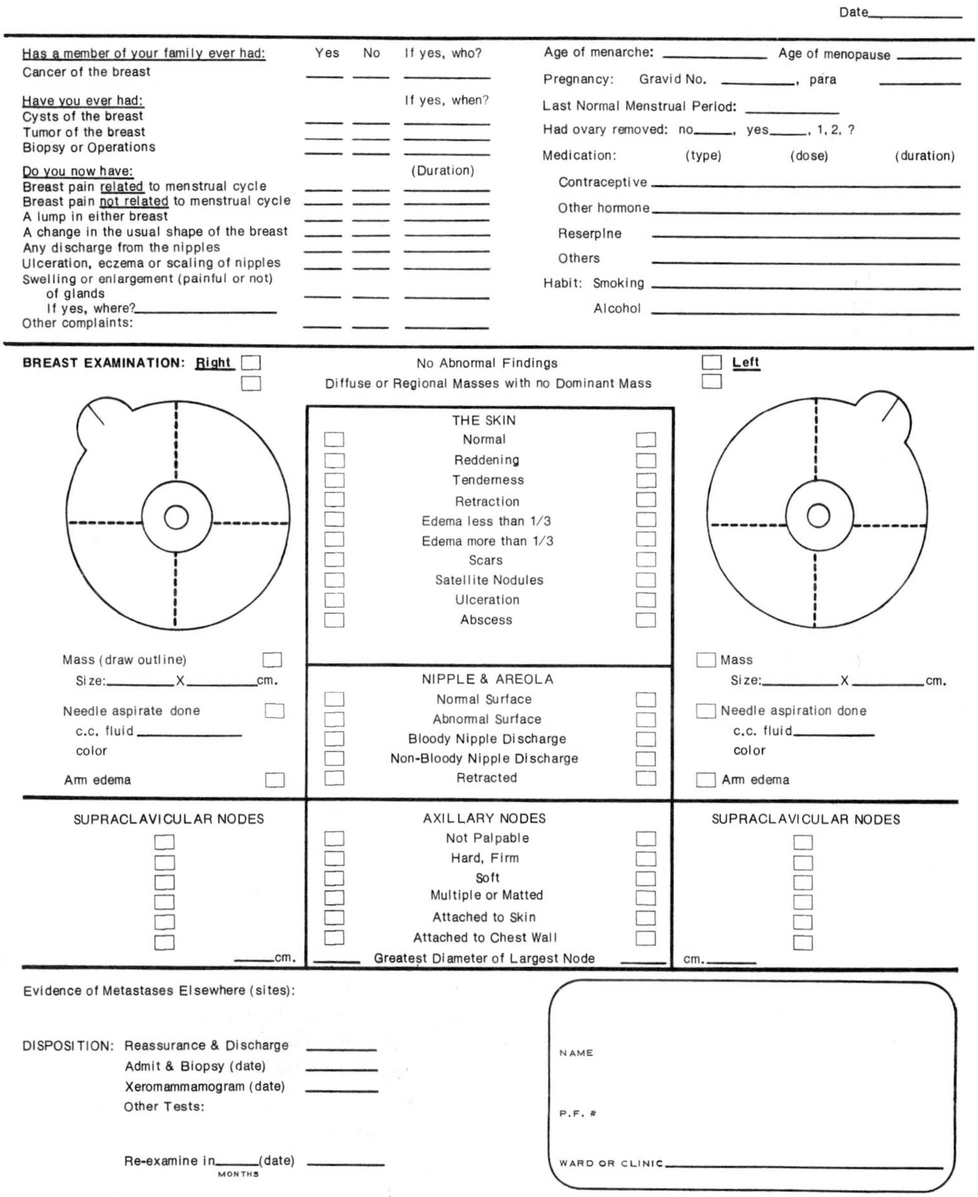
Date________

Has a member of your family ever had: — Yes — No — If yes, who?
Cancer of the breast

Have you ever had: — If yes, when?
Cysts of the breast
Tumor of the breast
Biopsy or Operations

Do you now have: — (Duration)
Breast pain related to menstrual cycle
Breast pain not related to menstrual cycle
A lump in either breast
A change in the usual shape of the breast
Any discharge from the nipples
Ulceration, eczema or scaling of nipples
Swelling or enlargement (painful or not) of glands
If yes, where?________
Other complaints:

Age of menarche: ______ Age of menopause ______
Pregnancy: Gravid No. ______, para ______
Last Normal Menstrual Period: ______
Had ovary removed: no____, yes____, 1, 2, ?
Medication: (type) (dose) (duration)
Contraceptive
Other hormone
Reserpine
Others
Habit: Smoking
Alcohol

BREAST EXAMINATION: Right — No Abnormal Findings — Left
Diffuse or Regional Masses with no Dominant Mass

THE SKIN
Normal
Reddening
Tenderness
Retraction
Edema less than 1/3
Edema more than 1/3
Scars
Satellite Nodules
Ulceration
Abscess

Mass (draw outline)
Size:______X______cm.
Needle aspirate done
c.c. fluid ______
color
Arm edema

NIPPLE & AREOLA
Normal Surface
Abnormal Surface
Bloody Nipple Discharge
Non-Bloody Nipple Discharge
Retracted

Mass
Size:______X______cm.
Needle aspiration done
c.c. fluid______
color
Arm edema

SUPRACLAVICULAR NODES
______cm.

AXILLARY NODES
Not Palpable
Hard, Firm
Soft
Multiple or Matted
Attached to Skin
Attached to Chest Wall
Greatest Diameter of Largest Node

SUPRACLAVICULAR NODES
cm.______

Evidence of Metastases Elsewhere (sites):

DISPOSITION: Reassurance & Discharge ______
Admit & Biopsy (date) ______
Xeromammamogram (date) ______
Other Tests:

Re-examine in______(date) ______
MONTHS

NAME
P.F. #
WARD OR CLINIC______

Figure 6–11 History and physical examination form for breast problems.

DATE:_____

DATE OF MASTECTOMY:_____   R_____   L_____

TYPE OF MASTECTOMY: Dx: Ductal Ca_____infiltrating_____, lobular Ca_____,
_____ Radical   other:_____
_____ Modified   No. of nodes _____   positive _____
_____ Simple   level I
_____ Tylectomy   level II   _____   _____
_____ Bx only   level III   _____   _____

TYPE OF RADIOTHERAPY: _____ Preop   _____ Postop   Dates: _____

        Site: _____ Axilla   _____ Sternal
                   _____ Breast   _____ Supraclavicular
                   _____ Others   _____ Chest Wall

        DOSE: _____

Baseline Xeromammagrom: _____ Preop   _____ Postop   Dates: _____

ROUTINE QUESTIONS FOR SYMPTOMS:
Bone Pain   site _____   duration _____   severity _____
Other Pain   site _____   duration _____   severity _____
Headache   site _____   duration _____   severity _____
Other complaints   site _____   duration _____   severity _____

ROUTINE EXAMINATION FOR FUNCTION:
Arm edema: Mid-arm   circumference_____   Normal side_____ cm.
Shoulder motion (abduction degrees):
Extremity function: excellent_____ good_____ partial_____ limited_____

ROUTINE EXAMINATION FOR TUMOR (palpation   ✓ = Checked, No abnormality)
                              R   L
Opposite breast   _____ _____
Chest wall   _____ _____

Axilla node   _____ _____
Supraclavicular   _____ _____
Parasternal   _____ _____
Liver edge   _____ _____

Exam for complaints:

IMPRESSION:
1. Cancer on this date   2. Other problems

        _____ none   _____
        _____ suspected   _____
        _____ positive

TESTS ORDERED:

FOLLOW-UP PLAN AFTER WOUND HEALED:
1. Clinic check every three months for the first two years, then annually.
2. Chest x-ray six months after operation, then annually.
3. Teach patient to do self-examination for breast mass and lymphadenopathy.
   Advise to return to clinic sooner if abnormality appears.
4. If recurrent disease is documented, please send patient to Friday's TSS
   clinic.

DISPOSITION: (Appointment Date)
Routine return visits   _____
Special return visits   _____
Refer to another clinic   _____
Discharge/hospitalized   _____

NAME

P.F. #

WARD OR CLINNC _____

Figure 6–12   Follow-up form for malignant breast lesions.

disseminated, systemic therapy should be instituted. For too long, the clinician's attention has been focused solely on the diagnosis of the presence of the tumor, whereas the assessment of extent of dissemination of the carcinoma has been ignored. With the availability of newer diagnostic tests and the acceptance of postsurgical adjuvant therapy, the pretreatment staging search for subclinical or occult metastasis has become a prerequisite in cancer management before applying specific therapy to a patient with an apparently early carcinoma.

After initial therapy, if there is any question of recurrence of the lesion, repeated tests may be required to restage the extent. When a single focus of recurrent tumor appears, restaging work-up is also indicated to rule out other foci of disease. If no other disseminated lesion is found by various staging tests, the solitary recurrence or metastasis may still be aggressively treated with resection or radiation therapy. During treatment of unresectable lesions, serial staging work-ups may be needed to assess response and to assist in making decisions concerning new treatment.

Among 1000 patients who died of malignant neoplasms of epithelial origin, the most common sites of dissemination at autopsy included lymph nodes, liver, lung (about 50 per cent each), bone, peritoneum and brain (about 25 per cent each).[1] The pattern and extent of metastasis varied greatly among malignancies originating from different organs. At present, roentgenograms of the chest and full lung tomograms are very accurate for detecting silent pulmonary metastases. For detecting occult metastatic disease of the bone, liver and brain, there are a number of sophisticated tests and procedures available. The carcinoembryonic antigen (CEA) test has been shown to be useful in monitoring the effects of therapy and as an aid in detecting recurrent or metastatic disease. However, none of these tests is perfect, and each test has its own limitations.*

---

*A *false negative* report means patients had the disease or condition but the diagnosis was missed by the particular test. Low false negative rate means that the test has high sensitivity. *Sensitivity* is calculated from the subpopulation of patients with documented disease: the number of patients with a positive test divided by the number of all those with disease. A *false positive* report means patients were diagnosed to have the disease by the test but actually did not have the particular disease. A low false positive rate means the test was very specific. *Specificity* is calculated from the subpopulation of patients or normal controls known to be without disease: the number of those with negative tests divided by the number of all those without disease. Accuracy rate refers to how good a test is in detecting the absence *or* presence of a particular disease. Overall *accuracy rate* is equal to the sum of patients correctly diagnosed by the test as having or not having the disease, divided by the total population tested.

Detection of Bony Metastases

Osseous metastases commonly are not demonstrable by radiological examination until they are approximately 1 to 1.5 cm in diameter or until 50 to 75 per cent of bone minerals have been lost. In a number of large series it has been shown that about 15 to 35 per cent of cancer patients with normal roentgenograms have abnormal radioisotopic scans.[17] Even in patients with positive x-rays, one-third to one-half of the cases had scans that showed more metastatic diseases than those revealed by x-rays.

However, none of the bone scan agents labels cancer cells specifically and skeletal scans have false positive and false negative rates of around 10 per cent each. In patients with early operable breast cancers, it has been reported that about 16 to 26 per cent had positive bone scans.[15, 31, 66] Other series showed that for patients with clinical stage I/II lesions, routine preoperative bone scans were positive in less than 5 per cent of the cases.[5, 22, 33] Even among patients with positive bone scans, 40 per cent survived eight years free of any recurrence.[66]

Clinically, there are factors that correlate with a higher risk of bony metastases, such as primary cancer greater than 5 cm in diameter and axillary metastases, especially of higher levels and with more than six nodes involved.[15, 18] After obtaining an initial normal bone scan, conversion to a positive scan on subsequent studies usually signifies bony metastases.[33] Thus, patients with a high risk for dissemination should have a "baseline" bone scan. And radiographs should be taken of abnormal areas in scans to rule out the presence of benign conditions.

Detection of Liver Metastasis

The early diagnosis of hepatic metastasis is extremely difficult. In cases in which a laparotomy is performed for a suspected hepatic tumor, there is a rather high incidence of abnormal liver function tests in patients found to have normal livers and a rather high incidence of normal test results in patients with a solitary liver tumor. Hepatic scintigraphy is more sensitive, and about 74 to 90 per cent of those with documented liver lesions have abnormal scans.[32] False positive diagnoses have been reported as low as 15 per cent and as high as 25 per cent, and false negative rates vary from 5 per cent to 42 per cent. The accuracy of liver scan can be increased if one correlates radioisotopic results with elevated alkaline phosphatase or carcinoembryonic antigen levels.[69]

Sears and associates[61] reviewed liver scans as part of the initial evaluation of 100 patients with potentially resectable carcinoma of the breast. Five positive scans were reported, and four of these were found to be falsely positive. For patients with small cell carcinoma of the lung, only one liver scan in 21 yielded new information suggesting organ involvement.[77] For patients with head and neck cancers, sarcoma, melanoma or pelvic malignancies, preoperative evaluation yields positive liver scans in less than 3 per cent of the cases. It appears that routine preoperative screening liver scan is not indicated for extra-abdominal malignancies.

Fee and associates[28] estimated the value of preoperative screening liver scans in 70 patients before operation for suspected intra-abdominal tumors (22 had documented hepatic metastasis). The overall accuracy of the liver scan was 84 per cent (13 per cent false positive and 23 per cent false negative results). For comparison, the accuracy of the serum alkaline phosphatase levels was 63 per cent (18 per cent false negative and 46 per cent false positive results). The authors commented that of all the single diagnostic tools, the liver scan, inaccurate as it is, is probably still the best. However, liver scanning is not as useful a screening test as cerebral or skeletal scintigraphy, in which the in-

cidence of false positive is relatively low.[32]

During the past few years, ultrasonography of the liver and whole body computed tomography (CT) have become clinically available. Bryan and colleagues[14] compared the ability of CT, ultrasonography and radionuclide image to detect and characterize space-occupying processes in the liver. The false positive rates for these three tests were 0 per cent, 2 per cent and 4 per cent, and the false negative rates were 12 per cent, 6 per cent and 4 per cent respectively. They concluded that these three tests appeared to be complementary studies. They recommended liver scan as the initial screening modality, except for patients with lymphoma, in whom ultrasonography was preferred. When a definite or suspected abnormality is observed by nuclear imaging, either ultrasonography or CT should be performed to obtain better anatomical definition and characterization of the process.

Carcinoembryonic Antigen

Carcinoembryonic antigen (CEA) is a glycoprotein that is normally secreted into the lumen by epithelial cells of the gastrointestinal tract. As the normal tissue architecture is disrupted, the CEA is released into underlying tissue and diffuses into the vascular or lymphatic channels. The common denominator of rapid cellular proliferation and disruption of basement membrane explains the presence of elevated circulating CEA levels in entodermal and nonentodermal malignancies, in various nonmalignant metabolic or inflammatory diseases, in surgical trauma and in cases of heavy smoking.

Among healthy nonsmoking subjects, 97 per cent have CEA titers of 2.5 ng/ml or below, none above 5 ng/ml. Among chronic smokers (more than one pack a day for at least 10 years), 4 per cent have CEA above 5 ng/ml and 1 per cent have a CEA level over 10 ng/ml. Among smokers, elevated CEA levels decline to the nonsmoker range within three months after cessation of smoking.[2] In general, high CEA levels (above 20 ng/ml) usually indicate metastatic disease, except for patients with primary pancreatic or colorectal carcinoma.

For patients with colon cancers, the CEA levels vary with the extent of the tumor. In one series, the assay was greater than 2.5 ng/ml in 14 per cent with Duke A lesions, in 54 per cent with B, in 60 per cent with C and in 79 per cent with D lesions.[48] Within any particular Duke's stage there is a tendency for higher values to carry a worse prognosis.[49] Preoperatively elevated CEA determinations usually fall to normal levels about one month after complete resection of the colonic cancer. Following potentially curative resections, progressively rising CEAs usually suggest relapses, up to 29 months before clinical evidence of recurrence.[67] However, about 10 per cent of patients with rising CEAs do not have evidence of relapse and another 10 per cent of the cases with extensive disease do not have elevated CEAs.[38]

At least two sequential elevated CEA values, the second being higher, should be obtained before considering that progression of disease has occurred.[38] Balz and associates[6] suggested that each laboratory should establish 95 per cent confidence limits at various CEA levels. Any patient with a CEA value greater than two standard deviations above his last level can then be said to have a significant elevation of CEA. In three reports utilizing second-look operations for patients with rising CEA, 39 out of 45 patients explored had recurrent disease. Some patients were convertible to a tumor-free state.[43] Rising serial CEA levels correlated with disease progression in patients with known metastatic gastrointestinal cancer who were treated with chemotherapy.[65] Persistently low or undetectable values was a favorable prognostic sign.

In patients with carcinoma of the breast, CEA levels are generally lower than those seen in patients with gastrointestinal cancer. The proportion of elevated CEA levels increases as the tumor spreads.[73] More patients with spread in lymph nodes have abnormal levels of CEA than those with lesions limited to the breast, and over 70 per cent of the patients with distant metastasis have increased concentrations. The rate of elevated CEA varies according to the site of metastasis, ranging from 41 per cent in patients with soft tissue metastasis to 64 per cent for osseous, 83 per cent for pulmonary, and 93 per cent for hepatic metastasis.[19]

Among patients with operable breast carcinomas, the actual levels of CEA before mastectomy do not accurately predict the risk of recurrence during follow-up. Wang and associates[74] showed that patients with elevated CEA ten days after mastectomy had a higher chance of recurrence, while Tormey and colleagues[73] found no direct correlation between postoperative CEA changes and the presence or absence of relapses. They obtained postoperative CEAs at one-month or longer intervals.

In patients with advanced lesions treated with chemotherapy or hormonal therapy, some investigators report a good clinical response to therapy mirrored by a fall of CEA to normal levels.[73] Others show good correlation among patients with marked regression or progression of the disease, but the overall correlation is not good.[19]

In summary, decreases in CEA titers are reported to be associated with effective therapy. Persistent increases in titer are associated with a lack of response to therapy or a recurrence of disease; in some cases, the titer rise precedes clinical signs. However, CEA titers are not an absolute test for malignancy. Just as with many other diagnostic tests in medicine, interpretations of CEA results should include consideration of the patient's clinical status.

Bone Marrow and Scalene Node Biopsies

In staging the patient with a lymphoreticular malignancy, the bone marrow biopsy has proven to be valuable. Since marrow biopsy can be done as an outpatient procedure, it has been included with increasing frequency as a part of the total clinical evaluation of patients with nonhematopoietic cancers. Metastasis may be present in the bone marrow without any abnormalities being recognized in bone scans, radiographic picture, serum chemistry or hematological parameters.[63]

In male patients with primarily unresectable cancers, about 31 per cent are reported to have tumor cells in marrow biopsies.[12] Lesions of lung and prostate had a positive rate of about 42 to 60 per cent. Of the patients with positive bone scans, only half had positive marrow biopsies, and of those with abnormal peripheral blood smears, about one third had documented marrow involvement. In another series of 101 patients with solid nonlymphomatous neoplasms and marrow involvement, probably all had relatively advanced lesions. Sixty per cent had negative roentgenographical or bone scan examinations or both.[63] Metastases from a primary tumor in the breast were the most frequent, followed by metastases from the prostate.

In 1949, Daniels described the technique of scalene fat pad biopsy for the diagnosis of intrathoracic diseases. Subsequent studies showed that scalene node biopsy was useful in detecting extrathoracic spread of intrathoracic neoplasms and in diagnosing obscure systemic conditions and diseases involving lymph nodes, even when they are not palpable. Some surgeons have included left scalene node biopsy as part of the routine pretreatment staging procedure for Hodgkin's disease to define further the extent of involvement.[45]

Ketcham and associates[39] included scalene lymph node biopsy as part of the preoperative work-up for patients before radical pelvic resections. Surprisingly, the scalene fat pad was the site of previously unrecognized metastasis in 13 per cent of individuals with locally advanced cancer of the uterine cervix.

Other Tests

Brain scans are often ordered as screening procedures in patients with carcinoma of the lung. However, even in patients with oat cell carcinoma of the lung, only one brain scan in 35 yields new information.[17] Among patients with recurrent breast cancers and symptoms of central nervous system involvement, only one third have positive brain scans.[54] Computed tomography (CT) of the head certainly has proved its superiority and may replace brain scan in the future.

Other invasive diagnostic procedures such as thoracoscopy, peritoneoscopy, minilaparotomy and so on require more than local anesthesia and are usually performed in the hospital. The impact of the CT scan on screening for occult metastasis remains to be seen. At the present time, the justification for using scans or other tests as routine screening for distant metastasis during the initial evaluation of patients with localized solid cancer remains to be delineated. All tests represent great expense to the patient and can delay initiation of therapy. Pending further reports, one should order all tests selectively and with specific indications.

Postoperative Adjuvant Therapy

In addition to routine postoperative care such as checking for wound healing, removal of drains and sutures and so on, administration of adjuvant therapy has become very important for the tumor outpatient clinic. It is well known that, despite the best surgical efforts, a distressing proportion of patients with clinically localized solid tumors already have subclinical metastatic foci, which appear late as disseminated lesions. Destruction of these tumor cells requires repetitive courses of treatment, usually lasting one to two years.

Although postsurgical adjuvant therapy has not become part of the standard medical practice, many institutions have been or will be participating in cooperative randomized studies searching for more effective therapeutic regimens. Some general guidelines and useful examples are presented here.

All protocol studies specifically define a patient population that has a high risk of developing recurrence. All adjuvant treatments demand regular comprehensive follow-up examinations, laboratory and x-ray tests to detect recrudescence of malignancy and careful monitoring of side effects of the specific therapeutic agent(s).

Myelosuppression is the most common side effect of chemotherapeutic drugs. General guidelines to modify the dosages of chemotherapy according to the degree of myelosuppression are as follows: If no toxicity was evident (WBC > 4000/mm^3 and platelets > 130,000/mm^3), 100 per cent of each drug is administered. For grade 1 toxicity (WBC = 3999–2500/mm^3 and/or platelets=129,000–75,000/mm^3) 50 per cent of the calculated dose is given. In the presence of grade 2 toxicity (WBC < 2500/mm^3 and/or platelets < 75,000/mm^3), no drug is administered until at least grade 1 toxicity is reached.

For patients who have had a mastectomy and whose breast cancers had metastasized to the axillary nodes, two studies have shown that postsurgical adjuvant chemotherapy is effective in delaying recurrence and possibly improving the rate of survival as well. One study randomized patients between placebo and cyclic single agent chemotherapy (L-PAM orally at 0.15 mg/kg/day × 5 every six weeks for two years).[29] In the other study, patients were randomly allocated to no further therapy or to CMF — cyclophosphamide (100 mg/m^2 PO on days 1–14), methotrexate (40 mg/m^2 IV on days 1 and 8) and 5-FU (600 mg/m^2 IV on days 1 and 8) every four weeks. In the absence of relapse, CMF was continued for 12 cycles (i.e., about 12 months).[9] The available data indicated that multiple drug treatment was superior to the single agent in decreasing the total failure rate after radical mastectomy in all subgroups of patients, with the exception that L-PAM and CMF were equally effective in premenopausal women.

Regarding drug tolerance in the L-PAM study, 60 per cent of the patients experienced decreased white cell count at some time during therapy. Forty per cent of the patients complained of nausea and vomiting during chemotherapy. Alopecia and stomatitis were rarely observed.

In the CMF study, side effects were more numerous. About 75 per cent of the patients had leukopenia, thrombocytopenia or both, but there were no episodes of infection or bleeding secondary to drug-induced hematosuppression. Stomatitis was rare (19 per cent). Hair loss occurred in 69 per cent of the patients, but pronounced alopecia was rare. Mild chemical cystitis secondary to cyclophosphamide was observed in 30 per cent of patients. Treatment produced amenorrhea in 78 per cent of premenopausal patients, and in 17 per cent the suppression of menses was temporary.

Most patients complained of nausea and vomiting within a few hours after drug injection. In more than two-thirds of the patients, the daily administration of cyclophosphamide caused prolonged nausea and loss of appetite. Unless encouraged to take the drug regularly, about one-third of the patients showed a repeated tendency to discontinue treatment or diminish the dose. Only 23 patients (11 per cent) refused to complete the chemotherapy, chiefly for psychological reasons rather than because of severe side effects.

In our clinic, each patient is given an information sheet describing the drug programs, side effects, schedules of laboratory tests and so on. Patients are told to take antiemetic medications one hour before they are given intravenous chemotherapy. Sometimes a suppository form of antiemetic is most effective. We have eliminated the severe nausea and vomiting episodes in a few very sensitive patients by giving the injections slowly over five minutes or by using intravenous infusion over 30 to 60 minutes.

In our tumor clinics, with or without protocol studies, each patient has a designated social worker who sees the patient for initial and follow-up visits. In order to enhance consistency and continuity of patient care, it is also essential to have well-trained nurse clinicians. Clerical associates can keep records or order the necessary tests according to schedule, but only the nurse can screen abnormal test reports, provide psychological support to the patient and administer the chemotherapeutic or immunotherapeutic treatment.

Long-Term Follow-up Care

Long-term follow-up care of all patients is mandatory following surgery for cancer. A registry of all tumor patients should be established in each hospital. Stable funding, secretarial assistance and staff coverage for these clinics are essential for successful recall of patients and intelligent, sequential recording of information. The general surgical Tumor Clinic in most hospitals will follow patients with cancers of the head and neck, breast, thyroid, lung, gastrointestinal tract, soft tissue sarcomas and skin. Most specialty clinics follow the patients with cancer who were operated upon by their inpatient services.

The nature of the follow-up examination varies with the type of tumor the patient had. Questions about general health and specific complaints should be evaluated. The patient's overall performance status and functional adjustment should be recorded. In all cases, the operative area and regional lymph nodes must be checked. The supraclavicular area and abdomen should be examined. A chest x-ray is usually indicated at six-month intervals for patients who have been operated upon for cancer, except cancers that recur locally almost exclusively, such as those of the skin. Melanomas and sarcomas frequently reappear as silent pulmonary metastases.

One important activity of tumor clinics should be patient education. All patients having cancers of the skin or breast should be trained to watch for and report promptly signs of new primary cancers, locally recrudescent disease and regional lymph node metastases. All patients should be advised that when they note unusual symptoms or findings they should return immediately and *not* wait for their regular appointments.

Incidence, pattern and time of appearance of recurrent carcinomas vary with the type and extent of primary lesions treated. For instance, for operable carcinoma of the breast, the incidence of recurrence is highest in the first three years after mastectomy — as much as 75 per cent of all initial recurrences are detected within three years.[60] The annual rate of recurrence is consistently higher among patients who have involved axillary nodes than among those who do not. The risk of recurrence falls off gradually to a low level, but even during 7 to 15 years after mastectomy the risk still is about 2 to 4 per cent per year. Contralateral breast cancers, an independent threat, appear at a constant rate of 1 per cent per year.[26] Before the days of radioisotopic scans, skeletal metastasis accounted for 44 per cent of initial recurrences, and nonskeletal sites accounted for the other 56 per cent. The latter included operative region

(19 per cent), supraclavicular area (8 per cent), lung (12 per cent), pleural effusion (6 per cent), liver (2 per cent) and others (11 per cent).[60]

Thus, the interval for follow-up varies, depending on the prognosis at surgery and the length of time since operation. For most cancers, monthly follow-up is indicated for three months, followed by visits at three-month intervals for the first two years. The visits may be at six-month intervals for the next three years and then at yearly intervals. For detailed information about following patients with all types of cancer, the Commission on Cancer of the American College of Surgeons has published a pamphlet entitled "The Patient With Cancer — Guidelines for Follow-up."[3]

REFERENCES

1. Abrams, H. L., Spiro, R. and Goldstein, N.: Metastases in carcinoma: Analysis of 1000 autopsied cases. Cancer, 3:74–85, 1950.
2. Alexander, J. C., Silverman, N. A. and Chretien, P. B.: Effect of age and cigarette smoking on carcinoembryonic antigen levels. J.A.M.A., 235:1975–1979, 1976.
3. American College of Surgeons' Commission on Cancer: The Patient with Cancer — Guidelines for Follow-up. 1976, pp. 1–60.
4. Ashikari, R., Rosen, P. P., Urban, J. A. et al.: Breast cancer presenting as axillary mass. Ann. Surg., 183:415–417, 1976.
5. Baker, R. R., Holmes, E. R., Alderson, P. O. et al.: An evaluation of bone scans as screening procedures for occult metastases in primary breast cancer. Ann. Surg., 186:363–368, 1977.
6. Balz, J. B., Martin, E. W. and Minton, J. P.: CEA as an early indicator for second-look procedure in colorectal carcinoma. Rev. Surg., 34:1–4, 1977.
7. Barrie, J. R., Knapper, W. H. and Strong, E. W.: Cervical nodal metastases of unknown origin. Am. J. Surg., 120:466–470, 1970.
8. Benjamin, R. S., Baker, L. H., O'Bryan, R. M. et al.: Advances in the chemotherapy of soft tissue sarcoma. Med. Clin. North Am., 61:1039–1043, 1977.
9. Bonadonna, G., Rossi, A., Valagussa, P. et al.: The CMF program for operable breast cancer with positive axillary nodes: Update analysis on the disease-free interval, site of relapse and drug tolerance. Cancer, 39:2904–2915, 1977.
10. Breslow, A.: Tumor thickness, level of invasion and node dissection in stage I cutaneous melanoma. Ann. Surg., 182:572–575, 1975.
11. Breslow, A. and Macht, S. D.: Optimal size of resection margin for thin cutaneous melanoma. Surg. Gynecol. Obstet., 145:691–692, 1977.
12. Broghamer, W. L. and Keeling, M. M.: The bone marrow biopsy, osteoscan and peripheral blood in non-hematopoietic cancer. Cancer, 40:836–840, 1977.
13. Brownstein, M. H. and Helwig, E. B.: Spread of tumors to the skin. Arch. Dermatol., 107:80–86, 1973.
14. Bryan, J. P., Dinn, W. M., Grossman, Z. D. et al.: Correlation of computed tomography, gray scale ultrasonography and radionuclide imaging of the liver in detecting space-occupying processes. Radiology, 124:387–393, 1977.
15. Campbell, D. J., Banks, A. J. and Oates, G. D.: The value of preliminary bone scanning in staging and assessing the prognosis of breast cancer. Br. J. Surg., 63:811–816, 1976.
16. Cantin, J., McNeer, G. P., Chu, F. C. et al.: The problem of local recurrence after treatment of soft tissue sarcoma. Ann. Surg., 168:47–53, 1968.
17. Charkes, N. D.: Bone and soft tissue sarcomas: Current status of radioisotopes in the diagnosis of bone cancer. In Proceedings of Seventh National Cancer Conference. Philadelphia, J. B. Lippincott Co., 1973, pp. 915–919.
18. Charkes, N. D., Malmud, L. S., Caswell, T. et al.: Preoperative bone scans; Use in women with early breast cancer. J.A.M.A., 233:516, 1975.
19. Chu, T. M. and Nemoto, T.: Evaluation of carcinoembryonic antigen in human mammary carcinoma. J. Nat. Cancer Inst., 51:1119–1122, 1973.
20. Clark, W. H., From, L., Bernardino, E. et al.: The histogenesis of biologic behavior of primary human malignant melanomas of the skin. Cancer Res., 29:705–727, 1969.
21. Copeland, E. M. and McBride, C. M.: Axillary metastases from unknown primary sites. Ann Surg., 178:25–27, 1973.
22. Davies, C. J., Griffiths, P. A., Preston, B. et al.: Staging breast cancer; Role of bone scanning. Br. Med. J., 2:603–605, 1977.
23. del Regato, J. A. and Spjut, H. J.: Ackerman and del Regato's Cancer — Diagnosis, Treatment and Prognosis, Ed. 5. St. Louis, C. V. Mosby Co. 1977, p. 918.
24. Didolkar, M. S., Fanous, N., Elias, E. G. et al.: Metastatic carcinomas from occult primary tumors: A study of 254 patients. Ann. Surg., 186:625–630, 1977.
25. Donegan, W. L.: Diagnosis of mammary cancer. In Spratt, J. S. and Donegan, W. L.: Cancer of the Breast, Vol. V in Major

Problems in Clinical Surgery. Philadelphia, W. B. Saunders Co., 1967, pp. 60–61.

26. Donegan, W. L.: Management of pregnancy and lactation. *In* B. A. Stoll (Ed.): Breast Cancer Management: Early and Late. Chicago, Year Book Medical Publishers, 1977, pp. 195–202.

27. Epstein, E., Bragg, K. and Linden, G.: Biopsy and prognosis of malignant melanoma. J.A.M.A., *208*:1369–1371, 1969.

28. Fee, H. J., Prokop, E. K., Cameron, J. L. et al.: Liver scanning in patients with suspected abdominal tumor. J.A.M.A., *230*:1675–1677, 1974.

29. Fisher, B., Glass, A., Redmond, C. et al.: L-Phenylalanine mustard (L-PAM) in the management of primary breast cancer; An update of earlier findings and a comparison with those utilizing L-PAM plus 5-fluorouracil (5-FU). Cancer, *39*:2883–2903, 1977.

30. Fu, Y. S., Gabbiani, G., Kaye, G. I. et al.: Malignant soft tissue tumors of probable histiocytic origin (malignant fibrous histiocytomas): General consideration and electron microscopic and tissue culture studies. Cancer, *35*:176–198, 1975.

31. Galasko, C. S. B.: The detection of skeletal metastases from carcinoma of the breast. Surg. Gynecol. Obstet., *132*:1019–1024, 1971.

32. Galasko, C. S. B.: The value of scintigraphy in malignant disease. Cancer Treat. Rev., 2:225–272, 1975.

33. Gerber, F. H., Goodreau, J. J., Kirchner, P. T. et al.: Efficacy of preoperative and postoperative bone scanning in the management of breast carcinoma. N. Engl. J. Med., *297*:300–303, 1977.

34. Glass, R. L. and Perez-Mesa, C. M.: Management of inadequately excised epidermoid carcinoma. Arch. Surg., *108*:50–51, 1974.

35. Gumport, S. L., Harris, M. N. and Kopf, A. W.: Diagnosis and management of common skin cancers. CA, *24*:218–228, 1974.

36. Helsper, J. T.: Staining techniques: Screening tests for oral cancer. CA, *22*:172–175, 1972.

37. Holmes, F. F. and Fouts, T. L.: Metastatic cancer of unknown primary site. Progress in Clinical Cancer, Vol. IV. New York, Grune & Stratton, 1973, pp. 21–24.

38. Holyoke, E. D., Chu, T. M. and Murphy, G. P.: CEA as a monitor of gastrointestinal malignancy. Cancer, *35*:830–836, 1975.

39. Ketcham, A. S., Hoye, R. C., Taylor, P. T. et al.: Radical hysterectomy and pelvic lymphadenectomy for carcinoma of the uterine cervix. Cancer, *28*:1272–1277, 1971.

40. Kline, T. S. and Neal, H. S.: Needle aspiration biopsy: A critical appraisal (eight years and 3,267 specimens later). J.A.M.A., *239*:36–39, 1978.

41. Knutson, C. O., Hori, J. M. and Spratt, J. S.: Melanoma. Curr. Probl. Surg., 3–55, December 1971.

42. Krementz, E. T., Cerise, E. J., Ciaravella, J. M. et al.: Metastases of undetermined source. CA, *27*:289–300, 1977.

43. Lee, Y-T.N.: Clinical use of carcinoembryonic antigen in patients with breast or colon carcinomas. West. J. Med., *129*:374–380, 1978.

44. Lee Y-T. N.: Malignant melanoma: To biopsy or not to biopsy. CA, *24*:104–105, 1974.

45. Lee, Y-T. N.: Surgery for diagnosis. *In* Lee, Y-T. N. and Spratt, J. S.: Malignant Lymphoma: Nodal and Extranodal Diseases. New York, Grune & Stratton, 1974, pp. 126–134.

46. Lee, Y-T. N. and Gold, R. H.: Localization of occult testicular tumor with scrotal thermography. J.A.M.A., *236*:1975–1976, 1976.

47. Lieberman, Z. and Ackerman, L. V.: Principles in management of soft tissue sarcomas. Surgery, *35*:350–365, 1954.

48. Livingstone, A. S., Hampson, L. G., Shuster, J. et al.: Carcinoembryonic antigen in the diagnosis and management of colorectal carcinoma. Arch. Surg., *109*:259–264, 1974.

49. LoGerfo, P. and Herter, F. P.: Carcinoembryonic antigen and prognosis in patients with colon cancer. Ann. Surg., *181*:81–84, 1975.

50. Lukes, R. J. and Collins, R. D.: Immunologic characterization of human malignant lymphomas. Cancer, *34*:1488–1503, 1974.

51. Macht, S. D. and Thompson, L. W.: Intraoral field block anesthesia for extra-oral lesions. Surg. Gynecol. Obstet., *146*:87–89, 1978.

52. Manual for Staging of Cancer, 1977. Published by American Joint Committee, 55 East Erie St., Chicago, Ill., 60611.

53. Moertel, C. G., Reitemeier, R. J., Schutt, A. J. et al.: Treatment of the patient with adenocarcinoma of unknown origin. Cancer, *30*:1469–1472, 1972.

54. Muss, H. B., White, D. R. and Cowan, R. J.: Brain scanning in patients with recurrent breast cancer. Cancer, *38*:1574–1576, 1976.

55. Nussbaum, M.: Carcinoma of prostatic origin. N. Y. State J. Med., *73*:2050–2054, 1973.

56. Parker, G. A. and Chretien, P. B.: Axillary lymph node biopsy. Arch. Surg., *112*:1124, 1977.

57. Pascal, R. R., Hobby, L. W., Lattes, R. et al.: Prognosis of "incompletely excised" versus "completely excised" basal cell carcinoma. Plast. Reconstr. Surg., *41*:328–332, 1968.

58. Perez, C. A., Jesse, R. H. and Fletcher, G. H.: Metastatic carcinoma in cervical lymph nodes: Unknown primary site. *In*

Neoplasia of Head and Neck. Clinical Conference in Cancer, M.D. Anderson Hospital and Tumor Institute. Chicago, Year Book Medical Publishers, 1974, pp. 289–302.

59. Pierce, E. H., Gray, H. K. and Dockerty, M. B.: Surgical significance of isolated axillary adenopathy. Ann. Surg., *145*:104–107, 1957.

60. Romsdahl, M. M., Sears, M. E. and Eckles, N. E.: Post-treatment evaluation of breast cancer. *In* Breast Cancer — Early and Late. Chicago, Year Book Medical Publishers, 1970, pp. 291–299.

61. Sears, H. F., Gerber, F. H., Sturtz, D. L. et al.: Liver scan and carcinoma of the breast. Surg. Gynecol. Obstet., *140*:409–411, 1975.

62. Shedd, D. P. and Gaeta, J. F.: In vivo staining of pharyngeal and laryngeal cancer. Arch. Surg., *102*:442–446, 1971.

63. Singh, G., Krause, J. R. and Breitfeld, V.: Bone marrow examination for metastatic tumor: Aspirate and biopsy. Cancer, *40*:2317–2321, 1977.

64. Skandalakis, J. E., Gray, S. W., Takakis, N. C. et al.: Tumors of the neck. Surgery, *48*:375—384, 1960.

65. Skarin, A. T., Delwiche, R., Zamcheck, N. et al.: Carcinoembryonic antigen: Clinical correlation with chemotherapy for metastatic gastrointestinal cancer. Cancer, *33*:1239–1245, 1974.

66. Sklaroff, R. B. and Sklaroff, D. M.: Bone metastases from breast cancer at the time of radical mastectomy as detected by bone scan: Eight year follow-up. Cancer, *38*:107–111, 1976.

67. Sorokin, J. J., Sugarbaker, P. H., Zamcheck, N. et al.: Serial carcinoembryonic antigen assays: Use in detection of cancer recurrence. J.A.M.A., *228*:49–53, 1974.

68. Spratt, J. S.: Multiple primary cancers — Review of clinical studies from two Missouri hospitals. Cancer, *40*:1806–1811, 1977.

69. Sugarbaker, P. H., Beard, J. O. and Drum, D. E.: Detection of hepatic metastases from cancer of the breast. Am. J. Surg., *133*:531–535, 1977.

70. Sugarbaker, E. V. and McBride, C. M.: Melanoma of the trunk: The results of surgical excision and anatomic guidelines for predicting nodal metastasis. Surgery, *80*:22–30, 1976.

71. Suit, H. D., Russel, W. O. and Martin, R. G.: Sarcoma of soft tissue — Clinical and histopathologic parameters and response to treatment. Cancer, *35*:1478–1483, 1975.

72. Swinton, N. W. and Scherer, W. P.: The value of proctosigmoidoscopic examinations. CA, *18*:88–91, 1968.

73. Tormey, D. C., Waalkes, T. P., Snyder, J. J. et al.: Biological markers in breast carcinoma, III — Clinical correlations with carcinoembryonic antigen. Cancer, *39*:2397–2404, 1977.

74. Wang, D. Y., Bulbrook, R. D., Hayward, J. L. et al.: Relationship between plasma carcinoembryonic antigen and prognosis in women with breast cancer. Eur. J. Cancer, *11*:615–618, 1975.

75. Weinberger, H. A. and Stetten, D.: Extensive secondary axillary lymph node carcinoma without clinical evidence of primary breast lesion. Surgery, *29*:217–222, 1951.

76. Winawer, S. J., Miller, D. G., Schottenfield, D. et al.: Feasibility of fecal occult-blood testing for detection of colorectal neoplasia. Cancer, *40*:2616–2619, 1977.

77. Wittes, R. E. and Yeh, S. D. J.: Indications for liver and brain scans: Screening tests for patients with oat cell carcinoma of the lung. J.A.M.A., *238*:506–507, 1977.

Metabolism and Endocrinology 7

GEORGE J. HILL, II, M.D.
and MENELAOS A. ALIAPOULIOS, M.D.

BIOCHEMISTRY AND PHYSIOLOGY FOR THE OUTPATIENT SURGEON

Body composition, metabolism and physiology are important aspects in the preoperative evaluation of patients. The surgeon should recognize deficiencies which can be corrected, for many patients can be prepared for surgery more economically as outpatients than as inpatients. Anemia, acid-base problems, obesity and chronic vitamin deficiencies are examples of metabolic lesions that can frequently be improved prior to hospitalization for elective surgery. Awareness of patients' biochemical and endocrine status will expedite their hospital course and lead to a more successful result from surgery.[26]

This chapter reviews the charac-

194

teristics of body composition which may be assessed in ambulatory patients. Metabolic defects commonly seen in outpatients will be discussed. The surgical aspects of the endocrine organs will be reviewed, with emphasis on the features that are pertinent in office and clinic outpatients.

BODY COMPOSITION AND METABOLISM

Normal Values (Table 7–1)

The mass of the different components of the body has been determined by a variety of indirect means. A considerable amount is now known about the composition of "typical" men, women and children in a variety of clinical situations. Important reports that are available in this field include those by such authorities as Moore (1959)[22], Shires (1971)[28] and Blackburn (1976).[3]

Although the hematocrit is the most readily and frequently used measure of anemia, the red cell mass and blood volume can be measured with more accuracy in outpatients using isotope dilution analysis of ^{51}Cr-labeled red blood cells. Most major hospitals offer this service in the hematology, diagnostic radiology or pathology departments. Dilution analysis of Evans blue dye is a cumbersome but accurate non-isotopic method for measuring plasma volume (and when hematocrit is known, calculation of total blood volume is then a simple arithmetical manipulation). A commercial device (Volemetron) that performs the same measurement rapidly is available, using ^{131}I-labeling of plasma proteins.

Abnormalities in physiology and

Text continued on page 199.

TABLE 7–1 Body Composition – Normal Values (Adult)*

Body water 47–80% of body weight (approximately 50% in healthy young people)
 Intracellular 30–40% of body weight
 Extracellular 20% (5% plasma volume; interstitial fluid 15%) of body weight
Serum osmolarity (the sum of anionic, cationic and nonionic molecules present) approximately
 300 mOsmoles (280–295)/liter
Blood volume 6.0–9.0% of body weight

BLOOD, SERUM AND PLASMA VALUES

Ammonia (B)		80–110 mcg/100 ml
Amylase (S)		4–25 units
Bicarbonate (P)		22–26 mE/L
Bilirubin (S)	Direct:	0.4 mg/100 ml
	Total:	0.7 mg/100 ml
	Indirect:	is total minus direct
Calcium (S)		8.5–10.5 mg/100 ml
		4.5–5.5 mEq/L
		(Approximately 50% is ionized)
Carcinoembryonic antigen (CEA) (P)		0–2.5 ng/ml
CO_2 capacity (S)		55–75 vol %
		20–33 mEq/L
CO_2 content (S)		24–30 mEq/L (20–27 in Denver)
Chloride (S)		100–106 mEq/L
Cortisone (P)		6–16 mcg/100 ml
Creatinine (S)		0.6–1.5 mg/100 ml
Ethanol (B)		0.3–0.4%, marked intoxication
		0.4–0.5%, alcoholic stupor
		0.5% or greater, alcoholic coma

Table continued on the following page.

TABLE 7-1   Body Composition — Normal Values (Adult)* *(Continued)*

BLOOD, SERUM AND PLASMA VALUES *(Continued)*

Fibrinogen (P)		160–420 mg/100 ml
Gastrin (P)		0–200 pcg/ml
Glucose (blood)		58–100 mg/100 ml (fasting)
Immunoglobulins (S)	IgG:	540–1663 mg/100 ml
	IgA:	66–344 mg/100 ml
	IgM:	39–290 mg/100 ml
Iodine, protein-bound (S)		3.5–8.0 mcg/100 ml
Iron (S)		75–175 mcg/100 ml (males)
		50–150 mcg/100 ml (females)
Lactic acid (B)		0.6–1.8 mEq/L
Lactic dehydrogenase (S)		60–120 U/ml
Lipase (S)		0–2 U/ml
Lipids		
Cholesterol (S)		120–220 mg/100 ml
Cholesterol esters (S)		60–75% of cholesterol
Phospholipids (S)		9–16 mg/100 ml as lipid phosphorus
Total fatty acids (S)		190–420 mg/100 ml
Total lipids (S)		450–1000 mg/100 ml
Triglycerides (S)		40–150 mg/100 ml
Magnesium (S)		1.5–2.0 mEq/L (1.8–3.8 mg/100 ml)
Phosphatase (S)	Acid:	0.13–0.63 Sigma units/ml (male)
	Alkaline:	13–39 IU/L
Phosphate, inorganic (S)		3.0–4.5 mg/100 ml (0.6–1.1 mEq/L)
Potassium		3.5–5.0 mEq/L
Protein, total (S)		6.0–8.4 gm/100 ml
Albumin		3.5–5.0
Globulin		2.3–3.5
$\alpha 1$ globulin	4.2–7.2% of total	
$\alpha 2$ globulin	6.8– 12% of total	
β globulin	9.3– 15% of total	
γ globulin	13– 23% of total	
Prothrombin time (blood)		50–100%
Sodium (S)		135–145 mEq/L
Sulfate (S)		0.5–1.5 mg/ml
Thyroid hormones		
Thyroid stimulating hormone (TSH) (S)		0.5–3.5 μU/ml
T3 by RIA		70–190 ngm/100 ml
T4 by RIA		4–12 μgm/100 ml
T3 resin uptake		25–35%
Free T4 I		1–4 ngm/100 ml
Transaminase (S)		
SGOT		10–40 U/ml
SGPT		0–17 IU/ml
Urea nitrogen (B)		8–25 mg/100 ml
Uric acid (S)		3.0–7.0 mg/100 ml
Vitamin A (S)		0.15–0.6 μgm/ml
Vitamin B$_{12}$ (S)		200–800 picograms/ml
Vitamin C (S)		0.4–1.5 mg/100 ml

TABLE 7–1 Body Composition – Normal Values (Adult) *(Continued)*

MCV	80–94 cu μ^3
MCH	33–38%
RBC Males	4.6–6.2 million/cu mm
Females	4.2–5.4 million/cu mm
WBC	4800–10,800/cu mm
PMNs	54–62%
Band forms	3–5%
Lymphocytes	25–33%
Monocytes	3–7%
Eosinophiles	1–3%
Basophiles	0.1%
Reticulocytes	0.5–1.5% of RBCs
Platelets	200,000–350,000/cu mm
Hematocrit	
Males	42–50%
Females	40–48%
Hemoglobin	
Males	13–16/100 ml
Females	12–15/100 ml

Ammonia	11–115 mEq/24 hrs
Amylase	24–76 U/ml
Calcium	150 mg/day or less
Catecholamines	Epinephrine: under 20 μgm per day Norepinephrine: under 100 μgm per day
Creatine	0–100 mg/24 hrs
Male and nonpregnant female	less than 6% of creatinine
Pregnant female	up to 12% of creatinine
Creatinine	0.4–2.6 gm/24 hrs (15–25 mg/kg/24 hrs)

Creatinine clearance	150–180 L/day
	  (104–125 ml/min) per 1.73 M^2 of
	  body surface area

5-hydroxyindoleacetic acid (5HIAA)	2–9 mgm/24 hrs (women less than men)
Lead	0.08 μgm/ml or 120 μgm or less per 24 hrs
Pituitary gonadotrophins	
Male	6.5–13 mouse units
Female	6.5–53 mouse units
Postmenopausal	>104 mouse units
Porphyrin, uro	0–60 mcg/24 hr
Copro	100–300 mcg/24 hrs (male)
Copro	75–275 mcg/24 hrs (female)
Potassium	30–150 mEq/24 hrs (66–90% of dietary intake)
Protein	0

Table continued on the following page.

TABLE 7–1   Body Compósition — Normal Values (Adult) (*Continued*)

Urine (*Continued*)

PSP

20 min	greater than 30% excretion
60 min	greater than 60% excretion

Sodium	40–350 mEq/24 hrs
	(88%–100% of dietary intake)

Steroids
17–ketosteroids (per day)

Age	Males	Females
10	1–4 mg	1–4 mg
20	6–21 mg	4–16 mg
30	8–26 mg	4–14 mg
50	5–18 mg	3–9 mg
70	2–10 mg	1–7 mg

17–hydroxysteroids (per day)	3–8 mg/day (women lower than men)
Titratable acidity	20–40 mEq/24 hrs
Urobilinogen	up to 1.0 Ehrlich units/2 hrs
Uroporphyrin	0
Vanillylmandelic acid (VMA)	up to 9 mg/24 hrs
Urea nitrogen	2.7–18.7 gm/24 hrs

*Adapted in part from Scully, R. E. (Ed.): Normal reference values, N.E.J.M., *298*:34–35, 1978.

TABLE 7–2   Respiratory Function and Blood Gas Values (Adults)

Arterial Blood Gas

pH	7.35–7.45
P_{CO_2}	35–45 mmHg
P_{O_2}	75–100 mmHg
Oxygen content	15–23 vol. %
Oxygen capacity	16–24 vol. %
Oxygen saturation	96–100%
CO_2 content	45–55 vol. %

Pulmonary Function (from Comroe[5])

Vital capacity
Male	[27.63–(0.122 × age in years)] × height in cm
Female	[21.78–(0.101 × age in years)] × height in cm

Respiratory rate	11–14/min
Tidal volume	450–600 ml

Minute volume
Males	3.1–3.9 × body surface area
Females	3.2–3.4 × body surface area

Basal oxygen consumption   135–145 ml/min/sq meter of body surface

Maximum breathing capacity
Males	[86.5–(0.522 × age in years)] × surface area in sq meters
Females	[71.3–(0.474 × age in years)] × surface area in sq meters

Forced expiratory volume
1 sec	75–83% of total vital capacity
3 sec	97% of total vital capacity

metabolism are frequently detected by chemical analysis of serum, body fluids, blood cells and cells of specific organs and tissues (Table 7–1). The acid-base balance of the individual is a reflection of overall metabolic compensation in health and disease. The most convenient tests of acid-base balance are the arterial blood gas studies and pulmonary function tests shown in Table 7–2. Body surface area may be estimated from the values listed in Table 7–3.

Health, Exercise, and Fitness

The general benefits of physical fitness have been increasingly apparent during the past several years. It seems likely that the gradual reduction in deaths in America from cardiovascular disease must be related in part to the awareness of health and fitness and to the improvements in personal health that have been displayed by literally hundreds of thousands of Americans. It has been estimated that a 14 per cent

TABLE 7–3   Body Surface Area (M^2) as a Function of Height and Weight*

Height (inches)	Weight (pounds)						
	90	100	110	120	130	140	150
48	1.21	1.27	1.34	1.40	1.46	1.51	1.57
50	1.23	1.30	1.36	1.42	1.48	1.54	1.60
52	1.25	1.32	1.38	1.45	1.51	1.57	1.62
54	1.27	1.34	1.41	1.47	1.53	1.59	1.65
56	1.29	1.36	1.43	1.49	1.55	1.62	1.67
58	1.31	1.38	1.45	1.51	1.58	1.64	1.69
60	1.32	1.40	1.47	1.54	1.60	1.66	1.72
62	1.34	1.42	1.49	1.56	1.62	1.69	1.75
64	1.36	1.44	1.51	1.58	1.65	1.71	1.77
66	1.38	1.46	1.53	1.60	1.67	1.73	1.79
68	1.40	1.47	1.55	1.62	1.69	1.75	1.82
70	1.41	1.49	1.57	1.64	1.71	1.78	1.84
72	1.43	1.51	1.59	1.66	1.73	1.80	1.86
74	1.45	1.53	1.61	1.68	1.75	1.82	1.88
76	1.46	1.55	1.62	1.70	1.77	1.84	1.90
78	1.48	1.56	1.64	1.72	1.79	1.86	1.93
Height (inches)	Weight (pounds)						
	160	170	180	190	200	210	220
60	1.78	1.84	1.89	1.95	2.00	2.05	2.10
62	1.81	1.86	1.92	1.97	2.03	2.08	2.13
64	1.83	1.89	1.94	2.00	2.05	2.11	2.16
66	1.85	1.91	1.97	2.03	2.08	2.13	2.18
68	1.88	1.94	2.00	2.05	2.11	2.16	2.21
70	1.90	1.96	2.02	2.08	2.13	2.19	2.24
72	1.92	1.98	2.04	2.10	2.16	2.21	2.27
74	1.95	2.01	2.07	2.13	2.18	2.24	2.29
76	1.97	2.03	2.09	2.15	2.21	2.26	2.32
78	1.99	2.05	2.11	2.17	2.23	2.29	2.34

*Values for intermediate heights and weights may be obtained by interpolation. (e.g., 125 lbs., 56″ = 1.52 M^2).

reduction in mortality from cardiovascular diseases has occurred in the past ten years. Healthy individuals of all ages are characterized by good cardiopulmonary function, good skeletal muscle strength and a relatively low fat to muscle ratio. A physically fit, well-muscled patient appears generally to be a better operative candidate than a patient who is overweight and physically weak. The hypertensive patient with marginal cardiac output, obese and exhausted after a normal day's activity, has a higher incidence of infection, postoperative thromboembolism and other complications than his contemporary who is in better general health.

One of the most useful programs emphasizing health and fitness is that described by Cooper, called "aerobics."[6] As explained by Cooper, aerobics refers to a variety of exercises that stimulate heart and lung activity for a time period sufficiently long to produce beneficial changes in the body. Cooper defines aerobic capacity as "the maximum amount of oxygen that the body can process within a given time." He points out that the training effect achieved by regular exercise strengthens muscles of respiration, improves strength and pumping efficiency in the heart, tones up muscles, improves circulation, lowers blood pressure, reduces the work required of the heart and increases the total amount of blood and red blood cells. Cooper suggests that participation in a regular progressive exercise program can be initiated by anyone under age 30 who is in generally good health and who has had a medical examination within the previous year. Between ages 30 and 39, a checkup and an exercise EKG should be obtained within the three month period before beginning the exercise program. Over age 39, a checkup plus an exercise EKG should be obtained immediately preceding entry into the exercise program.

The exercise program includes warm-up and stretching exercises; a brief walk; a cardiovascular stimulating exercise selected by the individual, such as jogging, running or swimming; and a cooling-down period. The exercise program should be performed at least three to four times per week. Following exercise the pulse should return to less than 120 beats per minute within five minutes, and to less than 100 beats per minute within ten minutes. Various fitness programs suggest that the heart rate during exercise (or immediately after exercise) should be pushed to a high fraction, for example, 75 per cent, of the "maximum heart rate." The maximum heart rate varies with age and fitness and should not be selected arbitrarily. Cooper suggests that patients with a cardiac history should not exceed a heart rate greater than 150 for those aged less than 30, 135 in the 45 to 49 year age group or a heart rate over 120 in the 65+ age group.

Cooper encourages his individuals to achieve at least 30 aerobic "points" per week, calculated on the basis of tables presented in his publications. For example, a 2.0 mile run performed in 13 to 16 minutes, three times per week, would give the individual 33 aerobic points per week. Cooper stresses motivation, based in part on a desire of the individual to achieve and maintain an appearance of health and fitness. He points out that the average expenditure of energy for an eight minute mile jog/run is only 100 Kcal, but a regular exercise program will achieve a substantial improvement in muscular tone, ligamentous strength and psychological well-being in most individuals.

An in-depth scientific review of aerobic and other exercise programs has been reported from several other laboratories and summarized in a report to the New York Academy of Sciences[21] which reviewed the physiological, medical, epidemiological and psychological aspects of the marathon and other intensive physical activities.

Abnormal Body Composition

Weight

The patient should always be weighed as the first step in an elective routine physical examination and in subsequent interval follow-up examinations. Obesity is common in the United States, so a loss in weight may be missed if weight is recorded only after weight loss has commenced. Unexplained weight loss of significant degree is frequently due to cancer, but a vast number of other diseases also cause loss in weight. Psychological factors may cause severe weight loss, even though the patients may not be aware of a decrease in appetite. The presence of a psychosis is usually recognized without undue difficulty by the physician or members of the patient's family. However, neuroses and external psychic stresses may require considerable probing to uncover. It is obviously important to be aware of these factors rather than to plunge directly into an expensive and possibly fruitless work-up for the cause of weight loss. Diuretics, chronic infection, metabolic diseases, arteriosclerosis, peptic ulcer and endocrinopathies are other common causes of weight loss which are seen in surgical clinics. Ideal weights for men and women of various ages are shown in Table 7–4.

Water

Retention or loss of body fluids should be detected and treated appro-

TABLE 7–4   Ideal Weights (Pounds)

| Height | | \multicolumn{7}{c}{MEN — Age} | | | | | | |
Feet	Inches	25–29	30–34	35–39	40–44	45–49	50–54	55 up
5	4	134	137	140	142	144	145	146
	5	138	141	144	146	148	149	150
	6	142	145	148	150	152	153	154
	7	146	149	152	154	156	157	158
	8	150	154	157	159	161	162	163
	9	154	158	162	164	166	167	168
	10	158	163	167	169	171	172	173
	11	163	168	172	175	177	178	179
6	0	169	174	178	181	183	184	185
	1	175	180	184	187	190	191	192
	2	181	186	191	194	197	198	199

| Height | | \multicolumn{7}{c}{WOMEN — Age} | | | | | | |
Feet	Inches	25–29	30–34	35–39	40–44	45–49	50–54	55 up
5	0	118	121	124	128	131	133	134
	1	120	123	126	130	133	135	137
	2	122	125	129	133	136	138	140
	3	125	128	132	136	139	141	143
	4	129	132	136	139	142	144	146
	5	132	136	140	143	146	148	150
	6	136	140	144	147	151	152	153
	7	140	144	148	151	155	157	158
	8	144	148	152	155	159	162	163
	9	148	152	156	159	163	166	167
	10	152	155	159	162	166	170	173
	11	155	158	162	166	170	174	177

priately prior to elective surgery. Net retention of water is usually the result of cardiac, renal or hepatic decompensation but may also result from the physical effects of blockage in lymphatic or venous drainage. Water intoxication can be self-induced, accidental or iatrogenic (through excessive intravenous fluid administration). Less common are endocrine disorders such as Cushing's syndrome, exogenous steroid hormone administration, inappropriate ADH secretion in oat cell cancer of the lung and other tumors as listed on page 241. Peripheral edema may occur in chronic anemia, such as that due to carcinoma of the cecum. Edema may also occur in patients with protein loss from polypoid lesions of stomach or colon. Excessive net water retention is usually manifested by Hct ↓, [Na] ↓, [Cl] ↓ in venous blood.

Water loss (dehydration) may occur from the gastrointestinal, genitourinary or respiratory tracts or through the skin. GI losses in surgical patients are exemplified by chronic diarrhea resulting from a partially obstructed intestine, from vomiting due to gastric outlet obstruction, from GI tract fistulas and from villous adenomas or hypertrophic gastritis. Loss of water from other causes is rarely seen in surgical outpatients, though patients with chronic high output renal failure, fever or permanent tracheostomies should be watched closely for signs of dehydration. Insensible loss of water through the skin is a serious problem in patients with burns and in unacclimatized persons in hot environments. Water loss is manifested by Hct ↑, [Na] ↑, and [Cl] ↑ in venous blood.

Acid-base Balance and Changes in Serum Electrolytes

Problems of acid-base balance and electrolytes, though more frequently seen in complicated hospitalized and intensive care unit patients, may also often be seen in office and clinic out-patients in whom rapid recognition may be more difficult but is no less critical and essential to the preservation of life.[23] The three major fluid compartments in the body are:

(1) the circulating intravascular fluid, i.e., blood;

(2) the interstitial fluid, which bathes the cells; and

(3) the intracellular fluid, i.e., cells themselves.

Nutrition in the form of oxygen, amino acids and glucose is brought to the cells by blood via the interstitial fluid, whereas cellular metabolic wastes such as carbon dioxide and urea enter the interstitial fluid, are removed by the blood and then excreted by the kidneys or lung. All of the body fluids and electrolytes are involved in the problem of acid-base balance and will be highlighted in this chapter. A recent comprehensive, concise, well-written book on this subject, by Rose[25] is highly recommended.

The clinical term "acid-base balance" refers to the chemical state of the body fluids as measured in arterial blood. The concentration of hydrogen ions [H^+] is of utmost importance in determining the acidity (hydrogen [i.e., proton] donor) or alkalinity (hydrogen [proton] acceptor) of a solution. pH is defined as the reciprocal logarithm of the hydrogen ion concentration:

$$pH = Log \frac{1}{[H^+]}$$

A hydrogen ion concentration of 10^{-7} grams per liter represents pH 7, which is neutrality, since that is the weight of ionized hydrogen in distilled water.

Optimal cellular metabolism requires a slightly alkaline pH, with the complex biochemical processes of the body operating within the narrow normal limits of *pH 7.35* to *pH 7.45*. The homeostatic maintenance of this delicately normal range of acid-base balance is primarily accomplished by three important systems: the blood buffers, the respiratory system and the kidneys.

Buffers react rapidly by neutralizing excess or releasing surplus hydrogen ions to prevent changes in pH. The most important of the many buffer systems in the body is the carbonic acid-sodium bicarbonate system and, therefore, disturbances of acid-base balance can be considered essentially as imbalances of this system.

Twenty parts bicarbonate to one part carbonic acid (20:1 ratio) is maintained as a constant ratio in arterial blood under normal circumstances. Excess body acid is converted to additional carbonic acid, which in turn separates into carbon dioxide and water, the CO_2 being eliminated through the lungs and the H_2O through the kidneys.

Carbonic acid is proportional to PCO_2 (partial pressure of carbon dioxide), which is controlled by the lungs, and the HCO_3^- (bicarbonate) is under primary control of the kidneys. Thus the Henderson Hasselbalch equation simply[1] and figuratively speaking becomes:

$$pH = pK \text{ (constant)} + \log \frac{\text{Kidney } (HCO_3^-) \text{ functions}}{\text{Lung } (PCO_2) \text{ functions}}$$

Substitution in the above equation reveals that acid pH ↓ (acidosis) is produced by ↓ HCO_3^-, whereupon renal adjustments take place by excretion of chloride and acidification of the urine and the buffer ratio returns to the original value of 20:1. Alkaline pH ↑ (alkalosis) results from ↑ HCO_3^-. Graphically, this can be shown in Figure 7–1, in which reducing bicar-

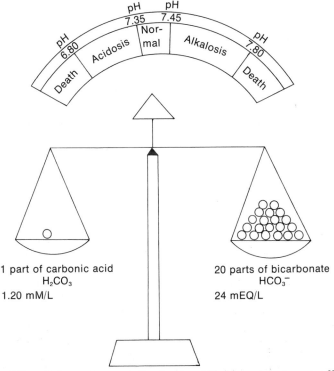

Figure 7–1 *Acid-Base Balance.* One part of carbonic acid balances twenty parts of bicarbonate salt under normal body pH conditions. Therefore, the pH changes whenever this proportion is altered. For instance, reducing the bicarbonate swings the pointer towards *Acidosis*, whereas increasing the bicarbonate swings the pointer towards *Alkalosis*.

bonate swings the pointer toward acidosis and increasing bicarbonate swings the pointer toward alkalosis. The usually reported blood gases and pH with their normal values are:

pH   7.35–7.45
PO_2 75–100 mm Hg
O_2 saturation $\geqq$95 per cent
PCO_2 35–45 mm Hg
HCO_3^- 22–26 mEq/L

For ease and convenience in delineation of acid-base:

$$pH = 7.4$$
$$PCO_2 = 40 \text{ mmHg}$$
$$HCO_3^- = 25 \text{ mEq/L}$$

The reason that interpretation of changes in pH, PCO_2 and HCO_3^- is not straightforward is because the values do not change independently; they are in a locked relationship, that is, if one changes, at least one other also changes.

The following chart summarizes the abnormalities that occur in the partially compensated, simple acid-base disturbances.

Primary ⬅ Compensatory ↑
Resultant pH ↑

	PCO_2	HCO_3^-	pH
Metabolic acidosis	↓	⬅	↓
Metabolic alkalosis	↑	⬆	↑
Respiratory acidosis	⬅	↑	↓
Respiratory alkalosis	⬅	↓	↑

Most alterations in acid-base balance in outpatients are compensated. They will not usually be detected unless the surgeon is alert to the possibilities and does the proper tests to detect the biochemical lesions.

1. RESPIRATORY ACIDOSIS. Chronic obstructive respiratory disease or acute airway obstructions produce hypoxia, hypercarbia and acidosis (arterial PO_2 ↓, PCO_2 ↑ and pH ↓, urinary pH usually acid). Treatment for severely decompensated patients includes placement of an endotracheal tube by the oral or nasal route, fol-

Causes of Respiratory Acidosis
(↑ PCO_2)

Obstructive lung disease
Oversedation and other causes of reduced function of the respiratory center even with normal lungs
Other causes of hypoventilation

lowed by creation of a tracheostomy with placement of a cuffed tracheostomy tube. Oxygen should be given only after the airway is controlled, since administration of oxygen may remove the only remaining respiratory drive. When the airway is controlled, a ventilating bag or respirator can be used to remove CO_2 by hyperventilation, and to administer an increased concentration of oxygen in inspired air. If the patient had shown bradycardia and obtundation prior to establishment of the airway, administration of $NaHCO_3$ intravenously (44–88 mEq) is advisable to correct the metabolic acidosis present due to hypoxemia. Arterial blood gases should be drawn before and after intubation and use of the respirator or ventilating bag. Patients with chronic respiratory acidosis frequently compensate successfully with metabolic alkalosis (through renal excretion of acid) and have a normal blood pH, in spite of the high PCO_2.

2. RESPIRATORY ALKALOSIS. Severely injured casualties frequently exhibit mild respiratory alkalosis on arrival in the Emergency Room.[2] Several causes are apparent: anxiety, chest wall injury and pulmonary contusion stimulate a high rate of breathing, and automatic respiratory compensation also occurs for the metabolic acidosis which results from tissue injury and poor perfusion. Arterial blood shows pH ↑ and PCO_2 ↓. PO_2 may be ↓ or normal. It is important to remember that the alkalosis of traumatized patients should not be treated with metabolic acids. Instead, the causes must be determined and treated specifically. In-

Causes of Respiratory Alkalosis
($\downarrow$ P_{CO_2})

Hypoxia
Nervousness and anxiety
Pulmonary embolus, fibrosis, etc
Pregnancy
Other causes of hyperventilation

creasing the concentration of inspired oxygen and judicious use of narcotics to alleviate pain will usually lead to a more appropriate rate and depth of respiration.

3. METABOLIC ACIDOSIS. Acute metabolic acidosis will occur from tissue injury and poor perfusion. This condition is seen in traumatized patients, patients with ischemic necrosis of limbs or intestines, after irregular rewarming following frostbite and in a variety of other situations with low blood flow. Tissue injury causes a measurable increase in circulating levels of lactic acid as the result of a shift from aerobic to anaerobic glycolysis in skeletal muscle. When recovery is delayed, aerobic conversion of lactate to pyruvate by the Krebs cycle does not occur at a normal rate, and an increase is seen in the ratio of lactate to pyruvate. A high or increasing lactate-pyruvate ratio in the blood is a poor prognostic sign in patients with acute metabolic acidosis.

Chronic metabolic acidosis may occur as the result of retention or addition of metabolic acid, or by loss of base. Renal retention of acid occurs in patients treated with carbonic anhydrase inhibitors such as topical Sulfamylon, and in patients with chronic renal failure. "Subtraction" acidosis is seen in patients with chronic diarrhea or fistulas distal to the stomach (pancreatic, biliary or small bowel). Chronic metabolic acidosis is associated with hyperchloremia and a decreased blood bicarbonate level, but blood pH is usually normal because of compensation by respiratory excretion of CO_2, and by renal excretion of acid, predominantly in NH_4^+ ions. Thus, venous blood shows [Cl] $\uparrow$, [HCO_3] $\downarrow$; arterial pH is normal; urine pH is acid. If an acidotic patient has a paradoxically alkaline urine, a renal acidifying defect should be suspected.

4. METABOLIC ALKALOSIS. The problem of acute post-traumatic metabolic alkalosis begins when the injured patient is first seen in the Emergency Room. Metabolic alkalosis does not become apparent until one to three days after severe injury, when the patients are under treatment on the inpatient wards. However, a major factor in the cause of post-traumatic alkalosis begins during the initial resuscitation, when large amounts of lactated saline solutions and citrated blood are administered. Lactate and citrate are metabolized during the next few days and provide a significant burden of base for the normal respiratory and renal excretory systems to handle. Alkalosis in these traumatized patients is detrimental because oxyhemoglobin disso-

Causes of Metabolic Acidosis
($\downarrow$ HCO_3^-)

Tissue injury—crush, frostbite, etc.	Poor perfusion—low cardiac output, arterial occlusion, venous occlusion
Diabetic ketoacidosis	Diarrhea
Poisonings	Drainage of pancreatic juice
salicylate	Ureterosigmoidostomy
ethylene glycol	Rx with Sulfamylon
methyl alcohol	Rx with Diamox
paraldehyde	
Lactic acidosis	Rx with NH_4Cl
Renal failure	Renal tubular acidosis

ciation is less effective, and cerebral perfusion is diminished in the presence of an elevated blood pH.

Peptic ulcer is the usual cause of chronic metabolic alkalosis in surgical patients. Chronic use of antacids produces "addition" alkalosis, which may cause the formation of renal calculi and secondary hyperparathyroidism — the "milk-alkali" syndrome. "Subtraction" alkalosis becomes a serious problem in patients with vomiting from chronic gastric outlet obstruction. Loss of gastric acid in these patients produces hypochloremic, hypokalemic alkalosis, measured by $[Cl^-]\downarrow$, $[K^+]\downarrow$ and $[HCO_3^-]\uparrow$ in venous blood. Acid-base balance is maintained by conservation of H^+ by renal excretion of K^+ as the predominant cation. If vomiting occurs over a long period of time, failure of the renal compensating mechanism eventually occurs, followed by a rapid increase in metabolic alkalosis. This dangerous situation can be detected because the urine becomes acid at this time, as the result of severe depletion of potassium, so that K^+ can no longer be excreted instead of H^+. A patient with long-standing gastric outlet obstruction who has a paradoxically acid urine is in precarious condition. Prompt therapy with intravenous saline and stronger acids (NH_4Cl, glutamic acid or arginine HCl) is usually required in such patients (see following section).

5. MIXED ACID-BASE IMBALANCE. An isolated defect such as respiratory acidosis or metabolic alkalosis is actually seen on only rare occasions in clinical medicine. As indicated above, compensatory mechanisms immediately begin to regulate each lesion in acid-base balance. Metabolic acidosis usually leads to increased respiratory rate (respiratory alkalosis); on the other hand, a lesion producing respiratory alkalosis is compensated for by retention of metabolic acids, and so forth.

In addition, it is common to encounter mixed acid-base imbalance clinically because patients frequently have lesions that tend to produce more than one type of acid-base disturbance. For example, a patient may present with severe chronic obstructive pulmonary disease (respiratory acidosis) and pyloric obstruction from peptic ulcer (metabolic alkalosis). Or a child may be seen on a hot summer's day with severe dehydration from fever and lack of water intake (metabolic acidosis), complicated by severe diarrhea (subtraction-type of metabolic alkalosis).

Obviously, a careful history, examination and use of good judgment regarding the etiology of the illness is of great importance in such patients. A simplistic view of treatment based on laboratory results alone would be devastating. Also, since errors occasionally occur in even the best laboratories, each piece of data should be examined in the total context of the patient and all other available information regarding his illness.

Body Fluid and Electrolytes

The cells of the body are bathed in tissue fluid, which is kept remarkably constant in composition.[9] Major ingre-

---

Causes of Metabolic Alkalosis
($\uparrow HCO_3-$)

Diuretic Rx — mercurhydrin, Edecrin, Lasix and thiazides
Rx with corticosteroids (prednisone, cortisone, etc.)
Cushing's disease
Aldosteronism
All above augment renal excretion of H+, K+ and Cl−
Fluid losses
    from upper GI tract with loss of acid (vomiting or NG tube)

Clinical Acid-Base Summary

Classification	pH	CO_2 Content	P_{CO_2}
Normal	normal	normal	normal
Metabolic alkalosis	high	high	normal–high
Unsuspected alkalosis	high	normal	low
Respiratory alkalosis	high	low	low
Compensated alkalosis or acidosis	normal	high	high
Compensated acidosis or alkalosis	normal	low	low
Metabolic acidosis	low	low	low
Unsuspected acidosis	low	normal	normal–high
Respiratory acidosis	low	high	high

dients of this fluid are water and certain electrolytes, as well as oxygen, carbon dioxide, hormones, enzymes and nonelectrolyte crystalloids such as urea, and nutrients such as sugar and proteins. Water is the basic solvent in which the chemical activities of the cell occur and is the largest single constituent of the body, representing approximately 60 per cent of the adult total body weight. The percentage varies with the proportion of fat; the fatter the individual, the less the proportion of water to total body weight, since fat is essentially water-free. The approximate distribtuion of this total body water is listed in the box diagram below.

The usual blood volume is estimated to be 8 per cent of the body weight in kilograms, since whole blood = plasma + red blood cells.

The body maintains a careful water balance via kidneys, lungs, skin and gastrointestinal tract. The kidneys, the major controllers of water balance, are under the control of antidiuretic hormone (ADH) from the posterior pituitary gland, which acts on the distal renal tubule to increase the reabsorption of water. Sodium ordinarily is the most important electrolyte being excreted and is controlled by aldosterone, which is secreted from the adrenal cortex. Elevated secretion of aldosterone will cause retention of sodium in the circulation by diminishing its excretion in the kidneys.

Renal sodium excretion (natriuresis), water excretion and reduction in blood pressure are apparently enhanced by the activity of certain vasodepressor renomedullary prostaglandins, particularly PGA and PGE.[30] Prostaglandins

**Total Body Water
(TBW)**

60% of body weight in Kg

$\frac{2}{3}$ = Intracellular fluid (ICF)

(40% body weight)

$\frac{1}{3}$ = Extracellular fluid (ECF)

(20% body weight)

$\frac{3}{4}$ = Interstitial

(15% body weight)

$\frac{1}{4}$ = Plasma

(5% body weight)

Average Daily Fluid Intake and Output for Adults

INTAKE			OUTPUT	
In food	= 1200 ml		Kidneys	= 1500 ml
As water	= 1000 ml		GI tract, skin, lungs	= 1000 ml
Water of oxidation	= 300 ml			
Totals	= 2500 ml			2500 ml

are 20-carbon fatty acids with a 5-membered cyclopentane ring. These hormones are found in many tissues of the body in addition to the prostate. The microsomal fraction of the renal medulla is rich in prostaglandin synthetase. Synthesis apparently occurs in the endoplasmic reticulum, but the prostaglandins are almost immediately released into the extracellular fluid. Synthesis of prostaglandins is markedly inhibited by nonsteroidal anti-inflammatory agents such as aspirin, indomethacin and phenylbutazone.

Mechanical and osmotic pressures control movement of water between body compartments — intestine and peritoneal cavity — whereas hydrostatic pressure and osmotic pressure of the blood influence movement of fluids in and out of the intravascular space, that is, arterioles and venules. Osmotic gradients govern the movement of water between extracellular and intracellular spaces as the electrolytes move back and forth across the cell membrane by active metabolic processes.

The simplest and most accurate way to monitor water balance is to determine accurate body weight daily. A weight change of 1 kilogram (2.2 pounds) reflects a fluid loss or gain of one liter with adjustments required for catabolic conditions. The measurement of central venous pressure or pulmonary artery wedge pressure by

means of a Swan-Ganz catheter can be an important guide in measurement of fluid replacement.

Chemical compounds in solution may behave as:

(1) electrolytes, i.e., compounds that dissociate into ions and thus conduct electrical current in solution, such as potassium (K^+) and chloride (Cl^-); or

(2) nonelectrolytes, i.e., compounds that remain intact, undissociated and not ionized in water solutions, such as dextrose, urea and creatinine.

Dissociated particles of an electrolyte are called "ions" and carry an electrical charge. Thus, electrolytes are compounds that undergo ionization and dissociate into ions. For example, sodium chloride dissolves in water, provides sodium ions (Na^+) and chloride (Cl^-). The sodium ion carries a positive charge and is referred to as a "cation" and the chloride carries a negative charge and is referred to as an "anion," since positively charged ions migrate to a cathode and negatively charged ions migrate to an anode in solution.

The physiological and chemical activity of electrolytes are proportional to:

(1) the *number* of particles present per unit volume (moles or millimoles); and

(2) more importantly, the number of

CATIONS	IONS OF INORGANIC ACIDS	ANIONS
Sodium (Na+)	Lactate	Chloride (Cl−)
Potassium (K+)	Pyruvate	Bicarbonate (HCO$_3$−)
Calcium (Ca++)	Acetoacetate	Phosphate (HPO$_4$−)
Magnesium (Mg++)	Proteinates	Sulphate (SO$_4$−)

Normal Electrolyte Concentrations in the Blood

In healthy individuals, the concentration of serum electrolytes falls within a fairly narrow range, as follows:

Sodium (Na)	135–145 mEq/L
Potassium (K)	3.5–5.0 mEq/L
Chloride (Cl)	100–106 mEq/L
Calcium (Ca)	4.5–5.5 mEq/L or 8.5–10.5 mg/100 ml
Magnesium (Mg)	1.5–2.0 mEq/L
Phosphate (PO_4)	3.0–4.5 mg/100 ml
Bicarbonate (HCO_3)	22–26 mEq/L

electrical charges per unit volume (equivalents or milliequivalents per liter).

The *weight* of the electrolyte per unit volume (grams or milligrams per 100 ml) gives no direct information as to the number of ions or the number of electrical charges they carry.

The electrolytes of body fluids must be expressed in terms of chemical activity, that is, "equivalents." The more suitable term is milliequivalents per liter (mEq/L). The number of milliequivalents per liter is derived from the milligrams per liter multiplied by valence and divided by atomic weight according to the following formula:

$$mEq/L = \frac{mg/100\ ml \times 10 \times valence}{atomic\ weight}$$

Routine laboratory procedures measure electrolytes within the intravascular compartment only. The intravascular and interstitial fluids are merely passageways to the cells themselves. Electrolyte measurements in the serum do not accurately measure the components within the huge cellular space *itself*, which is one of the major targets of therapy; however, they do *reflect* the cellular metabolism.

A substantial portion of the body's store of water and electrolytes is destined for secretions in the digestive tract. The volume and electrolyte composition of various gastrointestinal fluids are given on page 210. In the normal healthy individual, the water and electrolytes in these secretions are not lost from the body but are ultimately largely reabsorbed. However, with excessive diarrhea, vomiting, gastrointestinal suction, fistula drainage and so on, fluid and electrolyte losses through these secretions may represent a large and serious deficit. An awareness of the electrolyte composition of these fluids, along with the careful measurement of the patient's intake and output will obviate any serious clinical metabolic derangements. A more accurate assessment of the electrolyte losses in the secretions of any given patient may be better obtained by sending a portion of these secretions for electrolyte determination by the laboratory. Thereafter a simple calculation of con-

Urinary Electrolyte Concentrations

Urinary electrolyte concentrations can often be helpful in assessing the clinical situation but are more variable in accordance with the tubular activity as follows:

Tubular Function	Sodium (mEq/L)	Potassium (mEq/L)
Normal	40	40
Early conservation	10–30	20–30
Maximal conservation	5	15–25

Volume and Electrolyte Composition of Gastrointestinal Fluids

Fluid	Na+ (mEq/L)	K+ (mEq/L)	Cl− (mEq/L)	HCO₃− (mEq/L)	Volume per day (mL)
Gastric juice, high in acid	20 (10–30)	10 (5–40)	120 (80–150)	0	1000–9000
Gastric juice, low in acid	80 (70–140)	15 (5–40)	90 (40–120)	(5–25)	1000–2500
Pancreatic juice	140 (115–180)	5 (3–8)	75 (55–95)	80 (60–110)	500–1000
Bile	148 (130–160)	5 (3–12)	100 (90–120)	35 (30–40)	300–1000
Small-bowel drainage	110 (80–150)	5 (2–8)	105 (60–125)	30 (20–40)	1000–3000
Distal ileum and cecum drainage	80 (135–140)	8 (5–30)	45 (20–90)	30 (20–40)	1000–3000
Diarrheal stools	120 (20–160)	25 (10–40)	90 (30–120)	45 (30–50)	500–17,000

*Note: Average values per 24 hours are given; the range is in parentheses.
Reproduced with permission from: Krupp, M. A., and Chatton, M. J. (eds.): Current Medical Diagnosis, 1979. Copyright 1979 by Lange Medical Publications, Los Altos, California.

centration in mEq/L × volume in liters gives the mEq for any specific electrolyte that must be replaced.

1. SODIUM. Net retention and net loss of sodium ions both tend to produce a reduction in serum sodium concentration. *Loss* of sodium as a cause for hyponatremia is so rare in surgical patients that it should be documented before treatment is given with NaCl. In most cases hyponatremia is due to *retention* of both sodium and water. Occasionally, chronic GI loss or sodium-loss nephropathy will produce a deficit in sodium. Rarely, a severe dietary restriction of sodium, combined with chronic loss in perspiration, GI tract or urine will produce a sodium deficit. Diuretics will also cause loss of sodium ion, and the patient with puzzling hyponatremia should be queried carefully regarding his use of medications. The question of sodium-loss nephropathy may easily be studied in outpatients by collection of serial 24-hour urine samples for sodium. After

several days with a normal diet, the patient is placed on a diet severely restricted in NaCl. Normally, urine Na will immediately drop to 2–3 mEq per 24 hours. A salt-losing nephropathy will block this conservation in Na, and urinary Na excretion will continue unchanged.

Sodium retention is induced by adrenal cortical hormones, especially aldosterone. Sodium retention usually occurs from cardiac, hepatic or renal failure. It is usually treated with diuretics, especially furosemide (Lasix), Aldactone or hydrochlorthiazide (Hydrodiuril). Intractable sodium retention may also be treated successfully in some instances by diuresis induced with rapid infusion of 100–300 ml of 3 or 5 per cent of NaCl. The patient should be placed in the observation unit overnight for this treatment.

2. POTASSIUM. Relatively wide variations occur in serum levels of potassium, which is the predominant intracellular cation. Accuracy of meas-

urement is impaired by hemolysis of red cells, and the technique of analysis also has a relatively high absolute error. Potassium is an important ion in membrane function, especially in acid-base transfers in the kidney. The K^+ : Ca^{++} ratio is of great importance in myocardial function, especially in the presence of digitalis. Loss of K^+ subjects the heart to the danger of cardiac irritability and digitalis toxicity. Hyperkalemia $[K^+] \uparrow$, on the other hand, diminishes the strength of cardiac contraction, which can lead to asystole, followed by anoxic-induced ventricular fibrillation. The cardiac effects of potassium are essentially opposite to those of calcium.

Potassium loss is a serious problem in chronic diarrhea or GI fistulas. Hypokalemia is frequently produced by excessive use of diuretics, though this loss can be controlled by administration of liquid potassium salts (KCl elixir; K-Triplex) if the physician remembers to give the correct instructions to his patient. In patients who take diuretic tablets infrequently, potassium supplementation with a glass of orange juice is usually satisfactory. Urinary potassium loss also occurs from endogenous or exogenous adrenal cortical hormones, especially aldosterone. Hypokalemia $[K^+] \downarrow$ of unknown origin should therefore raise the question of an adrenal cortical tumor, whereas hyperkalemia $[K^+] \uparrow$ is seen in adrenal insufficiency. The body's stores of potassium can be estimated in outpatients by potassium determination on a solution of hemolyzed red cells in distilled water. If the volume of red blood cells and distilled water was accurately measured, the intracellular RBC potassium concentration can be calculated with ease by a simple algebraic relationship.

3. BICARBONATE. The bicarbonate-carbonic acid system is the major buffering apparatus of the body. Venous blood bicarbonate is determined by a variety of methods that have a wide range of normal values. The test is relatively inaccurate, depending on the laboratory and the method used. Since the purpose of measurement of HCO_3^- in patients is to assess the acid-base balance, we prefer to measure arterial pH, PCO_2 content directly and simultaneously with a polarographic gas electrode. The CO_2 content, HCO_3^- and pH are directly related to each other through the Henderson-Hasselbalch equation, as described in standard textbooks of biochemistry and outlined in Shires.[28] Regulation of bicarbonate was discussed in the previous section, *Acid-Base Balance*.

4. CALCIUM. The concentration of serum calcium is predominantly under the control of the parathyroid glands, the effect of parathyroid hormone being to increase serum calcium concentration, which thereby increases urinary excretion of calcium. Serum phosphate concentration is decreased by parathyroid hormone, which impairs renal tubular reabsorption of phosphate. Calcium is also regulated by thyrocalcitonin (also known as calcitonin), a hormone manufactured by the "C" cells of the thyroid gland, which lowers serum calcium. Thyrocalcitonin is ordinarily a major control mechanism for calcium in some patients (Figs. 7–2 through 7–5) with medullary carcinoma of the thyroid, a tumor derived from the "C" cells. Recent evidence also suggests that thyrocalcitonin may also be the cause of hypocalcemia in acute pancreatitis, since thyrocalcitonin is released from the thyroid gland by stimulation by glucagon, which can escape from the acutely inflamed pancreas.[27]

Figures 7–2 through 7–5 demonstrate the clinical manifestations of one of the more recently defined hormone secreting tumors (multiple endocrine anomalies, MEA) involving a patient with medullary carcinoma of the thyroid and multiple mucosal neuromas along with a typical body habitus. This young man was found not to have any of the other possible manifestations of this syndrome such as pheochromocy-

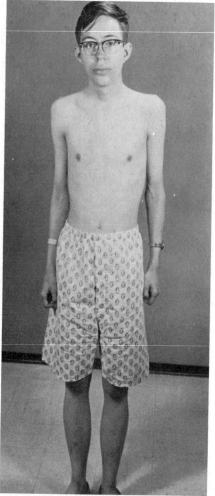

Figure 7-2 *Medullary Carcinoma of the Thyroid.* Body habitus—thin and tall, with long arms and legs (marphanoid).

noma of the breast with bony metastases. However, hypercalcemia can also occur in patients who have no demonstrable bony metastases, and in other cancers such as adenocarcinoma of the colon and lung. A parathyroid-like hormone secreted by the tumor has been implicated in some of these patients. Hypercalcemia also occurs in some patients with hyperthyroidism.

Hyperparathyroidism is caused by parathyroid adenoma, parathyroid hyperplasia and carcinoma of the parathyroid gland. Hypercalcemia produced by hyperparathyroidism may cause chronic illness or an acute crisis that warrants emergency parathyroidectomy. The chronic disease is associated with nonspecific and occasionally bizarre symptoms, including nausea, diarrhea, constipation and mental disturbances. Chronic hyper-

toma, carcinoid, diabetes, parathyroid tumors, increased prostaglandin secretion and so on. Serum (thyro) calcitonin levels are drawn regularly. The patient is well 10 years following his original surgery.

Hypercalcemia occurs in a variety of diseases in addition to hyperparathyroidism; sarcoidosis and metastatic cancers are the other major causes of hypercalcemia observed by surgeons. Of metastatic cancers, the most frequent cause of hypercalcemia is carci-

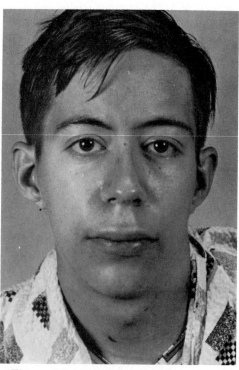

Figure 7-3 *Medullary Carcinoma of the Thyroid.* Facies – prominent lips, ears and eyes.

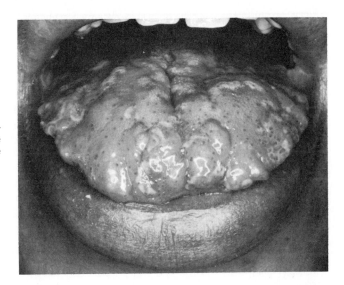

Figure 7–4 *Medullary Carcinoma of the Thyroid.* Multiple mucosal neuromas of the tongue and other mucous membranes.

parathyroidism also causes bony resorption (osteitis cystica) recognizable as cystic lesions of the bone, fractures and resorption of lamina dura, and renal calculi. The acute crisis is manifested by profound lethargy, coma, cardiac irritability, and can be fatal.[36] Although the symptoms of hyperparathyroidism are nonspecific and may be inconstant, a consistent finding of *hypercalcemia* should be considered due to hyperparathyroidism unless another cause for the abnormality can be found.

Hypocalcemia is frequently a difficult, long-term complication of radical surgery for carcinoma of the thyroid, and of jejunoileostomy performed for control of obesity. Mild hypocalcemia for one to six months is a frequent problem after other forms of thyroid surgery, especially when performed for hyperthyroidism. It can usually be controlled with oral tablets of calcium lactate or liquid calcium chloride, but may require the addition of vitamin D. Mental sluggishness, premature senility and constipation may occur in chronic hypoparathyroidism, even though serum calcium does not fall low enough to produce periorbital tingling, numbness in the fingers, muscle cramps or tetany. Subclinical hypocalcemia may be detected by the Chvos-

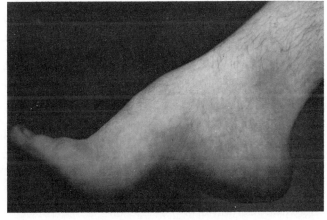

Figure 7–5 High metatarsal arch.

tek or Trousseau sign, or by rapid onset of paresthesias during voluntary hyperventilation. Approximately 50 per cent of the calcium in serum is bound to albumin, and it is the unbound (ionized) fraction which is responsible for most of the effects of calcium that are described in this portion of the text. In patients with significant degrees of hypoalbuminemia, the ionized calcium level obviously takes on greater significance; this determination formerly was usually made indirectly by the nomogram provided in standard textbooks of biochemistry, but increasing numbers of hospitals now provide the determination of ionized calcium as a routine laboratory procedure.

5. MAGNESIUM. The control mechanisms for magnesium in the body are poorly understood, but the level of this ion in the blood apparently follows that of calcium to a great extent. Magnesium is predominantly an intracellular cation, serum concentrations being only 1.5–2.5 mEq/L. Magnesium is of major importance in the long-term supplementation of patients with extensive small bowel resection, and jejunoileostomies for obesity. Hypomagnesemia produces muscular cramps, delirium, seizures and other mental changes. Magnesium sulfate or magnesium chloride is an effective emergency parenteral treatment for seizures due to eclampsia of pregnancy, and oral magnesium salts are given to supplement the diet of patients with chronic magnesium deficiency.

6. TRACE ELEMENTS. Other cations are of relatively less significance in surgical outpatients. The role of zinc in wound healing is still under investigation. It may have some role in local application for leg ulcers due to venous stasis, but these lesions have been treated with almost every poultice known to man and are still an unsolved problem. Iron is necessary for hemoglobin formation and should be given to surgical outpatients when deficiency exists. Anemia from chronic blood loss may not be correctible until the causal lesion is resected. However, if iron deficiency anemia is the result of menstrual bleeding in a woman, or lack of iron in the diet of a nursing infant, oral treatment with ferrous salts (gluconate or sulfate) should be administered for 30–45 days prior to admission for elective surgery. Iron must be given on an empty stomach, since it is not absorbed well in the presence of food or an alkaline pH.

7. PROTEINS. Serum proteins, which are predominantly anions, account for approximately 16 milliosmols (5 per cent) of the total ionic strength of plasma. Removal of fibrinogen as fibrin lowers the oncotic pressure in serum slightly, compared with plasma. Albumin, fibrinogen and the immunoglobulins make up approximately 75 per cent of the circulating plasma proteins. Conjugated globulins such as glycoproteins, lipoproteins, mucoproteins and metal-binding proteins constitute most of the final 25 per cent of the plasma proteins.

Albumin is synthesized only in the liver, at a rate of approximately 25–50 gm per day. The globulins are also all formed in the liver, except for gamma globulin which is formed by lymphocytes and plasma cells. Serum protein synthesis is impaired by a variety of diseases, including cirrhosis and cancer, and by antimetabolites. Serum protein can be lost from the GI tract by failure of digestion (loss of gastric or pancreatic enzymes) and by loss from diarrhea, from Menetrier's disease or villous adenoma of the colon. Massive losses of serum proteins (predominantly albumin, because of its relatively small size) may occur in the nephrotic syndrome, and moderate losses of gamma globulin may occur in multiple myeloma. Both of the latter diseases have surgical complications, so the surgeon may be forced to contend with serious hypoproteinemia in the postoperative period.

One of the most remarkable achievements of the past decade in surgical metabolism has been the use of intravenous administration of protein hydrolysate, glucose, lipids, vitamins, minerals and small amounts of plasma which permit dogs and humans to synthesize proteins, fat and skeleton. Dudrick[8] achieved positive nitrogen balance, weight gain and normal growth and development on a well-balanced intravenous "diet" administered through a central venous catheter. Dudrick's technique has been used widely and the results confirmed in many other laboratories and clinics. This alternative or supplement to oral feeding, termed "hyperalimentation," can be used for outpatients. The protein hydrolysate and hypertonic glucose solutions are commercially available, e.g., Aminosol and 50 per cent glucose ampoules. The surgeon who desires to use this technique must be experienced in the placement and maintenance of central venous catheters (see Chapter 4) and should also be familiar with the methods and hazards of hyperalimentation and give pertinent instructions to patients and the professional staff.[31]

Protein solutions of various types are available for intravenous therapy. All are expensive and, if not sterilized, they carry the risk of viral (serum) hepatitis. "Plasmanate" (5.0 gm protein per 100 ml in hypotonic saline) and concentrated serum albumin are the best proteins for intravenous administration to outpatients. Single units of type specific, frozen or fresh plasma may be used for specific indications on the recommendation of a hematologist.

8. OTHER ANIONS. Phosphates, sulfates and organic acids are present in a total of approximately 8 mEq/L in plasma. The concentration of these anions increases in a variety of metabolic diseases, especially renal failure. Since many are di- or tri-valent, they contribute significantly to the buffering power of the blood. Blood levels of these ions, are, however, of relatively little significance in the surgical outpatient clinic.

Nonelectrolyte Ions in Blood

1. GLUCOSE. Both hyperglycemia and hypoglycemia provide a multitude of problems for the surgeon. In most cases the diagnosis is known, and the patient has an internist who will advise and assist in the regulation of glucose metabolism during the pre- and post-operative period. It should be remembered that far more deaths occur in surgical patients from *hypo*glycemia due to overzealous use of insulin than result from *hyper*glycemia.

Hyperglycemia. It is of great importance for the surgeon to remember that occasionally patients appear in the surgical clinic because of complications of hitherto undiagnosed diabetes mellitus. Infection or diabetic foot ulcer with neuropathy are the most common problems of this type. A relatively painless but badly infected foot is a typical diabetic lesion. Any patient with an infection should, therefore, have his urine sugar checked, and all known diabetics must be watched closely for ketoacidosis when they develop infections. Let us emphasize that a *positive* urine sugar in an outpatient should be considered as an indication that the patient has diabetes mellitus unless some other cause can be found; there are very few false positives (e.g., IVP dye). Diabetics should in general receive more careful attention to cultures, antibiotics and follow-up than nondiabetics in all outpatient procedures. The diabetes mellitus which follows pancreaticoduodenectomy usually is relatively simple to manage, with 20–40 units of NPH insulin daily.

Hypoglycemia. Reactive hypoglycemia is a common, nonpathological accompaniment of the irregular and irrational dietary habits of many people. Nevertheless, the surgeon will be alert to the possibilities of beta cell (insulin-secreting) adenomas in all patients with symptoms of hypoglycemia. It is remarkable that many patients with these tumors are diagnosed only after a long history of psychiatric evaluations and fainting spells, even when hypoglycemia was suspected or known to exist. Liver glycogen stores become depleted in many chronic diseases. The outpatient surgeon should therefore be prepared to reduce insulin or oral hypoglycemic drug doses in diabetics who become emaciated because of cancer or complications of other diseases.

2. UREA AND CREATININE. Ordinarily urea is measured only in transit from the liver, where it is produced in protein catabolism, to the kidneys, where it is excreted. Urea is usually measured as blood urea nitrogen (BUN), although serum urea nitrogen (SUN) or total protein nitrogen (NPN) provide essentially the same information; all measure the degree of azotemia present. Urea accounts for most of the nitrogen excreted daily. The amount excreted fluctuates greatly with the nitrogen balance achieved by protein anabolism and catabolism. Approximately 30 grams of urea are excreted daily by normal adult humans. Urea accounts for approximately 90 per cent of the 24 gm of nitrogen excreted on a normal or high protein diet. The additional, relatively constant 3 gm of urinary nitrogen is accounted for by ammonia, uric acid, creatine and creatinine plus small amounts of amino acids, hippuric acid and indican. After injury or during starvation, protein catabolism releases nitrogen in the form of amino acids, which are utilized in energy consumption through gluconeogenesis. The outpouring of nitrogen, predominantly as urea, in the absence of protein intake is referred to as negative nitrogen balance. Positive nitrogen balance is an accompaniment of the convalescence from injury or operation, so patients who return to the surgical clinic for postoperative follow-up may have a relatively low urinary nitrogen output. Urinary nitrogen excretion may be as low as 3 gm per day for as long as one to two months in convalescence from major

trauma, depending on the length of the period of protein anabolism. Nitrogen excretion gradually rises as the patient regains his normal muscle mass and is normal in the final phase of convalescence, when adipose tissue is synthesized.

When urea is administered intravenously it acts as an osmotic diuretic and formerly was used extensively for this reason to reduce brain edema.

High levels of BUN may occur from prerenal lesions — most commonly dehydration, from intrinsic renal disease or from postrenal urinary tract obstruction. Azotemia is also a hallmark of decreased renal excretion of metabolic acids and of potassium, which causes lethal cardiac arrhythmia when present in high concentrations. As an indicator of renal function, BUN is not as specific as creatinine. However, BUN is quicker and easier to measure, and the determination of BUN is less subject to intrinsic error than creatinine. BUN is filtered through the glomerulus and is passively reabsorbed in the renal tubules, whereas creatinine — in man — is excreted almost solely by glomerular filtration.

Glomerular filtration rate (GFR) in man is approximately equal to the rate of creatinine clearance. GFR is therefore estimated by calculation of creatinine clearance (Ccr), using the equation:

$$Ccr = \frac{U \cdot V}{P}$$

C = Clearance (ml/min)
U = Urinary creatinine excretion (mg/100 ml)
V = Volume of urine (ml/min)
P = Plasma creatinine concentration (mg/100 ml)

The test is simple to perform in outpatients, requiring only a 24-hour urine collection and one (or preferably two) serum (plasma) creatinine determinations. The main problem is to perform the calculation properly! The normal rate of creatinine clearance in an adult man is approximately 100–150 ml/min. Creatinine excretion is relatively constant in a given individual, so a 24-hour output of creatinine should be used to assess the accuracy of 24-hour urine collections for other purposes, such as excretion of protein and hormone metabolites.

3. AMMONIA. NH_3 is produced in the gut by protein-splitting bacteria, in the liver (in the process of deamination of amino acids) and in the kidney, where it is used as a vehicle of H^+ excretion as NH_4^+. Excretion of NH_4^+ conserves other cautions, such as Na^+, K^+ and Ca^{++}. The hepatic production of NH_3 normally is followed promptly by conversion to urea, which is then excreted by the kidney. Ammonia produced by bacteria in the GI tract is also metabolized in the liver. This important function of the liver does not occur properly if the portal circulation is diverted from the liver or if hepatic failure is present. Portal-systemic shunts and cirrhosis are therefore common causes of increased blood levels of NH_3. These patients frequently exhibit asterixis, confusion and coma. It is believed that NH_3 is not the sole cause of hepatic coma, but a high or increasing blood ammonia level is usually a sign of impending coma. The coma-producing effects of a high protein diet in these patients can be improved or controlled by reduction of dietary protein to 70 gm or less, and by elimination of protein-splitting bacteria with nonabsorbable antibiotics such as neomycin.

4. LIPIDES. Blood lipides are particularly important in two types of surgical diseases: (1) the atherosclerotic-hypertensive diseases of aging, and (2) the familial hypercholesterolemias. The measurement and control of serum cholesterol in patients over age 50 is of relatively little surgical importance. The effects of dietary cholesterol are relatively irreversible by late middle age, except by massive alteration in diet. The surgical problems related to atherosclerosis in middle aged and older patients are the technical repair or removal of diseased vessels and organs, including plaques in coronary arteries, aorta, peripheral arteries of the trunk, limbs, kidneys and brain, and atherosclerotic aneurysms of great and small vessels. Patients with familial hypercholesterolemias frequently appear to be benefited by reduction in serum cholesterol by dietary means, by cholestyramine resin, or by ileal bypass.[4] When serum cholesterol is lowered significantly in these patients, plaques sometimes resorb from soft tissues, and coronary artery disease appears to be improved or stabilized. Portacaval shunts have been used successfully to reduce hyperlipidemia and produce resolution of subcutaneous plaques in patients with type II hyperlipidemia.

Cholesterol is excreted by the liver as one of the components of bile. It is formed by decomposition of RBCs, and it is also synthesized in the liver as a precursor of bile salts. Bile salts are the salts of glycocholic and taurocholic acids; they are of enormous importance in digestion: emulsifying fats, stimulating pancreatic enzymes and intestinal motility and aiding the absorption of fat-soluble vitamins, such as vitamin K. The bile salts are also responsible for solubilizing and transporting cholesterol. Bile is concentrated in the gallbladder, and it is here that cholesterol usually tends to precipitate and form stones. Gallstones are composed of precipitated cholesterol, pigment and calcium carbonate in various concentrations, but cholesterol accounts for more than 90 per cent of the weight of most human gallstones. Cholesterol and the bile salts are responsible for most of the color in feces, so acholic (white) stools are the classic sign of obstruction of the biliary tree. Cholesterol is normally reabsorbed in the distal ileum, along with vitamin B_{12}, and this vitamin must therefore be administered parenterally to patients who have undergone the ileal bypass operation for hypercholesterolemia.

Other blood lipides of surgical importance are the triglycerides, free fatty acids and alcohols. The triglycerides, known as neutral fats, are esters of glycerol with fatty acids. Fats and fatty acids are insoluble in water, transported in blood in chylomicrons as β-lipoprotein, and bound to albumin. The albumin-bound lipides are the nonesterified fatty acids (NEFA's), also known as free fatty acids (FFA's). NEFA's are a rapidly-transported form of energy, which have a half-life in plasma of only two or three minutes. Their level fluctuates greatly with various states of stress and disease. Epinephrine, norepinephrine, growth hormone and ACTH cause NEFA levels to rise, whereas glucose and insulin reduce blood NEFA levels. Natural fats are complex mixtures of triglycerides, which are in dynamic equilibrium in living tissues. Fats occur in a spectrum from oils and soft fats to hard fats and waxes. Softness is imparted by short length and desaturation in fatty acids. Oleic and linoleic acids are examples of relatively short, unsaturated fatty acids that contain 17 carbon atoms. It is still uncertain which of the fatty acids are essential for humans, but linoleic acid apparently cannot be synthesized by man, so small quantities of it should be provided for optimum maintenance on a totally artificial diet. Hydrolysis of fats to glycerol and fatty acids may occur by enzymatic degradation, or by saponification, as occurs when calcium soaps are precipitated in the peritoneal cavity in patients with acute pancreatitis.

Ethanol is an alcohol that is of considerable interest and importance in surgery. Like glycerol, it is classified as a lipide, but it is metabolized as a carbohydrate. Ethanol is the antecedent cause of many surgical lesions, including traumatic injuries, birth defects, cirrhosis of the liver and its complications, pancreatitis and acute hemorrhagic gastritis. Heavy long-term consumption of alcohol is associated with the development of various cancers, such as carcinoma of the esophagus and carcinoma of the oral cavity. Chronic addiction to alcohol interferes with proper preoperative preparation and postoperative convalescence — problems range from failure to return for scheduled appointments to acute delirium tremens. Acute intoxication with ethyl alcohol is a significant cause of automobile accidents, the leading single cause of traumatic deaths in this country. The National Institute on Alcohol and Drug Abuse estimates that ten million Americans are problem drinkers and that drinking may be responsible for 205,000 deaths a year in the United States. Drinking problems cost about $43 billion per year in medical bills, property damage and other expenses. Alcohol appears to be involved in half of all murders and traffic deaths, one third of suicides and one fourth of all other accidental deaths.

The "social" drinker may easily achieve a blood level of 0.1 per cent (100 mg/100 ml) of ethanol, which is the legal definition of intoxication for drivers in many states. Ethanol interferes with glucose tolerance, and conversely, glucose ingestion apparently lowers the blood level of ethanol. However, sweetened mixed drinks may produce a significant degree of reaction hypoglycemia, causing difficulty in cerebration. Although the "happy" state of inebriation is generally recognizable by physicians, the precise concentration of alcohol in the blood can only be determined by a laboratory test. Since the test is simple, inexpensive and accurate, we encourage more frequent use of blood alcohol determinations in evaluation of acutely ill patients, especially when the question of head injury, ketoacidosis or intoxication by other drugs has been raised. Alcohol must not be used for skin preparation when drawing a specimen for blood alcohol determination. It has been frequently pointed out that ethanol is a high energy-yielding substance, producing 7 cal. per gram when fully oxidized. Nevertheless, the side effects of alcohol are so undesirable that virtually the only therapeutic use of ethanol in surgical patients is to prevent the development of delirium tremens in patients with chronic alcoholism who require emergency operations.

Metabolism of fats consists of the utilization of glycerol and the fatty acids in the Krebs (tricarboxylic acid) cycle to form CO_2 and H_2O. Glycerol is handled directly as a carbohydrate. The fatty acids, on the other hand, are broken into 2-carbon units, bound to coenzyme A, and then metabolized in the Krebs cycle. When fatty acids are presented to the liver at an excessively high rate or in the presence of a diminished rate of glucose metabolism, the acetyl-co-A fragments accumulate and condense in pairs as acetoacetic acid. This is the first step in ketogenesis, which produces ketoacidosis in diabetics and starved patients who metabolize fat in the absence of glucose. It is of interest that although glucose is metabolized to form fats and proteins, and proteins can be utilized as a new source of glucose, the formation of fatty acids from glucose is a one-way street — for all practical purposes, fatty acids cannot be converted back to carbohydrates.

Blood Cells

1. RED BLOOD CELLS (RBCs). Red cells are responsible for 98 per cent of oxygen transport, and hemoglobin in the red cells is the most important buffer in the blood. Red cells contain large amounts of carbonic anhydrase, the enzyme that catalyzes the reversible reaction between CO_2 and H_2O to form carbonic acid, thus permitting easy transport of CO_2 in the blood. Synthesized in the bone marrow, RBCs normally lose their nuclei when released into peripheral blood. There they have a half-life of 28 days in normal individuals, and less than that in patients with a variety of diseases, including infection, trauma, defective heart valves and hemolytic diseases. Approximately 60 per cent of the red cell is water, and most of the rest (35 per cent) of its substance is hemoglobin.

Red cells are usually exceedingly uniform in appearance and are approximately 6μ in greatest diameter.

Hemoglobin is an iron-containing protein composed of four heme molecules joined to a specific globulin, globin. Each heme molecule consists of four substituted pyrrole rings bound to iron, which is in the ferrous (Fe^{++}) state. Pyrrole rings are five-membered rings, containing four carbons and one nitrogen atom; in hemoglobin the rings are substituted with methyl, vinyl and propionic acid groups. Hemoglobin is a medium-sized globulin, with a molecular weight of 66,700. It is approximately the same size as prothrombin and only half as large as most gamma globulins. Each globin molecule consists of two polypeptide subunits, the α-chain and the β-chain, which are important in the cause of sickle cell anemia (see below). Hemoglobin binds oxygen loosely, combining with oxygen in passage through the lungs. Part of the oxygen is released in transit through the tissues, where oxyhemoglobin dissociation is favored by the higher CO_2 pressure, lower pH and warmer temperature.

Red cell formation is controlled by erythropoietin, a hormone that is released by the kidneys. Hypoxia is the main stimulus to production of erythropoietin and thereby to formation of RBCs.

An excessive level of RBCs in the peripheral blood is referred to as polycythemia and is commonly seen in chronic obstructive airway disease and other diseases in which chronic hypoxemia occurs, such as tetralogy of Fallot. Polycythemia vera is a condition of unknown etiology in which excessive red cell formation occurs. Patients with this condition also have a high blood platelet count, sometimes in excess of 1,000,000 per cmm. The platelets are defective and may allow troublesome bleeding to occur in surgery. Preoperative preparation of patients with all types of polycythemia should include normalization of the hematocrit with venesection and replacement by saline or plasma (by plasmapheresis or Plasmanate). Patients with polycythemia should be bled regularly to keep the hematocrit at 55 per cent or less to prevent spontaneous thrombosis, pulmonary hemorrhage and hemochromatosis. ^{32}P is also used to poison medullary hematopoiesis in patients with polycythemia vera. Endogenous or exogenous androgens also stimulate erythropoiesis. Thus, an elevated hematocrit is seen in women who receive treatment with testosterone for breast cancer and in patients who have masculinizing tumors.

Autotransfusion is the ideal form of blood transfusion in elective surgical operations. For this reason, preoperative removal and storage of one to four pints of blood is recommended prior to major elective surgery. This blood can be withdrawn in the outpatient clinic or blood bank. The volume of each pint of blood removed should be replaced simultaneously with 500 ml of saline or lactated Ringer's solution. The patients will reconstitute their shed RBCs rapidly if iron stores are maintained with 5 ml of Imferon given IM at the time of each venesection. Removal of one to two pints per week will not deplete the red cell mass excessively in most patients. However, each patient should have a hematocrit performed on the day on which venesection is planned.

Congenital diseases of the red cells have important implications for surgery. Spherocytosis is a familial disease in which the normal biconcave shape of the red cells is absent, apparently as a result of a deficiency in enolase, the enzyme which converts 2-phosphoglycerate to phosphoenol pyruvate. This deficiency diminishes the energy production available in the red cell by anaerobic glycolysis. The spherocytic red cells are trapped and destroyed at an increased rate in the spleen. Anemia is observed in the patients, and they may also develop heme-pigment gallstones and jaundice. Splenectomy should be done when the diagnosis is made, and cholecystectomy, too, if stones are present.

Sickle cell anemia is one of many diseases due to abnormal hemoglobins. Sickle cell anemia is a congenital disease caused by the presence of hemoglobin S instead of normal hemoglobin (hemoglobin A). It is an autosomal (i.e., not sex-linked) genetic disease which occurs almost exclusively in blacks. Hemoglobin S, like other abnormal hemoglobins, is the result of amino acid substitution in one of the polypeptide chains of globin. In the case of hemoglobin S, valine is substituted for glutamic acid in the β-chain. Hemoglobin-S chains polymerize at low PO_2. The RBCs thereupon become sickle-shaped and move sluggishly in small vessels. Infarction may occur in viscera such as spleen, kidneys, bowel, brain and bone. Severe abdominal pain occurs in sickle "crisis" and may require laparotomy to rule out infarction. A careful family history should be taken prior to any elective surgery in blacks, searching for familial occurrence of sickle cell disease. Sickle cell disease (homozygous) or trait (heterozygous) can be diagnosed easily by hemoglobin electrophoresis. Patients with hemoglobin S should be advised to live at altitudes under 8000 feet, not to fly in unpressurized planes, and they should be kept particularly well-oxygenated during surgery. Although sickle cell crisis is more common and more severe in homozygous individuals, it has been reported in heterozygotes as well.

Acute intermittent porphyria is an hereditary disease in which severe crises of abdominal pain occur, related to a congenital defect in heme production. Patients with this disease have an excessive production of δ-amino levulinic acid (DAL) and porphobilinogen, probably because of excessive amounts of DAL synthetase and dehydrase in the liver. The patients excrete urine containing increased amounts of porphobilinogen and its precursor, δ-amino levulinic acid. The urine of these patients may turn red spontaneously or on exposure to light. Since the abdominal pain in porphyria usually is not caused by a lesion that can be remedied by surgery, and since porphyria is exacerbated by anesthetics such as the barbiturates, careful observation rather than immediate surgery is indicated in patients with acute porphyria who develop abdominal pain.

Hematin is the oxidized form of heme. It is relatively insoluble in acid, and precipitates in the renal tubules of patients who have free circulating hemoglobin due to hemolysis of a mismatched transfusion. The tubular necrosis that follows transfusion reaction may be alleviated in part by liberal administration of $NaHCO_3$ to alkalinize the urine and diminish the precipitation of acid hematin.

2. WHITE BLOOD CELLS (WBCs). Several types of circulating leukocytes exist, each with somewhat different functions, and all of which have implications for surgeons. The most numerous, *polymorphonuclear leukocytes* (PMN), are phagocytes which engulf and (usually) destroy bacteria and other small foreign bodies. Attracted by serum opsonins, they begin to arrive at the site of injury within minutes, and later are joined by mononuclear cells. PMNs have a short half-life, probably less than 24 hours, and become increasingly segmented as they age. Their numbers can be increased rapidly; when released in large numbers from bone marrow they appear as "band forms" which lack the usual segmentation of mature PMNs. The presence of "band forms" is frequently a good indication of the presence of infection in the body. This change in segmentation of PMNs is referred to as a "shift to the left" in the differential leukocyte count, because traditionally the PMNs and band forms are listed at the left side of the table of WBC percentages. The control of leukocyte maturation and release is under intense investigation at the present time, and present evidence suggests that a hormone (leukopoietin) may be important in this regard. Pyogenic bacteria are usually destroyed by PMNs. However, large numbers of intact intracellular gonococci are present in gonorrhea. This suggests that multiplication rather than destruction may be taking place. Intracellular multiplication also may occur in tuberculosis and leprosy.

Eosinophiles are PMNs containing eosinophilic granules. These cells increase greatly in allergic diseases — up to 40 to 50 per cent of peripheral leukocytes are eosinophiles in some cases. A high percentage of eosinophiles often points to a diagnosis of an allergenic disease, such as an infestation by amoebae or parasites. In patients with eosinophilia and abdominal pain who have a history of residence in areas where parasitic diseases are common, a cautious trial of drug treatment based on appropriate laboratory tests may be indicated instead of immediate exploratory surgery. It should be remembered that parasitic diseases are common in the tropics, and in many other areas where sanitation is inadequate. Poor hygiene is a problem in economically deprived subtropical and temperate communities and in the arctic, where perma-frost prevents filtration and disposal of waste. Echinococcal disease and trichinosis are widespread problems in dogs and other carnivores in the arctic and these diseases are easily transmitted to unwary humans.

Basophiles are PMNs containing black-staining granules, which are believed to be circulating mast cells, associated with heparin formation. Other than this, our knowledge of their exact function in health and disease is incomplete.

Mononuclear cells include lymphocytes and monocytes. *Lymphocytes* are small mononuclear cells with relatively little cytoplasm, which have a polyfunctional role in immunology. The circulating lymphocyte is one of a variety of lymphocytes that are histologically similar; others are present in spleen, marrow, thymus and lymph nodes. The age, life expectancy and exact function of the lymphocytes in each area are not known with certainty. It does, however, appear that some small lymphocytes are long-lived, multiplying cells. They play an important role in antibody synthesis, in transfer of antigenic information, and in the inflammation that occurs in chronic immunity. The lymphocyte appears to be the effector of rejection of homografts and of control of chronic infections such as tuberculosis. When properly stimulated by antigen, the small lymphocyte enlarges and acquires eosinophilic (pyroninophilic) staining material; it then synthesizes new DNA and may either divide or become multinucleated. Lymphocytes can be classified functionally into two main types – B and T lymphocytes. B lymphocytes are predominantly effectors of humoral immunity. They are bone marrow–derived in humans and arise in the bursa of Fabricius in birds. T cells are thymus-derived and are effectors of cellular immunity. B and T lymphocytes are histologically identical and must be differentiated by special tests, such as the sheep red cell "E rosette" test for T cells and the anti–gamma globulin immunofluorescence test for B cells. Some authorities also describe the existence of a third, functionally immature lymphocyte, the A cell type.

Monocytes are large mononuclear cells with round or kidney-bean–shaped nuclei. They appear to act as transferrers of antigenic information and are increased in numbers in patients with chronic infections.

Plasma cells are rarely observed in peripheral blood of normal individuals. The plasma cells have a distinctive nuclear conformation, segmented like the spokes on a wheel. Their function apparently is the synthesis of gamma globulin, and they are usually seen only in tissue sections.

3. PLATELETS. Megakaryocytes in bone marrow give rise to these tiny (2–3 microns), angular cytoplasmic fragments which are of vital importance in coagulation. Thromboplastin is released from platelets in the first stage of clotting. Platelets accumulate quickly at the site of any bleeding, and are present in tumor metastases. Deprivation of platelets may occur as the result of excessive loss in external or internal bleeding, or in bacteremia, parasitemia[14] and other types of consumption coagulopathy. A large number of serious acute illnesses have now been associated with disseminated intravascular coagulation (DIC). DIC is rarely encountered in outpatients, but may be seen in septicemia, massive trauma (especially with fat embolism) and metastatic cancer. When platelets are incorporated into microthrombi, the platelet count falls[13] and fibrin split products appear in the peripheral blood. Evaluation of a patient for possible presence of DIC should include platelet count, prothrombin time, clotting time, clot retraction, clot lysis at 37°C, fibrinogen and fibrin split products. If bleeding is due to DIC, heparinization may be required to control the consumption of platelets and fibrin. Hospitalization is required to initiate this treatment. On the other hand, if prothrombin deficiency is observed, outpatient treatment may be sufficient, using vitamin K and correction of the underlying cause for decreased prothrombin time. Platelets contain serotonin (5-hydroxy tryptamine), a potent vasoactive substance which is also secreted by carcinoid tumors.

Blood clotting is of obvious importance to the patient with a surgical lesion, such as an injury or a disease for which surgery will be needed. Briefly, normal clotting is a dynamic process in which clot formation and clot lysis occur constantly. The equilibrium normally leads to clot formation in the presence of tissue injury and bleeding, in a sequence which is outlined in Chapter 17. The most common conditions leading to increased bleeding in surgical outpatients are thrombocytopenia, prothrombin deficiency, capillary fragility, exogenous heparin administration and hemophilia (an hereditary deficiency in antihemophiliac globulin). Surgery should not be un-

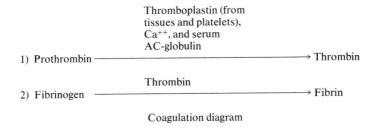

Coagulation diagram

dertaken electively in any of these patients in the Outpatient Department. If emergency surgery in a "bleeder" is required, consultation with experienced hematologists should be obtained immediately. Heparin is a mucoitin sulfuronic acid which is a powerful thrombin antagonist. It is ineffective by the oral route, and is given subcutaneously, IM, or IV. The usual daily dose is variable, depending on the effect desired and the patient's tolerance. Doses range from 2000–6000 international units (formerly termed 200–600 mg) per day. Depoheparin is the most commonly used heparin preparation in our Outpatient Clinic.

Diet and Nutrition

Although every physician quickly develops his own notions about the optimum diet and the value of specific foods, a review of some pertinent data may be of help to doctors in counseling their patients. A "balanced" diet will be discussed and illustrated. The suggested requirements for water, calories, carbohydrates, fats, proteins, minerals and vitamins will be outlined briefly. The composition of foods is presented in detail in Watt and Merrill.[34]

A Balanced Diet

An adequate diet should include foods in four main categories in addition to condiments, oils, sugars and other types of foods that are less essential. The essential aspects of the diet are:

(1) Milk and Dairy Products. Two cups daily for adults; three to four cups for children, teenagers and pregnant women; six cups for nursing mothers. Milk and other dairy products with low fat content should be favored.

(2) Meat and Eggs. At least two servings daily; soybeans and nuts can substitute if taken in large amounts. Consumption of fatty meats should be discouraged in favor of veal, poultry and fish. The proper caloric ratio of fats should be one third from unsaturated, one third from saturated and one third from cholesterol and other fats.

(3) Vegetables and Fruits. At least four servings daily, including: one serving of yellow or green leafy vegetables for vitamin A; one or more servings of citrus fruits or tomatoes for vitamin C; and one or more servings of potatoes or other vegetables and fruits.

(4) Cereals and Bread (whole grain). At least two servings daily.

Sugar and salt intake should be kept to a minimum. Take the sugar bowl and salt shaker off the table and add as little as possible when cooking.

The new national dietary goals suggest (1) increasing consumption of complex carbohydrates and naturally occurring sugars until they account for 48 per cent of caloric intake; (2) reduction of fat to approximately 30 per cent of dietary calories (10 per cent saturated, 10 per cent polyunsaturated and 10 per cent from cholesterol and other lipids); (3) cholesterol reduction to 300 mg per day (a large egg contains 250 mg); (4) sugar reduced to 10 per cent of total calories — about one-fourth cup including sugar used in cooking; and (5) salt reduced by as much as 85 per cent to 5 gm per day — about one teaspoon including the salt used in cooking and salt present in pre-prepared foods.

Water

The homeostatic economy of the body requires water for internal movement of substances by diffusion and circulation. Water is a necessary vehicle for transportation of food and for excretion of waste products by the gastrointestinal and urinary systems. Water must also be available for evaporation in regulation of body temperature. Conservation of water is assisted by the integument, by reabsorption in the air passages and by concentration in kidneys and gastrointestinal tract. Water conservation is highly developed in some species, such as the camel — which can obtain water by oxidation of its fatty "hump" — and the mouse, which can live almost indefinitely in closed burrows by obtaining water from seeds, and by its intense conservation in respiratory, renal and gastrointestinal systems. Adaptation also occurs in man, as seen in decreased water excretion in perspiration during adaptation to a hot environment.

The daily requirements for water are extremely variable, depending on age, general health, body surface area, and environmental conditions. Approximately 2000 ml is sufficient for normal adults in temperate climate zones. Increased respiratory rate, fever or diminished reabsorptive mechanisms will increase the need for water. Water requirement may be calculated precisely by metabolic balance, utilizing factors such as daily weight, serum osmolarity, urine specific gravity, deuterium-labeled water and hemato-crit. However, clinical signs of increasing or decreasing body water are also important. These signs include turgor of skin and soft tissues, moisture of the mucous membranes, and frequency of urination. In outpatients, clinical judgment regarding the patient's water balance must be skillfully rendered, since the laboratory tests are usually not requested or interpreted correctly until the physician suspects an abnormality on clinical grounds.

Water is available in the form of liquids, such as drinking water, other dietary fluids and intravenous fluids; in solid foods; and as water of oxidation released by combustion of foods or body tissues. A 3000 cal. diet contains approximately 450 ml of water in solid food and releases approximately 400 ml more during combustion. Water released by combustion includes approximately 0.3 ml per gram of protein, 0.5 ml per gram of carbohydrate and 1.0 ml per gram of fat.

Water content of solid food can generally be estimated from the relative moisture and texture of the food. Exact values are given in Watt and Merrill.[34] Values range from more than 90 per cent in many fresh and canned fruits and vegetables to values of 5 to 10 per cent in dried foods. Desiccated and powdered foods generally consist of less than 5 per cent water. Meats are approximately 50 per cent water; bread is about 30 per cent water; and fat is about 10 per cent water.

Calories

The usual caloric intake for a 70 kg male with moderate exercise should be approximately 3000 cal. per day. For heavy exercise, up to 6000 cal. may be required. A balanced diet providing 2000 cal. will be satisfactory for sedentary conditions, but if less is provided than is required, negative nitrogen balance will occur due to catabolism of muscle protein for energy. Oxidation provides 4 cal./gm of carbohydrates, 4 cal./gm of protein and 9 cal./gm of fat. In conversations with laymen we should emphasize that an ounce of fat yields 270 calories, while an ounce of carbohydrate or protein yields only 120 calories. Anaerobic glycolysis releases only 21 per cent of the energy of glucose, since it is less efficient than aerobic metabolism for energy production.

Caloric contents of 100 gm and 1 pound edible portions of foodstuffs are given in Watt and Merrill and summarized in Table 7–5. Energy available per 100 gm ranges from 783 cal. in salt pork to 1 cal. in black coffee. Foods with a high fat content provide the most energy, e.g., mayonnaise, bacon, butter and heavily sweetened dessert pastries. The energy available in nuts, seeds and soybean flour is remarkably high (421–598 cal./100 gm). Medium calorie yields are obtained from foods with high carbohydrate or protein content, such as beef, cheese, fish, sweetened fruits and breads. Low calorie yield is seen in raw or cooked, unsweetened fruits and vegetables and cooked cereals. For balanced diets with low calories, variety and sufficient protein can be obtained from such foods as milk, yoghurt, lobster, commercial stews and soybean "milk." Significant differences in calorie yield due to methods of preparation are illustrated by the various types of olives, cherries, potatoes and corn shown in Table 7–5. There appears to be little practical difference between the caloric content of various spirits, wines and beers, since the caloric content of 8 oz of beer is approximately the same as that of 4 oz of table wine and 1 oz of 80 proof whisky.

Carbohydrates

Simple sugars of six carbon atoms, (e.g., glucose, fructose and galactose), disaccharides (e.g., maltose, lactose and sucrose), or polysaccharides (e.g., starch) are subjected to oxidative phosphorylation in the Krebs cycle or are metabolized to lactic acid by anaerobic glycolysis. Pentoses such as ribose can be utilized but produce relatively little energy. In oxidative energy production, CO_2 and H_2O are produced. The anaerobic pathways lead to production of CO_2 and lactate. Lactate is ordinarily metabolized further when the temporary period of hypoxia is past and sufficient oxygen is again available. Carbohydrates are predominantly stored in the form of glucose, present in all of the body tissues, and in glycogen, which occurs mainly in liver and skeletal muscle but is also present in many other tissues.

Disaccharides must be hydrolyzed before they can be utilized, and intestinal lactase deficiency is considered to be a cause of milk intolerance in the postgastrectomy "dumping" syndrome.

Foods also include other carbohydrates such as D-xylose and cellulose, which cannot be assimilated by humans. D-xylose is therefore used as a tracer substance for GI tract function; it is absorbed by the GI tract but excreted through the kidneys without metabolic degradation. Cellulose is neither degraded nor absorbed and therefore serves as an important source of bulk in the diet, a factor which is necessary for normal function of the colon. Cellulose, or non-nutritive fiber, appears in the diet in various forms, the most potent form being bran.

A remarkable increase in bran consumption has been noted in the past decade, because of the obvious effects of bran on GI motility (larger, softer stools and decreased transit time) and the reports of associated decrease in colonic diseases in populations with high bran intake. The exact mechanism for the effect of bran on the GI tract is unknown; it may be in part a chemical effect and in part an effect caused by water absorbed to the cellulose.

Several other types of abnormal carbohydrate metabolism are important in surgery. These include: lactate accumulation in metabolic acidosis; glyco-

TABLE 7–5   Caloric Content of Some Common Foods*
(cal. per 100 grams edible portions)

High Calorie (>400 cal/100 gm)		Medium Calorie (100–400 cal/100 gm)		Low Calorie (<100 cal/100 gm)	
DAIRY PRODUCTS					
Butter	716	*Cheese*		*Milk*	
		Swiss	370	whole, cow	65
Chocolate				skimmed, cow	36
sweet	528	*Cheese*			
		Cottage, creamed	106	*Yoghurt*	
Salad dressing				from whole milk	62
Roquefort	504	*Cream*			
Mayonnaise	718	(half & half,			
		milk & cream)	134		
		Ice Cream			
		rich	222		
MEATS, EGGS AND NUTS					
Almonds	598	*Beef*, choice grade,		*Beef & vegetable stew*,	
		trimmed	301	canned	79
Bacon, cooked	611				
		Bluefish, fried	205	*Chow mein*, canned	38
Fat, cooked	729				
		Chicken pot pie	235	*Lobster*, cooked	95
Peanuts	564				
		Chicken, cooked		*Oyster stew*, commercial,	
Pork		light meat	166	with milk	84
total edible	553				
salt	783	*Eggs*, hard boiled	163	*Soup*, chicken,	
				consomme, canned	9
Pumpkin seeds	553	*Haddock*, fried	165	prepared with milk	73
				with rice, prepared	
Suet, beef kidney,		*Ham*, cooked	289	from dehydrated mix	20
fat, raw	854				
		Liver, beef, cooked	229		
VEGETABLES AND FRUITS					
Potato chips	568	*Cherries*, with extra		*Apples*, raw	58
		heavy syrup	112		
Popcorn, without oil				*Asparagus*, cooked	20
and salt	456	*Jelly*	273		
				Celery, raw	17
Soybean flour		*Olives*			
full fat	421	ripe	129	*Cherries*, raw	58
		ripe, Greek style	338		
				Corn, kernels, cooked	
		Potatoes, fried	268	on cob	91
		Prunes, raw, soft	255	*Fruit cocktail*,	
				canned, with light	
		Soybeans, cooked	130	syrup	59
				Onions, boiled	29
				Oranges, raw	49

TABLE 7-5   Caloric Content of Some Common Foods* (*Continued*)
(cal. per 100 grams edible portions)

High Calorie (>400 cal/100 gm)		Medium Calorie (100–400 cal/100 gm)		Low Calorie (<100 cal/100 gm)	
VEGETABLES AND FRUITS					
				Peas, cooked	71
				Potatoes, boiled in skin	76
				Soybean "milk"	33
				Tomatoes, raw	26
CEREALS AND BREADS					
Cookies, chocolate chip	516	*Baby food barley cereal*	348	*Farina*, cooked	42
Crackers, saltine	433	*Biscuits*	369	*Oat cereal*, cooked	62
Pie, pecan	418	*Bread*, whole wheat	243	*Wheat cereal*, cooked	45
Rolls, Danish	433	*Cake*, chocolate with icing	369		
		Crackers, graham	384		
		Macaroni, cooked, tender	111		
		Pancakes, made with egg and milk	225		
		Pie, apple	256		
		Pie, strawberry	198		
		Pudding, vanilla	111		
		Rice, white cooked	109		
		Rolls, whole wheat	257		
		Sugar, granulated	385		
BEVERAGES					
		Spirits, (gin, whisky, etc.) 80 proof	231	*Beer* (alcohol 4.5% by volume)	42
				Coffee	1
				Cola	39
				Wine, (table; alcohol 12% by volume)	85

*Adapted from Watt and Merrill.

gen storage disease with splenomegaly and hypersplenism; diabetes mellitus (with renal, vascular and ocular complications); and excessive production of insulin and glucagon in islet cell tumors of the pancreas.

Carbohydrate content of common foods ranges from 0 per cent in meat, fish and chicken to 99.5 per cent in granulated sugar. Low carbohydrate content is seen in eggs (1 per cent), cheese (2 to 3 per cent) and most cooked vegetables, which have less than 10 per cent, usually less than 5 per cent. Cow's milk is also low in carbohydrate (5 per cent), although of course sweetened condensed milk has a high carbohydrate content (54 per cent). Beer and wine are surprisingly low (4 per cent), compared with fresh fruits (10 to 15 per cent) and nuts (20 per cent). Custard is a low carbohydrate dessert (11 per cent), compared with cookies (60 to 80 per cent) and candy (up to 95 per cent in butterscotch). Nougat and caramel have the lowest carbohydrate content of the common candies (39 per cent). Prepared breads and cereals have a wide range of carbohydrate content (generally 50 to 80 per cent), with a maximum in corn flakes (91 per cent). The fiber content of our foods is remarkably low, being far less than 1 per cent in the common starchy foods, and only 1.6 to 2.6 per cent in such foods as soybeans, peanuts and almonds. The highest non-nutritive fiber content of commonly ingested food is in "all bran" or "100 per cent bran" breakfast cereals, which contain 7.5 per cent fiber by weight.

Proteins

Amino acids are joined together within the ribosomes to form polypeptides, which — when an arbitrary molecular weight of 5000 has been reached — are called proteins. The two major types of proteins synthesized in the body are enzymes and structural proteins. In addition, there are the plasma proteins, synthesized in the liver; the globulins, synthesized in the liver and in various hematological cells; and fibrinogen. The plasma proteins serve at least seven functions: (1) colloid osmotic pressure, especially albumin, which is responsible for 80 per cent of this role, (2) blood buffer, the pH stabilization by hemoglobin and the plasma proteins being equal in importance to HCO_3^- and the other inorganic buffers, (3) transportation of lipides, hormones and drugs, (4) nutrition, since albumin is a readily available source of amino acids, (5) coagulation, (6) immunity and (7) serum enzymes.

Protein anabolism is directed by a complex series of events stimulated by androgens and growth hormone, and catabolism occurs continuously. Catabolism releases amino acids for reuse, as well as for energy production in cases where fats and glycogen cannot be used at an adequate rate. Far more reserve energy is present in fat than in glycogen, since only 1600 cal. can be liberated by the glycogen in an adult human liver. On the other hand, each kilogram of muscle can yield 1000 cal. through gluconeogenesis from its content of protein. Of the approximately 22 naturally occurring amino acids, eight* are required in human diets and six others are "semidispensable."** The other amino acids are either nonessential in humans or can be synthesized in sufficient amounts from the essential amino acids if adequate protein intake is provided. Casein, the protein of milk and cheese, is an excellent source of all of the essential amino acids and is a well-balanced source of 18 others, lacking only hydroxyproline. A mixture of animal and vegetable proteins

---

*Isoleucine, leucine, lysine, methionine, phenylalanine, threonine, tryptophan and valine. However, recent evidence suggests that valine and phenylalanine may be synthesized in man from their ketoacids.
**Arginine, cystine, glycine, histidine, serine and tyrosine.

is generally preferable to a restricted diet, however.

The most convenient dietary sources of proteins are, of course, meats, poultry and fish. Cooked meats, including beef, bacon, chicken and cod, usually contain 30 to 35 per cent protein by weight. Raw whole eggs are 13 per cent protein, which is moderately higher than enriched breads (8–10 per cent). Baby food cereals are generally deficient in protein (6 per cent with rice cereal), although high-protein baby food cereal is available, containing 35 per cent protein. Cooked beans (8 per cent), soybeans (10 per cent), almonds (19 per cent) and peanuts (26 per cent) are all considerably higher than milk, cream and yogurt, each of which contains only 3.5 per cent protein. Saltine crackers (9 per cent) are surprisingly high in protein, compared to spaghetti (3 per cent). Medium raw pork is only 10 per cent protein, but is 52 per cent fat. Candy contains 2 per cent protein or less. Most fresh fruits and vegetables contain less than 1 per cent protein, although raisins are 2.5 per cent protein and the edible portion of breadfruit is 5.9 per cent protein.

A convenient source of amino acids for intravenous use in outpatients is 5 per cent dextrose in Aminosol. Dietary protein supplements are available commercially as Sustekal, various elemental diets such as Vivonex-100† and Instant Breakfast.

Protein formation is essential in surgical patients, with polymerization and cross-linking of collagen occurring to give strength to the healing wound. Specific deficiencies occur in diseases such as lathyrism and vitamin C deficiency. On the other hand, excessive formation of collagen causes a multitude of complications, including failure of tendon repairs, common duct strictures and recurrent bowel obstructions due to adhesions. High doses of corticosteroids have occasionally been reported to interfere with excessive formation of collagen, and for this reason dexamethasone has been used to prevent recurrent adhesions and fallopian tubal fibrosis.

Fats

The class of biochemical compounds that will dissolve in organic solvents is complex. It includes the triglycerides and their constituents (the fatty acids and glycerol); sterols, such as cholesterol and the steroid hormones; alcohols; and the lipides of the nervous system, such as sphingomyelin. The surgeon is particularly concerned with

---

†Vivonex-100 is an elemental, bulk-free diet that is stated by the manufacturer to contain in six 80 gm packets, each diluted with water to a total volume of 300 ml: *1800 ml of Vivonex — 1800 Kilocalorie:*

		Caloric contribution (%)
Available nitrogen, as purified amino acids, including all eight essential amino acids	5.88 gm	8.5
Fat (safflower oil–linoleic acid)	2.61 gm	1.3
Carbohydrate (glucose and glucose oligosaccharides)	407.4 gm	90.2
Calories	1800	

Vitamins–measured amounts of 15 vitamins, including A, B_{12} and C
Minerals–measured amounts of eight cations and six anions, including sodium (1548 mg), potassium (2105 mg), calcium (800 mg) and magnesium (350 mg). 1800 ml supplies 67 mEq of sodium and 54 mEq of potassium
(Eaton Laboratories, Division of Morton-Norwich Products, Inc. Norwich, N.Y. 13815)
Vivonex-100 HN has recently been released for use. It is stated to contain 3.4 times the nitrogen in the recommended daily intake of Vivonex-100 Standard Diet. Ten 80-gm packets are said by the manufacturer to provide 3000 KCal, 20 gm usable nitrogen (125 gm usable protein), and a full day's balanced nutrition in 3000 ml.

the most common of the fats, the triglycerides, for these are the main constituents of adipose tissue. Adipose tissue is poorly vascularized and is easily subject to infection, yet it is, per gram, the most important source of energy in the body. The free fatty acids are energy sources that are rapidly mobilized in response to stress, through hormonal systems utilizing insulin and epinephrine. Surgical diseases and operations specifically involving the fatty tissues include cosmetic removal of subcutaneous fat in excessively obese patients, jejunoileostomy for control of obesity, and hyperlipidemia, lipomas, liposarcomas and lipidystrophy of the mesentery. Fat interferes locally with wound healing, although the fatty tissues of the body are essential reserves in convalescence from severe injury.

Fat is usually thought of as the dietary derivation of certain meats such as pork and bacon, which are approximately 50 per cent fat. However, a similar proportion of fat is obtained from peanuts (48 per cent), almonds (54 per cent) and many other nuts. The largest proportion of fat in any common food is raw beef kidney fat (suet) which is 94 per cent fat. Cooked lean beef, on the other hand, contains only 7 per cent fat, which is considerably less than cake (9 to 20 per cent) and candy (10 to 40 per cent), or even cream (12 per cent in "half and half"). Whole milk contains 3.5–4.0 per cent fat, which is about the same as cooked chicken light meat (3 per cent), soybeans (5 per cent) or codfish (5 per cent). Saltine crackers are remarkably high in fat (12 per cent), which is the same as whole eggs. Most raw fruits and vegetables contain less than 1 per cent fat, but some cereals are considerably higher; bread contains up to 4 per cent fat and baby food oatmeal contains 5.5 per cent fat.

Considerable concern has recently been expressed regarding the potential danger of a high fat intake in the diet of normal adults, and the special danger of high fat intake in patients with hyperlipoproteinemia.

It is likely that little can be done to produce massive reversal in body fat distribution in most outpatients who are seen in surgical clinics with problems of obesity, atherosclerosis or xanthomas. Nevertheless, it is entirely reasonable to make dietary suggestions which may prevent progression of disease and which may reduce the likelihood of similar disease developing in younger members of the household who share the diet. If the patient has accepted dietary instructions with interest and follows the recommendations carefully, it is likely that he would profit by dietary counseling from a dietitian or an internist specializing in this field. On the other hand, if the patient shows little inclination to study his own problem objectively and to participate in the planning of his diet, it is unlikely that he will be able to exert sufficient self-discipline to alter his fat metabolism significantly.

It is generally believed that a high fat intake should be avoided and that the caloric contribution of fats in the diet should be no greater than 35 per cent. Dietary fats should be relatively high in unsaturated fatty acids, and cholesterol intake should be reduced as much as possible. It has been reported that multiple xanthomas were completely eliminated by eight years of careful dieting by a patient with type–2–hyperlipoproteinemia.[24] In this case, the unsaturated/saturated (U/S) fatty acid ratio in the diet was approximately 1.5/1.0, and the total caloric intake was maintained at 2500 cal. per day.

Table 7–6 shows the total fat, fatty acid and cholesterol content in several common foods. It is apparent from cursory examination of this table that many surprises are in store for those who begin to evaluate the fat content of their diet. A serious student of this problem should utilize a more complete reference such as Watt and Merrill.[34]

As would be expected, most fresh fruits and vegetables are extremely low in total fat, saturated fatty acids and cholesterol. Canned beans, for example, contain only 3 per cent fat. A higher fat content is available in some vegetables, such as avocados and soybeans, which still preserve a relatively high U/S fatty acid ratio. On the other hand, coconut meat has a *high* saturated fatty acid content (30 per cent). Meats range from a high of 85 per cent fat with salt pork and 52 per cent with whole pork or bacon to a low of 4 per cent with venison. Beef and lamb have 21–25 per cent fat and a U/S ratio of approximately 1.0. Chicken (12 per cent), veal (12 per cent) and fish are lower in fat content. But fish have considerable variation in fat content, as illustrated by the 4 per cent fat in humpback salmon and 16 per cent fat in Chinook salmon.

All "shortening" is high in fat, but considerable variation is possible in the U/S ratio by careful selection, as shown in Table 7–6. Vegetable oils have a high unsaturated fatty acid content, safflower oil being 11.0/1.0 and also providing the highest amount of the essential fatty acid, linoleic acid. On the other hand, butter, which is 81 per cent fat, has a U/S ratio of only 0.62. The use of fats and oils in cooking usually converts cooked breads and vegetables to a higher fat content, as illustrated by bread vs. biscuits (3 per cent vs. 17 per cent fat) and mashed vs. French fried potatoes (4 per cent vs. 14 per cent). Salad eaters can clearly see the difference in fat content of the ingredients, by noting that cottage cheese is 4 per cent fat, whereas most salad dressings are 50 per cent fat. However, dietary salad dressings provide significantly lower fat content (6 per cent).

Of all commonly eaten foods, the cholesterol content of egg yolks is highest — 1.5 per cent by weight. Only beef brains, with more than 2.0 per cent cholesterol, are higher than egg yolks. It is usually forgotten that egg *whites* have virtually *no* fat, however. Other foods with significantly high cholesterol are shellfish (0.2 per cent), liver (0.3 per cent) and butter (0.25 per cent). Margarine is much lower in cholesterol than butter, with no cholesterol in vegetable margarine, and only 0.065 per cent cholesterol in margarine which is two-thirds animal in origin. The common meat, fish and fowl are all approximately the same in cholesterol content, with 0.06 to 0.07 gm cholesterol per 100 gm of edible food.

Minerals

The importance of sodium, potassium, calcium, magnesium and iron was stressed above. Copper and cobalt are present in the enzymes which facilitate oxidative phosphorylation. On the other hand, lead and mercury are poisons that cause symptoms mimicking the acute surgical abdomen and brain tumors.

Few natural foods are truly high in content of sodium and potassium. Man has a profound craving for salt, however, and prepared foods are frequently salted to an astonishing degree. The concentration of sodium, potassium, phosphorus, iron and magnesium in common foods can be found in Watt and Merrill.[34] The summary presented in this text refers to concentration of these ions in mg per 100 gm of edible food.

It is generally recognized, of course, that sodium content is high in bacon, corned beef and saltine crackers. These foods have sodium contents of slightly more than 1000 mg/100 gm of food. It is, however, rarely remembered that many other common foods also have high sodium concentrations, although they do not taste particularly salty. Examples are cheddar cheeses (1136 mg), Italian-style salad dressing (2092 mg) and puffed oats dry cereal (1267 mg). Baby foods generally have high sodium concentrations that may reach 300-450 mg/100 gm in cereals and meats. Truly salty foods, of course, have expectedly high sodium concentration, with smoked herring (6231 mg), lightly salted dry cod (8100) and soy sauce (7325) leading the list. (For comparison, table salt contains 37,758 mg per 100 gm.)

TABLE 7-6   Fat Content of Some Common Foods
Total Fat; Saturated and Unsaturated Fatty Acids; Cholesterol

Food	Amount In 100 Gm of Edible Portion			
		Fatty Acids		
	Total fat (gm)	Saturated (gm)	Unsaturated (gm)	Cholesterol (gm)
Almonds, roasted	57	5	51	.070
Avocados	17	3	10	
Bacon, cooked	52	17	30	
Beans, canned	3	1	1	
Beef, choice, trimmed	25	12	12	
Biscuits				
made with lard	17	6	10	
made with vegetable				
shortening	17	4	12	
Bread, white	3	1	2	
Butter	81	46	29	.250
Chocolate candy	35	20	14	
Cheese				
Swiss style	28	15	10	
American style	32	18	12	.100
Cottage, creamed	4	2	1	.015
Chicken, cooked with				
vegetable shortening	12	3	8	.060
Coconut meat, fresh	35	30	2	
Crackers, saltine	12	3	8	
Eggs, chicken, raw				
whole	12	4	6	.550
whites	trace			0
yolks	31	10	15	1.5
Fat, cooking				
vegetable	100	23	72	
animal & vegetable	100	43	52	
Ice cream	13	7	4	
Lamb	21	12	9	.070
Lard	100	38	56	.095
Margarine	81	18	60	0–65
Oils				
corn	100	10	81	
cottonseed	100	25	71	
safflower	100	8	87	

Salt is usually added in preparation of most canned vegetables, raising the concentration from 1 mg or so to 200–300 mg/100 gm. Special diet-pack canned foods are available, with sodium concentrations of 3 mg or less per 100 gm. Most fresh fruits and nuts are also low in sodium, as illustrated by bananas (1 mg) and dried almonds (3 mg). Preparation of food in the home usually involves addition of either sugar or salt. For example, white bread contains 507 mg sodium per 100 gm, whereas chocolate cake contains only 294 mg. And whole milk contains 50 mg sodium whereas cottage cheese con-

TABLE 7–6 Fat Content of Some Common Foods
Total Fat; Saturated and Unsaturated Fatty Acids; Cholesterol *(Continued)*

Food	Amount In 100 Gm of Edible Portion			
		Fatty Acids		
	Total fat (gm)	*Saturated (gm)*	*Unsaturated (gm)*	*Cholesterol (gm)*
Milk				
whole	4	2	1	0.011
skimmed	2	1	1	
Pancakes made with				
egg and milk	7	3	5	
Peanuts	48	10	34	
Pork	52	19	27	
Potatoes				
mashed, with milk				
and butter	4	2	1	
french fried	14	3	10	
Salad dressing				
Roquefort, regular	52	11	39	
special dietary	6	3	2	
Salmon				
King (Chinook)	16	5	5	.070
humpback (pink)	4	1	1	
Salt pork	85	32	44	
Soup, creamed chicken,				
prepared with milk	4	1	2	
Soybean "milk"	20	6	5	
Veal	12	6	5	0.090
Venison	4	3	1	
Yoghurt, made with				
whole milk	3	2	1	
Zweibach	9	2	6	
Foods With High Cholesterol Content				
Brains				>2.000
Egg yolk				1.500
Liver				.300
Caviar				>.300
Lobster				.200
Oysters				>.200

tains 229. Lightly cooked meat, fish and fowl contain only 24–70 mg sodium per 100 gm, until it is "salted to taste." A moderately restricted sodium diet (2.0 gm; 87 mEq) is shown in Table 7–7. More stringent diets (500 or 1000 mg) are available in manuals published by the American Heart Association, 44 East 23 Street, New York City, New York 10010.

Potassium content of most foods is changed relatively little in the course of preparation. The naturally occurring potassium concentration, is, however, quite variable. For example, meats have potassium concentrations of 200–

TABLE 7–7   87 mEq Sodium Diet (2000 mg)

SALT SHOULD NOT BE USED ON ANY FOODS OR IN THE PREPARATION OF FOODS EXCEPT AS ALLOWED. ALL SALT SUBSTITUTES FOR PATIENTS MUST BE APPROVED BY THE PHYSICIAN.

	ALLOWED	AVOID
BEVERAGES:	Coffee, coffee substitutes, tea; 3 cups daily of whole or skim milk (if more milk is desired use low sodium milk), cocoa made from cocoa powder and milk allowance; fruit juices, lemonade, Kool-Aid, carbonated beverages in moderation	Cultured buttermilk, malted milk; low calorie carbonated beverages which use sodium base sweeteners; instant cocoa mixes
BREAD:	4 slices daily of salted yeast bread or rolls (if more bread is desired use low sodium bread); quick breads made with sodium-free baking powder or potassium bicarbonate and without salt, or made from low sodium dietetic mix; barley, cornmeal, cornstarch, flour; melba toast, graham crackers, low sodium crackers	Waffles, pancakes or quick breads made with baking powder, baking soda, or salt; commercial mixes; self-rising cornmeal or flour; any crackers except those allowed
CEREAL:	Unsalted cooked cereals; puffed rice, puffed wheat, shredded wheat; and any other low sodium dry cereal; cornmeal, barley	Dry cereals except those allowed
CHEESE:	Unsalted cottage cheese, unsalted American cheese	All other cheese
DESSERT:	Tapioca; unflavored gelatin (use fruit and fruit juices with gelatin), commercial low sodium gelatin, low sodium rennet dessert powder or tablets; unsalted fruit pies; desserts using milk allowance and other allowed food items	Commercial sweetened gelatins containing sodium; pudding mixes; other commercial desserts or dessert mixes
EGGS:	1 per day if desired, prepared any way without salt	No more than 1 per day
FATS:	4 teaspoons per day of salted butter or margarine (if more is desired use unsalted butter or margarine); 1/2 cup cream; unsalted fat or oil for cooking; unsalted salad dressing and unsalted mayonnaise; unsalted nuts	Bacon and bacon fat, salt pork; commercial salted salad dressings, salted nuts
FRUITS:	Fresh, canned, dried, or frozen fruits, fruit juices, unsalted tomato juice; apples, melons and berries may be used if they do not cause distress	Regular canned tomato juice; crystallized or glazed fruit, and those containing salt or sodium compounds
MEAT, FISH AND POULTRY:	5 ounces daily (2 servings) of fresh beef, chicken, duck, lamb, pork, quail, rabbit, fresh tongue, turkey, veal; beef or calf liver allowed not more than once in two weeks; fresh fish such as bass, bluefish, catfish, cod, eels, flounder, haddock, halibut, rockfish, salmon, sole, trout, tuna, whitefish; unsalted canned tuna or salmon	Brains or kidneys; canned, salted or smoked meat such as bacon, bologna, chipped or corned beef, frankfurters, ham, kosher meats, luncheon meats, salt pork, sausage, smoked tongue; packaged frozen fish; canned, salted or smoked fish such as anchovies, caviar, salted or fried cod, herring, canned salmon or tuna (except low sodium dietetic), sardines; shellfish such as clams, crabs, lobsters, oysters, scallops, shrimp

TABLE 7–7   87 mEq Sodium Diet (2000 mg) (*Continued*)

	ALLOWED	AVOID
POTATO AND SUBSTITUTE:	White or sweet potato, macaroni, noodles, spaghetti and rice	Instant mashed potato, commercial potato products, potato chips
SEASONINGS:	Most spices and herbs may be used including garlic powder, onion powder, and pepper	Regular salt at the table or in cooking (except as allowed); celery salt, garlic salt; onion salt; monosodium glutamate, meat tenderizers, Accent; dried parsley flakes, celery seeds
SOUPS:	Unsalted broth, unsalted cream soups made with milk allowance and allowed foods; low sodium canned soup	Bouillon cubes, salted commercial soups
SWEETS:	White sugar; home-made candy without salt, or special low sodium candy; jam, jelly or marmalade, honey; hard candy without salt or sodium compounds	Commercial candies made with salt or sodium compounds and milk or eggs; large amounts of brown sugar, molasses, syrups
VEGETABLES:	2 to 3 servings daily of any fresh, frozen, or canned vegetables	Sauerkraut and those which cause distress
MISCELLANEOUS:	Cream of tartar, sodium-free baking powder, potassium bicarbonate, yeast; cocoa, unsweetened baking chocolate; unsalted nuts, *salted* peanut butter, unsalted popcorn; unsalted catsup; lemon juice; extracts of almond, lemon, peppermint, and vanilla; vinegar	Regular baking powder, baking soda (soda bicarbonate); salted gravy or white sauce; Worcestershire sauce, Kitchen Bouquet, soy sauce, prepared mustard or horseradish, chili sauce, pickles, olives; Dutch processed chocolate; pretzels and snack foods; any foods prepared in a salt brine

General Rules:
1. *Read labels carefully* and avoid products containing salt, sodium, and NaCl unless allowed on your diet.
2. If snacks are desired between meals, use foods allowed on the diet not exceeding the amount permitted per day.
3. *Do not use* unprescribed medicines such as alkalizers, antibiotics, cough medicines, laxatives, pain relievers, and sedatives containing sodium.
4. *Do not use* water which has been treated in water-softening equipment with sodium compounds.

SUGGESTED MEAL PLAN

Breakfast	*Lunch*	*Supper*
Orange juice	Salt free chicken noodle	Salt free roast beef
Salt free Cream of Wheat	soup with salt free	Baked potato with 1 tsp.
with ½ cup cream	crackers	salted butter
Soft cooked egg	Salt free baked fish	Regular carrots
1 slice salted toast	Salt free potatoes	Lettuce and tomato salad
1 tsp. salted butter	Frozen peas	with salt free dressing
1 cup milk	1 slice salted bread	1 slice salted bread
Sugar–jelly	2 tsp. salted butter	1 tsp. salted butter
Coffee or tea	Canned peaches	Salt free vanilla pudding
	1 cup milk	(using ½ cup milk
	Sugar	allowance)
	Coffee or tea	2 squares graham crackers
		½ cup milk
		Sugar
		Coffee or tea

400 mg/100 gm. On the other hand, potassium concentration of eggs (129) and milk (144) is considerably less than that of meat. And almonds (773) are unexpectedly high. Most vegetables and fruits have potassium concentrations between 100 and 200 mg/100 ml, although some are higher — bananas contain 370 mg/100 gm, which is higher than cooked bacon! Some of the high sodium foods are comparatively low in potassium, as illustrated by Italian dressing (15) and smoked herring (157). Alcoholic beverages are generally low in both sodium and potassium, although table wine has 92 mg potassium per 100 gm.

Calcium is generally a well-tolerated and useful addition to diets, especially in children and lactating or pregnant women. Unfortunately, many of the foods with high calcium content also have high concentrations of substances that are generally not as valuable or well-tolerated — particularly sodium, saturated fats or cholesterol. However, for those who are in specific need of calcium, for bone formation or for treatment of hypoparathyroidism, it is important for the surgeon to know which foods provide significant amounts of calcium. In general, calcium content is good in dairy products, seafood, and foods prepared from these raw materials. Calcium concentration of milk is 118 mg/100 gm; biscuits contain 209 mg, white bread 98 mg, and caramel 148 mg/100 gm. Although most fruits and many vegetables are low in calcium (0.3–10 mg/100 gm), beans contain 50 mg/100 gm and collards 188 mg. Egg yolks are a good source of calcium (141 mg), although whole eggs are considerably less (54), since egg white contains only 9 mg/100 gm. Almonds are surprisingly rich in calcium (234 mg/100 gm). Seafood is especially rich in calcium, with sardines containing 437 mg/100 gm, and kelp 1093 mg. Fish flour contains the astonishing quantity of 4610 mg/100 gm. For those rare patients who must receive calcium deficient diets, the most useful foods will be fresh

fruits, vegetables such as potatoes (9 mg/100 gm), starches such as spaghetti (8) and most terrestrial meats and fowl (11 mg/100 gm).

Magnesium is abundant in many nuts (225–270 mg/100 gm), chocolate (292 mg) and soybeans (265). Moderate amounts are found in many other vegetables. Magnesium is relatively low in milk (13), meats (12–15) and fish (25–30).

Iron is generally found in sufficient quantities in meats (3–4 mg/100 gm) and seafood. Iron concentration is particularly high in braised kidneys (15 mg/100 gm) and egg yolk (5.5). As with many other substances needed in the human diet, almonds are rich in iron (4.7 mg/100 gm). On the other hand, milk contains only a trace of iron, and children who are fed predominantly on milk will develop a profound iron deficiency anemia.

Vitamins

Although vitamins are obviously of general importance to surgical patients, three are of particular interest: vitamins C, B_{12} and K.

Vitamin C (ascorbic acid) is a powerful reducing agent. It is essential for wound healing and must be supplemented vigorously in chronically neglected, debilitated patients or those who are undergoing a prolonged series of operations while receiving little dietary intake. Treatment may consist of 500–1000 mg per day. Scurvy is the classic disease produced by deficiency of this water soluble vitamin. Wound healing can be impaired by ascorbic acid deficiency in the absence of the classic signs of pyorrhea and cutaneous sores. Blood levels of ascorbic acid can be easily and accurately determined in any chemistry laboratory.

Citrus fruits are the most notable source of ascorbic acid, but many other fruits, berries and vegetables such as cabbage or kohlrabi are equally high in ascorbic acid content. Liver, onions and okra also provide substantial amounts of ascorbic acid. The ascorbic acid content of most foods is shown in Watt and Merrill.[34]

Vitamin B_{12} (cyanocobolamin) is a necessary coenzyme for synthesis of many amino acids. Vitamin B_{12} is widely distributed in meats and fish, especially in liver. It is not commonly found in fresh vegetables. Natural sources are documented in detail in a U.S. Government document on the subject (Home Economics Research Report[18]). It is believed that much of the Vitamin B_{12} utilized in human beings is synthesized by intestinal bacteria and absorbed in the terminal ileum.

In the absence of a specific glycoprotein ("intrinsic factor") secreted by the parietal cells of the stomach, B_{12} is not absorbed, and pernicious anemia develops. Pernicious anemia is a disease characterized by severe megaloblastic anemia and peripheral neuropathy. Patients with pernicious anemia have achlorhydria and a high incidence of carcinoma of the stomach. Unfortunately, they frequently have been given folic acid in the form of a multivitamin preparation. Folic acid will control the anemia, but it does not prevent development of neuropathy. It also masks the presence of pernicious anemia, so that the potential danger of gastric carcinoma is not recognized. It is important for surgeons to be aware of the dangers of B_{12} deficiency, and of the need for correction of this deficiency with B_{12} rather than with folic acid.

B_{12} must be given to patients who have had a total or nearly total gastrectomy, and to patients with ileal bypass (since B_{12} is absorbed in the terminal ileum). B_{12} deficiency develops slowly, occasionally becoming apparent only after many months or years. The patient may by then have moved to the care of another doctor. B_{12} is administered in injections of 100 mcg intramuscularly every month. Since only 1 mcg per day is required to maintain adequate levels of the vitamin, it has been said that

vitamin B_{12} is the most potent therapeutic agent known to man.

Vitamin K is synthesized by intestinal bacteria and obtained in the diet from green leafy vegetables. It is a fat-soluble vitamin that is absorbed from the GI tract and used as a coenzyme in hepatic production of prothrombin. Surgeons may unintentionally interfere with vitamin K formation by alteration of intestinal bacterial flora with nonabsorbable antibiotics. The coumarin drugs, warfarin (Coumadin) and Dicumarol, block hepatic synthesis of prothrombin. The action of these drugs is potentiated by phenylbutazone (Butazolidine), which is frequently used in treatment of superficial phlebitis, bursitis or muscular pain. Many other drugs increase or decrease the action of the coumarin drugs, so patients receiving these drugs should be cautioned to consult their physician before accepting any other medication. Prothrombin formation is also impaired in patients with a variety of biliary and hepatic diseases, including cirrhosis and common duct obstruction. Vitamin K may be replaced by oral (Synkayvite) or parenteral (Synkayvite, Aqua Mephyton, Konakion) therapy. In general, Aqua Mephyton (vitamin K_1 oxide) is preferred, because jaundice and nonicteric liver damage have been observed in infants treated with synthetic vitamin K (Synkayvite).

Fiber

Cummings and associates conducted a randomized prospective trial comparing purified dietary fiber obtained from various sources with respect to fecal weight and fecal transit time.[7] They observed that 20 gm per day of dietary bran produced a 127 per cent increase in fecal weight and proportional decrease in intestinal transit time. The changes in fecal weight and transit time were greater with bran as the source of dietary fiber than with any of the other sources tested. The change was related to the amount of pentose containing polysaccharides in the fiber, and thus was probably related to the water-holding capacity of the fiber. They noticed that 47 gm of an "average" English (35 per cent dietary fiber) bran would double the fecal weight. The change was proportional to the initial fecal weight. For purposes of comparison with a normal American diet, it should be noted that bran is most commonly available in the U.S. in breakfast cereals. Kellogg's "All Bran" contains 7.5 per cent non-nutritive fiber by weight, and 1 oz (1/4 cup) contains only 2 gm per serving. A 1–2 oz serving of All Bran, therefore, would not be expected to produce a major change in intestinal transit time or fecal weight, based on the studies of Cummings and associates. Nevertheless, a change in stool consistency is readily apparent when a bowl of bran cereal is added to the daily diet, and a substantial increase in dietary consumption of bran has occurred in the United States in recent years. Bran and other foods containing high dietary fiber have become more popular in the treatment of various colonic conditions such as diverticulosis and diverticulitis, in a complete reversal of the tendency two decades ago to prescribe a low dietary fiber content for such patients. Moderately large, relatively soft stools are produced by ingestion of only 1–2 oz of All Bran dry cereal per day, an intake of only 2–4 gm of bran — less than a teaspoon of pure bran. This is hardly more than a trace amount of this dietary constituent, representing less than 1 per cent by weight of the total food ingested per day, yet the effect on bowel habits is substantial.

Elemental Diets

For many patients, a low-residue, easily absorbed diet is desirable. These patients include individuals with a short or poorly functioning gastrointestinal tract, such as patients with enteric fistulas, enteritis, extensive small bowel resections for tumor, trauma or vascular occlusions, chronic pancreatitis, and various other malabsorption problems or enzyme deficiencies, as well as cancer of the head and neck. A variety of such chemically formulated, nutritionally complete diets, which need only to be absorbed, not digested, are now commercially available (Table 7–8). These diets are composed predominantly of L-amino acids, glucose and medium- and short-chain triglycerides and have varying amounts of specific additional vitamins and minerals. Collaborative support from a nutritionist is helpful in selecting the best product and the most palatable formulation for an individual patient.

Intravenous Therapy

A wide variety of replacement and supplemental solutions are commercially available and can be used in the Out-patient Clinic. Many institutions have reported cases of septicemia associated with the use of intravenous therapy. The solutions used should therefore be examined carefully to be certain that no sediment or particles are present, and questionable solutions should be cultured but not administered to patients. Meticulous aseptic technique should be used for venipunctures; plastic catheters should be used as a route for infusion only when necessary; and catheters and needles should be removed from the veins as soon as possible.

The components of intravenous solutions commonly used are outlined in Table 7–9. Additional information regarding intravenous fluids and blood substitutes can be obtained in the monographs by Shoemaker and Walker (1970)[29] and Gruber (1969).[12]

The selection of a site for intravenous infusion is dictated by the type of therapy to be used, by the urgency of the situation, and by the patient's anatomy. In general, we prefer to use peripheral

TABLE 7-8 Commercially Available Elemental Diet*

CONTENTS/ 1000 ML	VIVONEX HN®	VIVONEX®	FLEXICAL®	PRECISION LR®	ENSURE®	ISOCAL®	COMPLEAT B®	NUTRI-1000®	MERITENE®	SUSTACAL®
Grams										
Protein	45.6	20.4	19	23	37.1	32.5	38	37.8	55	60.3
Fat	0.9	1.4	34	0.77	37.1	42	40	52	33	23
CHO	202	226	154	240	144	125	120	100	115	137
Lactose	—	—	—	—	—	—	+	+	+	+
SOURCE										
Protein	L-amino acids	L-amino acids	Casein hydrolysate 3 amino acids	Egg albumin	Casein Soy	Casein Soy	Beef Milk	Skim milk	Nonfat milk	Milk Casein Soy
Fat	Safflower oil	Safflower oil	Soy oil MCT† oil	Vegetable oils	Corn oil	Soy oil MCT† oil	Corn oil Beef fat	Soy oil Coconut oil	Vegetable oils	Soy oil
mEq Na	33	37	15	36	31	22	68	22	40	39
mEq K	18	30	38	27	33	33	40	39	43	53
Trace Metals	+	+	+	+	+	+	—	—	—	—
Essential vitamins	+	+	—	—	+	+	—	—	—	—
M Osm/Liter	810	550	805	600	460	350	468	500	560	625

*From Meguid, M. M.: The enteral alternative. Contemp. Surg., *13:*41–52, 1978.
†MCT = Medium-chain triglyceride.

veins of the upper extremity for slow, elective infusions. The vein can thereby be watched closely for evidence of extravasation, phlebitis or infection, and the patient can assist with these observations.

A series of so-called "scalp vein" needles will take care of most of the needs for intravenous infusions in surgical outpatients. Phlebitis and infection do not appear to be as common or rapid in onset when needles are used as when plastic intravenous catheters are employed. A 19 gauge scalp vein needle in a hand or forearm vein is an excellent route for blood, plasma or isotonic glucose and electrolyte solutions. The internal bore of this needle is as large as a standard 18 gauge needle. The short length of a scalp vein needle actually allows flow to occur more rapidly than occurs through standard 1½ inch long needles, and much more rapidly than with plastic catheters, which are usually 3 to 36 inches long! The differential rate of flow is most apparent when viscous solutions such as packed red cells are being infused. When solutions run slowly because of spasm of peripheral veins, intravenous injection of 0.5–1.0 ml of 1 per cent procaine or lidocaine through the tubing will often speed things up nicely, and simultaneously relieve the patient's discomfort.

Intravenous catheters must occasionally be used, because a secure route is necessary if percutaneous venipuncture attempts have failed. When venous cannulation of this type is necessary, as short a catheter as possible is preferred, to avoid unnecessary trauma to the vein and to reduce the impediment to flow which is caused by long tubing. A medium (16) or large (14) gauge catheter is usually used, preferably of the needle-through-catheter type (Rochester, Buffalo, Angiocath, E-Z Cath, among others) instead of a catheter-through-needle (e.g., Intracath), to avoid the risk of shearing off the catheter with the needle. A silastic catheter is theoretically preferred, but it is difficult to advance this type of catheter very far in most peripheral veins, and silastic catheters have a tendency to kink or be cut easily. A polyethylene catheter is therefore usually best for most patients.

If a cutdown is needed on an elective basis, the basilic vein at the antecubital fossa is usually used, as shown in Hill.[16] For administration of hypertonic solutions, or in emergency placement of intravenous catheters, superior vena cava cannulation by the subclavian approach is usually more appropriate (see technique in Chapter 4).

ENDOCRINOLOGY

Endocrinology is the science of hormones — chemicals that are produced in the body, circulate through the blood stream and produce effects elsewhere in target organs. Hormones are produced in specific endocrine glands, in other organs and tissues and in some tumors. The surgeon is particularly interested in tumors of the endocrine glands, for these are frequently benign and are curable when operated upon early enough. The surgeon must be aware of the nature of hormones normally produced throughout the body and of the deficiency states that exist in the absence of these hormones. The hormones produced by malignant tumors of endocrine and nonendocrine tissues frequently present serious problems, since the patients may be in more distress from the effects of the hormones than from the tumors themselves.

The apudomas are a family of endocrine tumors that arise from APUD cells (amine, precursor uptake, decarboxylase), having common cytochemical characteristics and common embryological origins from the neuroectodermal cells of the neural crest (Tables 7–10 through 7–12).

It is not easy to recognize excess hormone production in its early stages. Many wise physicians have missed the early stages of conditions such as thyrotoxicosis, Cushing's syndrome, insulin-secreting adenomas of the pancreas, and hyperparathyroidism — all of which are obvious to medical students when in florid state. Yet each of these diseases and many others can be cured by surgery. It is therefore important to consider endocrine disorders in the differential diagnosis of a variety of seemingly routine complaints. Examples include changes in complexion, fatigue, headache, dizziness, weight gain, weight loss and so on. Since most of these complaints are screened initially by internists, surgeons are frequently spared the embarrassment of having erred in the initial assessment. But surgeons may be the first to have the opportunity to make the diagnosis of an endocrine disorder. Examples of several endocrine lesions in which the primary presentation has been a surgical problem are shown in Table 7–13.

It is wise to obtain prompt consultation with a competent internist or endocrinologist for each patient in whom an endocrine disorder is strongly suspected, whether it is excessive or insufficient hormone production.

Ectopic or Inappropriate Hormone Production by Tumors

Since many patients with cancer come to the Emergency Room with a variety of signs and symptoms, and since a variety of tumors have been uncovered which are hormone secreting, the following list to facilitate diagnosis has been prepared in conjunction with Dr. Merle A. Legg of the New England Deaconess Hospital, Department of Pathology.

ACTH
Lung carcinoma (small cell undifferentiated)
Pancreatic carcinoma (islet cell, almost exclusively)
Thymic carcinoid tumor
Carcinoid
Medullary carcinoma of thyroid

Pheochromocytoma
Ganglioneuroma
Neuroblastoma
Paraganglioma
Esophageal carcinoma
Hepatoma
Prostatic carcinoma
Parotid carcinoma
Parathyroid adenoma
ADH
Lung carcinoma (small cell undifferentiated)
Islet cell tumor
Pancreatic carcinoma
Duodenal carcinoma
Hodgkin's disease
Thymoma
Erythropoietin
Renal cell carcinoma (not inappropriate)
Cerebellar hemangioblastoma
Hepatoma
Leiomyoma of uterus
Pheochromocytoma
Gonadotropin
Hepatoblastoma
? Lung carcinoma, large cell and squamous
Growth Hormone
? Lung carcinoma
Hypoglycemia
(Hepatoma and adrenal cortical carcinoma — different mechanism)
Fibrosarcoma or spindle cell sarcoma
Mesothelioma
Fibroma
Rhabdomyofibroma
Liposarcoma
Leiomyosarcoma
Hemangiopericytoma
Pseudomyxoma peritonei
Reticulum cell sarcoma
Dermatofibrosarcoma
Cecal adenocarcinoma
Gastric adenocarcinoma
MSH
Lung carcinoma (small cell undifferentiated)
Islet cell carcinoma
Parathyroid Hormones
Renal cell and renal pelvic carcinoma
Lung carcinoma (mostly squamous cell)

Text continued on page 249.

TABLE 7-9 Composition of Intravenous Solutions*

INTRAVENOUS SOLUTION	GLUCOSE GM/100 ML	COMPOSITION					MILLIOSMOLS PER LITER	pH	COMMENT
		Na	K	Cl mEq/L	Ca	Lactate			
5% Dextrose injection U.S.P.	5	0	0	0	0	0		4.0	isotonic
10% Dextrose injection, U.S.P.	10	0	0	0	0	0		4.0	hypertonic
20% Dextrose injection, U.S.P.	20	0	0	0	0	0		4.0	hypertonic
50% Dextrose injection, U.S.P.	50	0	0	0	0	0	2532	4.0	hypertonic
5% Dextrose and 0.2% NaCl injection, U.S.P.	5	34	0	34	0	0		4.0	hypertonic
5% Dextrose and 0.45% NaCl injection, U.S.P.	5	77	0	77	0	0		4.0	hypertonic
5% Dextrose and 0.9% NaCl injection, U.S.P.	5	154	0	154	0	0		4.0	hypertonic
Lactated Ringer's (Hartman's) solution with 5% dextrose	5	130	4	109	3	28		5.0	hypertonic
Lactated Ringer's injection, U.S.P.	0	130	4	109	3	28		6.5	slightly hypotonic
Ringer's injection, U.S.P.	0	147.5	4	156	4.5	0		5.5	isotonic
Sodium chloride injection, U.S.P.	0	154	0	154	0	0	308	5.7	isotonic
0.45% Sodium chloride in water (1/2 normal saline)	0	77	0	77	0	0	154	5.5	hypotonic
3% Sodium chloride, U.S.P.	0	513	0	513	0	0	1026	5.0	hypertonic
5% Sodium chloride, U.S.P.	0	855	0	855	0	0	1711	5.6	hypertonic, pH adjusted with HCl, 1 mEq/L

Solution								pH	
Sodium lactate injection, U.S.P. (M/6 sodium lactate)	0	167	0	0	0	167		6.0	slightly hypertonic
5% alcohol, 5% dextrose	5.0	0	0	0	0	0		4.5	5.0 ml absolute ethyl alcohol per 100 ml
6% Dextran 75 in 0.9% sodium chloride solution	0	154	0	154	0	0	308	5.0	hypertonic Dextran mol. wt. 75,000, similar to colloid effect of albumin
10% Dextran 40 in 0.9% sodium chloride	0	154	0	154	0	0		5.0	hypertonic Dextran mol. wt. 40,000
10% Dextran 40 in dextrose	5	0	0	0	0	0		5.0	hypertonic
5% Sodium bicarbonate in water	0	595	0	0	0	0		7.5	HCO_3^- 595 mEq/L
Intralipid 10% 10% soybean oil, 1.2% egg yolk phospholipids, 2.5% glycerin and water for injection, and linoleic acid (54%), oleic (26%), palmitic (9%), linolenic (8%)							208		
5.5% Travasol (amino acid) injection	0	70	60	70	0	0		6.0	5.5 gm L-amino acids, 924 mg N, Mg 10 mEq/L, acetate 100 mEq/L, phosphate 60 mEq/L, hypertonic
8.5% Travasol (amino acid) injection	0	70	60	70	0	0		6.0	8.5 gm L-amino acids 1.42 gm N, Mg 10 mEq/L, acetate 135 mEq/L, phosphate 60 mEq/L, hypertonic

*Adapted in part from Brochure F23-50-11-74 of Travenol Laboratories, Deerfield, IL, 60015.

TABLE 7–10 Centrally Located APUD Cells, Their Products and Their Associated Apudomas and Clinical Syndromes[*]

| ORGANS | CELLS | PRODUCTS | | | APUDOMAS | ORTHOENDOCRINE SYNDROMES |
		POLYPEPTIDES	AMINES			
Hypothalamus	Neurones	Releasing and inhibiting hormones	Dopamine, Nor-epinephrine and 5-HT		?	?
Posterior pituitary	Neurones	ADH	—		?	?
		Oxytocin	—		?	?
Anterior pituitary	c	ACTH	? Tryptamine		Hyperplasia	Cushing's
	m	MSH	? Tryptamine		Adenoma	Pigmentation
	s	GH	—		Carcinoma	Acromegaly or gigantism
	l	Prolactin	—			Forbes-Albright
Pineal body	P	Melatonin	5-HT		Pinealoma	Hypogonadism

[*]Welbourn, R. B.: Current status of the apudomas. Ann. Surg., *185*:1–12, 1977.
Abbreviations: APUD = Amine, precursor uptake, decarboxylase; ACTH = (Adreno)corticotrophin; ADH = Antidiuretic hormone; GH = Growth hormone; 5-HT = 5-hydroxytryptamine; MSH = Melanocyte-stimulating hormone.

TABLE 7-11 Generally Distributed APUD Cells, Their Products and Their Associated Apudomas and Clinical Syndromes*

| ORGANS | CELLS | PRODUCTS | | APUDOMAS | ORTHO-ENDOCRINE SYNDROMES | PRINCIPAL PARAENDOCRINE SYNDROMES (AND HORMONES) |
		POLYPEPTIDES	AMINES			
Thyroid	C	Calcitonin	? 5-HT	Medullary carcinoma	Hypercalcitoninemia	Cushing's (ACTH)
Adrenal medulla	E	?	Epinephrine	Pheochromocytoma	Hypertension, etc.	Cushing's (ACTH) WDHA (VIP)
	NE	?	Norepinephrine	Ganglioneuroblastoma		
Carotid body	Type 1 (Glomus)	?	Catecholamines and 5-HT	Chemodectoma	Hypertension, etc.	?
Lungs	P (Feyrter)	? VLP	?	? Oat cell carcinoma	?	Cushing's, etc. (ACTH, MSH, 5-HT) Schwartz-Bartter (ADH)
	EC	?	? 5-HT / ? 5-HTP	Carcinoid	Atypical carcinoid	Cushing's (ACTH, 5-HT)
Urinary tract	U	? Urogastrone	?	?	?	?
	EC	?	? 5-HT	?	?	?
Skin	Melanocyte	?	?	Melanoma	?	Cushing's (ACTH)

*Welbourn, R. B.: Current status of the apudomas. Ann. Surg., *185*:1-12, 1977.
Abbreviations: 5-HTP = 5-hydroxytryptophan; VIP = Vasoactive intestinal polypeptide; VLP = Vasoactive lung peptide; others as in Table 10.

TABLE 7–12 APUD Cells of the Alimentary Tract, Their Products and Their Associated Apudomas and Clinical Syndromes*

ORGANS	CELLS	PRODUCTS		APUDOMAS	ORTHO-ENDOCRINE SYNDROMES	PRINCIPAL PARAENDOCRINE SYNDROMES (AND HORMONES)
		POLYPEPTIDES	AMINES			
Salivary glands	?	? Urogastrone	—	?	?	?
Stomach	G	Gastrin	—	Hyperplasia, carcinoma	Zollinger-Ellison	?
	D	Somatostatin	—	?	?	?
	EC	? Substance P	5-HT, ? 5-HTP	Carcinoid	Atypical carcinoid	?
Pancreas: islets	B (β)	Insulin	—	Hyperplasia	Hypoglycemia Diabetes, dermatitis, etc.	Zollinger-Ellison (gastrin) Cushing's (ACTH) WDHA (VIP) ? Malignant carcinoid (5-HT)
	A (α)	Glucagon	—	Adenoma		
	D (δ,α_1)	Somatostatin[10]	—	Carcinoma	?	?

inter-acinar cells	D_1	Pancreatic polypeptide	—	? Ditto	?	?
	EC	?	5-HT, ? 5-HTP	Carcinoid	Malignant carcinoid	?
Duodenum and small intestine	S	Secretin	—	?	?	?
	EC	Motilin, ? Substance P	5-HT	Carcinoid	Malignant carcinoid	Cushing's (ACTH)
	I	CCK	—	?	?	?
	K	GIP	—	?	?	?
	?	Gastrin	?	Adenoma or carcinoma	Zollinger-Ellison	?
	D	Somatostatin	—	?	?	?
	? H	VIP	—	?	?	?
Large intestine	? H	VIP	—	?	?	?
	EG	Enteroglucagon	—	?	?	?

*Welbourn, R. B.: Current status of the apudomas. Ann. Surg., *185*:1–12, 1977.
Abbreviations: CCK = Cholecystokinin-pancreozymin; GIP = Gastric inhibitory polypeptide; others as in Tables 7–10 and 7–11.

TABLE 7–13   Surgical Presentations of Endocrinopathies

Initial Presentations	Endocrine Lesions
Peptic ulcer Renal calculi Pancreatitis Kidney transplant recipient	Hyperparathyroidism
Mass in neck Excessive weight loss	Hyperthyroidism
Mass in neck	Calcitonin-secreting thyroid cancer
Orthopedic problems related to excessive bone growth	Pituitary eosinophilic adenoma
Urinary frequency from dysfunction of posterior pituitary and decreased release of ADH	Pituitary chromophobe adenoma
Compression fracture of spine Peptic ulcer Atrophy of skeletal muscle	Cushing's syndrome (adrenal hyperfunction or pituitary basophile adenoma)
Peptic ulcer, virulent (gastrin-secreting adenoma—the Zollinger-Ellison syndrome) Seizures (from hypoglycemia in insulin-secreting adenoma) Coma (insulin- or glucagon-secreting adenoma)	Pancreatic islet cell adenoma
Intestinal obstruction Gastrointestinal bleeding Abdominal mass, with or without abdominal pain	Carcinoid
Amenorrhea Sterility in females Clitoral hypertrophy	Androgen hypersecretion (adrenal or ovarian tumors; adrenal-genital syndrome; Stein-Leventhal ovaries)
Abdominal mass (males or females) Gynecomastia and nipple discharge (males or females) Question of pregnancy (females) Testicular mass (males)	Female gonadotrophin hypersecretion (choriocarcinoma of trophoblast or testis)
Cough, palpable lymph nodes, chest pain or abnormal chest x-ray	Antidiuretic hormone hypersecretion (oat cell carcinoma of lung)
Hypertension or fever in patients with neurofibromatosis or medullary carcinoma of thyroid	Pheochromocytoma

Ovarian adenocarcinoma and papillary
  adenocarcinoma
Pancreatic adenocarcinoma
Vulvar carcinoma
Leiomyosarcoma of uterus
Penile carcinoma
Lymphosarcoma
Bladder carcinoma
Colonic adenocarcinoma
Esophageal carcinoma
Hodgkin's disease
Bile duct adenocarcinoma
Hepatoma
Hemangiosarcoma
Gingival carcinoma
Mycosis fungoides
  Serotonin (not really inappropriate)
Gastrointestinal carcinoid
Bronchial carcinoid
Lung carcinoma, small cell undifferentiated
Thymic carcinoid tumor
Islet carcinoid
  TSH or LATS
Choriocarcinoma and hydatidiform
  mole (not really inappropriate)
? Embryonal carcinoma of testis
? Lung carcinoma, squamous cell

Pituitary

Chromophobe adenomas are the most frequent pituitary tumors, representing two thirds of the neoplasms of that gland. They usually do not cause excessive secretion of pituitary hormones. Enlargement of the sella turcica produces compression of the optic chiasm, bitemporal hemianopsia and headaches. Compression of the posterior pituitary lobe causes reduction in secretion of ADH and diabetes insipidus, which is manifested by increased urinary frequency and thirst. *Eosinophile adenomas* represent about one-third of anterior pituitary tumors. They secrete growth hormone, causing gigantism if they arise in childhood and acromegaly if they arise in adults. Enlargement of the sella occurs, though not as disproportionate to the size of the skull as is seen in chromophobe aden-

omas. *Basophile adenomas* represent only 1 to 2 per cent of pituitary tumors. They secrete ACTH and cause Cushing's syndrome. Most patients with Cushing's syndrome can be successfully treated with adrenalectomy, but up to one-fifth of these patients will later require pituitary irradiation or hypophysectomy.[11] Basophile adenoma should be particularly suspected in adrenalectomized patients who develop hyperpigmentation of the skin in spite of adequate steroid replacement therapy. Since these adenomas are slow growing and do not cause enlargement of the sella, they are difficult to detect except at surgery or at autopsy.

Tests of pituitary function that may be performed with accuracy in outpatients include:

(1) Urinary volume, concentrating power and 24-hour excretion of 17-ketosteroids and 17-hydroxycorticosteroids. All specimens should be checked for accuracy of collection by performance of creatinine excretion, which remains relatively constant. Concentrating power is assessed by measuring specific gravity on the first voided specimens in the morning, following deprivation of water overnight.

(2) ACTH and growth hormone bioassay.

(3) ACTH test. Four-, 6- or 8-hour infusion of 25–40 units of ACTH intravenously, with 24-hour collection for steroids the day before, during and after the day of ACTH infusion. Plasma cortisols can be obtained before and at the end of infusion and on the following day.

(4) Metopirone (metyrapone)· test. This drug blocks 11–beta hydroxylation of corticosteroids in the adrenal gland, and thereby leads to increased secretion of ACTH by normal individuals. The response in a patient with normal pituitary and adrenal glands is an increase in production of urinary metabolites measured as 17–ketosteroids and 17–hydroxycorticosteroids.

(5) Lateral skull x-ray with measurement of size of the sella turcica.

Radioimmunoassay techniques and other new methods have revealed a complex array of hypothalamic hormones that act as releasing or inhibiting agents for pituitary hormones. These new discoveries will undoubtedly provide a greater spectrum of therapeutic possibilities for the endocrine surgeon in the next decade.

Another interesting, newly discovered class of pituitary hormones is called "endorphins" (endogenous morphine-like substances). These polypeptide hormones appear to have pain-relieving capabilities and seizure-reducing activity, at least in the lower animals.

Thyroid

Hyperthyroidism does not commonly produce symptoms that bring the patient initially to a surgeon. If a surgeon suspects hyperthyroidism in a patient whom he is evaluating for some other reason, he should arrange for a full evaluation by an endocrinologist.

Thyrotoxicosis usually is the result of diffuse thyroid hyperplasia. Thyrotoxicosis from an adenoma is unusual, though "hot" nodules are occasionally seen on scan.

The usual initial therapy for most patients with hyperthyroidism is nonsurgical — destruction of the gland with ^{131}I or ^{125}I or reduction in circulating thyroxine levels with propylthiouracil. Surgery is usually reserved for those who do not accept propylthiouracil well (because of failure to take the drug or untoward side effects from the therapy), and in those who should not receive a therapeutic dose of radioactive iodine (such as prepubertal children and women in the child-bearing age group). Occasionally, patients are referred for surgery who cannot be controlled with medical therapy. These patients represent the group at highest risk from surgery. In general, however, most patients with thyrotoxicosis can be rendered euthyroid prior to surgery.

Final preparation for thyroid surgery is best performed by seven to ten days in the hospital, where the patient can be kept quiet, with sequential observations of pulse, weight, temperature and caloric intake. If desired, much of the preparation can be performed on an outpatient basis, however. The patient should receive his usual doses of propylthiouracil (approximately 50–100 mg/day), plus Lugol's solution, 30 drops per day in divided doses. The iodine and iodide in Lugol's solution reduce vascularity of the hyperactive gland. Exophthalmos is rarely benefited by thyroidectomy and usually becomes worse postoperatively. Every effort should therefore be made to treat exophthalmic goiter medically, including possible use of immunosuppressive agents to reduce secretion of the gamma globulin (long-acting thyroid stimulating hormone — LATS) recently incriminated in hyperthyroidism.

Colloid goiter in euthyroid patients is usually operated upon for cosmetic reasons or to rule out the presence of cancer. This disease is more common in geographical regions in which the diet is deficient in iodine. Since a goiter may extend posterior to the sternum, a chest x-ray must be obtained preoperatively.

The best management of a thyroid nodule is still debated between internists and surgeons. It has been reported that well-differentiated papillary or follicular carcinoma can be suppressed with high doses (180 mg or more) of thyroid hormone per day. Nevertheless, we believe that surgical treatment is preferable. A percutaneous Vim-Silverman needle biopsy can be performed in the Outpatient Clinic, with convalescence overnight in the observation ward. If the nodule is superficial and easily biopsied, report of an adenoma probably justifies medical therapy. But if carcinoma is found, surgery is indicated. We have seen two patients in recent years who had massive, slowly growing local recurrences of papillary carcinoma of the thyroid that were eventually fatal. The type of operation performed will vary with the gross and microscopic findings at exploration. For biopsy-proven follicular or papillary carcinoma, total lobectomy of the involved lobe and subtotal lobectomy of the contralateral lobe appear to be indicated. A careful neck exploration should be performed for metastases, and a modified neck dissection should be done if tumor is found in the nodes. In less well-differentiated tumors, a larger margin of surgical excision is necessary for success, although in undifferentiated cancer of the thyroid the results of excision are no better than are achieved by tracheostomy and radiation therapy. Medullary carcinoma, a functioning tumor of the thyroid "C" cells, may occur by itself or in familial diseases associated with pheochromocytoma (Sipple's syndrome) and other endocrine tumors.[32]

Patients may develop postoperative hypoparathyroidism of a significant degree, but it may be missed if it develops slowly. Chronic, severe hypoparathyroidism has been reported in a large percentage of patients following thyroidectomy for a variety of reasons. In such patients, mental sluggishness, constipation or premature aging should be signs that warrant obtaining serum calcium and urinary calcium determination.

Hypothyroidism should be recognized and treated prior to performance of elective surgery for other diseases. Since the signs may be subtle, it should be remembered that hypothyroidism is a common late complication of ^{131}I treatment for thyrotoxicosis, or of hypophysectomy — if the patient does not take thyroid hormone. Thickened tongue, mental sluggishness, viscid peripheral edema and heart disease should alert the surgeon to study his patient and to arrange for proper therapy to be given.

Tests of thyroid function in outpatients include:

(1) Basal metabolism. Used with decreasing frequency in recent years because of the relative ease and greater accuracy of other tests.

(2) Plasma bound iodine (PBI). This test is invalid in patients who have received iodine in any form in recent weeks, including ^{131}I, iodine surgical skin prep or iodine-containing radiopaque dyes, as in IVP or gallbladder x-rays.

(3) [131]I uptake in neck. The normal value is 30 per cent in 24 hours. Abnormal values range from greater than 40 per cent in hyperthyroidism to less than 10 per cent in hypothyroidism.

(4) [131]I scan (searching for differentiation between "hot" and "cold" areas in the gland and outside the gland — in which case metastatic cancer of the thyroid is suspected).

(5) Red cell T^3 and T^4 uptake.

(6) Chest x-ray: looking for metastases, substernal thyroid, or evidence of heart disease secondary to hyper- or hypothyroidism.

(7) Lateral x-ray of trachea.

(8) Barium swallow with view of larynx and trachea.

Parathyroid

Diagnosis of hyperparathyroidism has been made earlier in the course of the disease in recent years. It is now rare for patients to present with hypercalcemic crisis or terminal multisystem disease resulting from longstanding hyperparathyroidism. Consistent elevation of serum calcium is a sufficient indication for parathyroid exploration if other causes have been ruled out. Other causes include sarcoidosis, metastatic cancer, chronic renal disease, vitamin D intoxication, multiple myeloma, hyperthyroidism and milk-alkali syndrome. Obviously, a thorough general medical and endocrinological work-up should be done before parathyroid exploration is carried out. The surgeon should review the information and ask for confirmatory tests in questionable cases and for tests that will help localize the lesions if they are available. The most common of these additional tests are barium swallow (looking for impingement by a posteriorly situated adenoma), selective percutaneous thyrocervical arteriography and selective venous sampling for parathyroid hormone levels (probably the best technique now available for localization of an adenoma).

Tests that may be used in outpatients are:

(1) Serum calcium, repeated until at least three elevated values are obtained.

(2) Serum phosphorus (should be low; if both Ca and P are elevated, hyperparathyroidism due to adenoma is less likely than if P is subnormal).

(3) Serum parathyroid hormone.

(4) Serum alkaline phosphatase.

(5) Urinary calcium (24-hour excretion, while on 200 mg calcium diet). Excretion of more than 200 mg per day indicates an increased rate of turnover of calcium and is consistent with hyperparathyroidism. Excretion of more than 200 mg per day also will occur in other types of hypercalcemia, such as metastatic cancer and multiple myeloma.

(6) Barium swallow (look for indentation by adenoma).

(7) Chest x-ray (to rule out sarcoidosis and metastatic carcinoma).

(8) BUN and creatinine. If these values are elevated, consider the possibility of parathyroid hyperplasia due to chronic renal disease, rather than adenoma. But renal failure can also develop in long-standing hyperparathyroidism, owing to recurrent formation of calculi.

(9) Selective thyrocervical arteriography.

(10) X-rays of bones: long bones, hands and teeth. Look for cysts, fractures, reabsorption ("motheaten" bones), or absent lamina dura.

Hyperparathyroidism may be due to any of several pathological conditions. Parathyroid adenomas were formerly found as the cause in up to 80 per cent of patients, with hyperplasia occurring in most of the remainder. Parathyroid carcinoma ranges from 1 to 4 per cent in various hospitals. Hyperplasia is now found increasingly in hospitals that manage chronic renal failure and have a large number of renal transplant recipients. Of adenomas, three-fourths are tumors of chief cells (eosinophilic), and approximately half of the rest are water-clear cells. Adenomas may be multiple or recurrent, and patients must be followed permanently following parathyroidectomy for signs or symptoms of either recurrent hyperparathyroidism or other endocrine adenomas.

Pancreas

Abnormalities in carbohydrate metabolism may be dramatic in patients with hormone-secreting tumors of the pancreas. Most of these patients are seen initially by internists, psychiatrists or endocrinologists, and are referred to surgeons only after a long work-up has been performed. Since hyperactivity of normal islets may be difficult to distinguish from adenoma, patients are often remarkably late in undergoing laparotomy. It should be remembered that patients with β-cell (insulin-secreting) adenomas do not necessarily exhibit Whipple's triad. In Tompkins' series[33] of ten insulin-secreting adenomas, three did not have the classic pattern of (1) blood sugar less than 50 mg/100 ml, (2) with symptoms at the time of documented hypoglycemia and (3) relief of symptoms by administration of glucose. The accuracy and safety of selective celiac arteriography has increased remarkably in past years, and patients with a question of adenoma should undergo this study. Alpha cell glucagon-secreting adenomas are very rare, but can also be localized by arteriography. Patients with the Zollinger-Ellison syndrome (δ-cell adenoma) are usually seen early by surgeons because of the severity of their ulcer diathesis. If possible, patients suspected of this diagnosis should also undergo arteriography, although occasionally the complication of gastrointestinal perforation or hemorrhage requires emergency surgery. Most of the procedures for study of small functioning pancreatic tumors require inpatient care. However, arteriography can easily and safely be performed in outpatients if a period of close observation follows the procedure.

The tests that can be performed on outpatients include:

(1) Fasting blood sugar.
(2) Glucose tolerance test, with careful observation for reactive hypoglycemia. If symptoms of hypoglycemia develop, a blood sugar should be drawn immediately for documentation.
(3) Serum insulin (immunoreactive insulin or — less satisfactory — insulin-like activity).
(4) GI series, with small bowel follow through, looking for indentation into barium column, widened C-loop of duodenum, peptic ulcer or anterior displacement of duodenum.
(5) Selective celiac arteriography, with venous phase also studied for "tumor blush" in pancreas or liver, or displacement of arteries around a tumor nodule.
(6) Serum gastrin immunoassay.
(7) Retroperitoneal CT scan.

Adrenal

Functioning adrenal cortical tumors may produce Cushing's syndrome (glucocorticoids) or Conn's syndrome (al-dosterone). Adrenal medullary tumors — pheochromocytomas — secrete epinephrine and other catecholamines, causing episodic hypertension and fever. Pheochromocytomas can also occur in other areas of the body, especially in the retroperitoneum at the bifurcation of the aorta —the organ of Zuckerkandl. Arteriography is therefore an important part of their work-up. Patients with adrenal tumors are almost invariably referred to surgeons after a prolonged medical work-up, which usually involves a period of hospitalization for study.[20] If the possibility of one of these lesions arises in a surgical outpatient, a simple series of tests may be utilized for screening purposes. Most patients admitted for surgery will already have undergone these tests:

(1) Fasting blood sugar (elevated by epinephrine and corticosteroids).
(2) Urinary excretion of ketosteroids and ketogenic steroids (24-hour collections, with volume and creatinine recorded).
(3) Plasma cortisol.
(4) ACTH test (see Pituitary Gland).
(5) Decadron suppression; effect of 4–12 mg per day of decadron on steroid excretion. If ACTH-induced hyperplasia is present, steroid output will decrease to normal during decadron administration. If adenoma is present, output will usually decrease somewhat. Functioning adrenal cortical carcinoma usually does not alter output when decadron is given.
(6) Metopirone test to determine the effectiveness of adrenal-pituitary homeostatic balance. (See Pituitary Gland.)
(7) Glucose tolerance test.
(8) Serum Na and K. Sodium is variable and potassium is low in Cushing's syndrome; potassium is especially low in Conn's syndrome. The effect of adrenal steroids can also be seen in urine: sodium is retained and potassium is excreted in higher than normal amounts.
(9) Blood pressure (elevated in Cush-

ing's syndrome and pheochromocytoma).

(10) Urinary catecholamine and VMA
excretion for suspected adrenal
medullary tumor. False positive
is seen when bananas are present
in diet.

(11) Selective distal aortography and
adrenal arteriography and venography.

(12) Retroperitoneal CT scan.

The outpatient surgeon must be alert
to the possibility of a crisis of insufficient adrenal hormone production associated with any surgical procedure in
patients who have received therapy
with cortisone or its derivatives, in patients with tuberculosis or metastatic
cancer[15] and in patients treated with
Rauwolfia derivatives, which deplete
nerve ending granules of catecholamines.

Carcinoid

Patients with the carcinoid syndrome
exhibit, to a varying degree, one or
more of the following signs and symptoms: (1) cutaneous flushing —constant
or intermittent, (2) diarrhea, (3) dyspnea, with or without asthma, (4) palpita-
tions and cardiac arrythmias, (5) neurosis or psychosis, (6) fluid retention, (7)
abdominal mass and (8) abdominal
pain. Functioning carcinoid tumors
occur mainly in the midgut (ileum, appendix and cecum). They usually secrete serotonin, and occasionally other
hormones such as bradykinin, ACTH
and insulin. The diagnosis of a functioning carcinoid tumor is confirmed by
an elevated level of urinary 5-hydroxy
indole acetic acid (5 HIAA). The normal excretion of 5 HIAA is $\leq$ 16 mg per
day. Most patients with functioning
carcinoids will excrete amounts larger
than this — up to 1000 mg or more per
day in some cases. Occasionally 5
HIAA excretion is only slightly increased, 5 hydroxytryptophane being
the metabolite excreted by the tumor.
Not all patients with carcinoid tumors

develop the carcinoid syndrome, since
some carcinoids do not produce hormones. Serotonin is detoxified in the
liver, so hepatic or pulmonary metastases are usually present in patients
who have the syndrome. A rare exception to this rule exists with primary or
metastatic carcinoids of the ovary,
which can produce the syndrome because venous drainage of the ovary bypasses the liver. Carcinoids are slow-
growing tumors and usually metastasize late in the natural history of the
disease. Most patients are cured by resection of the primary tumor. The most
common site is the appendix; bronchial
adenomas of the carcinoid type are
usually cured by lobectomy or a sleeve
resection of the bronchus. Palliative resection of tumor metastases has been
performed in some patients with carcinoid syndrome, and cardiac surgery
has also been performed in cases where
the myxofibrous reaction produced pul-
monic stenosis. Usually the treatment
is pharmacological, using serotonin antagonists, cytotoxic agents or palliative
drugs.[17] Hepatic artery infusion with
5-fluorouracil should be considered in
patients who do not respond to systemic therapy.

Ovary and Placenta

The outpatient evaluation and treatment of lesions of the female organs is
discussed in detail in Chapter 20. The
endocrinological problems considered
are predominantly related to sterility,
amenorrhea and neoplasms. The studies that can conveniently and accurately be performed in outpatients to assess
function in the pituitary-ovary-placenta
relationships are:

(1) Pregnancy tests — qualitative.
    a. A-Z test.
    b. Gravidex test.
(2) Chorionic gonadotrophin (24-hour
    urine) — quantitative. If positive
    postpartum, choriocarcinoma must
    be ruled out.
(3) Vaginal cytology for per cent cornifi-

cation. Squamous cells denote estrogen effect. A routine pap smear is performed, and the differential count is made on this specimen: cornified cells, precornified cells and basal cells.

(4) Daily temperature record for estimation of date of ovulation.

(5) Vaginal mucous test for estimation of date of ovulation.

(6) Urinary ketosteroids and ketogenic steroids, to rule out adrenal tumor in patients with presumed polycystic (Stein-Leventhal) ovaries.

Testis

Tumors and questions of fertility are the major endocrinologic aspects evaluated regarding the testicles in outpatients. The diseases and studies are also discussed in Chapter 19. In summary, the studies appropriate in outpatients are:

(1) Semen analysis (for volume of semen, sperm count — done in a hemocytometer — sperm morphology on a stained, dry specimen, and sperm motility).

(2) Chorionic gonadotrophin — urinary. Should be performed in all males with gynecomastia. Unless an obvious, treatable cause is found for gynecomastia, a nonpalpable choriocarcinoma of the testis must be ruled out. Choriocarcinoma of testis may cause unilateral or bilateral gynecomastia. Other neoplasms, such as seminomas, teratomas and embryonal cancers of the testis may also secrete hormone and give positive CGT tests.

(3) Urinary ketosteroids and ketogenic steroids. Normal male production of ketosteroids is 10–20 mg per day.

(4) Buccal smear. Testicular atrophy is one sign of Kleinfelter's syndrome, which is due to the XXY chromosome abnormality. These patients have a buccal smear that shows Barr bodies (female chromatin pattern).

(5) Testicular biopsy. This test can be performed under local anesthesia with proper sedation in the operating room associated with the Emergency Room or in the main operating room. The patient can be released from the hospital later in the day.

Summary

Although definitive proof of an endocrinopathy usually requires hospitalization for completion of studies, endocrine diseases are usually first suspected in ambulatory patients. The proper screening tests must be obtained to determine if further studies are warranted. An alert surgeon is sure to have his curiosity rewarded by the occasional discovery of patients with thyrotoxicosis, hyperparathyroidism, Cushing's syndrome, the Stein-Leventhal syndrome, or other endocrine diseases. If the disease is discovered while it is still localized and curable, this diligence should permit restoration of the patient to a normal life.

REFERENCES

1. Beerel, F. R. and Vance, J. W.: A simplified method for presenting acid-base balance situations. Chest, 57: 480–484, 1970.

2. Berman, I. R., Moseley, R. V., Doty, D. B. and Gutierrez, V. S.: Post-traumatic alkalosis in young men with combat injuries. Surg. Gynecol. Obstet., 133:11–15, 1971.

3. Blackburn, G. L., Bistrian, B. R., Maini, B. S., Benotti, P., Bothe, A., Gibbons, G. and Smith, M. F.: Manual for nutritional/metabolic assessment of the hospitalized patient. 62nd Ann. Clin. Cong., ACS, Chicago, October 11–15, 1976.

4. Buchwald, H., Frantz, I. D., Jr. and Gebhard, R. L.: Effect of ileal bypass versus ileal excision on cholesterol synthesis and whole blood cholesterol concentration in the rabbit. Surgery, 64:126–133, 1968.

5. Comroe, J. H., et al.: The Lung: Clinical Physiology and Pulmonary Function Tests, 2nd ed. Chicago, Year Book Medical Publishers, Inc., 1962.

6. Cooper, K. H.: The New Aerobics. New York, Bantam Books, 1972.

7. Cummings, J. H., Southgate, D. A. T.,

Branch, W., Houston, H., Jenkins, J. D. A. and James, W. P. T.: Colonic response to dietary fiber from carrot, cabbage, apple, bran, guar gum. Lancet, *1*:5–8, 1978.

8. Dudrick, S. J., Wilmore, D. W., Vars, H. M. and Rhoads, J. E.: Long-term total parenteral nutrition with growth, development and positive nitrogen balance. Surgery, *64*:134–141, 1968.

9. Fitzpatrick, G.: Body composition: water, cells and salts; Surg. Biol. Seminars, U. Mass. Med. School, November 1976.

10. Ganda, O. P., Weir, G. C., Soeldner, J. S., Legg, M. A., Chick, W. L., Patel, Y. C., Ebeid, A. M., Gabbay, K. H. and Reichlin, S.: "Somatostatinoma": A somatostatin-containing tumor of the endocrine pancreas. N. Engl. J. Med., *296*:963–967, 1977.

11. Glenn, F., and Mannix, H., Jr.: Diagnosis and prognosis of Cushing's syndrome. Surg. Gynecol. Obstet., *126*:765–776, 1968.

12. Gruber, U. F.: Blood Replacement [Translated by L. Oxtoby and R. F. Armstrong]. New York, Springer, 1969.

13. Hill, G. J., II, and Longino, L. A.: Giant hemangioma with thrombocytopenia. Surg. Gynecol. Obstet., *114*:304–312, 1962.

14. Hill, G. J., II, Knight, V. and Jeffery, G. M.: Thrombocytopenia in vivax malaria. Lancet, *1*:240–241, 1964.

15. Hill, G. J., II, and Wheeler, H. B.: Adrenal insufficiency due to metastatic carcinoma of the lung: Case report and review of Addison's disease caused by adrenal metastases. Cancer, *18*:1467–1473, 1965.

16. Hill, G. J., II: Central venous pressure technique. Surg. Clin. N. Amer., *49*:1351–1359, 1969.

17. Hill, G. J., II: Carcinoid tumors: Pharmacological therapy. Oncology, 25:329–343, 1971.

18. Home Economics Research Report No. 13, "Vitamin B-12".

19. Lee, J. B., Patak, R. V. and Mookerjee, B. K.: Renal prostaglandins and the regulation of blood pressure and sodium and water homeostasis. Am. J. Med., *60*: 798–816, 1976.

20. Melby, J. C.: Assessment of adrenocortical function. N. Engl. J. Med., *285*:735–739, 1971.

21. Mildy, P. (Ed.): The marathon: physiological, medical, epidemiological, and psychological studies. Ann. N.Y. Acad. Sci., *301*, 1977.

22. Moore, F. D.: The Metabolic Care of the Surgical Patient. Philadelphia, W. B. Saunders Co., 1959.

23. Nusynowitz, M. L., McFadden, E. R., Decherd, J. F., Strader, W. J. and Hawkins, J. A.: Principles of acid-base balance. Med. Seminar, William Beaumont General Hospital, November 1969.

24. Palmer, A. J. and Blacket, R.: Regression of xanthomata of the eyelids with modified fat diet. Lancet, *1*:66–68, 1972.

25. Rose, B. D.: Clinical Physiology of Acid-Base and Electrolyte Disorders. New York, McGraw Hill, 1977.

26. Schumer, W.: Metabolic considerations in the preoperative evaluation of the surgical patient. Surg. Gynecol. Obstet., *121*:611–620, 1965.

27. Shieber, W., Kingsbury, R. and Baue, A. E.: The role of the thyroid gland in the hypocalcemia of acute pancreatitis. Surg. Forum, *22*:333–334, 1971.

28. Shires, G. T.: Fluid and electrolyte therapy. *In* Kinney, J. M., Egdahl, R. H. and Zuidema, G. D. (Eds.): Manual of Preoperative and Postoperative Care. Philadelphia, W. B. Saunders Co., 1971.

29. Shoemaker, W. C. and Walker, W. F.: Fluid-Electrolyte Therapy in Acute Illness. Chicago, Year Book Medical Publishers, Inc., 1970.

30. Skillman, J. J., Awwad, H. K. and Moore, F. D.: Plasma protein kinetics of early transcapillary refill after hemorrhage in man. Surg. Gynecol. Obstet., *125*:983–996, 1967.

31. Sorg, J. L.: A protocol for hyperalimentation in a community hospital. Am. Surg., *42*: 716–724, 1976.

32. Steiner, A. L., Goodman, A. D. and Powers, S. R.: Study of a kindred with pheochromocytoma, medullary thyroid carcinoma, hyperparathyroidism and Cushing's disease: multiple endocrine neoplasia, type 2. Medicine, *47*: 371–409, 1968.

33. Tompkins, R. K., Hardacre, J. M., Tzagournis, M. and Greider, M.: Definitive diagnosis of insulin-secreting tumors of the pancreas. Surg. Gynecol. Obstet., *125*: 1069–1074, 1967.

34. Watt, B. K. and Merrill, A.: Composition of foods; raw, processed, prepared. Washington: U. S. Dept. of Agriculture, 1963. (U. S. Dept. of Agriculture, Agriculture Handbook no. 8).

35. Welbourne, R. B.: Current status of the apudomas. Ann. Surg., *185*:1–12, 1977.

36. Wilson, R. E., Bernhard, W. F., Polet, H. and Moore, F. D.: Hyperparathyroidism: The problem of acute parathyroid intoxication. Ann. Surg., *159*:79–93, 1964.

8 The Skull and Nervous System

PHILIP R. WEINSTEIN, M.D.
and CHARLES B. WILSON, M.D.

INTRODUCTION

Except for uncomplicated procedures such as nerve and muscle biopsy, or excision of intradermal lesions such as sebaceous cysts situated in the scalp or adjacent to the spine, there are few neurosurgical operations that can be performed safely without hospitalization. However, initial diagnostic evaluation and preliminary nonoperative or preoperative treatment of some central nervous system disorders can and should be accomplished by outpatient or emergency room physicians, especially when a neurosurgical unit is not readily available or hospitalization for operative treatment is not indicated. In this manner, unnecessary hospitalization or transfer to a neurosurgical center for mild or reversible conditions can be avoided and appropriate definitive treatment of more serious disorders can be expedited by early diagnosis and prompt emergency intervention. With this goal in mind, a brief review of the clinical features and standard management of the most common neurosurgical problems will be presented. A more detailed discussion will follow of head, spine and peripheral nerve injuries, as well as scalp and paravertebral infections, cervical and lumbar disk disease and cerebral ischemia. Techniques and indications for certain diagnostic procedures that can be performed on an outpatient basis will be described. Emphasis will be placed upon initial management of the special problems presented by comatose and paralyzed patients. Indications for hospitalization and surgery will be outlined and prognosis will be discussed.

NEUROSURGICAL PROBLEMS: INITIAL DIAGNOSIS AND DISPOSITION

Head Injury

Head injuries are the most common neurosurgical outpatient or emergency room problems. Such injuries most often result from a motor vehicle accident, fall, altercation or industrial accident. Mild head trauma may result in scalp contusion or laceration without alteration of consciousness or evidence of injury to the skull or brain. A complete history, including immediate response to the injury, specific details of the mechanism of trauma as well as the extent of injury, instrument, location of impact or a description of any penetrating weapon must be obtained from the patient, an observer present at the time of the injury or any police officer and ambulance attendant involved in the case. The physician should perform a complete physical and neurological examination at once and carefully record the findings for comparison with data obtained from subsequent examination when indicated. Skull x-rays should be obtained in all cases of significant head injury. Since up to 10 per cent of severe head injuries may be associated with a fracture of the cervical spine, x-ray films of the cervical spine should also be obtained, especially after a fall or motor vehicle accident. In handling an unconscious patient, assume the possibility of a broken neck until its occurrence has been excluded by radiographic examination.

Although the majority of head injuries are not associated with complications, and complete recovery may usually be expected, it should not be assumed. Many such patients are candidates for initial outpatient management or early discharge after a 12 to 24 hour observation period in the emergency room. It is crucial to determine as early as possible which patients will require more extensive observation and testing.

The most important information needed for assessing the severity of a head injury is its effect on consciousness. Most victims of any but the mildest head injury are dazed for a few seconds after impact. It may therefore be difficult to determine whether or not traumatic unconsciousness has occurred. An accurate estimate of the duration of the unconscious period may be impossible to obtain.

The existence of amnesia in regard to the injury and the events that preceded it indicates that concussive unconsciousness has occurred. The extent of retrograde amnesia correlates with the degree of injury unless intoxication is an associated factor. Severe headache, dizziness, emesis or blurred vision suggest that a more severe injury has been sustained.

Patients with persistent alterations of consciousness or any neurological deficit following head injury must be hospitalized for observation. They are far more susceptible to development of serious complications such as intracranial hematoma. Likewise, those with penetrating injuries and compound or depressed skull fractures or extensive scalp lacerations require hospitalization for appropriate operative treatment. Those with simple linear skull fractures that are extensive or lie adjacent to vascular structures, such as the middle meningeal artery or sagittal sinus (Fig. 8–1), must be hospitalized or at least observed for 24 hours in the Emergency Room, even if there has been no loss of consciousness. All cases of skull fracture in the pediatric age group require hospitalization because of the difficulty of detecting subtle changes in neurological function in young children. Occurrence of seizures indicates brain injury and requires hospitalization. Hemotympanum and cerebrospinal fluid otorrhea and rhinorrhea indicate that basal skull fracture has occurred and hospitalization is required because of the danger of meningitis. Persistent CSF leaks require surgical repair.

After evaluating a clearly conscious and neurologically normal patient who has sustained a head injury without these complications, who has been merely dazed or momentarily unconscious without amnesia, the physician may choose outpatient management. The patient and his family must re-main nearby and accept responsibility for reporting delayed occurrence of headache, nausea, emesis, alterations of consciousness or neurological impairment which may herald the onset of complications due to intracranial injury. When the period of unconsciousness has been less than five minutes in an otherwise uncomplicated head injury, 6 to 12 hours observation in the Emergency Room prior to discharge for outpatient management may be appropriate. If the period of unconsciousness exceeds five minutes, hospitalization or a 24 hour emergency room observation period is indicated.

Details of the initial and subsequent neurological examinations and techniques for repair of scalp lacerations will be described later. Outpatient management of head injuries requires written instructions for the person who assumes responsibility for observing the patient, and follow-up examination by a physician within 24 to 72 hours, or sooner if symptoms develop or progress (Table 8–1). Delayed occurrence of an altered level of consciousness, diplopia, facial nerve palsy, hearing loss, dysarthria, dysphasia, focal or lateralizing numbness, weakness, loss of motor control or seizures require hospitalization for further evaluation and constant observation.

Headache or pain from other injuries may be treated with non-narcotic analgesics, but care must be taken to avoid medication that could interfere with accurate assessment of the level of consciousness and mental acuity. Patients with head injuries may show an increased sensitivity to analgesics or sedatives. If necessary, codeine (30 mg every six hours) can be safely prescribed after the initial 12 to 24 hour observation period has passed.

Persistent or episodic dysequilibrium, nausea, dizziness, vertigo, tinnitus, photophobia, blurred vision, memory lapses and drowsiness are common symptoms following head injuries. They may be provoked or aggravated by physical and emotional

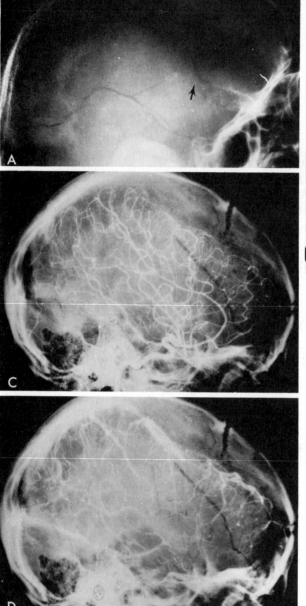

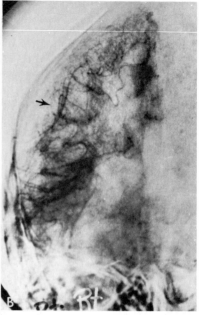

Figure 8–1 *A.* Lateral skull x-ray showing fracture crossing the middle meningeal artery groove (arrow) in a patient with acute epidural hematoma. *B.* Hematoma demonstrated on right carotid arteriogram (arrow). *C.* Lateral arteriogram showing a diastatic fracture in the coronal suture extending across the superior sagittal sinus, which caused a venous epidural hematoma requiring surgical evacuation. The venous phase *D.* shows depression of the sagittal sinus.

stress, fatigue or sudden changes in position, such as rolling over in bed or standing up. When nonprogressive and not associated with alterations in level of consciousness and mental status or any abnormality in the neuro-

logical examination, these complaints can be treated symptomatically on an outpatient basis. Antiemetics, such as Compazine, 10 mg (prochlorperazine) or antivertiginous agents, for example, Dramamine, 50 mg (dimenhydrinate),

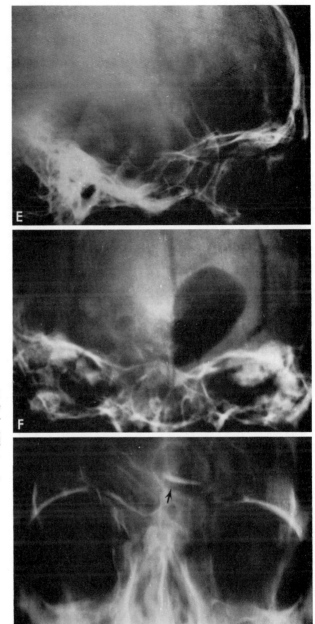

Figure 8-1 *Continued.* *E.* Lateral skull x-ray showing skull fracture entering the frontal sinus and resulting in cerebrospinal rhinorrhea. Two days later AP view showed pneumocephalus. *F.* Air has entered through the fistula. Tomogram *G.* shows fracture lines and bone fragments (arrow).

may be administered every six to eight hours. Such symptoms may reflect irritative effects of relatively mild subarachnoid or parenchymal hemorrhage or reversible traumatic irritation and edema that can affect cranial nerves, labyrinth, brain stem and cerebral cortex. Headache and cervical pain may persist because of contusion and hemorrhage in the dura, scalp and suboccipital muscles, as well as in association with concomitant cervical sprain.

TABLE 8-1 Head Injury Instructions

Following injury to the head, these symptoms should be watched for once the patient is at home. If any of them occur, call your doctor or bring the patient back to the hospital. Dr. _____
PHONE_____

(1) Unconsciousness that cannot be interrupted by awakening the patient or inability to remain awake
(2) Vomiting
(3) Severe or worsening headache
(4) Weakness or paralysis of arm or leg or loss of balance when walking
(5) Slurred speech; inability to speak or understand
(6) Blurry or double vision or blind spots
(7) Change in the size of one or both pupils
(8) Bleeding or fluid drainage from ear or nose
(9) Convulsions
(10) Abnormal behavior, mental confusion or memory loss
(11) In children under four years, allow the child to sleep but awaken and check every one to two hours for the first 24 hours after the injury

The following symptoms are normal and to be expected after any head injury:

(1) Mild headache
(2) Mild nausea
(3) Mild dizziness
(4) Mild unsteadiness

Any of these symptoms may linger or recur for days, weeks, months or even years, depending on the severity of injury. An association may be observed between persistence of the posttraumatic syndromes and litigation involving personal injury or workmen's compensation liability. However, possible emotional sequelae of mild or severe head injury and traumatic unconsciousness should be anticipated and taken into consideration by the attending physician, staff and the patient's family. Traumatic neurosis causing psychological disability due to anxiety, depression, phobias and loss of self confidence may be prevented by sympathetic reassurance and careful explanation of symptoms early in the course of recovery. Persistence of seemingly nonspecific and subjective symptoms such as headache, dizziness, dysequi-librium and memory lapse can be real, frightening and disabling experiences for the patient with head injuries in the recovery phase of a postconcussion syndrome.

Spinal Injury

Back pain, most often due to muscular and ligamentous injury or degenerative vertebral joint disease, is one of the most common acute problems encountered in medical practice. When it is associated with severe spinal impact or multiple injuries, rather than merely with strenuous physical activity, the risk of associated damage to the spinal cord and nerve roots is considerable. Again, a thorough and detailed history of the mechanism of injury must be obtained. Special attention should be given to the position of the spine, head and extremities before, during and after injury. The size and length of weapon involved in stab wounds or penetrating injuries, as well as caliber and velocity of bullets in missile injuries, should be determined if possible. Of greatest importance is information regarding the immediate and delayed neurological effects of spinal injury, again with special reference to the time course and distribution of progressive or resolving loss of sensation and motor function in the extremities. An accurate history may be difficult to obtain and interpret if consciousness is altered as a result of associated head injury. When the extremities cannot be moved by the patient because of excruciating back or extremity pain or severe anxiety, the neurological examination may be difficult to interpret.

Initial evaluation must begin with a complete neurological examination with the patient maintained in a supine position to avoid further dislocation of a potentially unstable spinal fracture. Neurological deficit may be localized according to level of spinal cord, nerve root or cauda equina injury. The physician may find it helpful to palpate along the spinal column, sliding the examining hand under the patient, in order to localize the injury site by eliciting focal tenderness or discovering malalignment of the spinous processes. Turning the patient for inspection of the spinal column or examination of spinal range of movement with the patient in a sitting or standing position should be deferred until after x-rays are obtained, if a fracture is suspected. Impairment of bladder function should be anticipated in association with either traumatic paraplegia or severe back pain without neurological deficit.

Appropriate x-rays should be obtained as soon as possible, and care should be taken to keep the spinal column immobilized during transfer for this examination. The mode of injury, location of pain and level of sensory deficit (if present) should indicate the probable site of injury and potential fracture. The cervicothoracic junction is especially difficult to visualize in the crucial lateral projection, and special transaxillary views may be required to eliminate overlying shoulder shadows. The vertebrae most often fractured are C5–C6 at the apex of the cervical lordosis in hyperflexion or hyperextension injuries; T7–T8 at the apex of the thoracic kyphosis; T12–L1 at the thoracolumbar junction in hyperflexion injuries; and L4–L5 at the fulcrum of the lumbar lordosis in compressive injuries (Fig. 8–2).

If unconscious, the patient with a spinal injury should undergo radiographic examination of the entire spinal column. Diagnosis of fracture or cord injury can easily be missed or delayed when the patient cannot give a history or cooperate during testing of sensation and motor strength. As in the patient with head injuries, observation of involuntary movements or elicited withdrawal to painful cutaneous or deep muscle stimuli may be the only method of neurological examination possible. Asymmetry or absence of deep tendon reflexes and the presence of pathological reflexes may be helpful. Interpretation of neurological findings may be complicated by any combination of cerebral and spinal cord lesions in a patient with multiple injuries.

Patients with penetrating or extensive lacerating spinal injuries, spinal fracture of any type and any neurological deficit, even of momentary duration, must be hospitalized either for observation, nonoperative fracture reduction and spinal immobilization or corrective surgery. A neurological classification of spinal cord injuries will be presented later with a detailed discussion of Emergency Room management. Outpatient management may be considered in cases of uncomplicated spinal column injury associated with pain and paraspinous muscle spasm, without evidence of fracture or neurological deficit. If pain can be controlled with oral analgesics, sedation and muscle relaxants, and if the home situation allows relatively complete bed rest with assistance from family, friends or visiting nurse, hospitalization may be unnecessary. Provision of a hospital bed, urinal, bed pan or commode for home use may be helpful initially. Relevant orthopedic principles will be discussed in Chapters 12 and 13.

Peripheral Nerve Injury

Peripheral nerves may be injured in association with blunt injury, compression, laceration, fracture or dislocation of the extremities. Management of lacerations or penetrating injuries of major peripheral nerves requires hospitalization. Relevant neuroanatomical and diagnostic principles will be outlined later. Neurological deficit due to closed injuries resulting from nerve stretch, contusion, compression or inadvertent hypodermic injection may disappear without surgical intervention. After appropriate orthopedic management of any associated fracture

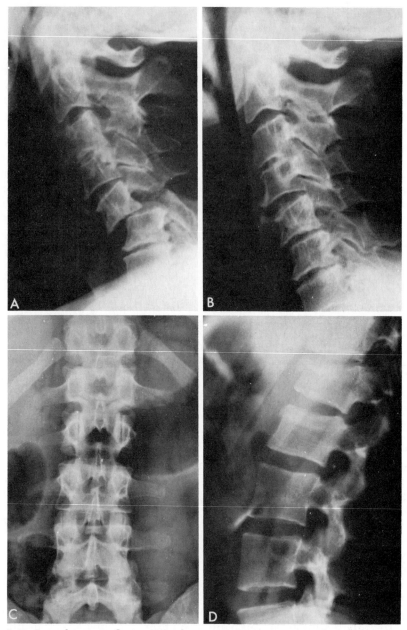

Figure 8–2   Lateral x-rays in flexion (A) and extension (B) in a patient with cervical fracture dislocation at C5–C6 that is unstable. Note almost complete subluxation of C5 over C6 in position of flexion.
There was no neurological deficit. *C., D.* Anteroposterior and lateral x-rays of a patient with lumbar
spinal compression fracture at L1 and mild paraparesis. Recovery and spontaneous fusion occurred
after treatment with immobilization.

or dislocation, outpatient management
consisting of weekly neurological examinations and periodical electrodiag-
nostic evaluation is appropriate (see
Neurosurgical Diagnostic Procedures).

Splinting or bracing is indicated for
wristdrop due to radial nerve injury or
foot drop due to peroneal or sciatic
nerve injury, to prevent sprain caused
by associated loss of muscular joint

support and to prevent overstretching of the paralyzed muscles. Patients must be warned of the possibility of dangerous burns, lacerations, or pressure sores that may occur in areas of anesthetic skin, especially when the hands or feet are affected. Meticulous skin care, including regular cleaning and lubrication with ointment, should be taught. Cervical root avulsion or stretch injuries of the brachial plexus can occur with severe shoulder dislocations. Little if any recovery can be expected in most cases, but evaluation and management should be carried out by a neurosurgeon.

Nontraumatic peripheral nerve palsies can occur as manifestations of diabetes, vasculitis and a variety of toxic, metabolic, inflammatory and degenerative disorders. Referral for outpatient medical and neurological evaluation is indicated.

Intervertebral Disk Disease

Displacement of the intervertebral disk or progressive vertebral spondylosis occurring in the cervical, lumbar and, uncommonly, thoracic spine is a frequent cause of pain, neurological deficit and disability. The disk, which develops embryologically from the primitive notochord, consists of central gelatinous nucleus pulposus, surrounded by concentric lamellae of fibrocartilage forming a capsule that is attached to the adjacent vertebral bodies as the annulus fibrosus. Degeneration, dehydration and loss of elasticity of the disk occur universally with advancing age, thereby increasing vulnerability to displacement either spontaneously or following the stress of repetitive minor trauma or major injury. Since the disks are situated on the floor of the spinal canal, posterior protrusions or proliferating osteophytes may impinge upon the spinal cord or nerve roots, causing symptoms and signs of myelopathy or radiculopathy (Fig. 8–3).

The history may be one of acute onset following stress or injury of the lower back or neck; pain may radiate into one or both legs or arms and be associated with symptoms of neurological dysfunction in a radicular distribution. Evidence of spinal cord or cauda equina involvement may also be elicited by neurological examination, if the disk has herniated extensively into the central rather than the lateral portion of the spinal canal at the appropriate level. Acute spinal injuries may produce neurological deficits due to displacement of the intervertebral disk without occurrence of detectable fracture or dislocation. Since the cartilaginous disk is not radiopaque, spinal x-rays may show little or no abnormality except for a slight decrease in height of the affected intervertebral space. Myelography is therefore required if a discogenic lesion is suspected.

More often the history obtained will be one of insidiously progressive or spontaneously occurring back or neck pain, followed by a variable delay in the onset of symptoms of radiculopathy or myelopathy over a period of days, weeks, months or even years. Spinal x-rays obtained in this setting may show diffuse or focal degenerative changes. Narrowing or collapse of the disk spaces with posterior proliferation of osteophytes on the floor of the spinal canal or neural foramena is the signature of degenerative spondylosis.

Radicular pain is usually sharp and lancinating, with rapid radiation all the way down the affected extremity to fingers or toes. It is often associated with paresthesias and numbness, and may be provoked by coughing, straining or turning and bending movements of the neck or back. Relief will characteristically follow spinal immobilization with bedrest.

Examination may reveal focal tenderness on palpation over the involved spinous process or facet joint and aggravation or triggering of radiating pain and paresthesias during palpation of the involved peripheral nerves in the upper or lower extremities. Spasm

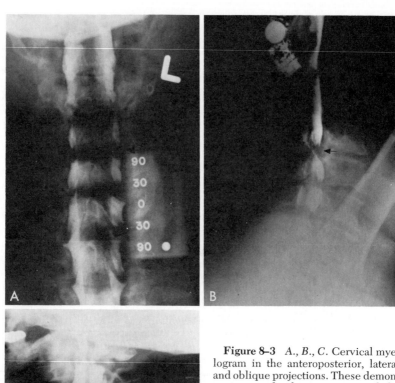

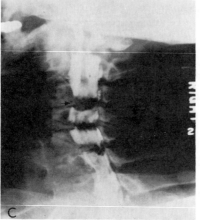

Figure 8–3 *A., B., C.* Cervical myelogram in the anteroposterior, lateral and oblique projections. These demonstrate extradural compression of the spinal cord and nerve roots at three levels by ventral and lateral osteophytic disc protrusions and dorsal thickening of the ligamentum flavum in a patient with progressive spastic quadriparesis due to cervical spondylosis. Arrows identify filling defects in the contrast column at C 3-4.

of the paraspinous muscles may occur in response to irritation of spinal nerve roots. Splinting and restriction of spinal movement, as well as loss of normal curvature and secondary scoliosis, may be observed. Other signs of nerve irritation include radiation of extremity pain during stretch of the sciatic or brachial roots following elevation of the leg with the knee extended (straight leg raising test), or contralateral tilting of the neck with the shoulder pulled down. Sensory loss over a radicular distribution and depression or loss of deep tendon reflexes with or without associated

muscle weakness may be helpful localizing signs. The neurological examination is far more helpful in the diagnosis of complicated disk disease than is x-ray examination of the spine. Degenerative changes are often diffuse and may be entirely asymptomatic; they are commonly identified on films taken for other indications. Pertinent neuroanatomical principles helpful in diagnosing these disorders will be reviewed in the section on Neurological Examination and Observation.

Myelography is essential for demonstrating and localizing disk lesions, but it is never recommended until surgical

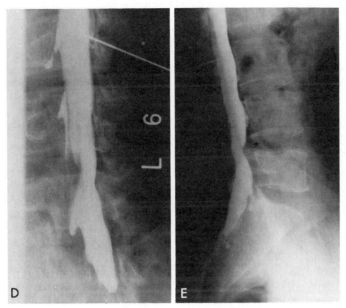

Figure 8–3 *Continued D., E.* Anteroposterior and lateral myelogram in a patient with intractable sciatica and right L-5 radiculopathy. Arrow indicates ventrolateral extradural defect. A large herniated L4 disk fragment was removed at surgery.

treatment becomes necessary after alternative methods of therapy have failed. Emergency surgical decompression is indicated only for acute onset of major radicular muscle weakness or myelopathic paralysis. It may be difficult to interpret findings of motor dysfunction in the presence of severe pain, since involuntary inhibition of muscle function may occur. Initial treatment of cases with chronic, acute but minor or rapidly resolving neurological deficit, requires spinal immobilization with bedrest, sedation, analgesics and muscle relaxants. Outpatient management, when practical, is often adequate. Pelvic or cervical traction may be easily arranged at home with the standard equipment that is available through orthopedic appliance outlets. Traction facilitates immobilization, enforces bedrest, corrects spinal posture and relieves muscle spasm. It is unlikely that significant distraction of the collapsed intervertebral space occurs. Weekly office visits for follow-up neurological evaluation

are advisable, especially since disappearance of radicular pain may not imply improvement, but may instead be associated with worsening of radicular motor deficit if further disk extrusion has caused complete ablation of nerve root function.

In the majority of cases gradual recovery will be observed during 10 to 20 days of bedrest at home. Resolution of edema and inflammation caused by transient nerve root stretch or entrapment associated with minor acute or chronic disk protrusion usually occurs. A gradual increase in activity in conjunction with a progressively more strenuous physical therapy and exercise program is then recommended during the next 10 to 20 days. Bending and lifting should be restricted and a cervical collar or lumbar corset may be helpful, to prevent excessive spinal movement during convalescence.

Failure to improve, recurrence of radicular symptoms after resumption of activity or progression of a neurological deficit at any time requires hospitalization for possible surgical treatment. Patients with chronic cervical or thoracic myelopathy or cauda equina radiculopathy due to progressive spondylosis are unlikely to respond to conservative therapy. Such cases are best managed with inpatient observation for evidence of subtle changes in neurological function during evaluation and consideration of definitive surgical therapy.

Hemorrhage and Hematoma

Nontraumatic hemorrhage within the central nervous system (CNS) may cause syncope, seizure or explosive onset of severe headache or back pain. It is often associated with physical or emotional stress, which is presumed to cause elevation of systemic blood pressure. In some cases, hemorrhage is followed by rapid progression of neurological deficit and alteration of consciousness. Hypertension, vasculitis or coagulopathies may be predisposing conditions.

Subarachnoid hemorrhage (SAH) may result after the rupture of an intracranial aneurysm or a congenital cerebral or spinal arteriovenous malformation (AVM) (Fig. 8–4). Extensive and devastating hemorrhage can be preceded by one or a series of minor episodes designated as "warning leaks," which provide an often overlooked opportunity for early diagnosis and prompt prophylactic surgical ligation of the lesion. Therefore, acute onset of severe and unusual nonmigrainous headache, even if transient and not associated with altered consciousness or neurological deficit, should be an indication for diagnostic lumbar puncture. Nuchal rigidity may not be present until 12 to 24 hours after SAH, and may never appear if minimal bleeding has occurred. If bloody fluid is obtained after an atraumatic spinal puncture, the patient should be hospitalized for cerebral arteriography. A traumatic tap should be suspected if the fluid clears after a few milliliters are drained or if the supernatant is not xanthochromic 12 to 24 hours after the ictus.

Intracerebral hemorrhage is frequently associated with hypertension, anticoagulation therapy, arteriovenous malformation or tumor. It may be difficult to distinguish clinically from hemorrhage into the subarachnoid space, since focal progressive neurological deficit can occur in both instances. After subarachnoid hemorrhage, hemi-

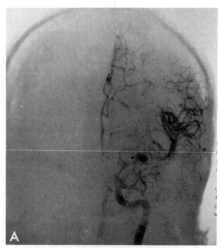

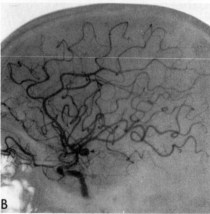

Figure 8–4 *A., B.* Anteroposterior and lateral carotid arteriogram demonstrating a large aneurysm (arrow) at the terminal bifurcation of the left middle cerebral artery in a patient with delayed onset of mild dysphasia and right hemiparesis after acute subarachnoid hemorrhage. Note lobular configuration of the aneurysm sac and extensive narrowing of the parent vessel due to vasospasm.

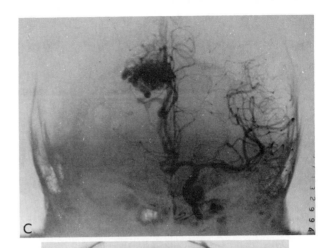

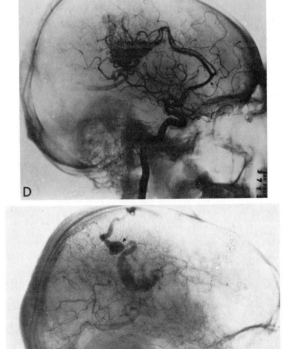

Figure 8–4 *Continued C., D., E.* Anteroposterior and lateral carotid arteriograms demonstrating a large arteriovenous malformation of the peri-callosal artery in a patient with recurrent subarachnoid hemorrhage. Note enlargement of the major feeding artery (arrow, *D*) and draining vein (arrow, *E*).

paresis is due to reactive vasospasm causing regional cerebral ischemia in the territory of the affected vessel. Chronic headache and recurrent seizures, with or without occurrence of repeated hemorrhage, are more commonly associated with AVM than with aneurysm. Although emergency surgical evacuation of acute spontaneous intracerebral hematomas is rarely beneficial because of their deep location, delayed removal may facilitate recovery after surrounding cerebral edema and ischemia have subsided. In any event, hospitalization is indicated for diagnostic evaluation and intensive supportive care. If available, computerized tomographic (CT) brain scans are of great value in the diagnosis and localization of intracranial hematoma. Cerebral arteriography is the standard examination for demonstrating these lesions.

Emergency neurosurgical intervention is rarely indicated following spontaneous intracranial hemorrhage unless definite progression, contralateral hemiparesis and occurrence of ipsilateral pupillary dilatation suggest that an expanding hematoma is causing transtentorial herniation. Patients with "warning leaks" are an exception at the opposite extreme of the clinical spectrum, and they should undergo early arteriography and surgery before major hemorrhage occurs from an aneurysm. However, in many cases bleeding ceases spontaneously and early neurological deficit, if present, does not progress. Level of consciousness may vary from normal to stupor or coma, depending on the extent and location of the hemorrhage and the severity of resultant vasospasm. Early craniotomy has been found to be associated with increased morbidity and mortality rates. Craniotomy is best tolerated from seven to ten days after SAH or intracerebral hemorrhage. Therefore, arteriography is usually performed electively within a day or two, after the patient's condition has stabilized and hypertension, if present, has been controlled. Transfer to a neurosurgical center can usually be accomplished under sedation by ambulance without undue risk of provoking recurrent hemorrhage. The incidence of recurrent bleeding within the first 14 days after initial hemorrhage has been reduced from 20 per cent to 10 per cent by administration of Amicar (epsilon-aminocaproic acid), 2 gm every 2 hours as an antifibrinolytic agent, which is thought to retard clot lysis. Dexamethasone (4 mg every 6 hours) may be helpful in control of reactive cerebral edema.

Operative treatment of aneurysms and AVM's continues to represent a major technical challenge to the neurosurgeon. In patients whose neurological condition is stable, lesions that are in anatomically favorable locations can be clipped, ligated, obliterated, resected, reinforced by encasement, thrombosed or even embolized with intravascular catheters. With the use of the operating microscope to facilitate exposure and dissection, and controlled hypotension to reduce the risk of intraoperative hemorrhage, surgical mortality rates of 5 per cent and neurological morbidity rates of 10 to 15 per cent can be expected. These results represent a significant improvement over the major risk of recurrent hemorrhage in untreated patients. Prevention of cerebral infarction due to pre- or postoperative vasospasm remains a major unsolved problem in aneurysm patients.

Ischemia and Infarction

After heart disease and cancer, stroke is the third most common cause of death in the United States. Many patients present with warning attacks of transient cerebral ischemia, providing an opportunity for surgical repair of preocclusive or ulcerating extracranial vascular lesions or bypass of intracranial lesions before completed stroke occurs. Any patient who presents with a single episode of a major transient neurological deficit, or recurrent minor deficits, should be hospitalized for a definitive diagnostic evaluation that will usually include cerebral angiography.

Symptoms of paralysis or sensory loss may be present upon awakening from sleep or may develop rapidly in seconds or minutes during sedentary activity. Premonitory headache is not characteristic and if present may be relatively mild. Absence of aura or tonic-clonic movements distinguishes stroke from seizure. Transient monocular visual blurring or blindness associated with contralateral hemiparesis is the signature of internal carotid artery embolism or thrombosis. Bilateral visual impairment and leg weakness or "drop attacks" associated with dysarthria, diplopia, dizziness, nausea or syncope may indicate the presence of vertebrobasilar occlusive disease. Transient neurological deficit may persist for minutes, hours or days. Complete recovery implies that infarction has not occurred or has affected small areas of functionally unimportant brain tissue.

Seizures, cerebral hemorrhage, brain tumors, systemic sources of cerebrovascular embolization and occurrence of cardiac arrhythmias should be considered in the differential diagnosis. Noninvasive diagnostic procedures, such as Doppler ultrasonography and ocular plethysmography, may be helpful as screening tests to identifying hemodynamically significant occlusive lesions of the carotid arteries. Brain scans may demonstrate a blood-brain barrier defect (increased vascular permeability to radioisotopes) within five to seven days after cerebral infarction. Arteriography is ultimately required for anatomical demonstration of the offending vascular lesion. Patients with steady or stepwise progression of neurological deficit (stroke in evolution) or "crescendo" transient ischemic episodes (increasing severity of deficit with each attack) should undergo emergency arteriography. If an appropriate lesion is demonstrated at the common carotid bifurcation, and the internal carotid artery remains patent, immediate endarterectomy is indicated.

Cases of completed stroke characterized by immediate onset of fixed neurological deficit, especially in elderly patients, can be considered for outpatient management. If level of consciousness remains adequate for maintenance of adequate alimentation and airway, cardiopulmonary function is intact and major paralysis does not prevent appropriate toilet and skin care and mobilization, home care arrangements can be made. A 24 hour period of observation in the Emergency Room is appropriate to determine that the patient's condition is stable. Where indicated, noninvasive diagnostic procedures can be obtained at a later date on an outpatient basis. Under such circumstances, general supportive care and intensive physiotherapy are the only treatments that are clearly indicated. Vasodilating agents have not been shown to be effective. The value of anticoagulation therapy remains controversial and, if indicated, it must be carefully managed by a neurologist or internist. Cerebral arteriography may be indicated at a later date, especially in younger patients who recover from a stroke. Identification of certain lesions may lead to prophylactic surgical therapy to prevent recurrent embolism, progression of stenosis or thrombosis.

Tumor

Tumors of the central nervous system cause signs and symptoms of increased intracranial pressure and mental deterioration or gradual progression of focal neurological deficit localizing the site of involvement of brain, spinal cord or nerve roots. A long history of headaches that are worse upon awakening may be obtained from patients harboring brain tumors. Back pain aggravated by the supine position may be a sign of intraspinal neoplasm. Papilledema may be present as a sign of increased intracranial pressure and should be an indication for immediate hospitalization, unless it is chronic and not associated with headache, nausea or neurological deficit. Slow growing meningiomas or gliomas of the anterior frontal or temporal lobes may become very large before symptoms or signs develop, especially if they involve the nondominant hemisphere. A danger of sudden decompensation exists owing to hemorrhage, infarction or brain herniation. Adult onset of seizures without a history of other causes such as trauma, infection, infarction or previous cranial surgery may be an early sign of brain tumor and is an indication for a thorough outpatient evaluation.

Initial noninvasive tests should include skull x-ray, electroencephalogram (EEG) and brain scan. Outpatient lumbar puncture (LP) should not be performed. LP may be dangerous if intracranial pressure (ICP) is elevated, or it may have to be repeated if contrast studies are needed. Ultimately, hospitalization for arteriography or myelography will be necessary. Chest x-rays should always be obtained because of the high incidence of cerebral and spinal metastases from lung carcinoma. Spinal x-rays may show evidence of bone erosion or destruction due to primary or metastatic tumors (Fig. 8–5). Resulting vertebral instability can lead to dislocation, causing further compromise of spinal cord func-

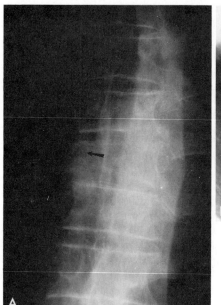
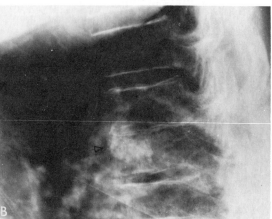
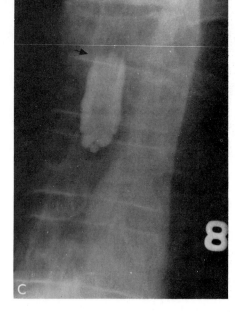

Figure 8–5 *A., B.* Anteroposterior and lateral thoracic spine x-rays in a patient with back pain and progressive leg weakness showing metastatic carcinoma eroding the pedicle and collapsing the vertebral body at T9 (arrows). *C.* AP myelogram in this patient demonstrating a complete extradural block due to a tumor at T9-10 that was decompressed by emergency laminectomy.

tion. Bone scans may be helpful in identifying metastatic cranial or spinal tumors.

Certain metastatic and reticuloendothelial spinal neoplasms presenting with pain and not associated with neurological deficit can be treated nonsurgically with radiation therapy. However, in this setting, onset of even the most subtle manifestation of spinal cord dysfunction, such as leg numbness or mild urinary retention, requires immediate hospitalization for emergency myelography unless the history is that of a benign, slow growing tumor. However, with any degree of spinal cord compression, progression to complete paraplegia or quadriplegia may be rapid. Severe or complete spinal cord deficit may be irreversible, especially if present for more than six to eight hours. Emergency surgery for spinal cord decompression in metastatic cancer patients with fixed total paraplegia may be a futile and life-threatening exercise. On occasion, laminectomy is indicated for biopsy if the primary malignancy cannot be otherwise identified, regardless of the presence or extent of neurological deficit.

Removal of solitary cerebral metastases, especially if situated in functionally unimportant areas, can produce significant palliation. Multiple metastatic lesions are usually treated with radiation therapy and the administration of steroids for control of cerebral edema. Benign CNS tumors arise from the meninges or nerve sheaths and frequently can be partially or completely resected. Peripheral nerve tumors are also mostly benign and can usually be identified by palpation and associated neurological deficit. Glial tumors of the brain and spinal cord tend to infiltrate diffusely but vary in malignant potential and growth rate. They are usually treated with biopsy and extensive internal decompression followed by radiation and chemotherapy, since complete removal is seldom possible

without further sacrifice of remaining neurological function.

Skull tumors, when circumscribed and intraosseous in location, may present with headache and focal scalp tenderness. Larger lesions may be evident on inspection or palpation. Tangential x-ray views are helpful for identifying exophytic growth and stereoscopic views may delineate the position of the lesion and demonstrate involvement of the inner table of the skull. Temptation to biopsy or excise even small skull tumors in the office or emergency room should be resisted. Although overnight hospitalization may not be necessary, full operating room facilities should be available. Prior brain scan and arteriography may be indicated to rule out intracranial extension. Profuse bleeding from tumor, skull or dura may be difficult to control without electrocautery, bone wax or wider resection. Sedation may be necessary as an adjuvant to local anesthesia. Surgical removal of soft tissue tumors of the scalp or paraspineous area will be discussed in the section on Outpatient Neurosurgical Procedures.

Infection and Abscess

Infections of the central nervous system that may require surgical treatment include scalp, subgaleal or paraspinous abscess, cranial or spinal osteomyelitis, epidural or subdural abscess, brain abscess and tuberculous or fungal granuloma. Although systemic antibiotics may be effective in arresting cases of extensive scalp or paraspinous cellulitis, hospitalization may be indicated for parenteral therapy and careful observation for signs of meningitis or abscess. Such problems usually represent post-traumatic or postoperative infections, and in the post-traumatic group a common cause of late infection is inadequate débridement or delayed closure of scalp or paraspinous lacerations. Because of transcranial venous drainage through diploic channels or pterygoid and condylar plexuses, the risk of secondary meningitis or brain abscess is high in the presence of scalp, orbital, facial or sinus infections.

Bacterial cerebritis may respond to appropriate antibiotic therapy without the necessity of surgical treatment, especially if the offending organism has been identified by culturing the blood or obtaining a specimen from the primary infection site. All cases of osteomyelitis or CNS abscess will require hospitalization for treatment, usually definitive surgical excision or drainage. Subdural empyema, a true neurosurgical emergency, may cause death within 24 hours unless radical surgical drainage is accomplished immediately. Diagnosis of intracranial abscess should be considered in patients presenting with headache, fever, confusion, signs of increased intracranial pressure and focal neurological deficit. Brain abscess may be associated with otitis, mastoiditis, sinusitis, compound or depressed skull fracture and bone or foreign body fragments retained after penetrating cranial injuries. If no obvious local source of infection is evident, one should suspect systemic disorders such as congenital cyanotic heart disease, pneumonia, bronchiectasis, pyelonephritis, abdominal or pelvic abscess and skeletal osteomyelitis. Spinal epidural abscess is a rare condition characterized by back pain, fever and paraparesis. Diabetes and immunoparetic or myeloproliferative disorders may be predisposing factors in cases of CNS infection. Brain abscess may be idiopathic in up to 20 per cent of cases.

Although lumbar puncture provides a definitive diagnosis in most cases of meningitis when cerebrospinal fluid contains bacteria, pleocytosis and lowered glucose concentration, it may be of little or no value in the diagnosis of brain abscess, since these parameters are more often normal and cultures may be negative. If signs of increased intracranial pressure are present, spinal tap should be deferred until after neurosurgical consultation and cerebral arteriography or CT brain scan has been performed, especially if papilledema is present or a mass lesion is suspected. Recurrent meningitis may be associated with congenital neurenteric cyst or occult CSF fistulae to the paranasal sinuses or middle ear. Excessive removal of CSF during LP may result in pneumocephalus under these circumstances, by allowing air to enter through the fistula.

Congenital Anomalies and Hydrocephalus

Rarely will the outpatient physician be called upon to diagnose hydrocephalus or congenital lesions of the nervous system. However, familiarity with certain aspects of these problems may be helpful, especially if clinical manifestations occur after birth or in association with acquired disorders.

Hydrocephalus is identified anatomically as either obstructive or communicating, according to whether the site of blockage of CSF circulation is within the ventricular system or in the subarachnoid space. Congenital hydrocephalus may arrest spontaneously or reach a state of physiological equilibrium. Symptoms of increased ICP or brain dysfunction may not be present or detectable until later childhood or adulthood. If their case is symptomatic, infants or young children may present with an abnormal increase in head circumference, tense fontanelle (if still open), dilated scalp veins, irritability and failure to thrive. Skull x-rays should demonstrate spreading of the cranial sutures. A history of difficult birth with forceps delivery or neonatal head injury may be obtained, presumably causing subarachnoid hemorrhage. Infantile meningitis may be followed by hydrocephalus or subdural hygroma. Association of hydrocephalus with spinal dysraphism and meningomyelocele is common. Hospitalization for diagnostic evaluation and ventricular shunt implantation is necessary.

Congenital or acquired hydrocephalus may present in adolescents or adults with headache, dementia, gait ataxia and urinary incontinence. Papilledema is rarely seen in communicating hydrocephalus or chronic cases of congenital aqueductal stenosis. Secondary hydrocephalus characteristically presents with papilledema in both adults and children. This condition is due to aqueductal or ventricular obstruction by tumors usually located in the posterior fossa. Since the size and position of the ventricles and subarachnoid cisterns, as well as their anatomical relationship to tumors, can be clearly demonstrated with computerized tomographic brain scans, this test is rapidly becoming the procedure of choice for pre- and postoperative evaluation of hydrocephalus.

The topic of subcutaneous lumps situated upon the cranium or spine requires special attention in this section, because they can be difficult to distinguish from meningocele, encephalocele, dermoid with intracranial involvement or lipoma with intraspinal extension. Skin and subcutaneous lesions, such as sebaceous cysts or circumscribed lipomas, can be removed with standard surgical techniques and do not require hospitalization. However, evidence of CNS involvement should be sought if the lesion is extensive or has unusual features. Examination of patients with even the smallest encephalocele or meningocele may disclose position-dependent alterations in the volume or pressure within the mass. Skull or spine x-rays may reveal a characteristic bone defect or anomaly. A cutaneous nevus or hemangioma, sometimes associated with an uncharacteristically colored tuft of hair, may be present on the skin of the back in association with a dermal sinus or "dumbbell" lipoma that has an intraspinal extension. A large sacral dural cyst may present as a pelvic mass. Thoracic neurofibroma, identi-

fied as a mediastinal mass on chest film, may grow into the spinal canal. If associated neurological deficit is detected under any of these circumstances, a thorough inpatient evaluation including myelography or pneumoencephalography is indicated. Treatment will then require neurosurgical removal of the intracranial or intraspinal extension of the lesion and watertight closure of the dura.

Headache and Neurogenic Pain Syndromes

Acute, recurrent or chronic pain syndromes are seen with great regularity in Emergency Room and office practice. These include tension headache, migraine, trigeminal neuralgia, post-herpetic neuralgia, painful diabetic neuropathy, post-traumatic and post-surgical neuralgia, chronic radiculopathy, incisional pain, phantom limb, paraplegic pain, causalgia, reflex sympathetic dystrophy and thalamic pain due to stroke. Most attacks or exacerbations of chronic pain syndromes can be managed with appropriate sedation or psychotropic medication, as a supplement to oral or parenteral analgesics administered as indicated, to control associated anxiety and depression. Hospitalization for pain control is rarely indicated and, in fact, may be psychologically detrimental if it sets a precedent for recurrent episodes of emotional decompensation and dependence on hospital treatment.

A variety of vasoactive medications are now available for treatment of vascular headache syndromes, and intractable cases that do not respond to routine treatment should be referred to a neurologist. Some neuralgias and central pain syndromes may respond to anticonvulsant drugs such as Dilantin (phenytoin) or Tegretol (carbamazepine). Injections of local anesthetic and steroid medications into or around musculoskeletal trigger areas, irritable nerves, scars or neuromas, spinal nerve roots or the lumbar theca may result in dramatic relief of pain, sometimes outlasting the effect of the anesthetic. Careful sterile technique and prior aspiration after needle positioning should be employed to avoid infection and intravascular injection. Neurosurgical treatment of intractable pain requires hospitalization, and may consist of neurectomy, rhizotomy, cordotomy, thalamotomy or electrical neurostimulation to activate pain inhibitory mechanisms. A thorough search for systemic or CNS disorders as an otherwise treatable cause of the pain is always indicated before neurosurgical treatment is considered.

NEUROLOGICAL EXAMINATION AND OBSERVATION

After any acute neurological illness or injury has occurred the earliest examination will indicate the extent and location of initial damage to the central nervous system. Although severed peripheral nerve axons can regrow, neuronal regeneration does not occur. Irreversible tissue destruction from infarction or necrosis will result in permanent neurological deficit unless compensatory function by other areas of the CNS is possible. On the other hand, progression of initial deficit or delayed onset of CNS dysfunction may indicate reversible impairment due to treatable lesions such as hematoma, dislocated fracture or rapidly enlarging tumor. Therefore, the importance of an accurately recorded and regularly repeated neurological examination to establish initial baselines and document subsequent changes cannot be overemphasized. Only in this manner can indications for hospitalization and emergency surgery or outpatient management be determined following an appropriate observation period.

Initial Evaluation

An accurate history is invaluable, and facts relating to an accident should be obtained from any witness. The patient's state immediately prior to an injury should be learned, if possible, as well as any past history of nervous system disease, alcoholism or major physical illness. If a history cannot be obtained, the only information available will be that acquired by examining the patient.

The physical examination should be thorough and systematic. Even in the unconscious patient the general examination should precede the neurological examination. The initial evaluation may be the only complete physical examination performed under emergency circumstances, and therefore its importance cannot be overemphasized. Vital signs will approximate normal values in the uncomplicated case of head injury. A rapid rise in intracranial pressure produces bradycardia, a rise in systolic blood pressure and a slowing or change in the character of respirations, in that sequence. Any deviation of the vital signs from the normal range is reason for concern and may be due to cerebral causes.

Particular attention should be given to an examination of the head and neck. The scalp is inspected for lacerations and contusions. Very early after injury, the course of a fracture may be accurately delineated by palpation of an overlying ridge of local scalp edema or hemorrhage. Crepitus beneath the scalp may be due to air forced through a laceration. A "doughnut-shaped" hematoma of the scalp can be mistaken for a depressed skull fracture. Regardless of the impression gained by palpation, the diagnosis of a depressed fracture should not be made without radiographic confirmation.

Fractures of the facial skeleton and jaws do not require immediate attention unless soft tissue swelling threatens the airway, but their presence should be determined before facial edema and hematoma preclude adequate examination. The orbits and zygomas should be palpated, the maxilla rocked by traction on the upper incisors, and the mandible examined for dental occlusion, mobility and crepitus. If facial edema is already present, it is wise to assume that facial fractures have occurred.

The ears should be examined for the presence of blood within the external canal or behind the tympanic membrane. This is a sign of basal skull fracture. Signs of damage to the eyeball or its adnexa should be sought before development of periorbital edema renders this more difficult. Epistaxis, in the absence of significant direct trauma to the nose, or cerebrospinal fluid rhinorrhea indicate the presence of a basal skull fracture extending into one of the paranasal sinuses.

The neck should be examined carefully. Local tenderness or displaced spinous processes may indicate a fracture of the cervical spine. Protective resistance to movement of the cervical spine, even in the face of painful injury, cannot occur in the unconscious patient. Therefore, in the unconscious patient, neck movement should not be tested and management should proceed as if there is a cervical fracture until x-ray films are obtained. Evidence of trauma to the anterior cervical region should alert the examiner to the possibility of injury to the trachea or carotid artery. Direct trauma to the carotid artery can induce thrombosis with infarction of a cerebral hemisphere, which may mimic a cerebral contusion.

An adequate examination of the abdomen is difficult to perform in the unconscious or uncooperative patient. If shock is present and its cause cannot be found, it must be assumed to be the result of intra-abdominal hemorrhage. Ruptured spleens occur commonly in patients with head injuries. Head injuries alone do not cause ileus. However, thoracolumbar fractures with or without spinal cord injury are associated with abdominal pain and are regularly followed by paralytic ileus.

As part of the initial treatment of an unconscious patient, a nasogastric tube should be passed for evacuation of the stomach. It makes vomiting less likely, thereby preventing aspiration. Swallowed blood is often found with extensive facial injuries and will usually be vomited if not removed. The tube may be left in place and attached to gravity drainage. An indwelling urethral catheter should also be passed in unconscious patients and in those unable to void voluntarily. Examination of the urine for blood should be carried out immediately to exclude injury to the urinary tract in the abdomen or pelvis.

Neurological Examination

The level of consciousness is best determined by noting the patient's response to a stimulus. Various intensities of stimuli activate the patient to different degrees depending on the severity of the injury. One tries the least potent stimulus first and then proceeds to more powerful stimuli until a response is achieved. Calling the patient's name may arouse him to alertness. If sound does not arouse the patient, light supraorbital pressure is applied and gradually increased to a maximum. Supraorbital pressure, which directly stimulates a branch of the trigeminal nerve in the supraorbital foramen, is a harmless, reproducible and powerful stimulus. It is important to note whether or not the patient tries meaningful defensive maneuvers to ward off the stimulus. It is equally important to note other types of movement, such as decerebrate posturing, during which the patient extends the elbows and internally rotates the shoulders. In decorticate posturing the elbows and fingers are flexed. Serial recording of the stimuli and the patient's responses represents a meaningful characterization of the patient's condition. One should avoid the unqualified use of the terms "coma," "semicoma," and "stupor," since these can be imprecise and therefore misleading.

The following example is used to emphasize this important point:

4 P.M. Slightly confused, awakens with verbal stimulus, thinks he is at home; moves extremities equally well, pupils equal and reactive.

5 P.M. Sleepy, won't talk unless supraorbital pressure is applied, then becomes combative; extremity movements and pupils unchanged.

This information may be recorded by a physician or a nurse. These observations clearly demonstrate to anyone seeing the patient that he has become less responsive and requires neurosurgical investigation. Obviously, no matter how carefully the observed changes are recorded, the information is of no use unless appropriate measures are undertaken when danger signs appear.

Another technique of characterizing the level of consciousness is caloric stimulation for testing of the vestibulo-ocular reflex. If otoscopic inspection reveals an intact tympanic membrane, a 50 cc syringe filled with ice water is used to irrigate the external auditory canal for three minutes, or until an ocular response is obtained. Four types of response are found, depending on the patient's level of consciousness. In deep coma ice water produces no eye movement. Oculocephalic reflexes ("doll's eye" response), elicited by turning the head back and forth, are also absent. As the patient becomes more responsive there is tonic conjugate deviation of the eyes toward the side of the ear being irrigated. As the level of consciousness lightens still further, there is tonic conjugate deviation with a fine nystagmus, the fast component of which is opposite the side being irrigated with ice water. As the patient becomes wakeful there is arousal associated with gross nystagmus, least prominent when the patient looks toward the side being irrigated and most prominent with gaze opposite the side

being irrigated. Oculocephalic reflexes are normally absent in awake individuals.

The pupils are checked for equal diameters and reaction to light (Table 8–2). Minor inequalities may come and go and are not important if they are transient. Direct trauma to the globe produces traumatic mydriasis, which may persist for hours or days. Sympathetic pupillary nerve involvement is uncommon, but an associated Horner's syndrome may account for pupillary inequality. This usually indicates injury to the cervical spinal cord or brachial plexus. With these exceptions, unilateral dilatation of a pupil indicates the presence of an intracranial mass lesion requiring surgical intervention. Bilateral dilated and fixed pupils indicate that the situation is grave, but not invariably fatal, since the loss of pupillary reflexes may be in response to hypoxia or postictal state. Mydriatics should not be used to facilitate the funduscopic examination, since the information gained does not warrant the loss of the important pupillary reaction. The value of examining the optic fundus lies in establishing a baseline for future observation. Papilledema rarely appears sooner than 48 hours following head injury or cerebral hemorrhage.

Cerebral function can be assessed by observing spontaneous or induced movements of the extremities. Sensation is evaluated simultaneously. Speech should be evaluated if the patient's level of consciousness permits. A minor aphasic disturbance may be a valuable initial observation. Hemianopic visual loss may indicate involvement of the optic tract, optic radiation or the occipital cortex. The early presence of decerebrate or decorticate rigidity indicates contusion injury in the brain stem. The late appearance of these responses is due to herniation. Decorticate posturing occurs when the cerebral lesion lies above the red nucleus in the midbrain. Decerebrate posturing results from a lesion below

TABLE 8-2 Changes in Size and Reactivity of the Pupils

Size	Response	Interpretation
3–5 mm bilaterally	Constrict: 2–3 mm	Normal, patient alert
Small (2–3 mm)	Constrict	Diencephalic or hypothalamic lesion (Cheyne-Stokes respiration)
Mid position or slightly enlarged	None (fixed)	Midbrain lesion; patient comatose (neurogenic hyperventilation)
Pinpoint (1–2 mm)	None	Pontine lesion; patient comatose (irregular breathing with inspiratory pause)
Small with ptosis (Horner's) unilateral or bilateral	Constrict	Medullary lesion; patient somnolent (ataxic breathing with irregular pauses and variable tidal volumes)
Dilated 5–7 mm; unilateral first, then bilateral	None (fixed)	III cranial nerve lesion: herniation, aneurysm, diabetic neuropathy. Oculomotor palsy may occur. (Consciousness and respiration depend on level of brain stem involvement)

the red nucleus and above the vestibular nuclei. Flaccid paralysis follows a lesion in the medulla below the vestibular nuclei.

Pupillary dilation associated with coma may be due to transtentorial temporal lobe herniation with secondary oculomotor nerve or brain stem compression (Fig. 8–6). Damage to the optic or oculomotor nerves can be determined by the direct and consensual pupillary reactions to light. The extraocular muscles are not examined individually, but the range and nature

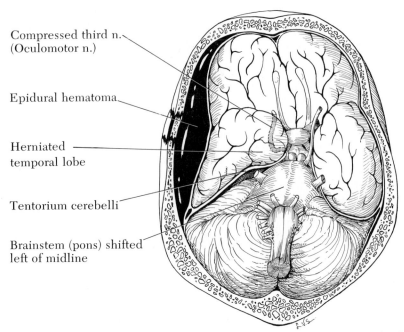

Compressed third n.
(Oculomotor n.)

Epidural hematoma

Herniated
temporal lobe

Tentorium cerebelli

Brainstem (pons) shifted
left of midline

Figure 8–6 Uncal herniation. Diagrammatic representation of compression of the third nerve along the medial edge of the tentorium caused by herniation of the medial temporal lobe (uncus) due to expanding mass lesion compressing and shifting the hemisphere. Clinical signs include ipsilateral dilated pupil, contralateral hemiparesis and deteriorating level of consciousness.

of spontaneous and induced eye movements should be recorded. Eye movements may be elicited by caloric testing or by rapidly turning the head first to one side and then the other (oculocephalic reflex). Dysconjugate eye movements may occur in deep coma or in cases of primary injury to the cerebellum or brain stem.

Facial nerve function is easily examined by observation of the facial response to painful stimuli; an asymmetrical grimace may be seen. Peripheral facial nerve palsy occurs with 20 per cent of basal skull fractures into the ear and may be immediate or delayed in onset. Since lid closure is impaired, the cornea requires protection by temporary closure of the eyelids with a strip of tape that can be removed periodically for inspection of the pupil. The eye should be kept moist if lacrimation is impaired.

Reflex activity has the advantage of neurological objectivity, since re-

sponses are involuntary. The deep tendon and pathological reflexes should be tested. Bilateral Babinski signs are not uncommon in patients with severe head injury, after subarachnoid hemorrhage and in the postseizure state.

Interpretation of Findings

CEREBRAL LESIONS. Hemiparesis with involvement of the lower facial muscles reflects a contralateral cerebral lesion in the corticospinal pathway above the pons. Often a lesion can be localized "by the company it keeps." For example, abrupt onset of such hemiparesis with a contralateral oculomotor palsy unassociated with trauma identifies a midbrain infarction involving the cerebral peduncle and the third cranial nerve. Associated sensory and reflex findings can also be helpful in this regard. Dementia and confusion are nonspecific and may reflect intoxication, metabolic or hypoxic encephalopathy, diffuse brain contusion, increased ICP, hydrocephalus or bilateral frontal lobe mass lesions. Aphasia indicates involvement of the left posterior frontal or anterior parietal regions and should not be mistaken for dementia. Lesions of the visual pathways can often be localized to optic nerve, chiasm, tract, radiation, or occipital cortex by tangent screen visual field examination.

BRAIN STEM LESIONS. Impairment of consciousness with unilateral or bilateral paralytic corticospinal tract lesions, decerebrate or decorticate posturing, cranial nerve involvement and loss of corneal, oculocephalic and gag reflexes may occur in patients with brain stem lesions. These syndromes may present as manifestations of primary hemorrhage, tumor or infarct or as a result of secondary brain stem impairment due to transtentorial herniation.

SPINAL CORD LESIONS. Hemiparesis without facial or trapezius and sternomastoid (XI cranial nerve) involvement indicates that an ipsilateral spinal cord lesion is present below the decussation of the pyramidal tracts. If associated with contralateral loss of pain and temperature sensation (spinothalamic tract), a hemicord lesion is present. The anterior cord syndrome is seen with anterior spinal artery thrombosis or ventral cord compression due to disk herniation, fracture dislocation or tumor. This condition is characterized by bilateral lesions of the corticospinal (motor) and spinothalamic (pain and temperature) tracts, with sparing of the dorsal columns (touch, joint position, vibration). The central cervical cord syndrome occurs in hyperextension injuries and is characterized by upper motor neuron type motor loss (spastic paralysis) in the legs and the lower motor neuron deficit (flaccid paralysis) in the arms, with a variable sensory level located somewhat below the lesion. Quadriplegia localizes the lesion in the cervical cord above the C7 segment, while paraplegia indicates that the lesion is somewhere below T1. Sphincter dysfunction may be present in either case.

A discrete sensory level detected on the trunk helps to localize a spinal fracture or tumor. It is usually found from one to three segments below the site of the lesion. Lesions below the T10 vertebra may present a mixed and predominantly upper or lower motor neuron picture, depending on the relative involvement of lumbosacral nerve roots and the conus medullaris, which is situated at about the L1 level.

NERVE ROOT LESIONS. Cervical and lumbar nerve root lesions are easily localized by sensory, motor and reflex deficit in the arms or legs (Table 8–3). Thoracic nerve roots give rise to the intercostal nerves. Lesions of these nerve roots can be identified by appropriate dermatomal sensory deficits on the thorax and abdomen.

PERIPHERAL NERVE LESIONS. Nerve lesions are most easily identi-

TABLE 8–3 Common Cervical and Lumbar Nerve Root Syndromes

ROOT	REFLEX	MOTOR	SENSORY
C5	Biceps, brachioradialis (slight decrease)	Deltoid	Lateral shoulder and arm
C6	Biceps, brachioradialis (depressed or absent)	Biceps	Thumb and index finger, lateral forearm
C7	Triceps	Triceps and wrist extensors	Index, middle and ring fingers, dorsal forearm
L4	Quadriceps	Quadriceps	Anteromedial thigh and calf
L5	None	Big toe and ankle extensors	Anterolateral calf, dorsum of foot to big toe
S1	Achilles	Triceps surae	Posterolateral calf to fifth toe

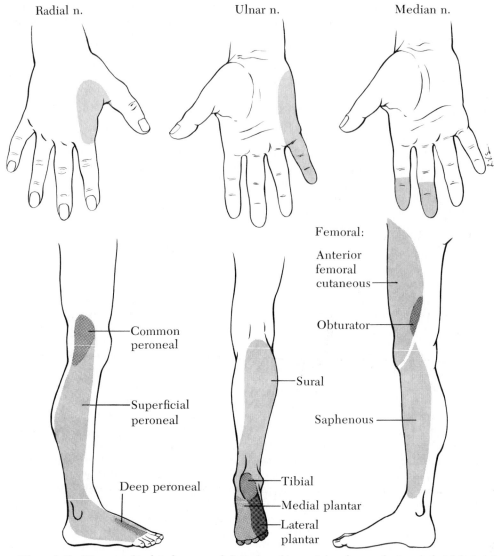

Figure 8–7   Diagram of isolated sensory deficits found in peripheral nerve lesions helpful for brief neurological examination following extremity injuries.

fied in the emergency room by searching for loss of sensation over the small areas of isolated sensory supply indicated in Figure 8–7. Associated motor and reflex deficits may also be present (Table 8–4). Characteristic lesions involve the radial nerve (Saturday night palsy), causing wristdrop, and the peroneal nerve (lotus position palsy), causing footdrop. Pressure-induced le-

sions may exhibit a predominantly motor deficit and are usually reversible.

Neurological Observation

Whenever there is historical, physical or radiographical evidence of head or spine injury, the patient should be

TABLE 8-4 Reflex, Motor and Sensory Deficits in Peripheral Nerve Lesions

Nerve	Reflex	Motor	Sensory
Musculocutaneous	Biceps	Unable to flex elbow	Anterolateral forearm
Axillary	None	Unable to abduct arm at shoulder	Anterolateral shoulder
Radial	Triceps	Unable to extend elbow, wrist, fingers	First dorsal interosseous space
Median	None	Unable to flex wrist, fingers or oppose thumb	Thumb, index, middle and lateral ring fingers
Ulnar	None	Unable to adduct or abduct fingers; claw hand	Little and medial ring finger
Femoral	Quadriceps	Unable to flex hip or extend knee	Anteromedial thigh and medial calf
Common peroneal	None	Unable to extend toes or ankle or evert foot	First dorsal interosseous space, dorsum of foot, lateral calf
Posterior tibial	Achilles	Unable to plantar-flex ankle and toes	Posterior calf and foot
Sciatic		Combination of common peroneal and posterior tibial deficits	

managed with expectant observation. This applies especially to patients who are alcoholics, epileptics and so called "stroke" patients. The following observations should be made and recorded at least every hour:

(1) level of consciousness, response to command and verbal response
(2) pupil size and response to light
(3) vital signs
(4) sensation and movement of extremities
(5) response to appropriate painful stimulus.

Orders should be given to notify the physician of any significant changes that might indicate deterioration. Bradycardia, increase in systolic blood pressure and irregular respirations (the Cushing reflex caused by medullary compression) are late and often irreversible signs of raised intracranial pressure, and thus they are not as helpful as early changes in the patient's level of consciousness, which can lead to beneficial therapeutic intervention.

The importance of neurological observation is understandable when one pauses to consider both the purpose and limitations of neurosurgical treatment. Brain damage occurring at the time of an injury results in immediate deficit that remains fixed. An operation can relieve increased pressure and terminate compression of contiguous structures produced by a hematoma. Fortunately, most hematomas are progressive and announce themselves by causing a gradual further deterioration in a patient's condition. Therefore, if a baseline is established soon after the injury, failure to improve or regression from the baseline status can be recognized as an indication for surgery. Thus any deterioration in a patient's neurological status is an indication to consider the diagnosis of a removable hematoma or mass lesion.

NEUROSURGICAL DIAGNOSTIC PROCEDURES

Radiographic Studies

Plain x-ray films of the skull and spine are valuable when calcification is present or bone changes have occurred, but they often provide only preliminary information. The examiner should then consider using one or more isotope or contrast studies in order to visualize nonradiopaque CNS structures. Skull or spinal tomography may identify or confirm subtle or suspected erosion or fracture in the sella turcica or vertebral pedicles.

In cases of head injury, skull films should be obtained immediately after physical examination and emergency treatment have been completed. Properly positioned films permit recognition of the following:

(1) pineal shift

(2) fracture into a cranial sinus

(3) intracranial air (pneumocephalus)

(4) fracture across the middle meningeal artery groove or a major venous sinus

(5) presence and extent of depressed skull fractures and foreign bodies

(6) evidence of a pre-existing contributory lesion (e.g., neoplastic or congenital).

Echoencephalography

By passing an electrical current through a crystal, a beam of ultrasound can be produced and directed from one side of the skull to the other. Some of the sound waves are deflected by midline structures in the area of the third ventricle, and a characteristic response is produced on the recording apparatus. This is a rapid, safe and noninvasive method of detecting a shift of midline structures — information that is particularly helpful in acute head injuries, especially when a calcified pineal gland cannot be visualized on plain skull x-rays.

Isotope Studies

Isotopes of mercury and other elements have been used for brain scanning, but technetium-99m pertechnetate has the most desirable characteristics. The intravenously injected isotope is preferentially taken up in the brain, where the blood-brain barrier has been disturbed owing to increased vascular permeability, and this area of isotope concentration shows up as a "hot spot" on the read-out of the scan. With high speed repetitive scanning, it is also possible to determine intracranial vascular blood flow patterns.

The flow characteristics of CSF can be studied by isotope cisternography, which involves the lumbar or upper cervical injection of radioiodinated serum albumin (RISA) and scanning during its course through the subarachnoid space. Such a study provides useful information in certain cases of hydrocephalus.

Regional cerebral blood flow can be measured quantitatively by injecting ^{133}xenon into the carotid artery. Such information may be helpful in the diagnosis and management of cerebrovascular disease and other conditions such as trauma, tumor and hemorrhage which indirectly cause cerebral hypoxia. Since puncture or catheterization of the carotid artery and computerized calculations are required, widespread application is not expected until newer intravenous isotope injection techniques are perfected.

Computerized Axial Tomography

A recently developed method of recording relative intracranial tissue densities by transmission through the head of x-ray photons focused from a rotating source provides a noninvasive technique for visualization of the brain, skull and CSF-containing spaces. Using a continuously scanning narrow collimated x-ray beam and system of crystal detectors, 28,000 computer analyzed density readings are obtained. The matrix can be displayed and photographed as a series of transverse axial sections of the cranium either 2.6 or 1.6 cm thick. This detailed anatomic representation often eliminates the need for angiography or pneumoencephalography. Because many lesions such as edema, infarct, hematoma, abscess, cyst and tumor — especially if calcified — have abnormal densities, information can be obtained about the nature and location of intracranial mass lesions. Repeat scanning after intravenous iodinated contrast injection often provides additional information. Ventricular size and position can be visualized in the diagnosis of hydrocephalus or cerebral atrophy.

Myelography

Myelography is useful principally in the study of the spinal canal, although injection of a contrast medium, such as isophendylate (Pantopaque), into the subarachnoid space is used to delineate the cerebellopontine angle and the internal auditory meatus in the posterior fossa. By this technique, contrast medium is introduced into the subarachnoid space via lumbar or cervical puncture. The patient is tilted at various angles, the contrast medium (heavier than CSF) flows by gravity and x-rays are obtained in desired projections at the appropriate level. The defects produced in the dye column by the various pathological entities, such as fracture, tumor, cyst or herniated disk, can be characterized, in general, as extradural, intradural-intramedullary, or intradural-extramedullary. Unless a complete block is present, the contrast medium should be removed (if feasible) at the completion of the study. Water-soluble contrast materials that are absorbed without removal are now becoming available. Air may be used instead of liquid contrast medium but is generally helpful only when hydromyelia is suspected. Contrast medium myelography should not be performed in the presence of a bloody spinal tap because of the increased risk of aseptic arachnoiditis. The finding of a complete myelographical block requires immediate surgical decompression, since rapid deterioration of spinal cord function may follow lumbar puncture below the level of the block owing to an altered pressure differential.

Angiography

The arterial and venous systems of the brain and spinal cord can be visualized by the intra-arterial injection of a water-soluble iodinated contrast medium. If angiography is indicated, it is generally performed before other contrast studies. The contrast material may be injected via a femoral catheter introduced through the aortic arch by the Seldinger technique. All of the extracranial cerebral vessels may be studied separately, including the external and internal carotid and vertebral arteries. Such a study may demonstrate displacement of vessels, anomalous vessels, occlusion or stenosis of vessels, abnormality of the vessel wall, aneurysms and masses. The risk of neurological sequelae following angiography has been reduced by the newer contrast media and improved techniques but has not been eliminated, particularly in elderly patients with cerebrovascular disease. Overnight hospitalization is usually recommended to permit observation for possible complications.

Pneumoencephalography

To perform pneumoencephalography, the basal subarachnoid cisterns and the ventricular system of the brain are gradually filled with increments of air introduced via a lumbar puncture needle as CSF is withdrawn. The study is hazardous in patients with increased intracranial pressure and may precipitate respiratory arrest. Such an occurrence is rare if, after the initial injection of a small volume of air, tomograms are taken to demonstrate the position of the cerebellar tonsils. If the tonsils are found to have herniated through the foramen magnum, the procedure should be terminated.

Pneumoencephalograms are particularly helpful in the study of posterior fossa lesions, sellar and suprasellar lesions, hydrocephalus and atrophic processes. Tomography performed during this study enhances its value. Pneumoencephalography may produce transient fever, headache, nausea, vomiting and vertigo, and a two to three day period of hospitalization is usually required.

Ventriculography

In the presence of papilledema as a sign of increased intracranial pressure, or cerebellar tonsillar herniation, direct study of the ventricular system with air or contrast material may be necessary in place of pneumoencephalography. Such a study is carried out via a burr hole made off the midline at the coronal or lambdoidal suture. Air may then be introduced by ventricular puncture in exchange for CSF. The lateral ventricles and the third ventricle can usually be filled quite satisfactorily by this technique, but visualization of the cerebral aqueduct and the fourth ventricle may be inadequate unless a positive contrast agent is used instead of air. As a rule, the basal cisterns and the subarachnoid space over the hemispheres are not satisfactorily visualized. Definitive surgical treatment nearly always follows immediately after ventriculography, because a patient with a demonstrable lesion may deteriorate rapidly from the effect of injected air on the intracranial dynamics. Ventricular puncture can produce intracerebral hemorrhage, porencephalic cysts, seizures or infection and should be done only when clearly necessary. Occasionally, ventricular taps are done for emergency decompression, for inserting ventricular shunts, for obtaining ventricular fluid for analysis, to introduce an antibiotic agent or to establish continuous monitoring and drainage for control of intracranial pressure.

Electrical Studies

Nervous system function can be evaluated on an outpatient basis by recording the electrical potentials generated in brain, nerve and muscle.

ELECTROMYOGRAPHY (EMG). EMG records muscle and nerve action potentials through needle or skin electrodes. It is helpful in the diagnosis of neuromuscular disorders, particularly in determining the anatomical site of a lesion on an individual peripheral nerve or in separating a diffuse peripheral neuropathy from a single root or nerve lesion. It is sometimes useful in identifying the specific nerve, root or cord segment involved. In conjunction with muscle biopsy, it is frequently helpful in the diagnosis of muscle diseases. In peripheral nerve lesions it can be used to identify the site of nerve compression, to determine whether injury has caused complete or partial loss of conduction and to document regeneration. Muscle denervation potentials may not appear for up to two weeks after nerve or neuronal injury. EMG studies should be normal if muscle weakness is due to an upper motor neuron lesion.

ELECTROENCEPHALOGRAPHY (EEG). EEG records the electrical activity of the cerebral cortex with electrodes placed on the scalp. It is perhaps most useful in identifying and localizing seizure disorders, but diffusely abnormal or localizing patterns may be seen in brain abscesses, subdural hematomas, brain tumors, metabolic disorders and degenerative diseases of the CNS. Although it is a diagnostic procedure without risk, it is useful to the neurosurgeon only as a screening procedure.

Lumbar Puncture

Lumbar puncture (LP) is indicated as an emergency procedure only when meningitis or spontaneous subarachnoid hemorrhage is suspected. It is of little if any value in the management of head injury, since the presence of blood in the CSF is a nonspecific finding that may occur after a mild concussion and be absent in cases of large subdural hematomas. Spinal tap in the presence of increased ICP due to a cerebral lesion may precipitate fatal transtentorial herniation. Unless performed for suspected meningitis or SAH, LP should be avoided or deferred until after arteriography or brain scan has been obtained to rule out the possibility of a large intracranial mass lesion. Performing LP in infants is difficult and should be done only by an experienced physician or pediatrician. Opening and closure pressures should always be measured and recorded and cell count should be performed immediately for accuracy. The Queckenstedt or jugular compression test as a sign of spinal subarachnoid block is not always reliable, but can be carried out as a screening procedure during myelography. The significance of certain CSF findings is presented in Table 8–5. The proper technique of spinal tap is illustrated in Figure 8–8.

EMERGENCY CARE OF THE UNCONSCIOUS OR PARALYZED PATIENT

Emergency Treatment

An adequate airway must be secured and maintained before anything else is done. No procedure takes precedence over the establishment of an adequate airway. Frequently this requires no more than elevation of the sagging mandible or placing the patient in the semiprone position to relieve soft tissue obstruction by tongue and pharynx. Often, especially in the seriously injured patient, insertion of a nasal airway, endotracheal tube or tracheostomy is the wisest course. An oral airway is poorly tolerated and may provoke emesis. The insertion of an endotracheal tube or tracheostomy is done as soon as possible and is recommended if there is any question about airway adequacy. Hypoxia produces cerebral edema, while hypercapnia produces increased intracranial pressure by vasodilatation. In critical situations these factors may tip the balance. It is well to remember that head injury alone usually does not produce dyspnea, cyanosis or stertorous breathing. These are more likely to be the result of injuries to the trachea, chest wall or lungs and require immediate correction. Brief anoxia produces irreversible cerebral damage, and therefore clearing the airway must be given first priority.

Second, active bleeding should be controlled. This generally means securing a lacerated major artery on the face or neck; considerable blood can be lost from a torn superficial temporal artery in the scalp. The bleeding scalp can be controlled temporarily by firm pressure with fingertips or a firm dressing. Persistent bleeding from the scalp is best managed by placing a hemostat upon the galea for retraction and turning it over the scalp edge. It is difficult to place a hemostat directly upon small bleeding vessels. In practice, scalp bleeding is seldom more than a troublesome ooze that usually can be managed by firmly applied sterile dressings.

The third urgent problem is shock, which must be treated immediately without regard for the head injury. Cerebral concussion may be accompanied by a "shock-like" state, the duration of which is a matter of minutes. Other than this, brain injury alone does not produce shock. Rarely is blood loss from the scalp sufficient to produce shock. If shock is present, its cause must be sought in the thorax, abdomen, pelvis or extremities. Administration of blood or blood substitutes is the only method of restoring the cerebral circulation. The Trendelenberg position does not improve cerebral blood flow in the normotensive patient, and venous congestion in the head-down position is deleterious. Conversely, elevation of the top of the patient's bed will improve venous drainage and help to control intracranial pressure.

TABLE 8–5 Significance of CSF Findings

Diagnosis	Pressure	Appearance	Cells	Protein	Glucose
Normal	70–180 (lateral recumbent position)	Clear, colorless	0–5 lymphocytes or monocytes	15–45 mg%	50–80 mg%
Brain tumor	Normal to markedly elevated	Clear	Normal	Normal to increased	Normal
Spine tumor	Normal to decreased	Clear to deep xantho-chromia	Normal or slight increase WBC's	Normal to marked elevation	Normal
Subarachnoid hemorrhage	Normal to extreme elevation	Pink to bloody or xanthochromic if LP delayed	Few RBC's to grossly bloody	Elevated relative to RBC count	Normal to reduced
Bacterial meningitis	Moderate to markedly elevated	Clear, cloudy or purulent	Marked increase (10–50,000 polys)	Moderate to marked elevation	Moderate to marked reduction
Viral meningo-encephalitis	Normal to moderately elevated	Clear, colorless	Slight to moderately increased (100–1,000 lymphs, monos)	Normal to slightly increased	Normal
Brain abscess	Slight to extreme elevation	Clear unless abscess ruptures	Normal to markedly increased WBC's	Normal to markedly increased	Normal or reduced if meningitis associated
Chronic subdural hematoma	Increased or decreased	Clear or xanthochromic	Normal to slightly increased	Normal to slightly increased	Normal
Herniated disk or spondylosis	Normal or decreased if sub-arachnoid block	Clear or xanthochromic below block	Normal	Normal to slight increase	Normal

Care of the Unconscious Patient

(1) Aspiration of vomitus can result in a fatal pneumonitis. Vomiting may be delayed until the second or third day after the ictus, especially when blood is in the stomach. In the unconscious patient it is good practice to insert a nasogastric tube periodically or at-

tach it to gravity drainage if gastric dilation or ileus occurs.

(2) The patient should be turned from side to side into the lateral or semiprone position every two hours. The supine position is best for examination but should not be maintained because of the rapid development of pressure damage to the skin and pulmonary atelec-

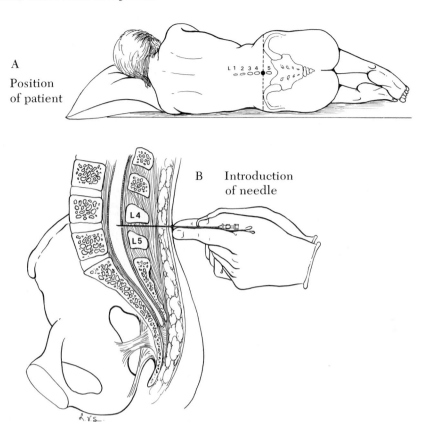

A
Position
of patient

B   Introduction
    of needle

Figure 8–8 *A.* Technique of lumbar puncture. The patient is placed in the knee-chest position on his side to flex the spine separating the spinous processes and enlarging the interlaminar space. *B.* After antiseptic scrub of the skin and injection of local anesthetic, the needle is passed between the L-4 and L-5 spinous processes in the midline, angled slightly superiorly. Letting go of the needle after penetration of the interspinous ligament provides a check of its midline orientation. Advancing the needle slowly may result in a palpable popping sensation as the dura is penetrated. The stylet should be withdrawn every few mm to check for CSF drainage in case dural penetration is not felt. If a bony surface is encountered (spinous process or lamina), the needle must be withdrawn to the subcutaneous layer and re-directed.

Once the dura is penetrated, the needle should be advanced 1 to 2 mm farther and rotated in order to be sure the tip is through the arachnoid. However, puncture of the ventral dura should be avoided, since its anterior surface is covered by epidural veins and a bloody tap may result.

With a stopcock and manometer in place the system's patency can be checked with a Valsalva maneuver or by applying pressure to the patient's abdomen to elevate CSF pressure. Fluid should be collected in two or three tubes for culture, chemistry and cell determinations and both opening and closing pressures measured. After the needle is withdrawn, the patient should be kept supine for six hours to prevent low pressure headaches due to persistent extradural CSF leakage.

tasis in dependent areas of the lungs.

(3) Unless respiratory insufficiency or shock contraindicates it, the top of the bed should be elevated at 20 to 30 degrees to encourage venous return from the head.

(4) The cornea should be protected from drying and abrasion. A strip of tape should be placed over the lid and methylcellulose eyedrops instilled into the conjunctival sac every four hours.

(5) Hyperpyrexia must be treated vigorously; it exhausts the patient's systemic metabolic reserves and adversely affects the damaged brain. A temperature of

100° F or above should be treated vigorously and specific directions provided for measures to reduce it. Hyperpyrexia may be delayed in onset from 12 to 36 hours after brain injury. The body should be kept normothermic by aspirin and cold sponging or hypothermia blanket. Causes of hyperpyrexia other than those directly related to hypothalamic injury should be sought. Systemic infections, such as aspiration pneumonitis, are common in unconscious patients.

(6) Tube feedings may be started at the end of 48 hours if the patient does not have ileus and has not vomited, and if gastric fluid volume recovered by periodic suction is not excessive.

(7) Intravenous fluids should permit a urinary output of about 1000 cc/day. A small number of brain injured patients will retain or lose salt because of hypothalamic damage. Serum electrolytes should be determined at least every other day for one week. Deliberate dehydration should be avoided despite the value of fluid restriction and hyperosmolar diuretics in controlling cerebral edema.

(8) An indwelling urinary catheter facilitates nursing and permits accurate determination of urinary output in the unconscious or uncooperative patient. However, an external condom catheter may be an effective alternative in males.

Special Problems After Head Injury

Seizures occur in 5 per cent of head injuries during the first week, often producing hypoxia. They should be controlled promptly. Many early seizures are focal, thereby indicating that a site of cerebral irritation is due to contusion or hematoma. The occurrence of seizures should be considered an indication for neurosurgical evaluation and CT brain scan or angiography. In the event that status epilepticus occurs, it must be treated vigorously to prevent severe hypoxia. Seizures are best managed with Dilantin (phenytoin). To be immediately effective, Dilantin must be given intravenously in a dosage of 500 mg over a 10 minute period, together with 500 mg by nasogastric tube. The maintenance dose is 300 mg daily. The route of administration and the drug used depend upon the urgency of the situation. Sodium amytal and pentobarbital are respiratory depressants and are poor drugs for emergency seizure control. Phenobarbital or paraldehyde may be used. Valium (diazepam) is also effective.

Restlessness to an extreme degree is uncommon after head injury, and possible reasons for its cause should be sought in a full bladder, an unrecognized extremity fracture, meningismus from subarachnoid hemorrhage or delerium tremens. Wrist and ankle restraints often aggravate the situation and should be used only as a last resort. Side rails and an attendant are preferable to any mechanical restraint. Sedation during the acute phase of cerebral injury depresses respiration and the level of consciousness, and is therefore contraindicated even in minor head injuries.

Basal skull fractures extending into the middle ear or paranasal air sinuses commonly accompany severe head injuries, although they may also be seen in association with relatively minor trauma. Those involving the temporal bone are readily diagnosed by otoscopic examination demonstrating hemotympanum, or by the observation of blood or cerebrospinal fluid draining from the ear. Fractures into the frontal and ethmoid sinuses should be suspected in all patients with facial injuries. The diagnosis is established by observing cerebrospinal fluid rhinorrhea. However, this may go undetected in the supine unconscious patient. Fractures into the frontal, ethmoid, sphenoid and mastoid sinuses may not be visible on radiographs. These are considered compound fractures by virtue of their communication through a torn mucous membrane into an air-containing cavity. Their treatment requires parenteral prophylactic antibiotic coverage for five to seven days, or longer if leakage of cerebrospinal fluid persists. The conscious patient with cerebrospinal fluid rhinorrhea should be cautioned not to blow his nose. Since pneumococcus is the pathogen in 80 per cent of cases of post-traumatic meningitis, penicillin (20 million units/day) is the antibiotic regimen of choice.

Respiratory and Vasomotor Dysfunction After Spinal Cord Injury

Patients with cord injuries at the C3 level may become apneic because of loss of phrenic nerve outflow to the diaphragm. Intubation or tracheostomy and controlled ventilation will be necessary. Lower cervical or thoracic cord lesions result in a typical rocking pattern of abdominal or diaphragmatic respiration. Innervation of the intercostal and chest wall muscles is lost, and respiratory excursions are accomplished only by contractions of the diaphragm. Tidal volume and arterial blood gases must be monitored at regular intervals. Vigorous pulmonary toilet is required to prevent atelectasis and pneumonia, because coughing may be ineffectual and pooling of bronchial and tracheal secretions may result.

Because sympathetic nervous system outflow may also be eliminated in cervical or upper thoracic cord injuries, hypotension and bradycardia may occur with loss of compensatory responses following change in position or posture. Systolic pressures of 60 mm Hg and pulse rates of 40 per minute may be observed. Perfusion, however, may be well maintained in a supine position. Treatment consists of intravenous volume supplement and administration of atropine (0.4 mg) to attenuate the release of parasympathetic inhibition. Great care must be exercised during turning and transportation of such patients. Elastic stockings should be used to improve venous return from the legs and to prevent stasis and thrombophlebitis leading to pulmonary embolism.

Transfer and Transportation

Trauma patients suspected of having a spinal fracture must be moved with as little change of spine position from neutral posture as possible, to avoid causing or aggravating dislocation. Often this requires having three or even four attendants present during transfer to ensure proper support for the head, spine and pelvis. Transfers should be minimized until appropriate x-rays have been obtained and this should be done if possible while the patient remains on a stretcher, either in the emergency room or in the x-ray department. If a cervical fracture is suspected, manual traction can be instituted during transfer, and halter traction can be applied during ambulance or air transportation if cranial tongs are not available. In either case, neutral posture should be maintained with traction applied in the line of spinal axis. Thoracic and lumbar spine fractures present less of a problem during transportation, since the ribs and abdominal musculature provide some stabilization.

A network of specialized regional spinal cord injury centers is now being established in the United States with federal government support. Helicopter transportation by trained paramedic teams, accompanied when necessary by the receiving physician, will become available in many areas of the country.

Insertion of Cranial Tongs

When a fracture, dislocation or potentially unstable fracture involving the cervical spine is identified by x-ray examination, insertion of cranial tongs may be indicated for skeletal traction. The fracture can be stabilized and closed reduction can often be accomplished with stepwise addition of increments of additional weight applied while changes in vertebral alignment are monitored with serial x-ray films. Closed reduction can be hazardous and should be carried out by an experienced orthopedist or neurosurgeon. If such consultation is not available, tongs can be readily inserted in any emergency facility, and the patient transported by ambulance or air transport on a Stryker frame or a stretcher especially equipped with traction pulley.

A set of Gardner cranial tongs should be available in any emergency facility organized to receive trauma cases. These tongs can be quickly and safely applied under local anesthesia without scalp incision or cranial drilling (Fig. 8–9). Simple instructions are printed on a metal tag attached to the tongs. The scalp should be widely shaved and thoroughly prepared above the ears. The skull prongs are positioned 3 cm above the pinnae in a vertical line with the external auditory canal and tightened down until firmly fixed to the skull with appropriate tension monitored by the indicator pins. Ten to fifteen pounds of weight can then be applied to maintain vertebral alignment. Additional weight should not be required unless closed reduction is being attempted.

Indications For Cranial Surgery

COMPOUND WOUNDS. Compound wounds require special consideration. These are injuries in which the intracranial or intraspinal contents are in communication with air through the scalp, sinuses or skin. Patients with open wounds seldom deteriorate rapidly unless they have been fatally injured; missile injuries account for most exceptions to this rule. They usually tolerate transfer by ambulance or by air to a hospital equipped for major cranial surgery. Compound or open wounds must be adequately debrided with watertight reapproximation of the dura and accurate closure of the scalp or skin. Unrecognized or inadequately treated compound skull or spinal fractures may lead to fatal infection.

Emergency treatment before transfer consists of applying a sterile dressing over the wound. Rarely will active bleeding from the scalp or exposed cerebral or paraspinous vessels constitute a problem. No attempt should be made to remove the clotted blood or exposed tissues since this will merely activate bleeding and produce further contamination. Initial surgery should be definitive; therefore, nothing beyond the application of a sterile dressing is indicated prior to transfer. Although treatment of compound cerebral or spinal cord injuries should not be delayed unnecessarily, these injuries do not take precedence over life-threatening catastrophes such as intra-abdominal hemorrhage. The patient should be observed until it is apparent that the vital signs are stable and that transfer for neurosurgical attention may be safely carried out. Definitive débridement may be delayed for up to 24 hours if circumstances warrant, provided that prophylactic antibiotic therapy is started promptly.

Depressed skull fractures with an intact scalp are treated as closed head injuries. The underlying brain damage occurs at the moment of impact and continued presence of the depressed bone fragments requires elective elevation only if the depression is greater than 5 mm. Spinal fracture dislocations with more than 2 mm subluxation require reduction with traction unless the presence of "locked" facets or comminuted bone fragments require operative realignment.

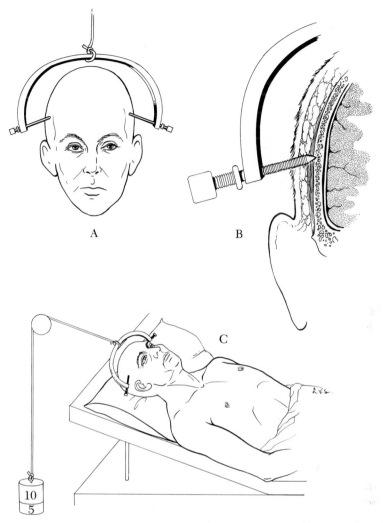

Figure 8–9 Diagram showing techniques of skeletal traction for cervical fracture. *A.* Gardner-Wells tongs are inserted under local anesthesia after shaving and scrubbing the scalp bilaterally above the ears. *B.* Pins are inserted 6 to 8 cm above the external auditory canal. *C.* 10 to 15-lb weights are attached over traction pulley and the head of the bed is elevated to provide counter-traction.

INTRACRANIAL HEMATOMAS. Subarachnoid hemorrhage, common even in trivial head injuries, is unimportant. However, blood in significant quantity can collect on either side of the dura mater or within the brain. Extradural and subdural hematomas are situated on the surface of the brain and are accessible through a trephine opening in the skull. Intracerebral hematoma is uncommon, and it is most often seen with compound depressed fractures.

Extradural hemorrhage is a true neurosurgical emergency. A typical case will have a history of minor trauma producing a short period of unconsciousness (concussion) followed by a lucid interval of one to six hours followed by signs of rapidly progressive compression of one cerebral hemisphere and oculomotor nerve and, ultimately, the brain stem. A fracture crossing the middle meningeal groove is often present. After an initial complaint of headache, weakness of one side of the body appears with dilation of the pupil on the opposite side. The evolution of extradural hematomas is rapid, because blood under arterial pressure is being pumped into the extradural compartment from a torn middle meningeal artery. Compression of the brain by hematoma must be relieved immediately. This patient cannot be transferred to another hospital; time is critical. The blood clot must be evacuated

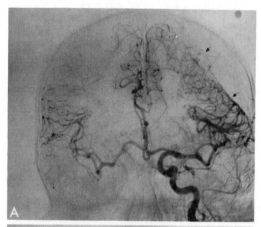

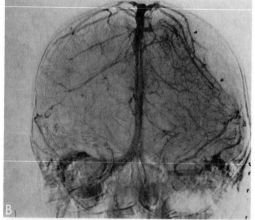

Figure 8–10 Anteroposterior left carotid arteriogram in the arterial *(A)* and venous *(B)* phases performed during manual compression of the right common carotid to visualize vessels of both cerebral hemispheres. The large extracerebral space (arrows) demonstrated over the left frontoparietal convexity causes little shift of the midline vessels. This liquefied subacute subdural hematoma was removed through burr holes. *C.* CT brain scan in another patient showing acute subdural hematoma (high density extracerebral space) causing shift of the ventricles and midline structures.

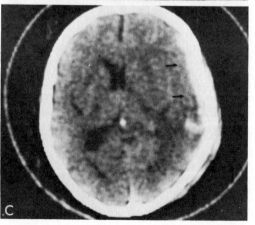

and this can be done through a low anterior temporal trephine that has been enlarged with rongeurs (see the section on Emergency Surgery of the Epidural Hematoma). It is important to make an opening in the skull large enough to allow the entire clot to extrude. The hematoma usually underlies the fracture site and the first burr hole should be made there. The torn meningeal artery can be coagulated, clipped or transfixed with sutures. In order to prevent irreversible brain damage, the surgeon on the spot must operate as soon as the diagnosis is suggested. A neurosurgeon can be summoned, but evacuation of the hematoma should not be delayed until he arrives.

Subdural hemorrhage can also be acute, causing rapid deterioration and necessitating surgery in the first few hours after injury (Fig. 8–10). Here the problem is different. The bleeding is arterial but is caused by laceration of the brain, with tearing of cerebral arteries. Brain damage is characteristically severe and the acute subdural bleeding is coincidental. Following evacuation of these hematomas, the lacerated and contused brain swells rapidly, and he-

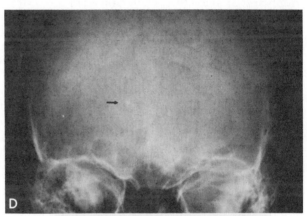

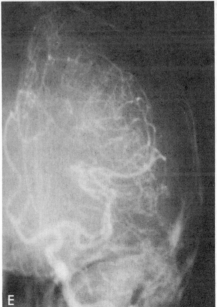

Figure 8–10 *Continued.* Acute subdural hematoma. Calcified pineal (arrow) is shifted to the right on the AP skull x-ray and extradural space (*D*) is seen on the left carotid arteriogram (*E*).

matoma removal may be of little value. The mortality rate for acute subdural hematoma is over 80 per cent. Often a subacute subdural hematoma with minimal associated brain damage is encountered. The source of bleeding is usually a torn sinus or bridging cerebral vein. Treatment here requires extensive craniotomy for hematoma removal and results may be gratifying.

Chronic subdural hematomas manifest themselves 3 to 12 weeks after injury. A vein bridging from the cortex to the superior sagittal sinus is torn; resultant venous bleeding is slow and it arrests spontaneously. Encapsulation, clot liquefaction and secondary enlargement produce the delayed onset of signs and symptoms. Drainage through exploratory burr holes is curative.

Subacute subdural hematomas are intermediate between acute and chronic hematomas. Headache, progressive somnolence and a generally unfavorable course prompt investigation at some time beyond the third day after injury. In this instance, the outlook is more favorable for satisfactory recovery. Sometimes, particularly with a subacute evolution, one encounters a subdural hygroma rather than a hematoma. A hygroma consists of xanthochromic cerebrospinal fluid, probably resulting from a tear in the arachnoid, permitting one way flow of CSF into the subdural space. A hygroma cannot clinically be differentiated from a hematoma and it also responds to drainage through burr holes.

Corticosteroids, hyperventilation and the use of a hyperosmolar mannitol solution to decrease cerebral edema have a place in the treatment of closed head injuries causing diffuse cerebral contusion and edema. In the patient with a severe head injury who has increased intracranial pressure produced by cerebral edema, rather than a hematoma, Decadron (dexamethasone), 10 mg IV, may be given initially, with 4 mg repeated every four hours. The only means for excluding a hematoma as the cause of increased pressure are angiography, CT brain scan, ventriculography or burr holes and craniotomy. A ventricular cannula introduced through a burr hole or a twist drill opening will permit monitoring of intracranial pressure and removal of CSF. Controlled ventilation with arterial pCO$_2$ levels of 24 mm Hg may significantly reduce intracranial pressure. Mannitol, 25 per cent, given intravenously (1 gm per kg) may rapidly reverse signs of tentorial herniation while the patient is being taken to surgery for evacuation of a hematoma. Given repeatedly in smaller doses, it may be helpful in controlling ICP in diffuse brain injury.

In summary, an adequate airway, maintenance of blood volume, recognition and treatment of associated injuries and the provision of supportive and protective care for an unconscious patient are the principles on which to base management of this problem. Regression from initial baselines indicates a dynamic process that warrants investigation to exclude or establish the existence of a surgically correctable lesion.

Indications for Spinal Surgery

Other than for débridement and dural closure in compound or penetrating spinal cord injuries, emergency surgical decompression and open fracture reduction are indicated only under the following circumstances:

(1) bone fragments present in the spinal canal
(2) failure of closed spinal reduction
(3) progressive neurological deficit suggesting intraspinal hematoma or cord swelling
(4) partial or incomplete neurological deficit with a myelographic block at the site of injury.

Careful neurological observation is also required following severe spinal injuries in which neurological deficit is present or anticipated.

Prognosis

Mortality rates for epidural hematomas remain in the 25 to 30 per cent range for patients who are unconscious at the time of surgery, but drop to 3 per cent for those who are verbally responsive preoperatively.[1] The mortality rate climbs to 80 per cent if an associated subdural hematoma is found at a different location. Acute subdural hematoma is associated with a mortality rate of 60 to 90 per cent.[3] The outcome of a closed head injury causing major cerebral contusion with or without removal of hematoma is poor. Only a 20 to 30 per cent survival rate can be expected after prolonged traumatic unconsciousness.[2] Concomitant occurrence of coma, pupillary dilatation, decorticate or decerebrate posturing and loss of oculocephalic and other brain stem reflexes is associated with little chance of recovery.

Recovery from spinal cord injury depends upon the extent of initial irreversible tissue damage and the effectiveness and rapidity of treatment in preventing further loss of neurological function. Immediate onset of complete paraplegia or quadriplegia usually is indicative of a spinal cord laceration or major contusion, and significant recovery cannot be expected. Patients with partial deficits, especially when the onset is delayed, have a good to fair prognosis. This is particularly true when spinal cord decompression, if present, is relieved. Prognosis of lesions involving the cauda equina, spinal nerve roots and peripheral nerves is better, since they are less vulnerable to injury and have a potential for regeneration.

EMERGENCY SURGERY FOR EPIDURAL HEMATOMA

Instruments

Any hospital with facilities for major surgery should be equipped to perform burr holes for epidural hematoma. The following instruments should be available, in addition to the standard surgical set:

Hudson brace
McKenzie perforator
Cushing burr
Periosteal elevator
Penfield #3 dissector
Mastoid retractor or Weitlaner self-retaining tissue retractor
Angled double action rongeur
Frazier suction tip
Bone wax
Electrocautery unit

Surgical Procedure (Figure 8–11)

1. The skin incision is vertically placed 1 inch in front of the ear, extending from the superior extent of the temporalis muscle to the zygomatic arch. Do not go below the zygoma, or the upper facial nerve will be transected.
2. The temporalis muscle is stripped from its attachment and a self-retaining retractor is positioned.
3. A burr hole is made in the temporal bone directly above the zygomatic arch and enlarged with a rongeur. The middle meningeal artery will be exposed as the hematoma is evacuated. Bleeding is controlled with electrocautery, ligatures and bone wax; oozing from the dura can be controlled with Gelfoam and gentle pressure. If bleeding cannot be stopped the wound may be packed, and the patient can then be transferred to a neurosurgical center.
4. If no hematoma is present at the first site of exploration, a second hole should be made over any existing fracture line.
5. Closure is carried out in layers with interrupted sutures placed in the temporalis muscle, fascia and scalp.

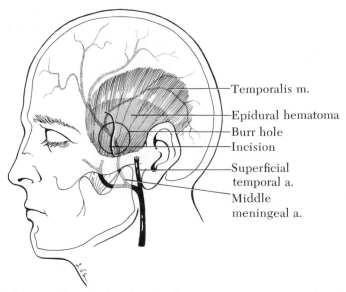

Temporalis m.
Epidural hematoma
Burr hole
Incision
Superficial
temporal a.
Middle
meningeal a.

Figure 8–11 Diagram of surgical technique for emergency evacuation of epidural hematoma showing scalp and temporalis muscle incision as well as burr hole and craniectomy in relation to the lacerated middle meningeal artery (see text).

REPAIR OF SCALP LACERATIONS

Adequate repair of scalp lacerations requires special attention to basic surgical principles of wound care as well as familiarity with certain unique anatomical features of this crucial cranial covering. The scalp is vascular, vulnerable and hidden under hair. It overlies cranial bone and brain. Infection of a scalp wound can lead to osteomyelitis, meningitis and brain abscess, any one of which can be fatal. However, in most cases scalp lacerations can be treated safely and definitively on an outpatient basis.

The scalp must be examined carefully and systematically, especially in individuals with long hair. Not all deep lacerations bleed profusely enough to become obvious during casual inspection. Once located, even a relatively superficial laceration should be exposed by clipping and shaving the hair from an adequate area of surrounding scalp. If the laceration is extensive it is best to shave the entire scalp. In our experience, inadequate shaving is the most common factor responsible for late scalp wound infection.

Cleansing by profuse irrigation, using one to three liters of sterile saline solution, is essential. Fragments of hair, hat, glass, road dust or cinders must be removed with a sterile hemostat or forceps. Obviously devitalized tissue should be debrided. However, débridement should be accomplished sparingly because closure of large defects may be difficult and tension on the wound edges must be avoided. Buried glass or metallic fragments can be located by x-ray. Routine closure of linear scalp lacerations can usually be accomplished in the emergency room under local anesthesia. However, pain or associated intoxication may result in unmanageable restlessness and agitation when effective sedation is contraindicated because of the patient's head injury. Often such problems can be more easily taken care of after a few hours' delay. Otherwise, small lacerations must be left unsutured and large ones repaired under general anesthesia in the operating room. As a rule, infants and young children can be adequately managed with reassurance and the use of moderate restraints.

Use of local anesthesia containing epinephrine may be helpful both in controlling troublesome scalp bleeding and in prolonging anesthesia. Cutaneous innervation of the scalp occurs through the supraorbital, temporal, auricular and occipital nerves, as illustrated in Figure 8–12. Regional and field blocks are useful for larger injuries but direct infiltration of the margins of a small laceration will suffice.

The layers of the scalp include the integument, subcutaneous layer, galea aponeurotica, subaponeurotic areolar layer and pericranium (Fig. 8–13). Larger scalp vessels such as the supraorbital, superficial temporal and occipital arteries and veins course through the galea and may require ligation (Fig. 8–14). Often they retract several millimeters back from the laceration after injury and begin bleeding

again during irrigation, débridement or suturing. Although major bleeding from scalp injuries usually ceases spontaneously, it is important to recall that subgaleal hematoma in infants can result in significant hypovolemia requiring blood replacement.

Contaminated scalp lacerations are best closed with a single layer of deep interrupted vertical mattress sutures using a nonabsorbable material such as 3-0 or 4-0 nylon or stainless steel wire. Care must be taken to include the galea in the deeper needle passage to assure hemostasis and provide support to the closure by reapproximating this strong fascial layer (Fig. 8–15). Use of skin tapes or fine superficially placed sutures alone for delicate plastic closure, even in front of the hairline, is contraindicated unless the laceration is superficial and the deep layers remain intact. To prevent infection, buried suture material should be avoided. Closure in a single layer is to be contrasted with the customary two layer closure of clean

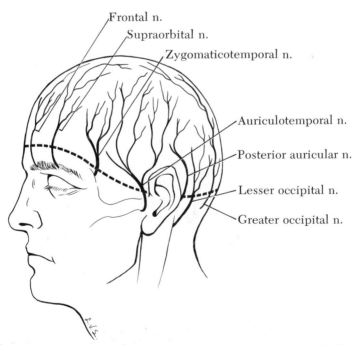

Figure 8–12 Diagram illustrating cutaneous nerve supply of the scalp. Infiltration along the dotted line provides regional anesthesia suitable for repair of large scalp lacerations.

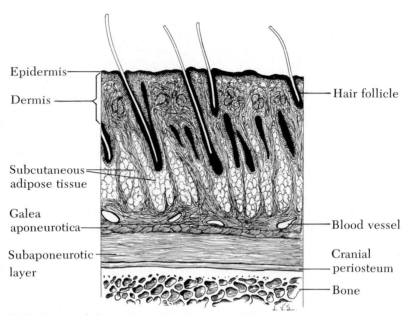

Figure 8–13 Layers of the scalp. Attention to anatomical details demonstrated is essential for accurate repair of scalp lacerations (see text). Note that depth of galea varies, depending on the thickness of the subcutaneous layer.

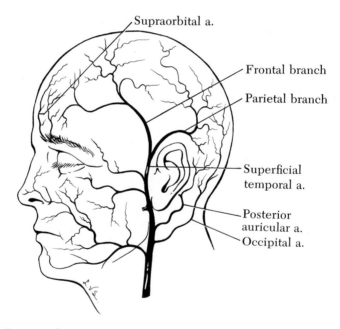

Figure 8–14 Diagram of arterial supply of the scalp. Cutaneous bleeding can be controlled with proximal pressure over appropriate vessel. Survival of scalp flap or graft depends on relation to nutrient arteries.

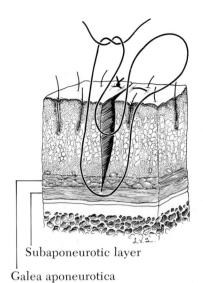

Subaponeurotic layer

Galea aponeurotica

Figure 8–15 Technique for placement of vertical mattress sutures. Including the galea in each stitch is facilitated by grasping and everting it with teeth forceps (see text).

surgical scalp incisions, in which the galea is appropriately closed with buried inverted interrupted sutures. Small patch dressings can be applied with collodion, tincture of benzoin or other adhesives, followed by a stockinet cap or rolled gauze bandage when the patient's scalp has not been shaved extensively. Sutures should not be removed until 10 to 14 days after a single layer scalp closure.

Small stellate scalp lacerations are commonly seen after scalp injuries by a blunt object or surface. If skin tags remain viable, they should not be excised but rather should be sutured loosely, approximated with sterile skin tapes or left to heal by secondary intention (Fig. 8–16).

Because of generous vascularity and extensive collateral blood supply, scalp injuries generally heal well. Although delayed primary closure of a grossly contaminated or devitalized wound is always hazardous, relatively clean and sharp scalp lacerations can be closed primarily without undue risk of complication even if six to eight hours have elapsed since the time of injury. This is especially true if the wound was

cleaned and dressed initially. However, such patients should be hospitalized for observation or seen daily for dressing change.

Avulsion or crush injuries leaving large scalp defects require hospitalization for repair in the operating room by the neurosurgeon or plastic surgeon. Rotation of scalp flaps or extensive undermining with relaxing incisions may be required for adequate coverage of any areas of exposed cranium. Granulation for adequate secondary healing or later skin grafting will occur only if the scalp avulsion is not of full thickness or if pericranium has been spared. When coverage is not possible because of the large size of a defect, as seen following scalp burns, removal of the outer cranial cortical bone may stimulate granulation from the diploë. Craniectomy may be necessary to promote granulation from the underlying dura, especially if the situation has been complicated by scalp infection or osteomyelitis.

Large hemicranial or cranial scalp flaps can be elevated or avulsed in unusual injuries caused by broken auto windshields, long hair caught in wheels, propellers, rotating farm or in-

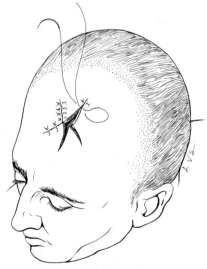

Figure 8–16 Stellate scalp laceration. These can usually be closed loosely after cautious débridement (see text).

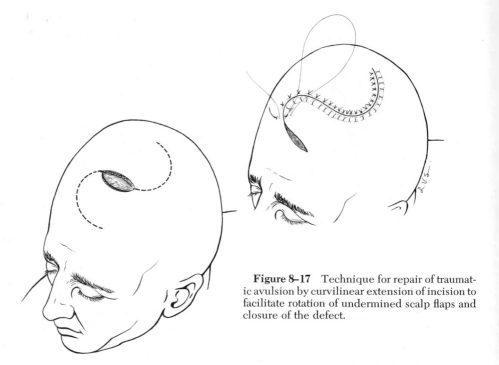

Figure 8–17 Technique for repair of traumatic avulsion by curvilinear extension of incision to facilitate rotation of undermined scalp flaps and closure of the defect.

dustrial equipment or machete attack. Using microsurgical techniques for anastomosis of several scalp arteries and veins, even completely free scalp flaps can be reimplanted successfully. Therefore, large avulsed scalp segments should be cleansed, packed in iced saline and transported to the neurosurgical center with the patient.

Small areas (2 to 3 cm) of scalp avulsion can be covered primarily by extending short curvilinear incisions in either direction, as shown in Figure 8–17. Hospitalization may be required for only 24 to 48 hours under such circumstances, if the wound was not unduly contaminated.

ELECTIVE OUTPATIENT NEUROSURGICAL PROCEDURES

Nerve and Muscle Biopsy

Nerve and muscle biopsy may be requested for diagnostic purposes by the neurologist, pediatrician or internist evaluating a case of suspected degenerative or inflammatory neuropathy or myopathy. Sural nerve and gastrocnemius muscle tissue are best obtained under local anesthesia through a 4 to 6 cm vertical incision extending superiorly above the lateral malleolus, lateral to and parallel with the Achilles tendon (Fig. 8–18). The nerve can be identified lying upon the fascia and must be carefully isolated from the vein it accompanies. Branching occurs at the ankle level. The proximal nerve end should be amputated by undermining above the incision to prevent painful neuroma formation within the incisional scar. Postoperatively, only minimal sensory deficit will be detectable along the lateral aspect of the foot.

Excision of Dermal Lesions

Most intra- or subdermal lesions, such as sebaceous cysts or lipomas, can be removed in an outpatient surgical facility (but see "Congenital Anomal-

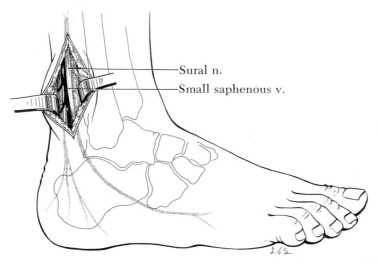

Sural n.
Small saphenous v.

Figure 8–18 Diagram of exposure for sural nerve biopsy. Note that the nerve parallels the lesser saphenous vein, which must be carefully isolated and divided without injuring the nerve.

ies and Hydrocephalus" for differential diagnosis of congenital dysplasias, spina bifida and encephalocele). Scalp and paraspinous skin incisions should be closed in two layers. Large scalp lesions may not be easily exposed and isolated through a straight linear incision. An "S" shaped curvilinear incision or an inverted "U" shaped flap placed over the lesion and based toward the source of blood supply may facilitate retraction, exposure, hemostasis and wound healing. Integrity of the pericranium is maintained by sharply undermining the scalp in the subgaleal plane of areolar tissue. Removable metal skin clips (Michel) are helpful for controlling cranial or spinal skin bleeding, as are small self-retaining retractors (mastoid or Weitlaner).

Peripheral Nerve Decompression

Certain operations for decompression of subcutaneously located peripheral nerves can be carried out safely with a 24 to 48 hour hospital stay. Transverse carpal ligament section for median nerve entrapment (carpal tunnel syndrome) and ulnar nerve transposition for ulnar nerve entrapment (tardy ulnar palsy) can be performed under local or regional anesthesia. If neurological function is improved or stable within one or two days after surgery, no wound complications have developed, and incisional pain is not excessive, early discharge for outpatient postoperative care is in order.

REFERENCES

1. Jamieson, K. G., and Yelland, J. D. N.: Extradural hematoma. J. Neurosurg., 29:13–23, 1968.
2. Jennett, B., and Teasdale, G.: Aspects of coma after severe head injury. Lancet, April 23, 1977, pp. 878–881.
3. Richards, T., and Hoff, J.: Factors affecting survival from acute subdural hematoma. Surgery, 75:253–258, 1974.

GENERAL REFERENCES FOR ADDITIONAL READING

Jamieson, K. G.: A First Notebook of Head Injury. Boston, Butterworths, 1971.
Youmans, J. R. (Ed.): Neurological Surgery. Philadelphia, W. B. Saunders, 1973.

The Integument 9

R. C. A. WEATHERLEY-WHITE, M.D.,
and MALCOLM A. LESAVOY, M.D.

THE REPAIR OF INJURIES

Principles of Wound Healing

The fundamental aim of the surgeon faced with a disruption of the integument is to ensure that the wound heals as rapidly as possible and with the minimum of complications. This axiom, seemingly self-evident, is valid for the optimum care of all injuries, whether they are simple incised lacerations or major wounds involving loss of tissue, crushing or burns. Too often, however, in the emergency situation, principles of tissue management are neglected, with the predictable consequences of decreased tensile strength and unsightly hypertrophic scarring.

The process of wound healing is complicated, and a detailed description would be out of place in this context. For a review of the intricate responses of the body to injury, Schilling's monograph is complete and up to date.[16] However, a brief summary is pertinent to a discussion of the factors known to inhibit wound healing.

Immediately following injury and surgical repair, a nonspecific inflammatory response takes place, the object of which is to enhance the circulation to the wound. Phagocytes remove clot, necrotic tissue and bacterial inhabitants of the injured skin, and undifferentiated cells from the circulation migrate into the injury to undergo metamorphosis into fibroblasts. Endothelial budding takes place in the capillaries adjacent to the injury, and these anastomose across the interface of the wound to produce microvascular continuity. At this stage (one to three days following injury) the only tensile strength to the repair resides in the sutures holding the wound edges together, with some weak assistance from fibrin and mucopolysaccharide ground substance deposited at the interface.

The main constituent giving strength to the healed wound is collagen, produced by the proliferating fibroblasts in three to ten days following injury. Although collagen production is at a maximum at the end of this period, there is still relatively little strength to the wound. It is the covalent cross-linking of single strands of tropocollagen into the triple helices of mature collagen and the orientation of these molecules that provide the ultimate tensile strength to the healed wound. This alignment process takes several weeks and is dependent largely upon tension. Finally, the scar tissue produced by this sequence of events softens and matures over a number of months until there is little histological evidence of previous injury.

In our present state of knowledge, it can be stated that there is an optimum rate of wound healing. Apart from some controversial studies involving the deposition of powdered cartilage in the wound,[15] there is no evidence that the surgeon's dream — the acceleration of wound healing — can be accomplished. All we can do is avoid known inhibitory factors.

These inhibitory factors may be conveniently subdivided into systemic and local influences. There will be little time in the acute care of the injured patient to diagnose, let alone restore to normal, systemic deficiencies known to affect adversely the normal progress of wound healing. In elective outpatient procedures, however, these deficiencies should be investigated and treated as carefully as they are before major operations, for they will have an equivalent adverse effect.

The two main systemic factors involved in the inhibition of wound healing are anemia and protein deficiency. It is known that skin grafts rarely "take" when the hematocrit is less than 35 per cent. This specific clinical situation serves well as an experimental model for wound healing in general. Dunphy[5] has pointed out that the principal cause of delayed wound healing is a decreased oxygen tension at the site of the wound; certainly correction of a pre-existing anemia is necessary to avoid this situation. Hypoproteinemia will result in a decreased number of proliferating fibroblasts, with a consequent shortage of collagen, the single most important constituent of the healed wound. Other systemic factors known to be implicated in healing include the deficiency of vitamin C and the trace element zinc, and recently Peacock has given us insight into the biomechanics of collagen cross-linking through his experimental use of beta-amino-proprionitrile, the active agent in lathyrism, a connective tissue disease.[14]

It is, however, the local factors that are most directly under the control of the operating surgeon and are, unfortunately, the most abused. Of these, infection is the prime offender. In the presence of infection, not only will cellular proliferation of all types cease, but tissue already laid down will necrotize. The recurrence rate of repaired inguinal hernias is over 50 per cent when there has been an operative infection; many times the surgeon involved in the care of burns has seen apparently well-taken skin grafts "melt" when adjacent granulating tissue becomes grossly infected.

Hematoma in the wound not only

will provide the substrate for bacterial growth, but will in itself, by virtue of its space-occupying nature, produce tension on the wound edges and attenuate the capillary blood supply to the interface, thus causing a decreased tissue Po_2 at the critical location. Hematoma must be recognized immediately, drained and irrigated, and if possible any active bleeding should be identified and terminated.

Undue tension on the wound per se will unquestionably harm the quality of healing. Its short-term effect is the jeopardy of blood supply; it has long-term effects on the cross-linking and alignment of mature collagen fibers. Not only will the wound brought together under tension and held in place only by means of tight constricting sutures heal with an unsightly spread scar (an important factor on the face), but the tensile strength in the wound will be measurably decreased.

Arterial insufficiency and venous stasis (both resulting in decreased tissue Po_2) are most commonly seen by the plastic surgeon engaged in the preparation of a skin flap for transfer. Frequently, injured patients will manifest a "flap" partially separated from its source of blood supply; in this case, an individual surgical judgment will have to be made as to the viability of the tissue.

Control of local factors known to inhibit wound healing involve the Halstedian principles of surgical technique first introduced to the medical student in the "dog lab" and reinforced, it is hoped, throughout surgical residence. These include rigid asepsis, immaculate hemostasis and gentle handling of tissue.

There is no excuse for slipping a pair of gloves over unwashed hands and, with face unadorned by a mask, suturing a laceration whose edges have been perfunctorily dabbed with antiseptic solution. These techniques would not be tolerated in the operating room, and outpatient care should be no less immaculate.

A thorough (five minute) wash of the adjacent skin with pHisoHex or any of the surgical soap solutions can be regarded as an adequate skin preparation. Copious irrigation of the wound itself with sterile saline solution will serve to flush out debris carried into the wound at the time of injury. Following injection of a local anesthetic, the wound should be inspected carefully and any foreign material not removed by irrigation picked out. Retained foreign bodies (glass fragments, shreds of clothing, road dirt, and so on) will either cause immediate infection or, if walled off by a fibrous capsule, may necessitate secondary removal.

Ragged wound edges are best trimmed to straight lines to effect a neat linear scar, and any devitalized or grossly contaminated tissue must be debrided to prevent infection (Fig. 9–1). These measures may result in a

A

B

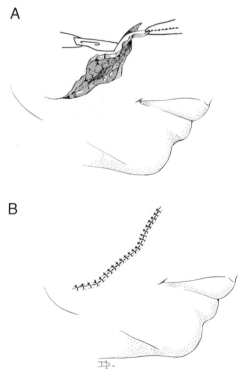

Figure 9–1 Trimming the ragged or devitalized skin edge to produce a clean linear closure.

modest tissue deficit, the suturing of which would be possible only under some tension. This undesirable situation may be averted by the judicious undermining of adjacent skin for a centimeter or so at a level between the underside of the dermis and the subjacent fat, separating the fibrous septa that are holding the wound edges apart. The laceration may then be closed in layers (to minimize dead space) and the skin sutured with fine silk or nylon under little or no tension. When a major loss of tissue has occurred, the surgeon will have to decide whether wide undermining will allow the wound to be closed directly or whether a skin graft will be needed to resurface the defect. In general, if the skin sutures are seen to blanch the skin when it is brought together, closure is under *too great tension,* and alternative methods must be sought.

Hemostasis must be absolute, and particular care must be paid to potentially serious bleeders when epinephrine has been used in the local anesthetic injected. Severed vessels that are constricted under the influence of the agent and do not show obvious bleeding at the time of repair may well "cut loose" several hours after the patient has been discharged from the Emergency Room. Immobilization and a firm pressure dressing will help prevent hematoma formation. All sutured lacerations should be inspected the following day to detect hematoma or infection so that appropriate measures may be taken to forestall their known inhibitory effect on healing.

Handling of tissue should be gentle and should superimpose no additional necrosis to that of the injury itself. The use of skin hooks rather than forceps on skin edges is recommended, and after a little practice this useful instrument can be handled with a surprising dexterity. Placement of hemostats on bleeders should be accurate and precise and as little tissue taken with the open vessel as possible. Fine catgut ligature is preferred to the use of cau-

tery. Skin suture should be of as fine a material as will hold the apposition securely and should be placed close to the wound edge. Many fine sutures are preferable to a few gross "bites."

When these simple measures, which occupy little additional time and effort, are taken, the optimum rate of wound healing will be attained and both surgeon and patient will be rewarded by the development of an unobtrusive and firmly healed scar. When these measures are neglected, such a favorable result will be fortuitous, and more commonly the end-point will be either an infected wound or at the very least an unsightly hypertrophic scar with little tensile strength.

Common Emergency Room Situations

The first responsibility of the surgeon called to examine an injured patient in the Emergency Room is *not* to treat the region apparently injured, but to ensure that there are no associated injuries that threaten the well-being of the patient or even pose a hazard to life. The history of the means by which injury occurred, if available, is of paramount importance. Facial abrasions sustained by a patient who was thrown 50 feet by a speeding car carry more obvious implications of associated injury than do the same abrasions incurred in a fist fight.

Measurement of vital signs should be a routine procedure on admission to the Emergency Room, and it should be noted that soft tissue injuries to the head and face rarely, if ever, cause circulatory collapse, even when bleeding is profuse. If shock is apparent, a diligent search for causative factors, such as pelvic fractures, blunt abdominal trauma causing lacerations to liver or spleen, or pneumothorax, should be undertaken before proceeding with repair of facial lacerations. Physical examination should be complete and, in cases of injury to the face and scalp, should include a neurological evaluation.

Facial Lacerations

It is in dealing with facial lacerations that the technical skills and patience of the reparative surgeon are perhaps most obviously rewarded, for deforming scars that might be acceptable in other locations are always "on display" for the constant inspection of the patient and his or her associates. Such scars may be a source of psychological disturbance to the patient, and they are frequently avoidable by attention to details of wound healing as outlined in the foregoing section.

The adequacy of blood supply to the face is an advantage from two standpoints, both related to wound healing. The incidence of infection is lessened to the point of being a rarity unless there have been gross errors of technique, and the entire healing process takes place in a shorter time than occurs in areas where the blood supply is less abundant.

The so-called "golden period" (within which lacerations can be safely sutured) of three to four hours following injury is at least doubled, allowing time for evaluation of more serious associated injuries. There is no reason, however, why facial lacerations should not be repaired meticulously under local anesthesia while the patient is being observed for signs of intraperitoneal bleeding; or a combined surgical approach to multiple injuries can be taken so that the plastic surgeon deals with the face while another team is operating on a different area. Where circumstances absolutely preclude the early repair of facial lacerations, these injuries may be dressed with frequently changed moist compresses until surgery is accomplished, preferably within 48 hours. In such cases, broadspectrum antibiotic coverage is used and a rather more extensive débridement of the wound edges employed.

Fine suture (5-0, 6-0, or 7-0 silk or nylon) is for the repair of the skin, and owing to the rapid healing response it may be removed earlier than is customary to prevent "stitch marks." One acceptable approach is to remove alternate sutures three days following repair and the remainder 48 hours later; a bolder method is to remove all of the sutures at three days, and to support wound edges with Steri-strips or muslin soaked in collodion.

When a facial injury is necessarily closed under some tension because of tissue loss, the most advantageous method of repair is the intradermal subcuticular "pull-out" suture (Fig. 9–2). Either nylon or fine monofilament wire may be used and the free ends taped to the skin rather than employing lead shot or heavy knots. This suture may be left for two or three weeks to hold the edges together until the reparative processes, delayed by tension, take over; yet it will not cause the ugly scarring that would inevitably accompany conventional skin sutures if left in place for that length of time. This technique, however, does not allow for perfect wound approximation, and it should not be used unless the surgeon feels that regular cuticular sutures cannot be removed after three or four days.

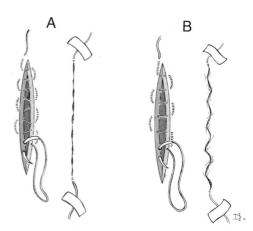

Figure 9–2 The technique of a subcuticular pull-out closure, using wire or nylon. To obtain a straight scar it is necessary to go back slightly with each suture.

Automobile Accidents

Some of the most technically awkward lacerations of the face come about as the result of automobile and motorcycle accidents. The force of injury may well cause fractures of the facial skeleton that are obscured by the rapid onset of edema; stereoscopic x-ray in the Waters position (a 30-degree occipitomental view) will best show such fractures. Management of these fractures requires a general anesthetic and operating room care, in which case the soft tissue injuries can be repaired simultaneously. Many injuries involving soft tissue alone are so extensive that admission of the patient to the hospital is appropriate; a good rule of thumb is that if the repair will take two hours or more, or if skin grafting for tissue loss is required, then the situation is best handled on an inpatient basis.

Even those limited injuries suitable for outpatient repair may well pose a reconstructive challenge. Lacerations will frequently be of a "bursting" nature, in which soft tissue has been rapidly compressed over a bony prominence. Such lacerations will be jagged, irregular, and accompanied by massive contusion of adjacent tissue, not seen in incised injuries. Contamination of the wound with foreign material is common, and road dirt may be "ground in" to such an extent that irrigation alone will not remove it. Such potential contaminants must be removed by firm scrubbing with a brush or even by cutting away the involved tissue.

It is readily apparent that injuries of this nature require more extensive débridement than usual to accomplish primary healing without infection; loss of tissue will consequently be greater. It may be possible by undermining and mobilization of adjacent tissue to restore continuity without undue tension; if not, a skin graft will be necessary.

The temptation to achieve primary reconstruction with the use of an ingeniously planned flap must be resisted. When a wound is contused and contaminated, the most meticulous surgical reparative technique may result in the development of an unsightly hypertrophic scar. If the use of the knife has been limited to the injured area, such disfigurement is amenable to a secondary revision several months later. If the wound has been extended by "relaxing incisions," or the creation of a flap, these incisions may also undergo hypertrophy, making a subsequent revision infinitely harder.

In general, surgical débridement and repair of complex injuries to the soft tissue of the face should be adequate and simple, aimed at achieving healing as quickly as possible. Elaborate reconstructions have no place in the primary treatment of such injuries, for these procedures are best performed electively in the well-healed wound, where there is no accompanying tissue destruction.

Bites

The ordinary dog bite is an extremely common injury, and it is estimated that approximately one-half million persons are treated yearly in Emergency Rooms throughout the U.S.A. for this problem. Such injuries are seen most frequently on the hands or face and commonly occur in children, who are more prone to pet or tease unfamiliar dogs than are adults. In fact, a completely unprovoked attack by a dog is a rarity and should arouse grave suspicions of rabies infection in the animal.

Dog bites may range in severity from small punctures to major avulsions of tissue requiring general anesthesia and operating room care; however, the majority are quite suitable for treatment in the Emergency Room. Many surgeons have advocated leaving these wounds open to heal by granulation, but it is this author's firmly held opinion that a dog bite is relatively clean, and if strict attention is paid to the principles of wound débridement and copious irrigation, they may all be closed primarily. Following a thorough skin prep as described, the wound is sutured loosely and dressed with moist compresses that can be changed at home, and the patient is given tetanus toxoid and antibiotic coverage. It must be acknowledged that even with meticulous care about 10 to 15 per cent of dog bites become infected, with the consequent necessity of opening the repair to relieve purulent collection; however, to condemn 85 to 90 per cent of these people to slow granulation and a mandatory scar revision would seem an unnecessarily conservative approach. Awkward bites on the face in small children have customarily been handled on an inpatient basis with a general anesthetic used to secure an immobile operating field; however, the recent advent and use of ketamine anesthesia has extended the scope of outpatient repair.

The most serious complication of a dog bite is, of course, rabies, a reportable disease that kills 10 to 25 individuals in this country yearly. Every physician involved in Emergency Room care should understand the indications for initiating prophylactic treatment against this disease. The World Health Organization has published guidelines to assist in making this decision. (See also Chapter 4, Table 4–1, and Chapter 28, Table 28–2.) The WHO guidelines may be abstracted as follows:

(1) When the attacking dog is shown by postmortem examination to have the disease.

(2) When a clinical diagnosis of rabies is made by a veterinarian.

(3) When an unprovoked attack is made, and the dog escapes or is killed without postmortem.

Treatment consists of *not* suturing the wound but injecting hyperimmune rabies serum in the adjacent tissue, while commencing a 14- to 21-day course of rabies vaccine. It must be remembered that wild animals such as bats, skunks, foxes and squirrels may also carry rabies.

Human bites generally occur in the heat of passion, either amorous or belligerent, and should include, by definition, knuckles skinned on the teeth of an adversary. The principal complication of such bites is massive secondary infection due to the large quantities of pathogenic bacteria — streptococcus, staphylococcus and spirochetes — which are normal inhabitants of the human, as opposed to the canine, mouth. Such injuries should never be sutured primarily, but the patient should be admitted to the hospital where intensive local and systemic treatment aimed at eradicating infection may be instituted.

The growth in popularity of camping and related outdoor activities has led to an increased incidence of snakebite. Several thousand people a year are bitten by poisonous snakes, and whereas the actual mortality is low (10 to 20 per year), the local complications, such as tissue necrosis, are severe. The vast majority of poisonous snakes belong to the Crotalidae family, which includes the rattlesnake, the cottonmouth moccasin and the copperhead. Such snakes are residents of almost every state but have not to date been found in Alaska, Hawaii or Maine or at altitudes above 7,000 feet.[13]

The principal problem is to decide whether the patient has been bitten by a poisonous or an innocuous snake. Ideally the snake should be killed and brought in for identification using the charts available in most Emergency Rooms. Poisonous snakes have fangs, and a double puncture rather than the marks of serrated teeth is pathognomonic of the bite of a crotalida. Local reaction — pain and swelling — is severe and instantaneous, and systemic symptoms such as nausea, vomiting, chills, fever, dizziness and tachycardia develop rapidly.

Treatment consists of the application of a loose tourniquet to impede lymphatic flow, cruciate incisions through the bite with suction, and the local and systemic injection of polyvalent antivenin. Packing the injured extremity in ice has received unfortunate publicity and is to be condemned as an extremely hazardous and ineffective procedure. The systemic absorption of venom is delayed rather than prevented by this procedure, and several serious injuries (including the complete loss of an arm below the elbow) have been reported as a direct result of injudicious hypothermia.

The coral snake, found in the Gulf states, Arizona and New Mexico, is the most deadly of all snakes found in the U.S.A. This snake produces a lethal neurotoxin, and although an antivenin is manufactured in Brazil, it is not generally available in this country. Consequently its bite is invariably fatal.

The most common biting spider is the black widow, found principally in outhouses, garages and basements. Only the female is dangerous, and she may be recognized by her globular jet-black body and characteristic red or yellow "hourglass" mark on the belly. There is usually some local discomfort at the time of the bite; this is rapidly followed by generalized muscle spasms. These patients may present in the Emergency Room with belly pain and spasm, and the differential diagnosis of an acute abdominal crisis such as a perforated duodenal ulcer may be hard to rule out. Treatment consists of relief of pain, injection of antivenin and the use of intravenous calcium gluconate and other muscle relaxants.

Specific Problem Situations

There are certain regions of the face which, due to their unique anatomical or functional characteristics, require special consideration when injured.

1. EYEBROWS AND EYELIDS. Facial lacerations, particularly those resulting from automobile accidents in which the unbelted rider may be ejected through a shattered windshield, will frequently involve the adnexal structures of the eye. The globe itself, owing to the protective "blink reflex," is less commonly injured; however, in any through-and-through laceration of the eyelid the globe should be examined by an ophthalmological surgeon. The sequelae of unrecognized and untreated injuries to the globe are disastrous, and if only for medicolegal reasons consultation should always be obtained in these situations.

Lacerations through the eyebrows are repaired in the customary manner appropriate for facial lacerations. The brow itself should not be shaved, less from the standpoint of hair not growing back (a rarity) than from the fact that correct alignment of the laceration will be easier with the hairs in place to serve as a guide. However, when hair adjacent to a laceration is deliberately left *in situ,* not only must the area be prepped with additional thoroughness to prevent infection but care must also be taken not to invert hair-bearing skin into the repair.

Lacerations of the lids themselves may be superficial or through-and-through, involving skin, orbicularis muscle, tarsal plate and conjunctiva. When these lacerations do not involve any absolute loss of tissue they are simply repaired in layers, care being taken to reapproximate each anatomical structure separately and in correct position. The "key" suture is in the gray line immediately behind the lashes; correct positioning of this stitch will align with other structures. The conjunctiva is repaired next using fine (6-0) catgut with the knots away from the globe; the other structures are sutured in sequence from inside out with the skin repair last (Fig. 9–3).

Two adnexal structures deserve special mention. A deep horizontal laceration of the upper lid may divide the levator palpebrae muscle or its tendinous attachment to the tarsal plate. This filmy muscle may be hard to identify in

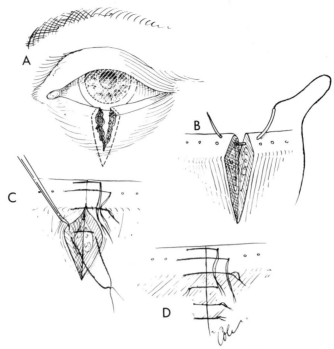

Figure 9–3 Repair of laceration of the eyelid.

the bloody mess of an acute injury, yet a diligent search must be made, for if left unrepaired, ptosis of the upper lid, requiring an elaborate secondary procedure for its correction, may develop. Lacerations through the medial portions of the lid margins may divide the canalicular system providing drainage of tears. An injury to the upper canaliculus may be fairly safely ignored, as it contributes only 10 per cent of the drainage of lacrimal secretions. If, however, a laceration through the margin of the lower lid is seen to be medial to the punctum, a search must be made for the cut ends of the divided inferior canaliculus. A fine polyethylene or Silastic catheter is threaded through the punctum, across the divided canaliculus, and into the lacrimal sac just below the attachment of the medial canthal ligament to the periosteum of the nasal bones. If this precaution is ignored and soft tissue is repaired without regard to the canaliculus, scarring of this structure

will prevent proper internal drainage of tears, with consequent epiphora.

Tissue losses of up to one quarter of the lid margin may be repaired directly without distortion of the palpebral fissure.[12] Both skin and conjunctiva must be undermined laterally in order to move the residual tissue in a medial direction; too much pull on the canalicular system is undesirable. Losses of up to one third of the margin of either upper or lower lid may be similarly repaired, with the added maneuver of dividing the appropriate branch of the lateral canthal ligament. A small horizontal incision is made just lateral to the eye and the Y-shaped ligament exposed (Fig. 9–4). Division of the upper bifurcation for tissue losses of the upper lid and of the lower branch for losses of the lower lid will permit additional mobilization of the entire lid for tension-free closure. The main attachment of the ligament to the lateral orbital rim should not be incised before it divides into upper and lower portions, for a major deformity of the palpebral fissure will result. Losses of greater than one third of either lid will require a more elaborate reconstruction than should be performed in the Emergency Room. Major losses of skin alone will require either a graft or a local flap for their resurfacing; such reconstructions are described in a subsequent section of this chapter.

2. THE EARS. The pinna of the ear is a subtle structure characterized by three-dimensional curves. Reconstruction is hard and frequently disappointing because of the inability to restore surgically the original delicacy of contour. Lacerations of the ear will commonly be jagged and irregular, and avulsing injuries may cause exposure of the cartilage owing to loss of surface skin.

Simple lacerations are repaired in layers with fine chromic catgut for the cartilage, using the folds of the ear as landmarks to achieve anatomical alignment. The ear is dressed with moderate pressure, using moist cotton or gauze fluffs packed both in front of and behind the ear itself to reduce the possibility of hematoma formation. Hematoma is a common sequel of ear injuries whether or not the skin has been lacerated and should be aspirated promptly and the ear redressed with a pressure dressing as described. If hematoma occurs following aspiration, a formal incision and drainage using a

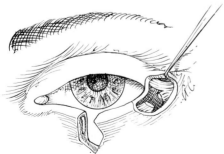

Figure 9–4 Exposure of lateral canthal ligament during procedure for repair of tissue loss of the lower eyelid.

short length of rubber band for the drain will be needed. Recognition of the problem is essential, for undrained hematoma of the pinna will result in destruction of cartilage and a "cauliflower ear," a deforming and preventable condition.

When more serious injuries necessitate débridement of devitalized skin, cartilage will be exposed. There is little laxity to the skin of the ear; consequently a decision will have to be made whether to excise the exposed cartilage to achieve tension-free closure or to employ alternative means of achieving coverage. Cartilage denuded of its nutrient skin should never be left exposed, for the inevitable consequence will be progressive chondritis resulting in a major destruction of the architecture of the ear. Depending on the location of the exposed cartilage and the deformity that would result from its excision, as much as half a centimeter may be removed. Otherwise a primary skin graft will be needed for coverage.

Major losses of a portion of the pinna may be dealt with in the following manner (Fig. 9–5 A, B and C). The ear is debrided to viable and uncontaminated tissue and "laid back" against the adjacent postauricular scalp. An incision is made in this area directly under the cut margin of the ear and is spread slightly, and the skin of the ear is sutured in two layers to the postauricular scalp. This may be elevated in a later stage and a skin graft placed behind the pinna to replace lost tissue. If the loss has been relatively small, the scar tissue may be enough to provide adequate "stiffness" to the ear. If the loss has been greater, added structural support in the form of carved costal cartilage or a Silastic prosthesis may have to be implanted before raising the ear. Such a reconstructive procedure will require a general anesthetic and inpatient care, but the preparatory maneuvers can be carried out in the Emergency Room.

3. THE LIPS. Lacerations of both

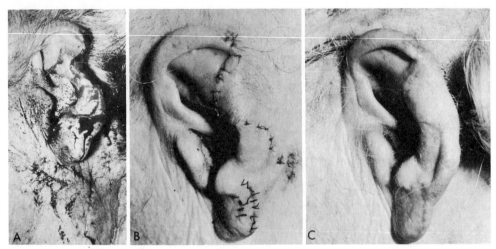

Figure 9-5   *A.* Raccoon bite of the ear with multiple lacerations and loss of a major portion of the pinna. *B.* Debrided and with a postaural skin flap sutured to defect. *C.* Flap divided and ear elevated from scalp with split-thickness skin graft.

upper and lower lip are common and frequently involve loss of tissue. Small lacerations on the inner aspect of the lips do not require suturing, but with a clear liquid diet and frequent peroxide mouthwashes they will heal spontaneously and rapidly. Through-and-through injuries must be repaired in layers; if the laceration crosses the skin-vermilion border, correct anatomical alignment of this feature is highly important. The vermilion margin is marked with a dye (methylene blue, brilliant green or India ink) *prior* to injection of the local anesthetic, for this will blanch and distort both skin and mucosa and make recognition of the border difficult. The initial suture is placed at the pre-marked border (Fig. 9-6); alignment of other sutures, mucosa, muscles and skin, follows in

sequence. Failure to observe this precaution will frequently result in a "step deformity," which will need a later revision.

When tissue is missing because of the injury, losses of up to one quarter of the lip may be sutured primarily without significant deformity; greater degrees of loss will require a reconstructive procedure too elaborate for the Emergency Room.

4. INJURIES TO THE FACIAL NERVE AND PAROTID DUCT. Deep lacerations of the cheek will frequently involve two important structures, the facial nerve and the parotid duct.

A careful preoperative examination of muscular activity of the face will reveal any injury to the branches of the facial nerve. This examination must be completed prior to infiltration with

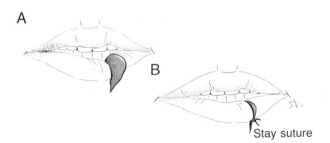

Stay suture

Figure 9-6   When the lip is lacerated through and through, the key stitch aligns the skin vermilion border correctly.

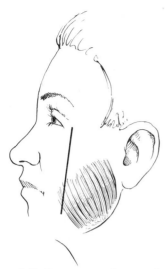

Figure 9–7 Laceration of nerve branches anterior to an imaginary vertical line drawn from the lateral canthus of the eye need not be repaired.

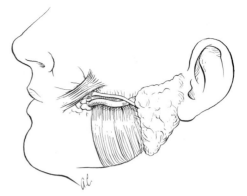

Figure 9–8 Location of parotid duct.

local anesthesia. All too often, patients are transferred from outlying Emergency Rooms after being examined by primary physicians who have infiltrated the wounds with Xylocaine to relieve pain. This makes the definitive identification of nerve injury impossible at the time of secondary examination. However, once the operating surgeon has performed a physical examination and documented nerve continuity or discontinuity, local anesthetic infiltration can be commenced. If the laceration is anterior to a line dropped from the lateral canthus of the eye, then only fine peripheral branches are involved (Fig. 9–7). These need not be repaired, as their function will almost always regenerate. When major branches of the facial nerve appear to be interrupted on the basis of the neurological examination, only operative exploration will identify a loss of continuity. It is the author's conviction that repair of these structures should be carried out primarily — however, a procedure of this type requires lighting, equipment and teamwork best supplied by the Operating Room.

Failure to identify and repair a divided parotid duct will result in persistent leakage of saliva through the skin repair. The duct runs in a straight line between the tragus of the ear and the commissure of the lips (Fig. 9–8); a deep laceration of the cheek across this line should raise the suspicion of an injury to this structure. Intraoral probing of Stensen's duct will determine whether there has been an interruption of continuity; if so, it should be repaired with fine catgut over a polyethylene catheter extending into the oral cavity and fixed to the buccal mucosa (Fig. 9–9). This may be withdrawn after a week.

Lacerations of the parotid gland it-

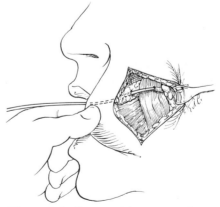

Figure 9–9 Repair of laceration of parotid duct using fine catgut over a polyethylene catheter. See text for details.

self (located between the lobule of the ear and the angle of the mandible) may cause a temporary fistulous leak; these, however, usually subside spontaneously, although a collection of salivary fluid will occasionally require aspiration. Radiation therapy has been recommended to suppress parotid activity if the accumulation is persistent.

Thermal Injuries

Burns have been classified traditionally according to the depth of injury into first degree, second degree and third degree; a more descriptive term for the latter two categories would be "partial-thickness" and "full-thickness" burns. In partial-thickness burns, only the more superficial layers of the dermis are destroyed, and if kept free from infection they will heal spontaneously with skin of good quality. Full-thickness burns have by definition lost the entire depth of the dermis, including the stratum germinativum, and if ungrafted they will heal only by scarring and contracture. Thus an early recognition of the depth of the burn should be attempted, for on this factor will depend not only the prognosis but the eventual management of the burn.

If the skin is charred or dead white, with thrombosed capillaries evident on the de-epithelialized surface, then the burn is almost certainly full-thickness in depth. If intracutaneous blebs are present, implying that the dermal circulation is intact, then the burn is probably only of partial thickness. Not all burns are so clear-cut, however, and in addition there may be a mosaic pattern of areas of mixed partial- and full-thickness burns present. Although supravital dyes and thermography have been used experimentally to determine the depth of a burn, the single most useful clinical test remains the retention of sensation to pinprick in a burn of partial thickness.

In addition to recognition of the

depth of the burn, assessment of the body surface area (BSA) involved is crucial, for on this will depend, among other things, the program of fluid replacement therapy. The "rule of nines" is a reasonably accurate guide for the relative areas of different parts of the body: the head is 9 per cent, each surface of the trunk is 18 per cent, each arm is 9 per cent and each leg is 18 per cent (Fig. 9–10). The proportions in the infant or small child are different in that the head is relatively larger and the legs smaller.

An important decision facing the examining physician in the Emergency Room is, "Can the burn be treated on an outpatient basis or is it serious enough to warrant admission to the hospital?" In general, our criteria for admission are as follows:

(1) Any burn of greater extent than

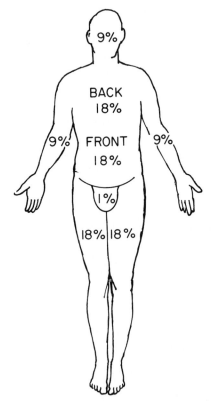

Figure 9–10   Schematic representation of the "rule of nines" for assessment of body surface area burned.

10 per cent, or 5 per cent in a small child or old person (burns are tolerated poorly on the extreme ends of the age spectrum), represents a threat to life on the basis of fluid loss, and such patients should be admitted.

(2) Any full-thickness burn will require grafting and should be admitted, although with limited areas of loss, admission need not be effected until the dead eschar is separated and the burn ready for surgical coverage.

(3) Burns of the hands, face or perineal region are hard to care for at home and should all be admitted to the hospital.

Standards for admission will be more liberal in the case of children, and if there is the suspicion that the parents are not equipped to deliver conscientious and effective care at home, the child should always be taken into the hospital.

Minor burns not meeting the above criteria may be treated on an outpatient basis. First-degree burns manifesting erythema only may be quite painful and can be treated with an analgesic ointment, and the patient may be discharged. Partial-thickness burns of limited extent should be washed gently but thoroughly with pHisoHex, all contaminants removed from the surface, blisters aspirated and cultured and the areas dressed with a fairly bulky dressing. There is some controversy, however, about the aspiration or débridement of skin blisters. Work has been done in the laboratory and good evidence is available that a blister provides an excellent biologic dressing. If this blister is intact, some surgeons feel today that these blisters should not be debrided or aspirated. If, however, the blister is not intact, then it should be debrided. If débridement is carried out on an intact blister, one essentially opens this wound to air and other contaminants, and this may lead to superficial infection. An instance where an intact blister should be decompressed is when this bullous deformity interferes with movable functional parts — i.e., limiting flexion of the metacarpal phalangeal joints or extension of the interphalangeal joints of the fingers, limiting eyelid closure, or obstructing airways about the nostrils or mouth. Furacin mesh-gauze is a very suitable material to place next to the wound itself. It must be remembered that the arbitrary classifications of burns are *not* static, and that if a partial-thickness burn becomes infected, it may well be converted into a full-thickness loss which will require a skin graft for coverage. Consequently the burn should be inspected and redressed daily until there is evidence of healthy re-epithelialization. Sterile technique should always be used for the dressing changes, and prophylactic penicillin should be employed systemically for the same reason, that of prevention of infection.

The remainder of this section will deal with the important sequence of measures to be taken when an acute major burn is first brought into the Emergency Room. Burn centers will have their own standard operating procedures for the receiving area; in the Emergency Rooms of the average general hospital the admission of a major burn is an event associated with some degree of urgency and excitement; consequently, a "check list" is vital to ensure that therapeutic and diagnostic measures follow a logical sequence without forgetting any important aspects of management.

These measures are listed as follows:

1. AIRWAY. The integrity of the airway is of prime importance in any acute injury, and burns are no exception. Flashburns to the face, neck or upper chest should always suggest the possibility of an intraoral burn which may involve the glottis and vocal cords. Stridor, retraction and rising respiratory rate will confirm these suspicions, and if there is upper airway obstruction due to the burn, then a tracheostomy or nasotracheal intubation should be performed. It must also

be remembered that small children have not only narrower tracheas but also more reactive laryngeal mucosas than adults; consequently, the sequence of events leading to total obstruction occurs in an accelerated manner requiring greater alertness on the part of the responsible physician.

2. FLUIDS. Any burn of greater than 10 per cent of the body surface area (BSA) is potentially hazardous on the basis of fluid loss and hypovolemic shock. Consequently, the early administration of fluid replacement is mandatory. Insertion of a polyethylene catheter into the subclavian vein not only will allow a convenient route for rapid fluid administration but will also allow constant monitoring of the central venous pressure. Either normal saline or lactated Ringer's solution in dextrose may be used for initial treatment until the exact fluid requirements are derived. All fluids should be administered by the intravenous route at this early stage, for oral fluids may merely dilate the stomach to be vomited later.

3. URINE OUTPUT. Hourly measurement of the urine output and specific gravity is the most useful way to assess the effectiveness of fluid replacement as well as to detect at the earliest possible moment impending renal failure. If the urine output begins to dwindle and the specific gravity to rise, then the patient is being underhydrated and will need an increased rate of fluid administration. Changes in the urine will provide proof of impending hypovolemic shock well before any change in the pulse or blood pressure. Consequently, insertion of a Foley catheter to allow easy measurement of these indices is one of the important early measures to take in the acute management of the severely burned patient.

4. CHARTING. Having assured the patency of the airway, established an intravenous line and urinary drainage, a more leisurely assessment of the burn itself can be made. A detailed description of both depth and extent should be charted in the permanent record using the criteria outlined previously. On the basis of the severity of the burn a fluid plan should be evolved, recognizing that this will always need modification according to the individual's unique response to the burn as measured by urinary output, specific gravity, hematocrit and central venous pressure. However, the Brooke Army Formula:

0.5 cc plasma × body weight in kg ×
% of the burn (up to 50%)
+
1.5 cc electrolyte (saline or Ringer's)
× weight × % burn
+
Daily maintenance fluids

for the first 24 hours' needs has proved successful in preventing gross mismanagement of fluid therapy and serves as a useful preliminary plan.[1]

More recently, burn physicians have been using other formulas for the first 24 hours after severe burns to correct hypovolemia. The Parkland (Baxter) Formula has gained wide acceptance recently because no colloid is administered in the first 24 hours. It is felt that the massive burn wound creates capillary fragility and alterations in arteriovenous shunts. Colloid or albumin therefore will not be retained within the intravascular spaces and subsequently will be of little use to the cardiovascular system. Using this rationale, colloid is used after capillary and cell membrane stabilization occurs (usually after 24 hours). The Parkland Formula is 4 cc of electrolyte solution times the body weight in kilograms times the percent of the body surface area burned. This amount of intravenous fluid is administered in the same time intervals as those of previous formulas, i.e., one half of the calculated 24 hour dose in the first 8 hours and the remaining half of the calculated 24 hour dose in the remaining 16 hours (see Table 9–1). Obviously this is a dy-

TABLE 9–1   Parkland (Baxter) Formula for Fluid Requirements in Major Burns

To calculate the first 24-hour dose of intravenous electrolyte solution:

4 cc × body weight (kg) × % BSA burned

Dosage:
  1/2 the calculated amount in first 8 hours
  1/2 the calculated amount in next 16 hours

---

namic situation and has to be monitored constantly. Subsequent therapy and revision of the rate of fluid administration is ordered for the patient after hospitalization.

5. OTHER MEASURES. Before transferral from the Emergency Room to the burn or intensive care unit, the patient should be sedated, the burned areas should be cleansed, and whichever form of topical antibacterial is currently popular should be commenced. In our unit we use dressings soaked in 0.5 per cent silver nitrate, as described by Moyer,[11] by sulfamylon, gentamicin and silver sulfadiazine all have their devotees. A discussion of the relative merits of these agents is out of place in this context, except to say that none of them will substitute for devoted and laborious wound care. Prophylactic penicillin is added to the intravenous fluids until cultures of specific organisms dictate a change of antibiotic.

However, controversy exists about the use of prophylactic penicillin therapy. Some surgeons feel that giving prophylactic penicillin eliminates the gram-positive organisms and allows gram-negative organisms to flourish. If these injured patients then develop septicemia, it will be of the gram-negative type, which is a more lethal infection. Some burn physicians feel that penicillin should be given only if there is evidence of superficial infection; however, all feel that prevention of infection is important so that extension of the burn wound does not occur.

If these measures are taken promptly and in sequence, culpable disasters due to errors of omission can be avoided, and the patient can be admitted to the hospital in optimal condition for appropriate inpatient care.

6. COLD INJURY. Injury by cold represents the opposite end of the thermal spectrum, and in civilian practice frostbite is not as common, nor are the sequelae as devastating, as burn injuries.

Our experience at the University of Colorado Medical Center is based on the review of 113 patients admitted over the past ten years[8] and implies that the physical appearance of the acutely injured part bears no correlation whatsoever with the extent of tissue ultimately lost. Thus no "first, second or third degree" system can be evolved on the basis of physical examination; of greater value as a prognostic indicator is a detailed knowledge of the duration of exposure, the ambient temperature and wind speed during exposure, (Table 9–2) and the type of protective clothing worn. The injury is a product of the tissue temperature reached and the time period that the tissue remains frozen. The rate of heat loss will determine the ability of the body to "self-warm" a cooled part with increased blood flow; hence an individual protected by insulated clothing will sustain a lesser injury than the same individual whose socks and feet are soaked by tramping through the snow in indoor shoes, or who has removed his gloves in an effort to start his car stalled on an isolated mountain pass.

TABLE 9-2   Chill Factor Chart

WIND SPEED (MILES/HOUR)	THERMOMETER READING (°F)									
	40	30	20	10	0	−10	−20	−30	−40	−50
	EQUIVALENT TEMPERATURE (°F)—THE CHILL FACTOR									
calm	40	30	20	10	0	−10	−20	−30	−40	−50
5	37	27	16	6	−5	−15	−26	−36	−47	−57
10	28	16	4	−9	−21	−33	−46	−58	−70	−83
15	22	9	−5	−18	−36	−45	−58	−72	−85	−99
20	18	4	−10	−25	−39	−53	−67	−82	−96	−110
25	16	0	−15	−29	−44	−59	−74	−88	−104	−118
30	13	−2	−18	−33	−48	−63	−79	−94	−109	−125
35	11	−4	−20	−35	−49	−67	−82	−98	−113	−129
40	10	−6	−21	−37	−53	−69	−85	−100	−116	−132
		Least Danger			*Greater Danger*			*Great Danger*		

When patients present in the Emergency Room with an acutely frozen extremity, the part is usually white, hard and lacking in sensation. If enough time has passed for the part to be partially thawed out, there may be edema, cyanosis, blisters and a varying degree of return of sensation.

Emergency Room treatment consists of immediate rewarming of the part in a water bath whose temperature is precisely 40° C. A cooler bath will not be as effective, and a hotter one will increase the metabolic demand on the tissue and cause additional necrosis. Narcotics may be necessary during this often painful procedure, which should be prolonged until return of blood flow to the part is seen. Rapid rewarming reduces the duration of time during which the tissue is at subviable temperatures and is the *only* therapeutic maneuver that has to date been shown clinically effective in reducing or preventing the gangrene of frostbite. It should be accomplished in the Emergency Room.

All patients in whom tissue damage is suspected should be admitted to the hospital, where the subsequent treatment will depend on whether one believes the necrosis of cold injury to be a direct result of thermal cellular assault, immediate and irreversible, or a slow process due primarily to intravascular aggregation and infarction. Our own laboratory studies imply that frostbite injury is potentially reversible if the microcirculation is kept patent. We are currently using intravenous infusion of Pluronic F-68 (a copolymer of polyoxyethylene and polyoxypropylene glycol), which is a nontoxic surface-active agent known to stabilize both the endothelial lining and the red cell membrane as an adjuvant to rapid rewarming. Use of this agent is still in the experimental stage.

Whether or not drugs are used in an attempt to augment the capillary circulation, the treatment for frostbite consists of supportive measures designed to prevent infection. The extremities are elevated, the patient kept on bed rest, and sterile dressings changed daily. *No* attempt at surgical débridement should be made, for it is preferable that nonviable tissue should separate spontaneously.

ELECTIVE RECONSTRUCTIVE PROCEDURES

The ascending spiral of hospital costs in recent years has forced conscientious physicians to consider a wider use of the Outpatient Department rather than inpatient operating room care for certain elective surgical procedures. "Unnecessary" hospitalizations should be avoided as long as this can be done without jeopardizing the optimal care of the patient. Many reconstructive procedures of limited extent are performed under local anesthesia and thus lend themselves ideally to outpatient care; in some institutions brief procedures under a general anesthetic are performed and the patients discharged after a period of observation in the recovery room.

What are some of the types of procedures most suited to surgery on an outpatient basis? They include excision of skin lesions, both benign and malignant.

Skin Lesions

Basal Cell Carcinoma

Basal cell carcinoma is the commonest skin malignancy and arises in the connective tissue beneath the dermis. Its etiology is related to solar radiation and consequently is found most frequently on the exposed portions of the body — face and the dorsum of the hands — of fair-skinned persons of middle age who spend a great deal of time out-of-doors. It is rarely, if ever, found in blacks and in general, the darker the complexion the less prone the individual is to basal cell carcinoma (presumably a protective genetic adaptation). It is more common in males than in females and very rare in adolescents, the youngest case in the author's experience being 15 years of age.

Basal cell carcinomas are divided both clinically and histologically into several types, but all have in common masses of deeply staining basophilic round cells with palisading of their nuclei at the periphery. The most common form is the papular basal cell carcinoma, which may present as a nodule or a small ulcer with a rolled pearly edge (Fig. 9–11). It is slow-growing and circumscribed and may be ignored for several years by the patient, since it is painless. Other types of basal cell carcinoma include the cystic lesion and the sclerosing and morpheic types, which manifest an ill-defined indurated surface and marked subdermal extension. The rare pigmented basal cell carcinoma is important in that is hard to differentiate clinically from a malignant melanoma.

Basal cell carcinoma is a local lesion and extends only by direct invasion, never by metastasis via the blood stream or lymphatics. Consequently, the treating physician is required only to ensure adequate local removal.

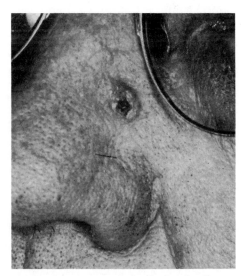

Figure 9–11 Typical papular basal cell carcinoma, with pearly rolled edges. (From the collection of S. E. Blandford, Jr., M.D.)

Treatment modalities have included surgical excision, radiation therapy, electrodesiccation and topical chemotherapy. The recurrence rate following adequate treatment from any of these means is low (2 to 5 per cent); however, for the following reasons it is strongly recommended that surgical excision be employed:

(1) A surgical specimen will be obtained from which may be defined not only histological confirmation of the diagnosis but, most important, the adequacy of surgical resection. Some of these tumors are multifocal, and some manifest subdermal extension not apparent to clinical examination. When the pathological specimen reveals tumor extending to the margin of resection, a re-excision must be performed with complete clearance from the pathologists of a margin adequately free of tumor.

(2) When recurrence of basal cell carcinoma is noted following surgical resection, the re-excision may be limited to the area of recurrence; when recurrence occurs following radiation, the entire radiated area must be re-excised. This will often involve removal of a great deal of tissue with the consequent necessity of performing an elaborate reconstruction to prevent a major deformity.

(3) Surgery is preferred to radiotherapy when adjacent structures may be damaged by radionecrosis. These regions include the lids and canthal regions, the nose, the external ear, the lips and the hands.

An adequate surgical excision usually entails a 5 mm margin around the clinically evident lesion; *all* specimens should be submitted for histological examination, and a re-excision should be performed if sectioning shows evidence of inadequate resection. All patients in whom basal cell carcinomas have been removed should be examined at six-month intervals for the rest of their lives — to recognize recurrence and to diagnose the appearance of new lesions. The patient with

one basal cell carcinoma is constitutionally and environmentally liable to develop others. For the same reason such patients should be advised to avoid deliberate sun-bathing and to protect the exposed parts with clothing or an ultraviolet screening lotion when solar exposure is inevitable.

Most basal cell carcinomas are small, and excision and direct closure can be accomplished without deformity by placing the long axis of the elliptical incision in the natural tension lines of the face when this is the region involved (Fig. 9–12). However, when the lesion is larger owing to patient neglect, the resection may entail sacrifice of so much skin that simple closure under tension would result in a major disfigurement. In these cases, there is controversy over whether merely to resurface the area with a skin graft or to employ a local flap for immediate reconstruction of the deformity. The proponents of grafting hold that, while the cosmetic appearance is less satisfactory, recurrence is easier to detect than when tissue adjacent to the tumor is "buried" under a flap. Those, including the author, who prefer direct re-

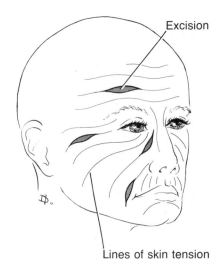

Figure 9–12 Elliptical excisions of facial lesions are made with their long axes in the direction of wrinkles in the aged or lines of tension in the younger patient.

construction of the deformity, feel that with a histologically adequate margin of resection, the recurrence rate of basal cell carcinoma is so low that the best possible means of achieving a normal appearance should be employed. Specific examples of local flaps will be described in a later part of this section.

Squamous Cell Carcinoma

Squamous cell carcinoma, also occurring commonly on the face and hands, is hard to differentiate clinically in its initial stages from basal cell carcinoma (Fig. 9–13). It is, however, rapidly growing, highly invasive and liable to metastasize through lymphatic channels, and therefore it requires a more aggressive surgical approach. Prone to occur in radiated tissue, it is a

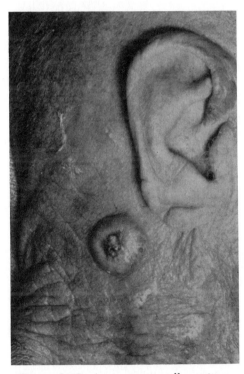

Figure 9–13 A squamous cell carcinoma, rapidly growing and with marked adjacent induration. (From the collection of S. E. Blandford, Jr., M.D.)

frequent and tragic aftermath of injudicious radiotherapy for benign lesions such as acne and hemangioma. The tumor is usually less well defined than a basal cell carcinoma, and local induration is marked. Growth is rapid and may be characterized by ulceration and bleeding or by the development of an irregular cauliflower-like excrescence.

The majority of squamous cell carcinomas can, if diagnosed early, be excised locally with primary closure. Because of the higher degree of invasiveness noted in these tumors, the margin of excision should be wider than for basal cell carcinoma and should include at least 1 cm of histologically clear tissue. For the same reason, the extent of the resection is best judged by frozen section.

Lymph node dissection, which is outside the scope of outpatient surgery, should be carried out in continuity when nodes are clinically involved. Serious consideration should be given to a delayed prophylactic node dissection when the lesion is recurrent or has an anaplastic histological appearance or when the patient is under 45 years of age.

When the extent of resection makes primary closure a deforming procedure, the same controversy exists as to whether to perform a primary reconstruction or to resurface the defect with a skin graft. Each case must be judged entirely on its own merits; the early and well-circumscribed lesion can be safely reconstructed when frozen section gives evidence of adequate resection. In long-standing lesions with diffuse indurated edges it would seem more prudent to accept the temporary deformity of a skin graft; if there is no evidence of recurrence within a year the grafted area can be excised and a delayed reconstruction performed if frozen section demonstrates no further tumor cells in the specimen removed. Lifetime follow-up of each patient is of course mandatory.

Keratoacanthoma is a rapidly grow-

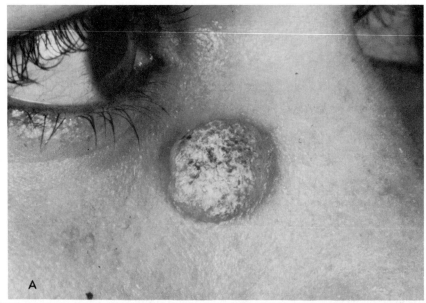

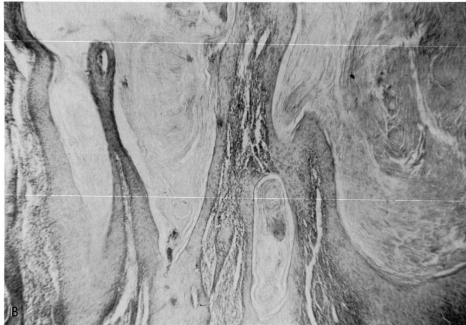

Figure 9-14 *A.* Keratoacanthoma clinically resembles squamous cell carcinoma. *B.* Microscopically it is easily distinguished by the lack of mitotic cells and the hyperkeratotic plugs. (From the collection of S. E. Blandford, Jr., M.D.)

ing benign lesion that greatly resembles squamous cell carcinoma in its physical appearance; however, its rapid growth is followed by equally rapid resolution. The experienced clinician may be able to make the differential diagnosis and await disappearance of the tumor with equanimity; others less confident of their acumen (including the author) prefer the security engendered by excisional biopsy and histological section (Fig. 9–14 *A* and *B*).

Nevus and Malignant Melanoma

Nevi, or moles, are pigmented skin lesions that may be flat or elevated, hairless or hair-bearing. Although the exact etiology of these lesions is controversial, the most generally accepted theory is that they arise from neural elements within the dermis. They are extremely common, it being estimated that each individual bears an average of 15 nevi on his or her body.

Nevi are classified histologically into intradermal, junctional and compound nevi.[3] The intradermal nevus is the common mole of adulthood and characteristically is brown or black, with a raised surface that frequently bears hairs (Fig. 9–15). The clinical importance of this physical description is that melanoma rarely if ever arises from an intradermal nevus.

The junctional nevus, common in childhood, is so named because the mass of melanotic cells comprising the lesion resides at the junction between the dermis and the epidermis. Most preadolescent junctional nevi mature at puberty into adult intradermal nevi; however, as malignant melanomata arise almost exclusively from junctional nevi, it is important to recognize their physical characteristics. Junctional nevi are flat or only slightly raised, may vary in color from light brown to black, are hairless and commonly have a less well-defined edge than the intradermal nevus, the margin "blending" into the adjacent skin.

Compound nevi are a histological combination of the two with a darker raised central intradermal portion surrounded by a flat "areola," usually paler in color and representing the junctional part of the lesion.

The indications for removal of nevi are twofold, cosmetic and prophylactic. An obvious intradermal nevus of the face, dark, raised and hairy, represents a disfigurement that can well be improved by careful surgical excision. A small ellipse is planned aligning the long axis with the known tension lines (see Fig. 9–12) and, after undermining the incisional edges to relieve tension, is sutured with fine silk or nylon, the sutures being removed on the third or fourth postoperative day to prevent stitch marks. As the principal object of this procedure is cosmetic, care must be taken to ensure an inconspicuous scar less offensive than the original lesion. The specimen should, of course, be consigned to the pathology department for section and histologic confirmation of the benign nature of the lesion.

The junctional nevus, because of its malignant potential, should be watched carefully. In addition, it would seem proper to excise prophylactically junctional nevi in areas of chafing and potential irritation from belt, collar, or brassiere, for it has been shown that continued trauma may precipitate melanomatous change in the junctional or, rarely, the compound

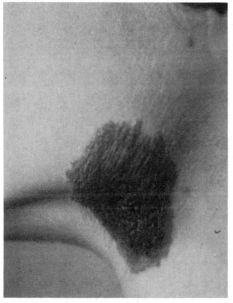

Figure 9–15 A typical intradermal nevus: raised, hairy and with a uniform color.

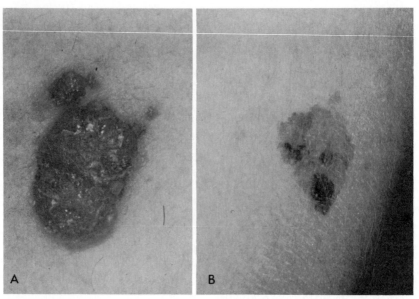

Figure 9–16   Malignant melanomas: (*A*) showing satellite formation and adjacent inflammation and (*B*) showing typical irregularity of both edges and pigmentation. (From the collection of S. E. Blandford, Jr., M.D.)

nevus. For the same reason, measures other than formal surgical excision should *never* be employed. Electrodesiccation or cryotherapy must not be performed. A high proportion of patients with malignant melanoma will present a history of previous improper treatment of this type, the trauma quite possibly precipitating the malignant change.

Malignant melanoma (Fig. 9–16 *A* and *B*) is a highly malignant lesion that frequently metastasizes early. Definitive treatment consists of wide and deep excision (a margin of 5 to 10 cm is acceptable) and en-bloc lymphatic dissection in continuity, if possible. This procedure cannot be done satisfactorily on an outpatient basis. The poor prognosis of the patient can, however, be improved by the early recognition of malignant changes in an established pigmented lesion. These signs include:

(1) Enlargement of the lesion or satellite formation

(2) A change in pigmentation — either lighter or darker

(3) Crusting, ulceration or bleeding

(4) Pain or itching, and local inflammation

(5) Melanuria

Any new or established pigmented lesion that demonstrates one or more of these physical changes should undergo excisional biopsy with a margin of at least 1 cm and be submitted for frozen section to determine if melanoma is present. Pigmented lesions of the soles of the feet, the palms and genitalia should be excised, for these lesions have a distinct predilection for junctional activity and melanoma formation.

Hemangioma and Lymphangioma

Hemangiomas are benign tumors of vascular origin, principally occurring in or just beneath the skin. They are common, with an overall incidence of 10 per cent, and the sex ratio shows a predisposition for females over males by 3:1. As 50 per cent of these tumors occur in the head and neck region, mostly evident at or just after birth, they are highly visible and commonly a source of great anxiety to the parents. Consequently an understanding of their natural history is important for planning effective and logical treatment. Hemangiomas are divided both clinically and pathologically into two principal types — capillary hemangiomas and cavernous hemangiomas. Occasionally lesions show features of each type.

Capillary hemangiomas (port-wine stain, nevus flammeus, angioma simplex) are characterized histologically by masses of densely packed abnormal capillaries, usually lined with adult endothelial cells, located within or immediately below the dermis. Clinically they present as a smooth discoloration, ranging from deep pink to livid purple, with a sharp margin cleanly delineated from the adjacent normal skin. They occur principally on the face, located usually on only one side and following the distribution of one or more branches of the trigeminal nevus. The congenital nature of these lesions, together with an anatomical distribution limited to one of the fetal facial processes, suggests that it is a developmental rather than a neoplastic entity.

Although some faint capillary hemangiomas spontaneously resolve during the first few years of life, the majority remain unchanged, growing with the other facial structures and retaining their color. Malignant degeneration has never been reported and the problem is entirely cosmetic. However, the disfiguring nature of these lesions is such that merely ignoring capillary hemangiomas as a harmless accident of birth is an inadequate approach.

Various methods of treatment have been employed. Radiation of any kind is to be condemned absolutely, for not only is it entirely ineffective against the mature endothelial cells, but the short-term hazards of alteration of growth of facial structures and the long-term sequelae of radiodermatitis and skin cancer are well known.

An opaque make-up may be used with great success in camouflaging the lesion where it is of similar texture to the adjacent skin. This is psychologically more suited to the female than the male patient and has the disadvantage of requiring constant reapplication, especially when the individual tends to sweat with activity.

Relatively small lesions may be excised and closed either directly, using the lines of skin tension, or with the aid of a local flap. The majority of these hemangiomas are, however, quite extensive, and the resurfacing involved might well lead to a greater disfigurement than the original lesion.

A unique and successful approach to the problem was evolved by Conway.[4] This consists of the tattooing of pigment into the superficial layers of the dermis to conceal the underlying angioma. Inorganic pigment is sterilized and carefully mixed to match the individual complexion of the patient. The principal pigment used is white (titanium oxide) and small amounts of red, yellow, brown and green are added judiciously by trial and error to achieve an exact color match. A surgical instrument — the Dermajector — has been modified from the crude equipment of the tattoo parlor, and this can be attached to the cord of a conventional Stryker motor. Following induction of local anesthesia, the pigment, mixed with sterile saline, is "painted" onto the skin surface and driven into the dermis by the repeated needle punctures of the Dermajector. The entire operation should, of course, be conducted as a sterile surgical procedure.

Frequently, two or three procedures, several months apart, are necessary to achieve the desired degree of opacity for camouflage of the hemangioma. Never perfect, the results are usually satisfactory, particularly to the male who does not wish to be seen applying make-up in the men's room.

A few authors have had fairly extensive experience using the Argon Laser to photocoagulate port-wine hemangiomata. Evidently, the physical properties of the blue Argon Laser light are attracted to the red of hemoglobin, and the light can pass through intact skin without much damage. Much work is still being done on this technique of "erasing" large port-wine hemangiomata that are not amenable to operative extirpation without producing worse deformities.

Rarely, a capillary hemangioma of the face is accompanied by hemangiomas of the cerebral cortex and retinal vascular lesions. This syndrome — Sturge-Weber's disease — should be thought of whenever a patient with a facial hemangioma demonstrates seizure activity.

Cavernous hemangiomas are the commonest benign tumors of childhood and are histologically characterized by vascular channels of large size lined with embryonal endothelium. They will present as raised, compressible lesions with a bluish or red discoloration and may range in size from a small nodule to a gross lesion involving most of the face or an extremity. Also of embryonal rather than neoplastic origin, they may not become evident until the latent vascular "lakes" become continuous with the systemic circulation, usually by the end of the first month of life.

The surgical treatment of cavernous hemangioma is almost never an emergency, and when possible a course of "watchful waiting" should be adopted by the surgeon and urged on the patients.

Statistically, 80 per cent of cavernous hemangiomas will undergo spontaneous involution (even when growth of the lesion in the early months of life occurs at an alarming rate); 10 per cent will regress to the point where surgical resection is limited and relatively easy; and 10 per cent, usually fed by a major vessel, will require early operation. Involution usually occurs during the second or third year of life, is has-

tened by infection or the injection of sclerosing agents such as sodium morrhuate, hot water, or hypertonic saline solution, and is heralded by the appearance of gray atrophic patches in the epithelium overlying the hemangioma.

It is readily apparent that conservative treatment of these lesions is justified in the majority of cases. Radiation is again to be condemned in the young child, and the indications for surgery should be clearly understood. These include recurrent bleeding (an uncommon problem usually due to the child picking at the lesion), pain caused by a phlebolith, and persistent ulceration. If a bruit is heard within a rapidly growing lesion, it usually signifies the presence of an arteriovenous fistula of significant size. This will preclude spontaneous involution and is an indication for early surgery.

In general only the smallest hemangiomas, or those which have incompletely resolved, are amenable to outpatient care. In these cases, the principles of excision of skin lesions as previously described apply; most hemangiomas are so richly vascular that effective hemostasis is the preeminent surgical consideration; this is best obtained in the operating room.

Cavernous hemangiomas appearing after infancy should be resected, for not only are they unlikely to involute but they are hard to distinguish from hemangiopericytoma, a malignant lesion which must be widely excised for control of local spread.

Lymphangioma is a true neoplasm of lymph vessels, and resembles hemangioma in that it is compressible and frequently exhibits a bluish discoloration of the overlying skin. It frequently involves the tongue and lips, causing macroglossia and macrocheilia respectively, and is common anywhere on the upper half of the body. It may be noticeable at birth or acquired in later life, and it will not involute. When noted, it should be excised in order to make a definitive diagnosis ruling out lymphangiosarcoma, from which it cannot be clinically distinguished.

Scars and Keloids

The ideal scar is an unobtrusive fine line, supple in texture, and producing no functional or esthetic deformity. When a surgical incision is properly planned with regard to lines of skin tension and executed with gentle handling of tissue, and the normal wound healing sequence proceeds without complication, the end result will usually be an acceptable scar. Injuries requiring suture may well, owing to circumstances such as tissue crushing or contamination, produce a scar that is thick, red and unsightly. When a scar has been infected or allowed to granulate slowly, a hypertrophic scar will be the rule rather than the exception. Scars of this nature, particularly on the face where they are a source of embarrassment to the individual, will be referred for elective reconstruction frequently suitable for the Outpatient Department.

The natural tendency for a scar is to contract somewhat along its longitudinal axis. For this reason an incision should never be planned directly across a flexion crease, for it will usually form a "bridle" which either limits full extension or at the least gives rise to an objectionably noticeable scar. Areas where this precaution should be noted include the inguinal crease, the antecubital, volar wrist and popliteal regions, the axilla, the neck and the nasolabial folds. Injuries are not as discriminating as the wise surgeon, and lacerations in the "wrong direction" may cause scar contractures even when repaired perfectly.

Massive contractures, such as commonly follow burns that have been allowed to granulate, will frequently require release and a skin graft to resurface the resultant bare area. Contractures of a lesser degree will respond well to a Z-plasty, one of the basic techniques in the plastic surgeon's armamentarium.

The Z-plasty, whose origins are obscure,[9] consists essentially of the transposition of two triangular flaps (Fig. 9–17). The principal functional purpose of the Z-plasty is to increase the length of the skin in a desired direction at the expense of the width. The central portion of the Z is the contracture, which may be excised or incised depending on the characteristics of the

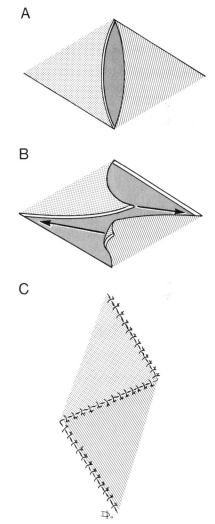

Figure 9–17 The Z-plasty, consisting of the transposition of two triangular flaps to lengthen the axis or change the direction of a contracted scar.

tissue. Two side incisions of the same length as the central portion are made, generally at an angle of 60 degrees to the axis of the scar, creating two triangular flaps which, after undermining, are transposed. It is the interposition of the width of these triangles that provides lengthening of the previous axis of the scar and thus release of the contracture. The simple Z-plasty is suitable for the release of all contractures of modest dimensions, the greatest elongation possible being one third of the original scar. When the bridle to be released is lengthy, requiring the transposition of large flaps, a series of Z-plasties along the length of the excised scar may be effectively employed with a less obtrusive result.

Another justifiable use for the Z-plasty is to change the direction of a scar. Lacerations of the face across the lines of tension may be thrown into prominence because their immobility in the presence of expressive muscular activity is noticeable. Examples are vertical scars of the forehead, scars across the nasolabial crease, and vertical scars between lower lip and chin. Their egregious characteristics may be reduced by a carefully planned Z-plasty, switching the main axis of the scar through 90 degrees as shown in the illustration. The degree of cosmetic improvement resulting from this simple maneuver is often remarkable.

Linear scars of the face, even when well healed, are highly visible and in certain cultures carry unfortunate social connotations. The long scar of an innocently acquired "windshield laceration" may suggest the stigma of knife-fighting and prostitution in an adolescent Spanish-American girl. Breaking up this scar by means of multiple Z-plasties not only will reduce the visual impact of the scar but will imply surgical intervention rather than that of the wielder of a switchblade knife or razor.

An alternative method of breaking up the straight line of a long linear scar to render it less conspicuous is the "W-

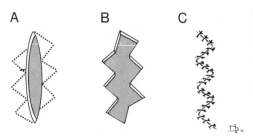

Figure 9–18 The W-plasty, an effective method of breaking up a prominent linear scar.

plasty."[2] If camouflage is required, rather than change of direction per se, then this is probably a better method than the multiple Z-plasty. W-plasty subjects the adjacent tissue to less pull than does multiple Z-plasty. Triangular sections, equilateral and with the sides 1 cm in length, are taken along with the scar to be removed (Fig. 9–18). Sections larger than 1 cm will be too conspicuous, and smaller sections will be ineffective. This may be done by eye or by means of a preset pattern; if done by eye, the ends must be carefully plotted and the same number of triangles cut on each side. This procedure, first described by Borges, is a very valuable means of scar revision.

The degree of hypertrophy of a scar usually depends on the length of time taken for the wound to heal. Infected or granulating wounds or incisions closed under extreme tension will nearly always become thick, reddened and subject to breakdown and itching. Maturation of these scars into a flat, supple structure that is asymptomatic is always delayed and may never occur, in which case surgical revision will be necessary. However, the intense reaction of these scars may be suppressed and maturation hastened by the local use of steroids.

Steroid-impregnated adhesive tape (Cordran tape), when applied directly to the scar and left in place 24 hours a day, will often, over the course of months, achieve a fair degree of improvement. For the more troublesome scar, triamcinolone (Aristocort, 15 mg per cc) may be injected directly into the scar tissue at monthly intervals until regression has taken place.[7] The same agent may be deposited into the superficial 5 mm of the scar without pain by the use of the French-designed Dermajet, which works on an "air-rifle" principle and blasts a bolus of fluid into the skin by pressure alone. When 1.5 cc of triamcinolone is mixed with 0.5 cc of 1 per cent Xylocaine and 0.5 cc of Wydase, the administration is painless and effective. This is the method preferred by the author for the suppression of the moderately hypertrophic scar.

The most objectionable type of scar tissue formation is keloid. Commonest in blacks and swarthy whites, but by no means limited to them, it is regarded by some as the ultimate degree of scar hypertrophy. As the true keloid will not respond to the limited measures described above for suppression of hypertrophic scar, a distinction would be practical. Keloid scar exists when:

(1) The scar tissue extends beyond the confines of the original injury and invades the adjacent normal skin.

(2) There has been no precipitating cause for scar hypertrophy such as infection or tension, or when the reaction is out of proportion to the stimulus.

(3) A similar reaction has occurred before in the same individual — the "keloid former."

(4) Histological or tissue culture differentiation can be made.

Whereas a scar, hypertrophic from a known causative factor, can frequently be excised and closed meticulously to achieve a permanent "hairline incision," the keloid treated in this manner will tend to recur. Treatment of keloids in the past has generally consisted of excision of the lesion, direct suture and immediate radiotherapy (2000 R in four daily divided doses), commencing the day of surgery. However, as this level of irradiation will produce dermal atrophy in the adjacent normal skin, the author prefers an intermediate and less hazardous step — that is, excision of

the keloid and closure after deposition of triamcinolone into the edges of the wound. Treated in this manner, over 50 per cent of keloid scars are significantly improved; the remainder will need re-excision and the more powerfully suppressive effect of radiation as outlined.

Mowlem[10] has pointed out that retained foreign bodies often serve as a nucleus for keloid formation. For this reason, no buried suture material is used; the layers are closed with pull-out sutures of nylon or wire. Ideally, neither ligatures nor the cautery should be used for hemostasis, cessation of flow being obtained by leaving clamps longer than usual on the cut ends of blood vessels and then "twisting" them, or by the use of compresses soaked in dilute (1:200,000) epinephrine solution.

General principles of plastic and reconstructive surgery teach us that tension is the big culprit in scar hypertrophy. A good method to alleviate direct tension on the skin scar is the "vest over pants" technique (Fig. 9–19 A to E). Using this method, tension is placed on the subepidermal and subdermal tissues. Theoretically, no tension is placed on the dermal and epidermal visible scar. However, a hypertrophic scar of the presternal or the deltoid region still remains a problem.

Skin Grafting in the Outpatient Department

The taking of a skin graft is generally regarded as a fairly major procedure requiring a general anesthetic and admission to the hospital. Certainly the successful coverage of large areas of skin loss can best be attained by the close attention to the patient and his wound that this environment provides. However, within certain limitations, it is entirely possible to resurface smaller areas of loss with a skin graft taken under local anesthesia and followed on an ambulatory basis.

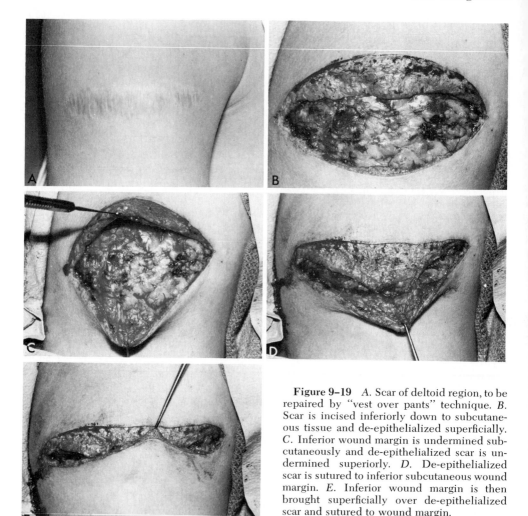

Figure 9–19 *A.* Scar of deltoid region, to be repaired by "vest over pants" technique. *B.* Scar is incised inferiorly down to subcutaneous tissue and de-epithelialized superficially. *C.* Inferior wound margin is undermined subcutaneously and de-epithelialized scar is undermined superiorly. *D.* De-epithelialized scar is sutured to inferior subcutaneous wound margin. *E.* Inferior wound margin is then brought superficially over de-epithelialized scar and sutured to wound margin.

Certain areas of the body lend themselves better than others to this economical approach. Grafts on the trunk are hard to immobilize, owing to constant motion, and need to be observed closely; grafts on the lower extremities should *never* be treated in an ambulatory manner, for the poor venous return of the legs dictates that the grafts be immobilized with a pressure dressing and the legs elevated for at least ten days. Relatively limited areas of skin loss on the head, neck and upper extremities are ideally suited for coverage by skin grafting on an outpatient basis.

Skin grafts are classified anatomically according to the thickness of the graft. Split-thickness skin grafts consist of the epidermis and part of the dermis. As the deeper layers of the dermis are left behind, the donor site will heal spontaneously by epidermal regeneration. They may be cut either freehand, using a skin grafting knife, or by a mechanical dermatome (Fig. 9–20 *A* and *B*). The Davol battery-powered dermatome is suitable for use in the Outpatient Department. The entire cutting head is sterile and disposable, and the motor unit may be wrapped in a sterile polyethylene bag provided with each head piece. A suitable donor site for the split-thickness skin graft is the inner aspect of the upper arm, which is anesthetized by field block. The soft tissues of the arm are pressed taut against the humerus to present a flat surface to the blade, and the graft is taken. The donor site is dressed with scarlet-red gauze next to the raw surface, and covered with sponges and a Kling bandage.

The full-thickness skin graft consists of the epidermis and the entire thickness of the dermis. Cut by hand, it requires that the donor site be sutured closed, thus limiting the extent of the graft. Favorable locations for taking a full-thickness skin graft include the postauricular region, the upper eyelid in elderly people and the supraclavicular skin. The full-thickness skin graft will neither contract nor develop unsightly pigmentation; hence it is an ideal graft to resurface skin loss on the face. This is particularly so when the raw area involves the lower lid or the skin adjacent to the mouth. In these areas, minor degrees of contracture meet no resistance and thus cause significant distortion.

The survival and successful healing of skin grafts depend on the develop-ment of vascular communications between the graft and its recipient bed. The graft is initially sustained by diffusion alone. Capillary endothelial budding occurs at the interface to restore blood flow between recipient site and skin graft within 36 hours. Any factor which tends to disrupt these tenuous early vascular anastomoses will predispose to failure of the graft. The most important of these are "shearing," or sliding of the graft on its bed, hematoma formation which will elevate the graft, and infection.

Dressing techniques must therefore minimize these factors, providing both compression and immobilization to ensure rapid adherence of the graft. The "tie-over bolus dressing" (Fig. 9–21) has stood the test of time and is particularly suited for outpatient care, as it will immobilize the graft while allowing movement in the grafted part.

The skin graft, taken as described, is laid in place on the recipient site and tacked at its four corners. Silk sutures are placed at one-inch intervals, the ends being left long enough to tie over the dressing. The graft is then trimmed so as to fit the defect exactly, and a fine running nylon suture is used to approximate the edge of the graft to the bor-

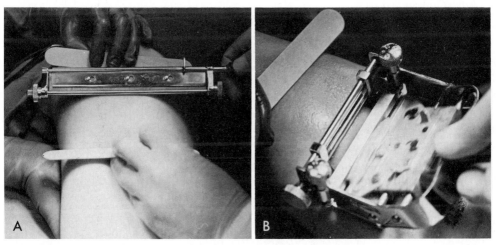

Figure 9–20 *A.* The freehand cutting of a split-thickness skin graft; immobilization of the donor part by an assistant is essential. *B.* Use of the Brown electric dermatome.

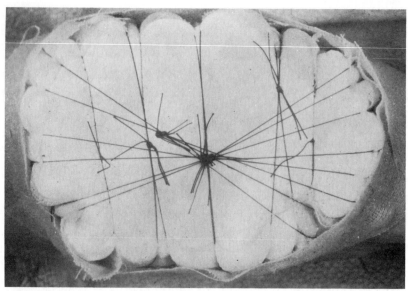

Figure 9-21   The tie-over bolus dressing that both immobilizes a skin graft and provides firm compression to minimize hematoma.

ders of the defect, after irrigation under the graft. The dressing is then built up, using wet cotton, fluffs or sterile foam rubber (Reston, manufactured by the 3M Company, is a very suitable material). The long ends of the sutures are then laid over the dressing to secure firm coaptation of the graft to its bed and yet allow motion in the grafted part without shearing. The whole area is wrapped in a bulky compression dressing. Pain, fever, purulent odors or bleeding imply the necessity of a dressing change and may salvage a jeopardized graft.

The Reverdin or "pinch-graft" is popularly taught to surgical trainees as a simple method of obtaining skin under local anesthesia. However, the resultant scarring of both donor site and grafted area make it an unacceptable substitute for the methods described above.

The Use of Local Flaps

The other method of resurfacing a defect, alluded to many times in the preceding portion of this chapter, is by means of a flap. The flap, sometimes

referred to as a "pedicle graft," is the earliest known reconstructive procedure, and originated with the Hindu tile cutters, who used forehead tissue to replace noses punitively amputated for adultery. The free graft (usually skin) is transplanted without blood supply and depends for its survival upon development of vascular anastomoses with the recipient site. The flap, in contrast, carries with it its own blood supply. The flap consists of skin, dermis and fat, and is always left attached (at least temporarily) with a vascular pedicle to maintain tissue respiration. The skillful design of a flap retains great fascination for the plastic surgeon, for when artistically executed the results are usually far superior to the more pedestrian and easily executed free skin graft. Sir Harold Gillies characterized this appeal when he titled one of the chapters in his outstanding text, "Flap Happy."[6]

Indications

The use of a flap rather than a graft for resurfacing a defect is indicated in the following instances:

(1) When a weight-bearing surface, or an area constantly subjected to minor trauma, is involved.

(2) When a further reconstructive procedure, for example, tendon transfer or bone graft, is contemplated at the site.

(3) When major vessels, nerves, bone without periosteum or tendon denuded of paratenon are exposed.

(4) Where a bulky defect would leave significant deformity if merely resurfaced with skin alone.

(5) Where the recipient site is of poor vascularity — for example, in radiated tissue.

(6) When resurfacing defects of the lower half of the face (i.e., below the level of the eyes) where a graft, subject to changes of pigmentation and texture, would tend to present a "patchy" appearance.

Classification

Flaps are usually classified under two principal headings: local flaps where the tissue to be transferred lies adjacent to the defect, and flaps from a distant source. Distant flaps — the cross-leg flap and those flaps transferred by means of an intermediary carrier such as the wrist — are operative procedures outside the scope of a discussion of outpatient surgery and properly belong in the operating room. Many local flaps are entirely suited to outpatient care, for immobilization and frequent inspection will not be as critical in determining the outcome.

Advancement Flap

The simplest flap is the advancement flap, where incisions in the axis of the desired tissue shift, undermining to provide mobility, and the natural elasticity of the skin will permit movement of tissue into an adjacent location (Fig. 9–22). Frequently "back-cuts" into the base of the pedicle will be required to allow the tissue to expand pantographically, or small triangles can be excised lateral to the flap to compensate for the disparity of length along the axis of closure. An example of the advancement flap is where the tissue of the cheek, incised and undermined generously, is advanced to resurface a defect at the side of the nose (Fig. 9–23 A and B).

Rotation Flap

The rotation flap utilizes a long, curving incision to allow the tissue to rotate about a pivot point (Fig. 9–24 A, B, C). Where the adjacent tissue is lax, as in the glabellar region between the eyebrows, the resultant defect may be closed primarily. Where easy closure of the defect is precluded by unyielding tissue, it is best resurfaced with a skin graft of appropriate size.

Interpolation Flap

The interpolation flap again is rotated about a pivot point, but it is taken from a suitable region near, but not immediately adjacent to, the defect (Fig. 9–25 A, B, C). The flap must therefore be "jumped" over intervening tissue and should be planned so that the defect created by elevation and transfer of the flap can be closed directly. This requires a careful selection of donor sites in which the axis lies in a natural crease and the tissue is lax enough to permit nondistorting closure. Common sites for the interpolation flap include the use of lax upper lid skin to resurface defects of the lower lid, as in the canthal flap (Fig. 9–26 A, B and C), and of the nasolabial region to restore defects of the lower part of the nose (Fig. 9–27 A, B and C).

Technique

Most local flaps are applied directly with the raw surface of the flap laid on

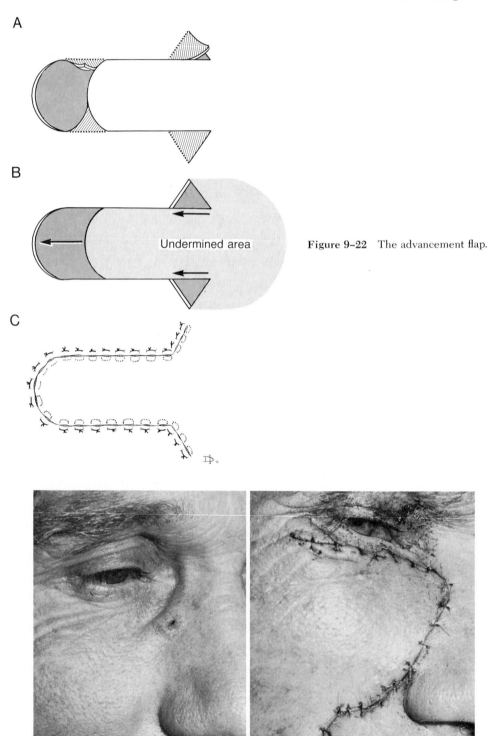

A

B

Undermined area

Figure 9–22   The advancement flap.

C

A   B

Figure 9–23   Use of an advancement cheek flap to resurface a defect on the side of the nose.

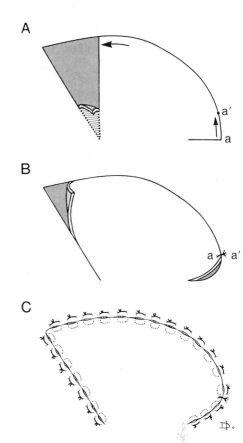

Figure 9–24 The rotation flap pivots tissue about a fixed point.

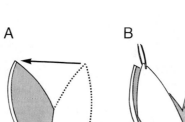

Figure 9–25 The interpolation flap, which is jumped over intervening tissue.

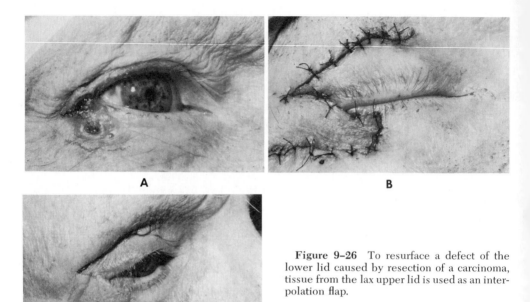

A

B

C

Figure 9–26 To resurface a defect of the lower lid caused by resection of a carcinoma, tissue from the lax upper lid is used as an interpolation flap.

the defect. Where the base of the flap lies at some distance from the defect, part of the flap will serve as a bridge, which if unsurfaced will provide a raw area liable to infection. A closed system can be provided either by grafting the underside of the flap or "tubing" the pedicle by sewing the edges of the flap together to provide a seam down the axis of the pedicle. Care must be taken

not to do this under too great tension, causing compression of the nutrient vessels, and the underside of the flap may be defatted to allow easy closure of the tube. An example of this technique is shown in Figure 9–28 (*A* to *E*) where a small tube pedicle from the forehead is used to reconstruct a defect of the medial canthus involving both upper and lower lids.

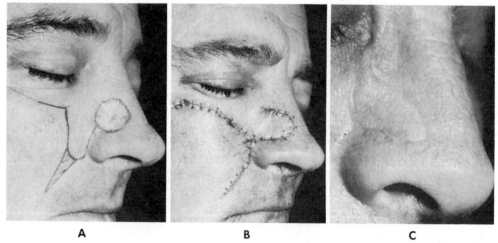

A   **B**   **C**

Figure 9–27 Defects of the lower nose may be replaced effectively by means of a nasolabial interpolation flap.

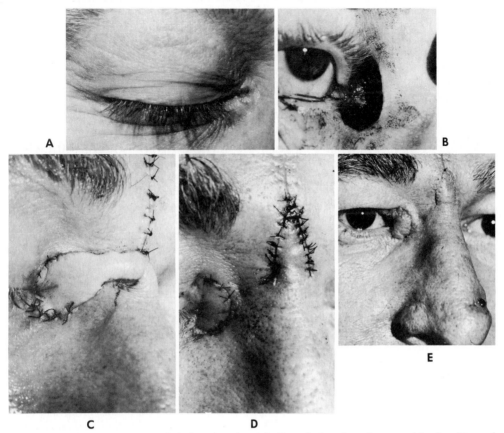

Figure 9–28 A small tube pedicle based on the glabella and taken from the central forehead is used to reconstruct a sizeable defect of the medial canthus caused by removal of a recurrent basal cell carcinoma.

All flaps of whatever type have this in common: the secret of success lies in meticulous planning. Ideally, a pattern of the defect is made and the operative steps are planned in reverse until a template corresponding to the outline of the tissue to be transferred is traced on the skin of the donor site. Care must be taken to include the base of the pedicle in the pattern, which must be cut a little longer and wider than the defect to allow for shrinkage of the transferred tissue.

"Delaying" a Flap

Much has been written about the supposed ideal dimensions of flaps in an attempt to introduce mathematical certainties into an imprecise field. The vagaries of individual circulatory patterns depend on the age of the individual and the location and direction of the flap. "Safe" length:width ratios are therefore almost meaningless. Rather than incise the whole of a planned flap, and upon undermining find that the tip is avascular, it is better to incise and undermine only part of the flap and determine whether the circulation is sufficient to allow extension of the flap. If at any time during the preparation of the flap for transfer, dermal bleeding is dark and capillary filling slow, it is mandatory to return the flap to its original site in order for it to recover from circulatory assault. The oxygen debt in the tissue will enhance collateral circulation through the base of the pedicle — the principle of "delaying" a flap — which will permit eventual transfer of a pedicle too long and narrow to be formed in a single stage.

Enemies of flap survival other than incorrect planning include hematoma, which will "balloon" the flap and stretch the already marginal blood supply. For this reason, hemostasis must be precise, and gentle pressure must be applied to the flap, although pressure must not be so great as to further embarrass the circulation. Various modalities have been used experimentally to enhance the circulation in a flap of dubious viability. These include hypothermia, hyperbaric O_2, and antisludging agents such as low molecular weight Dextran. None will substitute for correct planning.

Tissue handling must be gentle in the extreme, the tip of the flap being held with skin hooks or stay sutures through the dermis rather than with crushing forceps. Suture technique of the flap to the recipient site is important and must cut off as little of the dermal circulation as possible. The "half-buried mattress suture," being parallel to the dermal plexus, is the least noxious in this regard (Fig. 9–29) and should be employed in preference to other sutures.

When these considerations are followed with care, the successful preparation and transfer of flaps become routine, and the dismaying sight of a partially necrotic flap, incapable of fulfilling the reconstructive role for which it was designed, may be avoided. Gillies defines plastic surgery as a "con-stant battle between beauty and blood supply," and nowhere is this more pertinent than in the design and execution of flaps.

Surgery of the Hand

With the astute use of intravenous sedatives and analgesics and the skilled methodology of local and regional anesthesia, many surgical procedures of the hand may be performed in the Outpatient Department. Many plastic surgeons and other hand surgeons perform daily outpatient operations on both elective and traumatic hand injuries. Excision and incision of paronychias, felons and other common hand infections that do not require hospitalization can be performed on an outpatient basis. This is not to minimize the operative intervention but to emphasize the need for a well-equipped outpatient operating room, good lighting, good instrumentation, good assistance and, above all, good judgment. The repair of extensor tendons, flexor tendons and simple or compound fractures in the hand can also be handled in a well-equipped outpatient operating room. If tourniquet exsanguination is used during these procedures, if complicated or prolonged dissection is carried out or if postoperative observation is necessary, then the outpatient operating room can be used and the patient kept in the hospital overnight. The financial impact to patients, insurance companies and, in terms of space utilization, to hospitals is staggering. This is not to mention the rapidity with which hand injuries can be managed conveniently by the surgeon. Obviously, the sooner a hand injury can be operated upon the better the result, and time in the inpatient operating room is always at a premium.

Carpal Tunnel Syndrome

Occasionally, surgeons dealing with the problems of the hand will correct the carpal tunnel syndrome on an out-

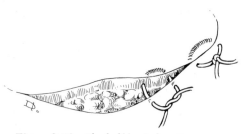

Figure 9–29 The half-buried mattress suture described by Halsted; this technique is most appropriate when blood supply to the skin edge is jeopardized.

patient basis. This syndrome, which involves compression of the median nerve at the wrist, usually occurs in patients of middle age and is more frequently found in females than in males. There are no particular etiological factors in carpal tunnel syndrome, for any obvious anatomical impingement within the carpal tunnel will cause compression of the median nerve and subsequent symptoms and signs. Paresthesia over the distribution of sensibility of the median nerve is usually first seen. Paresthesias can also be associated with thenar muscular atrophy, and symptoms can be reproduced by hyperextending the wrist. If conservative management has failed, exploration of the median nerve and decompression within the carpal canal is indicated.

Carpal tunnel release can be done on an outpatient basis, but exploration of the median nerve and intraneural neurolysis should be accomplished in the main operating room with good lighting, assistance, adequate instrumentation and magnification. Intravenous double tourniquet arm block or brachial block provides satisfactory anesthesia with adequate sedation. A curvilinear incision with angulation at the wrist is accomplished to avoid scar contracture and a flexion posture of the wrist (Fig. 9–30). One should take great care to identify and preserve the palmar cutaneous branch of the median nerve, which may lie anterior to the transverse carpal ligament. Similarly, once the volar aspect of the carpal canal is identified (the transverse carpal ligament) one should completely incise this ligament in its entirety from the proximal to the distal ends. The incisional line should be in the ligament's most ulnar position so that the recurrent branch of the median nerve is not damaged and motor innervation of the thenar eminence is preserved. At this point, identification of the median nerve is carried out. There is some controversy about whether intraneural neurolysis should be commenced. After the tourniquet is released and hemostasis is achieved, the skin only is closed over the wound, the hand is placed in a compression dressing and a volar splint is applied. The hand is elevated at all times, both during awakening in the outpatient recovery room and during convalescence at home. The patient is followed closely in the following days.

Reconstructive Procedures of the Breast

In recent years, the outpatient operating room has been used for many elective reconstructive and cosmetic procedures. Probably the most frequent of these is the augmentation

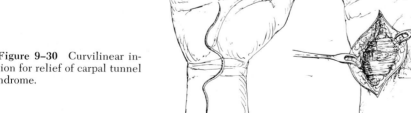

Figure 9–30 Curvilinear incision for relief of carpal tunnel syndrome.

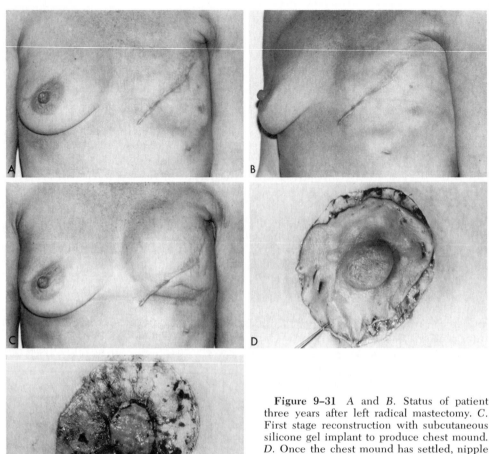

Figure 9–31 *A* and *B*. Status of patient three years after left radical mastectomy. *C.* First stage reconstruction with subcutaneous silicone gel implant to produce chest mound. *D.* Once the chest mound has settled, nipple reconstruction is commenced by harvesting a tangential contralateral areola and nipple from the right breast. *E.* Donor site of harvested nipple and areola.

mammoplasty. This procedure is done for cosmetic increase in the profile of small breasts and for the staged reconstruction following mastectomy (Fig. 9–31).

For augmentation mammoplasty the patient generally arrives in the outpatient department at 7 A.M., having fasted the night before, is given intramuscular premedication and is prepped and draped on the outpatient operating room table. Cardiovascular monitoring is imperative. Augmentation of sedation and analgesia is given intravenously, and local infiltration of ½ per cent Xylocaine with epinephrine (1:200,000) is administered. A retromammary dis-

section can be carried out either through an inframammary crease incision, a periareolar incision or a transaxillary incision. After adequate local anesthesia, a retromammary-suprapectoral pocket is developed, and either a silicone gel–filled or saline-filled mammary prosthesis is inserted. The size and shape of these implants are determined by the judgment of the surgeon and the patient's body and skin profiles. Following irrigation and hemostasis, closure of the wounds is appropriately commenced and a brassiere is then fitted. The patient is allowed to recover for two or three hours in an adjacent recovery room and then dis-

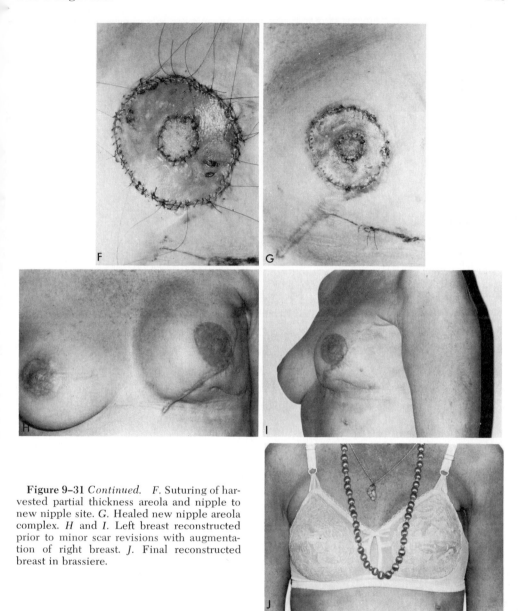

Figure 9–31 *Continued.* *F.* Suturing of harvested partial thickness areola and nipple to new nipple site. *G.* Healed new nipple areola complex. *H* and *I.* Left breast reconstructed prior to minor scar revisions with augmentation of right breast. *J.* Final reconstructed breast in brassiere.

charged with a companion to her home (Fig. 9–32).

Reconstructive Procedures of the Face

Blepharoplasty

Cosmetic outpatient procedures are also performed on the face, the most common being an upper or lower lid blepharoplasty. This operation is done for both cosmetic and functional deformities of the eyelids, to reduce excessive or herniating periorbital fat and excess skin about the eyelids. After appropriate preoperative examination of the eye, the lacrimal drainage system and the muscle tone of the orbicularis oculi, after funduscopic examination,

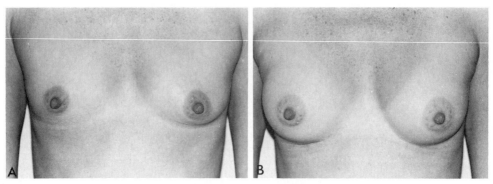

Figure 9–32   *A.* Preoperative micromastia with mild asymmetry. *B.* Postoperative bilateral trans-axillary augmentation mammoplasty.

and possibly after ophthalmological consultation, the patient is sedated and preoperative eyelid markings are made. Infiltration with 1 per cent Xylocaine with epinephrine (1:100,000) is accomplished, and the previously determined skin and periorbital fat is removed.

Some plastic surgeons feel that removal of a small portion of upper lid orbicularis oculi is necessary in order to expose the orbital septum, which is then incised, allowing easy dissection of upper lid periorbital fat. By placing slight atraumatic pressure on the globe, one can judge the amount of periorbital fat to be removed. Hemostasis is achieved and the wounds are closed with fine suture material. Occasionally, supratarsal fixation or anchor blepharoplasty may be desired to give the supratarsal fold more definition. Cold compresses are applied in the postoperative recovery room and the patient is discharged with a companion.

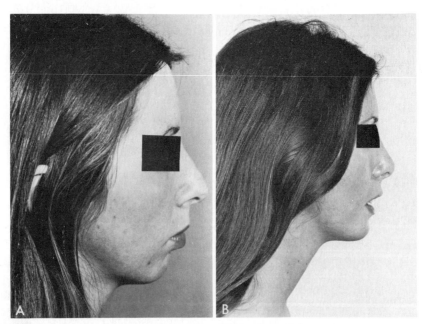

Figure 9–33   *A.* Preoperative nasal deformity and hypoplasia of chin. *B.* Postoperative rhinoplasty and intraoral augmentation mentoplasty.

Rhinoplasty

Occasionally, plastic surgeons perform rhinoplasty and septoplasty on patients as an outpatient procedure. Simply stated, sedation and local and regional anesthesia is used to anesthetize the nose with intranasal packing with a mixture of cocaine and Xylocaine with epinephrine. After adequate nasopharyngeal packing, this operation is carried out entirely within the nasal vestibules. Bilateral intranasal mucosal incisions are made, the lower lateral cartilages are excised to refine a bulbous nasal tip, anterior and inferior cartilaginous septal excisions are made to reduce the height and length of the nose, and lateral nasal osteotomies are performed intranasally to narrow the nasal bridge and reduce the anterior nasal hump. Active cautery hemostasis is generally not needed because of the excellent vasoconstriction provided by cocaine and epinephrine. Mucosal incisions are closed with absorbable fine sutures and the intranasal compartment is then repacked and a plaster or aluminum splint is applied for bony stabilization. The patient can then be discharged with a companion. A rhinoplasty procedure can be technically difficult, and good lighting, assistance and instruments are necessary.

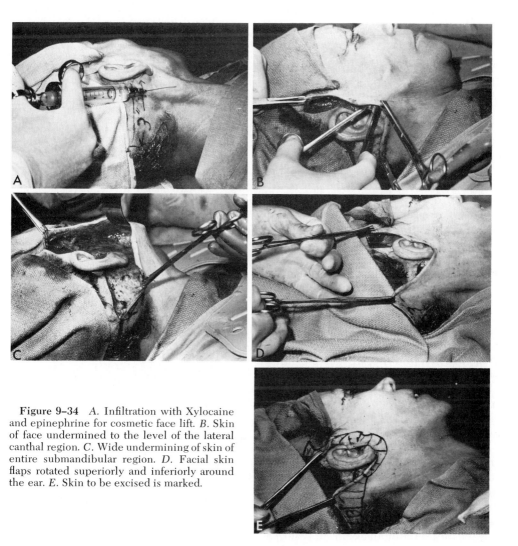

Figure 9–34   *A.* Infiltration with Xylocaine and epinephrine for cosmetic face lift. *B.* Skin of face undermined to the level of the lateral canthal region. *C.* Wide undermining of skin of entire submandibular region. *D.* Facial skin flaps rotated superiorly and inferiorly around the ear. *E.* Skin to be excised is marked.

These can be supplied by an adequately staffed outpatient operating room (Fig. 9–33).

Cosmetic Face Lift

Cosmetic face lift (meloplasty, rhytidectomy) is performed on an outpatient basis by some plastic surgeons. This operation, however, requires a large amount of cutaneous undermining and has the possible complications of facial nerve trauma and postoperative hematoma. Because of the latter complication, most plastic surgeons ask their patients to stay in the hospital at least one postoperative night to try to minimize motion and Valsalva's maneuvers in the early postoperative phase. This operation can be and is being performed in outpatient operating rooms. It utilizes incisions that start in the temporal region behind the hairline, come down inferiorly in a preauricular fashion (some surgeons prefer to incise posterior to the tragus), traverse the contour of the ear lobule, continue superiorly in the postauricular sulcus and then end behind the hairline in the mastoid region. With adequate sedation and infiltration of Xylocaine with epinephrine (Fig. 9–34A), the skin of the face is undermined to the level of the lateral canthal region (Fig. 9–34B), just lateral to the nasolabial fold, the midportion of the body of the mandible and the posterior lateral neck. Frequently, the entire submandibular region is undermined, and excision or plication of the platysma muscle is carried out in these areas for better neck contour. After this wide undermining (Fig. 9–34C) and possibly after submental lipectomy through a separate submental incision, hemostasis is achieved with care, and these facial flaps are rotated both superiorly and inferiorly around the ear (Fig. 9–34D). The excess skin is excised (Fig. 9–34E), and the wounds are closed. Gentle compression dressings are applied, and the patient is either kept overnight in the hospital or discharged with a companion. These patients must be well relaxed and sedated to avoid increasing blood pressure with facial pain or discomfort in order to minimize postoperative hematoma formation that will require re-exploration and evacuation.

REFERENCES

1. Artz, C. P., and Reiss, E.: The Treatment of Burns. Philadelphia, W. B. Saunders Co., 1957.
2. Borges, A. F.: Improvement of anti-tension scar lines by the W-Plasty operation. Br. J. Plast. Surg., 12:29–33, 1959.
3. Conway, H. C., Hugo, N. E., and Tulenko, J. F.: Surgery of Tumors of the Skin. Springfield, Ill., C. C Thomas, 1966.
4. Conway, H. C., and Montroy, R. E.: Permanent camouflage of capillary hemangiomas of face by intradermal injection of insoluble pigments (tattooing): indications for surgery. N. Y. State J. Med., 65:876–885, 1965.
5. Dunphy, J. E.: On the nature and care of wounds. Ann. R. Coll. Surg. Engl., 26:69–87, 1960.
6. Gillies, H. D., and Millard, D. R.: The Principles and Art of Plastic Surgery. Boston, Little, Brown and Co., 1957.
7. Griffith, B. H.: The treatment of keloids with triamcinolone acetonide. Plast. Reconstr. Surg., 38:202–208, 1966.
8. Knize, D. M., Weatherley-White, R. C. A., Paton, B. C., et al.: Prognostic factors in the management of frostbite. J. Trauma, 9:749–759, 1969.
9. McGregor, I. A.: Fundamental Techniques of Plastic Surgery. Baltimore, Williams & Wilkins Co., 1962.
10. Mowlem, R.: Hypertrophic scars. Br. J. Plast. Surg., 4:113–120, 1951.
11. Moyer, C. A., Brentano, L., Gravens, D. L., et al.: Treatment of large human burns with 0.5% silver nitrate solution. Arch. Surg., 90:812–867, 1965.
12. Mustardé, J. C.: Reconstruction of eyelids and eyebrows. In Grabb, W. C., and Smith, J. W.: Plastic Surgery. Boston, Little, Brown and Co., 1957.
13. Paton, B. C.: Bites — Human, dog, spider and snake. Surg. Clin. North Am., 43(2):537–553, April 1963.
14. Peacock, E. E., and Madden, J. W.: Some studies on the effects of B-aminopropionitrile in patients with injured flexor tendons. Surgery, 66:215–222, 1969.
15. Prudden, J. F., Wolarsky, E. R., and Balassa, L.: The acceleration of healing. Surg. Gynecol. Obstet., 128:1321–1326, 1969.
16. Schilling, J. A.: Wound healing. Physiol. Rev., 48(2):374–423, 1968.
17. Stark, R. B.: Plastic Surgery. New York, Harper and Row, 1962.

10 The Eye

JAMES R. CERASOLI, M.D.

INTRODUCTION

The ability of the physician to formulate a diagnosis and proceed with treatment is the basis for training in all fields of clinical medicine, but it is especially difficult in ophthalmology because physicians tend to feel awkward when treating eye problems. As in other specialties, a methodical approach is necessary in ophthalmology to arrive at a proper diagnosis. This will include a history, examination and appropriate laboratory tests. This chapter will describe the evaluation and treatment of eye conditions in the Outpatient Clinic or office. For a more complete review of ophthalmology and methods of treatment utilized in hospitalized patients, a definitive text such as that of Newell[3] should be consulted.

ANATOMY

Seven bones form the bony orbit (Fig. 10–1A). The zygoma, maxilla and frontal bones form the orbital rim, which is the strongest part; the thin bones of the inner walls fracture easily, especially those in the floor and medial wall. The sphenoid bone contains the optic canal through which the ophthalmic artery and the optic nerve pass. Located temporally to this canal is the supraorbital fissure through which cranial nerves III and IV and first division of V and VI pass into the orbit. In the orbital apex syndrome, cranial nerve II and part or all of the cranial nerves passing through the superior orbital fissure may be affected (Fig. 10–1B). In contrast to this syndrome, the superior orbital fissure syndrome does not involve cranial

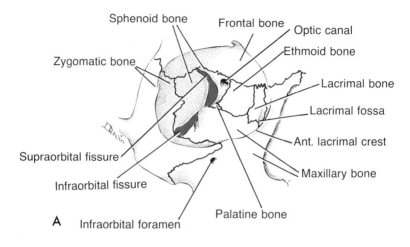

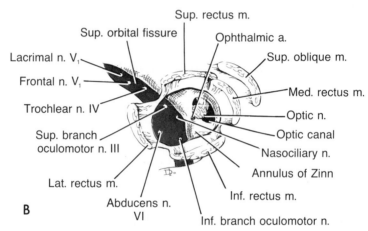

Figure 10–1 *A. Bony orbit. B. Posterior orbit.*

nerve II. If the second division of cranial nerve V is involved along with the other cranial nerves passing through this area, a localization can be made in the cavernous sinus.

Periosteum (periorbita) lines the orbit as a continuation of the dura mater. Originating from the annulus of Zinn, which encircles the optic canal and part of the superior orbital fissure, are the four rectus muscles (medial and lateral, superior and inferior). Pain caused by movement of the eye in patients with optic neuritis may be explained by the proximity of the origin of these muscles to the optic canal. The rectus muscles insert in the globe anteriorly to the equator approximately 5.5 to 7 mm from the limbus. The superior oblique and levator palpebrae muscles originate above the annulus of Zinn, while the inferior oblique muscle takes its origin from the inferior orbital rim near the anterior lacrimal crest. The two oblique muscles insert posteriorly to the equator on the temporal aspect of the globe. A cone-shaped compartment is formed by the recti muscle sheaths behind the globe where the injection of local anesthetic is placed for a local block of the orbit. Adipose tissue fills in the posterior orbit.

The eyeball measures approximately 24 mm in all diameters and has three layers composed of sclera, uvea and retina (Fig. 10–2). The outer scleral layer is a protective shell with a corneal window anteriorly. The middle vascular layer, or uvea, consists of choroid, ciliary body and iris, while the retina makes up the third inner layer. The lens lies behind the iris suspended by zonules. The ciliary body epithelium secretes aqueous humor into the posterior chamber and flows into the anterior chamber between the lens and iris through the pupil, exiting from the eye through the trabecular meshwork located in the angle of the anterior chamber and finally into Schlemm's canal.

A loose layer of connective tissue called Tenon's capsule encloses the eye from the limbus to the optic nerve. Conjunctiva lies external to Tenon's and reflects from the eyeball onto the lids in the upper and lower fornices. It contains mucous, sebaceous and accessory lacrimal glands which secrete the tear layers. Located upper temporally in the orbit near the rim, the lacrimal gland secretes tears reflexly that flow into the superior and inferior punctum at the inner canthus with each blink. Tears exit into the nose via the canaliculi, into the lacrimal sac and then into the lacrimal duct, and from there into the inferior meatal area in the nose (Fig. 10–3). Blockage of this system can occur at any point from the puncta to the lacrimal duct. The most common area of blockage is in the lacrimal duct. Management of this problem will be discussed under the section on inflammation.

The orbit is separated into anterior and posterior compartments by the orbital septum, which extends as a connective tissue layer from the bony rim to the tarsus of the upper and lower lids. A defect in the orbital septum allows posterior orbital fat to prolapse into the anterior compartment. A fibrous tarsal plate provides stability to the lids when blinking (Fig. 10–4). The

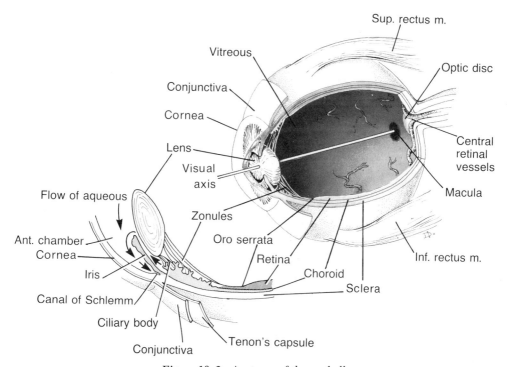

Figure 10–2   Anatomy of the eyeball.

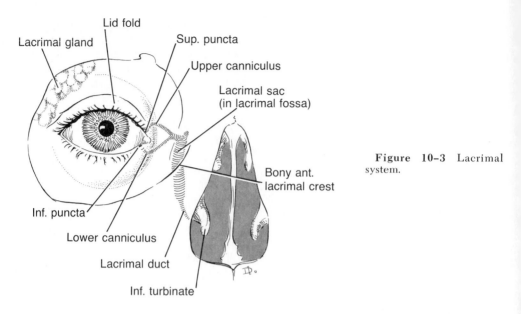

Lid fold
Lacrimal gland
Sup. puncta
Upper canniculus
Lacrimal sac
(in lacrimal fossa)
Bony ant.
lacrimal crest
Inf. puncta
Lower canniculus
Lacrimal duct
Inf. turbinate

Figure 10-3 Lacrimal system.

upper tarsal plate measures approximately 10–12 mm in width as opposed to 5–6 mm in the lower lid. The levator palpebrae muscle inserts largely into the upper tarsus and the strands that extend into the skin form a lid fold in the upper lid. Mueller's muscle, a sympathetically innervated smooth muscle, lies between the palpebral conjunctiva and the levator palpebrae muscle.

PHARMACOLOGY

Some of the following medications should be readily available for diagnosis and treatment (Fig. 10–5):

1. TOPICAL ANESTHETICS. Proparacaine (Alcaine, Ophthaine, Ophthetic) is a minimally irritating topical corneal anesthetic with a rapid onset of action (15 seconds) that lasts approximately 15 minutes. Pain, photophobia and blepharospasm from a superficial foreign body or corneal irritation are relieved with one topical application, allowing the physician to examine the eye comfortably. Most eye injuries or conditions are not adversely affected by the diagnostic use of proparacaine. Its repeated therapeutic use to coun-

teract the pain of an eye injury is contraindicated. Repeated use retards corneal healing and may allow further corneal injury or a corneal ulcer to develop without warning symptoms. Proparacaine should be refrigerated when used infrequently. Tetracaine causes more initial irritation than proparacaine but its advantage is that refrigeration is not needed.

2. TOPICAL ANTIBIOTICS. A broad-spectrum preparation of neomycin, bacitracin and polymycin (Neo-polycin, Neosporin) is used prophylactically after the removal of foreign

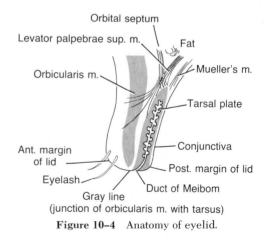

Orbital septum
Levator palpebrae sup. m.
Fat
Orbicularis m.
Mueller's m.
Tarsal plate
Ant. margin
of lid
Conjunctiva
Post. margin of lid
Eyelash
Duct of Meibom
Gray line
(junction of orbicularis m. with tarsus)

Figure 10–4 Anatomy of eyelid.

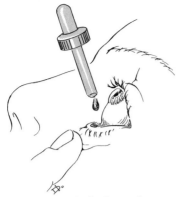

Figure 10–5 Method of introducing topical medications: (1) Have patient look up. (2) Slightly evert lower lid. (3) Place drop in lower cul-de-sac. (4) Do not touch eye or lashes with dropper.

bodies and in the treatment of unknown conjunctival infections while awaiting a culture report. A local allergic reaction to neomycin may occur.

This can be avoided by using a polymyxin B–bacitracin combination (Polysporin), which has an almost identical broad spectrum.

3. CYCLOPLEGICS. Homatropine (2 and 5 per cent) is a parasympatholytic drug that paralyzes the ciliary body and dilates the pupil. Its action relieves pain from ciliary body spasm such as that which occurs in traumatic iritis from an injury or after removal of a corneal foreign body. Its duration of action (24 hours) does not inconvenience the patient as do the longer acting cycloplegics atropine and scopolamine. Uncommonly in older patients an attack of acute narrow angle glaucoma may be precipitated.

The dangers of precipitating angle closure glaucoma by dilating the pupil are frequently impressed on the physician who is not an ophthalmologist. The typical patient with a predisposition to angle closure glaucoma is over 50 years of age, is hyperopic or farsighted (typically wears a convex glass prescription that gives a magnified image) and has a cataract in some stage of development. The combination of these factors in one patient should alert the physician to the possibility of angle closure glaucoma. The anatomical predisposition can sometimes be recognized by a penlight test. A penlight directed onto the eye from the temporal aspect allows the examiner to judge the depth of the anterior chamber. If the iris appears flat and the anterior chamber well illuminated both temporally and nasally, then the anterior chamber is of adequate depth and can be safely dilated. However, if the iris appears bowed forward and the illumination of the anterior chamber is basically limited to the temporal half, then this patient should be dilated with caution. A consultation should probably be obtained. Sometimes the patient will give a history of intermittent eye pain when in a dark room, such as when he is watching television or movies. This pain usually lasts for several hours. In any event, it is advisable to inform the patient to call or return if severe eye pain occurs in the twelve hours following dilation. This warning will usually bring back the patient who has pain from an angle closure attack (see section on Glaucoma).

4. MYDRIATICS. Phenylephrine 10 per cent is a sympathomimetic drug that dilates the pupil and is useful for examining the fundus. Its effect begins in approximately 30 minutes and lasts approximately 3 hours. It also may precipitate an attack of narrow angle glaucoma (see section on Glaucoma).

5. GLAUCOMA TREATMENT. Ophthalmologists use parasympathomimetic drugs (pilocarpine and echothiophate iodide) which constrict the pupil, lower intraocular pressure and facilitate accommodation. Only echothiophate iodide (Phospholine Iodide) is used in the treatment of accommodative esotropia, but both medications are used for chronic glaucoma.

Glycerol, Diamox and mannitol lower the intraocular pressure by an osmotic action. One of these osmotic agents (preferably IV mannitol, 20 per cent, 1 gm/Kg) combined with the frequent topical use of pilocarpine 4 per cent usually breaks an attack of narrow angle glaucoma. The pupil becomes miotic and the intraocular pressure normal.

6. STEROIDS. The use of topical steroid preparations should be avoided because of the ocular side effects of glaucoma, cataracts and corneal ulcers. Patients tend to use these preparations unsupervised for the treatment of viral conjunctivitis and nonspecific corneal irritation because of the symptomatic relief provided.

7. FLUORESCEIN. Fluorescein is a water-soluble dye that stains a corneal abrasion. It fluoresces a brilliant green with ultraviolet illumination (Wood's lamp or a bright light directed through a cobalt blue filter). Many times a fluorescein stain may be recognized with a very bright handlight alone, but this is not always reliable. The use of fluorescein-impregnated paper strips (Fluor-I-Strip-A.T.) is a simple and useful clinical technique to determine if the corneal epithelium has been damaged by trauma, chemicals or exposure to ultraviolet light. The fluorescein paper strip is moistened by the tears from the patient's eye or tap water. It is then touched to the conjunctiva on the lower lid to stain the tear film. The excess fluorescein will be removed in a short time by the normal tear action of the eye. The cornea then is examined for brightly stained green areas, which indicate that the epithelium has been abraded or injured.

LOCAL ANESTHESIA

The first division of the trigeminal nerve enters the orbit through the superior orbital fissure and provides the sensory innervation to the orbit and upper lid (Fig. 10–1 *B* and 10–6). The supraorbital nerve is a branch of the ophthalmic division and exits through the supraorbital foramen in the superi-

or rim. The infraorbital nerve, a branch of the maxillary division, exits through the infraorbital foramen in the lower rim. Xylocaine (1 or 2 per cent) with epinephrine infiltrated in either area gives excellent local anesthesia for the upper or lower lid. Sometimes the medial and lateral canthal areas of the upper and lower lids may require additional infiltration because of overlapped innervation from other branches of the ophthalmic and maxillary division of V. Xylocaine injected into the muscle cone gives akinesia and anesthesia for globe and orbital structures. This type of retrobulbar injection may be complicated by a hemorrhage and rarely by occlusion of the central retinal artery.

EYE EXAMINATION

Any physician can examine the eye with a visual acuity chart, a bright handlight, an ophthalmoscope and a Schiøtz tonometer. If the problem cannot be diagnosed, the patient should be referred to an ophthalmologist for consultation.

The three most common complaints encountered are: (1) a red eye, (2) a painful eye and (3) a change in vision. This section will outline the steps in the evaluation of these and all eye complaints. The history alone many times leads to the correct diagnosis, even though it may be difficult or impossible to verify the diagnosis by the eye examination. However, in all cases a thorough eye examination is necessary to help establish the correct diagnosis.

A common complaint is pain in the eye. Many times this complaint is secondary to trauma and the patient's history is all that is needed. At other times trauma may have occurred but the patient does not recall the injury or the foreign body. A typical example of such an occurrence is eye pain secondary to ultraviolet light radiation which can occur from a welder's arc or

Figure 10–6 Methods of local anesthetic blocks. *A.* Technique for local anesthesia for upper and lower lids: (1) Use a 25 gauge needle to infiltrate 1–2 cc of 2 per cent Xylocaine in the area of the supraorbital or infraorbital nerve near periosteum. (2) To block the VIIth nerve innervation of the orbicularis muscle, an additional injection must be given temporally by infiltrating an area from the brow to the zygomatic eminence.

B and *C.* Technique for retrobulbar block: (1) Palpate lower temporal orbital rim as patient looks up and toward nose. (2) Insert 23 gauge needle of less than 2 inches length in the space between the eyeball and bony rim. (3) Once the eyeball is cleared by the needle tip, direct the needle toward the center of the annulus of Zinn, which is approximately the middle of the posterior orbit. This will place the needle in the muscle cone. (4) Never insert the needle a full 2 inches into the orbit because the anesthetic agent can be accidentally injected into the bony optic canal and compress the optic nerve. (5) Approximately 2 cc of 2 per cent Xylocaine injected into this space will give excellent orbital anesthesia and akinesia.

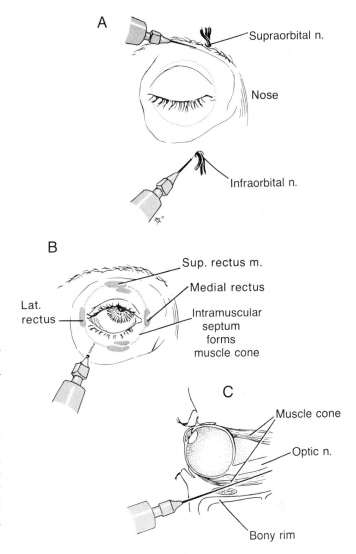

bright sunlight many hours after the insult. Delayed symptoms from trauma secondary to small corneal foreign bodies, contact lens abrasions and ultraviolet radiation are very common.

If trauma is not the cause of a patient's eye pain the examiner must look for other causes, such as infection, inflammation and acute narrow angle glaucoma. Each of these entities will be discussed later in the chapter. This section will outline the step by step process in the eye examination.

1. VISION. The corrected visual acuity is the most important part of the eye examination. For acute eye problems, the examiner must rely on the patient's glass prescription as the best correction. If the patient's glasses are not available, refractive errors may be partially overcome by having the patient read the eye chart through a pinhole device. This may be a commercially available one or a 1.5 mm round hole punched in an index card. The vision may be checked on a Snellen chart at 20 feet. Another handy alternative is to use a Rosenbaum Pocket Vision Screener, which is shown in Figure 10–7. Instructions for the use of

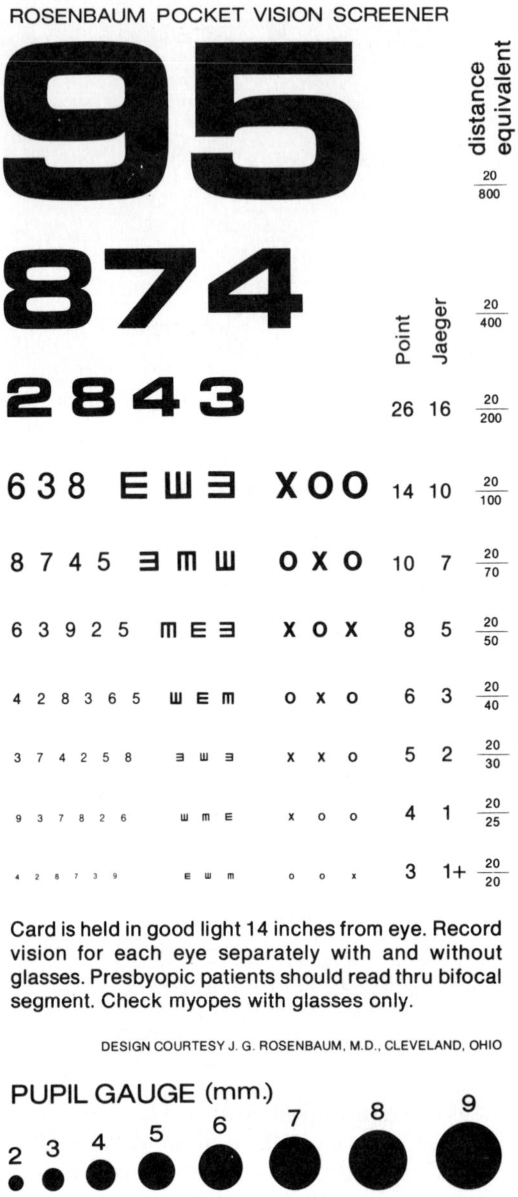

ROSENBAUM POCKET VISION SCREENER

	distance equivalent
95	$\frac{20}{800}$
874	$\frac{20}{400}$
2843	26 16 $\frac{20}{200}$
638 EШƎ XOO	14 10 $\frac{20}{100}$
8745 ƎmШ OXO	10 7 $\frac{20}{70}$
63925 mEƎ XOX	8 5 $\frac{20}{50}$
428365 ШEm OXO	6 3 $\frac{20}{40}$
374258 ƎШƎ XXO	5 2 $\frac{20}{30}$
937826 ШmE XOO	4 1 $\frac{20}{25}$
428739 EШm OOX	3 1+ $\frac{20}{20}$

Point Jaeger

Figure 10-7 Rosenbaum Pocket Vision Screener.

Card is held in good light 14 inches from eye. Record vision for each eye separately with and without glasses. Presbyopic patients should read thru bifocal segment. Check myopes with glasses only.

DESIGN COURTESY J. G. ROSENBAUM, M.D., CLEVELAND, OHIO

PUPIL GAUGE (mm.)

2 3 4 5 6 7 8 9

this handy card are included in the illustration. It should be emphasized that in a patient over 45 years of age a reading glass is necessary.

A difference in acuity between the two eyes or poor vision in both eyes requires an explanation. Normal vision (20/20 in both eyes) indicates the central visual apparatus is intact, including the cornea, lens, vitreous, macula and the visual pathway to the lateral geniculate nuclei. The peripheral vision is tested monocularly by a finger-counting confrontation technique as part of the vision exam. Each quadrant is examined as the patient fixes on the examiner's eye. The patient and the examiner should see the fingers in approximately the same peripheral position. A gross field defect should have quantitative perimetry and its cause should be explained by the eye examination or a neurological examination.

2. PUPILS. The afferent and efferent pathways of the light reflex include the iris, visual apparatus and autonomic nervous system. The light reflex is intact if the pupils are equal in size and react briskly and equally to a light stimulus when tested both directly and consensually. Consider the pupils abnormal if they are unequal in size or if the light reaction is poor or absent. The cause must be explained, since the prognostic significance of these findings varies greatly. Some common causes of abnormal pupils are eye medications, third nerve paralysis, Horner's syndrome, Adie's tonic pupil, tertiary syphilis and trauma to the iris. Horner's syndrome consists of ptosis, miosis and anhidrosis with apparent enophthalmos, resulting from a lesion in any one of the three neurons forming the sympathetic pathway from the hypothalamus to the eye. In Horner's syndrome the pupil responds like a postganglionic, sympathetically denervated structure which is hypersensitive to weak dilutions of topical epinephrine (1:1000) and will dilate, whereas the normal pupil will not. Topical cocaine dilates the normal pupil by preventing the re-uptake of norepinephrine at the effector site. In Horner's syndrome, topical cocaine will not dilate the affected pupil, since norepinephrine is not secreted in the denervated situation. Cocaine (4 per cent) gives more reliable results than epinephrine (1:1000) in the test for Horner's syndrome.

Another reliable chemical test for Horner's pupil is the use of hydroxyamphetamine 1 per cent (Paredrine), which indirectly stimulates the release of norepinephrine from the effector site. It dilates the normal pupil but not the Horner's pupil in a postganglionic lesion, because norepinephrine is available at the effector site. It is useful in differentiating a postganglionic Horner's lesion from a preganglionic lesion. The subject of the physiology of the eye is discussed in detail by Moses.[2]

In the tonic pupil or Adie's syndrome, parasympathetic denervation of the pupil occurs because of a lesion in ciliary ganglion. Clinically the abnormal pupil is larger than normal and the reaction to a light stimulus is poor or absent. Topical application of a weak cholinergic agent (methacoline 2.5 per cent) constricts the affected pupil but not the normal pupil. Recognition of this common syndrome is important because it is a benign condition and should be differentiated from a third nerve paralysis.

In most cases the history and other neurological findings help differentiate a third nerve paralysis from other causes of abnormal pupils. Pilocarpine (4 per cent) will constrict a pupil that is dilated because of third nerve paralysis. Many patients have unilateral or bilateral dilated, poorly reacting pupils caused by mydriatic medication placed in the eye that a patient usually fails to relate to the examiner. Pilocarpine (4 per cent) will not constrict these pupils.

The Argyll Robertson pupil seen in tertiary syphilis consists of an intact near-reaction while the light reaction is poor or absent. Both pupils are usually miotic and irregular in shape. They may dilate very poorly in response to any mydriatic. In paresis or in latent lues, the patient may have, instead of an Argyll Robertson pupil, a fixed dilated pupil.

Abnormal pupils secondary to trauma can usually be recognized. A small defect in the pupillary sphincter causes a partially dilated pupil with a very irregular margin. In some cases, a defect in the iris stroma (iridodialysis) may occur. The history, examination and use of appropriate topical medications help differentiate these causes of abnormal pupils.

3. EXTRAOCULAR MUSCLES (Fig. 10–8). The third, fourth and sixth cranial nerves are evaluated when a

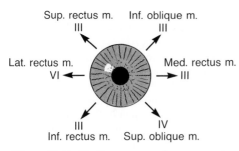

Sup. rectus m.   Inf. oblique m.
III   III

Lat. rectus m.   Med. rectus m.
VI   III

III   IV
Inf. rectus m.   Sup. oblique m.

Figure 10–8   Testing eye muscle movements.

patient follows a light into the eight fields of gaze. Old photographs and the history help distinguish an acute external ophthalmoplegia (extraocular muscle paresis) from a decompensated congenital muscle imbalance. The degree of diplopia increases in the field of action of the acutely paretic muscle. Mechanical limitation from an orbital floor fracture or mass may simulate a muscle paresis. A forced duction test consists of moving the eye in all positions of gaze with a tooth forceps to determine if mechanical limitation is present. This test is easily performed after several drops of topical anesthesia with proparacaine or cocaine. The eye is grasped with a 0.5 mm tooth forceps near the limbus in front of the muscle tested. The test is positive (mechanical limitation is present) when the eye cannot be moved fully with the forceps.

4. ANTERIOR SEGMENT OF THE EYE. The lids, lacrimal apparatus, conjunctiva, cornea, anterior chamber, iris and lens may be grossly evaluated with a bright hand light. Fluorescein dye placed in the tears helps in locating small foreign bodies and corneal epithelial abrasions. The dye stains the disturbed corneal epithelium a bright green after the excess is blinked away with the tears as described previously in the section on Pharmacology.

Blood in the anterior chamber (hyphema) may settle inferiorly as a red clot or may, if extensive, obscure the iris detail. Usually inflammatory cells in the anterior chamber, like those in an iritis, cannot be seen with a hand light, but a flush of the perilimbal vessels is usually present. Tremulous movements of the iris (iridodonesis) occur when the lens partially dislocates (subluxation) or totally dislocates (luxation). Also, the depth of the anterior chamber appears deeper or irregular compared to its normal fellow eye.

5. POSTERIOR SEGMENT OF THE EYE. Ophthalmoscopic evaluation of the vitreous, disc, macula, retina and retinal vessels should be done through a dilated pupil. One drop of neosynephrine (10 per cent) works well. After the pupil is dilated, the examiner should begin the evaluation approximately 8 to 12 inches in front of the patient's eye, with the direct ophthalmoscope set on approximately + ten focus. This allows the examiner to focus on the anterior segment and observe a red reflex through the dilated pupil. Against this background, opacities such as corneal scars, cataracts and vitreous floaters can be recognized. As the examiner moves closer to the patient, the focus of the ophthalmoscope must be changed toward zero in order to focus the optic disk, retina and blood vessels.

It is important to recognize a red reflex through the dilated pupil. If a black or gray reflex is seen, this usually indicates a dense opacity in the media. The differential diagnosis includes (1) dense cataract, (2) dense vitreous hemorrhage, (3) intraocular infection, (4) retinal detachment, (5) retinal tumor, (6) large chorioretinal scars and (7) retinal exudate.

A monocular visual loss or central scotoma may be explained by changes in any of the posterior structures. Scars, hemorrhages or tumors in the macular area can cause a marked visual loss. Abnormalities in the peripheral area such as hemorrhages, inflammation, scars, vascular abnormalities, tumors and retinal detachments are other common causes of monocular visual loss.

Vitreous floaters are a common complaint and are usually benign. Small spots are seen that move and float with eye movements. These usually have been present for some time without other visual complaints. Numerous vitreous floaters may occur suddenly and be associated with symptoms of photopsia (flashing lights) and scotomas (shadows or curtains). These patients should be evaluated for a vitreous hemorrhage, a retinal hemorrhage, retinal tears or a retinal detachment.

Early signs of papilledema are bilateral blurring of the disk margins, hyperemia of the disk and loss of venous pulsation. The presence of splinter hemorrhages and elevation of the disk margins establish the diagnosis. The vision remains normal but the blind spot enlarges on testing the central fields. In optic neuritis the disk may appear similar to that seen in papilledema, but it is usually unilateral and vision is decreased with the presence of a field defect.

6. GLAUCOMA. A screening measurement of the intraocular pressure with a Schiøtz tonometer for glaucoma should be done routinely on patients who have had trauma or possible acute angle closure glaucoma attack (Fig. 10–9 and Table 10–1). An intraocular pressure of 10–22 mm of mercury that approximately is equal in both eyes is normal. A low intraocular pressure may be the only clue to a posterior rupture of the globe.

A large irregular central cup should alert the examiner to possible chronic glaucoma (Fig. 10–10). A comparison of the diameter of the central cup to

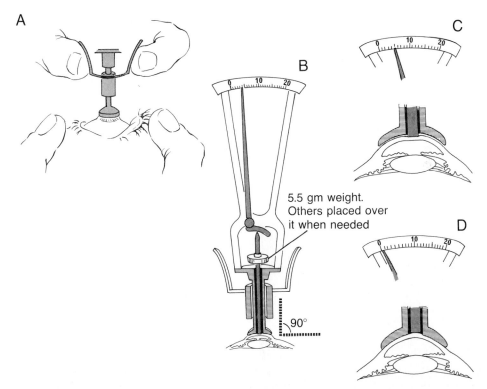

Figure 10–9 Use of Schiøtz tonometer. For conversion numbers see Table 10–1. (1) Patient recumbent. (2) Cornea anesthetized. (3) Patient fixates with opposite eye. (4) Lids held open with no pressure on eyeball. (5) Tonometer reading is converted to mm of mercury by chart supplied with instrument (see Table 10–1). (6) Tonometer readings 0–2.5 with 5.5 gm or any weight are inaccurate and additional weights must be added until the tonometer reading is greater than 2.5.

TABLE 10–1   Schiøtz Conversion Table*

Schiøtz Reading	5.5 gm	7.5 gm	10 gm	15 gm
0.0	41.5 mm Hg	59.1 mm Hg	81.7 mm Hg	127.5 mm Hg
0.5	37.8	54.2	75.1	117.9
1.0	34.5	49.8	69.3	109.3
1.5	31.6	45.8	64.0	101.4
2.0	29.0	42.1	59.1	94.3
2.5	26.6	38.8	54.7	88.0
3.0	24.4	35.8	50.6	81.8
3.5	22.4	33.0	46.9	76.2
4.0	20.6	30.4	43.4	71.0
4.5	18.9	28.0	40.2	66.2
5.0	17.3	25.8	37.2	61.8
5.5	15.9	23.8	34.4	57.6
6.0	14.6	21.9	31.8	53.6
6.5	13.4	20.1	29.4	49.9
7.0	12.2	18.5	27.2	46.5
7.5	11.2	17.0	25.1	43.2
8.0	10.2	15.6	23.1	40.2
8.5	9.4	14.3	21.3	38.1
9.0	8.5	13.1	19.6	34.6
9.5	7.8	12.0	18.0	32.0
10.0	7.1	10.9	16.5	29.6

*To use the Table:
 1. Determine scale reading on Schiøtz tonometer.
 2. Find reading on Conversion Table under column titled Schiøtz Reading.
 3. Determine intraocular pressure in mm Hg by reading under column with appropriate wt. used.

the diameter of the disk gives a cup/disk ratio (C/D). If the cup/disk ratio is 0.3 or greater, the intraocular pressure should be checked for possible chronic glaucoma.

Acute or narrow angle glaucoma is

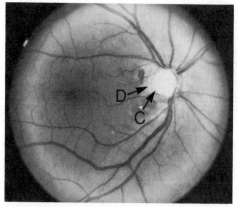

Figure 10–10. Glaucoma cupping of optic nerve. *C.* Optic cup. *D.* Optic disc.

differentiated from chronic or open angle glaucoma by gonioscopy. An ophthalmologist must make this evaluation by examining the appearance of the angle of the anterior chamber. In acute glaucoma there is a sudden rise in the intraocular pressure (usually greater than 50 mm of mercury) associated with sudden severe pain, loss of vision and an injected irritable eye with a dilated pupil. Usually the clinical diagnosis is easily made. Delay in treatment of the glaucoma may result in permanent loss of vision (see section on Pharmacology). In contrast, chronic glaucoma occurs bilaterally with an insidious loss of the peripheral fields over many years while good central acuity is maintained with few symptoms. Patients sometimes complain of halos around lights. On examination the vision is normal and intraocular pressure is usually greater than 30 mm Hg. In advanced cases, glaucoma cupping is seen, as demonstrated in Fig. 10–10.

TRAUMA

For a definitive review of the problems of trauma to the eye and its supporting structures, the reader is referred to the standard text by Paton and Goldberg.[4]

1. FOREIGN BODIES. Foreign body complaints from flying metal fragments and blast injuries require orbital x-rays. To distinguish an intraocular from an orbital foreign body, a localization may be performed using a Sweet's radiological technique[5] or a radiopaque contact lens may be placed on the cornea. Most inaccessible orbital foreign bodies need not be removed, but an intraocular foreign body should be referred to an ophthalmologist for management. It is helpful to know the kind of metal composing the foreign body, since iron and copper are extremely toxic to the eye while some inert materials are best left undisturbed. Magnetic foreign bodies are easier to remove and therefore have a better prognosis than other types.

Superficial foreign bodies of the tarsal conjunctiva and cornea may be located by use of fluorescein staining, a bright light and magnification. After topical corneal anesthesia, the foreign body may be wiped away with a moist, sterile cotton-tip applicator. This may be unsuccessful if the foreign body is a rust ring or is deeply imbedded in the corneal stroma. In this case it should be referred to an ophthalmologist who can remove it under high magnification with a sharp needle or spud.

Sand and dirt particles lodge in the tarsal conjunctiva of the upper lid and, to the patient, feel like corneal foreign bodies. They cause streaklike, diffuse staining of the cornea and can be removed by everting the upper lid and wiping away with a sterile, moist, cotton-tip applicator (Fig. 10–11). A topical broad-spectrum antibiotic should be used prophylactically on the eye. Follow-up examinations are necessary until the corneal epithelium no longer stains with fluorescein, because these abrasions frequently result in corneal ulcers which require emergency management. An untreated corneal ulcer may perforate the cornea with loss of the eye. These infections are difficult to treat because of corneal avascularity.

Large corneal abrasions, whether due to a foreign body or other trauma, require the same precautions as outlined above. Two oval eye pads should be taped firmly with seven strips of 1 inch tape approximately 5 to 6 inches long. The tape should be applied from the center of the forehead across the patch toward the angle of the mandible to splint the lid so the patient cannot

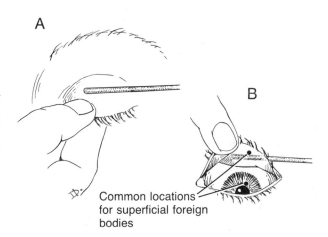

Figure 10–11 Technique of everting lid and removing foreign body. (1) Anesthetize cornea. (2) Patient looks down. (3) Lid everted as shown. (4) Foreign body located and removed.

A

B

Common locations for superficial foreign bodies

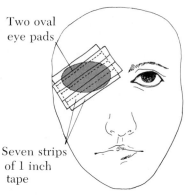

Two oval
eye pads

Seven strips
of 1 inch
tape

Figure 10–12 Modified pressure patch for the eye.

blink. This will relieve symptoms and allow the corneal epithelium to regenerate more quickly. The epithelial defect usually heals in 24 to 48 hours. Figure 10–12 demonstrates the proper patching of the eye.

2. LACERATIONS OF THE LIDS. A lid laceration should alert the physician to possible intraocular damage. Multiple lid lacerations may appear as avulsed tissue. Usually little or no tissue loss occurs and the lid fits together like a jigsaw puzzle. The physician should copiously irrigate the debris from the laceration, but try not to debride tissue unless it is truly necrotic (the excellent blood supply to the lid usually prevents necrosis). Superficial lid lacerations that do not involve the lid margin or canalicular area are easily repaired with interrupted 6–0 silk sutures. A deep laceration involving the orbital septum can be recognized when orbital fat prolapses into the wound; the deep layers should be closed anatomically with 5–0 or 6–0 absorbable sutures. If skin avulsion does occur, the most satisfactory sites from which to take a skin graft are the opposite upper lid or the site behind the ear. Extensive loss of tissue requires a bridge flap from the uninvolved lid.[1] Jeweler's loupes or other magnifying lenses are helpful in performing this type of surgery.

Exposure and tearing problems may result from poorly repaired lid lacerations through the margin. Since the lower canaliculus drains the majority of tears into the nose, lacerations through this area require meticulous repair and are best referred to an ophthalmologist. Lacerations through the upper canaliculus and lid margins are repaired as diagrammed (Fig. 10–13). Lid notches may occur if these lacerations are not exactly approximated, and corneal irritation with pain and decreased vision may develop.

3. LACERATION OF THE EYEBALL. Pigmented uveal tissue found in a corneal or scleral laceration establishes this diagnosis (Fig. 10–14). The laceration requires immediate repair by the ophthalmologist. Both eyes should be patched lightly without further manipulation and the patient instructed to remain quiet. Squeezing of the lid, coughing and unnecessary movements will increase the intraocular pressure and cause further prolapse of the intraocular contents.

4. CONTUSION INJURIES TO THE EYE. Blunt trauma about the eye causes serious intraocular injury in ap-

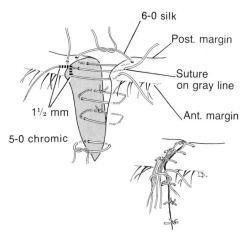

6-0 silk

Post. margin

Suture on gray line

Ant. margin

1½ mm

5-0 chromic

Figure 10–13 Repair of laceration of lid. (1) Place the posterior lid margin suture first and leave its ends long for traction while placing the other sutures. (2) Repair the tarsal and orbicularis laceration with 5-0 chromic. (3) Complete the gray line and anterior margin suturing with long ends so that the knots can be pulled away from the cornea as illustrated.

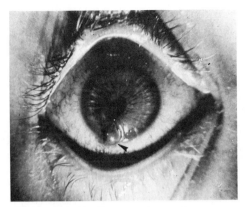

Figure 10–14 Pigmented uveal tissue in corneal laceration.

proximately 15 per cent of all cases. A methodical examination differentiates the routine "black eye" from one that has a serious intraocular injury. Rupture of the sclera, traumatic glaucoma, blood in the vitreous or anterior chamber (hyphema), dislocation of the lens, traumatic cataracts, retinal detachment, retinal hemorrhage and injury to the optic nerve with permanent loss of vision can occur if not properly treated.

It may be difficult to examine a swollen eye after blunt trauma. A drop of topical anesthetic should be placed on the cornea. Lid retractors are then introduced if needed to open the swollen lids so no pressure is exerted on the possibly injured eye. A subconjunctival hemorrhage is usually pres-

ent. Figure 10–15 demonstrates a layer of blood between the conjunctiva and sclera. The subconjunctival hemorrhage alone requires no treatment. If the remainder of the examination is normal, the patient may be assured that no permanent damage has occurred to the eye and the blood will slowly clear.

Frequently a hyphema occurs with a contusion injury as seen in Figure 10–16. The blood in the anterior chamber may layer out in the deepened position or entirely fill the anterior portion of the eye. The blood generally obscures details of the iris to some degree. Immediate treatment for hyphema is to patch both eyes and sedate the patient. Re-bleeds usually occur three to five days after the initial injury. The patient should be watched daily for clearing of the blood and checked for secondary glaucoma. In most cases the blood clears spontaneously over several days. Usually topical steroids are used to decrease the traumatic iritis.

5. ORBITAL FRACTURES. Proper x-ray examination helps make the diagnosis when orbital fractures are suspected. A routine orbital series of x-rays should include an anterior-posterior view, a lateral view, a Waters' projection and a submental view. These views may be interpreted as normal even when there is clinical evidence of a fracture, in which case further study by tomography should be

Figure 10–15 Subconjunctival hemorrhage.

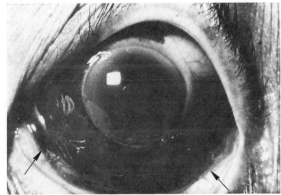

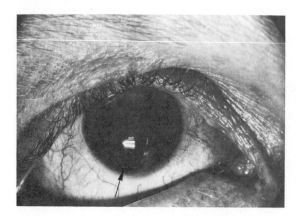

Figure 10–16 Hyphema obscures iris details.

done. A blow-out fracture incarcerates the inferior orbital contents into the floor defect (Fig. 10–17), thus mechanically limiting elevation and depression of the eye and causing vertical diplopia (Fig. 10–18). Injury to the infraorbital nerve in this area causes hypesthesia to the lower lid area. The fracture should be repaired within one or two weeks after injury, when the swelling has subsided. If misdiagnosed, organization of the tissues in the fracture site occurs and makes repair difficult. A blow-out fracture is best repaired through an orbital approach with a silastic or methylmethacrylate implant inserted to cover the defect after the incarcerated tissue is retracted.

The trimalar fracture usually involves the zygomatic-maxillary suture, zygomatic-frontal suture and arch of the zygoma. A nondisplaced trimalar

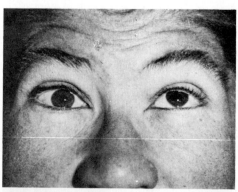

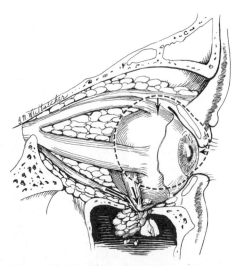

Figure 10–17 Diagram of blow-out fracture of orbit. From Paton, D. and Goldberg, M. F.: Management of Ocular Injuries, Philadelphia, W. B. Saunders Co., 1976.

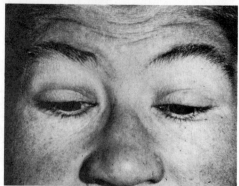

Figure 10–18 Loss of upgaze in right eye in blow-out fracture.

fracture requires no further treatment; however, displacement causes flattening of the cheek bone and occasionally temporomandibular joint problems. Repair is accomplished by wiring two legs of the tripod at the zygomatic-frontal and zygomatic-maxillary sutures after open reduction of the displacement. Isolated fractures involving only the orbital rim do not require repair. Orbital emphysema may occur from a fracture in the ethmoid sinus or the orbital floor, and treatment requires time for the orbital air to slowly reabsorb, during which time the patient should be given a broad-spectrum antibiotic and instructed not to blow his nose for several weeks.

A fracture in the optic canal is difficut to diagnose using x-rays alone. Tomograms sometimes help. Edema of the intraosseous portion of the optic nerve occurs and may result in permanent visual loss if not decompressed early by a neurosurgical approach. Surgical treatment of this edema should not be undertaken if vision is poor on the initial examination; this diagnosis should be considered and surgery contemplated only if the vision has been reported on an initial examination and later deteriorates.

6. RADIATION. Ultraviolet light from an arc welder's machine or prolonged exposure to the snow or sandy beaches causes corneal epithelial changes. Severe pain, photophobia and blurred vision occur five to ten hours after the insult. Fluorescein stains the cornea in a stippled pattern. One application of a topical anesthetic gives instant relief; however, its chronic use can inhibit epithelial regeneration and can cause corneal scarring. A firm dressing on both eyes (Fig. 10–12) and mild sedation provide relief for the patient until the epithelium regenerates. Usually no residual corneal problems occur.

7. CHEMICAL BURNS. Any caustic material in the eye requires rapid and copious irrigation with any solution at hand. The patient should immediately blink his eyes under water as an initial treatment at home or at work. Thereafter, the physician should use a topical anesthetic and irrigate the eye with 2 to 3 liters of normal saline or balanced Ringer's lactate using a bulb syringe or IV tubing. To remove particular matter in the cul-de-sacs of the upper and lower lids, a cotton-tip applicator may be used. The damage resulting to the eye from a chemical burn depends upon the type, concentration and duration of the chemical in the eye; lye burns heal poorly while acid burns cause relatively less damage.

Mace and tear gas corneal injuries are self-limiting and usually leave no residual corneal defects. The eye may be irrigated with 0.4 per cent sodium sulfite solution or normal saline after application of a topical anesthetic. The propellant used in mace may cause a contusion injury if ejected near the patient's eye.

INFLAMMATION OF THE EYE

In the differential diagnosis of a red eye, conjunctivitis, iritis, scleritis and acute glaucoma must be considered, although there are many other causes that are too numerous to be considered. Certain guidelines for these entities can be set (Table 10–2), although their differentiation may puzzle the examiner if a methodical history and eye examination are not done. Acute glaucoma requires emergency treatment, and a delay in diagnosis can result in permanent loss of vision (Fig. 10–19). Corneal ulcers cause the patient to complain of pain and a foreign body sensation, and vision is usually decreased; on examination a corneal opacity is usually noted (Fig. 10–20). A dendritic ulcer of herpes simplex may be seen only after staining the cornea with fluorescein (Fig. 10–21). All corneal ulcers require scrapings for gram stains, culture and sensitivities to establish the diagnosis. Treatment with

TABLE 10–2　Differential Diagnosis of a Nontraumatic Inflamed Eye

	CONJUNCTIVITIS	IRITIS	SCLERITIS	ACUTE GLAUCOMA
VISION	Normal	Normal or mild blur	Normal	Decreased
DISCHARGE	Mucoid or pus	Tearing from photophobia	Tearing from photophobia	Tearing from photophobia
CONGESTION	Lids and superficial conjunctival vessels	Circumcorneal and conjunctival	Deep scleral vessels	All vessels
PAIN	Foreign body sensation, sandy or mild	Moderate to severe	Severe	Severe
CORNEA	Normal	Probably clear Keratic precipitate present*	Normal	Cloudy
ANTERIOR CHAMBER	Normal	Probably clear Cells present*	Normal	Shallow
PUPIL	Normal	Usually miotic	Normal	Dilated
INTRAOCULAR TENSION	Normal	Usually decreased	Normal	Increased (50 mm Hg)
TREATMENT	Culture and smear Appropriate topical antibiotics	Cycloplegia Topical steroids qhs Treat systemic disease	Cycloplegia Treat systemic disease Analgesia Topical steroids qhs	Osmotic agents 1) Intravenous: Diamox, mannitol, urea 2) Oral: glycerol (1 cc/kg) 3) Pilocarpine 4% topically q 15 min Surgery q 15 min

*Can be seen with biomicroscope.

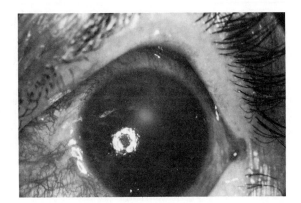

Figure 10–19 Acute glaucoma.

antibiotics is started according to the results of the bacteriology studies.

Orbital cellulitis usually is caused by a sinus infection or trauma, and the inflammation can quickly spread to the cavernous sinus because of the orbital venous drainage into this area. These patients should be hospitalized and treated with appropriate antibiotics after culture and sensitivity studies.

In dacryocystitis inflammation occurs over the lacrimal sac (Fig. 10–22), and with pressure over this area, pus can be expressed through the lower punctum. These infections tend to be chronic because of obstruction in the nasal lacrimal system due usually to a congenital anomaly or trauma. Obstruction may occur at any point in the lacrimal drainage system. Tearing usually precedes the appearance of recurrent episodes of infection. This

condition is frequently seen in infants because of a blockage in the area of the inferior turbinate (see Fig. 10–3). Most of these infants can be cured by pressure applied over the inner canthus in the area overlying the lacrimal sac. This forces the tears present in the sac into the nose and cures the obstruction. If after several weeks there is no improvement in the tearing, the lacrimal duct should be probed. Children over six months of age usually move too much for this procedure to be done safely without a general anesthesia.

The anatomy of the lacrimal drainage system must be understood thoroughly prior to attempting prob-

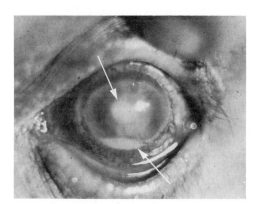

Figure 10–20 Bacterial corneal ulcer.

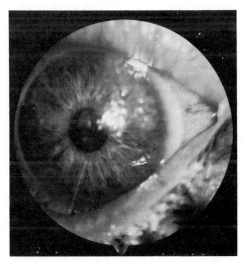

Figure 10–21 Dendritic herpetic corneal ulcer, stained.

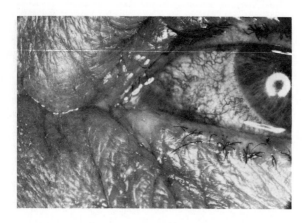

Figure 10–22   Infection of lacrimal sac.

ing. The instruments needed are (1) a lacrimal punctal dilator, (2) a lacrimal irrigating cannula and (3) a lacrimal probe, size 00. The infant is mummified with a blanket and held firmly by the assistant if general anesthesia is not used. A topical anesthetic is placed in the eye. The superior (never the inferior) puncta is dilated adequately so the irrigating cannula attached to a 5 cc syringe filled with water can be introduced into the dilated puncta. Many times gentle irrigation alone will open the obstruction. If this is not successful, a 00-sized Bowman lacrimal probe is introduced through the dilated upper puncta into the sac through the lacrimal duct into the inferior meatus of the nose. The probe is never forced at any point during this procedure. If force is exerted there is an error in technique (Fig. 10–23). A dacryocystorhinostomy will re-establish a drainage system into the nose which cures the epiphora and prevents recurrent infection, if probing is unsuccessful.

CATARACTS

Cataract surgery has become an outpatient procedure in many institutions. With a good home situation this is often desirable. Most cataract surgery is performed under local anesthesia with mild sedation. The procedures should be performed only by those trained and skilled in the techniques. After surgery the patient is observed in the recovery room and then discharged to be followed in the office. Not too many years ago the patient was not allowed to move postoperatively because few if any sutures were used to close the cataract incision. With presently available sutures, the cataract incision can be securely closed with small chance of a wound dehiscence. This is true in all cataract surgery, whether there is a standard incision of 180 degrees or a small incision of 10 degrees as used in phacoemulsification.

Generally speaking, ultrasonic phacoemulsification (breaking the cataract with ultrasound and aspiration of the fragments) works well in the patient under 45 years of age, because the cataract is "soft" and can be aspirated easily by this technique. Cataracts tend to be very hard in older patients, and therefore this procedure is less successful in the elderly. With the advent of intraocular lens implants, the advantages of a small incision as used in ultrasonic phacoemulsification are lost, since the incision must be enlarged to insert a lens implant (pseudophakos). In either case, the patient can be discharged home from the recovery room.

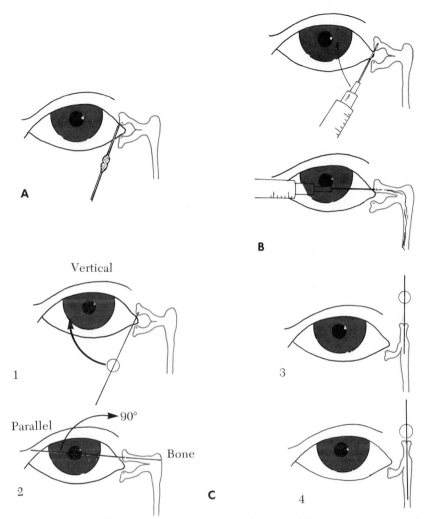

Figure 10–23 Dilatation and irrigation of the lacrimal duct. *A.* Dilate upper puncta vertical to the lid margin. *B.* Irrigate through the upper puncta. Insert irrigating cannula vertical to the lid margin for 2 mm and then direct parallel for 2–4 mm and irrigate. *C.* If still obstructed after irrigation, probe with a 000 Bowman lacrimal probe. Again enter the puncta vertical to the lid margin 2 mm, then direct the probe parallel and slightly inferior to the lid margin until the nasal bone is reached. Change the direction of the probe 90° and direct inferiorly and slightly anterior. The probe should enter the lacrimal duct without force. Advance 1.5 cm to relieve obstruction.

COMMON LID PROBLEMS IN THE OUTPATIENT CLINIC

Lagophthalmos or inability to close the lids usually results in corneal exposure and occurs after a seventh nerve paresis or proptosis of the globe. Short-term management with frequent topical methyl cellulose drops, ointment and patching at night works very well. If corneal exposure problems develop during long-term management, partial closure of the lids is necessary with a tarsorrhaphy. A temporary tarsorrhaphy is accomplished by excising a thin layer of both lid margins in the lateral canthus and placing a 4–0 silk

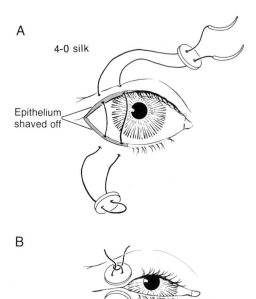

A

4-0 silk

Epithelium
shaved off

B

Figure 10-24   Temporary tarsorrhaphy.

mattress suture through the lid, as demonstrated in the diagram (Fig. 10–24).

Lid margin carcinomas require pathological diagnosis prior to surgical management. A basal cell carcinoma is removed en bloc with frozen sections at the time of surgery to show clear margins. Small lesions that involve less than 30 per cent of the lid can usually be closed primarily (see Fig. 10–13). A lateral cantholysis may be necessary to close larger lesions.[6] Very large defects must be closed with bridge flaps from the upper or lower lid (see Chapter 9). Squamous cell carcinoma of the lid is uncommon and may require extensive surgery with a node dissection, although small squamous cell carcinomas of the lid are usually treated with radiation therapy.

Subconjunctival hemorrhages alarm the patient but usually cause no eye damage. They may indicate systemic problems such as hypertension or clotting deficiencies and should alert the physician to investigate these possi-

bilities if the history and physical examination warrant it.

Chalazions are chronic granulomatous inflammations of the meibomian gland of which the cause has not been established. Hordeolums are acute inflammations of glands of the lid margin. Both can be managed with frequent warm soaks and topical antibiotics. A hordeolum may be incised if pointing. If the chalazion does not regress with conservative management it may be curetted through an incision that overlies it. No sutures are necessary.

Conclusion

A methodical history, eye examination and appropriate laboratory tests are essential in evaluating any eye problem. Commonly overlooked in this procedure is the test for visual acuity, which undoubtedly is the most important part of the examination. It is difficult to advise the physician which eye problems to treat and which to refer to an ophthalmologist, since this depends on so many factors, but one of the most important of these is a correct diagnosis.

REFERENCES

1. Hughes, W. L.: Reconstructive Surgery of the Eyelids. St. Louis, C. V. Mosby Co., 1954.
2. Moses, R. A.: Adler's Physiology of the Eye: Clinical Application. St. Louis, C. V. Mosby Co., 1970.
3. Newell, F. W.: Ophthalmology: Prinicples and Concepts. St. Louis, C. V. Mosby Co., 1965.
4. Paton, D. and Goldberg, M. F.: Injuries of the Eye, the Lids and the Orbit: Diagnosis and Management. Philadelphia, W. B. Saunders Co., 1968.
5. Pendergrass, E. P.: The Head and Neck in Roentgen Diagnosis. Springfield, Ill. C. C Thomas, 1956.
6. Smith, B. and Cherubini, T. (Eds.): Ophthalmic Plastic Surgery. International Ophthalmology Clinics: *10*(1), Spring, 1970.

11 Ear, Nose, Throat and Sinuses

GERALD M. ENGLISH, M.D.

369

INTRODUCTION

This chapter contains a discussion of those surgical procedures that can be performed on patients either in the Emergency Department, outpatient surgery or in the office. Many of the problems encountered in the daily practice of otolaryngology can be treated in these facilities.

Diagnosis depends upon the ability to examine the head and neck carefully and accurately, and often the success or failure of therapy depends upon these clinical skills.

THE EAR

Examination

A good history is especially important in deciding what is relevant in the patient's account of his otologic problem. Hearing loss, tinnitus, vertigo, pain and drainage are the symptoms that lead patients to seek help. These symptoms may either distress the patient or be ignored, depending upon the age, intelligence, psychologic state, education and occupation of the patient.

Hearing loss may be sudden or slow in onset, unilateral or bilateral, and progressive or stable. Wax occluding the ear canal or pressing against the tympanic membrane produces a sudden deafness that leads the patient to seek help *quickly.* On the other hand, the insidious, progressive hearing loss produced by otosclerosis may not stimulate the patient to consult a physician until deafness is well advanced. Questioning a close relative may help in establishing the time of onset and rate of progression of hearing loss when the patient is vague in his replies. The association of deafness with symptoms of pain, vertigo, tinnitus and otorrhea may be helpful in making the proper diagnosis. Common causes of hearing loss such as noise, trauma and ototoxic drugs should be included in the history. A fluctuating hearing loss with

episodes of vertigo followed by symptom-free intervals is characteristic of Meniere's disease.

Pain may be due to diseases within the ear or it may be referred from other structures (Fig. 11–1). Most inflammatory disease affecting the external or middle ear will produce pain, and often the most severe pain will be caused by inflammations of the external ear. Pain arising from otitis media is also severe and it usually subsides dramatically when there is a release of the inflammatory exudate from the middle ear space. Relief of pain is just as dramatic with a rupture of the tympanic membrane as with a myringotomy, or spontaneous drainage through the eustachian tube. Continuing pain, in spite of therapy, or recurring pain after a symptom-free interval, often indicates a more serious problem. Referred ear pain may arise

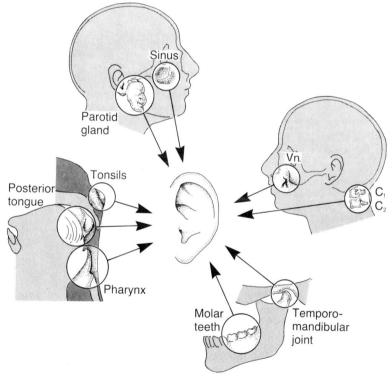

Figure 11–1 Referred otalgia. Referred otalgia is a common problem. Several diseases involving the maxillary sinus, parotid gland, pharyngeal tonsil, base of the tongue, hypopharynx, larynx, molar teeth, upper cervical nerves and the maxillary division of the trigeminal nerve are depicted. These areas must be carefully examined in any patient who complains of ear pain but has no apparent ear disease.

from the molar teeth, the pharynx, the posterior tongue, the palatal tonsils, the paranasal sinuses, the parotid gland, the temporomandibular joint and lesions of the fifth cranial nerve or upper cervical nerves.

The term vertigo should be reserved for the symptom of an hallucination of motion. When the environment moves and the patient feels stationary, it is "objective vertigo," and when the patient feels he is turning in a stationary environment, it is "subjective vertigo." Symptoms of dizziness, light headedness, unsteadiness or fainting are usually associated with nonvestibular (cardiovascular or psychoneurotic) disorders; they rarely arise from inner ear diseases.

The relationship of the attack of vertigo to various activities may give some clue to its cause. Vestibular diseases often cause an attack of vertigo when the patient is quiet or when the head is placed in certain positions. Sudden changes in posture may produce momentary attacks of unsteadiness or dysequilibrium in patients with cardiovascular insufficiency. The duration of the attack will often help determine its cause. Vertigo that lasts several minutes to hours and subsides to recur again after a symptom-free interval is characteristic of Meniere's disease. The prolonged attack that subsides after several days or weeks, followed by vertigo with certain head positions, often indicates irreversible vestibular damage. When both vestibular end organs are damaged slowly (as with streptomycin) the patient may have only a slight balance disturbance, but he will have great difficulty walking in the dark or on uneven surfaces. Nausea and vomiting often accompany an acute vestibular disturbance, and these symptoms may direct the patient's or physician's attention away from the vestibular disorder.

The symptom of tinnitus indicates a subjective symptom of ear or head noise. These sounds are often charac-terized as whistling, blowing wind, bells, sea shell sounds and throbbing or pulsating noises. Tinnitus may be associated with many ear disorders and it is often increased when the patient is tired or under stress. It is usually more troublesome at night when the patient is trying to sleep. Objective or audible tinnitus may arise from tumors within the ear, vascular lesions, foreign bodies and temporomandibular joint disease.

Otorrhea is associated with many ear problems. Any inflammatory condition in the ear canal or middle ear, whether acute or chronic, can cause a variable amount of ear drainage. The appearance, odor and amount should be noted. Watery or mucoid secretions are produced by chronic inflammations of the middle ear or inflammation of the ear canal. Purulent drainage is associated with acute inflammatory diseases, and foul-smelling material may indicate suppuration of bone.

Careful examination of the ear will help avoid errors in diagnosis. The pinna must be gently palpated and inspected before inserting the speculum into the ear canal. Superficial lesions, small pits, areas of swelling and tenderness, excoriation of the epithelium and scars should not be overlooked. By gently pulling the pinna upward and backward and stretching the tragus forward, the external meatus and canal can be seen. In many children and in most adults this simple maneuver will expose the meatus, external canal and tympanic membrane. Reflected light from the headmirror is a good source of illumination. An aural speculum large enough to avoid unnecessary pain and possible trauma to the ear is required for this part of the examination (Fig. 11–2). The battery-powered otoscope or reflected light from the headmirror may be used for examining the ear. Cerumen or other debris must be carefully removed to allow complete inspection of the entire canal and tympanic membrane. A cerumen curette, a Day hook or a Baron suction are useful instruments for this purpose.

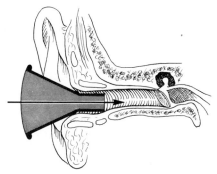

Figure 11-2 Examination of the ear. An aural speculum and head mirror reflecting light into the ear can be used for illuminating the ear canal.

Eustachian tube patency can be determined by altering air pressure in the ear canal with a pneumatic speculum or by having the patient perform a Valsalva maneuver to inflate the middle ear. Movement of the tympanic membrane with either technique indicates a patent eustachian tube.

Hearing tests are essential for the evaluation of ear disorders. An audiometric examination performed in a sound room is ideal; however, this is not always possible. Tuning fork tests are dependable when performed correctly. They are easy to perform and will help distinguish a conductive from a sensorineural hearing loss (Table 11–1). The 512, 1024, and 2048 cycle per second forks are the most practical for these tests. These tuning forks correspond to the speech frequencies and provide data concerning the patient's functional hearing levels. All tuning fork tests should be performed as closely as possible to the patient's hearing thresholds.

Air conduction and bone conduction can be tested with a tuning fork. The test for air conduction measures the ability of the ear to transmit an airborne sound through the entire ear to the temporal lobe of the brain, and is performed by holding a vibrating tuning fork near the external auditory canal. The test for bone conduction measures the ability of the inner ear and hearing nerve to receive and utilize a sound stimulus without air sound transmission. This test does not require the external auditory canal or the middle ear. The handle of the tuning fork is held directly on a portion of the skull. The vibrations reach the inner ear directly through the bones of the skull. The tuning fork can be placed on the mastoid bone, the forehead, the closed mandible or the upper teeth.

A number of tuning fork tests have been described, and several are quite useful. The two most common tests are the Rinne and Weber. The Weber test is performed by holding the handle of the vibrating tuning fork against a midline point of the patient's forehead or the upper incisor teeth (Fig. 11–3). The patient is then asked where he thinks the sound is loudest. The patient with a conductive hearing loss will usually hear the louder sound in the ear with poorer hearing. As an example, plugging the external auditory canal with a finger produces a conductive hearing loss and the tuning fork will be heard better in this ear. This technique may be used by the examiner to determine the reliability of this test. The Weber test will refer to the patient's better hearing ear when there is a nerve or perceptual deafness and when there is a significant difference between the nerve functions of the two ears.

TABLE 11-1   Summary of Tuning Fork Tests

TEST	NORMAL HEARING	CONDUCTIVE HEARING LOSS	SENSORINEURAL HEARING LOSS
Weber	Equal	Loudest in poor ear	Loudest in better ear
Rinne	*AC better than BC**	BC better than AC	AC better than BC

*AC – Air conduction
**BC – Bone conduction

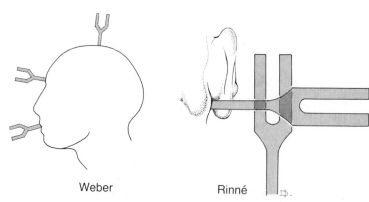

Weber   Rinné

Figure 11–3   Tuning fork tests, such as the Weber and the Rinne, are useful in differentiating and detecting the various types of hearing loss.

The Rinne test is used to detect either a conductive or a perceptual hearing loss and is performed in the following manner. A vibrating tuning fork is held in front of the ear and then placed behind the ear over the mastoid bone (Fig. 11–3). The patient is asked whether the sound is louder in front of the ear or behind it. When the fork is heard louder behind the ear, that is, on the mastoid bone, bone conduction is better than air conduction, and the patient has a conductive hearing loss. When the tuning fork sound is heard louder in front of the ear than behind the ear, the patient either has normal hearing or a nerve deafness.

Tests for vestibular function should be performed when there is a symptom of vertigo. Spontaneous and positional nystagmus should not be overlooked. Frenzel glasses may help the examiner detect the nystagmus. The caloric test is a simple method of determining vestibular function, requiring little equipment, and allowing the physician to test the two ears separately. Before these tests are performed, the ears should be examined for perforations of the tympanic membrane; if present, the ears must not be irrigated with water. Foreign bodies or cerumen plugs should be removed to insure proper stimulation of the labyrinth. It is preferable to start with a mild stimulus because this produces little subjective vertigo and no nausea and vomiting. Stronger stimulation may be required

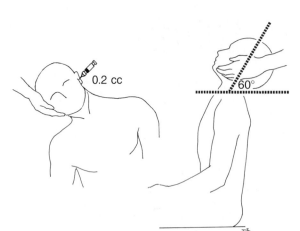

0.2 cc

60°

Figure 11–4   Caloric test. Vestibular function can be tested by placing a small quantity (0.2 cc) of cold or hot water near the tympanic membrane for 30 seconds. Horizontal nystagmus lasting for 60 seconds indicates a reacting vestibular system.

for the patient with a relatively insensitive labyrinth. The patient's head is tilted back (Fig. 11–4) at an angle of 60° and 0.2 cc of ice water (0° C) is placed in the external canal. The eyes are observed for nystagmus. The direction and duration of nystagmus should be recorded. The direction of the nystagmus is recorded as the direction of the quick component, which is normally away from the stimulated ear. The duration should be one and a half to two minutes. After a five minute interval the opposite ear is stimulated, and the response from this side recorded. The direction of nystagmus should be away from this ear and the duration of nystagmus comparable to the other side. When no response is detected, a larger volume of ice water (5 cc) is injected into the ear canal and the responses recorded. If there is still no response, 30 cc of ice water are injected into each ear canal over a 30 second period, and if this stimulus produces no nystagmus it may be concluded that the vestibular system is not functioning. Those patients with vestibular disorders will usually report that the vertigo produced by caloric testing is similar to their symptom of vertigo.

Nystagmus can be documented and recorded with electronystagmography(ENG).[5, 30] This technique is dependent upon the detection and amplification of the resting electro-potential of the eyes. The retina has a negative charge as compared with the positive charge on the cornea. The tracing (electronystagmogram) can be analyzed and an assessment of vestibular function made. The tracing serves as a permanent record for comparison with future tracings. Another advantage of ENG is that a much higher percentage of patients with either spontaneous or positional nystagmus can be detected. There are estimates that 80 per cent of the nystagmus exhibited in these patients will not be seen without an ENG. There are very few contraindications for the test (perforated or very thin tympanic membrane is one), and it should be performed on any patient in whom there is a vestibular problem that might lead to litigation.

Congenital Lesions

Minor variations in the size and shape of the auricle are fairly common. These are simply variations from the normal and require no treatment. True malformations are often associated with other anomalies of the ear and face. These patients should have a careful evaluation before any surgical therapy is undertaken.

Preauricular Cysts

The preauricular cyst or fistula (Fig. 11–5) is a congenital lesion arising from a defective union of the first and second branchial arches that form the auricle. Usually, a small opening can be identified anterior to the helix or tragus. From this opening, a long branched tract extends under the skin. If the tract becomes obstructed or infected a mass may develop. Many are asymptomatic and require no treatment; however, pain, drainage or an enlarging mass are indications for surgical excision. The operation can be performed with general or local anesthesia, and a small segment of skin surrounding the open-

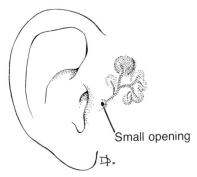

Small opening

Figure 11–5 Preauricular sinus or cyst. A small opening in the preauricular area may be an indication of an extensive preauricular sinus and cyst. Multiple branches are quite common and all of these must be excised if surgical treatment is to be successful.

ing should be included. Branching tracts make it difficult to define the extent of the fistula, and an injection of methylene blue stains the tracts and makes it easier to excise them. One should remember that the methylene blue might not enter the smaller branches of the tract and these small unstained channels must also be removed. The dye may spread into surrounding normal tissue and this should be spared. The operation must be performed with care because the tract may extend deep into the soft tissue of the face and lie close to branches of the facial nerve. When the cyst is infected, antibiotics should be used before and after surgery.

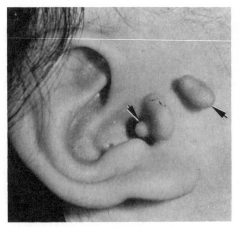

Figure 11–6   Accessory auricles (arrows).

Accessory Auricles

These small firm skin elevations often contain elastic cartilage (Fig. 11–6). They may be either single or multiple and may occur anterior to the tragus along the ascending crus of the helix or on the cheek along a line between the tragus and the angle of the mouth. Accessory auricles may be excised with local anesthesia, and the dissection should include the elastic cartilage that extends into the underlying soft tissues. Branches of the facial nerve may be closely related to these structures and these branches must not be injured or excised during surgery (Fig. 11–7).

Angioma

These congenital tumors are rather common, often involving the auricle and other areas of the face and neck. Two types of angiomas occur in the auricle. Capillary hemangiomas consist of capillary-sized vessels in the form of a spider nevus or flat mass with a port wine stain appearance. The spider nevus is usually not a problem and either no treatment or coagulation of the central vessel is all that is necessary. Because large, flat port wine stain tumors may increase in size and become disfiguring, these patients require extensive treatment and should

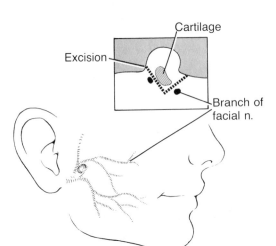

Figure 11–7   Accessory auricle. Accessory auricles usually contain a small piece of cartilage and may be close to the facial nerve. Excision must be performed carefully to avoid facial nerve injury.

be sent to a specialist in plastic surgery (see Chapter 9).

Cavernous hemangiomas or "strawberry tumors" consist of raised masses of large blood-filled spaces. They enlarge rapidly during the first years of life and produce severe cosmetic deformities. These patients should be referred for treatment (Chapter 9).

Lop Ears

Protruding auricles are not uncommon. Minor degrees of protrusion require no treatment, but the markedly protruding auricle causes embarrassment and it should be corrected (Fig. 11–8). The operation can be performed on outpatients but complications of infection, hematoma and perichondritis must be avoided.

Traumatic Conditions

The auricle is frequently injured, and these injuries must be treated promptly and adequately to reduce subsequent deformities.

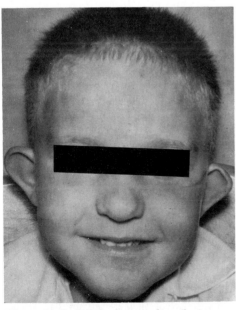

Figure 11–8 Bilateral protruding (lop) ears.

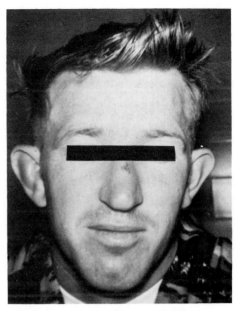

Figure 11–9 A right auricular hematoma. (From: English, G. M.: Common injuries to the ear. Primary Care, 3(3):509, 1976.)

Hematoma

A large, bluish swelling involving the auricle is the characteristic appearance of this problem (Fig. 11–9). Extravasation of blood between the perichondrium and cartilage will result in cartilage necrosis and severe deformities. Ischemic necrosis of cartilage results from the interference with the blood supply to the cartilage from vessels within the perichondrium. "Cauliflower ear" is the deformity produced by this process.

Treatment consists of evacuating the blood from the hematoma as soon as possible (Fig. 11–10). When a patient with a small hematoma is seen shortly after the injury, needle aspiration may be all that is necessary. Larger hematomas and those of longer duration will require an incision and evacuation of the hematoma. This procedure should be performed with careful aseptic technique because any bacterial contamination may produce a severe perichondritis. Antibiotics are useful in preventing this complication. A tight

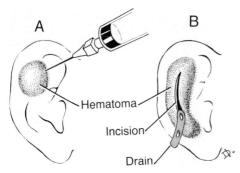

Figure 11–10 Treatment of hematoma of the auricle. Subperichondrial hematomas of the auricle can be (A) aspirated or (B) incised and drained. Aspiration may have to be repeated several times and should be used for small hematomas. The incision of a hematoma must be adequate in length and should be made through the perichondrium. Drainage can be obtained by placing a small rubber drain beneath the perichondrium. A pressure dressing should be placed on the ear for at least 48 hours.

pressure dressing is placed over the ear for 48 hours to prevent accumulations of blood. Moistened cotton can be molded to the contours of the ear to insure adequate pressure. Drains must not be left in the incision more than 48 hours because they increase the risk of infection. Local or general anesthesia may be used, depending upon the age of the patient and the extent of the injury.

Lacerations

These injuries may extend through the skin, the perichondrium and the cartilage, and occasionally the entire auricle is severed from the head. These injuries require meticulous surgical repair. Control of bleeding, cautious débridement of devitalized tissue and removal of all foreign materials are essential. Careful approximation of tissues with fine sutures is important, and these sutures should not pass through the cartilage. Exposed cartilage must be covered and skin flaps from the postauricular area can be used for this purpose (Fig. 11–11). When open injuries are not treated, infection invariably occurs, resulting in severe cosmetic deformities and possible loss of the entire auricle. Antibiotics will help prevent infection and pressure dressings will help prevent accumulations of blood or serum. The auricle has been successfully resutured to the head in a number of patients with severe injuries.[9, 22] Even a partial success is well worth the time and the effort involved (Fig. 11–12).

Frostbite and Burns

The unprotected position of the auricle and its lack of subcutaneous tissue predispose it to this injury. Severity of trauma is dependent on the duration and degree of exposure (Table 11–2). At first the auricle has a white appearance and is cold to the touch. Later, a stage of hyperemia and edema follows. The ear becomes swollen, with fluid-filled "blebs" forming beneath the skin.

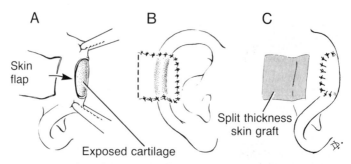

Figure 11–11 Protection of cartilage. Exposed cartilage must be covered to prevent perichondritis and loss of the cartilage. A. A full-thickness postauricular skin flap has been elevated. B. The skin flap is then sutured to the skin edges of the auricular defect. C. After adequate healing, the auricle is freed from the flap and any postauricular defect covered with a split-thickness skin graft.

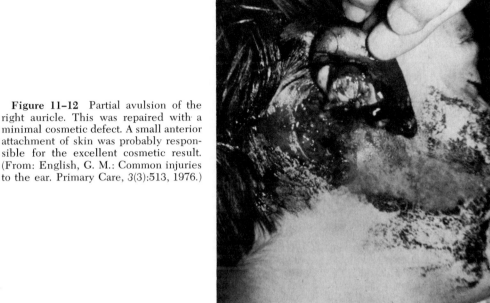

Figure 11–12 Partial avulsion of the right auricle. This was repaired with a minimal cosmetic defect. A small anterior attachment of skin was probably responsible for the excellent cosmetic result. (From: English, G. M.: Common injuries to the ear. Primary Care, 3(3):513, 1976.)

Treatment consists of allowing the ear to return to body temperature and the admininistration of analgesics for pain. Dressings and other manipulations of the auricle must be avoided because they may cause further injury. Should gangrene or aseptic necrosis develop, the patient should be hospitalized and referred to a specialist for treatment.

Foreign Bodies

A wide variety of objects have been removed from the ear canal (Fig. 11–13). Children are more apt to insert a

TABLE 11–2   Classification of Frostbite of the Auricle

SUPERFICIAL
   1st degree — Erythema and edema of the skin
   2nd degree — Bulla formation
DEEP
   3rd degree — Necrosis of skin and subcutaneous
            tissue
   4th degree — Necrosis, gangrene, loss of tissue

(Adapted from English, G. M.: Common injuries of the ear. Primary Care, 3:507–520, 1976.)

foreign body than are adults. Small stones, beads, cotton balls, beans and erasers are the objects most frequently found in the ear. Insects may fly or crawl into the ear canal and cause great discomfort while they are alive.

All foreign materials should be removed from the ear, and the major difficulties of this procedure can be overcome by using a few simple techniques. First, the patient must be comfortable, and he must remain immobile. Injuries to the tympanic membrane or ossicular chain can occur when the patient moves. A local anesthetic injected around the external meatus will provide excellent anesthesia, although children who are very apprehensive may require a general anesthetic. Second, insects that are alive must be killed before attempting to remove them. A small cotton tampon moistened with ether and placed in the ear canal for 5 to 10 minutes will stupefy the insect and sterile mineral oil instilled into the canal will kill it.

Either a small cerumen curette or a Day hook is a useful instrument for

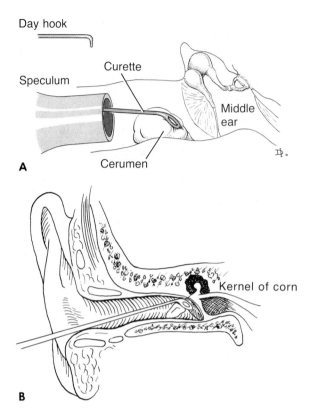

Figure 11–13 Minor procedures performed on the ear. *A.* Cerumen removal from external auditory canal. Cerumen or foreign bodies (*B*) should be removed with a curette under direct vision. A Day hook may be used instead of a curette.

removing foreign bodies. A Baron finger control suction and Hartmann alligator forceps also may be used. Any manipulations in the external canal may elicit a cough reflex making removal of the foreign body difficult. A local anesthetic will block this reflex in addition to relieving pain.

Removing foreign bodies by irrigation is risky. If there is a pre-existing perforation of the tympanic membrane, the irrigating solution may enter the middle ear and produce an infection. Occasionally the force of the irrigating solution will rupture a thin tympanic membrane and cause a conductive hearing loss and middle ear infection. When the tympanic membrane cannot be seen, it is best to remove foreign bodies without irrigation. The trauma of extracting a foreign body is preferable to the complications of irrigation.

There is sometimes a place in an outpatient practice for removal of wax by irrigation. The principal concern is not to irrigate an ear with

a pre-existing perforation of the tympanic membrane or with a tympanic membrane that is very thin and atrophic. When the irrigating solution enters the middle ear, a severe infection usually occurs. Unfortunately, the wax often obscures the tympanic membrane, and the irrigation is performed in a "blind" fashion. If the patient has had wax removed successfully in the past by this technique, then it can probably be performed without too much danger. The proper technique consists of using a warm solution (37°C.) and an irrigation syringe without applying too much pressure. Symptoms of pain, bleeding, hearing loss or dizziness should alert the physician to discontinue the irrigation immediately. Another technique should be used in that particular situation. This often indicates that the middle ear has been contaminated by the irrigation.

Foreign bodies that are large or in contact with the tympanic membrane are more difficult to extract. Some foreign bodies are hygroscopic and swell to completely occlude the ear canal. Edema and inflammation of the external canal may make it nearly impossible to remove the foreign body, and occasionally these patients require a general anesthetic and an endaural incision before the foreign body can be removed.

Excessive cerumen is a problem for some patients. Soft moist cerumen can be removed with the curette without too much difficulty. Cotton-tipped metal applicators can be used to cleanse the ear canal of debris. Hard impacted cerumen can be softened by using a few drops of mineral oil in the ear two or three times each day for a day or two before removal. The hard wax plug can be removed with instruments, but occasionally a local anesthetic is necessary to insure the patient's cooperation and comfort.

Traumatic Rupture of Tympanic Membrane

These injuries result from blows to the ear with a cupped hand, instrumentation of the ear, blast injuries, diving, water skiing, forceful inflation of the eustachian tube when the membrane is thin, rapid descent in unpressurized aircraft and basal skull fractures. Welders can develop a perforation from hot metal fragments flying into the ear canal. These perforations fail to heal because there is cauterization of the edges of the perforation. The symptoms are pain, hearing loss, tinnitus and occasionally bleeding from the ear.

Treatment is quite simple and consists of aspirating the blood and debris from the ear canal. This is necessary to determine if there are injuries to the tympanic membrane. The ear should not be irrigated nor the clot in the middle ear disturbed. Ear drops have little value and may do some harm. Usually the perforation heals slowly over a period of weeks and the patient's hearing returns to normal. During this inter-

val the patient should be advised to avoid water in the ear. Swimming should be discontinued and the external meatus filled with cotton. Vaseline should be smeared over the cotton and auricle before showering and shampooing the hair. This simple technique will prevent water from entering the middle ear and will help prevent acute otitis media. Infection will delay healing of the perforation and perhaps lead to more serious problems. If the perforation has not closed in 10 to 12 weeks, the patient should be sent to an otologist for surgical repair of the tympanic membrane.

Tumors

Most ear tumors arise from the skin or its appendages; however, bone, cartilage or neural tissues may be involved. Early diagnosis and prompt treatment are important to avoid extensive tissue loss, functional impairment or death. Both benign and malignant tumors occur in the ear, and the diagnosis will depend upon a histopathologic examination of a biopsy specimen.

Sebaceous Cysts

These cysts (Fig. 11–14) are common around the ear. They are usually locat-

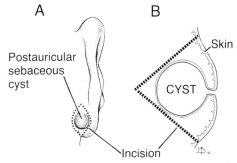

Figure 11–14 Sebaceous cyst of the ear. The postauricular sulcus and lobule (A) are the most common sites for sebaceous cysts near the ear. The incision should include a margin of normal tissue (B) and should be placed in the postauricular sulcus.

ed on the posterior surface of the lobule, the postauricular sulcus and the skin overlying the mastoid process. Soft and nontender, they are easy to diagnose, though they may become infected and confused with a furuncle. Treatment consists of total excision of the cyst with its walls intact. This will insure complete removal. A margin of skin about the external opening should be removed with the cyst. Local anesthesia is usually adequate for this surgical procedure.

Fibroma

Fibromas are firm, discrete tumors that are nontender. They grow slowly and occasionally occlude the external meatus. Surgical excision is indicated when the mass occludes the canal or

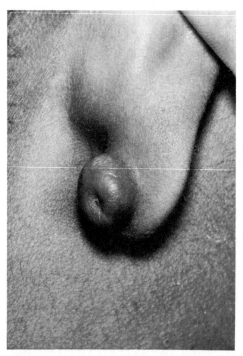

Figure 11–15 Keloid of the ear lobe. This lesion developed after the ear lobe was pierced for an earring. (From: Baker, B. B.: Neoplasms of the external ear. *In* English, G. M. (ed.): Otolaryngology, A Textbook. Hagerstown, Harper & Row, 1976, Chapter 14.)

creates a cosmetic problem. Keloids result from trauma to the ear and are a form of fibroma. They occur most frequently in dark-skinned people, particularly blacks. They arise as tumors on the lobule often after ear piercing (Fig. 11–15). Surgical excision followed by 500 R of irradiation to prevent recurrence is the most satisfactory treatment.

Cutaneous Horn

This rough, hard, brownish colored tumor occurs on the rim of the helix in older patients who have a long history of exposure to inclement weather. Surgical excision of this hornlike tumor will improve the patient's appearance. These tumors rarely recur.

Senile Keratoses

These flat, raised, yellowish-brown lesions appear on the auricle in elderly persons. They produce few if any symptoms and are treated much the same as they are anywhere else on the body (topical lanolin cream or excision).

Keratoacanthoma

This rare lesion is potentially malignant. The tumor may grow rapidly at first and then slowly regress in size to leave a retracted scar. Excisional biopsy is necessary to be certain that a carcinoma is not developing.

Papilloma

Papillomas occur on the auricle and in the external canal. The etiology may be viral or a response to chronic irritation of the skin. They may become malignant and should be excised completely. Obstruction of the external canal with a conductive hearing loss may result from these tumors.

Exostoses

These are common benign tumors of the external canal. They are usually symptomless unless they obstruct the external canal or interfere with wax and epithelial debris passing from the canal. Many patients with this tumor have a history of swimming in cold water.[12] This sessile tumor arises from the canal wall near the tympanic membrane, and there may be more than one tumor mass. When they interfere with hearing or are associated with repeated infections from retained debris, surgical excision is necessary and the patient must be referred to an otologist for treatment.

Although osteomas have a similar histopathologic appearance to exostoses, they are somewhat different clinically. They arise at the bony cartilaginous junction of the ear canal. Osteomas are usually solitary and pedunculated. They may obstruct the canal or allow an accumulation of debris within the canal that leads to repeated infections. Surgical excision should be performed by an otologist.

Adenoma

These tumors arise from the cerumen glands of the canal skin. They have a marked tendency to recur and may become frankly malignant. Wide surgical excision is necessary to prevent recurrence and this should be done by a specialist in ear surgery.

Carcinoma

Squamous cell carcinoma, basal cell carcinoma and adenocarcinomas occur on the auricle. The squamous carcinomas are the most common and comprise about 75 per cent of malignant tumors of the auricle. Fifteen per cent are basal cell carcinomas and 10 per cent are adenocarcinomas. The clinical course of these tumors varies, but 20 per cent of patients with these tumors will have metastatic disease when they are first seen. The diagnosis is not difficult to make if a biopsy is obtained.

The treatment of carcinoma of the auricle depends upon the location and size of the tumor. Very small lesions may be excised in the clinic; however, larger lesions should be treated by more radical surgery. This may entail excision of the underlying cartilage or amputation of the entire auricle. These procedures are beyond the scope of this text.

Inflammatory Conditions

Perichondritis

Inflammation of the perichondrium (Fig. 11–16) may occur when the cartilage has been exposed or injured by trauma, surgery, frostbite, burns or infection introduced during aspiration or incision of a hematoma. Occasionally a superficial infection of the auricle or canal will spread to the perichondrium. Pus collecting between the perichondrium and the cartilage causes a necro-

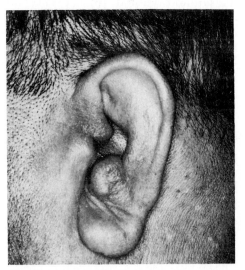

Figure 11–16 Acute perichondritis of the left auricle. There is swelling, erythema and edema of the concha, helix and tragus. These areas are very tender to palpation.

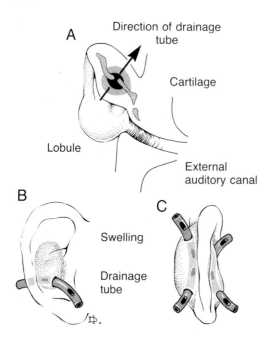

Figure 11–17 Perichondritis. Perichondritis should be treated by incision and drainage. *A.* When there has been destruction of the cartilage, the tube should be inserted through the auricle. (*B*). Drainage tubes placed on both sides of the auricle beneath the perichondrium (*C*) can be used to evacuate an abscess.

sis of the cartilage resulting in a marked deformity of the ear. This infection should be treated promptly with a broad-spectrum antibiotic. Any purulent drainage should be sent to the laboratory for culture and sensitivity tests. When an abscess forms it should be incised and drained (Fig. 11–17). The incision should be delayed until definite fluctuation is detected. Premature incisions will only spread the infection. In a few patients, the pain and swelling may continue despite these measures and more extensive surgical therapy will be required. Most of these patients require intravenous antibiotics, and hospitalization is necessary.

Chondrodermatitis Nodularis Helicis Chronicis

This small, painful, tender nodule arises from the upper margin of the auricle (Fig. 11–18). It is more common in men than in women and is thought to arise from exposure to cold temperatures. Patients often have difficulty sleeping because of the pain when the ear comes in contact with a pillow. A

local anesthetic is sufficient for the excision of the lesion with a small wedge of underlying cartilage, which usually results in a cure.

External Otitis

Furunculosis is a circumscribed external otitis that arises from a staphylococcal infection of a hair follicle.

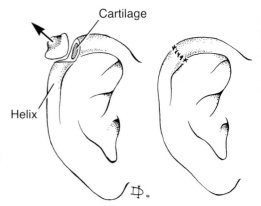

Figure 11–18 Chondrodermatitis nodularis helicis chronicis. Surgical excision of this painful helical nodule must include part of the underlying cartilage.

These infections may be multiple and may recur over long periods of time. The first symptoms are tenderness in the external meatus and pain that is increased with jaw movements. As the infection progresses, the pain becomes more severe and hearing loss results from edema occluding the external meatus. Examination reveals a red swollen area in the cartilaginous part of the ear canal. Manipulations of the auricle will cause a great deal of pain. Enlarged tender postauricular lymph nodes may simulate an acute mastoiditis. These nodes may displace the auricle forward and make it difficult to differentiate this condition from a mastoid infection. A mastoid x-ray will usually help clarify the problem. However, it is unusual for mastoiditis to cause pain and tenderness of the auricle unless there is an associated perichondritis. Lymphadenitis is unusual in acute mastoiditis and ordinarily the tenderness in mastoiditis is localized over the mastoid process. When the tympanic membrane can be seen, it will appear normal in furunculosis and it is abnormal in mastoiditis. Antibiotics should be used and the furuncle incised and drained when it localizes. A wick moistened with an antibiotic (bacitracin) ointment may be gently inserted into the external canal. This will allow drainage and prevent the accumulation of purulent debris in the canal.

Diffuse external otitis is quite common and may be associated with skin disorders such as eczema, neurodermatitis and seborrheic dermatitis. Hot, humid climates and bathing or swimming are often associated with this disorder. Trauma is an important factor and scratching the ears, unskilled irrigations of the canal, and vigorous drying with a soiled towel must be avoided. Occasionally, pus draining from a chronic otitis media will produce a diffuse inflammation of the canal, and this possibility can be excluded by a careful examination of the tympanic membrane. Meticulous cleaning of the canal is essential when treating this problem. Cotton-tipped metal applicators, suction, and small curettes are useful for this purpose. The patient must keep his ear dry during shampooing and showering by occluding the external canal with cotton and applying Vaseline over the meatus and auricle. Ear drops are of little value when debris in the canal does not allow the medication to reach the inflamed areas. Antibiotic ear drops may sensitize the canal and aggravate the problem. Topical steroids are of some value. Burrow's solution (1:17) or a saturated solution of boric acid in ethyl alcohol helps relieve the itching and pain. A cotton or ribbon gauze wick placed in the canal will facilitate drainage and allow the ear drops to reach inflamed areas.

Those patients who fail to respond to this regimen should be referred to an otologist for treatment.

Acute Otitis Media

Acute otitis media is one of the commonest diseases in children. In general, this disease results from a bacterial infection of the middle ear (72.8 per cent). The remainder of cases (27.2 per cent) are thought to be viral in etiology. Hemenway and Smith[16] have reviewed the etiologic agents in acute otitis media, and their data are presented in Table 11–3.

The patient's age must be considered in the etiology of this disease. Children under the age of six often have *Hemophilus influenzae* cultured from the ear; whereas patients over age six rarely have this organism. Children under six should receive an antibiotic that will eradicate *D. pneumoniae*, *H. influenzae* and a group A β-hemolytic streptococcus. The antibiotics of choice in this situation are ampicillin, tetracycline or erythromycin with sulfisoxazole. Those over six respond well to oral potassium-phenoxymethyl-penicillin or erythro-

TABLE 11–3   Etiologic Agents in Acute Otitis Media (1048 Specimens)

Organism	Positive Cultures	Per Cent*
Diplococcus pneumoniae	451	43.0
Hemophilus influenzae	273	26.1
β-Hemolytic streptococcus	118	11.3
Staphylococcus aureus	24	2.3
Streptococcus viridans	12	1.1
Neisseria catarrhalis	7	0.7
Other	4	0.4
Negative for bacteria	285	27.2

*Infrequently more than one organism was cultured from the same specimen.

mycin. *Hemophilus influenzae* is rarely involved in these patients.

When pus is present in the ear canal, this should be obtained for culture and sensitivity tests. A gram stain will help determine the best antibiotic for immediate use.

Myringotomy is indicated in those patients with severe pain, marked bulging of the tympanic membrane, severe toxemia, poor response to antibiotic therapy, a persistent conductive hearing loss and apparent or impending complications. This simple procedure involves little risk to the patient when performed skillfully. Adequate anesthesia is essential and sedation is frequently necessary in small children. Meperidine and phenobarbital (1 mgm of each per pound of body weight) is injected 30 minutes before the procedure is begun. A local anesthetic solution of 1 per cent lidocaine HCl (Xylocaine), and epinephrine (1:100,000) is infiltrated around the external canal at 12, 3, 6 and 9 o'clock positions (Fig. 11–19). About 0.5 cc of the solution is slowly injected at each site. Blanching of the canal occurs with the injection due to the vasoconstrictive action of epinephrine. The myringotomy incision is made in the inferior portion of the drum (Fig. 11–20). The anterior-inferior quadrant is farthest from the middle ear ossicles and the facial nerve. Injuries to these structures can have serious consequences and must be avoided. A circular incision is better than a radical one because the latter may extend into the

annulus of the tympanic membrane and cause troublesome bleeding. Magnification of the ear will help prevent accidents during the operation and a Zeiss operation microscope is quite useful for this purpose.

After myringotomy, the patient should be instructed to keep water out of the ear until the membrane has healed. Cotton placed in the ear and changed frequently when soiled will prevent pus draining out of the ear onto the face and clothing.

Analgesics, bed rest, mild sedation and antipyretics will make the patient more comfortable during convales-

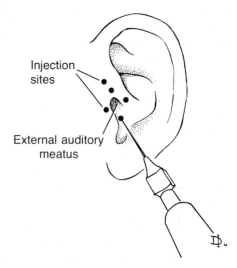

Figure 11–19 Anesthesia of the ear. Local anesthesia of the external auditory canal, tympanic membrane and middle ear can be obtained by injecting the external meatus and canal with a local anesthetic.

RIGHT EAR

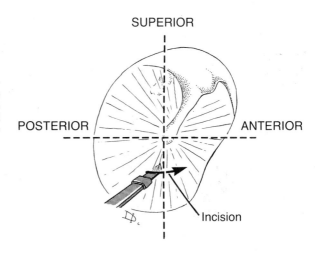

Figure 11–20 Myringotomy. Incision of the tympanic membrane (myringotomy) can be performed with local anesthesia. The incision should be made in the inferior-anterior portion of the drum head.

cence. The patient should return in 72 hours. If symptoms persist, a change in antibiotic may be indicated on the basis of sensitivity tests. This patient should be examined again in three or four days. Fever after seven days of treatment is nearly always an indication for myringotomy. A middle ear fluid specimen should be cultured and sensitivity tests performed. If the patient is doing well after 72 hours, he can be examined in 10 or 12 days and then periodically until the eardrum and the hearing are normal. Any patient with signs or symptoms of continuing infection must be hospitalized and observed for the complications of otitis media.

Serous Otitis Media

This clinical condition is characterized by an accumulation of nonpurulent fluid in the middle ear. The only consistent symptom is a conductive hearing loss. The onset of hearing loss may be gradual or sudden, in one or both ears. Hearing may be better in the supine position than when the patient is erect.

Several etiologic factors have been implicated in this disease. Unresolved acute otitis media from either inade-

quate therapy or a failure to develop immunity is a common cause of middle ear fluid. Obstruction of the eustachian tube from enlarged adenoids, infection, neoplasm, trauma, or allergy may result in a middle ear effusion. Diseases of the palate including clefts, submucous clefts, paralysis or trauma are frequently complicated by serous otitis media.[3]

Examination reveals a dull, retracted tympanic membrane with a prominent malleus. An air-fluid meniscus or bubbles may be seen in the middle ear. Pneumatic otoscopy reveals a tympanic membrane that moves poorly or not at all. Audiometry and tuning fork tests will indicate a conductive hearing loss.

Treatment is directed at removing the fluid from the middle ear. Catheterization of the eustachian tube may produce edema in the tube and cause more fluid accumulation. Autoinflation of the middle ear may be helpful, and this should be repeated several times each day for several days. Myringotomy and insertion of a polyethylene tube (Fig. 11–21) through the tympanic membrane are effective means of treatment. The anesthetic and technique are the same as described for acute otitis media. A small polyethylene tube inserted through the myringo-

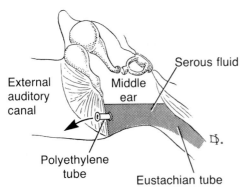

External auditory canal

Middle ear

Serous fluid

Polyethylene tube

Eustachian tube

Figure 11–21 Insertion of polyethylene tube. A flanged tube is inserted through the tympanic membrane into the middle ear space. This tube drains the serous fluid from the middle ear and allows air to enter the middle ear.

tomy after evacuation of the fluid allows ventilation of the middle ear. Local anesthesia is usually sufficient except for small children or uncooperative patients. The polyethylene tube can be removed after several weeks and during this time the patient must avoid any water in the ear. Oral decongestant therapy of pseudoephedrine HCl (Sudafed) is useful in many patients. Patients who do not respond to these techniques must be reexamined to be sure that an unsuspected etiologic factor has not been overlooked. This is particularly true in the adult with serous otitis media. An unsuspected nasopharyngeal tumor may be responsible for the problem and a mistake in diagnosis will produce serious consequences. Occasionally, mastoidectomy will be required in some of those patients who do not respond to treatment.

Chronic Otitis Media

There are two distinct types of chronic otitis media.[26] Each has a somewhat different etiology, clinical course and potential for serious complications. The benign form is due to recurrent or continuing infection in the middle ear and is associated with a perforation of the pars tensa portion of the tympanic membrane. The more dangerous variety is associated with cholesteatoma formation in the pars flaccida area of the tympanic membrane. The pars tensa may be normal in these patients and a small perforation or retraction pocket in the pars flaccida overlooked. Because serious complications (hearing loss, facial paralysis and CNS infections) may develop from this condition, these patients should be referred to an otologist.

The middle ear mucosa can be inspected through the perforation. Its appearance changes during various stages of the disease — in acute infections, it will appear thickened and edematous, and during quiescent periods it will appear normal. These changes are important indicators for the various methods of treatment. Patients with mucosal changes and otorrhea suggesting an infection should be treated with antibiotics. Culture and sensitivity tests are important in this situation because the bacterial flora may vary with each infection. Resistant organisms may develop with prolonged use of antibiotics. Swimming must be avoided and care should be taken to avoid water entering the ear during bathing and hair washing. Occlusion of the external meatus with cotton followed by a liberal application of Vaseline will effectively prevent water from entering the middle ear. Many perforations will close if recurrent infections can be prevented. Those perforations that do not heal may require tympanoplasty and reconstruction of the sound conducting mechanism (Fig. 11–22).[11] Cholesteatomas are potentially dangerous and should be treated by an otologist. Failure to recognize this problem could result in irreversible deafness, facial nerve palsy, meningitis and intracranial abscesses.

Ear-piercing for Earrings

The popularity of pierced ears varies considerably, but many women ask

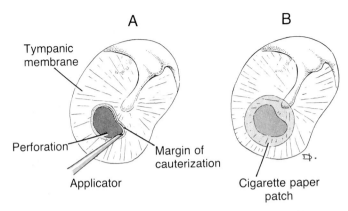

Figure 11–22 Patching the drum. A central perforation will often heal with cauterization of the edges of the perforation (A) and application of a paper patch (B). A small amount of trichloroacetic acid on a metal applicator is touched to the perforation margins (A).

their physicians to perform this minor procedure (Fig. 11–23). The operation should be inexpensive, simple, safe and effective. A 16 gauge needle with the hub removed is an ideal instrument for piercing the ear lobe. The needle and a plain gold "stud" are placed in ethyl alcohol for 15 minutes. The ear lobe is washed thoroughly with germicidal soap and water. An antiseptic solution is then applied to the ear and the lobe is anesthetized with lidocaine HCl and epinephrine (1:100,000) solution. After piercing sites are selected and the 16 gauge needle is pushed through the ear lobe, the earring is threaded into the barrel of the needle and pulled into proper position. The patient should be instructed to clean the ear lobes with ethyl alcohol moistened swabs three to four times each day for several days. A topical antibiotic ointment also will help prevent infections. The earring should not be removed or changed for 7 to 10 days. At this time, a well-epithelialized tract is present, and the earrings can be removed or changed as

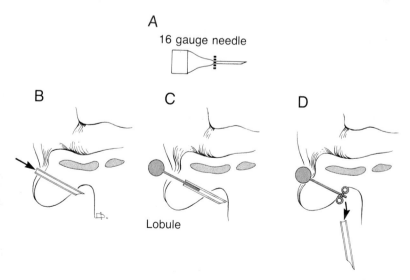

Figure 11–23 A simple method of ear-piercing with a 16 gauge needle.

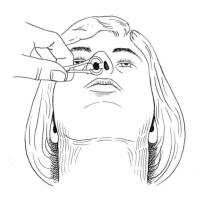

Figure 11–24 Examination of the nasal interior. Reflected light from a head mirror and a nasal speculum are used for this examination.

desired. Should infection occur, the earring must be removed immediately and systemic antibiotics prescribed. Keloids may occur and require treatment, particularly in dark-skinned persons.

NOSE

Examination

Inspection and palpation of the nose during the nasal examination will yield a great deal of information that might otherwise be missed. This is particularly true when trauma is involved. Palpation can reveal a fracture that might not be detected with an x-ray examination. When a deformity is suspected, a previous photograph is used for comparison.

Several basic instruments are necessary for examining the interior of the nose. Reflected light from a head mirror gives excellent illumination of the nasal cavity and allows the use of both hands for various manipulations. A nasal speculum inserted into the nares can be used to dilate the nares without discomfort for the patient. Tilting the patient's head from side to side and upward and downward will give a good view of the entire interior of the nose (Fig. 11–24).

When mucosal edema or congestion hampers the examination, a decongestant should be used. A solution of cocaine HCl (0.5 per cent) and ephedrine SO_4 (1 per cent) sprayed into the nasal cavity or inserted on cotton pledgets shrinks the mucous membrane. A bayonet forceps is a good instrument for accurate placement of cotton pledgets (Fig. 11–25). The cotton pack should be left in place for four to five minutes. This is not uncomfortable for the patient. When the cotton is removed, the examiner will have good visualization of the nasal cavity. The cocaine HCl solution will also anesthetize the nasal membrane and make subsequent intranasal manipulations less painful.

Secretions or blood may interfere with the examination and should be removed by a Fraser suction.

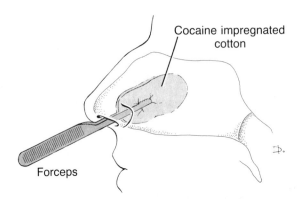

Cocaine impregnated cotton

Forceps

Figure 11–25 Nasal decongestion. Nasal decongestion can be obtained by inserting a cotton pledget saturated with an appropriate material, such as ephedrine sulfate 1 percent or cocaine hydrochloride 0.5 percent.

Congenital Lesions

Dermoid Cysts

These cysts often indicate their presence by a small moist sinus opening in the midline of the nose near its bone-cartilaginous junction. Caseous material may discharge from this opening from time to time. The cyst often extends into the nasal septum, and excision of the superficial portion will only lead to a recurrence of the cyst. Because an adequate excision often includes an exploration of the septum to insure complete removal of the cyst, the operation should not be performed in the office or Outpatient Department.

Obstructed sebaceous glands cause cysts and these may be excised using local (Xylocaine) anesthesia. A small ellipse of skin should be excised with the cyst.

Inclusion Cysts

These cysts occur along the lines of junction of segments of the face, at the sides of the nose and the philtrum of the upper lip. they can be excised with the use of local anesthesia. The incisions should be placed in natural skin lines to minimize unsightly scars.

Nasoalveolar Cysts

A smooth swelling in the floor of the nose is the usual presentation for these lesions. Unerupted incisor teeth may be confused with a cyst. An x-ray of this area will help to clarify the situation. These lesions should be removed in the operating room and the patients should be hospitalized.

Choanal Atresia

This condition consists of a closure of one or both nasal openings. It may be partial or complete, congenital or acquired. Atresias may occur at either the anterior or posterior choanae.

Anterior

Congenital atresia of the anterior apertures of the nasal passage is a rare condition. This situation occurs when the medial and lateral nasal folds fail to absorb in the embryo. More frequently, anterior atresia is an acquired condition caused by destruction of the normal cartilage and skin. Injury or chronic inflammatory diseases such as lupus, syphilis or leprosy are the most common causes. Scar tissue contracts to decrease one or both nasal openings. Cosmetic deformities are often associated with the atresia, and these defects may be very disfiguring. Reconstructive procedures should not be performed until the underlying disease has been eradicated. A surgeon trained in rhinoplasty should be consulted for repair of these problems.

Posterior

Atresia of the posterior choanae (Fig. 11–26) is not very common and is congenital in origin, although it may not be recognized immediately after delivery. The infant may have serious respiratory difficulties when sucking at the breast or bottle, and he usually keeps the mouth open continually during sleep.

Congenital atresia may be unilateral or bilateral. When it is unilateral, the infant will have less difficulty during feeding. This problem can be corrected later in life; however, the patient with bilateral atresia must be detected as soon as possible and treated immediately. Some method of providing an airway during feeding is essential because the child may suffocate if the problem is not detected. The diagnosis can be made by: (1) observing persistent nasal obstruction that does not improve with suctioning of secretions or the use of decongestant drops; (2) at-

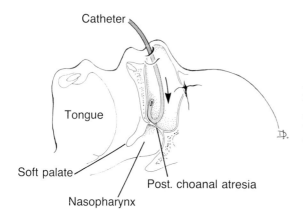

Figure 11-26 Posterior choanal atresia. Posterior choanal atresia can be detected by passing a small rubber catheter into the nose. The obstruction will be apparent when the catheter reaches the posterior choana.

tempting to pass a small catheter through the baby's nose into the pharynx; and (3) obtaining x-rays of the newborn infant's nose. A radiopaque liquid instilled into the nose can be seen on the x-ray against the occluding membrane.

In 90 per cent of cases, the atresia will consist of a bony occlusion. This bony obstruction must be completely removed along with a portion of the posterior septum. This operation should be performed by an experienced surgeon.

Traumatic Conditions

Injuries to the nose are very common and usually result from blows or falls. Abrasions and contusions from subcutaneous hemorrhage may obscure an underlying injury and make the diagnosis difficult. External lacerations (Fig. 11-27 and 11-28) often extend through the bone and cartilage into the nasal cavity. Inspection and palpation are important diagnostic techniques when evaluating a patient with nasal trauma. Nasal deformity,

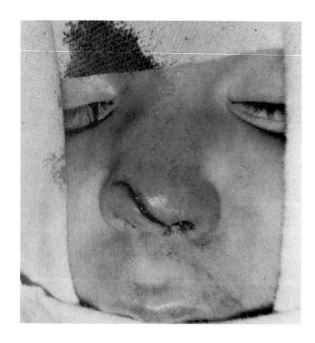

Figure 11-27 Laceration of the nose that extends through the lower cartilage into the nasal chamber.

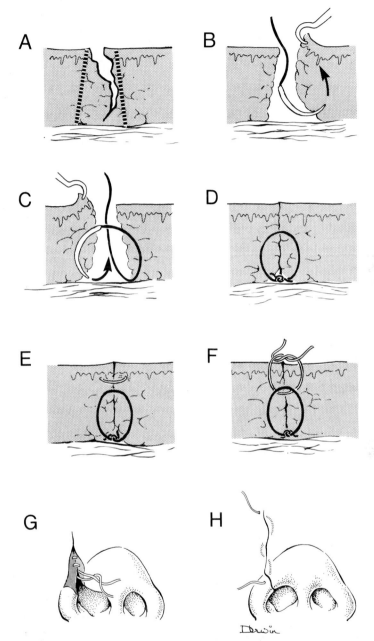

Figure 11–28   Repair of superficial laceration. Wounds should be debrided by slightly undercutting the skin edges (*A*). This provides the optimal surface for suture repair. The wounds are undermined slightly and the deep layers approximated with fine nylon subcuticular sutures (*E*) or interrupted sutures (*F*). The interrupted sutures should be removed in three days, but the subcuticular suture may be left in place much longer. A laceration of the nose is repaired using these techniques (*G* and *H*).

subcutaneous emphysema or crepitus, and mobility of the nasal bones indicate a fracture. Examination of the nasal interior is often unsuccessful because edema or blood clots obscure the chambers. The clots should be removed by suction and the edema reduced with a decongesting solution. Dislocations, fractures or subperichondral hematomas (Fig. 11–29) of the nasal septum may produce deformities that obstruct the airway or alter the appearance of the nasal contour. These septal problems must not be overlooked.

Fractures

Fractures of the nose may be either simple or compound with varying degrees of deformity. Often, the mucous membrane has been torn by depressed bone fragments penetrating the interior of the nose. There may be associated injuries to the orbit and its contents, the lacrimal apparatus, the

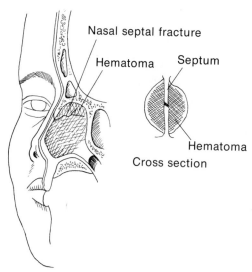

Figure 11–29 Septal hematoma, which should be incised and drained. After adequate anesthesia, a vertical incision is made into the area of swelling under direct vision. The incision is made through the mucosa and perichondrium and the blood or pus evacuated. A small rubber drain is inserted through the incision beneath the perichondrium and a pack inserted into the nose.

ethmoid sinuses and brain, the maxillary sinus and the teeth. A roentgen examination will aid in the diagnosis and the choice of therapy. Complicated nasal fractures should always be treated by a surgeon who is familiar with these problems.

Anesthesia must be obtained before reducing the fracture. Cotton packs moistened with 4 per cent cocaine HCl are inserted into the nose to anesthetize and shrink the mucous membrane. These packs should be placed along the course of the anterior nerves, over the sphenopalatine ganglion and along the floor of the nose. Infiltration anesthesia with 1 per cent Xylocaine containing epinephrine HCl (1:100,000) is started by raising a wheal beside each ala (Fig. 11–30). A 2 inch 25 gauge needle is inserted through the wheal along the lateral wall of the nose to its root just medial to the inner canthus of the eye. The solution is deposited along this tract as the needle is withdrawn. This injection will anesthetize fibers of the infratrochlear, infraorbital and anterior alveolar nerves. The second injection is made through the nostril by passing the needle through the intercartilaginous sulcus between the upper and lower lateral cartilages. The needle is passed upward over the lateral dorsal portion of the nasal bone to the root of the nose, and the anesthetic solution is deposited in the subcutaneous tissue as the needle is withdrawn. This injection anesthetizes the external nasal nerve and the terminal branches of the nasociliary nerve. Similar injections are made on the opposite side. The membranous septum and nasal spine are injected on each side, and the previously inserted nasal packs are removed. This technique, when performed properly, will give excellent anesthesia and allow the surgeon to manipulate the nose with little discomfort for the patient.

The Asch forceps is ideal for reducing nasal fractures; however, a small hemostat or bayonet forceps can be used (Fig. 11–31). Fragments can be

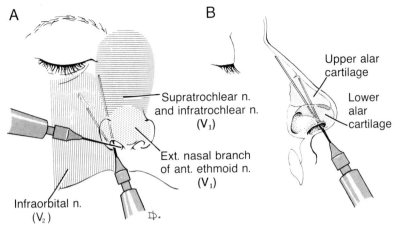

Figure 11–30 Anesthesia of the nose. The nose is anesthetized by injecting a local anesthetic solution as shown in this illustration. The infraorbital branch (1) of V_2 is injected by inserting the needle beneath the lower alar cartilage and passing it close to the infraorbital foramen. This foramen can be located by palpating the cheek. The supratrochlear and infratrochlear branches of V_1 can be anesthetized by inserting the needle along the base of the nasal pyramid up to the medial canthus of the eye (2). As the needle is withdrawn a small amount of anesthetic is deposited between the skin and periosteum of the nasal bones. The base of the columela can be anesthetized (3) by inserting the needle into the subcutaneous tissues about the anterior maxillary spine. This is particularly important for reducing fractures of the floor of the nose and anterior nasal spine. The external nasal branch of the anterior ethmoid nerve is blocked by inserting the needle through the groove between the upper and lower alar cartilages (4). Additional anesthesia of the supratrochlear and infratrochlear nerves is obtained by passing the needle over the dorsum of the nose between the skin and periosteum of the nose up to the root (glabella) of the nose and depositing anesthetic solution in this area.

pushed into alignment with the intranasal lever action of the forceps while the other hand molds the bones into proper position. An upward anterior force applied to the undersurface of the nasal bones with the forceps with external manipulation will usually produce the desired reduction of the fracture. Normally, it is necessary to insert the forceps into both nasal cavities, one blade on each side of the septum, to obtain a satisfactory reduction. When there is a unilateral displaced fracture, one blade of the forceps is inserted intranasally with the other blade on the external surface of the nose. External molding is usually required to obtain a good reduction.

Injuries of the nasal septum must not be overlooked. Alignment of fragments and drainage of hematomas will prevent serious deformities at a later date. A dislocated septum can be straightened with the Asch forceps by applying pressure against the two sides of the septum. An incision through the mucosa and perichondrium with evacuation of the blood and clots will prevent ischemic necrosis of the septal cartilage. These incisions should be left open to allow drainage, but packing material should not be inserted in them.

After the fractures have been aligned, any external lacerations should be carefully inspected, irrigated with a sterile normal saline solution, and all foreign material removed. The wound edges should be carefully approximated with fine nonabsorbable sutures such as 5–0 monofilament nylon.

Intranasal packs of one-half inch petroleum (Vaseline) gauze impregnated with an antibiotic ointment (bacitracin) are inserted after reduction of the fracture (Fig. 11–31C). This pack should be removed in 48 to 72 hours.

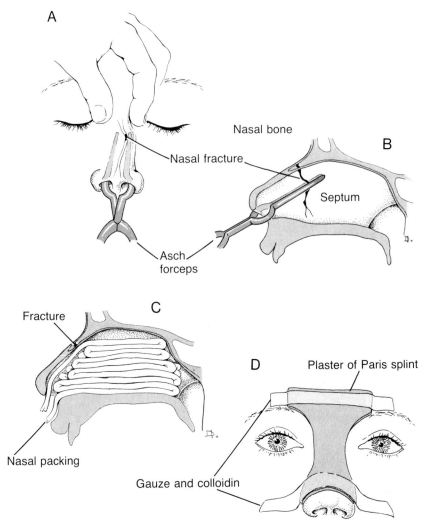

Figure 11–31 Nasal fracture reduction. *A.* The Asch forceps is inserted carefully into the nose on each side of the nasal septum. Using an upward and anterior force and palpation of the nose, the fractured segments can be guided into accurate realignment. *B.* The nasal septum can also be straightened by applying pressure on both sides with the Asch forceps. When extreme comminution is not present, the bones and cartilages will remain reduced so that intranasal packs (*C*) and an external splint (*D*) can be applied for adequate support. *C.* The nasal pack is placed gently and carefully into the nose from the nasal floor to its roof. Vaseline gauze ½" impregnated with an antibiotic is used. Both ends of the pack are brought out through the anterior naris to avoid dislodgement of the end of the pack into the pharynx. Placement of the pack into the fracture line or beneath the nasal mucosa can be avoided by inserting it with direct visualization. *D.* Plaster of Paris is trimmed and gently molded to the nasal pyramid. This lightweight splint is then held in position over the forehead and cheek with gauze strips and colloidin.

Plaster of Paris gauze is one of the best materials that can be used to make an external nasal splint (Fig. 11–31D). It can be easily molded over the skin and provides support for the nasal bones while preventing hematoma and edema formation. A layer of coarse mesh gauze impregnated with nonflexible colloidin placed across the forehead and the cheeks holds the splint in place. A small piece of folded gauze is placed under the nares and held with adhesive tape to absorb blood or mucus draining from the nasal openings.

This "snuffer" should be changed frequently.

While the nose is packed, antibiotics should be given to prevent infection. An orally administered decongestant and appropriate analgesics will increase the patient's comfort.

Splints should be removed in five to ten days depending upon the degree of comminution and displacement of the fracture. Edema and ecchymosis subside slowly and may require three or four weeks to disappear completely. The nasal skeleton is rather unstable and vulnerable to injury during the first eight or ten weeks after fracture and the patient should be advised to avoid any activities that could result in trauma to the nose.

Rhinoplasty can sometimes be performed for the correction of nasal deformities in conjunction with reduction of a nasal fracture. This procedure has a greater risk for complications than a simple reduction of the fracture, and it should not be performed on outpatients. Those nasal fractures that are seen too late for reduction or those for which the reduction has been unsatisfactory should wait until all reaction has subsided. At some future time a formal endonasal rhinoplasty can be considered.

Epistaxis

Nasal bleeding is always disturbing to the patient and may become serious when not treated promptly and adequately. Hemorrhage usually results from a rupture of the small vessels that lie within the mucous membrane of the nose. Epistaxis can be classified into four types: anterior, posterior, superior and generalized. Localizing the bleeding point helps to determine the bleeding vessel. The anterior ethmoid artery supplies the anterior and anterosuperior portion of the nose, whereas the remainder of the nose is supplied by the sphenopalatine and posterior ethmoid arteries (Fig. 11–32). Kiessel-

bach's plexus, located at Little's area in the anterior septum, is composed of vessels from both sources as well as labial branches from the upper lip.

Epistaxis has a varied etiology, a large number of local and systemic conditions contributing to the problem (Table 11–4). Trauma, infection, hypertension and other circulatory disorders, as well as neoplasms, coagulopathies and many miscellaneous conditions are some of the important causes.

Almost all epistaxis in children occurs in the anterior septum in Little's area, whereas about 50 per cent of adults bleed from the posterior nose. Posterior bleeding is usually caused by a spontaneous rupture of a blood vessel and is not associated with trauma. Many of these patients have a systemic disease that contributes to the nasal bleeding.

A history of the duration and amount of blood loss is important when evaluating a patient with epistaxis. When there is a small blood loss, it is usually easily controlled, and little treatment will be required. However, most patients will have had epistaxis for some time and quite often they have been bleeding intermittently for several days before they seek help. The patient is often frightened and an injection of morphine sulfate or diazepam (Valium) will help calm him. During this time, the patient must be questioned about any history of illness, trauma, medications, or bleeding disorders. A good indication of the bleeding site can be obtained by asking whether the blood was first noticed coming from the anterior nose or posteriorly into the pharynx.

When both patient and doctor are gowned, the patient should sit up and lean slightly forward to prevent blood running down his throat and to make the examination easier. The instruments needed for the examination and treatment of patients with epistaxis are shown in Figure 11–33. The clots can be removed from the nose with suction

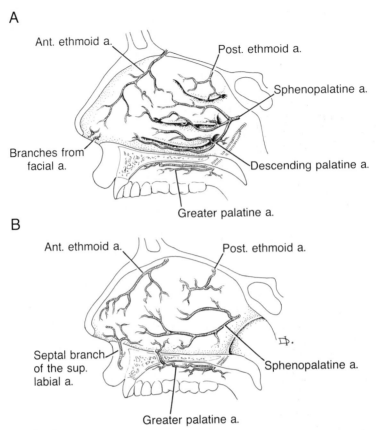

Figure 11–32 Blood supply of the nose. There is a rich blood supply to the interior of the nose, the vessels arising from several sources and entering the nose in various locations. The posterior portion of the lateral nasal wall is supplied by the sphenopalatine artery from the maxillary artery and the posterior ethmoid artery from the ophthalmic artery (*A*). The anterior lateral nasal wall receives its blood from the anterior ethmoid, which is also a branch of the ophthalmic artery. The vestibule is supplied by small branches from the facial artery and the nasal septum (*B*) is supplied by essentially the same vessels. The anterior septum also receives a branch from the superior labial artery. A very vascular area (Little's) on the anterior septum is supplied by all the vessels that supply the nose except the posterior ethmoid artery. This site is often injured and is a common site of bleeding.

or by having the patient gently blow his nose. If the bleeding is profuse it may be necessary to insert a cotton pledget soaked with 4 per cent cocaine HCl solution. Gentle pinching of the alae for 10 to 15 minutes will usually reduce the bleeding sufficiently to allow examination and the localization of its site of origin. Most often the blood will be coming from a small vessel on the anterior septum (Kiesselbach's plexus). Lidocaine HCl 1 per cent (Xylocaine) with 1:100,000 epinephrine U.S.P. injected into the sub-

mucosa with a 25 gauge needle will provide the anesthesia and vasoconstriction that are necessary for further manipulations. Cotton moistened with 1:1000 epinephrine solution applied to this area will often stop the bleeding. This cotton pack should be left in place for at least five minutes and pressure on the ala will increase its effectiveness. Such techniques may have to be repeated one or more times before the bleeding is controlled. Usually the vessel involved will be standing out from the mucosa and the next step is to

TABLE 11-4   Differential Diagnosis of Epistaxis

I. TRAUMA
  A. Blows to the nose with or without fractures
  B. Nose picking
  C. Surgical trauma
  D. Nasogastric tubes
  E. Foreign bodies
  F. Septal perforations

II. INFLAMMATION
  A. Acute rhinitis and sinusitis
  B. Chronic or atrophic rhinitis
  C. Acute systemic infections
    1. Rheumatic fever
    2. Scarlet fever
    3. Measles
    4. Typhoid and paratyphoid fever
    5. Rickettsial diseases
    6. Pertussis
    7. Diphtheria
    8. Leprosy
    9. Malaria
  D. Granulomatous diseases
    1. Syphilis
    2. Rhinoscleroma
    3. Tuberculosis
    4. Lupus erythematosus
    5. Sarcoidosis
    6. Wegener's granulomatosis and lethal midline granuloma
  E. Allergic disorders
    1. Henoch-Schönlein's purpura
    2. Allergic polyps

III. CARDIOVASCULAR AND CIRCULATORY
  A. Hypertension
  B. Atherosclerosis
  C. Hereditary hemorrhagic telangiectasis
    (Rendu-Osler-Weber disease)
  D. Increased venous pressure
    1. Bronchitis, asthma or other chronic lung disease
    2. Cardiac failure
    3. Pulmonary or neck tumors

IV. NEOPLASMS
  A. Carcinoma of the nose, sinuses or nasopharynx
  B. Papilloma
  C. Angiofibroma

V. COAGULOPATHIES
  A. Anticoagulant therapy
  B. Hemophilia
  C. Thrombocytopenia
  D. Prothrombin deficiency—alcoholic cirrhosis of the liver
  E. Leukemia
  F. Aplastic anemia
  G. Polycythemia

VI. MISCELLANEOUS
  A. Rhinoliths
  B. Irradiation
  C. Parasites and myiasis
  D. Chemical and drug poisoning
    1. Salicylates
    2. Phosphorus
    3. Cyanide gas
  E. Caisson disease
  F. Violent exertion

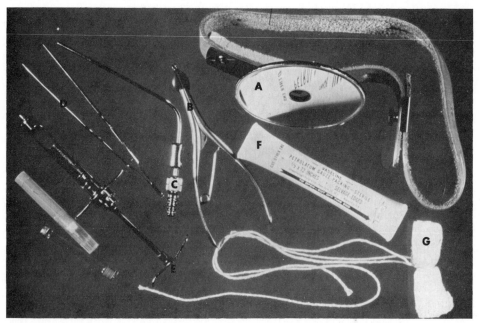

Figure 11–33   The instruments used for the treatment of epistaxis. A. Head mirror; B. nasal speculum; C. Fraser suction; D. bayonet forceps; E. dental syringe with 27 gauge needle and local anesthetic; F. Vaseline gauze; G. posterior nasal pack.

permanently thrombose this vessel.
After anesthetizing the area with a topical application of cocaine HCl solution or an injection of lidocaine HCl
(Xylocaine), electrocautery or chemical
cautery with trichloroacetic acid (10
per cent) can be used. Occasionally,
the attempts to coagulate the vessel
will start the nose bleeding again and
the whole process will have to be
repeated.

Epistaxis originating from the posterior part of the nose is more difficult to
evaluate and treat. This variety of epistaxis is often caused by a systemic
disease, and these patients should be
admitted to the hospital for an investigation of these problems.

To determine the bleeding site, the
mucous membranes must be shrunk
with a cocaine-ephedrine or epinephrine solution and the interior of the
nose carefully inspected. Decongestant solutions must be used with care
in patients with hypertension or other
cardiovascular diseases. A suction tip
inserted along the floor of the nose will

help to locate the bleeding site. When
the bleeding vessel is approached by
the suction tip, blood will cease to flow
into the nasal cavity. The most common bleeding site is located beneath
the inferior turbinate on the lateral
nasal wall. A small pledget of cotton
saturated with a decongesting solution, and placed beneath the inferior
turbinate at this site will often stop the
bleeding.

Occasionally, this small pack will
solve the problem; however, a larger
pack is usually necessary. Several
types of posterior nasal packs can be
used (Fig. 11–34). Packs made of gauze
or a vaginal tampon work quite well.
The pack should be held securely in
place by tying strings from the pack
across the columella of the septum.
Pressure necrosis of the columella can
be prevented by using a small gauze
pad beneath the knotted strings. A
number 12 or 14 French Foley catheter with a 30 cc bag makes a good
posterior nasal pack. After inserting
the catheter through the naris until the

tip has passed beyond the posterior naris into the nasopharynx, the bag is filled with 5–10 cc of water or air. The catheter is gently pulled forward until the inflated bag is lodged in the posterior choana. The catheter should be secured to the cheek with adhesive tape. Too much traction may pull the catheter from the nose and this trauma may increase the amount of bleeding.

An anterior pack usually must be inserted when a posterior pack is used (Fig. 11–31C). The most suitable material is one-half inch Vaseline gauze. An antibiotic ointment (bacitracin) applied to the gauze, oral antibiotics, and an oral decongesting agent will reduce the odor, rhinorrhea and the danger of infection associated with these packs.

Nasal packs should be removed after 48 to 72 hours. This period should be adequate for the control of the bleeding and allow enough time to investigate the patient's illness. Hypertension or a coagulopathy must be treated before removing the packs.

Padrnos[21] advocates the use of a pterygomaxillary injection for the treatment of epistaxis (Fig. 11–35). This technique is quite useful in the patient with a posterior nose bleed and will reduce the necessity for packs. The greater palatine foramen is located medial and adjacent to the last molar tooth. A 25 or 27 gauge needle one and a half to two inches in length can be inserted through the foramen one-half to three-fourths of an inch into the pterygomaxillary canal. An injection of 1 to 1.5 cc (1 per cent lidocaine with 1:100,000 solution of epinephrine) into the canal will compress the vessels and reduce the amount of circulating blood to the nose. Quite often this injection will control the bleeding and packing will be unnecessary.

When these measures fail to control nasal bleeding, appropriate vessel ligation may be indicated. The anterior ethmoid, sphenopalatine and external carotid arteries may be ligated.[24] Localizing the bleeding site is important when deciding which vessel should be ligated. Allen[1] has used a transmaxillary approach for ligating branches of the sphenopalatine artery. This opera-

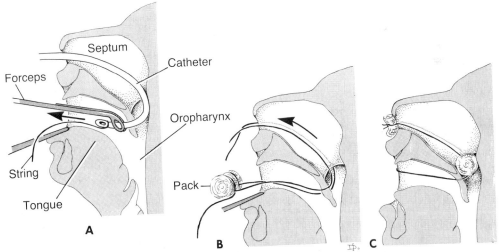

Figure 11–34 Posterior nasal pack. A posterior pack is inserted after anesthetizing the nose. A small rubber catheter (No. 10 French) is passed through the nose into the oropharynx, where it is grasped and pulled through the mouth with a forceps (A). A pack is fashioned from a roll of gauze with three 18 inch lengths of string tied about it. The pack is then tied to the catheter with one of the strings and the catheter and string pulled through the nasopharynx, nasal cavity and external naris. This procedure is repeated on the opposite side. With steady traction on the nasal strings and pressure from the index finger, the pack is directed into the nasopharynx (B). The third string is left hanging from the mouth and taped to the cheek to allow easy removal of the pack (C).

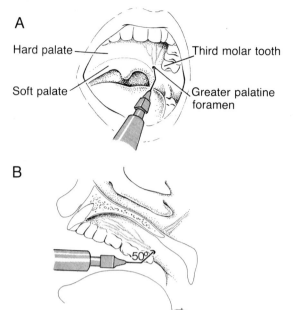

Figure 11–35 Pterygopalatine injection. A pterygopalatine (pterygomaxillary) injection is a useful technique for controlling posterior epistaxis and obtaining anesthesia of the posterior nose, palate and parts of the nasopharynx. A shallow dimple is usually visible next to the third molar tooth. This serves as a convenient landmark for inserting a 25 gauge needle 2½ inches in length, which can be inserted easily at an angle of 50°. The needle is passed into the pterygopalatine fossa about 1 inch, and 1 to 1.5 cc of anesthetic solution with 1:100,000 units of epinephrine is deposited before the needle is withdrawn. This solution will temporarily tamponade the descending palatine artery and frequently control a posterior epistaxis. If this injection fails to stop bleeding, it provides anesthesia for the insertion of a posterior nasal pack.

tion has been successful in a large number of patients in whom nasal packs were ineffective. Those patients who need vessel ligation should be hospitalized and referred to an otolaryngologist for surgery.

Nasal Polyps

These non-neoplastic tumors are composed of edematous hypertrophied nasal mucosa that arises from a chronic inflammatory process. Often bilateral, these masses occur singly or in numbers and may be either pedunculated or sessile. A smooth, glistening, grapelike lesion that is grey-white in color is the typical appearance of the nasal polyp. They must be differentiated from a squamous carcinoma, papilloma, angiofibroma, hemangioma, glioma, meningioma or encephaloceles.

Successful treatment must include therapy for the underlying allergic or infectious problems. Polyps can be removed with a snare and Green or Takahashi forceps (Fig. 11–36A). Unless the above etiologic factors are controlled, however, the polyps will in-

evitably recur. Underlying chronic sinus infections may require hospitalization and surgical treatment.

Allergy treatment requires a thorough investigation of the patient's hypersensitivity status and referral of these patients to an allergist is usually necessary.

Unilateral polyps should always be approached with caution. These lesions have many of the characteristics of an allergic or inflammatory polyp but biopsy often reveals a more serious condition. Injudicious excision may lead to severe bleeding, CSF rhinorrhea or failure to diagnose a neoplasm. All tissue removed should be sent to a pathologist for histopathologic diagnosis.

Injections of polyps with a depository steroid preparation will control many of them for long periods of time. Depo-Medrol (0.5–1.0 cc) injected directly into the polyp (Fig. 11–36B) frequently produces a marked reduction in size with subsequent improvement in the nasal airway. This procedure may have to be repeated at weekly intervals before a more or less permanent resolution of the polyp occurs.

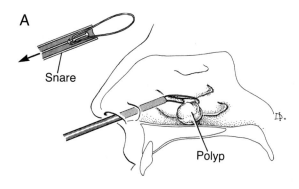

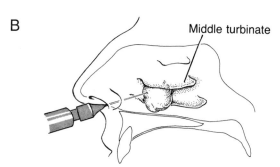

Figure 11–36 Treatment of nasal polyp. *A.* After anesthetizing the nose with tetracaine 2 percent or cocaine 10 percent, a nasal snare is slipped around the polyp. The polyp is transected and then removed with a forceps. Usually more polyps will be seen after the initial ones have been removed. These should be excised in a similar fashion. *B.* The nasal polyp is visualized and a 25 gauge needle inserted into the polyp. A small amount of steroid solution (Depo-Medrol) is injected into the polyp. Usually 0.25 to 0.5 cc is sufficient for this purpose.

Topical anesthesia with cocaine HCl solution (4 per cent) is all that is necessary for this procedure, and often the injection can be performed without anesthesia.

Antrochoanal Polyp

Antrochoanal polyps arise from abnormal mucosa within the maxillary sinus. The gradually enlarging polyp passes through the natural ostium of the sinus into the middle meatus of the nose. It extends backward into the posterior choana where it can be seen quite easily with a mirror. Occasionally, the polyp will become large and present below the soft palate. The polyp will have a smooth, translucent, slightly yellowish appearance and is associated with a radiopaque maxillary sinus from which it arises.

Once the diagnosis is made, the treatment consists of surgical excision of the maxillary sinus disease through a Caldwell-Luc incision, an operation that should not be performed in the Outpatient Department. Squamous cell carcinoma must be suspected until the entire specimen has been examined microscopically, because most carcinomas of the maxillary antrum are associated with squamous hyperplasia, and biopsy of the surface is frequently reported as benign.

Foreign Bodies

Many animate and inanimate foreign bodies, including anything small enough to enter the nares, have been found in the nose. Because most foreign bodies are placed in the nose by the patient, children are the most frequent offenders. Foreign bodies are usually easy to localize; however, x-rays may be of value in some instances. The exact location should be ascertained before any attempts are made to remove it. Usually the foreign body can be removed through the anterior naris without a general anesthetic, although in some cases this is inadvisable.

A forceps may be used to grasp an object with a rough surface. A curved probe may be adapted to remove smooth objects such as beads or marbles (Fig. 11–37) by passing the curved part of the probe behind the object and gently pulling it forward. When objects such as beans or peas have been in the nose long enough to swell and soften, a suction tip is a useful instrument to use for removing them. Enlarged objects may have to be fragmented before removal. The uncooperative patient may require a general anesthetic before the foreign body can be removed. There is always the danger that a foreign body can be dislodged from the nose and aspirated. A cuffed endotracheal tube or a finger in the nasopharynx will help prevent such a disaster. Quite often, small children will insert several objects into the nose and multiple foreign bodies should always be suspected.

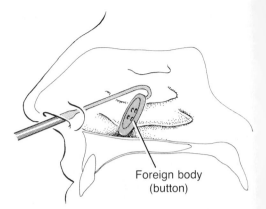

Figure 11–37 Nasal foreign body. Foreign bodies are frequently inserted into the nose. Such objects should be removed with care under direct vision or else they can be dislodged into the nasopharynx, larynx, trachea or bronchi. A small hook is a useful instrument for removing some objects, but a suction or a forceps may also be used. Topical anesthesia can be obtained with either a cocaine or tetracaine solution.

Nasal Myiasis

Nasal myiasis occurs when the common blow fly (screw worm) or the green bottle fly deposits its eggs in the nasal cavity. Such flies inhabit warm dry climates at low altitudes, with the screw worm fly *(Cochliomyia americana)* predominating in North America. The eggs hatch within 24 hours after being deposited in the nose. Mucous membranes may be destroyed, exposing bone and cartilage. This condition is usually associated with local nasal disease or systemic diseases (diabetes mellitus) in patients living in unsanitary conditions. The symptoms are those of an acute rhinitis or sinusitis and include rhinorrhea with an offensive odor, pain or headache. Rhinorrhea may be quite profuse and unilateral with a bloody mucopurulent appearance. The worms cling tenaciously to the tissues of the nose, but must be removed. Any associated

pyogenic infection should be treated with antibiotics.

Nasal Furunculosis

These superficial abscesses may occur in any part of the nose, but the most common site is the nasal vestibule. *Staphylococcus aureus* is the most common infecting organism. Bacteria may enter through minor injuries to the tissues produced by picking the nose or plucking the hairs from the vestibule of the nose. Diabetes mellitus may be associated with recurrent furunculosis.

Furuncles in the nasal vestibule, nasal apex or upper lip are potentially dangerous because the infection may spread into the cavernous sinus through veins that drain directly into the sinus from these areas. This serious complication will be evident by conjunctival chemosis, edema of the lids, proptosis, limitation of extraocular movement, papilledema, and decreased visual acuity.

Most abscesses around the nose will respond to systemic antibiotic therapy.

Cultures from the area will reveal the infecting organism and sensitivity studies will indicate the antibiotic best suited for the infection. Oxacillin or methicillin are the antibiotics of choice for a *Staphyloccus aureus* infection. Heat and topical bacitracin-neomycin ointment will relieve much of the discomfort. The abscess should not be squeezed or manipulated because these maneuvers may enhance the possibility of intracranial spread of infection. When the abscess becomes localized with an obvious fluctuant "head," it should be incised (Fig. 11–38) carefully and gently to avoid a cavernous sinus extension of the infection.

Rhinoliths

This term is applied to foreign bodies that have remained in the nose for some time and have become coated with calcium and magnesium salts. The nucleus may consist of bacteria, blood, pus, inspissated mucus or a small undetected foreign body. A mass with a rough exterior and a brown color is characteristic of these foreign bodies. They are often unilateral and vary considerably in size. The consistency may be either soft, crumbly, hard or brittle. A unilateral fetid nasal discharge and airway obstruction are the usual symptoms. The treatment is removal with topical, local or general anesthesia.

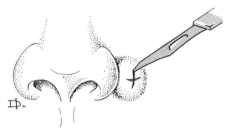

Figure 11–38 Incision of facial abscess. An area of cellulitis or an abscess of the face should be drained through a cruciate incision. Manipulation of these infections may allow pus to enter the cavernous sinus and produce thrombosis of this structure.

Epithelial Papilloma

Papillomas of the nose may be single or multiple. They are pink in color, firm, pliable, and tend to bleed when manipulated. The septum and inferior turbinate are the commonest sites of origin and the diagnosis may be missed if the specimen is not submitted for histopathologic examination.

A pedunculated mass of papilloma can be removed with a snare. Multiple papillomas require wide surgical excision and any recurrences should have complete excision followed by radiation therapy. Malignant degeneration is common.

Nasopharyngeal Angiofibroma

Angiofibromas arise in the posterior nose and nasopharynx of the preadolescent male.[10] They are firm, bluish red tumors that produce symptoms of nasal obstruction, rhinorrhea and epistaxis. These benign tumors may become very large and extend into adjacent areas such as the maxillary sinus, pterygomaxillary fossa, infratemporal fossa, sphenoid sinus, orbit and middle cranial fossa. Patients with large tumors may complain of failing vision, exophthalmos, proptosis, swelling of the cheek and nasal deformity. A biopsy of the tumor may produce disastrous consequences in the patient from massive bleeding. A patient suspected of having this tumor should be admitted to the hospital for diagnosis and treatment.

Nasal Carcinoma

Squamous cell carcinoma is the most common malignant neoplasm of the nose and paranasal sinuses. Unilateral nasal obstruction and a sensation of pressure and rhinorrhea may be the only symptoms. The discharge can be serous, serosanguinous or purulent. Pain, when present, is apt to be worse at night or when the patient is lying down.

Careful examination of the nose will often reveal a tumor, and a biopsy with histopathologic examination of the specimen will assure the diagnosis. Such a carcinoma requires carefully planned surgical and irradiation therapy.

Esthesioneuroblastoma is an unusual tumor arising from the olfactory epithelium high in the nasal cavity. Common symptoms are a one-sided nasal obstruction with associated rhinorrhea and epistaxis. A history of repeated polypectomy is quite common. Usually there is a rapid recurrence of the "polyp," and if this tissue has not been examined by a pathologist, the diagnosis will be missed.

Small tumors may be difficult to see. They are usually located on the septum or the superior turbinate. The tumor may spread by infiltration or metastasis. Large lesions often extend into the ethmoid and frontal sinuses, the orbit, and the face through the nasal bones. Exophthalmos, increased lacrimation, headache and masses about the nose occur when the tumor extends in these areas. Treatment consists of irradiation and surgery.

Several other malignant tumors may arise in the nose. Lymphoma, adenoid cystic carcinoma, malignant melanoma, chondrosarcoma, liposarcoma and fibrosarcoma have all been detected in the nose. Biopsy is essential to make the diagnosis and even the innocent "polyp" should be submitted for histopathologic examination. Many patients have not received prompt treatment for a serious disease because tissues removed from the nose were discarded, a practice to be avoided.

PARANASAL SINUSES

These spaces consist of the maxillary, ethmoidal, frontal and sphenoidal air cavities on each side of the head. The specific functions of the sinuses are unknown. They often harbor diseases that are overlooked.

Examination

Direct inspection of the sinuses is not ordinarily possible and some indirect method of examination is required when a disease is suspected.

The signs and symptoms of sinus disease are often subtle and easily missed. Disease may be restricted to a single sinus or it may be present in several on either one or both sides.

Pain is usually located over the affected sinus and is often increased with coughing, sneezing, bending over or walking. It may be referred to other areas and often decreases with rest in bed. The locations for sinus pains and the distribution of referred pains from the sinuses are presented in Figure 11–39.

Maxillary sinus pain is characteristically localized over the cheek and occasionally radiates along the upper alveolus, teeth or gums near the affected sinus. It also may be referred to the supraorbital nerve and mistakenly interpreted as arising from the frontal sinus. Occasionally the pain will be referred to the ear, and this pain is usually located in front of the ear. Ethmoidal pain is located over the bridge of the nose and inner canthus of the eye, and may be associated with a feeling of tenderness of the globe that is aggravated by moving the eye. This pain is often referred to a small area on the parietal eminence of the skull. Sphenoid disease usually produces an occipital or vertex headache; there may be pain behind the eye but the globe itself is not tender. Sometimes this pain is referred to the mastoid process. Frontal pain is localized to the forehead and is usually associated with a generalized headache. This pain often starts an hour or two after arising in the morning and decreases later in the afternoon. So-called "sinus head-

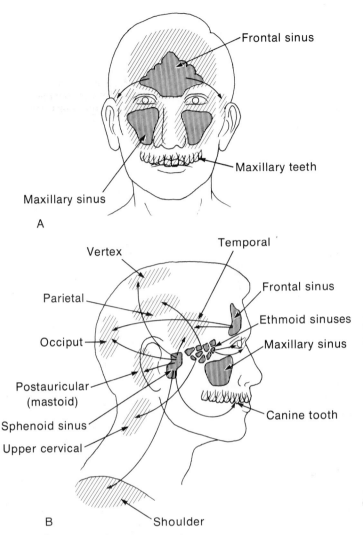

Figure 11–39 *A* and *B.* Areas of sinus pain and the distribution of referred sinus pains. (From: English, G. M.: Otolaryngology, A Textbook. Hagerstown, Harper & Row, 1976, Chapter 68.)

aches" are usually not associated with sinus disease.

Other symptoms of sinus disease include malaise, anorexia, mental dullness, forgetfulness and a slight elevation of temperature. In acute inflammations, rhinorrhea consisting of mucoid or mucopurulent material is seen. These patients usually have nasal airway obstruction. Chronic inflammations produce few nasal symptoms. The sense of smell is usually lost

and vocal resonance may be altered. Epistaxis is mild and may occur repeatedly, especially when the maxillary sinus is involved. An unpleasant-tasting postnasal drip may be noticed by the patient when the inflammation becomes less acute.

Flushing and swelling of the cheek, eyelids and forehead is sometimes seen in maxillary, ethmoid and frontal sinus infections. Swelling of the eyelids is more often associated with ethmoiditis in children. Tenderness in these areas is usually associated with a closed infection or abscess formation. Supraorbital nerve tenderness is often associated with maxillary sinus infections, whereas gentle tapping over the frontal sinus or pressure on its floor just above the inner canthus causes exquisite pain when the frontal sinus is involved.

Examination of the nose often reveals a generalized redness and swelling of the mucous membrane. Shrinking this congested membrane with a topical decongestant will make it much easier to detect the signs of sinusitis. A localized area of swelling and redness with pus coming from the drainage area of the sinus usually means disease in that sinus. Chronic sinusitis may be accompanied by a hypertrophic or atrophic rhinitis.

Nasopharyngeal examination with a small mirror or nasopharyngoscope will often reveal a pool of pus on the upper surface of the palate or pus trickling over the posterior end of the inferior turbinate. Pus coming from the region of the sphenoid ostium or sphenoethmoid recess indicates an infection in these sinuses.

Swelling of the lateral pharyngeal lymphoid tissue or pus coming down the lateral pharyngeal gutter indicates a sinus infection on that side. These findings also may be detected in patients who have a carcinoma of the paranasal sinuses with a superimposed infection.

Transillumination of the sinuses as a method of examination has been recommended for many years, but in my experience it has not been very reliable. Standard x-ray views are more valuable, but they must be taken with proper positioning of the head. All radiopaque articles must be removed, including dentures, hairpins, wigs or "pony tails" of hair. A textbook of radiology or otolaryngology should be consulted for the proper radiographic techniques. Air fluid levels, opacification, mucosal thickening and bone de-

struction may be seen on the x-ray and these findings, when correlated with the patient's symptoms and signs, are of great value in making a diagnosis.

Nasoantral Irrigation

This simple procedure (Fig. 11–40) is used for treating maxillary sinusitis and for obtaining purulent secretions from the sinus for culture and sensitivity tests. There are two routes for cannulation and irrigation of the maxillary sinuses. The inferior meatus of the nose and the canine fossa have a thin wall that can be easily punctured with a needle.

The preferred route is through the thin bone separating the maxillary sinus and nasal cavity in the inferior meatus. This area is anesthetized by packing the meatus with cotton soaked in 4 per cent cocaine HCl solution. A small amount of lidocaine HCl with 1:100,000 solution of epinephrine HCl can be injected into the nasal vestibule near the pyriform crest and the anterior end of the inferior turbinate. This injection will provide good anesthesia and decrease the amount of bleeding when the sinus is punctured. A 2½ inch disposable 16 gauge spinal needle can be used for this procedure. This needle is placed beneath the inferior turbinate approximately 1.0 centimeter behind its anterior tip. Steady pressure on the needle will force it through the antronasal wall into the sinus. The needle should be directed slightly upward, but it should not be inserted with such force that it traverses the sinus and enters the orbit or the lateral sinus wall.

The canine fossa approach is sometimes easier, particularly when the inferior meatus has been used previously and the bone has become thick and hard. The upper lip is retracted and a small amount of anesthetic solution is injected into the mucosa of the gingivobuccal sulcus. When the anesthetic solution reaches the infraorbital

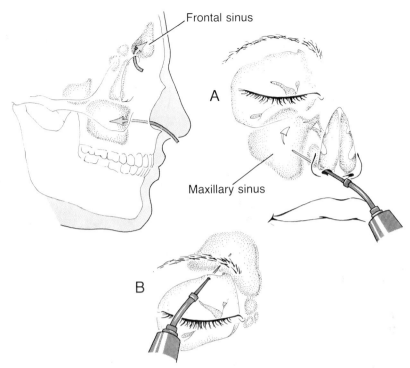

Figure 11–40 Sinus trephination. A. Irrigation of the maxillary sinus is a technique that can be performed with local anesthesia. The interior of the nose is packed with cotton saturated with cocaine hydrochloride solution (4 percent). A small amount (0.5 to 1.0 cc) of local anesthetic (Xylocaine) with 1:100,000 of epinephrine is then injected into the floor of the nasal vestibule and anterior end of the inferior turbinate. Within a few minutes the inferior meatus of the nose will be anesthetized and a 2 inch, 16 gauge disposable needle can be pushed through the inferior nasoantral wall into the maxillary sinus. The needle must be carefully controlled to avoid its misplacement into the orbit or lateral wall of the antrum. A syringe is then attached to the needle and the sinus aspirated. Air or pus entering the syringe usually indicates entry into the sinus. Warmed sterile saline is injected in the sinus. Excessive pressure may cause severe pain or may fracture the roof of the sinus into the orbit. Air should not be injected into the sinus, since it may cause an air embolus.

B. Trephination of the frontal sinus can be performed with local anesthetic. Xylocaine with epinephrine is injected along the medial floor of the frontal sinus. The sinus floor is usually quite thin and easily punctured. A small incision is made through the skin, subcutaneous tissue, muscle and periosteum. A trocar or a 16 gauge needle is then forced through the bone into the frontal sinus. When the bone is too thick, a small drill may be used to enter the sinus. Aspiration with a syringe will usually reveal purulent material when the sinus is infected. A small polyethylene tube is then inserted through the wound into the sinus to allow drainage of secretions.

The canine fossa route may be used for irrigating the maxillary sinus. A small amount of local anesthetic is injected into the mucosa and a 16 gauge needle is passed through the anterior wall of the maxillary bone. When the needle enters the sinus a small amount of air or pus can be aspirated.

canal or its nerve, a wide area of anesthesia (upper lip, maxillary teeth and cheek) will be obtained. The needle (2½ inch, 16 gauge spinal needle) is pushed through the thin bone of the anterior wall of the maxillary sinus. The needle must be placed well above the tooth roots. Firm pressure or a tap with a mallet is usually sufficient for entering the sinus. A 50 cc glass syringe is then attached to the needle with a rubber tube and adapter. It is essential to aspirate before irrigating the sinus. Either pus or air will indicate proper placement of the needle. When air or pus cannot be aspirated, this indicates that the needle tip either is not in the sinus or that the sinus is filled with solid material such as poly-poid mucosa or neoplasm. Warmed sterile normal saline solution is then injected into the sinus and collected in a basin as it flows from the nose. Excessive syringe pressure must be avoided when irrigating the sinus, and it is important to avoid injecting air into the sinus because this can cause an air embolism. Secretions from the sinus should be cultured. The irrigations may have to be repeated every two or three days before the infection is controlled, and subsequent irrigations should yield less purulent material.

In patients with chronic sinusitis, a small polyethylene tube can be placed in the sinus through the lavage needle and left in place for two to three days. It can be attached to the cheek with adhesive tape and an appropriate antibiotic injected into the sinus three or four times a day. These locally applied antibotics may help eradicate an infection that otherwise might not improve with the usual medical treatment. Systemic antibiotics, decongestants, heat, humidification of the air, bed rest and analgesics are all helpful. I usually treat the acute sinusitis patient with systemic antibiotics for 24 hours before attempting an antral irrigation; this reduces the risk of the irrigation spreading the infection.

Uncomplicated acute frontal sinusitis should be treated medically for 24 to 48 hours before any surgical intervention is considered. When the infection is not controlled by medical therapy or there are signs and symptoms of complications, it may be necessary to drain the sinus surgically (Fig. 11–39 C). Drainage can be accomplished through an external incision ¼ of an inch below and parallel to the medial end of the eyebrow. This incision should be made straight through to the bone. The superficial tissues are retracted away and a small hole is made with a drill or trocar. This opening into the sinus should be large enough to accommodate a small polyethylene tube. A suture placed through the skin

and around the tube will hold it securely in position. Pus from the sinus should be submitted to the laboratory for culture and sensitivity tests. Gentle irrigation of the sinus with warmed sterile normal saline will help relieve the patient's symptoms. The irrigating solution should drain through the nasofrontal duct if mucosal edema or inspissation secretions do not obstruct it. The operation can be performed with either local or general anesthesia.

Before antibiotics were available, numerous complications developed from even minor operations on the frontal sinus. Therefore it is important that frontal sinus trephination be performed with concomitant antibiotic therapy. Frontal sinus infections usually respond rapidly to this treatment and the drainage tube can be removed after four or five days. Patency of the nasofrontal duct can be determined by injecting a small quantity of sterile colored fluid into the sinus and observing whether or not this fluid passes through the duct into the nose.

Oromaxillary Fistula

Several of the upper molars are in intimate contact with the floor of the maxillary sinus. Large sinus cavities are separated from the apices of these teeth by a thin plate of bone, and in some instances the root of the tooth may extend into the sinus. Extraction of these teeth may produce an oromaxillary fistula (Fig. 11–41).

Blood in the nasal cavity and air escaping from the tooth socket are the initial symptoms of an oromaxillary fistula. Oral liquids may escape from the nose. Oral infection will become apparent in a few days and this problem produces pain and tenderness over the sinus and a profuse, foul-smelling rhinorrhea. Pus draining from the extraction site and a foul taste are characteristic of this problem.

Many fistulae will heal rapidly with conservative therapy, especially when they are detected early. Culture and

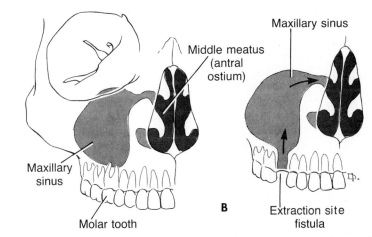

Figure 11–41 Oroantral fistula. The roots of molar teeth may project into the maxillary sinus (A). Extraction of such a tooth may result in an oroantral (oromaxillary) fistula with food particles and other foreign material entering the sinus. An infection usually develops, causing profuse rhinorrhea (B).

sensitivity tests of secretions will help determine the choice of antibiotics. Systemic and local antibiotic therapy with nasal decongestants for a two week period will often allow the fistula to close.

Several surgical procedures have been devised for the treatment of large or persistent fistulae. A buccal or palatal mucosal flap combined with resection of part of the alveolus may be required to close a fistula. These operations should not be performed on outpatients.

Nonsecreting Cyst

The floor of the maxillary sinus is the most common site for these cysts, which are smooth and round and contain a small amount of clear yellow fluid. These cysts are usually asymptomatic and have little significance. Surgical treatment is usually not indicated unless there is an associated problem.

Carcinoma

Squamous cell carcinoma is the most common malignant neoplasm of the paranasal sinuses. This tumor accounts for almost 60 percent of these problems. Adenocarcinomas, cylindromas, various sarcomas, lymphomas, intracranial tumors (meningiomas) and the occasional metastatic tumors account for the remainder. Carcinomas of the paranasal sinuses do not produce consistent clinical manifestations, and quite often the diagnosis is not made until the disease is in an advanced stage. These patients are often treated for an inflammatory disease that does not respond to medical therapy (Fig. 11–42). A high index of suspicion that an underlying malignant process may be involved will help to avoid this delay in diagnosis. A biopsy is necessary to make a diagnosis, and it should be performed as early as possible. The management of these tumors is beyond the scope of this text, because these patients cannot be treated in the Outpatient Department. They must be admitted to the hospital and treated by a physician familiar with these problems.

FACE

The most common congenital lesions, tumors and infections of the face

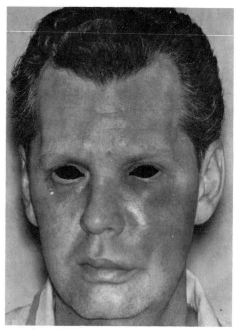

Figure 11-42 A patient with squamous cell carcinoma of the left maxillary sinus. There is edema and erythema of the left cheek. This was originally diagnosed as sinusitis.

treated with local anesthesia. Meticulous cleansing and débridement of the wound should be performed before repairing the laceration. A nonabsorbable suture such as 5–0 monofilament nylon or silk should be used on the skin (Fig. 11–44). A few vertical mattress sutures will help prevent inversion of the wound edges. The deeper layers of the wound should be carefully approximated with fine catgut sutures. Small rubber drains or a piece of sterilized rubber band inserted into the wound will prevent fluid accumulations and subsequent infection; a light pressure dressing that is left undisturbed for three or four days is usually sufficient. Pain and swelling usually indicate an infection, and the dressing should be removed and inspected. Antibiotics, hot compresses and improved drainage of the wound will usually control any infection.

BURNS. Thermal, electrical and

in general are similar to the problems described for the lips.

Injuries

LACERATIONS. These wounds bleed freely and heal rapidly because of the rich blood supply to the face. Infections will not be a problem if the wound is carefully cleaned and debrided before repair. Several structures that may be involved in facial lacerations will require consideration. The seventh cranial nerve may be transected, the parotid duct severed, the paranasal sinuses entered, the medial canthal ligament detached or the lacrimal apparatus injured with a facial laceration (Fig. 11–43). Failure to recognize such coexistent injuries can lead to serious complications. These problems require immediate attention and should not be handled in the Outpatient Department by an inexperienced surgeon.

Uncomplicated lacerations can be

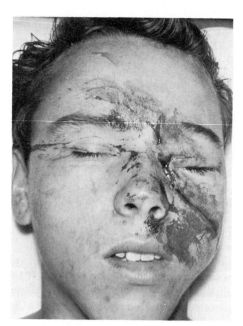

Figure 11-43 This patient's facial lacerations involved the left maxillary, ethmoid and frontal sinuses. The left medial canthal ligament was severed. The associated injuries were not readily apparent until the wounds were explored before repair.

A

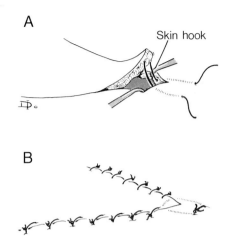

Skin hook

B

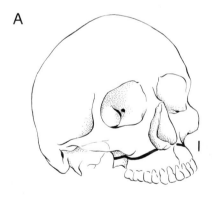

Figure 11–44 Gilles' corner suture for facial laceration.

chemical agents cause burns of the face. These are handled in the same way as burns involving other areas of the body. See Chapter 9.

FRACTURES OF THE MAXILLA AND ZYGOMA (Figure 11–45). Fractures of the maxilla and zygoma are caused by blows to the cheek from a fall, a fist or a hard object. Moderately severe blows may produce a separation of the zygomaticofrontal suture. Severe blows can produce a fracture of the zygoma, maxilla and orbit.[8, 25]

Pain, swelling, anesthesia of the distribution of the infraorbital nerve (lower lid, lateral nose and upper lip), diplopia and pain on opening the mouth are the usual symptoms of these fractures. Comparison of both sides of the face will reveal flattening of the involved cheek; displacement of the lateral palpebral ligament; retraction of the lower lid; ecchymosis of the cheek, lids, conjunctiva and sclera; and decreased mobility of the globe. Bimanual palpation will reveal depressions and irregularities that are not present on the opposite side of the face.

The Waters' view is the most useful x-ray for evaluating fractures of the zygomaticomaxillary complex. The stereoscopic method is of value. This view shows the outlines and contours of the zygomaticomaxillary complex

A

B

C

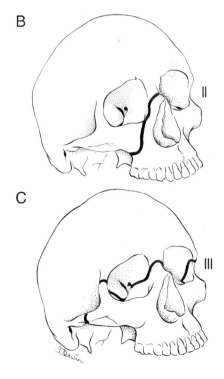

Figure 11–45 LeFort classification of midface fractures and fractures of the maxilla. LeFort I (transverse or Guérin fracture). LeFort II (pyramidal fracture). LeFort III (craniofacial disjunction.)

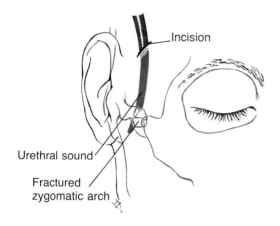

Figure 11–46 Reduction of fractured zygomatic arch. An incision is made through the skin, subcutaneous tissue and temporalis fascia. A small urethral sound is passed through this incision beneath the fracture and the fragments are manipulated into position with the other hand.

with a minimal superimposition of other structures. A submento-vertex view will demonstrate the zygomatic arches quite well. Planograms may be required to demonstrate irregularities of the orbital floor. Irregularities of the infraorbital margin and lateral wall of the maxilla, separation of the zygomaticofrontal suture, and clouding of the maxillary sinus are present in almost all of these fractures.

Zygomatic arch fractures can usually be reduced with the Gilles' operation (Fig. 11–46). After shaving the hair from the temporal area a small (2 cm) vertical incision is made behind the hair line. The incision is carried through the subcutaneous tissue and the temporal fascia overlying the temporalis muscles. A heavy elevator is inserted between the temporalis fascia and the muscle in the temporal fossa medial to the zygomatic arch. A roll of bandages placed on the skull above the incision serves as the fulcrum. The elevator is used as a lever. The arch is then guided into position. The opposite hand should be used to palpate the arch through the skin and assist in the reduction. Gentle pressure on the arch will demonstrate its stability after reduction. The wound is then closed in layers. The patient and his attendants should be instructed to avoid any pressure on the side of the fracture. If there are no complications, the patient can be discharged from the hospital in two

or three days; however, even minimal trauma or pressure may dislocate the fracture.

Pain, flattening of the cheek, diplopia, enophthalmos and a recurrence of trismus usually mean that the fracture has been dislocated (Fig. 11–47).

FRACTURES OF THE MANDIBLE. Fractures of the mandible make up about two-thirds of all facial fractures. Dingman and Natvig[8] have classified mandible fractures according to location (Fig. 11–48). Most of these result from automobile accidents, fights, or sports trauma. The common symptoms

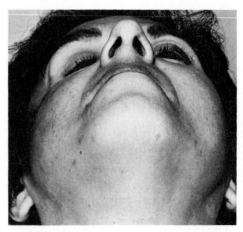

Figure 11–47 The appearance of a patient with a right zygomaxillary fracture that has not been repaired adequately. There is flattening of the right cheek, enophthalmos, diplopia, anesthesia of the infraorbital nerve and trismus.

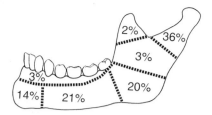

Figure 11–48 Frequency of fractures in various parts of the mandible. Midline fractures occur in less than 1 percent of these injuries. (Adapted from Dingman, R. O., and Natvig, P.: Surgery of Facial Fractures. Philadelphia, W. B. Saunders Co., 1964.)

of fractures of the mandible are pain on motion of the jaw; tenderness over the fracture site; inability to open the mouth; swelling and facial asymmetry; discoloration of adjacent tissues; deformity of the mandible; abnormal mobility of the jaw; grating, cracking and grinding sounds as the jaw is moved; drooling of saliva from the mouth; and offensive breath.

When one or more of the characteristic findings are evident, a tentative diagnosis of mandibular fracture should be made. Malocclusion is a reliable sign in patients with teeth. This may be more apparent with marked dislocation of the fracture and less evident with minimal dislocations. Bimanual manipulation of the mandible will usually produce movement and pain at the fracture site. Crepitus is not a very reliable sign for the diagnosis of a fracture. However, abnormal mobility of the mandible with deviation to one side when opening the mouth is a reliable indication of a fracture. Difficulties with eating and speech and swelling at the fracture site are quite common, but they do not necessarily indicate the presence of a fracture.

X-rays should be obtained in all patients with suspected fractures of the mandible. Fractures of the body and angle are usually detected on standard films, but the condylar processes are quite difficult to see and special stereoscopic views or tomograms may

be necessary to delineate fractures of these processes (Fig. 11–49). Dental x-rays and occlusal films sometimes help locate fractures of the symphysis, alveolus or the teeth. Postreduction x-rays are necessary to determine the effectiveness of reduction.

Fractures of the mandible are not emergencies, but the patient should have reduction and immobilization as early as his general condition permits. If treatment is delayed too long (seven to ten days) healing processes may make reduction more difficult.

Fractures of the mandible are often associated with intraoral lacerations. The oral cavity should be suctioned free of blood clots and secretions and then carefully inspected for foreign bodies such as teeth, fragments of bone and other debris. Aspiration of foreign bodies or gastric secretions may produce serious complications. Tracheostomy may be necessary to insure an adequate airway and it should be performed immediately whenever it is indicated. Nearly all patients with a mandible fracture will require hospitalization and surgical reduction of the fracture. A Barton bandage (Fig. 11–50) can be applied to hold the mandible in position until the patient can be moved to a hospital or until his general condition permits reduction.

MULTIPLE FACIAL FRACTURES. Multiple facial injuries are usually quite obvious. The clinical findings are those associated with the various facial bones involved in the fracture. Severe edema, periorbital ecchymosis, malocclusion, lacerations of the skin and oral mucosa, partial or complete airway obstruction and mobility of the fragments on palpation may be present, depending upon the severity of the fracture. Clear fluid coming from the nostrils or wounds should always be suspected as spinal fluid. Pulsation of the fluid, an increased flow with the head in a dependent position or compression of both jugular veins will help identify a cerebral spinal fluid leak. A simple chemical test for sugar will

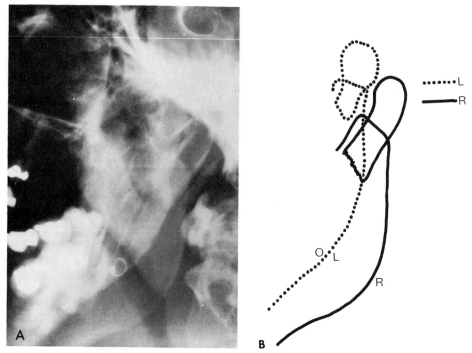

Figure 11–49 *A.* X-ray of a patient with bilateral condylar fractures. *B.* Line drawing depicting the fractures.

help confirm the diagnosis of this problem.

Radiographic examinations will help to determine the severity and location of these fractures. Patients with these fractures must be admitted to the hospital for treatment. The treatment of facial fractures may be safely delayed

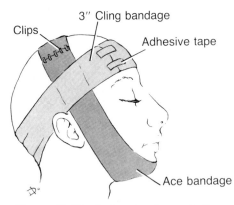

Figure 11–50 Barton bandage. A Barton dressing is an effective means of immobilizing a fractured mandible.

for several days; however, treatment should not be postponed after the patient's condition stabilizes.

DENTAL INJURIES. Dental trauma is common, but injuries to the teeth are rare until a child begins to walk. From that time on, these injuries increase in frequency. Preschool children sustain injuries to the teeth primarily from falls. During the early school years, bicycle and school playground accidents are the most common causes of dental injuries (Fig. 11–51). Contact sports, automobile accidents and fights are the causes of most dental injuries in teenagers and adults. Properly fitted intraoral mouth guards will reduce the incidence of trauma to the teeth incurred during participation in sports.

Most of the injuries involve the anterior teeth. The central incisors of the maxilla are the most often injured. Crown fractures are more common in the permanent teeth and luxation injuries are more common in the primary teeth.

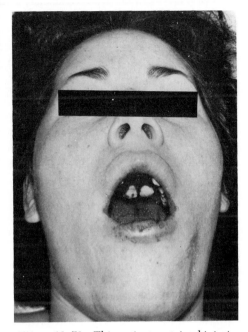

Figure 11-51 This patient sustained injuries to the maxillary incisor teeth from a bicycle accident. There was a fracture of the alveolar socket and posterior displacement of the incisors. This injury was treated satisfactorily with reduction of the fracture.

A variety of injury patterns have been described. These injuries have been classified by the World Health Organization and that classification is presented in Figure 11-52.

Dental injuries should always be considered as emergencies and treated promptly. The objectives of treatment are to reduce pain, to conserve the teeth whenever possible and to prevent complications. The specifics of treatment for each group of injuries will be discussed separately.

Uncomplicated crown fractures that involve only the enamel may not need treatment. If a sharp edge is present, it can be smoothed with a dental drill. A fractured mesial border of the central incisors produces a marked cosmetic defect. These fractures should be capped. When the dentin is exposed, it must be covered to protect the pulp. Exposed dentin has small tubules that have a potential connection between the oral cavity flora and the pulp tissues. This may lead to an infection and loss of the pulp and tooth.

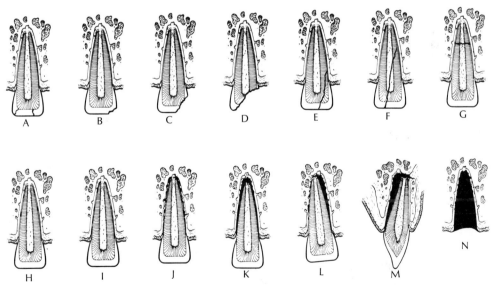

Figure 11-52 The classes of dental injuries. *A, B, C.* Uncomplicated crown fractures. *D.* Complicated crown fracture with exposure of the pulp. *E, F.* Crown-root fractures. *G.* Root fracture. *H.* Concussion of tooth without loosening. *I.* Subluxation with loosening but no displacement. *J, K.* Degrees of dislocation. *L, M.* Displacement with fracture of the alveolar socket. *N.* Complete avulsion of the tooth.

Complicated crown fractures with exposed pulp must be treated in a way that preserves and protects the pulp. Pulp capping, partial pulpotomy and pulpectomy are techniques that a dentist may use to preserve the tooth. Complicated crown fractures of primary teeth can be extracted. They usually cannot be preserved.

Uncomplicated crown–root fractures are treated in a manner similar to uncomplicated crown fractures. Complicated crown–root fractures that extend more than 3 to 4 mm below the gingiva should be extracted and replaced with a false tooth or bridge. Other dental techniques include pulpectomy and crowns of various types. Crown–root fractures of primary teeth are nearly always extracted.

The relationship between the fracture and the gingival margin determines the treatment of root fractures. As a general rule, the closer the fracture line is to the gingival margin the poorer the results of treatment. When the fracture is deep in the root, a reduction of the fracture and immobilization is a conservative method of treatment that is quite successful (Fig. 11–53). The average follow-up period should be one year. X-rays and viability tests will reveal pulp necrosis in 20 to 40 per cent of patients. This situation requires extensive endodontic and restorative procedures to save the tooth.

Concussion and subluxation injuries in primary and permanent teeth usually require no treatment. Follow-up examinations are necessary, however, to determine the need for future treatment.

Intruded teeth can be left to re-erupt spontaneously. Follow-up examination may reveal the need for other treatment.

Extrusion and lateral luxation injuries can be treated conservatively with a reduction of the fracture by digital pressure. Pulp necrosis occurs in 25 to 60 percent of these injuries. Markedly extruded teeth should be extracted.

Complete avulsion of a primary tooth does not require any specific treatment. The permanent tooth will erupt in its normal desired location. An avulsed permanent tooth can sometimes be reimplanted. The tooth should be free of caries and fractures, and the socket must be clean and not involved in the injury. Implantation is not successful if the injury is more than two hours old. The reimplanted tooth must be immobilized and observed carefully. There is a high incidence of root absorption in these teeth. These patients require long-term dental care (Fig. 11–54A, B).

TOOTHACHE. The afferent impulses from the teeth are carried by branches of the second and third divisions of the trigeminal nerve (fifth cranial nerve). There is a rich supply of unmyelinated and small myelinated nerve fibers in the pulp and periodontal tissues of the teeth. In addition to pain and touch, pressure and thermal sensations originate from these tissues.

Many of the diseases and disorders

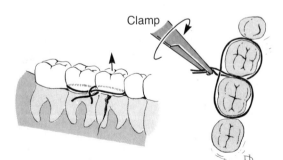

Clamp

Figure 11–53 Dental wiring. Stainless steel 20–30 gauge wire is passed around two teeth and the ends twisted together. This is an excellent method for holding one or two teeth in alignment.

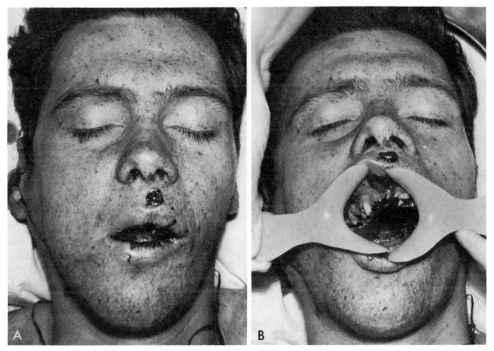

Figure 11–54 *A.* A penetrating injury of the upper lip without apparent dental injuries. *B.* Dental injuries are apparent when the lips are retracted. The maxillary incisor teeth on the right have been avulsed. There is a corresponding fracture of the maxillary alveolar process.

that cause toothache or referred head pains can be diagnosed with a few simple techniques. Other more complex problems may require the special skills of a dentist.

The history of the pain is important. The onset of pain may be sudden or insidious and the pain may be intermittent or continuous. Stimuli of various types may precipitate the pain, including opening and closing the mouth, thermal changes, a history of trauma or recent dental procedures and poor dental care. The pain may have its onset at night and it usually becomes more severe when the patient attempts to sleep. Various home remedies, including alcohol, aspirin and oil of cloves may have been used with varying degrees of success.

The head pains that arise from dental diseases are presented in Figure 11–55.

Inspection of the teeth will reveal many problems. The examination must be thorough. A small dental or laryngeal mirror is a useful instrument for inspecting the teeth. It will provide the examiner with an excellent view of the lingual surfaces of the teeth and can also be used as a retractor of the lips and tongue. The handle of the mirror is used to palpate and percuss the teeth.

Digital palpation may reveal swelling and tenderness of the gingival, lingual and buccal soft tissues. An x-ray examination is essential for any suspicious lesions and is particularly important before a tooth is extracted.

When the vitality of a tooth is in question, vitalometry should be obtained. These instruments may not be available in the office, emergency room or outpatient surgery, but the test is an important part of the evaluation.

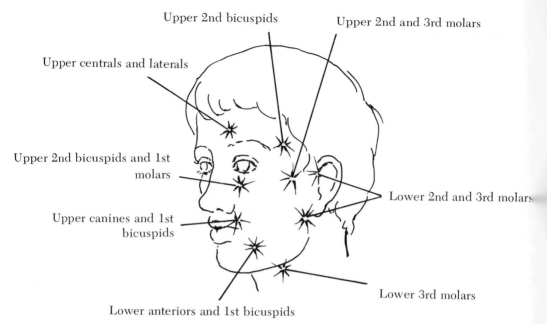

Upper 2nd bicuspids

Upper 2nd and 3rd molars

Upper centrals and laterals

Upper 2nd bicuspids and 1st molars

Upper canines and 1st bicuspids

Lower 2nd and 3rd molars

Lower 3rd molars

Lower anteriors and 1st bicuspids

Figure 11–55   Areas of referred dental pain. (From English, G. M.: Otolaryngology, A Textbook. Hagerstown, Harper & Row, 1976, Chapter 68.)

A dentist can usually assist with this procedure.

Caries and inflammation of the teeth and supporting structures are the most common causes of toothache. These processes must be differentiated from several other disorders. This can almost always be determined by direct palpation, inspection or x-rays of the tooth. Erupting teeth in young children may not be evident on direct inspection or palpation but x-rays will usually assist in making the diagnosis. Abrasions from grinding the teeth, pipe-stem friction, denture clasps, improper brushing of the teeth and malocclusion can cause toothache. When the cementum is exposed owing to recession of the gums, pain will be experienced during eating, drinking and deep inspiration through parted lips, and it will subside when the mouth is closed. Noxious stimuli from the interaction of a bright amalgam and gold filling may cause considerable discomfort. A traumatized tooth may lose its

blood supply with a resultant thrombosis, gangrene and discoloration of the tooth. Pain in this instance will occur at the site of the damaged tooth. Trauma of the pericementum from malocclusion, improper bite or poorly fitting dentures may induce a moderately severe pain. Rapid changes in barometric pressure associated with high-altitude flying when fluids or air are forced beneath a filling will cause a severe pain in an otherwise painless tooth. Very large metallic fillings may transmit extremes in temperature to the very sensitive underlying pulp. After secondary dentin has been deposited (2 years or more), the pain will disapper.

A number of disorders are associated with local tenderness and swelling of gum margin. The diagnosis is made by the absence of pathologic findings on the x-ray. Malpositioned teeth (notably the 3rd molars) sometimes cause pain. This pain is usually intermittent but occasionally is continuous. Malpositioned teeth may result in erosion and ultimate devitalization of teeth. The devitalized tooth is not painful, but a sterile cyst may arise and pressure and distortion of pain-sensitive structures will cause pain. Pulp nodules of calcific material may be associated with pain, although many of these are asymptomatic. Dentigerous cysts can cause pain, particularly when the cyst fluid becomes infected. Adamantinomas rarely cause pain unless there is an associated inflammation, degeneration from the pressure on necrotic tooth pulp or secondary abscess formation. Odontomas that press upon pain-sensitive structures give rise to pain of mild to moderate severity.

After thorough inspection, palpation and x-ray examination of the teeth, a diagnosis usually can be made. Treatment consists of relief of pain with appropriate analgesics and eradication of the dental disease. Aspirin, acetaminophen, codeine, Talwin and occasionally narcotics are the analgesics of choice. The extraction of suspicious or diseased teeth for the relief of headache or toothache is not justified until it can be demonstrated that the tooth is responsible for the pain. A local infiltration of 2 percent Xylocaine with a 27 gauge needle will usually give prompt relief of the toothache and relief of the head pain. Topical application of oil of cloves has long been a traditional remedy for temporary relief of toothache.

Temporomandibular Joint Pain

Temporomandibular joint pain can arise from grinding the teeth, poorly fitting dentures, dental diseases and, in pipe smokers, from habitually holding the stem of the pipe between the teeth. Gum chewers have a high incidence of this problem. Most of these patients find relief by discontinuing the practice that produces the problem. Occasionally, patients will require dental treatment for underlying dental pathology.

Dislocation of the Mandible

Dislocation of the mandible, particularly the first occurrence, may be very distressing to the patient. It usually results from yawning, although recurrent dislocations may occur during the acts of eating, speaking or laughing. These spontaneous dislocations may be unilateral or bilateral with the mandible protruded in an anterior open bite position. Physical violence or trauma usually produces medial or lateral dislocation and is nearly always associated with fractures or severe temporomandibular joint injuries. Chronic dislocation results in deformity and malfunction of the mandible. These problems can be avoided by prompt diagnosis and treatment. X-ray examination of the temporomandibular joint and condyles before and after reduction will reduce the risk of missing an associated fracture.

Moderate sedation to relieve apprehension and relax the muscles of mastication will help the operator manipulate the dislocated mandible into its proper position (Fig. 11–56A). With the patient in a sitting position and the head supported, the operator faces the patient and places the thumbs inside the mouth on the occlusal surfaces of the teeth or the alveolar ridges if the patient is edentulous. Pressing downward on the posterior area, elevating the anterior area and pushing the mandible backward allows the condyle to slip over the articular eminence into its normal position. This usually gives the patient immediate relief. When there is severe muscle spasm or the patient is unable to cooperate, a general anesthetic and muscle-relaxing drug will be required.

Johnson[19] described another method of reducing acute dislocations of the temporomandibular joint (Fig. 11–56B). This method consists of preparing either preauricular area of the face with an antiseptic solution. These are the sites for injection. Although the dislocation is bilateral, usually only

A

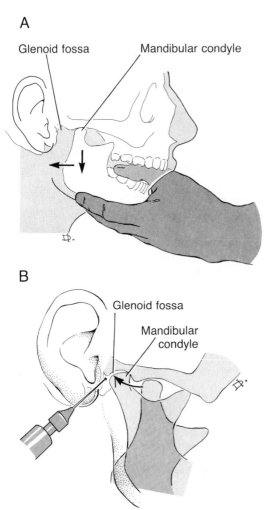

Glenoid fossa   Mandibular condyle

B

Glenoid fossa

Mandibular
condyle

Figure 11–56 Reduction of dislocated mandible. *A.* Reducing a dislocated mandible can be accomplished by inserting the thumbs over the last molar teeth and exerting a downward force. When the condyle is below the anterior tubercle, a slight posterior force will complete the reduction.

B. Johnson's technique for reducing a dislocation of the condyle is a simple and often effective method of treatment. A small 25 gauge needle is inserted through the skin and subcutaneous tissue in the shallow depression creased by the anteriorly displaced condylar head. Xylocaine is injected into this site (1.5 to 2.0 cc) and the needle withdrawn. Within a few minutes the dislocated mandible will return to its normal position.

one side requires injection. A depression over the glenoid fossa is readily apparent because the heads of the condyles are locked anterior to the articular eminences. About 2.0 cc of lidocaine HCl solution is drawn into a syringe with a 25 gauge needle, which is then injected into the subcutaneous tissue over the glenoid fossa depression. This anesthetic solution is injected slowly as the needle is directed inward and slightly anterior toward the head of the condyle. When the head of the condyloid process is contacted, the needle is withdrawn slightly and the remaining solution injected into the tissues surrounding the glenoid fossa.

Johnson[19] reported that the dislocations were reduced spontaneously without manipulation in about one minute. I have used this technique in many patients and found it satisfactory. Occasionally, I have injected both sides and found that spontaneous reduction occurred in some patients in whom a single injection had failed. After an acute dislocation, patients may be unable to occlude the posterior teeth for several days. The patient should avoid overextending the joint for several months because repeated injury of the joint may cause permanent damage and produce a recurring or chronic dislocation.

LIPS

Congenital Lesions

CLEFT LIP. Cleft lip is the most common congenital defect in this area. These abnormalities are frequently associated with an alveolar cleft or cleft palate. The surgical treatment of these defects is beyond the scope of this book and such problems should be referred to a specialist for treatment.

LABIAL PITS. These small slits usually occur in the lower lip and are thought to arise from improper development of the mucocutaneous junction of the lip. They produce a partial double lip and can be treated by local excision and advancement of labial mucosa. Careful approximation of the tissues with fine sutures to reduce scar formation is important.

HEMANGIOMA. These tumors may produce gross deformities and require intensive therapy. Only the smaller lesions should be treated by local excision in the office, clinic or outpatient department.

Traumatic Lesions

Injuries of the face are quite common, and the lips may be involved separately or in conjunction with other areas. Tissues in these areas usually heal rapidly and are relatively resistant to infection because they have a rich blood supply. Careful repair reduces scar formation and cosmetic deformities.

ABRASIONS. These injuries usually require a minimum of treatment. All foreign material must be removed and simple cleansing with soap and water will often suffice. When foreign particles of dirt, stones or other debris are imbedded in the tissues, they must be removed mechanically. A fine forceps or number 11 Bard-Parker knife blade may be used to remove implanted foreign material. Antibiotics are usually not necessary, but tetanus toxoid should be administered.

LACERATIONS. Puncture wounds of the lips that are made by the teeth are common. Two important considerations should be kept in mind: first, thorough cleansing of the wound to avoid infection, and second, careful approximation of tissues to prevent excessive scar tissue. These wounds usually bleed freely and hemostasis may require ligation of larger vessels. Lacerations through the entire thickness of the lip must be repaired by carefully approximating each layer. Mucosa, muscle, subcutaneous tissue and skin should be approximated in layers and irregular edges carefully removed before the repair is started. The vermilion border and mucocutaneous border should be aligned as accurately as possible (Fig. 11–57). Failure to accomplish this will result in an obvious cosmetic defect. Avulsion injuries may require flaps or grafts for closure of the defect and these injuries should be treated in the operating room by an experienced surgeon.

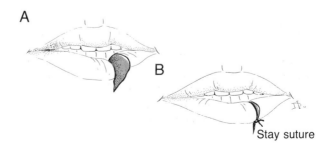

Figure 11–57 The vermilion border of the lip must be carefully approximated when lacerations of the lip are repaired.

A

B

Stay suture

Electric Burns

Most electrical burns of the head and neck occur in the perioral region of children between the ages of nine months to four years. The peak incidence is between the ages of one and two years. At this age, the electric cord is an object of curiosity, and the creeping child will often play with it. The cord is inevitably placed in the mouth, where moisture completes an electric circuit and the resulting arc burns the tissues. If the child is wet or touching a grounded metal object, the current may result in electrocution.[21a]

Thompson, Juckes and Farmer reviewed 43 children with perioral electrical burns.[29a] In that series, 28 of the 43 children were under the age of two years, and 12 were between the ages of two and four years. Thirty-seven of the 43 children sucked on or bit into the free end of a live extension cord. Four patients bit directly into the wire; one patient sucked on an electrical outlet and another bit the cord of an electric fireplace. The mucosa was involved in 10 patients and the entire lip in 33 patients. A commissure deformity occurred in 10 patients. Both the upper and lower lips were involved in 13 patients, the lower lip only in two, and the upper lip only in six. The tongue and buccal mucosa, without lip involvement, were burned in two cases. There were associated burns of the tongue in 18, of the buccal sulcus in 13, of the alveolus in 10 and of the teeth in four.

Examination usually discloses a third degree burn with a centrally depressed crater. There is a pale gray color to the surrounding slightly elevated tissues. The sensory nerves are destroyed, and this produces a relatively painless injury. The media of the blood vessels are disintegrated, which occasionally leads to severe secondary hemorrhage during the sloughing process. The healing of the burn is a relatively slow process with a minimum of surrounding tissue reaction.

The lips, alveolar processes and tongue are most often involved in electrical burns. The lips are damaged most severely, and the lower lip is usually more severely burned than the upper lip. The entire thickness of the lip is affected from the mucosa of its inner surface to the skin or vermilion. The adjacent alveolar process is also often involved.

Burns of the alveolar process and teeth are common, with a resulting sequestration of the teeth or bone. This may cause a loss of deciduous teeth, but the permanent teeth are not affected unless there is a deep injury to the alveolar process.

Damage to the tongue is usually not severe; however, the tip may be ulcerated in the initial stage of the injury. There may be an impairment of tongue mobility if the floor of the mouth is involved. This results in scar tissue that decreases the mobility of the tongue.

TREATMENT. Electrical burns are usually full-thickness in nature. The extent of the injury often can be determined within a few hours after the accident. Unfortunately, many burns of the lips and cheeks are not seen early, and they may involve areas that are not amenable to primary therapy. Occasionally, reconstruction can be performed at an early stage of the injury after the involved tissue has been excised. This approach prevents contraction deformities that are otherwise inevitable. It also reduces the prolonged healing period that is associated with these injuries.

When the burn involves the corner of the mouth (commissure), it is preferable to await separation of the eschar and the healing and softening of the wound before beginning a definitive repair of the resulting defect. Early excision of damaged tissue increases the risk of sacrificing valuable uninvolved tissue. A final reconstruction is best achieved after healing of the burn and after a significant period during which the scars begin to soften. This waiting period can extend for a year or more. There is a tendency for children to develop hypertrophic scarring, and reconstructive procedures that are performed while the scars are hypertrophic may lead to additional scarring. After a year or more, the scars begin to flatten and soften and there is less tendency for hypertrophic scarring.

Reconstruction of lip, commissure and the other defects of electrical burns is beyond the scope of this chapter.

Tumors

Small ulcers are quite common on the lower lip, particularly in individuals who are exposed to intensive sunlight. Because it is virtually impossible to differentiate a benign or a malignant lesion from the clinical appearance alone, a biopsy of the lesion is often necessary to make a diagnosis. A small lesion (under 1 cm in diameter) can be excised with a margin of normal tissue, whereas in larger lesions, biopsies should be performed in several areas with a small cup forceps. Malignant lesions (squamous cell carcinoma) can be treated with surgery or irradiation, and benign lesions should be treated with a bland ointment and avoidance of local trauma.

MUCOCELE. Mucous retention cysts present as small, circumscribed, elevated translucent lesions of the mucosa. They may rupture, drain a small amount of thick mucoid material, collapse, and then slowly reform. They develop from an obstruction or injury of the duct of a small accessory salivary gland with a subsequent accumulation of saliva within the tissues. Local anesthesia and surgical excision usually result in a cure.

VERRUCA VULGARIS. These soft, sessile, papillary lesions are usually only a few millimeters in size. Local excision results in a cure, but spontaneous regression may occur. A virus infection is thought to be the cause of this lesion.

PAPILLOMA. A papilloma is a benign epithelial neoplasm that can occur anywhere in the oral cavity. When it develops on exposed surfaces it is rough and scaly, whereas if it develops within the oral cavity it is soft and pliable. Papillomas do not undergo malignant transformation and rarely recur when adequately excised.

FIBROMA. These are elevated pedunculated or sessile lesions that occur as a response to local trauma. They vary in size from a few millimeters to a few centimeters. Lip biting is a common cause of this lesion, and local excision is the preferred treatment; however, when contributing factors are not removed, the tumor often recurs.

Inflammatory Conditions

FURUNCLES. Furuncles about the lips and face are usually due to staphylococcal infections and differ little from furuncles elsewhere on the body. Facial movements and an individual's tendency to squeeze these lesions often result in a spread of infection with a larger area of cellulitis. The "danger zone" of the face consists of the upper lip and nose, and infections from this area may spread into the cavernous sinus, resulting in thrombosis. This serious problem must be constantly borne in mind when treating infections arising in this area.

CARBUNCLES. A large area of swelling from cellulitis with pus draining from many small openings is characteristic of this problem. The lips are frequently involved. After culture and sensitivity studies, antibiotics should be administered in large doses. Heat, rest, intravenous fluids and analgesics will give the patient relief from his symptoms.

CELLULITIS. Streptococci or other pathogens may enter the skin through a small wound to produce the redness, swelling and tenderness that are characteristic of cellulitis. An underlying sinus or dental disease should be suspected when these findings are located in an appropriate area. Treatment consists of bed rest, hot moist compresses and antibiotics. Penicillin is the most effective antibiotic for this infection and it should be used routinely unless the patient is allergic to it.

ERYSIPELAS. The lips and face are common sites for erysipelas. Streptococci enter through small openings in the skin to produce a rather characteristic lesion. Often, the nose is the primary site of infection, with the lesion gradually extending onto the cheek, lips and forehead. The lesion may have a "butterfly" configuration with elevated red edges. Older people are most frequently affected during the spring and fall months of the year. This infection responds very rapidly to penicillin therapy. Most of the patients can remain active during the treatment.

MOUTH

Congenital Lesions

FORDYCE'S SPOTS. These small yellowish white granules may occur in clusters or plaquelike areas. The buccal mucosa along the occlusal planes, the lips and the retromolar areas are the most common sites. Almost 80 per cent of the population have these harmless developmental lesions, consisting of submucosal sebaceous glands that increase in size with age. These should not be excised.

"TONGUE TIE." Although this condition is known to exist, it is quite rare and almost never interferes with speech. The lingual frenulum appears short or taut and restricts movement of the tongue upward to the lower alveolar ridge. Surgical correction of a shortened frenulum can be accomplished in a number of ways. A child who is uncooperative or frightened may require a general anesthetic, but most children can be operated upon with a local anesthetic and physical restraints. A small wedge excision of the frenulum (Fig. 11–58) will increase the mobility of the tongue in these children. Hemostasis may require ligation of vessels. An absorbable suture material is preferred because it loosens and falls free in a few days. The child's articulation problems usually continue after frenulectomy unless his tongue and speech habits are retrained.

GLOSSOPTOSIS. Pierre Robin syndrome consists of micrognathia, glossoptosis and cleft palate. Micrognathia and glossoptosis are responsible for episodic respiratory obstruction in some newborn infants. There are cyanosis and stridor during feeding or when the infant is supine. The airway usually can be improved by placing the infant in the prone position. Glossoptosis interferes with deglutition,

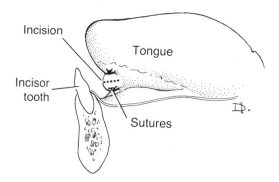

Figure 11–58 "Tongue tie." This procedure should be performed only on those patients who cannot protrude the tongue beyond the incisor teeth. The operation will not benefit patients with paresis or paralysis of the tongue. Local anesthesia is usually sufficient. Sutures are placed above and below the anticipated incision without obstructing the submaxillary duct orifices and the frenulum is incised.

Figure 11-59 Glossopexy. The glossoptosis associated with micrognathism (Pierre Robin syndrome) may cause severe respiratory distress. A simple and effective method of supporting the tongue in an anterior position is illustrated. A small rubber or polyethylene tube is threaded over a large (No. 1 or 2) nonabsorbable suture. This tube should be placed at the base of the tongue and each end of the suture passed through the floor of the mouth under the mandible and tied securely. The position of the tongue can be altered by the amount of tension on the sutures.

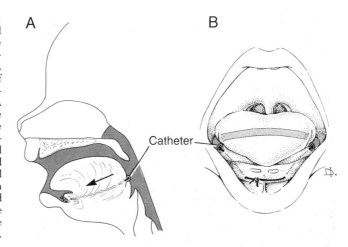

and aspiration during feeding is common. These infants fail to thrive and have repeated respiratory infections. As the infant becomes weaker from feeding problems, the respiratory obstruction becomes more severe and may result in death unless treatment is instituted early.

The most satisfactory method of treatment utilizes feeding by gavage or gastrostomy and fixing the tongue in an anterior position until the mandible develops sufficiently. A temporary glossopexy is the most effective method of relieving the airway obstruction and improving oral feeding. The micrognathic mandible usually catches up with the other facial structures by the end of the first year of life and spontaneous improvement results.

The Duhamel[20] operation has been a most satisfactory method of treatment (Fig. 11–59). It is a simple procedure that can be performed at the bedside and gives immediate results.

A 2-0 silk suture is passed through each side of the posterior tongue and threaded through a small caliber silicone tube resting across the base of the tongue. This tube prevents the suture from pulling through the tongue. Each end of the suture is brought out along the floor of the mouth beside the tongue and passed through the anterior mandible with a cutting needle. The ends of the suture are tied snugly

across the front of the mandible, holding the tongue in the desired position. They may be left in place for several weeks.

CYSTS. Many cysts occur in the oral cavity, mandible or maxilla, and some of these arise in the area of fusion of the facial processes. The median palatal, median alveolar, globulomaxillary and nasoalveolar cysts are examples of such developmental cysts. The nasopalatine cyst arises from remnants of the nasopalatine duct. Follicular cysts arise from the enamel organ or tooth follicle, and epithelial rests adjacent to a tooth may produce a radicular or residual cyst. Because these cysts involve the maxilla and mandible most of them should be treated in a hospital.

Salivary Glands

RANULAS (Figure 11–60). These cysts develop in the sublingual salivary gland from an obstruction of the ducts of the gland. They are usually located on one side of the frenum of the tongue and may become quite large. Aspiration or incision and drainage will give temporary relief (Fig. 11–61), but recurrences are common. Total excision through a neck incision may be necessary for recurrent cysts.

SALIVARY CALCULI. Calculi can

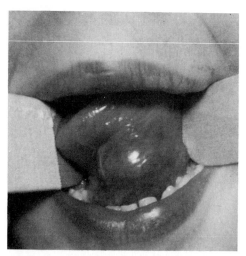

Figure 11–60 A ranula of the left floor of the mouth. The patient's only symptom was abnormal speech from the displacement of the tongue.

form in all the salivary glands or ducts. The submaxillary gland and its ducts are the most common sites with 80 to 85 per cent of stones occurring in these areas. The remaining 15 to 20 per cent occur in the parotid and sublingual glands or ducts.

The cause of these calculi is unknown, but they probably develop around a small nidus of bacteria or other foreign material. Composed mostly of calcium carbonate and phosphate, they can be either single or multiple.

They will cause symptoms when they become large enough to block the duct or induce stasis of secretions with a subsequent infection of the gland. The involved gland becomes swollen and tender and the mouth becomes drier than usual, especially after eating. Pressure on the swollen gland may force saliva or pus around the stone through the duct opening into the mouth. Frequently, the calculus can be felt during palpation of the involved duct. A lacrimal probe inserted into the duct will often help localize the exact position of the calculus by the rough grating sensation that will be apparent when the probe comes into

contact with the calculus. Care must be taken not to force the calculus further back into the duct or gland with the probe. Since about 20 per cent of calculi are radiolucent and are not visible on x-rays, a sialogram should be obtained in these patients.

Occasionally, a calculus will pass from the duct spontaneously. Dilating the orifice of the duct with a lacrimal probe and gently dislodging the calculus may allow the stone to pass into the mouth. When the stone does not pass spontaneously or cannot be removed with dilatation and a probe, surgical extirpation is necessary (Fig. 11–62). Local anesthesia is usually sufficient for this procedure. The calculus must be fixed by grasping either it or the duct distal to the stone with a forceps. A suture around the duct will prevent the stone from passing further back into inaccessible areas of the duct or the gland. An incision is made along the long axis of the duct. This allows exposure of the calculus and its extraction. Pressure on the gland often makes this procedure easier by bringing the stone into a more accessible position. Multiple stones are common in the submaxillary duct and should not be overlooked. The sublingual artery, lingual nerve, lingual vein and hypoglossal nerve are in close proximity to the submaxillary duct and must be avoided during surgery. Stones that

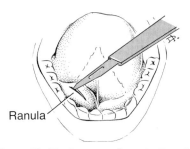

Ranula

Figure 11–61 Incision of ranula. Ranulas are cystic structures located in the floor of the mouth on each side of the tongue. After incising the cyst and evacuating the seromucus contents, part of the dome should be removed and the cyst marsupialized. A shallow gutter beside the tongue may persist after treatment.

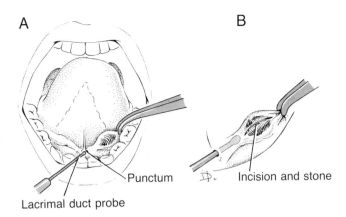

Figure 11–62 Submaxillary duct stone. Submaxillary duct stones can be removed with local anesthesia. The duct is occluded with a clamp or forceps (*A*) and a lacrimal duct probe inserted through the punctum into the duct. The stone is located and a small linear incision is made directly over the stone (*B*). One or more stones can be removed in this manner.

lie near the hilum of the submaxillary gland require an external incision, dissection and removal. Recurrent stones, dilatation of the duct system, calculi within the gland or chronic inflammation of the gland are the indications for gland excision. These procedures should not be performed on outpatients.

SALIVARY GLAND TUMORS. The parotid gland is the salivary gland most frequently involved by both benign and malignant tumors. The submaxillary gland and sublingual gland are less often affected, but tumors in these glands are more likely to be malignant than those that occur in the parotid gland.

Mixed tumor and papillary cystadenoma lymphomatosum (Warthin's tumor) are the two most common benign tumors of the salivary glands. Mucoepidermoid carcinomas, squamous cell carcinomas, adenocarcinomas, and malignant melanomas are the usual malignant tumors of these glands.

These neoplasms also are occasionally found in the minor salivary glands located in the mucosa of the pharynx, palate and larynx.

A biopsy is necessary for diagnosis; however, sialography is an important technique that will often determine the exact location of the tumor, and it should be performed before a biopsy is made. Very often the biopsy will entail an extensive operative procedure and

these operations should not be performed on outpatients.

Traumatic Lesions

HEMATOMA. Submucosal collections of blood are quite common. Clotting disorders are occasionally associated with hematoma formation. However, trauma is a more common etiology. Unless the hematoma interferes with respiration or swallowing it should be left alone. Respiratory distress may necessitate a tracheostomy.

LACERATIONS. Small lacerations usually require no surgical treatment. More extensive injuries should be carefully debrided of devitalized tissue, irrigated with sterile saline and repaired with fine sutures. Palatal, lingual and tonsillar lacerations are common in children who fall with a toy or "stick" in the mouth. Copious bleeding is common, and the injury may involve the internal carotid artery, causing hemorrhage or thrombosis of that vessel. These children are usually frightened, and a general anesthetic may be needed to repair the laceration. Careful approximation of the tissues will help prevent scar formation and loss of function.

Bleeding from around a tooth usually stops spontaneously. A loose tooth should not be disturbed, but partially extracted or fractured teeth should be removed, particularly when there is any danger that they may be aspirated by the patient. Lacerations of alveolar mucosa should be repaired with fine sutures.

Oral hygiene is important after any injury to the mouth. Hydrogen peroxide 1½ per cent or buffered sodium peroxyborate monohydrate (Amosan) solutions should be used within the oral cavity every two hours. Normal saline and a pleasant tasting mouthwash (Cēpacol) will make the patient more comfortable.

BURNS. Mucosal injuries may result from thermal, chemical or electrical agents. Chemical agents such as lye, ammonia, Clorox, Lysol, potassium permanganate and iodine solutions may be accidentally ingested or used in a suicide attempt. Children under age 5 make up 60 per cent of these patients and 80 per cent are under age 15.[7] The extent and degree of injury are important and may not be apparent when the patient is first examined. Oral burns without an esophageal injury occur in 25 per cent of these injuries and esophageal burns without an oral injury occur in 75 per cent of patients. The level of injury must be determined accurately. Esophagoscopy should be performed, although the esophagoscope should not be inserted beyond the area where the burn is first seen.

All these patients must be admitted to the hospital. They require intravenous fluid therapy and should receive nothing by mouth until the extent and the degree of injury have been determined. A nasogastric tube or beaded string should be carefully inserted into the stomach. Induced vomiting may produce aspiration pneumonia, particularly in the comatose or obtunded patient. Neutralizing substances such as dilute acetic acid, aqueous sodium bicarbonate (2 per cent) or milk may be of value but must be administered within three hours of ingestion to be effective. Shock is not uncommon and must be corrected with IV fluid thera-

py. Antibiotics and steroids help to reduce stricture formation.[18] Esophageal dilation may be required, but should never be performed by someone who is not completely familiar with the technique and its hazards.

FOREIGN BODIES. Accidental ingestion or inhalation is the most common cause of a foreign body in the food and air passages, although a disturbed person occasionally may attempt suicide by this means. Some foreign materials may be imbedded as a result of trauma and all patients with injuries of the oral cavity should be examined carefully to be certain that a foreign body is not overlooked. Usually a foreign body lodged in the gastrointestinal tract is not an emergency, whereas a laryngeal, tracheal or bronchial foreign body may cause severe respiratory distress. These latter patients may require tracheostomy or bronchoscopy for relief of this problem; however, ill-advised attempts to remove a foreign body may cause more trouble than the foreign body itself.

Small sharp foreign bodies usually lodge in the tonsil or lateral pharyngeal wall. These are usually obvious and can be removed with a forceps or clamp under direct vision. A topical anesthetic spray such as lidocaine HCl 4 per cent will relieve some of the discomfort, reduce the gag reflex and make extraction easier. Larger articles may become lodged in the valleculae, lingual tonsils or pyriform recesses. The ones that can be seen without the use of special instruments should be removed.

Foods may contain bones or other objects. Adults who chew poorly, swallow hastily and have poor dentition may accidentally ingest such objects. This may cause acute distress that simulates an acute coronary occlusion. Children may swallow an object that is carried in the mouth and this may go unnoticed for some time. Vegetable objects such as nuts and seeds are the most common objects aspirated in children.

Foreign bodies that enter the esophagus, larynx or tracheobronchial tree should be removed carefully and as promptly as possible. These procedures usually require hospitalization and endoscopic treatment.

Benign Tumors

Many benign and malignant tumors occur in the oral cavity, pharynx, esophagus, larynx or tracheobronchial tree. Biopsy and histopathologic diagnosis are essential before starting any form of therapy. Small lesions should be excised with a margin of normal tissue, and biopsy of several areas should be performed on the larger ones (see Chapter 6). Some of the tumors not discussed in that chapter are presented here. Carcinoma of the mouth is discussed in Chapter 6.

EPULIS. These growths of the hard palate are usually associated with ill-fitting dentures, extraction wounds or small extruding sequestra of bone. They are soft, red, painful masses of granulation tissue that bleed easily when manipulated. A surface ulcer is quite common, but usually the surface is covered with stratified squamous epithelium. Excision or curettage is necessary for the larger tumors, however, the origin of the problem should be treated directly by correcting the denture, removing a sequestrum of bone or closing the mucosa over an extraction site to prevent recurrence of the lesion.

GIANT CELL REPARATIVE GRANULOMA. These tumors occur most frequently on the gingiva or soft tissue of an edentulous ridge. The mandible is more often involved than the maxilla, and most of the patients are over age 20. Males are affected slightly more often than females and a history of trauma such as tooth extraction is quite common. Pedunculated or broad-based, these tumors have a smooth surface and are bluish-red in color. They are sometimes lobulated and bleed quite easily when manipulated. X-rays are usually negative, but occasionally the underlying bone may be radiolucent. Local excision with a small margin of normal tissue will prevent recurrence of the tumor.

PYOGENIC GRANULOMA. These tumors occur in both sexes and in nearly all age groups. The gingiva is the most common location, but the lips, tongue, oral mucosa and nasal mucosa may be involved. They may be pedunculated or broad-based and an ulceration of the smooth surface is common. The tumor bleeds easily when manipulated. Treatment of this benign tumor consists of surgical excision which should include a small margin of healthy tissue.

GRANULOMA GRAVIDARUM. Gingivitis of pregnancy is a common condition and a small number of these patients develop this tumor on the gingival surface. These tumors are histologically identical to the pyogenic granuloma. They appear during the first trimester of pregnancy and often regress spontaneously after delivery. Recurrence at the same site during subsequent pregnancies is not uncommon. Those tumors that do not regress should be excised after delivery. Excision may be necessary during pregnancy when the tumor becomes large or when bleeding is a problem.

IRRITATION FIBROMA. This is probably the most common tumor of the oral cavity and is identical to the fibroma involving the lip. Characteristically, it is an elevated, pedunculated or sessile lesion paler than the surrounding tissue and varying in size from a few millimeters to a few centimeters. These tumors are often associated with local trauma or irritation. Treatment consists of excision of the tumor and eradication of the source of irritation.

HEMANGIOMAS. Capillary and cavernous hemangiomas may be seen at any age in either sex. Most of them arise from congenital malformations that become apparent at a later age.

They may be elevated or submerged, circumscribed or diffuse, and red or bluish in color. They are characterized by a smooth surface and vary considerably in size. They are normally soft and compressible and may blanch with pressure. The tongue and cheek are the most common sites, but hemangiomas may occur anywhere in the oral cavity. Although large tumors may interfere with speech and mastication, and minimal trauma may cause considerable bleeding, they grow very slowly or not at all, and rarely become malignant.

Fibrosis and spontaneous regression may occur with internal bleeding or thrombosis of vessels. Superficial lesions should be removed surgically; cryosurgery has been found useful for larger or deeply seated tumors.

The juvenile hemangioma occurs in children shortly after birth up to about three years of age. The lip, oral cavity, parotid, and submaxillary glands are the most frequent sites of involvement. They usually present a clinical picture of a firm, slowly growing mass with a normal mucosal surface. Surgical excision is the treatment of choice, but spontaneous regression may occur and a period of observation is indicated before attempting any treatment. Small superficial lesions may be excised in the clinic or Outpatient Department, but if the hemangioma is large, the patient should be hospitalized and surgery performed in the operating room by an experienced surgeon.

LYMPHANGIOMAS. The oral cavity and tongue are common sites for these tumors. Superficial tumors present as a cluster of colorless, soft masses on the mucosa. Deeper tumors cause a diffuse enlargement and, when the tongue is involved, there may be a loss of surface structures such as the papillae. These tumors rarely undergo malignant degeneration. Because they do not respond to radiation, surgical excision is the treatment of choice.

NEUROFIBROMA AND SCHWANNOMA (NEURILEMOMA). These two tumors

are distinct entities, but because of their many similarities they will be considered together. The tongue, lips, palate and cheek are the usual sites for these tumors. Small, sessile, smooth-surfaced tumors or circumscribed nodules that grow slowly and produce few if any symptoms are the usual presentation of these tumors. Local excision is the preferred treatment.

GRANULAR CELL MYOBLASTOMA. This benign soft tissue tumor may occur anywhere on the skin or mucous membranes or in the gastrointestinal tract. In the oral cavity, one of the more common sites of origin, the dorsal and lateral surfaces of the tongue are the usual locations. A small, slightly elevated, smooth-surfaced growth under the mucous membrane is characteristic of this lesion. Surgical excision of the lesion produces a cure.

PLASMACYTOMA. This extramedullary plasma cell tumor occurs most frequently in males. The usual sites of occurrence are the nasal cavity, nasopharynx, tonsil, pharynx, tongue, paranasal sinuses and larynx. There is no distinctive clinical feature for this tumor; it may be characterized by a diffuse or pedunculated swelling. Bone involvement (multiple myeloma) may not develop until years after the soft tissue tumor has been discovered, but this problem is so frequent that a bone survey should be made when a soft tissue tumor has been diagnosed. Local recurrence without development of multiple myeloma is not uncommon.

Surgical excision or electrocoagulation are usually adequate to eradicate the local lesions.

LEIOMYOMA. This rare tumor composed of smooth muscle cells can occur in the oral cavity. It is usually small and grows very slowly. Excision results in a cure in most patients.

BENIGN MIXED TUMORS. These tumors arise from accessory salivary glands or mucous glands in the oral cavity, palate, pharynx, nose or nasopharynx.[28] Males are more often affected than females, and these tumors are most common between the fourth and sixth decades of life. About half remain localized and grow quite slowly; the others may grow rapidly and require a major surgical resection. Small tumors can be locally exised, but these patients must be followed carefully for a long period of time because the tumor often exhibits a greater malignant potential than when it occurs in a major salivary gland.

Inflammatory Conditions

Oral infections are very common and most of them can be treated medically. Only those infections that require surgical therapy are included in this section.

PERIAPICAL ABSCESS. These abscesses develop suddenly and are associated with swelling, pain, redness of the overlying mucosa or skin, elevation of the tooth, sensitivity of the tooth on percussion and occasionally an elevated temperature. The tooth may appear normal or it may have a deep carious lesion. Duration and location of the abscess will determine where the abscess "points." When it points within the mouth, it may appear on either the buccal or lingual surfaces.

X-rays may reveal either no abnormalities or a radiolucent area about one or more teeth.

Treatment consists of surgical drainage and antibiotics. Extraction of the tooth or surgical incision will allow drainage of the pus and relief of pain. When the tooth has not been removed, dental consultation should be requested.

LUDWIG'S ANGINA (Fig. 11–63). Cellulitis of the floor of the mouth and neck due to an infection with a hemolytic streptococcus is a serious complication of acute pharyngitis or inflammation of the mouth. The patient is usually in great distress.

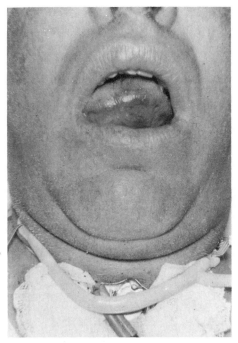

Figure 11–63. A sublingual abscess with an associated airway obstruction from glossal edema. A tracheostomy was required to correct the patient's distress.

Movements of the tongue cause severe pain and the patient often stops eating and drinking. Speaking and breathing may become almost impossible. Salivation is increased and the inability to swallow causes saliva to run freely from the mouth. The most striking clinical feature is a hard, brawny swelling between the chin and the neck. Bimanual palpation reveals that this swelling occupies the floor of the mouth and sublingual spaces. Fluctuation is rarely noted because the pus is located deep below the surface.

Intravenous antibiotics are indicated during the acute stage. When the condition does not respond to this treatment, incision and drainage must be considered. General anesthesia and oral-tracheal intubation are necessary (Fig. 11–64). A midline submental incision or sublingual oral incision will usually expose the abscess which should be opened widely with a blunt

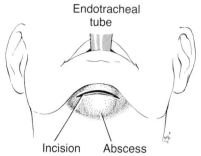

Figure 11–64 Ludwig's angina. A submental abscess should be incised, the pus evacuated, and a drain inserted. The incision is made beneath the mandible and a small hemostat is inserted into the abscess cavity and opened gently.

instrument. Rubber drains should be inserted and left in place until drainage ceases, the swelling has subsided and there is no danger of respiratory obstruction. Fever and toxemia usually subside after draining the abscess and the patient recovers quite rapidly. Cultures of the abscess will assist in the selection of appropriate antibiotics. Intravenous fluids should be continued until the patient can take adequate oral feedings, and antibiotics should be administered until the drains have been removed and the signs of inflammation have subsided. A total of ten days of antibiotic therapy is usually sufficient.

OROPHARYNX AND NASOPHARYNX

Most of the diseases occuring in this region can be diagnosed with simple techniques and inexpensive equipment. With a little practice and experience, a clinician can become quite adept at these procedures. A thorough systematic approach will help the examiner avoid costly mistakes. In general, it is best to begin with the lips and proceed backward, including the buccal-oral mucosal surfaces, teeth, tongue, floor of the mouth, tonsils, palate and pharynx. The nasopharynx, hypopharynx and larynx must also be in-

cluded. Materials necessary for the examination are a head mirror, tongue blades, and several hand mirrors for the nasopharynx and larynx.

Good light is essential for examining these areas and the best light source is a head mirror. First, place the mirror with its opening over the left eye and focus the beam of light on the patient's forehead. Movements of the mirror direct the light to the desired location and both hands remain free for manipulation. Inspect the lips, then have the patient open his mouth and examine all buccal and oral surfaces. Either a metal or disposable wooden tongue blade can be used for this purpose. I have found the large number 9 laryngeal mirror an effective "retractor" for exposing areas of the oral cavity that are ordinarily difficult to see. Do not forget to inspect the openings of the salivary ducts. Have the patient extend his tongue and carefully examine all of its surfaces as well as the gum margins and teeth. If active dental disease is suspected, a sharp tap on the questioned teeth will usually indicate which are involved. Movements of the palate should be symmetrical and an active gag reflex should occur when the base of the tongue, soft palate and pharynx are stimulated. Much of the pharynx can be seen by gently pulling the patient's tongue forward with a gauze pad. Instructing the patient to "relax" his tongue helps with this part of the examination. The nasopharynx, hypopharynx and larynx are examined after the inspection of the oropharynx. Mirrors of the proper size are required to reflect light into these areas.

Nasopharyngeal Examination

An indirect mirror technique is used for this examination (Fig. 11–65). A head mirror and lamp serve as the light sources. Gentleness and the patient's cooperation are essential for success.

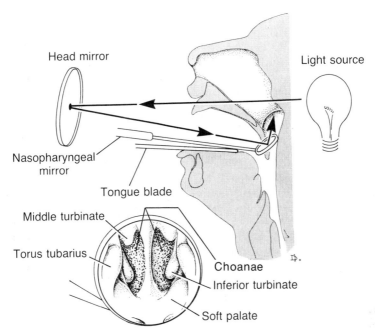

Figure 11-65 Nasopharyngeal examination.

A small mirror introduced through the mouth behind the palate gives a good view of the nasopharynx and posterior choanae of the nasal cavity. A tongue blade is introduced into the mouth and the tongue gently pushed downward. A warmed mirror is then slipped along the tongue blade behind the uvula and palate. Light can be reflected from the head mirror into the nasopharynx. Rotation of the mirror by moving the handle along its long axis gives a panoramic view of the nasopharynx.

When the palate interferes with examination, small catheters should be inserted through the nose into the pharynx, grasped and pulled forward to retract the palate. This allows better visualization of the nasopharynx with the mirror.

An electrically lighted nasopharyngoscope can be used when the other techniques fail; however, it should be used only by an examiner who is familiar with the instrument.

Tonsillectomy and Adenoidectomy

Tonsillectomy

Tonsillectomy, either alone or with adenoidectomy, is performed on outpatients in some hospitals and clinics.[27] However, this practice has not been adopted by all surgeons. There are many situations in which the operation can only be performed safely on a patient who has been admitted and subjected to a thorough investigation. Patients with heart diseases, pulmonary problems, coagulopathies, abscesses of the tonsils or peritonsillar tissues, renal diseases or any chronic debilitating illness should be hospitalized.

INDICATIONS. There is some difference of opinion regarding the indications for tonsillectomy. During the past decade or two, there has been a general trend toward conservatism in selecting patients for tonsillectomy.

Most agree that the operation is indicated in patients with a peritonsillar or intratonsillar abscess, enlarged tonsils that obstruct swallowing and breathing or a suspected malignant neoplasm of the tonsils. Chronic tonsillitis, a carrier state of streptococci and diphtheria, recurrent rheumatic fever, repeated upper respiratory infections, recurrent bronchitis and sinusitis, and cervical adenitis are less well accepted indications. Enlarged tonsils are not necessarily an indication for surgery, but an asymmetric enlargement may indicate a tumor. Unfortunately, there were too many deaths associated with this operation in which the indications for surgery were not well established.

There are several contraindications to surgery. Any patient who has an illness that increases the risk in using a general anesthetic should be carefully evaluated before surgery. In many instances, these patients can be treated quite adequately with medications. Patients with asthma, active respiratory infections, clotting disorders, immune deficiency states and chronic pulmonary, renal or cardiovascular disorders may respond better to medical than surgical treatment.[27]

A history, physical examination and laboratory studies are necessary before tonsillectomy. In most hospitals a CBC, urinalysis, chest x-ray and coagulation panel are required. If these tests reveal any significant abnormality, the operation should be postponed and the problem corrected before proceeding.

Either a general or a local anesthetic can be used. Local anesthesia should be used only in adults and patients who are emotionally stable and cooperative. If for any reason the local anesthetic fails, it is difficult to interrupt the operation, insert an endotracheal tube, administer a general anesthetic and complete the operation. The general rule is to use a general anesthetic unless there is a strong contraindication for its use and to reserve local anesthesia for carefully selected patients. The patient is placed on the operating table in the supine position for a general anesthetic and is seated upright for a local anesthetic.

There are two basic techniques for removing the tonsils. The dissection method is the most widely used and is the most effective (Fig. 11–66). The tonsil is grasped with a tenaculum and pulled toward the midline of the pharynx. An incision is made with a knife blade (No. 12) through the mucosa of the anterior tonsillar pillar. This incision is placed medial to the medial edge of the palatoglossus muscle. It must not extend into the capsule or tonsil. The capsule of the tonsil can then be identified by gently separating the mucosa and capsule with a Hurd dissector. After the capsule has been identified, the tenaculum should be reapplied, including both the capsule and tonsil in its grasp. This gives the surgeon a more secure control of the tonsil and allows more forceful traction. The capsule should remain intact

---

Figure 11–66 Tonsillectomy. *A.* Patient is in the Rose position. An oral retractor (Brown-Davis) gives an excellent view of the tonsils. *B.* An Allis clamp is applied to the tonsil and it is retracted medially. An incision is made through the mucous membrane of the anterior tonsillar pillar and the superior end of the tonsillar fossa. *C* and *D.* The mucosa of the anterior and posterior tonsillar pillars is incised with the tonsil knife. *E.* The Allis clamp is reapplied to include the superior pole of the tonsil, and the tonsil is dissected free of the fossa with either a curved scissors or a tonsil dissector. The tonsil is enucleated from the fossa by this method of dissection. *F.* A wire tonsil snare is placed over the tonsil and closed as the tonsil is pulled superiorly. The tonsil is then snared free and removed. Hemostasis is obtained by electrocoagulation or suture ligature of open blood vessels. A pack placed in the tonsillar fossa for a few minutes will reduce bleeding.

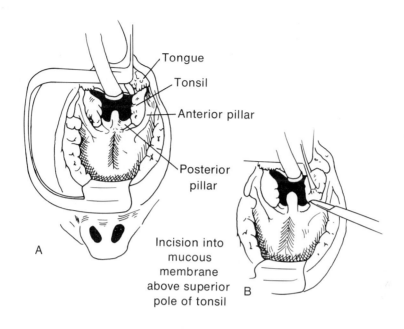

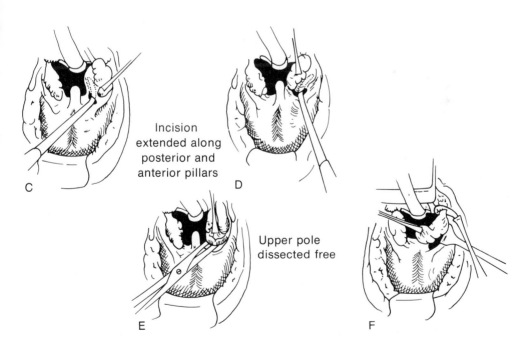

A — Tongue / Tonsil / Anterior pillar / Posterior pillar

Incision into mucous membrane above superior pole of tonsil

B

Incision extended along posterior and anterior pillars

Upper pole dissected free

Figure 11–66 *See legend on opposite page.*

and when the tonsil is freed from the fossa it can be cut or snared off at its base.

The guillotine technique is less precise than the dissection method, and there is a greater chance of leaving tissue behind. The lower pole and free portion of the tonsil are engaged in the opening of the guillotine instrument. The surgeon places an index finger on the anterior pillar to force the tonsil into the instrument. After the entire tonsil has been forced into the ring of the guillotine, the blade of the instrument is closed. This, in effect, avulses the tonsil from its attachments in the fossa.

Packs are inserted into the fossae after the tonsils have been removed. When the packs are removed any bleeding points are apparent and they must be controlled. Several techniques can be used. Suction coagulation is an effective method for controlling low pressure bleeding areas. Larger vessels that bleed briskly or that retract into the soft tissues of the fossa usually require a ligature. A free ligature of 4-0 chromic suture or a suture-ligature can be used. When bleeding is so severe that it cannot be controlled with these techniques, the anterior and posterior pillars can be stitched together. This is an effective method for controlling bleeding but should be used only as a last resort.

Bleeding is a difficult problem in some patients. The causes of bleeding are multiple and vary from failure to ligate all bleeding vessels to a rise in blood pressure, coughing, straining, anoxia or a bleeding diathesis. Patients who swallow large amounts of blood may vomit and aspirate. This can be a serious problem if not recognized and treated promptly. Obviously, prevention is preferred in this situation. Occasionally, submucosal bleeding may extend into the pharynx or larynx and obstruct the airway. Veins are less capable of retraction than arteries, especially when there is fibrosis of the capsule. A large clot will keep these vessels open and blood will ooze from beneath the clot. Copious blood may suddenly appear in the mouth when the clot breaks loose from the fossa. There is always the danger that the clot will enter the larynx and cause an airway obstruction.

Patients with a bleeding problem should be placed in a lateral position with the head hanging down. The airway must be protected at all times. The clot should be removed from the fossa with a suction tip. After the clot is out, a sponge, held firmly in the fossa for several minutes, may stop the bleeding. This may be all that is necessary to control the bleeding in some patients. Hydrogen peroxide or a weak solution of epinephrine (1:100,000 units) on the pack will often increase its effectiveness. These steps are especially important in children. If the pack is not effective, the offending vessel or vessels must be ligated. A general anesthetic may be necessary, and when there is any question of the airway status, an awake intubation is the preferred method. An intravenous solution of 5 per cent dextrose in lactated Ringer's solution should be started and maintained until all bleeding is controlled. Blood transfusions may be necessary in some patients. It is important to remember that the amount of bleeding may be misleading in small children or when the blood is being swallowed. These patients may suddenly exhibit the signs and symptoms of shock. Insertion of a gastric tube and removal of the blood from the stomach may be necessary. Occasionally, bronchoscopy is indicated, particularly when there is respiratory distress from aspirated blood or emesis.

Secondary bleeding is a complication that appears between the fifth and tenth day after surgery. Although it is much rarer than primary bleeding and usually less severe, it can be troublesome. It usually follows separation of the eschar from the fossa and a secondary infection of the fossa. Granulation tissue is exposed and this friable vascular tissue bleeds readily. The bleeding can usually be controlled with a pressure pack in the fossa, but when that technique fails more aggressive treatment is necessary. A local anesthetic can be obtained with an infiltration of Xylocaine containing epinephrine (1:100,000 units). This solution must not be injected directly into a major vessel. Cauterization is of considerable value in patients who have a superficial bleeding problem. If that fails, a suture ligature can be used. The tissues of the fossa are friable at this particular time, and they do not withstand trauma or manipulation very well. Bed rest, mild sedation, analgesics, antibiotics and reassurance are important in these patients. Patients who have more than a mild blood loss should be hospitalized.

Other complications of tonsillectomy include acute otitis media, cervical lymphadenitis, parapharyngeal abscess, septicemia, pneumonia, lung abscess, dental injuries, neck injuries and anesthetic complications. These problems, although less common than bleeding, must be detected promptly and treatment started early to avoid more serious problems.

Adenoidectomy

Adenoidectomy is indicated in patients with nasal obstruction and serous otitis media who have not responded to nasal decongestant therapy. Occasionally patients with chronic sinusitis or rhinitis will respond to adenoidectomy.

The usual symptoms of hypertrophied adenoids are nasal obstruction, mouth breathing, difficulty in eating, drooling, snoring and toneless (denasal) speech. Eustachian tube obstruction will produce deafness from retraction of the tympanic membrane and a middle ear effusion of fluid. Recurrent rhinitis, sinusitis, nasopharyngitis, cervical adenitis and pulmonary problems also have been attributed to adenoidal infections and hypertrophy.

Enlarged adenoids can be detected by an indirect mirror examination of the nasopharynx or palpation of the nasopharynx through the soft palate. Occasionally, direct palpation of the nasopharynx with a general anesthetic will be necessary. A lateral soft tissue x-ray examination of the nasopharynx will reveal the presence of enlarged adenoids. Xeroradiography is an excellent technique for this examination.

Before proceeding with adenoidectomy, it is important to determine whether or not a submucous cleft palate is present. When this abnormality is not detected and the adenoids are removed, a relative velopharyngeal insufficiency will ensue with a marked speech deformity (hypernasal) and regurgitation of fluids from the nose during feeding. These are distressing complications. A submucous cleft should be suspected when the posterior nasal spine cannot be felt and there is a bifid-appearing uvula.

Adenoidectomy can be performed on outpatients, either as an independent operation or in conjunction with tympanotomy and insertion of ventilating tubes into the middle ear. It is most often performed with tonsillectomy.

The preoperative evaluation should include a complete blood count, urinalysis, chest x-ray, and appropriate tests for any suspected coagulopathies. It is important to include in the history an accurate appraisal of the aspirin intake for two weeks preceding the operation. Aspirin used for pain or fever may have an adverse effect on blood clotting. If there is doubt about the patient's accuracy or veracity, the operation should be cancelled or a blood salicylate level obtained.

SURGICAL TECHNIQUE. A general endotracheal anesthetic is required for the operation. The endotracheal tube is inserted through the mouth and its cuff inflated to protect the lower airway. The patient is placed supine on the operating table. A slight Trendelenburg position is desirable to reduce the flow of blood and secretions into the hypopharynx. The pharynx can be packed with a slightly moistened gauze sponge that will absorb blood and secretions and protect the airway. Two techniques of adenoidectomy have been used. Both methods require exposure of the nasopharynx by retraction of the soft palate. This can be accomplished with a Love palate retractor. Two small (No. 8) rubber catheters are passed into the pharynx through the nose and used as retractors. These retractors also protect the palate during the operation. Either an adenotome or a curette can be used. The curette (Barnhill) is used to shave off the adenoids from the roof and posterior wall of the nasopharynx. The adenotome is shaped to the general configuration of the posterior wall and roof of the nasopharynx (Fig. 11–67). After the adenoids are engaged in the instrument, its sharp blade is closed over the mass upward from below. The adenoids must be removed completely. Any residual tissue will bleed and perhaps obstruct the eustachian tube or posterior nasal choanae.

Small bleeding points can be controlled with an electrocoagulation-suction unit. If the bleeding does not stop, a nasopharyngeal pack will be necessary. This pack is fashioned and inserted as described for epistaxis on page 400 and in Figure 11–34. An intravenous solution should be administered when the blood loss has been more than expected or the bleeding is difficult to control. The patient should never be taken from the operating room until all bleeding has been controlled. Patients who have bleeding that is excessive or difficult to control or who require a transfusion will require hospitalization. There will be moderate nasal congestion and drainage for a few days after surgery. The temperature should not be elevated unless there is a complication, such as an infection of the nose, nasopharynx, ears or sinuses. Atelectasis is another cause of fever in these patients. Antibiotics are used pre- and postoperatively by some surgeons. There is little evidence that the routine use of antibiotics materially affects the complications or results of surgery.

Bleeding is the most common complication of the operation. It can usually be prevented by following the procedures outlined above. In addition, sharp curettes and removal of all tags of adenoid tissue will prevent much of this problem.

Acute otitis media may follow adenoidectomy. Antibiotics, incision and drainage of the middle ear and analgesics are the methods of treatment for this problem.

Recurrence of the adenoid hypertrophy is not an uncommon occurrence. This can be minimized by a complete removal at the initial operation.

Trauma to the uvula, soft palate and eustachian tube orifices are all too common with adenoidectomy. Retropharyngeal abscess, cervical cellulitis,

Figure 11–67 Adenoidectomy. *A.* Patient is placed in the Rose position and the oral cavity and pharynx are exposed with an oral retractor (Brown-Davis). The relationship of the palate, adenoids and eustachian tube is illustrated. *B.* An adenotome is inserted into the nasopharynx in the closed position. It is often necessary to retract the palate before inserting the adenotome. *C.* Lateral view of the nasopharynx, adenoids and the adenotome. The adenotome is opened and pushed posteriorly to engage the adenoids. The blade is then closed. If too much pressure is used or the head is hyperextended, the fascia of the nasopharynx may be injured. *D.* Adenoid tissue that lies in the posterior superior nasopharynx is removed by inserting the index finger into the nasopharynx. This finger guides the tissue into a small adenotome that is then opened and closed. *E.* After retraction of the soft palate, the eustachian tube orifices can be seen and a ring punch can be used to remove any lymphoid tissue located in these areas.

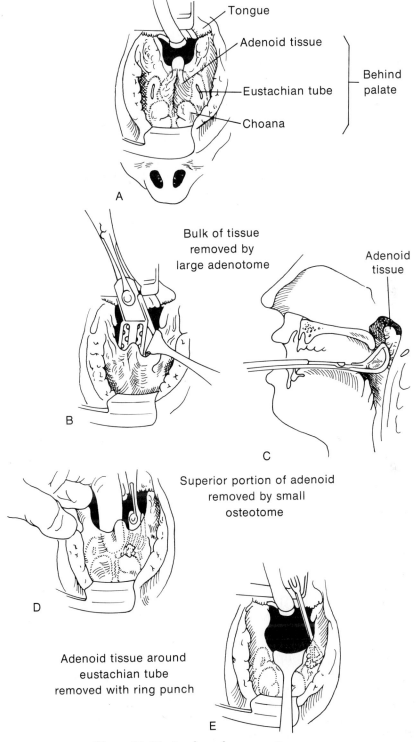

Figure 11–67 *See legend on opposite page.*

A

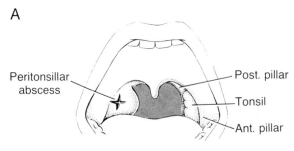

Peritonsillar abscess

Post. pillar

Tonsil

Ant. pillar

Figure 11–68 Peritonsillar abscess. The incision is made near the anterior pillar through the area of greatest fluctuance. Local anesthesia is usually quite adequate for this operation.

B

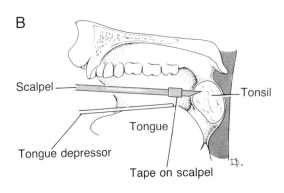

Scalpel

Tonsil

Tongue

Tongue depressor

Tape on scalpel

sinusitis and septicemia have also been reported.

Peritonsillar Abscess

Quinsy (peritonsillar abscess) (Fig. 11–68) usually arises during the third or fourth day after the onset of an acute follicular tonsillitis; occasionally there is no antecedent tonsillar infection. Most of the patients are adults; however, peritonsillar abscesses are more common in children than is generally recognized.

When there is a preceding acute tonsilitis, the patient reports that all his former symptoms are intensified. The pain becomes almost unbearable and radiates to the ear. Malaise, fever, dysphagia, indistinct speech, trismus, drooling of saliva and a foul breath are common symptoms. Examination reveals the whole chain of cervical lymph nodes to be enlarged and tender on the involved side. The soft palate and uvula are often edematous

and deviated to the opposite side. The affected tonsil may appear to be displaced backward and inward with an exudate or large necrotic ulcer on its surface. The surrounding mucosa is usually red and markedly thickened with edema. Fluctuation or softening can sometimes be detected with a probe or tongue blade. A yellow spot on the anterior pillar may indicate that the abscess is ready to rupture, but more often the abscess is too deep and its capsule too thick for this sign to be evident.

When the abscess has not ruptured spontaneously, it should be incised and drained. Antibiotics should be used, but they do not take the place of surgical therapy. If these patients are hospitalized and treated with intravenous fluids and antibiotics, most of them will be ready for discharge 24 to 48 hours after surgical treatment.

Good illumination is absolutely essential. The patient should be placed in an upright position with the head supported. General anesthesia may be quite hazardous because of the risk of aspirating pus into the trachea and it should be used with care. A surface anesthetic of cocaine HCl solution or 2 per cent lidocaine HCl is often sufficient. An incision should be made at the center of the most edematous portion of the anterior pillar after depressing the tongue as much as possible; a small clamp with sharp points is then thrust one-half to three-quarters of an inch into the chosen site. The blades of the clamp are opened widely to allow the pus to escape. A knife may be used for this procedure, but the blade should be covered with adhesive tape except for the terminal one-half inch. A gush of pus from the abscess indicates success. However, the first attempt occasionally fails when the incision enters the tonsil rather than the abscess, and another incision in a more lateral position is indicated. There is a dramatic relief of pain within a few hours after a successful incision.

Recurrent peritonsillar abscesses are common and in general it is advisable to perform a tonsillectomy four to six weeks after the infection has subsided.

Tonsillectomy for peritonsillar abscess has been advocated by some authors.[13] The operation removes the infected tonsils and also effectively drains the abscess. There is a greater risk of complications from the procedure and the anesthetic, and this procedure should probably be reserved for those patients with an impending pharyngomaxillary infection.

Retropharyngeal Abscess

Most of these infections (Fig. 11–69) occur during the first year of life. Infected adenoids or a nasopharyngitis are the usual sources of infection. Hemolytic and nonhemolytic streptococci or *Staphylococcus aureus* are often responsible for these abscesses.

A history of a preceding upper respiration infection in a child who refuses to take food, holds the neck stiffly and has a moderate elevation of temperature should alert the physician to the possibility of a retropharyngeal abscess. Slight swelling of the posterior pharyngeal wall a little to one side of the midline may be the only indication of this condition. As the abscess increases in size, the breathing becomes noisy, the cry muffled and a croupy cough develops. A lateral x-ray

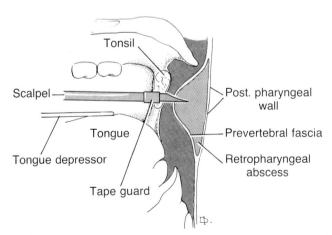

Figure 11–69 Retropharyngeal abscess, which may cause severe respiratory distress. A scalpel with a "tape guard" is used to incise the abscess. The guard prevents laceration of the prevertebral wall, and the incision is made vertically in the midline. If pus does not escape from the wound, a small pointed hemostat is inserted into the wound and the tissues spread apart.

of the neck will help in making the diagnosis, because widening of the retropharyngeal space is usually apparent. Palpation of the posterior pharyngeal wall may reveal fluctuation.

After applying restraints, the child's head should be lowered and a mouth gag inserted. A vertical incision is made over the point of maximum swelling. The procedure can be made much easier by the use of good illumination, suction and assistants who help hold the child. A sharply pointed clamp should be inserted into the abscess and opened. The opening must be made large enough to allow drainage and prevent a reaccumulation of pus. Good suction will prevent aspiration of the pus. Surgical treatment should be supplemented with antibiotic therapy. The patient usually recovers quite rapidly after treatment; however, severe dyspnea may ensue and tracheostomy may become essential.

Carcinoma

Malignant neoplasms should always be suspected whenever a mass or ulcerated lesion is detected in the pharynx or nasopharynx. A biopsy will usually assist in making the diagnosis; however, those tumors that arise in the nasopharynx are difficult to see and are often missed. These patients often have impaired hearing from obstruction of the eustachian tube and a secretory otitis media. They also may have pain over the distribution of the second division of the fifth cranial nerve and asymmetry of the palate.

Irradiation and surgery are usually required for these tumors and these procedures are beyond the scope of this text.

LARYNX

Indirect Laryngoscopy

A laryngeal mirror and head mirror are used for this examination (Fig. 11–

70). The most common light source is a standard lamp placed at the patient's left side. The examiner and patient sit facing each other, the patient sitting all the way back in his chair with his head and shoulders forward and his back straight. The patient should point his chin up, open his mouth and protrude the tongue. Either the examiner or patient should grasp the tongue with a piece of gauze and pull it out as far as possible without causing pain. Gentleness, patience and reassurance will make the examination much easier for both the examiner and the patient. A laryngeal mirror of the proper size, warmed so that it will not fog from the patient's breath, is passed into the pharynx without touching the tongue. If gagging occurs, the mirror should be withdrawn and the pharynx sprayed with a topical anesthetic such as Cetacaine. After the back of the mirror has been placed against the uvula and palate, it should be tilted slightly forward and the uvula and soft palate pushed backward. These maneuvers will allow visualization of the base of the tongue, the valleculae, the epiglottis and the larynx. Movements of the mirror will give a good view of all parts of the larynx. The patient should be asked to say "Eee" and this should bring the vocal cords into apposition in the midline. All parts of the larynx must be visualized or the examination is not complete. It must be remembered that the structures seen on the mirror are reversed in position.

Direct Laryngoscopy

Direct laryngoscopy (Fig. 11–71) is indicated in the following cases: in young children and in adults in whom the indirect examination is unsuccessful; for biopsy of lesions; for removal of foreign bodies; and for insertion of an oral endotracheal tube. Either general, local or topical anesthesia can be used. Preoperative sedation should be given one hour before the procedure is car-

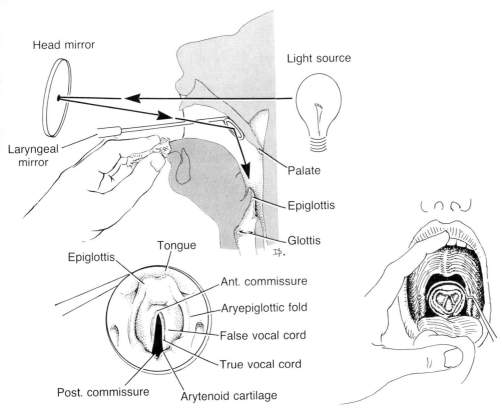

Figure 11–70 Indirect laryngoscopy. Indirect laryngoscopy can be mastered with the proper equipment, a little patience and practice. The patient's back should be straight, the body bent slightly forward at the waist. The mouth is opened wide and the tongue pulled forward with the fingers. A warmed mirror is then inserted into the oropharynx and directed downward. The base of the tongue, epiglottis, oropharynx, hypopharynx and larynx should be visualized. If the entire larynx is not seen the examination is not complete. This is particularly true of the anterior commissure, and a direct examination may be indicated.

ried out. A combination of a barbiturate (Nembutal), narcotic (morphine sulfate), and tranquilizer (Vistaril) will give good relaxation and sedation. Intravenous Innovar drip has been used successfully, but should never be used by an inexperienced physician. The examination should be conducted in a quiet darkened room. Relaxation and cooperation of the patient is very important and a calm, reassuring, unhurried and gentle approach by the examiner will facilitate the procedure.

The patient is placed on the operating table in the supine position with the head and shoulders extending beyond the end of the table. An assis-

tant sits on the right side of the patient, his right arm placed underneath the patient's neck with the right hand on the left side of the patient's face and his left hand placed on the occiput and vertex of the patient's head. This technique stabilizes the patient's head and allows controlled movement of the head into the various positions necessary for the examination. By extending the head, the mouth, pharynx, larynx and trachea are brought into a straight line that facilitates insertion of the laryngoscope. Either a battery-powered or fiberoptic light source can be used and the light should be checked before inserting the laryngo-

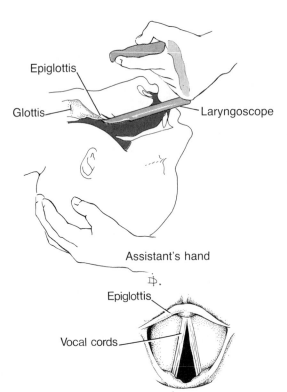

Epiglottis

Glottis — Laryngoscope

Assistant's hand

Epiglottis

Vocal cords

Figure 11-71 Direct laryngoscopy. Topical anesthesia or a superior laryngeal nerve-block is usually adequate for this procedure. The laryngoscope is inserted on one side of the mouth and directed to the base of the tongue. The tongue is retracted upward without exerting any pressure on the incisor teeth. The base of the tongue and epiglottis should be carefully inspected before inserting the laryngoscope into the larynx. The laryngoscope is then brought gently onto the midline of the tongue and the tip of the epiglottis. The posterior commissure, arytenoids, aryepiglottic folds, pyriform sinuses and hypopharynx are visualized. With extension of the head, the tip of the laryngoscope is advanced toward the base of the epiglottis. When the epiglottis is elevated, the entire glottis will be seen. A methodical, unhurried and relaxed approach to this procedure will make it much more comfortable for the patient and more rewarding for the examiner.

scope. Insert the laryngoscope under direct vision over the dorsum of the tongue, placing a finger between the barrel of the laryngoscope and the patient's teeth to avoid an injury to the teeth or lips. The tip of the laryngoscope should be placed beneath the edge of the epiglottis and the entire scope lifted forward. Do not tilt the laryngoscope on the teeth. Advance the laryngoscope forward beneath the epiglottis until the larynx is in view. If the larynx is not completely anesthetized it will be in spasm. A 10 per cent cocaine solution introduced through the scope as a spray or on a swab will reduce the spasm. After carefully inspecting all parts of the larynx, slowly withdraw the laryngoscope under direct vision. A biopsy should be performed on any suspicious lesions. Failure to visualize all areas of the larynx, hypopharynx or base of the tongue can lead to serious mistakes in diagnosis.

Vocal Cord Paralysis

Paralysis of the vocal cords is caused by an injury to one of the laryngeal nerves along its route from the nucleus ambiguous to the intrinsic muscles of the larynx. The inferior laryngeal (recurrent) nerves have a different course on the two sides of the neck, and this anatomic difference is important in the etiologic possibilities of the paralysis. On the left, the nerve curves around the arch of the aorta, and on the right it curves around the subclavian artery. In a small number of individuals (0.3 per cent) the right nerve does not reach the subclavian artery but enters the larynx directly from the vagus nerve. The nerves lie in a groove between the trachea and esophagus. They pass upward behind the thyroid ala and the cricothyroid joint. There are two branches (motor and sensory) which then enter the larynx. All the intrinsic muscles of the larynx are supplied by the motor branch. None of the fibers cross the midline, and there is no differentiation between the fibers that supply the adductors and those that supply the abductors. The sensory branch supplies the area beneath the vocal cords and a small loop of this nerve (Galen's) connects with the sensory branch from the superior laryngeal nerve.

Several important etiologies must be included in the differential diagnosis of these problems. Thyroid surgery is a relatively common cause of vocal cord paralysis. Paralysis of one or both vocal cords has been reported in from 0.3 to 9.4 per cent of thyroid operations.[23] The relationship of the inferior (recurrent) laryngeal nerve to the inferior thyroid artery is the most important factor in the development of paralysis from thyroid surgery. The nerve is deep to the artery in 46 per cent of patients, superficial to the artery in 10 per cent and passes between branches of the artery in 35 percent. Dissection about the artery and clamps or ligatures on the inferior thyroid artery may injure the nerve.

Cardiovascular surgery in the area of the right subclavian artery, the ductus arteriosus or the left aortic arch have a high incidence of vocal cord paralysis.

The anterior surgical approach to a cervical disk or cervical vertebrae is associated with an 11 per cent incidence of injury to the inferior (recurrent) laryngeal nerve.

Neoplasms of the thyroid gland, parathyroid glands, cervical esophagus and left upper lung are associated with vocal cord paralysis. Vocal cord paralysis has been reported in patients who have a toxic manifestation from vinblastine therapy for malignant diseases.

A viral etiology has been suggested as a cause of vocal cord paralysis. This occurs with epidemics of influenza.

Hydrocephalus and meningomyelocele may produce a bilateral vocal cord paralysis with severe stridor and respiratory obstruction. This is thought to arise from compression of the nucleus ambiguous in the medulla.

Laryngeal trauma, particularly when there is displacement of the skeleton of the thyroid and cricoid cartilages, can produce a vocal cord paralysis that is either temporary or permanent. This depends upon whether or not the nerves are contused, stretched or lacerated.

Tracheal intubation during general anesthesia has produced a vocal cord paralysis. This is thought to arise from stretching of the inferior (recurrent) nerve. There is usually spontaneous recovery of vocal cord function.

Idiopathic paralysis should be the diagnosis only after a thorough search has been made for another cause. Approximately 50 per cent of these will recede. The earliest recoveries occur within two months, and there is little chance of recovery after nine months.

CLINICAL FEATURES. Three symptoms are produced from vocal cord paralysis; laryngeal obstruction (bilateral paralysis), aspiration of liquids from glottic incompetence and voice changes are the usual complaints. There are more or less specific clinical findings for each specific vocal cord paralysis.

Unilateral inferior (recurrent) nerve paralysis is the most common. The only muscle functioning is the cricothyroid that is supplied by the superior laryngeal nerve. The vocal cord is immobile and positioned near the midline. The opposite cord can approximate the paralyzed one during phonation, and there is an adequate voice and airway (Fig. 11–72A).

A unilateral inferior (recurrent) and superior nerve paralysis produces a vocal cord that lies in a neutral position 3 to 5 mm lateral to the midline. The opposite cord may be unable to approximate the paralyzed vocal cord. These patients have a very weak voice, and they aspirate during swallowing of liquids (Fig. 11–72B).

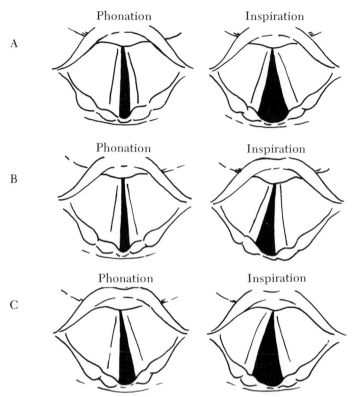

Figure 11-72 Vocal cord positions during phonation and inspiration. *A.* A unilateral inferior (recurrent) laryngeal nerve paralysis. *B.* A unilateral superior laryngeal nerve paralysis. *C.* A unilateral superior laryngeal and inferior (recurrent) laryngeal nerve paralysis. (Adapted from: Weaver, M.: Neurologic disorders of the larynx. *In* English, G. M. [ed.]: Otolaryngology, A Textbook. Hagerstown, Harper & Row, 1976, Chapter 51.)

A unilateral superior nerve paralysis produces a loss of function of the cricothyroid muscle, which is a tensor and adductor of the vocal cord. The other intrinsic muscles are functioning, and there is very little difficulty with respiration, vocalization or swallowing. This type of paralysis is usually not diagnosed (Fig. 11-72C).

A bilateral inferior (recurrent) nerve paralysis causes a decrease in the glottic airway, because the only functioning intrinsic muscle is the cricothyroid that adducts the cords into the midline. These patients may have a good voice if air can reach the lower airway through a tracheostomy.

A bilateral inferior (recurrent) and superior nerve paralysis cause the vocal cords to assume a position lateral to the midline. These patients have a good airway but a very poor voice and a marked tendency to aspirate during swallowing.

The most important step in the diagnosis of a vocal cord paralysis is indirect laryngoscopy. This technique gives more information regarding laryngeal function than any other procedure. A topical anesthetic (Cetacaine) and intravenous diazepam (Valium) may facilitate the examination. The vocal cord involved and its position are of great importance. Direct laryngoscopy is necessary when an intralaryngeal disorder or disease is a diagnostic possibility. A general or local anesthetic can be used, depending upon the patient and the particular problems involved. A biopsy of any suspicious lesion should be made at that time. A laryngogram might be useful in some patients. An air contrast or a radiopaque examination can be used. The x-ray serves as a permanent record of the disease and may demonstrate unsuspected lesions, particularly in the subglottic area. It is important to include inspiration, expiration and vocalization as parts of the examination.

TREATMENT. There are different objectives for different varieties of vocal cord paralysis. When there is a disease (carcinoma) that affects the vocal cord, the treatment is directed toward eradication of that disease. When there is a unilateral inferior (recurrent) nerve paralysis with the cord near the midline and an adequate voice and airway, treatment is probably unnecessary. When there is a bilateral inferior (recurrent) nerve paralysis with the cords adducted in the midline and associated stridor, a tracheostomy may be necessary to sustain the airway.

Several specific modalities of treatment are available. Many of these are not procedures that can be performed on outpatients. These include nerve repairs, arytenoidectomy, cricothyroid arthrodesis and transplantation of a nerve-muscle pedicle. Tracheostomy for airway obstruction may be required, and this operation can be performed on outpatients. A Teflon injection can be used for an incompetent larynx when the vocal cord is in the lateral position, as in unilateral superior and inferior (recurrent) nerve paralysis. These patients have a poor voice and they aspirate fluids. Teflon granules, 50 μ in diameter, suspended in glycerine, are injected into the soft tissues of the paralyzed vocal cord with a high pressure (Bruening) syringe. This increases the mass of the vocal cord and allows the opposite cord to approximate with it during vocalization and swallowing. The injected paralyzed vocal cord is permanently immobilized and should remain permanently fixed. This improves laryngeal func-

tion.[4] Some of these patients have respiratory distress after the injection, and they must be observed for several hours after the procedure.

Other Laryngeal Disorders

A wide variety of laryngeal problems can simulate vocal cord paralysis. Laryngospasm is not rare after endotracheal intubation, particularly in children. It may occur as a spontaneous problem and must be distinguished from croup in children and from angioneurotic edema in adults. Breath-holding and aspiration of foreign materials can also cause laryngospasm in children. Some children occasionally awaken from sleep with laryngeal spasm. No treatment is required.

Hysterical aphonia, spastic dysphonia, myasthenia gravis, muscular dystrophy and amyotrophic lateral sclerosis can simulate vocal cord paralysis. An indirect laryngeal examination of these patients will demonstrate that the vocal cords are not paralyzed.[31]

Larynx Fractures

The most common cause of a laryngeal fracture is blunt trauma to the neck from automobile accidents.[29] Quite often, multiple injuries result from such accidents and the laryngeal injury may be overlooked. The patient who has an airway problem may undergo a tracheostomy and no further thought is given to the possibility of a laryngeal injury until decannulation is attempted. By this time, it may be too late for a definitive repair. The patient will have to accept either poor laryngeal function or further corrective surgery. A laryngeal injury should be suspected in any patient who needs a tracheostomy or who has a history of neck trauma.

The symptoms most often produced by a laryngeal injury are increasing airway obstruction with dyspnea and stridor, dysphonia or aphonia, cough, hemoptysis or hematemesis, neck pain, and dysphagia or odynophagia. The clinical signs of an injury involving the upper airway are deformities of the neck (including swelling), subcutaneous emphysema, laryngeal tenderness and crepitus of the thyroid and cricoid cartilage or hyoid bone. X-rays of the neck and chest must be obtained to detect laryngeal fractures, tracheal injuries or pneumothorax.

A diagnosis of fractured larynx should be made as early as possible. Indirect and direct laryngoscopy are essential in any patient in whom laryngeal injury is suspected. An endotracheal tube must be inserted with great care because it may be misplaced through a fracture site into the neck and completely obstruct the airway. A careful tracheostomy placed below the second tracheal ring is a much better way to insure a competent airway. If a cricothyrotomy has been done, it should be replaced with a tracheostomy as soon as the patient's condition permits. Laryngeal fractures should be reduced and immobilized as soon as the patient's condition has stabilized. Chronic stenosis can be avoided if reduction and fixation are carried out

within seven to ten days. The various types of injuries to the larynx and cervical trachea and the methods of treatment of these injuries are presented in Table 11–5. These procedures should not be performed on outpatients by surgeons unfamiliar with the principles and techniques of laryngeal surgery.

Tracheostomy

Obstruction of the airway is one of the most common medical emergencies. Any available physician should be able to act quickly and expertly to prevent a death or the complications that may occur when a tracheostomy is needed. Bronchoscopy, oral-tracheal intubation, laryngotomy, and tracheostomy are the four techniques that can be used to establish an airway, and the indications for each technique depend upon the circumstances in which the emergency is encountered.

Bronchoscopy and oral-tracheal intubation require special skills and equipment, but either technique will alleviate the immediate problem and allow the physician to perform a tracheostomy under more favorable circumstances. The techniques for these

TABLE 11–5   Classification and Treatment of Trauma to the Larynx and Cervical Trachea

CLASSIFICATION	TREATMENT
Hematoma, edema or small mucosal lacerations	Voice rest, moist air, steroids and tracheostomy for airway obstruction
Extensive lacerations, exposed cartilage with the skeleton intact or easily repairable. No loss of mucosa	Above . . . Open repair of the lacerations. Silastic keel for injuries to the anterior vocal cords. Stents not necessary
Above . . . Loss of skeletal support. Extensive loss of mucosa	Above . . . Mucosal replacement with grafts. Stents
Tracheal-laryngeal separation or severed trachea	End to end anastamosis. Tracheostomy
Injuries in small children	Open reduction for displaced skeleton. Short term stents and dilation
Late cicatricial stenosis	Open exploration, excision of scar tissue, mucosal grafts and stents

(Adapted from Templer, J. W.: Trauma to the larynx and cervical trachea. *In* G. M. English (Ed.): Otolaryngology — A Textbook. Hagerstown, Harper & Row, 1976, p. 558.)

two procedures are presented in Chapters 16 and 26. When these methods are not possible, a tracheostomy or laryngotomy may be required as the initial method of therapy, and a knowledge of these surgical techniques is essential.

Although most of the diseases causing airway obstruction are reversible with appropriate therapy, the airway must be established first. The physician's attention should not deviate from the primary goal of a patent airway that will sustain life. Several broad categories of diseases causing upper airway obstruction are presented in Table 11–6. Because the glottic aperture of the larynx is the narrowest part of the upper airway, many diseases in this area cause some degree of respiratory distress.

The diagnosis of airway obstruction is usually apparent. Inspiratory dyspnea and stridor result from air passing through the narrowed airway. Retractions of the suprasternal notch, epigastrium, supraclavicular areas and intercostal spaces arise from the increased effort needed to pull air through the restricted airway. Such retractions serve as cardinal signs of airway obstruction and are not usually associated with cardiac or pulmonary diseases. Hoarseness or a "croupy" cough may be present. The respiratory and cardiac rates will be increased, and restlessness, apprehension and uncooperative behavior are common. Cyanosis occurs rather late and unless the airway is improved, unconsciousness and respiratory-cardiac failure will develop. This may indicate a terminal situation.

LARYNGOTOMY. Superior tracheostomy or coniotomy (Fig. 11–73) is a very useful technique for severe obstruction of the airway. Hemenway[15] has enumerated the advantages of this technique. No special training or equipment is required and the procedure can be performed almost anywhere. An adequate airway can be established in a few seconds with this innocuous procedure at any time the patient's condition indicates an obstruction.

SURGICAL TECHNIQUE. When the patient's condition is deteriorating rapidly, no anesthesia, skin preparation or draping is necessary. Otherwise a small amount of local anesthesia (lidocaine HC1) can be injected, the skin cleansed with alcohol and a few drapes applied around the neck. The face should not be covered because the surgeon must constantly observe it for signs of deterioration during the operation. After the space between the cricoid and thyroid cartilages is identified, the neck is extended. The neck is not extended until the surgeon is ready to make his incision, because extension of the neck may cut off the only remaining airway. A vertical skin incision is made over the cricothyroid membrane if time permits and a knife is available, but this incision is not always necessary. Any sharp object (knife, nail file, screwdriver or piece of glass) is forcefully inserted between the thyroid and cricoid cartilages into the larynx. The instrument is then turned 90 degrees to hold the incision open. This hole is well below the vocal cords and is usually below most obstructive lesions. The instruments may be left in place or replaced with a rigid tube if one is available. A permanent airway, usually by tracheostomy, should be established as soon as possible, but can be deferred until the proper facilities are available. Some bleeding will be encountered but this is usually not excessive and will not endanger the patient's life. Injuries to the cricoid cartilage and subsequent laryngeal stenosis have been overemphasized. Hemenway[15] emphasizes that large cricoid lacerations heal well with antibiotic treatment.

Tracheostomy is the procedure of choice when time and adequate facilities are available. Success depends upon a reasonable degree of surgical skill, a knowledge of neck anatomy, adequate surgical instruments, competent assistants and good light and suc-

TABLE 11–6 Differential Diagnosis of Airway Obstruction

I. CONGENITAL ANOMALIES
  A. Glossoptosis—Pierre Robin syndrome
  B. Laryngotracheomalacia
  C. Laryngocele
  D. Laryngoesophageal clefts

II. INFLAMMATIONS
  A. Laryngotracheobronchitis
  B. Epiglottitis
  C. Parapharyngeal abscesses
  D. Angioneurotic edema

III. TRAUMA
  A. Fractures
    1. Facial
    2. Laryngeal
    3. Cervical
    4. Chest
  B. Hematoma
    1. Oral
    2. Pharyngeal
    3. Laryngeal
    4. Cervical
  C. Burns
    1. Ingestion of caustics
    2. Inhalation of fumes, chemicals, smoke, steam.
  D. Postoperative
    1. Endoscopic injury
    2. Intubation injury
    3. Abdominal surgery
  E. Postirradiation
    1. Perichondritis
  F. Nasogastric intubation
  G. Foreign bodies

IV. NEOPLASMS
  A. Oral
  B. Pharyngeal
  C. Laryngeal
  D. Thyroid
  E. Cervical

V. NEUROLOGIC
  A. Cerebrovascular accidents
  B. CNS depressants
    1. Barbiturates
  C. Skull trauma
    1. Hematoma
    2. Fractures
  D. Arnold-Chiari malformation
  E. Myasthenia gravis
  F. Eclampsia
  G. Cervical cord tumors and injuries

VI. MISCELLANEOUS
  A. Laryngospasm
  B. Cricoarytenoid arthritis

A

B

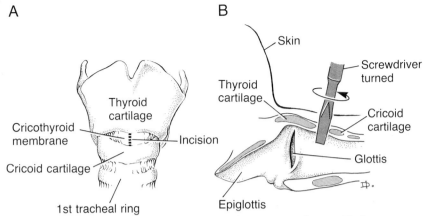

1st tracheal ring

Figure 11–73 Coniotomy. Coniotomy or cricothyroidotomy is used to establish an airway quickly when a tracheostomy is not possible. The cricothyroid membrane is located by palpating the thyroid and cricoid cartilages. A sharp object is then guided between these two structures to perforate the membrane into the upper trachea. This simple procedure will provide an adequate airway until tracheostomy can be performed.

tion. Whenever possible the procedure should be performed in the operating room. Insertion of an oral-tracheal tube or bronchoscope will usually alleviate the airway obstruction and create more favorable conditions for the operation (Fig. 11–74). Quite often, it is necessary to perform a tracheostomy on the ward or in the Emergency Room, and under these circumstances the surgeon should be very careful that the necessary equipment and assistants are available to prevent a serious complication or disaster.

TRACHEOSTOMY: SURGICAL TECHNIQUE (Fig. 11–75). Oxygen should be administered if available and sedatives or premedications should *not* be given to the patient. A few words of explanation and reassurance will often relieve the patient's apprehension and increase his cooperation during the operation. Even small children become more cooperative because they seem to realize how desperately ill they are.

The skin of the neck is painted with a suitable antiseptic and the area draped with sterile towels. The face must be left uncovered so that the patient's condition can be constantly observed throughout the procedure. If a

respiratory crisis develops before the tracheostomy is completed, a laryngotomy should be performed immediately and the tracheostomy completed when the patient's condition improves.

General anesthesia should not be

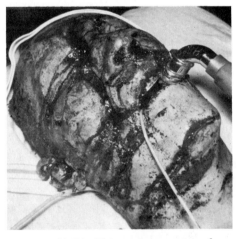

Figure 11–74 This patient sustained extensive facial and head injuries from an automobile accident. The airway became obstructed shortly after he arrived in the emergency room. An endotracheal tube was inserted to re-establish the airway and a tracheostomy was performed later in the operating room under more advantageous circumstances.

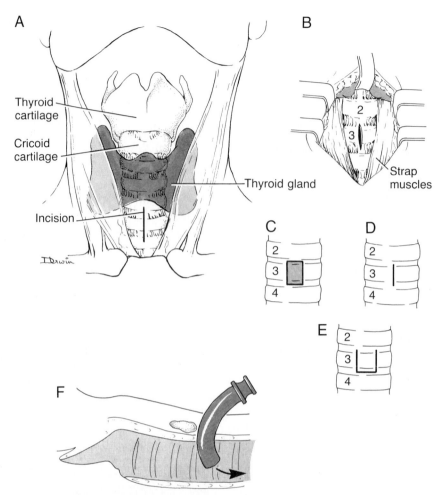

Figure 11–75   Tracheostomy. A vertical incision is made in the midline between the sternomastoid muscles (*A*). The "strap" muscles are separated and the thyroid gland elevated and retracted superiorly (*B*). The tracheal rings must be identified and an incision is made through the third tracheal ring. Several different tracheal incisions can be made (*C, D* and *E*) and a tracheostomy tube inserted (*F*).

administered unless an endotracheal tube or bronchoscope is in place. Local anesthesia is adequate when injected subcutaneously between the suprasternal notch and the lower border of the thyroid cartilage. Anesthesia is not necessary in patients with advanced stages of asphyxia.

Both the transverse and vertical midline incisions have been used in the past. The transverse incision has been recommended as the better tracheostomy incision for cosmetic reasons. However, when tracheostomy is an emergency procedure and is being done under less than ideal circumstances, the vertical midline incision is best. There will be less bleeding from this incision, and coughing and swallowing will produce less shearing force on the tube with resulting extubation. If desired, a vertical scar can be revised later with a Z-plasty. The vertical midline incision should extend from the inferior border of the cricoid cartilage to just above the suprasternal notch. All dissection must be kept strictly in the midline. The skin edges should be retracted and the incision deepened until the isthmus of the thyroid gland is exposed. Sometimes the isthmus may be retracted upward or downward by cutting the fibrous connective tissue between the gland and the trachea — Cooper's ligament. When the isthmus cannot be retracted sufficiently, it must be cut between clamps and each side of the incised gland then must be ligated with a silk suture. These techniques result in good exposure of the trachea. *Lateral dissection must be avoided.* Tracheal rings are easily identified by palpation; however, in infants and small children the trachea is small, soft and difficult to recognize. In this case, the soft tissues are dissected from the upper tracheal rings.

A tracheal hook is helpful at this stage of the operation. This instrument should be used to stabilize the trachea and pull it more superficially for better exposure. An incision into the trachea is then made with a No. 11 Bard-Parker blade at least one tracheal ring below the cricoid cartilage and above the fifth tracheal ring. Large 1–0 or 1 silk sutures can be placed on each side of the tracheal cartilage selected for incision. These sutures make good tracheal retractors during incision and insertion of the tube. They should be left in place and taped to the chest for the first 72 hours after surgery or until a tract between the trachea and skin has developed. If the tube should be coughed out or accidentally misplaced, these sutures can be used to pull the trachea up into the wound and guide the tube back into the trachea. The patient usually coughs when the trachea is incised and the surgeon must not allow the knife blade to penetrate the posterior tracheal wall and enter the esophagus. A cruciate incision may be made or a small piece of tracheal cartilage removed to facilitate insertion of the tracheostomy tube. A Trousseau dilator or hemostat may be used to hold the incision open while the tube is inserted. A tracheostomy tube of appropriate size should be selected and carefully checked for any

defects before it is inserted. The tube must be held securely in place with a finger until a tape is well tied about the neck. This will prevent the patient from coughing the tube out of the trachea. Hemostasis can be obtained during the procedure if time permits; however, bleeding vessels can be clamped and tied after the tube is in place. When there are more pressing circumstances many of the preceding steps may be omitted if absolutely necessary, but serious complications are more common when the operation is done too quickly.

The wound should never be sutured tightly about the tracheostomy tube, because a tight closure will predispose the patient to develop subcutaneous emphysema. Two or three 4–0 silk sutures can be used to approximate the lateral portion of the skin edges. However, one-half or two-thirds of the wound should be left open. A four-by-four gauze pad dressing should be placed beneath the flanges of the tube over the wound to collect secretions.

The postoperative management of a patient with a tracheostomy is very important. Careful, continuous observation is mandatory and special nurses may be necessary. Antibiotics should be given because an open wound often becomes infected and the operation may have been performed without sterile techniques. The tube should be checked repeatedly to be certain that it remains in the trachea. An extra tube of the same size should be taped to the patient's bed as an available replacement for a dislodged or obstructed tube. If it cannot be reinserted immediately another tracheostomy set should be obtained, the wound opened quickly and the tube reinserted. The outer tube should not be changed for three to five days. During this time granulation tissue will form about the tube, creating a fistula that makes reintroduction of a tube relatively easy. The inner cannula should be removed and cleaned as often as necessary.

Frequent suctioning is very important to keep the tube and tracheobronchial tree free of secretions. Secretions may accumulate that obstruct the airway or dry out to form crusts. This problem may cause or aggravate existing pulmonary difficulties. A sterile suction catheter of suitable size with a finger control should be inserted into the lower trachea. This usually stimulates coughing, and as the catheter is withdrawn the finger control is occluded. This technique will effectively remove secretions and cause a minimal amount of distress for the patient.

Humidification of the patient's room will help keep tracheal secretions thin and reduce crusting. Oxygen may be needed if the patient's pulmonary function is impaired.

A simple explanation of the procedure and a little reassurance will help reduce many of the patient's anxieties. The patient should be told that he can talk by occluding the tube with a finger and that help is available when needed.

There are several special problems associated with airway obstruction in infants and children. Congenital anomalies, certain inflammatory conditions and foreign bodies are common in these patients. Holinger and Johnson[17] have discussed the significance of the small glottic aperture in infants. They emphasize that 1.0 mm of mucosal swelling can reduce the infant's glottic airway by 65 per cent! Perhaps the best way to handle an airway problem in an infant or small child is to insert a bronchoscope into the trachea. This relieves the immediate problem and allows a tracheostomy to be performed in a more routine manner. Also, some infants are too weak to withstand tracheostomy as a primary operation and these patients should have their anoxia corrected before any operative procedure is attempted. The rigid bronchoscope makes the trachea much easier to identify and reduces some of the risks of surgery. Postoperative care must be carried out more carefully than with adults because tubes are often dislodged and the child is helpless when such difficulties occur. In addition, the small lumen of the tracheostomy tube is easily occluded with crusts and secretions.

COMPLICATIONS. Tracheostomy is not an innocuous operation.[6, 14] Many complications have been reported and these are generally classified as occurring during the procedure, during the postoperative period or later during convalescence. The patient may suddenly deteriorate before the airway is established. This situation must be recognized and an immediate laryngotomy performed. Many of these patients can be revived and the tracheostomy completed after resuscitation. Severe bleeding may occur from engorged neck veins, the thyroid isthmus, an anomalous vessel (thyroid ima) or a high innominate vein. Careful dissection in the midline will help the surgeon avoid the carotid sheath and vessels. Laceration of an innominate vein can lead to death from an air embolus. Improper positioning of the tube outside the trachea will increase the patient's respiratory distress. An incision into the posterior wall of the trachea and esophagus can lead to mediastinitis and a tracheoesophageal fistula. Sudden cardiac arrest or respiratory failure must be treated with immediate resuscitation measures. A rapid reduction of blood carbon dioxide levels may produce apnea. This problem can be reversed by artificial respiration until the carbon dioxide and oxygen levels are adjusted. Pneumothorax is not uncommon, especially in children, and results from cutting the dome of the pleura or from interstitial emphysema. Infections of the wound, neck, and mediastinum will usually respond to appropriate antibiotic therapy and good postoperative care. Expulsion of the tube from coughing or improper handling should be promptly recognized and managed. Pulmonary atelectasis can be prevented by frequent suctioning, and the crusting of blood or mucus reduced by adequate humidification, hydration of the patient and cleansing of the inner tube.

Tumors

Papillomas, chondromas, myomas, myxomas, chemodectomas, neurofibromas and angiomas are the usual benign neoplasms that occur in the larynx. These tumors usually produce hoarseness if they occur on the vocal cords; however, the patient may remain asymptomatic until the tumor becomes large enough to cause dyspnea or swallowing difficulties. The diagnosis can often be made by an indirect mirror examination of the larynx. The tissue type of the tumor can be determined only by a biopsy. These patients should be treated by a laryngologist.

Most malignant neoplasms of the larynx are squamous cell carcinomas. These tumors are curable when detected early and treated aggressively. Hoarseness, airway obstruction, sore throat, difficulties with swallowing or referred otalgia are the symptoms produced by these tumors. The diagnosis usually can be made by mirror examination of the larynx plus direct examination and biopsy. Treatment varies from irradiation therapy to surgical excision of the tumor or a combination of these two methods of treatment. There are several surgical procedures that are used for these tumors. In many instances a conservative operation can be used that will preserve the functions of the larynx. These operations should be performed only by a surgeon familiar with the techniques and problems these procedures entail.

ESOPHAGOSCOPY

The patient who is to have esophagoscopy should have an empty stomach. Preoperative sedation should be given at least one hour before esophagoscopy. For the average adult, a narcotic (morphine SO_4, 10 mg), atropine (0.4 mg) and a barbiturate (Nembutal 100 mg) are satisfactory. General or topical anesthesia can be used. Cocaine HCl (10 per cent solution) or tetracaine (2 per cent solution of Pentocaine) should be administered 5 to 10 minutes before inserting the esophagoscope. The patient's position is the same as that described for laryngoscopy. The assistant should elevate and extend the head at the beginning of the procedure. The esophagoscope should be held with the right hand. The upper lip is retracted with the third and fourth fingers of the left hand while the tube is stabilized with the thumb and index fingers of the same hand. The esophagoscope is passed over the tongue into the oropharynx under direct vision. The tip is pushed along the right pharyngeal wall behind the right arytenoid cartilage into the right piriform sinus. At the bottom of the piriform sinus the instrument comes to a full stop. The cricopharyngeus muscle usually remains closed and opens only with swallowing. By raising the tip of the esophagoscope anteriorly with the left thumb and pointing it at the suprasternal notch, a small lumen will appear. If the patient is asked to swallow, sometimes a small opening will be revealed through which the esophagoscope can be inserted. The danger of perforation is greatest at this point and great care must be exercised to avoid this complication. A small flexible lumen (Fig. 11–76) finder gently passed through the esophagoscope will often elicit a swallow reflex and facilitate descent into the esophagus. This instrument also serves as a valuable guide for inserting the esophagoscope. A nasogastric tube swallowed by the patient before anesthesia is induced will also provide a useful guide for the endoscopist. Once the lumen appears, the esophagoscope can be easily inserted into the upper esophagus. Patient cooperation and re-

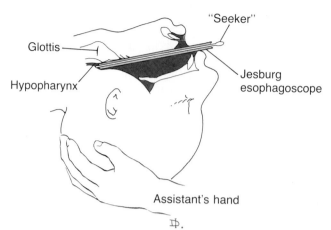

Figure 11–76 Esophagoscopy. Esophagoscopy is performed with the patient in the supine position, using either local or general anesthesia. The technique is relatively simple, but should be learned by performance under the guidance of an experienced surgeon.

laxation are extremely important and will make the procedure much easier and less dangerous. After the esophagoscope reaches the upper esophagus, the patient's head is lowered so that the lumen is in view and does not disappear. The esophagoscope is passed into the thoracic esophagus and the head is moved slightly to the right. The esophagoscope is aimed at the patient's left anterior iliac spine as the surgeon looks for the hiatal opening. A small slit in an oblique line between 4 and 10 o'clock or a small rosette indicates the opening. The lumen finder may be used to identify the esophageal hiatus and a moderate amount of pressure with the end of the tube will allow passage of the esophagoscope into the stomach. A change in the color of the mucosa, a gush of gastric fluid and the appearance of gastric rugae will be apparent when the esophagoscope enters the stomach. As the esophagoscope is withdrawn the esophagus should be carefully inspected and a biopsy should be performed on any suspicious lesions.

No oral feedings should be allowed for at least four hours after the procedure, and the patient must be examined for neck tenderness and subcutaneous emphysema. The immediate onset of pain that radiates into the upper mediastimum or back often indicates a perforation. A white blood count will reveal a marked leukocyto-sis before fever develops. Perforations of the esophagus are serious and should never be overlooked, for immediate hospitalization is required for definitive care.

REFERENCES

1. Allen, G. W.: Ligation of the internal maxillary artery for epistaxis. Laryngoscope, 80:915–923, 1970.
2. Andreason, J. O.: Traumatic Injuries of the Teeth. St. Louis, C.V. Mosby Co., 1972.
3. Armstrong, B. W.: Chronic secretory otitis media: Diagnosis and treatment. South Med. J., 50:540–545, 1957.
4. Arnold, G.: Technique of intrachordal injection. Arch. Otolaryngol., 76:358–368, 1962.
5. Barber, H. O. and Stockwell, C. W.: Manual of Electronystagmography. St. Louis, C. V. Mosby Co., 1976.
6. Beatrous, W. P.: Tracheostomy (tracheotomy). Its expanded indications and its present status. Based on an analysis of 1,000 consecutive operations and a review of the recent literature. Laryngoscope, 78:3–55, 1968.
7. Daly, J. F. and Cardona, J. C.: Acute corrosive esophagitis. Arch. Otolaryngol., 74:629–634, 1961.
8. Dingman, R. O. and Natvig, P.: Surgery of facial fractures. Philadelphia, W. B. Saunders Co., 1964.
9. English, G. M.: Common injuries to the ear. Primary Care, 3(3): 507–520, 1976.
10. English, G. M., Hemenway, W. G. and Cundy, R. W.: Surgical treatment of invasive angiofibroma. Arch. Otolaryngol., 96:312–318, 1972.
11. English, G. M., and Hildyard, V. H., Hemenway, W. G. and Davidson, S.: Autograft

and homograft incus transpositions in chronic otitis media. Laryngoscope, 81:1434–1447, 1971.

12. Fowler, E. P., Jr. and Osmun, P. M.: New bone growth due to cold water in the ears. Arch. Otolaryngol., 36:455–566, 1942.

13. Grahne, B.: Abscess tonsillectomy: Seven hundred twenty-five cases. Arch. Otolaryngol., 68:332–336, 1958.

14. Head, J. M.: Tracheostomy in the management of respiratory problems. N. Engl. J. Med., 264:587–591, 1961.

15. Hemenway, W. G.: The management of severe obstruction of the upper air passages. Surg. Clin. North Am., 41(1):201–212, 1961.

16. Hemenway, W. G. and Smith, R. O.: Treating acute otitis media. Postgrad. Med., 47:110–115, 1970.

17. Holinger, P. H. and Johnstone, K. C.: Factors responsible for laryngeal obstruction in infants. J.A.M.A., 143:1229–1232, 1950.

18. Johnson, E.: A study of corrosive esophagitis. Laryngoscope, 73:1651–1696, 1963.

19. Johnson, W. B.: New method for reduction of acute dislocation of the temporomandibular articulations. J. Oral Surg., 16:501–504, 1958.

20. Oeconomopoulos, C. T.: The value of glossopexy in the Pierre Robin syndrome. N. Engl. J. Med. 262:1267–1268, 1960.

21. Padrnos, R. E.: A method for control of posterior nasal hemorrhage. Arch. Otolaryngol., 87:181–187, 1968.

21a. Pitts, W., Pickrell, K., Quinn, G., et al.: Electric burns of lips and mouth in infants and children. Plast. Reconstr. Surg., 44: 471, 1969.

22. Potsic, W. P., and Naunton, R. F.: The implantation of an amputated pinna. Arch. Otolaryngol., 100:73–75, 1974.

23. Riddell, V.: Thyroidectomy, prevention of bilateral recurrent nerve palsy. Br. J. Surg., 57(1):1–11, 1970.

24. Rosnagle, R. S., Yanagisawa, E. and Smith, H. W.: Specific vessel ligation for epistaxis: Survey of 60 cases. Laryngoscope, 83(4):512–525, 1973.

25. Rowe, N. L. and Killey, H. C.: Fractures of the facial skeleton. Baltimore, Williams & Wilkins, 1968.

26. Shambaugh, G. E.: Surgery of the ear. Philadelphia, W. B. Saunders Co., 1967.

27. Sprinkle, P. M. and Veltri, R. W.: The tonsil and adenoid dilemma: Medical or surgical treatment? Otolaryngol. Clin. North Am., 7(3):909–925, 1974.

28. Stuteville, O. H. and Corley, R. D.: Surgical management of tumors of intraoral minor salivary glands: Report of eighty cases. Cancer, 20:1578–1586, 1967.

29. Templer, J. W.: Trauma to the larynx and cervical trachea. *In* G. M. English (Ed.: Otolaryngology, A Textbook. Hagerstown, Harper & Row, 1976.

29a. Thompson, H. G., Juckes, A. W., and Farmer, A. W.: Electric burns to the mouth in children. Plast. Reconstr. Surg., 35:466, 1965.

30. Toglia, J. U.: Electronystagmography: Technical Aspects and Atlas. Springfield, Charles C Thomas, 1976.

31. Weaver, M.: Neurologic disorders of the larynx. *In* G. M. English (Ed.): Otolaryngology, A Textbook. Hagerstown, Harper & Row, 1976.

Musculoskeletal System: Fractures and Dislocations

12

LELAND G. HAWKINS, M.D.

C. *Retention*
    1. Hanging arm plaster
    2. Plaster leg cylinder
    3. Short leg walking plaster dressing
    4. Long leg walking plaster dressing
    5. Overhead olecranon skeletal traction
    6. Buck's extension traction and split Russell's traction for children
D. *Restoration of function*

X. SPECIFIC FRACTURES
  A. *Scapula*
  B. *Clavicle*
  C. *Humerus*

D. *Forearm*
E. *Wrist*
    1. Navicular
    2. Hamate
    3. Triquetrum
F. *Femur*
G. *Patella*
H. *Tibia*
    1. Tibial plateau
    2. Tibial shaft
I. *Ankle*
    1. Lateral malleolus
    2. Posterior malleolus
    3. Medial malleolus
J. *Foot*
    1. Calcaneal fractures
    2. Talus
    3. Metatarsal

INTRODUCTION

This chapter is primarily concerned with fractures and dislocations that are treated on an outpatient basis. It is based on the author's experience as chief of a fracture service at a city hospital and now as a private practicing orthopedist. The author's recommendations are based on typical experience with fractures and dislocations, as shown in Tables 12–1 and 12–2.

In our health care system many different specialists and paramedical personnel are called upon to assist the acutely injured patient. This chapter is designed to enlarge their appreciation of extremity trauma. Emergency Room physicians are the nucleus at the beginning of this care. They may give prompt recognition of tissue injury, assign patients to the proper community physician and are often asked to initiate treatment. This chapter will increase their understanding and improve their skills.

The primary physician is responsible for all tissues of the extremities including skin, tendons, ligaments, muscles, joints, nerves, veins and arteries. To isolate the management of the bone injury would be a disservice to the patient, because the end results depend upon restoration of function of each of the tissues of any extremity.

It is recommended that an encounter form be completed in duplicate when a new trauma patient with an extremity problem is treated. This type of form (Table 12–3) emphasizes a thorough examination and, when completed, is a useful record for both hospital and office. Ideally, the extremity physician should be trained to handle each tissue included on the encounter form.

This chapter is designed to be a practical reference for physicians who may not be fully acquainted with these types of injuries or their management but who must nevertheless treat patients with injured extremities. The initial pages emphasize the soft tissue injuries that frequently accompany fractures and dislocations. Commonly missed fractures and dislocations are then discussed. Instructions for the application of several types of plaster dressings are included. The techniques for insertion of pins and wires utilized

TABLE 12–1   Distribution and Management of 1820 Consecutive Fractures*

UPPER EXTREMITY	Closed	Open	Admission
Clavicle and scapula	115	2	19
Shoulder	90	0	11
Humerus	64	3	12
Elbow	50	4	8
Forearm	260	1	41
Wrist	51	0	10
Hand	322	17	26
Total	952	27	127

LOWER EXTREMITY	Closed	Open	Admission
Pelvis	57	2	40
Hip	104	1	96
Femur	66	2	60
Knee	95	7	35
Tibia and fibula	144	9	59
Ankle	190	4	37
Foot	157	3	5
Total	813	28	332

*Open fractures associated with gunshot wounds are not included.

TABLE 12–2   Location of 181 Consecutive Dislocations

UPPER EXTREMITY		Number
Sternoclavicular Acromioclavicular }		20
Shoulder		59
Elbow		40
Wrist		6
Hand		20
	Total	145

LOWER EXTREMITY		Number
Hip		6
Knee		8
Ankle		17
Foot		5
	Total	36

TABLE 12–3 Orthopedic Health Care Visit Form

PRIORITY								
I								
II								
III								

Age — Ht. — Wt. — T — BP — P

Accident Date / Time

Type / Place

History, Exam, Present Problem

Confidential or additional information on back.

— DIAGNOSIS/PROBLEM —

FRACTURE Location
1.   ☐ Simple   ☐ Comminuted
2.   ☐ Open   ☐ Closed
3.   ☐ Stable   ☐ Unstable

Type of Reduction — Degrees Angulated

Type of Retention — Percent Displaced

Type of Anesthesia

Skin

Nerve

Artery

Joint

Ligament

Tendon

ADDITIONAL PROCEDURES
☐ Crutches   ☐ Sling   ☐ Cast Instruction Sheet

— LAB & X-RAY ORDERS —

— DRUG ORDERS — STRENGTH — SIG. — QUAN. —

REFER/ DESTINATION   EST. LENGTH OF DISABILITY

RETURN VISIT   DYS.   MOS.   Clinic
WKS.   PRN

Signature   No.

Current Address   Phone

Medicaid/Insurance Ident.

Medicare   Rate

Stat. | Site | Outc.

☐ Comp. ☐ Liab. ☐ BC ☐ BS ☐ CI

ORTHOPEDIC HEALTH CARE VISIT FORM

Date

Name

D.H.H. No.

Facility Cl./Serv.

Sex

Birthdate

Responsible Party

Appt. Time   D.H.H. No.

Clerk and Time

in skeletal traction are reviewed. The drawings will permit prompt access to the information. Although outpatient management is frequently not as convenient as inpatient treatment, and shortages of operating room time and bed space may often be encountered, it is nevertheless possible to maintain a high level of medical care, and it may greatly expedite patient care.

SKIN INJURY

The condition of the skin overlying a fracture or dislocation may dictate a course of management which will appear to be at variance with standard orthopedic practice. The primary physician must recognize the common associated skin injuries accompanying fractures and dislocations and appreciate, from the outset, how they may alter fracture management. All patients with skin injuries should receive tetanus protection (Table 12–4). Most wounds can be handled in the Outpatient Department except those that require formal débridement in the operating room or that overlie a fracture requiring hospital management.

Abrasions

Abrasions (Fig. 12–1) overlying midshaft fractures of both bones of the forearm in an adult illustrate the way skin damage may alter management of the fracture. This bone injury usually requires open reduction and internal fixation, but the multiple tears in the epidermis make a perfect medium for superficial infection. It is too risky to proceed with any type of surgery through this potentially contaminated area. Infection may follow the open reduction. Therefore, initially I take great care in obtaining a satisfactory reduction and maintaining the reduction with length and alignment because I may never be able to fix the fracture internally. Wound care requires repeated dressing changes to prevent further skin necrosis and allow early skin healing. Anesthesia may be required to avoid pain during the initial débridement to remove road tar and for the removal of the plaster and rescrubbing of the wound with iodophor sponges (Table 12–5). Repeated careful reduction and application of plaster are usually necessary. Before the plaster is applied, the abrasion is scrubbed vigorously and covered with a sterile fine

TABLE 12–4   Tetanus Protection

Previous Immunization	No Immunization
Tetanus toxoid	Hypertet
0.5 cc IM	250–500 units IM
Booster needed every ten years	

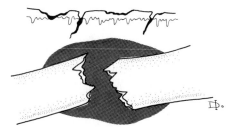

Figure 12–1   Abrasions overlying fracture.

TABLE 12–5   Betadine Solution

Betadine solution is the most effective topical germicide for use in treating open fractures. It kills bacteria (including antibiotic-resistant organisms), fungi, viruses, protozoa and yeasts. It is bactericidal, not merely bacteriostatic, and maintains germicidal activity in the presence of blood, pus, serum and necrotic tissue. It has a more prolonged germicidal action than ordinary iodine solutions, and forms a golden-brown film when topically applied that delineates treated areas. It can easily be washed off skin and natural fabrics. (Editor's note: The superiority of Betadine brand iodophor over other topical organic iodine preparations has not been conclusively demonstrated.)

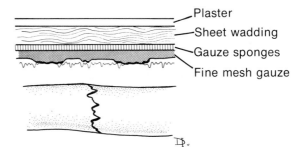

Figure 12–2 Circular dressings for abrasions.

mesh gauze, followed by a layer of gauze sponges. Finally, a circular dressing of Webrile, Kling or Kerlex bias-cut stockinette or sheet wadding is lightly applied (Fig. 12–2). In one week these dressings are removed, using anesthesia if necessary. Drainage or superficial infection alters the above routine. More frequent dressing changes may be necessary until the wound is clean, with continuous Bunnell's soaks that are changed every eight hours (Table 12–6). Once the skin is entirely healed the surgeon can consider open reduction and internal fixation of the fracture.

Tension on Overlying Skin

The fracture or dislocation that has placed *tension on overlying skin* (Fig. 12–3) should be reduced promptly to prevent necrosis. The lateral displacement and external rotation of the foot associated with a trimalleolar fracture often stretches the skin over the irregular fracture surface of the distal tibia. Simple linear traction and internal rotation of the foot relieve this tension. Another example is the tension on skin over the dislocated body of the talus after a fracture dislocation of the talus. Simple fingertip pressure moves the talar body into a position that reduces the skin tension.

Blisters

Fracture *blisters* (Fig. 12–4) are usually avoided by covering the ex-

TABLE 12–6 **Bunnell's Solution**
(MODIFIED)

Benzalkonium chloride 10%	200 cc
Glacial acetic acid	212 cc
Glycerin	8000 cc
Water, distilled qs ad	10 gal
D & C Red #39	1.0 gm

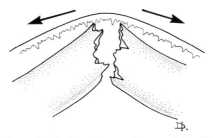

Figure 12–3 Tension on skin overlying fracture.

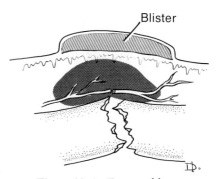

Figure 12–4 Fracture blister.

tremity promptly with a well-molded firm circumferential dressing. Blisters should be covered by a sterile dressing and well-molded plaster. The presence of blisters indicates poor venous out-flow and edema due to widespread underlying subcutaneous hemorrhage. They are not a contraindication to surgery unless they rupture and become secondarily infected.

Contusions

Complete necrosis of skin and adjacent subcutaneous tissue occasionally develops after a *severe contusion* (Fig. 12–5). The precarious circulation at the periphery of the contusion may be compromised if precautions are not taken to prevent pressure and swelling. These developments may cause or increase the area of necrosis by further compromising the circulation. Elevation, soft dressings and a water mattress or flotation bed are necessary in these circumstances.

Wound Flaps

Wounds about the lower leg and foot that leave undermined *skin flaps* separating the skin from underlying fat and fascia frequently undergo creeping necrosis. Over a period of several days to a week, progressive necrosis is noted, beginning at the incision edge and moving peripherally. Repeated débridement and later skin grafting may be necessary. Tight skin closures and venous stasis contribute to this problem.

Missile Wounds

A low-velocity *missile wound* with associated fracture such as that inflict-

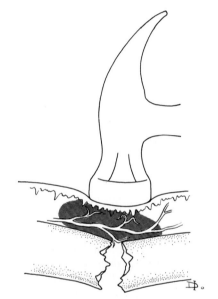

Figure 12–5 Contusion with skin necrosis associated with fracture.

ed by a .22, .38 or .45 caliber pistol bullet (Fig. 12–6) needs simple skin débridement, soft dressings and antibiotics. By following this routine one rarely encounters a deep infection. The tract need not be debrided nor the missile removed initially. When the fracture is comminuted, plaster dressings and nonoperative methods of treatment are frequently satisfactory.

High-velocity missile wounds usually require extensive débridement, open treatment and secondary explorations, unless the missiles are "spent rounds" no longer travelling at high velocity. Hunting rifles (.30 caliber or greater) and military rifles of all calibers produce high-velocity wounds with considerable tissue destruction. Shotgun wounds are extremely variable in their destructive power. At short range, particularly with a single missile or "buckshot," the shotgun produces great damage and even complete removal of soft tissue and bone from the victim. Shotgun blasts frequently contaminate wounds with nonradiopaque material, such as clothing, shell wadding or other secondary missiles blown into the wound, for example, dirt, sand or fragments of other injured persons.

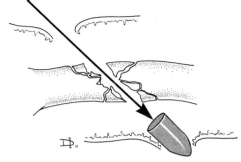

Figure 12–6 Missile wound with associated fracture.

Lacerations and Puncture Wounds

All *lacerations or puncture wounds* (Fig. 12–7) in the area of a fracture which result in communication between the skin surface and fracture hematoma are considered open fractures. The most frequent open fracture is the open distal fingertip injury, and open fracture of the tibial shaft is next in frequency. Intravenous antibiotics

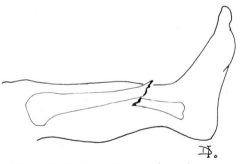

Figure 12–7 Laceration overlying fracture.

TABLE 12–7   Recommended Antibiotic Coverage for Open Fractures

ORGANISM	ROUTE	PATIENT DRUG SENSITIVITY	DRUG	RECOMMENDED DOSE FOR 70 kgm PATIENT
Gram +	Intra-venous	Sensitive to penicillin	cephalothin (Keflin)	1–2 gm IV piggy-back q 4 hrs
		None	nafcillin (Unipen)	1–2 gm IV piggy-back q 4 hrs
	Oral	Sensitive to penicillin	cephalexin (Keflex); or	250–500 mg tabs q 6 hrs
			erythromycin (Erythrocin, Ilotycin)	250–500 mg tabs q 6 hrs
		None	dicloxacillin (Dynapen)	250–500 mg tabs q 6 hrs
Gram −	Intra-muscular	None	kanamycin (Kantrex)	15 mg/Kg/day divided q 12 hr doses
			gentamicin (Garamycin)	2.5–4.5 mg/Kg/day divided q 8 hr doses
	Oral	Sensitive to penicillin	cephalothin (Keflex)	250–500 mg tabs q 6 hrs
		None	ampicillin (Omnipen, Penibritin, Polycillin, etc.)	250–500 mg tabs q 6 hrs

(Table 12–7) must immediately be started in the Emergency Room, and continued intraoperatively and post-operatively. Betadine-soaked sterile dressings are applied to the open fracture prior to the patient's arrival in the operating room. The incidence of infection is low if the wound débridement is carried out in the operating room within two to three hours after the injury. Antibiotics are administered for ten days and primary wound closure is accomplished when possible. A laceration or puncture wound in continuity with a fracture that is debrided in the Emergency Room should not be closed with sutures.

VASCULAR INJURY

Vascular injury (Fig. 12–8) is the single most important aspect of trauma to

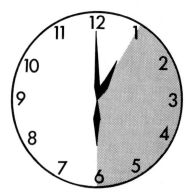

Figure 12–8 Vascular injury associated with fracture must be treated within five hours.

the extremities, and it demands immediate recognition by the primary physician. An extremity can be deprived of
arterial blood supply for only five
hours. Irreversible changes then occur
in the muscles, nerves, arteries and
skin. A vascular surgeon should be
called before arteriograms are obtained, so that precious time is not lost.
We do not usually attempt to repair
arteries distal to the bifurcation of the
brachial artery nor distal to the trifurcation of the popliteal artery (Fig. 12–
9).

Several medical centers scattered
over the United States now have
trained surgeons capable of reimplantation surgery utilizing the operating
microscope. These repairs have met
with success in restoring blood supply
to a part. We are now awaiting the functional results of this microsurgery. The
patient and the primary physician must
decide the need for consultation at one
of these centers.

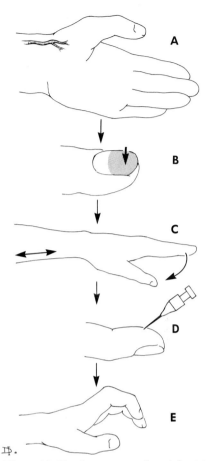

Figure 12–10 Assessment of vascular injury.
A. Pulse. *B.* Capillary refill. *C.* Passive stretch.
D. Sensory loss. *E.* Motor loss.

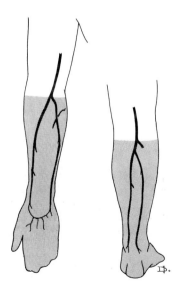

Figure 12–9 Injuries distal to bifurcation of
brachial and trifurcation of popliteal arteries are
not usually repaired.

Vascular Insufficiency

Vascular insufficiency is recognized
by the following aspects of the physical
examination:

First, the peripheral pulses of one
extremity are quickly compared to the
pulses of the opposite extremity.

Second and more important, the
promptness of capillary refill after pressure on the nail beds is assessed (Fig.
12–10).

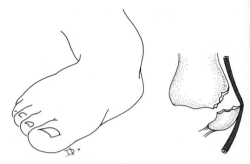

Figure 12–11   Arterial compression from fracture dislocation causes temporary ischemia.

Third, early ischemia to muscles causes severe pain when the muscle belly is stretched, while early nerve ischemia causes progressive distal sensory loss and paralysis in the extremity. An artery that is under tension as in a fracture dislocation of the ankle, may leave the foot cold and pulseless until the dislocation is reduced (Fig. 12–11). A rapidly expanding hematoma or persistent arterial bleeding suggests partial laceration of an artery (Fig. 12–12). The completely transected artery will often close spontaneously, preventing continued blood loss. An intimal tear obstructs the arterial flow. No extravasation of blood is noted, but peripheral signs of ischemia are evident. Arteriovenous fistula (Fig. 12–13) is rare; it is most frequently associated with stab wounds and low velocity gunshot wounds. A stethoscope may detect a bruit in these cases.

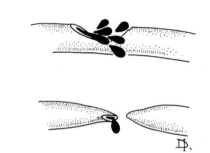

Figure 12–12   Rapidly expanding hematoma suggests partial laceration of artery.

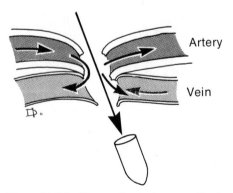

Artery

Vein

Figure 12–13   Traumatic arteriovenous fistula.

Aseptic Necrosis

In most cases, loss of arterial blood supply to bone cannot be recognized at the time of the fracture. *Aseptic necrosis* can be seen later by careful scrutiny of the x-ray. The three common fractures associated with a significant incidence of aseptic necrosis are the intra-articular fractures of the neck of the femur, the waist of the carpal navicular and the neck of the talus (Fig. 12–14). In each case the proximal fragment partially or completely loses its blood supply at the time of injury. The long-range prognosis is guarded as related to the union of the fracture, the degree of pain and the loss of function of the involved joint. Smaller areas of bone necrosis are noted at the edges of all fracture sites and bone fragments that have been stripped from their soft tissue attachments.

Fractures and Dislocations Commonly Associated With Vascular Injury

1. *A patient with a crush injury of the proximal tibia or knee*, with or without a significant tibial fracture, must not be treated as an outpatient because in 6 to 24 hours local hemorrhage and swelling may (Fig. 12–15) necessitate fasciotomy and arterial exploration.

2. *Dislocation of the knee* is a rare but significant injury, since it is associated with a tear or contusion of the popliteal artery in 50 per cent of cases. Ligamentous damage is of secondary importance to the arterial injury. Unnecessary delay in reduction and recognition of popliteal artery damage will result in amputation (Fig. 12–16). Restoration of blood supply must be prompt and effective.

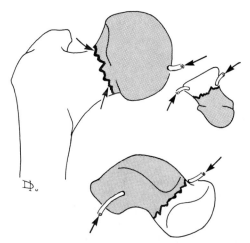

Figure 12–14 Common fractures associated with aseptic necrosis: femur, carpal navicular, and talus.

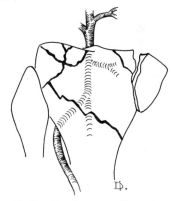

Figure 12–15 Crush injury of knee (proximal tibia), which frequently requires fasciotomy and arterial exploration.

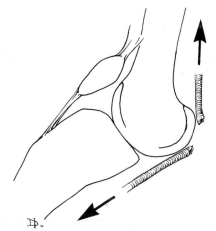

Figure 12–16 Dislocated knee is associated with popliteal artery injury in 50 per cent of cases.

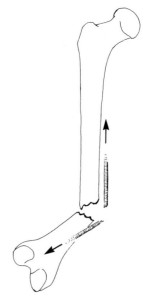

3. The superficial femoral artery may be partially or completely lacerated or have an intimal tear at the time of *fracture of the mid or distal shaft of the femur.* Major arterial and venous injuries also accompany fractures of the pelvis. These injuries necessitate prompt surgical repair (Fig. 12–17).

4. A child who has fallen on an outstretched arm and presents with marked deformity about the elbow is also likely to have an arterial injury. The deformity may be due to a *supracondylar fracture* of the humerus (Fig. 12–18). This has a high incidence of vascular spasm and intimal damage and associated fracture hemorrhage which will usually not become significant during the emergency transport and splinting phase if the physician keeps the elbow extended and the forearm aligned and elevated. Signs of ischemia frequently develop after closed reduction. Immobilization is afforded by a posterior plaster splint and short collar and cuff. Venous drainage and arterial blood flow are then blocked by swelling and the flexed position of the elbow. The radial pulse is obliterated

Figure 12–17 Other arterial injuries are associated with fractures and dislocation of the femur (shown here), pelvis and upper extremity.

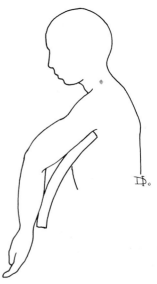

Figure 12–18 Arterial injury is also associated with a supracondylar fracture of the humerus (shown here).

(Fig. 12–19). When reduction and a good radial pulse cannot be maintained with the elbow in more than 90 degrees of flexion, the brachial artery may be torn, divided or in spasm. In this situation, skeletal overhead olecranon traction is immediately initiated.. If capillary filling is good, and if straightening the thumb, index and long finger does not cause pain in the forearm, the child can be observed closely, and exploration will not usually be needed. The pulse will return in a few days or weeks. The fracture can safely be reduced and retained during this period by overhead traction on a skeletal pin placed through the olecranon.

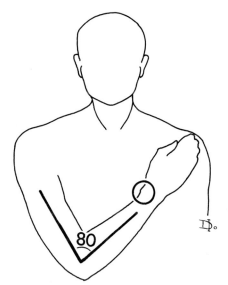

Figure 12–19 Postreduction immobilization of supracondylar fracture.

NERVE INJURY

The peripheral nerves are occasionally injured at the time of fractures and dislocations of the extremities. The primary physician needs to do little more than take all possible tension or angular forces off the nerves by reducing the fracture or dislocation. The nerve that is under tension or is ischemic benefits immediately by reduction, and function returns within minutes, hours or days. A nerve contused by a direct blow or stretching (Fig. 12–20) has disrupted axons and requires weeks or months before peripheral function returns. If either motor or sensory function persists after a mixed peripheral nerve is contused, the prognosis for return of function is more optimistic. Motor or sensory loss appearing after a closed reduction may necessitate surgical exploration to visualize the involved nerve and secure internal fixation of the fracture. After contusion, stretching or laceration of a nerve, the use of plaster dressings, passive motion, elevation and splints will maintain the extremity

Figure 12–20 Peroneal nerve injury by external trauma (A) and during lateral collateral ligament injury (B).

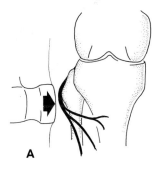
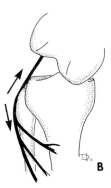

A   B

free of contractures (Fig. 12–21). If there is no return of function after a reasonable time has elapsed to allow for nerve regeneration, neurolysis or neurorrhaphy may be necessary. If no function or only partial function returns after surgery, tendon transfers may be used to eliminate the need for splints or braces. Function can be greatly improved in this way for patients with injury to the radial nerve, the peroneal nerve, the median nerve and the ulnar nerve.

Dermatomes and Peripheral Nerve Distribution

A review of the peripheral sensory and motor losses associated with the nerves that are commonly damaged at the time of fractures and dislocations seems appropriate. Occasionally the peripheral losses do not coincide with the patterns of distribution shown for the separate peripheral nerves. Consideration must then be given to more central injuries. The peripheral distribution of the dermatomes is shown in Figure 12–22. A brachial plexus injury

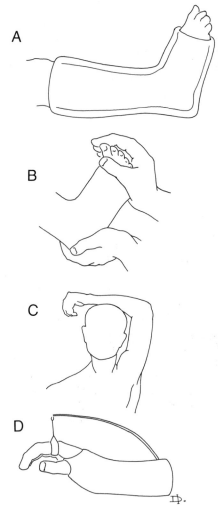

Figure 12–21 Prevention and treatment of peripheral nerve injuries associated with fractures by (A) plaster dressings, (B) passive motion, (C) elevation and (D) splints.

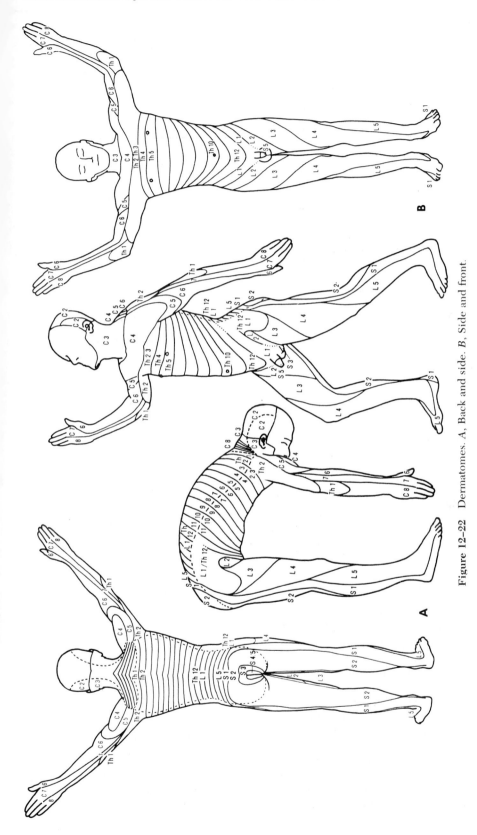

Figure 12–22   Dermatomes. *A,* Back and side. *B,* Side and front.

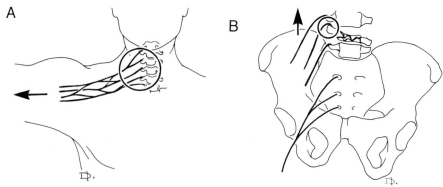

Figure 12–23   Brachial plexus and sciatic nerve injury.

(Fig. 12–23 *A, B*) can result from a severe stretch of the nerve roots as they
exit from the neural canal. A single
nerve root may be damaged in lumbar
and sacral fractures. Knowledge of dermatome sensory distribution may
therefore be useful in diagnosis.

Radial Nerve

The most frequent peripheral nerve
injury is *radial sensory and motor
palsy* associated with closed fractures
of the shaft of the humerus. The nerve
rests on the posterior surface of the
humerus, winding around distally to
pass anterior to the elbow. It is
stretched or contused at the time of the
fracture (Fig. 12–24), but it is unusual
for this nerve to be lacerated. Therefore, sensory and motor function can be
expected to return within three to four
months. The *radial nerve* is also susceptible to contusion in children with
supracondylar fractures of the humerus. Observation for several weeks
to three months is usually all that is
necessary, since peripheral function
will return in that time. The deep radial
nerve passing through the supinator
muscle is occasionally contused in fractures of the proximal radius. It also can
be stretched when the radial head is
dislocated at the time of a Monteggia
fracture of the ulnar shaft. Outrigger
wrist and finger extensor splints are
needed in adult patients to keep the
hand free from edema and contracture
while nerve regeneration occurs.

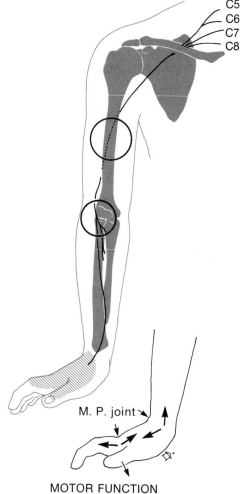

MOTOR FUNCTION
(EXTENSION WRIST AND THUMB)

Figure 12–24   Radial nerve injury in fracture
of the humerus.

Ulnar Nerve

The ulnar nerve courses deep in the muscles of the arm and forearm and is exposed to trauma primarily at the shoulder, elbow and wrist (Fig. 12–25). A patient with an anterior dislocation of the shoulder will occasionally complain of paresthesias in the ulnar distribution. Normal motor and sensory functions usually return promptly after reduction of the dislocation. The nerve is more frequently traumatized by external forces at the elbow where it rests subcutaneously in the ulnar groove on the distal humerus. At the wrist, a volar dislocation of the distal ulna associated with a radial shaft fracture (the Galeazzi's fracture) may stretch or contuse the ulnar nerve.

Frequently ulnar motor function is lost in the hand after a patient with a Colles' fracture is placed in excessive flexion. The problem can be avoided by limiting flexion at the wrist when the plaster is applied.

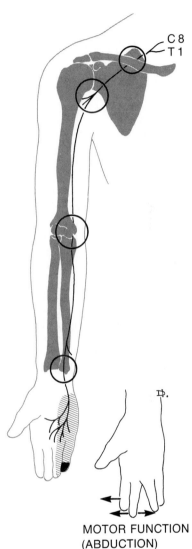

MOTOR FUNCTION
(ABDUCTION)

Figure 12–25   Ulnar nerve injury.

Median Nerve

The flexor muscle group in the arm and forearm usually affords good protection to the median nerve from injury by bone fragments at the time of fracture and dislocation (Fig. 12–26). The proximal humeral fragment of a supracondylar fracture may tear through the intervening brachialis muscle and contuse the median nerve. A more common median nerve injury occurs from hemorrhage, swelling and extreme flexion of the wrist in a reduced Colles' fracture. Prompt recognition and release of dressings may prevent an avoidable ischemic and neuropathic contracture of the hand. After leaving the forearm the nerve enters the limited space of the carpal canal. Volar displacement of the lunate into the carpal canal at the time of dislocation routinely creates pressure and ischemia in the median nerve. Prompt reduction will usually eliminate permanent nerve deficit.

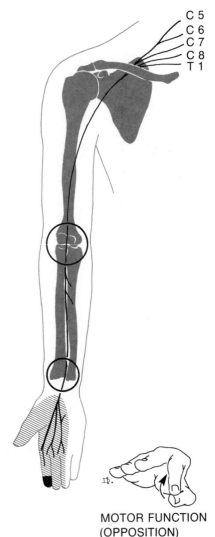

C 5
C 6
C 7
C 8
T 1

MOTOR FUNCTION
(OPPOSITION)

Figure 12–26   Median nerve injury.

Sciatic Nerve

The sciatic nerve rests on the acetabulum posterior to the hip joint (Fig. 12–27). In a posterior dislocation of the hip the femoral head breaks through the joint capsule and frequently stretches or contuses the adjacent nerve. The nerve may be lacerated if a posterior acetabular lip fracture fragment accompanies the dislocation. When recognized, prompt reduction of the dislocation is mandatory. Frequently the peroneal portion of the sciatic nerve is contused, while the adjacent posterior tibial portion is spared. If function does not return immediately after reduction, a prolonged period of disability is anticipated. This may necessitate a double upright brace with ankle spring assists or a tendon transfer at a later date.

Posterior Tibial Nerve

The sciatic nerve divides at the junction of the middle and distal third of the femur into the posterior tibial and peroneal nerves (Fig. 12–27). Signs and symptoms of injury to this nerve frequently occur with subtalar dislocations and fracture dislocations of the ankle. Prompt reduction of these injuries usually results in early return of function.

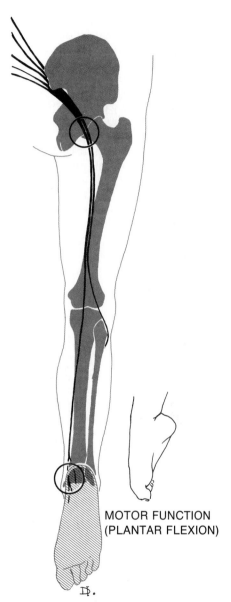

MOTOR FUNCTION
(PLANTAR FLEXION)

Figure 12–27   Sciatic nerve injury.

Peroneal Nerve

This nerve passes lateral to the knee joint in contact with the biceps tendon which inserts into the proximal fibula. It winds around the subcutaneous surface of the fibula until it reaches the anterior compartment. The peroneal nerve is particularly vulnerable to trauma (Fig. 12–28) in its subcutaneous position adjacent to the head of the fibula. The nerve is stretched when the knee joint opens into a varus position, tearing the lateral collateral ligament, the biceps tendon and the fascia lata from their insertion into the tibia. In its subcutaneous position the nerve is also exposed to direct external trauma, such as pressure from a mattress, an elastic bandage securing traction on the skin or a poorly padded plaster dressing. A direct blow causing a proximal fracture of the fibula may also damage the peroneal nerve.

LIGAMENTS AND CAPSULES

Certain ligamentous and capsular tears are frequently overlooked when there has been an associated fracture and dislocation. Once a spontaneous or manual reduction has been accomplished, the soft tissue damage is too often forgotten or not recognized. The local joint is painful and swollen with blood, and careful examination is difficult because of the patient's discomfort. In this situation, intra-articular injection of lidocaine may be used to produce satisfactory analgesia for examination. Thorough aspiration of the joint must be performed before lidocaine is injected. Uptake by the synovial membrane is prompt, and the total dose injected intrasynovially must be below toxic levels (1 mg per pound). A stress x-ray view provides verification and a permanent record of associated ligamentous damage or instability.

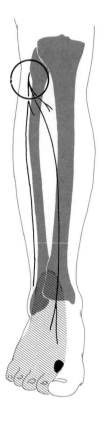

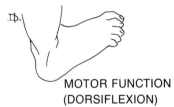

MOTOR FUNCTION
(DORSIFLEXION)

Figure 12–28   Peroneal nerve injury.

Common Ligamentous Injuries Associated with Fractures and Dislocations

A *tibial plateau fracture* (Fig. 12–29) can be associated with a torn collateral ligament on the opposite side of the knee from the fracture site. *Fracture of the lateral malleolus or distal fibula* (Fig. 12–30) may be associated with a torn medial collateral ligament of the ankle. Loss of stability may occur from avulsion of ligaments at their bony attachments. This is frequently seen when the anterior cruciate ligament avulses the *anterior tibial spine* (Fig. 12–31). The posterior cruciate ligament avulses bone from the posterior tibial surface. The medial and lateral ankle ligaments avulse bone from the *tips of the malleolus*. The collateral knee ligaments avulse bone from the *femur*, and *tibia* and *fibula*. The patellar ligament avulses bone from the *lower pole of the patella* and the *tibial tubercle* (Fig. 12–32). The quadriceps tendon may avulse bone from the superior pole of the patella. Radial deviation of the wrist

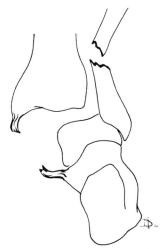

Figure 12–30   Lateral malleolus or distal fibula fracture associated with medial collateral ligament injury at the ankle.

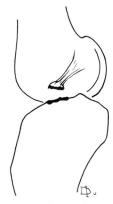

Figure 12–31   Avulsion of posterior tibial surface by posterior cruciate ligament.

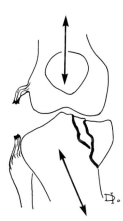

Figure 12–29   Stress x-ray for verification of instability and ligamentous injury associated with injury to a joint: tibial plateau fracture and associated collateral ligament injury.

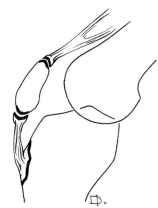

Figure 12–32   Patellar ligament avulses bone from patella and tibia.

avulses the *ulnar* styloid (Fig. 12–33). A fracture of the *shaft of the radius* may be associated with damage to the distal radial ulnar and ulnar carpal joints. A fracture of the *shaft of the ulna* may be associated with damage to the more proximal radial ulnar and radial humerus joints.

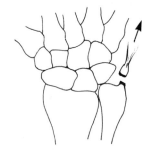

Figure 12–33   Ulnar styloid avulsion.

Treatment

The cartilaginous surfaces of the joints and intact soft parts usually lend enough stability to allow longitudinal capsular tears to heal with immobilization alone. The torn ligament or capsule may return to an anatomical position after reduction. Three weeks of immobilization is usually adequate for these injuries.

When transverse ligament and capsular tears heal there may be an increase in their length. This lengthening may be observed in the cruciate and medial collateral ligaments of the knee, the capsule of the elbow, thumb MP joint capsule and lateral ankle ligaments. All of these injuries may therefore be followed by recurrent dislocation or instability if the torn edges of the ligaments are not approximated surgically. Experimental ligament and capsule tears heal without laxity when their edges are anatomically repaired and adequately immobilized. Clinically, experience has demonstrated that treatment with adequate prolonged immobilization generally gives satisfactory results. Since a merely "satisfactory" result is not acceptable in young or athletic individuals, in these patients open surgical repairs of torn ligaments are routinely performed to assure that the ligament ends are approximated before immobilization is instituted.

MUSCLE TENDON UNIT INJURY AND ASSOCIATED FRACTURES

An interesting group of injuries occurs from violent muscle contraction or stress transmitted through the musculotendinous unit. The muscle tendon unit can rupture in various locations under such stresses. It is usually taught that the weakest point in this unit is the musculotendinous junction, as seen with ruptures of the Achilles tendon. Injuries classified as muscle strains occur when muscle fibers tear during violent muscle contraction. The pulled hamstring is a good example. However, avulsion fractures do occur at the origin or insertion of muscles. In the years prior to epiphyseal closure, avulsion fractures occur at the weak junction between an apophysis and adjacent metaphysis. An apophysis is a traction epiphysis not containing an articulating surface, and it appears as a secondary ossification center on the roentgenogram. The force of muscular contraction is transmitted across the muscle origin or insertion to the adjacent epiphyseal plate. The epiphyseal plate contains a band of growing cartilage which then separates, allowing the apophysis to displace with the shortened muscle.

Medial Epicondyle of the Humerus

The *medial epicondyle of the humerus* (Fig. 12–34) is a small apophysis or secondary ossification center at the elbow. The medial epicondyle prior to epiphyseal plate closure may be displaced distally by the forearm flexor muscle mass which originates from it. Nonunion without impairment of function is the expected result when treated in plaster.

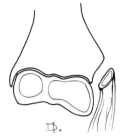

Figure 12–34 Avulsion of the medial epicondyle of the humerus by forearm flexors.

Anterior Inferior and Superior Iliac Spine

One of the four muscles in the quadriceps mechanism is the rectus femoris muscle, which takes origin from the *anterior inferior iliac spine* and inserts into the superior pole of the patella. A violent contraction of the quadriceps may avulse the anterior inferior spine and drag it into position anterior to the hip joint (Fig. 12–35). This may later lead to ossification anterior to the capsule of the hip, producing limitation of flexion of the hip. The sartorius or tensor fascia lata may avulse the *anterior superior iliac spine* or the leading edge of the anterior portion of the iliac crest. Both of these injuries are seen in young persons.

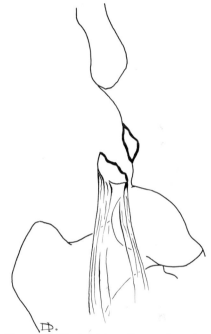

Figure 12–35 Avulsion of rectus femoris muscle origin from the anterior inferior iliac spine.

Ischial Tuberosity

The origin of the hamstrings is from the apophysis or secondary ossification center of the *ischial tuberosity*. This may be avulsed (Fig. 12–36). Nonunion can result from inadequate immobilization.

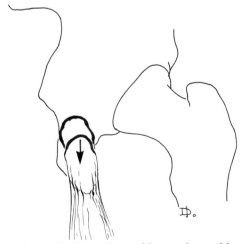

Figure 12–36 Avulsion of the apophysis of the ischial tuberosity by hamstrings.

Lesser Trochanter

An avulsion may occur at the insertion of the iliopsoas tendon into the
lesser trochanter of the femur (Fig. 12–
37), and is called an apophysis. The
lesser trochanter is displaced proximally, anterior to the head and neck of
the femur.

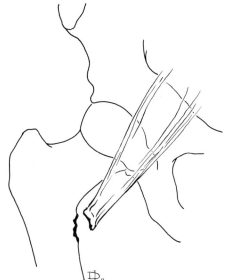

Figure 12–37 Avulsion of the lesser trochanter by iliopsoas tendon.

Other Avulsion Fractures

In the adult large fragments of bone
may be avulsed by violent muscle contraction; examples are seen in (Fig. 12–
38) the transverse fracture of the *pa-*

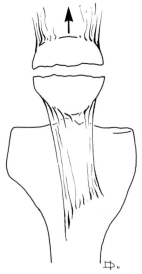

Figure 12–38 Transverse fracture of the patella.

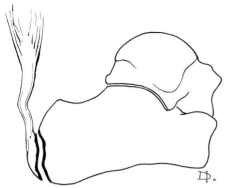

Figure 12–39 Displacement of the insertion of the Achilles tendon from os calcis.

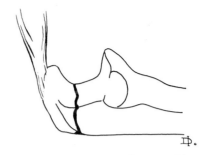

Figure 12–40 Transverse fracture of the proximal and middle olecranon.

tella, (Fig. 12–39) the upward displacement of the region about the insection of the tendon Achilles on the *os calcis* and (Fig. 12–40) the transverse fracture of the proximal and middle *olecranon*. These fractures frequently enter a joint and internal fixation of the displaced fragments may be necessary. However, minimally displaced avulsion fractures are best treated by immobilization and rest.

Muscle Strain and Rupture

Muscle strains are intramuscular fiber tears associated with overlying fascial tears. They are simply treated by rest for two weeks, followed by progressive return to normal activity. The origin of muscle fibers from the periosteum of long bones is occasionally torn from the bone. This condition may be followed by the development of myositis ossificans, a condition that is poorly understood. The most common serious disease of the muscle-tendon unit in the older adult is rupture of the musculotendinous junction. This occurs at the junction of the Achilles tendon and the gastrocnemius and soleus muscle fibers (Fig. 12–41). Rupture also occurs in the quadriceps group just above the patella and in the long head of the biceps distal to its exit from the bicipital groove of the humerus (Fig. 12–42). Surgical intervention is usually indicated in these cases.

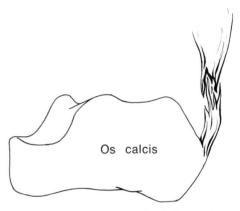

Os calcis

Figure 12–41 Disruption of Achilles tendon.

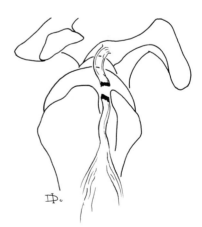

Figure 12–42 Disruption of tendon of long head of biceps.

SOFT TISSUE INJURIES ACCOMPANYING PELVIC FRACTURES

The patient with a fracture of the pelvis has usually sustained major blunt trauma which requires confinement in the hospital for an extended period of time. Prompt blood replacement is essential. The primary physician must be alert to the types of soft tissue damage which occur in these patients, requiring immediate recognition and surgical care. In 35 patients with pelvic fractures who required laparotomy (Table 12–8), the average blood replacement required was 4000 ml. Thirty of these patients had major injuries of intra-abdominal organs.[3] The only patient with a pelvic fracture who can safely rest at home is a patient who has had relatively minor trauma. Examples include a minimally displaced fracture of the ischial or pubic ramus with a normal hematocrit, a urine free of red blood cells and stable vital signs. In these cases as the pain decreases activity is increased. Nonunion is distinctly unusual (Fig. 12–43).

DISLOCATIONS

Dislocations of the joints in the extremities are usually easily recognized. Most of these injuries can be reduced by closed methods. Exceptions exist when it is necessary to remove soft parts or remove fracture fragments interposed between joint surfaces prior to the reestablishment of the normal articular surfaces. This situation is commonly encountered after a metacarpal phalangeal dislocation of the little and index finger and thumb in which the proximal phalanx is dorsally dislocated (Fig. 12–44). A successful closed reduction is prevented in these patients by volar plate interposition, and open reduction is therefore required.

TABLE 12–8   Abdominal Injuries Associated With Pelvic Fractures in 35 Patients Who Underwent Laparotomy

Urinary tract		19
Ruptured bladder	13	
Ruptured urethra	6	
Gastrointestinal tract		13
Ruptured spleen	4	
Liver laceration	4	
Bowel laceration	3	
Ruptured gallbladder	1	
Pancreatic laceration	1	
Vascular injury		5
No major associated injury		5

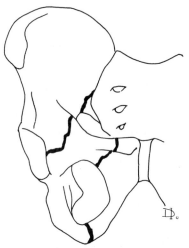

Figure 12–43   Pelvic fracture lines.

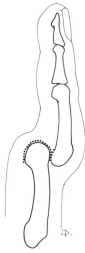

Figure 12–44   The irreducible metacarpal phalangeal dislocation.

Prompt reduction is recommended for all dislocations. The patient's severe pain is thus alleviated, and pressure and tension on the adjacent neurovascular bundle is relieved, preventing permanent distal vascular and neurologic loss. A long delay makes reduction more difficult because of local tissue edema and fibrosis, further hemorrhage, muscle spasm and contracture. Bone necrosis may occur if there is delay in reduction.

The primary physician can reduce most dislocated joints by placing manual traction on the extremity distal to the dislocation. Muscle spasm and local pain must be adequately controlled by sufficient analgesia. Relaxation then allows muscle and tissue stretching after traction is applied. After reduction, stability is obtained by the articular surfaces and soft parts. Surgical intervention may be required if the joint is unstable after reduction. Methods used include wire fixation across the joint, skeletal traction, ligament repair and plaster dressings.

Commonly Missed Dislocations

Every primary physician should be aware of the *commonly missed* disloca-tions. These include: posterior dislocation of the shoulder, volar dislocation of the carpal lunate, dislocation of the radial head associated with an ulnar shaft fracture and posterior dislocation of the hip associated with a femoral shaft fracture.

POSTERIOR SHOULDER DISLOCA-TION (Fig. 12–45). This condition should be suspected in a patient who presents with limited motion, crepitation and pain about the shoulder and who has a history of a recent seizure or a fall on the shoulder. The examination may be equivocal because of swelling and hemorrhage and because the glenoid may be caught by the infracture which is present on the anterior aspect of the humeral head. The standard anterior-posterior and lateral shoulder x-ray may be reported as normal. The diagnosis is made by an axillary x-ray view of the shoulder, in which the posterior dislocation and the extent of the associated anterior infracture of the humeral head are recognized. Closed reduction and immobilization for three weeks are satisfactory for most patients if the diagnosis and reduction are accomplished promptly. When a large infracture of the humeral head is present, surgical intervention can prevent recurrent dislocations.

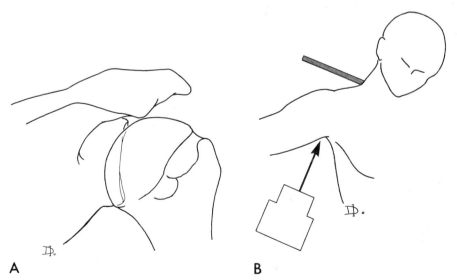

A   **B**

Figure 12–45 Posterior shoulder dislocation. *A.* Anatomy. *B.* Axillary x-ray technique.

VOLAR DISLOCATION OF THE LU-
NATE. Primary physicians examining
x-rays of the wrist need a review of the
normal relationships of the carpal
bones to avoid missing volar dislocation of the lunate. The diagrams demonstrate the normal position and the
dislocated position of the lunate as
seen on the lateral roentgenogram
(Fig. 12–46). This bone can be reduced
by placing traction on the hand with
the wrist dorsiflexed. Pressure is then
applied over the volar surface of the
displaced lunate. The wrist is flexed
while traction continues. The relationship between the lunate and the
navicular may be disrupted and separated after reduction. Median nerve
symptoms may be present, but they
usually disappear after a prompt reduction. Another easily missed injury
of the wrist is the transnavicular
perilunar dislocation (Fig. 12–47). The
capitate and distal pole of the navicular
are dorsally displaced, leaving the lunate and proximal pole of the navicular
articulating with the distal radius.
After reduction by straight traction the
proximal and distal fragments of the
navicular may be unstable and in unsatisfactory alignment. In this case
open reduction and internal fixation
are indicated to align and maintain the
fragments. Malalignment of the carpal
navicular fragment regularly results
in nonunion.

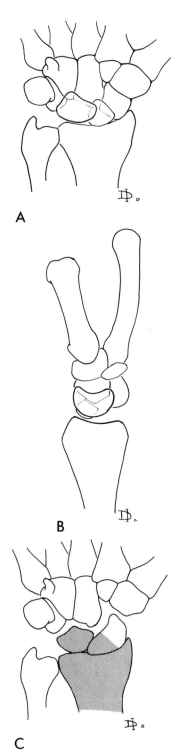

B

C

Figure 12–47   Transnavicular perilunar dislocation. *A.* AP view before reduction. *B.* Lateral
prereduction view. *C.* Postreduction.

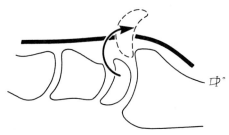

Figure 12–46   Dislocation of the lunate.

DISLOCATION OF THE RADIAL HEAD. Dislocation of the radial head is often associated with a fracture of the ulnar shaft (Fig. 12–48). The primary physician will not miss this diagnosis if he or she obtains an x-ray of the joints proximal and distal to the fracture. X-ray of the elbow demonstrates volar or dorsal displacement of the radial head. Reduction is usually obtained easily and is begun by applying longitudinal traction to the extended elbow. Direct force is then placed over the radial head. Reduction is completed and maintained by flexing the elbow and keeping it flexed. The associated ulnar shaft fracture requires internal fixation.

An isolated subluxation of the radial head ("nursemaid's elbow") cannot be recognized by x-ray. The patient presents with a history of having recently been lifted up in the air by the hand. The child keeps the hand in pronation and complains of pain in the extremity. He refuses to move the elbow. Treatment is simple. The physician grasps the child's hand and gently supinates the child's forearm. Immediate relief is obtained when reduction is completed and no further treatment is indicated.

The isolated displaced angulated fractured radius in an adult is accompanied by varying degrees of disruption of the distal radial ulnar joint (Fig. 12–49). X-rays of the joints below the fracture are needed to recognize the distal injury. Internal fixation of the radius may aid in reduction of the distal radial ulnar joint but does not protect against late development of painful degenerative arthritis.

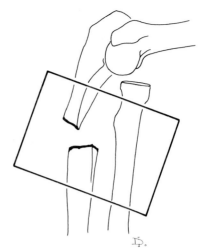

Figure 12–48 Dislocation of the radial head associated with fracture of ulna.

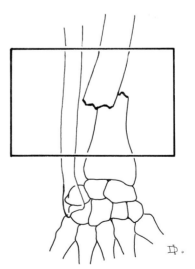

Figure 12–49 Displaced angulated fractured radius associated with disruption of distal radial ulnar joint.

POSTERIOR DISLOCATION OF THE HIP (Fig. 12–50). This is frequently associated with a femoral shaft fracture and with automobile injuries in which the knee strikes the dashboard. The patella and acetabulum may also be fractured in these patients, although the acetabular fracture may be difficult to see on x-ray. The proximal femoral shaft fragment will be adducted in these cases. An x-ray of the joint above the fracture confirms the dislocation. Open reduction of the hip is performed because traction applied to the distal femoral fragment and leg may not be sufficient to obtain a reduction.

Common, Easily Recognized Dislocations

The common, easily recognized dislocations of the elbow, shoulder, hip, knee, subtalar and metatarsal tarsal joints will be considered next.

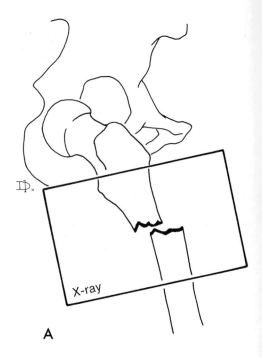

A

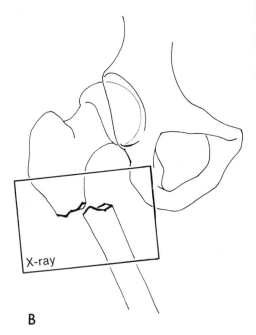

B

Figure 12–50 Posterior dislocation of the hip associated with femoral shaft fracture. A. Lateral view. B. AP view.

POSTERIOR LATERAL DISLOCATION OF THE ELBOW (Fig. 12–51). This is a rather alarming deformity when seen initially. It may occur in all age groups following forced hyperextension of the elbow. There may also be an associated fracture of the radial head or coronoid process, and in the younger age groups, an avulsion fracture of the medial epicondyle. If the median nerve is stretched while the elbow is dislocated paresthesias occur which resolve with reduction. Intravenous lidocaine is excellent analgesia to aid the reduction. Traction is first applied on the forearm, with countertraction on the arm. The elbow is brought into extension and out of varus or vulgus alignment to a neutral position. The reduction is accomplished by pressure applied over the olecranon while traction is maintained and flexion of the elbow is carried out. Further flexion to 90 degrees maintains the reduction. A posterior splint with cuff and collar is applied for three weeks. This allows capsular healing and prevents a lesser force from redislocating the joint. Return of normal motion may be slow, and residual loss of extension of the elbow may occur owing to capsular scarring. Recurrent dislocation is unusual.

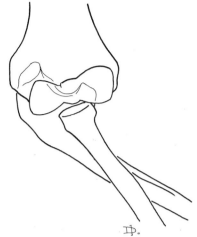

Figure 12–51 Posterior lateral dislocation of the elbow.

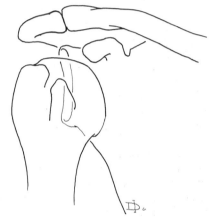

Figure 12–52 Anterior dislocation of the shoulder.

ANTERIOR DISLOCATION OF THE SHOULDER. The most common dislocation seen on our service is anterior dislocation of the shoulder (Fig. 12–52). The patient comes to the Emergency Room holding the involved arm with his opposite hand, with the dislocated shoulder in a few degrees of internal rotation. Pain and muscle spasm are present. The glenoid is palpated through the deltoid muscle and the humeral head is palpated anterior and inferior to its usual position. The ulnar nerve and axillary nerve are commonly stretched in the axilla. The patient is placed supine on a cart (Fig. 12–53). Traction and counter traction are applied by securing the patient to the cart with a sheet wrapped around the axilla. Traction is gradually applied to the arm and maintained with the

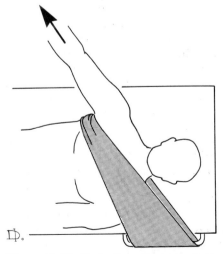

Figure 12–53 Reduction of anterior dislocation of shoulder.

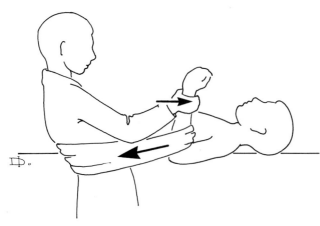

Figure 12–54 Alternate technique for reduction of anterior shoulder dislocation.

shoulder in about 30 degrees of abduction. If prolonged traction is required, it is helpful to wrap a sheet around the waist of the surgeon and the forearm of the patient (Fig. 12–54). Sufficient analgesia to relieve muscle spasm is accomplished with IV Valium and Demerol. Occasionally the glenoid rim will become an obstruction to reduction in a strong, muscular patient or in a patient with a large impacted fracture or infracture of the posterior aspect of the humeral head. In these cases, an interscalene block or general anesthesia is required. A sling and swathe or stockinette to prevent external rotation is advised for three weeks after the first dislocation. Any sensory and motor loss, if present, usually subsides after prompt reduction.

POSTERIOR DISLOCATION OF THE HIP. A person sitting in a car that is involved in an accident frequently strikes his knee on the dashboard and dislocates his hip posteriorly (Fig 12–55). The force of the impact is transmitted along the shaft of the femur to the posterior aspect of the hip joint. The posterior capsule tears or the posterior acetabular lip fractures and the femoral head exits from the joint. As this happens an unknown amount of the articular cartilage of the femoral head is damaged (Fig. 12–56). When the patient is seen in the Emergency Room he is usually lying supine on a cart. He refuses to extend the involved hip, which is held in flexion, adduction and internal rotation. Sciatic nerve symp-

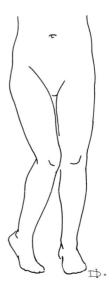

Figure 12–55 Posterior dislocation of the hip — position of the patient.

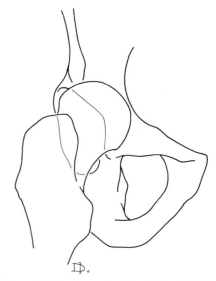

Figure 12–56 Posterior dislocation of the hip anatomy (AP view).

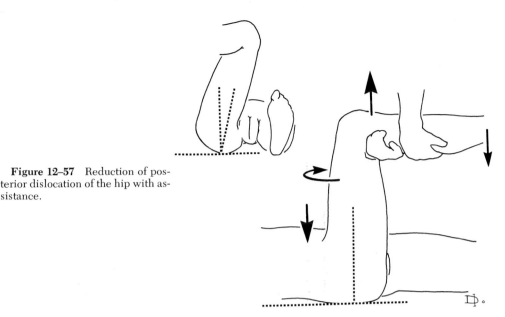

Figure 12–57 Reduction of posterior dislocation of the hip with assistance.

toms and signs may be present, and frequently do not resolve after reduction. Prompt reduction is indicated. Intravenous Valium and Demerol may be sufficient for analgesia and relaxation. Reduction is accomplished simply if the primary physician can enlist the help of other personnel (Fig. 12–57). The pelvis is held on a stretcher while traction is applied to the femur with the hip flexed 90 degrees, adducted 10 to 20 degrees, and internally rotated 5 to 10 degrees. The knee is flexed to allow for a better hold on the leg when traction is applied. If no strong assistants are available, turn the patient prone, allowing the hips to flex

over the side of the cart (Fig. 12–58). The knee is flexed and pressure applied to the posterior calf. This produces traction along the shaft of the femur. A reduction can then be obtained by rotating the femur slightly. Occasionally these methods fail, and a muscle relaxant and general anesthesia are required. After reduction, active exercises are initiated, avoiding extremes of flexion. While resting, the patient maintains the hip in extension until the capsule is healed. Aseptic necrosis of the femoral head may follow this injury, so the patient should be followed closely for at least three years.

Figure 12–58 Reduction of posterior dislocation of the hip without assistance.

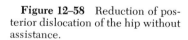

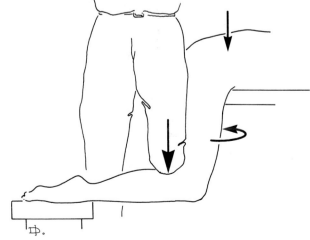

KNEE DISLOCATION. The problem of knee dislocation is discussed in some detail so that the primary physician will not miss the associated vascular injury. *Anterior dislocation* (Fig. 12–59) follows hyperextension of the knee. First, the posterior capsule tears, followed by a tear of the posterior cruciate ligament. The tibia then slides forward on the femur and comes to rest anterior to the distal femur. *A posterior dislocation of the knee* (Fig. 12–60) occurs when force displaces the proximal tibia posterior to the femoral condyles. Complete dislocations may occur in both medial and lateral positions. The cruciate ligaments are torn in all of these injuries, although one collateral ligament may remain intact owing to rotation. Closed reduction of these dislocations is usually possible except in a posterior lateral dislocation when the femoral condyle buttonholes throught the retinaculum and extensor mechanism. Open reduction is then required. The primary physician applies longitudinal traction which results in reduction, and then is immediately concerned with the associated vascular injury. Immediate exploration of the popliteal space is recommended to verify and repair arterial damage if there is any question of the blood supply distal to the recently dislocated knee. In these cases the collateral ligaments are usually torn from their femoral insertion. Closed treatment of the collateral ligaments is adequate if the surgical repair is delayed. However, residual instability in the anterior posterior plane will leave the patient with an unstable knee.

DISLOCATION OF THE TALOCALCANEAL OR SUBTALAR JOINT (Fig. 12–61). Usually medial in position, this dislocation produces marked deformity of the foot. Traction applied to the heel and forefoot in alignment with the tibial shaft brings about the reduction. If the reduction is stable a weight-bearing short leg plaster dressing should be worn for four weeks.

TALONAVICULAR DISLOCATION. The talonavicular dislocation is un-

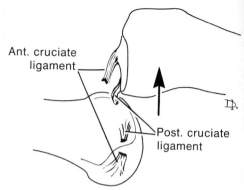

Figure 12–59 Anterior dislocation of the knee.

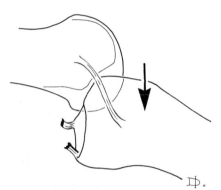

Figure 12–60 Posterior dislocation of the knee.

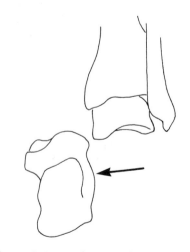

Figure 12–61 Dislocation of the talocalcaneal or subtalar joint.

stable after reduction (Fig. 12–62). A K-wire across the joint is usually required to maintain the reduction. The navicular is frequently fractured. A short, nonweight-bearing plaster dressing is recommended for six weeks prior to removal of the K-wire. The early presence of residual pain directs the physician to recommend fusion of the joint.

TARSAL-METATARSAL DISLOCATIONS (Fig. 12–63). Dislocation between the base of the metatarsals and the tarsal bones is occasionally accompanied by a fracture at the base of one of the metatarsals. The associated tearing of the dorsalis pedis artery and gross swelling may obscure the deformity. Adequate roentgenograms are essential to establish the diagnosis. A closed reduction is obtained by traction and inversion force on the forefoot and local pressure over the base of the metatarsal. Steinmann pin fixation may be necessary to hold the reduction. Painful degenerative arthritis may follow this injury.

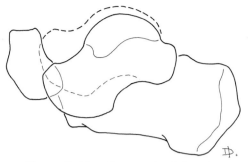

Figure 12–62   Talonavicular dislocation.

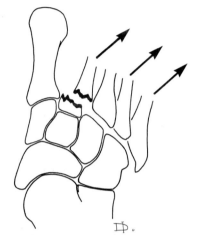

Figure 12–63   Dislocation between the base of metatarsals and tarsal bones.

FRACTURES

The physician treating a patient with a fracture should follow a logical course of thinking. We utilize an approach which we refer to as the *"four R's" of fracture therapy.*[5]
1. Recognition
2. Reduction
3. Retention
4. Restoration of Function

Different problems occur during each step in the patient's management. Additional information regarding the management of fractures may be obtained in the texts prepared by Blount[1] and Charnley.[2]

Recognition of the fracture includes a description of the anatomic site, not merely the name of the bone. The fracture geography is outlined from roentgenograms. Is the fracture transverse, oblique, spiral or comminuted (Fig. 12–64)? Is there a butterfly fragment?

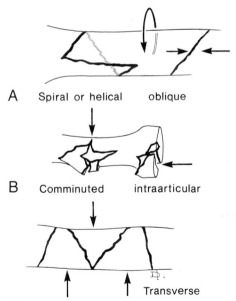

A   Spiral or helical   oblique

B   Comminuted   intraarticular

C   Butterfly fragment   Transverse

Figure 12–64   Recognition of the fracture geography – types of fractures.

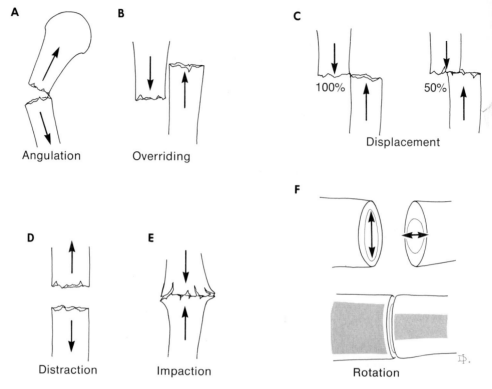

Figure 12–65   Recognition of fracture deformity.

The fracture deformity is illustrated by the roentgenogram. Is there angulation, overriding, displacement, distraction, impaction or rotation (Fig. 12–65)? *Reduction* or the removal of fracture deformity is planned in relation to the physican's plan for *retention* or maintenance of reduction. The final phase of fracture management is *retention* of function, which is also the responsibility of the physician who treats a patient with a fracture. Fracture management is not complete when fracture union has occured but should continue until maximal rehabilitation of function is achieved.

Recognition

If the patient has multiple injuries, is unconsicous, has a language barrier or is influenced by drugs or extreme pain, the doctor depends on a good physical and roentgenographical examination. Appropriate splinting is necessary before x-rays are taken, to prevent excessive pain and further damage to soft tissue. The splint must be applied in such a way that adequate x-ray can be obtained with the splint in place, and the splinting material must be easily penetrated by x-rays so that a fracture line will not be obscured. Well-padded balsa held to the extremity by a soft circular dressing is adequate for most fractures. A telescoping aluminum Thomas splint with Velcro straps and a windlass for traction is used for a fracture of the femur. This becomes extremely useful when a patient must be moved several times before arriving in his own bed.

The proper x-rays must be ordered to allow the radiologist and the primary physician to maintain a good diagnostic average. Anterior-posterior, lateral and oblique view of bones and joints are routinely obtained. I have also found that additional views often reveal a fracture or dislocation not seen on the routine roentgenogram.

Special x-rays to detect fractures include:

1. AXILLARY VIEW OF THE SHOULDER (Fig. 12–66). Abduction of the shoulder in the supine or sitting position may be painful for the patient after injury to the shoulder, but the physician usually can gain adequate abduction for this film. It allows visualization and localization of fractures of the humeral head as well as clearly demonstrating the presence or absence of a dislocation.

2. MULTIPLE VIEWS OF THE RADIAL HEAD (Fig. 12–67 A and B). If routine films are normal in a patient with localized pain over the radial head, multiple views from full pronation to full supination may be helpful in identifying an undisplaced fracture.

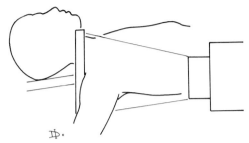

Figure 12–66   Axillary view of the shoulder.

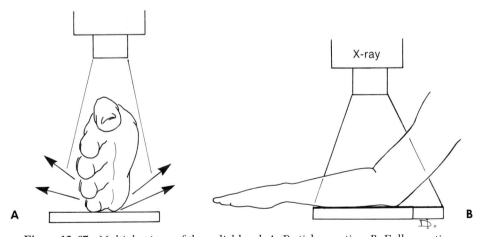

Figure 12–67   Multiple views of the radial head. *A*. Partial pronation. *B*. Full pronation.

3. NAVICULAR VIEW OF THE WRIST (Fig. 12–68). Fracture of the navicular is regularly overlooked on standard AP, lateral and oblique views of the wrist. Localized tenderness over the navicular should alert the primary physician to avoid the casual diagnosis of sprained wrist. The long axis of the navicular is brought into view in the special x-ray technique shown here. When a diagnosis of fracture of the carpal navicular is suspected, the patient should be treated in plaster for two to four weeks. A repeat navicular view is then obtained. If a fracture is present, resorption of the fracture site will have begun and recognition is no longer a problem. A prolonged period in a cast is required for healing, and surgery is occasionally required for nonunion.

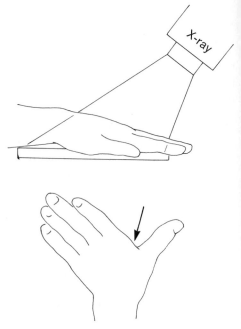

Figure 12–68 Navicular view of the wrist.

4. CARPAL TUNNEL VIEW OF THE WRIST (Fig. 12–69). The bony margins of the carpal canal can be clearly visualized on a roentgenogram by requesting a carpal tunnel view. Fractures of the hook of the hamate and the distal pole of the navicular come into view with this technique. The carpal tunnel view should be obtained in patients with pain localized in this area.

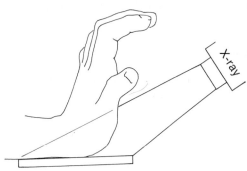

Figure 12–69 Carpal tunnel view of the wrist.

5. POSTERIOR OBLIQUE VIEW OF THE ACETABULUM (Fig. 12–70). This view aids in visualization of the posterior rim of the acetabulum when tomograms are not available to visualize a fracture dislocation of the hip.

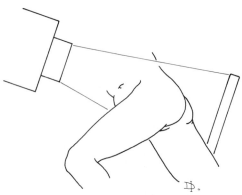

Figure 12–70 Posterior oblique view of the acetabulum.

6. PATELLAR OR SUNRISE VIEW OF THE KNEE (Fig. 12–71). A critical problem, after an acute dislocation of the patella, is the recognition of an osteochondral fracture of the medial facet of the patella. The relationship of the patella to the femoral condyle may also be useful in establishing the etiology of recurrent subluxation of the patella.

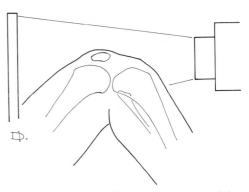

Figure 12–71 Patellar or sunrise view of the knee.

7. NOTCH VIEW OF THE KNEE (Fig. 12–72). The femoral condyles extend below and posterior to the intercondylar notch. Therefore, a loose body lodged in this area may block the motion of the knee but may not be seen clearly until the notch view is obtained.

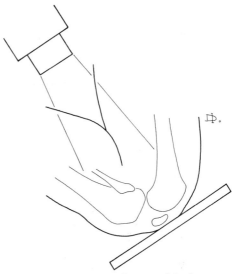

Figure 12–72 Notch view of the knee.

8. ANKLE MORTISE VIEW (Fig 12–73). This may be a routine view of the ankle in some hospitals. It demonstrates the relationship of the medial malleolus with the comma-shaped medial articular surface of the talus and the relationship of the distal tibial-fibular joint. An oblique view of the ankle nicely demonstrates the inferior sag of the anterior portion of a medial malleolus fracture.

9. X-RAY OF THE UNINJURED EXTREMITY. In children one must not forget that an x-ray of the uninjured extremity will show the normal relationship of the epiphysis, secondary ossification centers, apophysis and patterns of the epiphyseal plates, if there is any doubt about the normal anatomy.

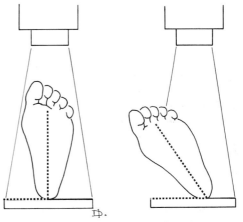

Figure 12–73 Ankle mortise view and oblique view of the ankle.

10. "FAT PAD SIGN" OF FRAC-
TURED ELBOW. A lateral x-ray of the
elbow that demonstrates a positive "fat
pad sign" (radiolucency posterior to
the olecranon fossa) (Fig. 12–74) indicates a bloody synovial effusion and
raises the physician's index of suspicion regarding fracture. If no fracture
is seen, repeat films two to three weeks
later may reveal the previously undetected fracture line.

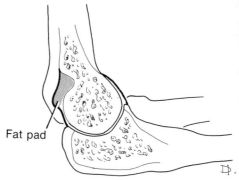

Figure 12–74   Lateral x-ray of the elbow.

Reduction

The second "R" of fracture therapy
refers to reduction of the fracture. The
primary physician must decide if reduction is necessary or possible. Obviously, the undisplaced fracture
needs no reduction, only protection
from loss of reduction.

FRACTURES NOT REQUIRING RE-
DUCTION. The following fractures
rarely need a formal reduction. The
first is a *comminuted fracture of the
calcaneus* which can rarely be reduced
satisfactorily.   Immediate   weight-
bearing is begun in a short leg walking
plaster, and triple arthrodesis is performed later if symptoms are prolonged and severe. The *metatarsal
shaft fracture* rarely requires reduction, because the soft tissues of the foot
maintain a satisfactory alignment and
rotation. The *clavicle fracture* maintains an intact sleeve of periosteum
and, though widely displaced, union is
expected to occur. The most common
fracture of the forearm of children, *a
torus fracture*, or outward buckling of
the cortex, does not require reduction.
This is also true of many *avulsion fractures* not involving the adjacent joint
function. Nondisplaced *stress fractures* do not require reduction.

INDICATIONS FOR OPEN REDUC-
TION. At the other end of the spectrum, generally speaking, fractures
that enter a joint cartilage surface or
cross a growing epiphyseal plate require not only reduction but open reduction. Open reduction and internal
fixation are required in many cases to
obtain and maintain an anatomical position.

METHODS. Traction in line with
the longitudinal axis of the long bone
is the most common method of reduction used in overcoming fracture deformity. This may cause the fracture to
lose its intrinsic stability, and retention of this position becomes difficult.

Analgesia is usually important in the
manipulations required to remove
fracture deformity. In many cases intravenous meperidine (Demerol) will
give satisfactory analgesia. Intravenous diazepam (Valium) depresses a patient to the point where some muscle
relaxation is obtained. Valium also produces temporary amnesia. This method is helpful in fractured tibia and
ankle fractures in the adult.

Fractures in the hand and foot are-
managed by digital block or injection
of lidocaine directly into the fracture
site.

I would like to suggest strongly that
IV block is a prompt, safe method of
anesthesia in the management of almost all closed upper extremity fractures in children and many adults.[4] It
is very satisfactory for outpatient use
(Fig. 12–75).

INTRAVENOUS BLOCK TECHNIQUE

A blood pressure cuff is secured to the arm. A small scalp vein needle with attached five cubic centimeter saline syringe is inserted into the most distal vein that can be found and taped into place, usually on the dorsum of the hand. The arm is elevated for two minutes, the tourniquet elevated to 200 millimeters of mercury. Lidocaine one-third per cent is then injected in a dose of 0.25 cc per pound of body weight (Fig. 12–75). The needle is removed. After five minutes anesthesia is complete. The fracture or dislocation is reduced and the plaster applied. The tourniquet is released. Normal sensation and motor function return within five minutes.

When there is adequate analgesia and a reduction is to be performed a primary physician must understand and be able to overcome fracture deformities that are not relieved with simple traction. I have found that, in a young child, the periosteum is torn at the apex of the fracture deformity and may remain intact on the concave surface (Fig. 12–76). In a completely overriding, displaced *forearm fracture* this intact periosteum prevents a reduction when longitudinal traction is used alone. It is essential to exaggerate the deformity, push the distal fragment until the intact periosteum is tight and bring the distal fragment into alignment with the proximal fragment. The fracture then hinges about the intact periosteum.

Metaphyseal fractures in the distal forearm or distal tibia in children commonly have rotational components. These require a specific rotational stress to bring about an anatomical reduction.

Intact collateral ligaments may stabilize a fracture fragment close to a joint. In the case of a transverse fracture of a proximal phalanx, the collateral ligaments of the metacarpal phalangeal joint of the index, long, ring or little finger allow no rotation or further flex-

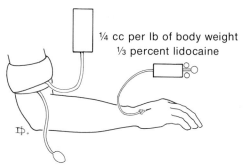

¼ cc per lb of body weight
⅓ percent lidocaine

Figure 12–75 IV bloc (intravenous lidocaine with arterial tourniquet).

ion of the proximal fragments when held in 90 degrees of flexion. The distal fragments can now be brought into alignment with it. The dressing can be applied and immobilization maintained in this position until the fracture is stable.

The use of *Chinese finger traps* on the thumb and index finger or great toe can be useful when no assistance is available to hold an arm or leg while a carefully molded plaster is applied.

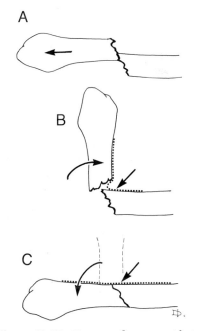

A

B

C

Figure 12–76 Forearm fracture with intact periosteum interfering with reduction.

Retention

The third "*R*" of fracture therapy includes the various methods of stabilizing the reduced fracture while healing takes place. Any immobilized part atrophies and new plaster dressings are indicated when looseness is apparent. The following types of retention are applied in the Emergency Room and are utilized until the fracture is stable enough to allow active exercises.

1. HANGING ARM PLASTER, MATERIALS:
    1. Two rolls of 4″ plaster of Paris
    2. Webril or sheet wadding
    3. Stockinette for cuff and collar
    4. Four safety pins

Application. (Fig. 12–77). The upper limit of the plaster does not have to reach the axilla or even extend above the fracture site but must immobilize the elbow at 90 degrees of flexion. The plaster extends distally across the wrist and palm but allows full metacarpal phalangeal motion. By shortening or lengthening the collar the angulation of the fracture is corrected in one plane. In the other plane angulation is corrected by moving the ring toward the palm or dorsal surface of the plaster. If more than two rolls of plaster are applied the weight may be excessive. This may serve to distract the fracture and is an undesirable feature of this technique. The patient must sleep sitting up in a chair the first few nights. Circumduction exercises are allowed early as pain subsides. When associated radial nerve palsies are present, active assist splints are applied to the plaster, helping to maintain contracture-free metacarpal phalangeal joints.

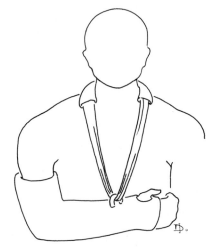

Figure 12–77   Hanging arm plaster.

2. PLASTER LEG CYLINDER. MATERIALS:
    1. Benzoin or Ace adherent spray to secure tape to skin
    2. 3″ white tape rolls
    3. Stockinette to fit closely over the leg from groin to ankle
    4. Webril or sheet wadding to pad and protect the leg
    5. Three rolls of 6″ or 8″ plastic dressing

Application (Fig. 12–78). The stockinette is applied from the groin to the
ankle. The lower half is turned and
pulled above the knee, exposing the
skin for application of the medial and
lateral tapes. The tape, cut long
enough to be turned back into the plaster when it is applied, prevents piston-
ing of the cylinder, a key feature in the
successful use of this dressing.

3. SHORT LEG WALKING PLASTER
DRESSING. MATERIALS:
1. Stockinette
2. Sheet wadding or Webril to
   protect bony prominences
3. Three rolls of 4″ plaster and
   two rolls of 4″ plaster
4. Walking rubber heel

Application (Fig. 12–79). Stockinette is first applied from the knee to the
toes. This is covered by additional
sheet wadding or Webril to protect the
malleolus, the heel and the peroneal
nerve as it crosses superficial to the
head of the fibula. This is uniformly
covered with the rolls of plaster dressing from the tibial tubercle to the metatarsal phalangeal joint of the foot. A
support under the forefoot during the
application of the plaster helps maintain the ankle in neutral position and
allows additional molding while the
plaster is setting. The stockinette is
folded back over the upper and lower
margins of the plaster and these margins are buried in plaster. The walking
heel is applied to the plaster in a line
extending from the anterior surface of
the tibia distally. Twenty-four hours
later the plaster is dry and weight-
bearing can be allowed. This utility
dressing is safe in wet climates if a
plastic bag is put over the entire cast
and secured just below the knee.

4. LONG LEG WALKING PLASTER
DRESSING. MATERIALS:
1. Stockinette
2. Sheet wadding or Webril to
   protect bony prominences
3. Three rolls of 4″ plaster, two
   rolls of 6″ plaster and two rolls
   of 8″ plaster
4. Walking rubber heel

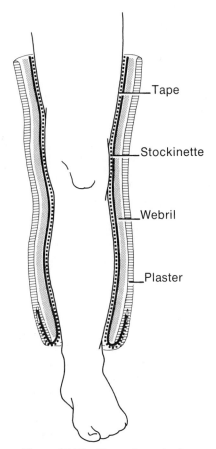

Figure 12–78   Plaster leg cylinder.

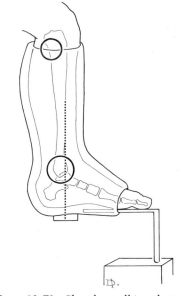

Figure 12–79   Short leg walking plaster dressing.

Application (Fig. 12–80). While the plaster is being applied for an acute tibial shaft fracture, reduction and retention of the fracture can be obtained if the knee is flexed 90 degrees and the leg hangs over the end of the table with gravity assisting in aligning the fragments. While the plaster hardens, the upper limits of this portion of the plaster can be narrowed and compressed in the AP direction. The knee is then extended to neutral and the thigh portion added with a smooth junction between upper and lower segments. Anterior-posterior molding at the knee while the upper portion hardens assures good contact and the immobilization that is needed for the comfortable early weight-bearing. A heel and sole lift on the opposite shoe adds to a more balanced gait. When the leg is to be protected from weight-bearing a bent knee plaster is recommended. This type of dressing makes crutch walking and sitting more comfortable. The emphasis, in either case, must be to extend the stockinette, padding and plaster high on the thigh to assure adequate immobilization of the knee.

5. OVERHEAD OLECRANON SKELE-
TAL TRACTION. MATERIALS:
1. Sterile Steinmann pin set, gloves and towel
2. Sling
3. Traction bow
4. Ropes, pulley, weights
5. Syringes and needles for lidocaine injection

Application (Fig. 12–81). The primary physician frequently must initiate skeletal traction in the Emergency Room, particularly in the widely displaced humeral fracture and the supracondylar fracture of the humerus in children. This technique will both reduce and retain the fracture. The insertion of wires for skeletal traction is carried out under sterile conditions. The skin is prepped with iodophor and draped with four towels, and the skin, muscles and periosteum are infiltrated with lidocaine. The Steinmann pin is

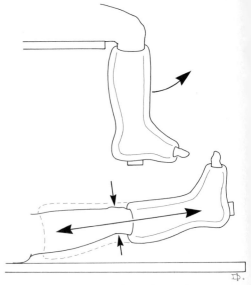

Figure 12–80 Long leg walking plaster dressing.

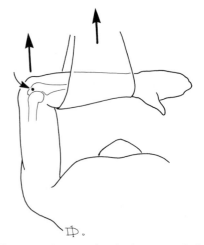

Figure 12–81 Overhead olecranon skeletal traction.

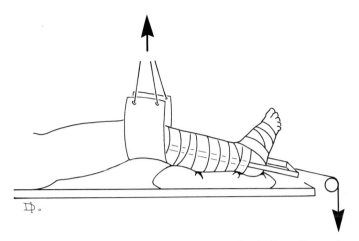

Figure 12–82   Buck's extension traction and split Russel's traction.

inserted from the ulnar side to avoid damaging the ulnar nerve, drilling the wire across two cortexes and the medullary canal and placing it close to the long axis of the humerus to avoid extending the elbow when traction is applied. A soft sling balances the forearm and supports the wrist. The elevation obviously aids in reducing swelling.

6. BUCK'S EXTENSION TRACTION AND SPLIT RUSSELL'S TRACTION FOR CHILDREN. MATERIALS:
    1. Ace wrap
    2. Moleskin and ventform traction tape
    3. Ropes, pulleys, weights, slings

Application (Fig. 12–82). Skin traction is applied in the Emergency Room prior to admitting the patient to the ward. In an adult with an intertrochanteric fracture or femoral neck fracture, Buck's extension traction will help reduce pain and muscle spasm when the leg is secured by the traction. The traction should not exceed five or six pounds because the skin will blister or the traction become loosened from the leg and slide down around the ankle.

The knee sling is added for children with femoral shaft fractures, lifting the thigh from the bed. This allows a vector force to come directly in line with the femur. Reduction of the fracture will then gradually occur.

The application of skin traction is successful if moleskin or a ventilated, spongy, hard-backed tape is available. This material is secured to the skin by an elastic wrap applied carefully, protecting the skin from blistering over the malleolus and the heel. The elastic bandage is wrapped gently over the proximal fibula to avoid a peroneal palsy.

Restoration of Function

Restoration of function begins immediately after retention is applied. Edema and excessive swelling can be averted by elevating the extremity, decreasing risk of ischemia in the muscles of the hands and feet. Constant, prolonged elevation of the injured extremity is most important. Adequate elevation at night is assured with a simple sling applied on the upper extremity (Fig. 12–83). For elevation during the day the ambulatory patient is instructed to carry his hand on top of his head (Fig. 12–84). This is done for approximately one week. It frequently averts the need for bivalving the plaster. In the lower extremity a sling is suspended from the overhead bed frame (Fig.12–85) which supports the plaster dressing. This supports the leg and foot at least two feet above the level of the chest.

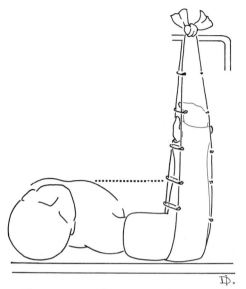

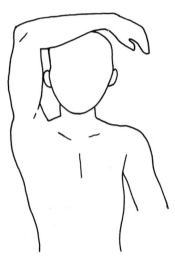

Figure 12–83 Elevation at night with a simple sling.

Figure 12–84 Elevation during the day with hand on head.

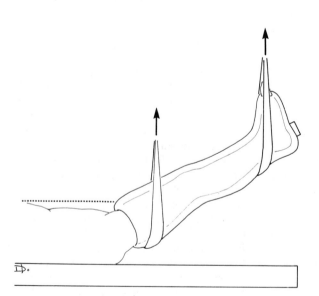

Figure 12–85 Elevation of the lower extremity from the bed frame.

Active motion of the muscles in an injured extremity should begin as soon as possible. When possible, circumduction or pendulum exercises should be used in all upper extremity fractures to obviate shoulder stiffness by preventing adhesions in the subdeltoid bursa (Fig. 12–86). In the lower extremity a walking plaster allows continued and constant motion of muscles and joints. This has been dramatically useful in the closed walking management of fractured tibia, as described in the tibial fracture section.

In the extremity with nerve deficit, full passive motion of joints is useful to prevent edema and contractures. Joint immobility is maintained and paralyzed muscles are not excessively stressed.

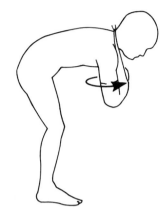

Figure 12–86 Circumduction or pendulum exercises for upper extremity fractures.

The duration of immobilization of a fracture is not decided on the first day. Changes in the plaster are necessary as swelling or atrophy progress. I use direct palpation of the fracture site for assistance in the decision as to when to discard the plaster. Local motion, pain or edema indicates replacement of the plaster. The roentgenogram cannot be relied upon completely because frequently only minimal callus can be seen when the fracture is stable enough to begin adjacent joint motion. Fractures of the clavicle, olecranon, carpal navicular and phalanges are typical examples of fractures in which clinical judgment dictates the length of immobilization in plaster.

SPECIFIC FRACTURES

Scapula (Fig. 12–87)

A severe, direct blow to the shoulder region is required to fracture the scapula. This bone is mobile and well protected by the 17 muscles that originate or insert here. Underlying rib fractures must not be overlooked. Few fractures of the scapula require more than sling immobilization and early active exercises for the shoulder girdle. The return of function is usually quicker than expected. On the other hand, a down-

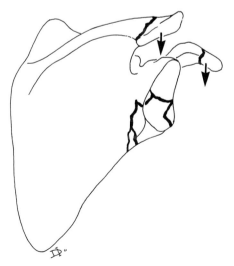

Figure 12–87 Scapula fractures.

ward displaced fracture of the acromial process may impede function of the rotator cuff. This will require elevation and internal fixation. The widely displaced intra-articular (glenoid) fracture is a rare injury, occurring mainly in young patients, and may necessitate reduction.

Clavicle (Fig. 12–88 A)

The fractured clavicle in children may be severely displaced but will usually retain a sleeve of periosteum between the proximal and distal fragment. Union proceeds without incident along this periosteal sleeve if the patient is treated symptomatically with a figure-of-eight dressing (Fig. 12–88 B) until the fracture is stable by clinical examination. The roentgenographical evidence of solid union requires a prolonged period of time.

In the adult the displaced fracture of the clavicle has classically been managed by a figure-of-eight dressing. Open reduction has been followed by a high rate of nonunion. Damage to the closely approximated neurovascular bundle is rare, but the possibility is greater when the first and second ribs are also fractured. A fracture extending obliquely through the distal third of the clavicle requires open reduction. The distal clavical fragment is held securely in the acromioclavicular joint by the coracoclavicular ligaments. The proximal fragment swings into severe elevation through the trapezius and lies beneath the skin, simulating an acromioclavicular separation. In children the distal clavicle may break out of its periosteal sleeve and rest beneath the skin. Closure of this periosteum about the displaced clavicle is sufficient treatment for this condition.

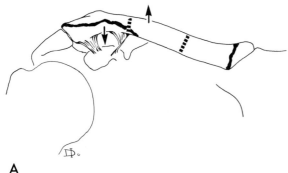

A

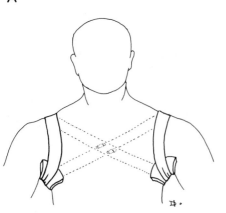

B

Figure 12–88 Clavicle fracture. *A*. Fracture lines. *B*. Figure-of-eight dressing.

Humerus (Fig. 12–89)

The *greater tuberosity* may be displaced by the glenoid rim at the time of an anterior dislocation or subluxation of the shoulder. The attached portion of the rotator cuff containing teres minor, infraspinatus and supraspinatus will also be displaced. After reduction of the shoulder, a return of the tuberosity to its normal position should be demonstrated on two x-ray views. This proves that the cuff is not significantly torn. The injury is managed with a stockinette sling for four to six weeks, allowing bone and soft tissue healing to take place. On the other hand, the rotator cuff may be torn significantly in the direction of its fibers, beginning at the bicipital groove and extending toward the muscle fibers of the supraspinatus. In this case, the displaced greater tuberosity fracture does not return to an anatomical position, but remains posterior to the humerus. This requires open reduction and suturing of the rotator cuff.

The *lesser tuberosity fracture* of the humerus with its attached portion of the rotator cuff containing the subscapularis is occasionally displaced with posterior dislocation of the shoulder. If the displaced fragment is satisfactorily reduced a stockinette sling is the recommended treatment.

The *humeral head* is subject to anterior and posterior infractures, in conjunction with anterior and posterior dislocations of the shoulder. The glenoid rim, after producing this infracture, may become locked in the defect and make reduction of the shoulder more difficult. The axillary x-ray view is helpful in recognizing this injury. Operative treatment is not suggested for these defects unless the patient develops recurrent dislocations of the shoulder. The rare isolated *anatomical neck fracture* which leaves the head free of its attachments may require reduction if displacement is significant.

SURGICAL NECK OF HUMERUS. A stable fracture without displacement is

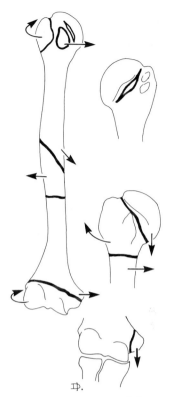

Figure 12–89 Humeral fractures.

frequently seen in the osteoporotic patient. A simple sling and early circumduction exercises are encouraged in these patients. If there is angulation and only 50 per cent displacement I place the patient in a light, hanging arm plaster. This is done because attempts at closed reduction often fail or create an unstable situation. Complete range of motion is not expected after union of the fracture, but pain is minimized by active early circumduction and external rotation exercises. Angular deformities frequently recur after closed reduction. If there is complete displacement the pectoralis major muscle is the deforming force and cannot often be dealt with except by olecranon skeletal overhead traction or open reduction.

A shoulder spica may be adequate when applied by those experienced in plaster work but this method is not recommended for routine outpatient use.

The correct alignment of a metaphyseal slip cannot be determined by x-ray in children younger than about four years of age, before the proximal secondary ossification centers of the humerus appear. In these patients the physician must depend upon the rotator cuff locking the epiphysis in an elevated position. The shoulder is swung into the pivotal position by lifting the humerus 180 degrees to a point where the arm is touching the ear and the forearm is rested on top of the head. Traction is applied. Reduction is obtained and the previously placed olecranon skeletal traction wire maintains the arm and shoulder slightly above the salute position. The child is kept in a supine position for two weeks.

The teenager with a mildly proximal angulated metaphyseal slip can be treated comfortably with a hanging arm plaster. Complete reduction is not expected. The double shadow of the epiphyseal plate in a young child may be mistaken for a fracture.

HUMERUS SHAFT FRACTURES. Fractures in the proximal, middle and distal thirds of the humerus need not be classified as to their complexity. Gentle traction will reduce the angulation and a light, hanging arm plaster will maintain a satisfactory reduction if applied and managed correctly. (See section on hanging arm plaster technique.) Soft tissue interposition may prevent reduction of displacement. Inferior subluxation of the head of the humerus is commonly recognized during treatment but resolves itself when immobilization is discontinued. Mild angular deformities can be accepted. Two to three months may be required for adequate callus to mature and stabilize the fracture before immobilization is discontinued.

SUPRACONDYLAR FRACTURE. The minimally displaced or angulated supracondylar fracture is frequently accompanied by an inordinate amount of swelling. Outpatient care is indicated only when an adequately applied posterior splint with a tight collar and cuff can be used. The displaced fracture is dramatic because of the deformity and hemorrhage which follow the injury. The radial and median nerves are frequently contused and the radial pulse may be absent. An axillary block or general anesthesia is utilized when swelling is not excessive. Reduction is accomplished by holding the patient's hand as if to shake it and then extending the elbow and applying longitudinal traction to dislodge the proximal humeral fragment from the brachialis muscle. The physician's fingertips are placed on the distal humeral fragment. Traction is maintained, the elbow is flexed and the distal fragment is pushed forward. The elbow is held in at least 110 degrees of flexion to stabilize the fracture and an x-ray is obtained. Rotation allows unacceptable varus and valgus angulation at the fracture site. If manual reduction is not anatomical or if swelling is excessive, overhead olecranon pin traction is applied to accomplish reduction and maintain a satisfactory alignment. Many of these fractures can be reduced and maintained using a posterior splint with short collar and cuff. At least 24 hours of observation in the hospital will usually permit an early detection of vascular insufficiency to the forearm. Prompt extension of the elbow and consideration of vascular exploration follows. Similar guidelines are appropriate in the adult patient with a displaced fracture.

The *medial epicondyle* is a traction apophysis which serves not only as the origin of the superficial forearm flexor muscle group but also as the proximal attachment of the medial collateral ligament of the elbow. Simple distal displacement of the fragment should be treated by immobilization. It will heal with a fibrous union which is free of epiphyseal plate disturbance and ulnar nerve symptoms. If the medial aspect of the joint is opened, as in a dislocation or extreme valgus deformity of the elbow, the fragment may come to rest in the joint. Removal is then required.

The adjacent trochlea with its irregular ossification center can be mistaken for a fracture. The opposite elbow should be x-rayed for comparison.

The lateral condylar fracture extends into the articular surface of the capitellum or as far medially as the trochlea. It requires an anatomical reduction to prevent permanent deformity of the elbow. Closed reductions usually fail and are not recommended.

Forearm (Fig. 12–90)

The outpatient care of radial or ulnar shaft fractures in adults is recommended only for stable undisplaced fractures. A long arm plaster is applied to prevent pronation and supination of the forearm which may lead to loss of reduction.

A displaced, unstable fracture of both bones of the forearm in an adult cannot be managed on an outpatient basis because reduction cannot be maintained in plaster. Open reduction and internal fixation with compression plates is recommended.

The rule about obtaining roentgenograms of the joint above and below the fracture applies also in the forearm. Dislocation of the radial head with an ulnar shaft fracture and dislocation of the distal ulna with an isolated fracture of the radius must not be overlooked. These associated dislocations necessitate internal fixation of single bone fractures in the forearm.

The isolated significantly displaced fracture of either the radial shaft or ulnar shaft is best treated by plate fixation, as union of the ulna may be delayed and nonunion of the radius leaves the forearm with significant loss of function.

The *Colles' fracture* (Fig. 12–91) with its associated ulnar styloid avulsion presents a challenge in the last "R" of fracture therapy, restoration of function. In the elderly osteoporotic patient the reduction is gained under IV lidocaine block, by traction and volar displacement of the comminuted distal radial fragment. Then, with the elbow flexed to 90 degrees, a ten-layer

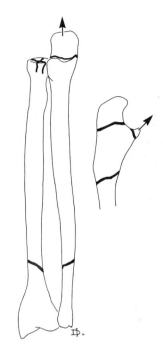

Figure 12–90   Forearm fractures.

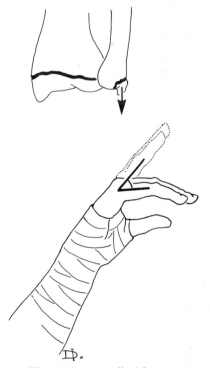

Figure 12–91   Colles' fracture.

splint, previously measured, cut and moistened, is placed inside a stockinette. The splint extends to the metacarpal phalangeal joint on the dorsum of the hand. It is brought around the elbow and then up along the volar surface of the forearm to reach the midpalmar area. The thumb and metacarpal phalangeal joints have complete freedom for active and passive motion. The wrist is in twenty degrees of flexion and ten degrees of ulnar deviation; too much flexion precipitates a median nerve compression. A mildly tight elastic wrap secures the splints to the arm and hand, which must be immediately and continuously elevated. The patient is given a night splint to maintain hand elevation during the sleeping hours. The Ace wrap is adjusted to secure uniform pressure as the hand and forearm swell or edema subsides. Immediate active finger and shoulder motion is started.

Perfect initial reduction may be lost in the elderly patient owing to the comminuted metaphyseal fragments. As swelling decreases better immobilization is obtained by a short arm circular plaster that is removed after five or six weeks. Restoration of function is stressed to the patient at all times. The young patient who has this fracture extending into the wrist joint needs a careful anatomical reduction maintained by skeletal wires in the second and third metacarpal and proximal ulna or radius. Open reduction may be indicated

FOREARM FRACTURES IN CHILDREN. The undisplaced fracture without angulation becomes a simple matter of applying a short arm, well-molded plaster dressing and waiting for sufficient mature callus formation before removal of the plaster. A torus fracture or outward buckling of the cortex falls into the above category. It is the most frequent forearm fracture in children.

Children with angulated and displaced forearm fractures are managed as outpatients. Satisfactory reductions are obtained if analgesia is complete.

This has been accomplished in our Emergency Room by the use of IV lidocaine block in closed fractures and dislocations of the forearm.

The *distal radial epiphyseal slip* in a child's forearm is a fracture along the zone of provisional calcification, frequently with a small metaphyseal fragment remaining attached to the dorsal surface of the epiphysis. The physician must use some care to avoid further damage to the epiphyseal plate. After satisfactory dense anesthesia, traction is applied in the direction of the distal fragment to loosen the two fragments. Increasing the deformity may be necessary. Then with direct pressure over the distal radial epiphysis (Fig. 12–92)

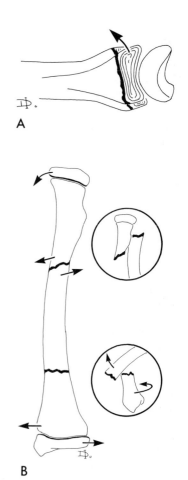

Figure 12–92   Radial fractures. *A.* Distal radial epiphyseal fracture in children. *B.* Other fractures of the radius.

and traction on the hand, the wrist is brought into extreme flexion. Usually the epiphysis then slides back toward its normal position. Mild angular deformity and displacement are acceptable and are often advisable, since repeated manipulation may injure the epiphyseal plate. A well-molded short arm plaster will maintain this stable reduction. Immobilization for four to six weeks allows stable healing.

FRACTURE OF BOTH BONES OF THE FOREARM. Marked deformity is observed in angulated and completely displaced fractures at the middle and distal thirds of the forearm. After dense analgesia by IV lidocaine, a series of three maneuvers is performed. First, the fracture deformity is increased to 90 degrees of angulation. Second, mild traction is applied and the physician's thumb is placed at the apex or concavity of the deformity. The distal fragment is then moved distally to correct displacement and obtain adequate length. Third, the distal fragment is brought into alignment with the proximal fragment, the intact portion of the periosteum being used here as a hinge. After reduction it lends some stability to the fracture. The postreduction roentgenogram allows comparison of the thickness of the cortex proximal and distal to the fracture site, a discrepancy indicating rotational deformity that is unacceptable. Then the patient is placed in a long arm plaster with the forearm in a neutral position regarding pronation and supination. Eight to twelve weeks is usually an adequate period of immobilization. Weekly roentgenograms are obtained to check for recurrence of angular deformity.

Fractures of both bones in the proximal one third of the forearm in children tend to angulate and open reduction may be required.

The volarly angulated undisplaced *fracture of the junction of the middle and distal one third of the radius* in a child can present a problem in retention. Reduction is easily performed

with IV block analgesia but often the fracture will tend to reangulate when the reducing force is removed. By overcorrecting the deformity the physician can snap the intact periosteum, or may place the forearm in full pronation and apply a well-molded long arm plaster. Both may aid in preventing recurrence of deformity. Weekly check films alert the physician to recurrence of deformity.

A radial neck fracture in a child with an angular deformity of less than 20 degrees is usually acceptable. Reduction is accomplished by direct pressure on the head of the radius associated with pronation and supination of the forearm. When the angular deformity is more than 50 degrees open reduction is necessary. Do not remove the radial head in children.

Wrist (Fig. 12–93)

NAVICULAR. A young adult who has fallen on his outstretched hand will frequently present with pain in the wrist. A normal x-ray may lead to the erroneous diagnosis of a "sprained wrist." This patient should be placed in a short arm plaster for two to three weeks and the x-ray repeated out of plaster. Navicular views should be obtained. If a fracture is present, bone resorption will have occurred and the fracture will be visible for the first time. After the fracture has been recognized and the absence of displacement has been verified, a short arm plaster should be applied with thumb, index

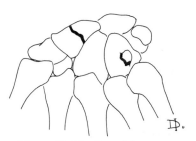

Figure 12–93 Carpal fractures.

and long finger immobilized. This will give adequate stability for healing. Prolonged plaster immobilization may be required to establish union. Aseptic necrosis of the proximal fragment usually leads to limited wrist motion with pain at extremes if it is not promptly replaced by living bone. Wrist fusion may follow if symptoms are severe. Navicular fracture, when associated with a perilunar dislocation, may require internal fixation to stabilize the fracture during healing.

HAMATE. The hook of the hamate can be fractured at its base. The carpal tunnel view will demonstrate the fracture. Simple recognition and immobilization are all that is usually required.

TRIQUETRUM. A fracture of this bone results from a direct blow or in association with a transnavicular perilunar dislocation. Simple plaster immobilization is suggested.

Femur (Fig. 12–94)

Fractures of the femur in children and adults are not routinely handled on an outpatient basis. These fractures have a large associated blood loss and considerable pain with motion. It is almost mandatory to handle them in a hospital, where portable x-rays are easily obtained and prolonged traction and bed care are available.

Small chip or avulsion fractures are the only femoral fractures that can be treated in the outpatient department.

Patella (Fig. 12–95)

Most *patella fractures* result from a direct blow to the anterior aspect of the knee. If the articular surface is undisplaced and the adjacent extensor retinaculum is intact we place these patients in plaster cylinders and start early weight-bearing. After four to five weeks the fracture is united and qua-

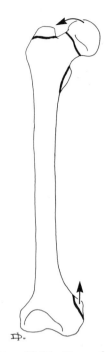

Figure 12–94   Femur fractures.

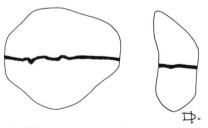

Figure 12–95   Patella fracture.

driceps exercises are begun. The bipartate patella may be mistaken for a fresh fracture when there is a fibrous union in the upper outer quadrant between the patella and smaller secondary ossification center.

Widely displaced or highly comminuted fractures are treated by patellectomy, plaster and early weight-bearing.

Tibia (Fig. 12–96)

TIBIAL PLATEAU. Anterior tibial spine fractures result from avulsion of bone by the anterior cruciate ligament. If extension of the knee brings the fragment back to its normal position a plaster cylinder is adequate treatment. Open reduction may be advisable if displacement is not reduced. The posterior cruciate ligament occasionally avulses a piece of bone from the posterior aspect of the tibial plateau, but more often the ligament is torn at its tibial attachment.

A fracture downward from the tibial articular surface into the *tibial plateau* without significant displacement is protected by a plaster cylinder dressing until soft tissues heal. Progressive active motion is then initiated. Protection from weight-bearing is necessary for six weeks in an unstable fracture. Since minimally displaced, simple fractures can be associated with extreme swelling and hemorrhage, careful observation is most important.

Associated collateral ligament injuries of the knee are common with tibial plateau fractures. A small avulsion chip fragment along the lateral tibial plateau and on the proximal fibula suggests a disruption of the lateral collateral ligament and iliotibial band. The younger patient with spreading of the plateaus or downward displacement of one plateau is treated by open reduction, followed by a cast brace to allow early motion and weight-bearing.

TIBIAL SHAFT. Closed fracture of

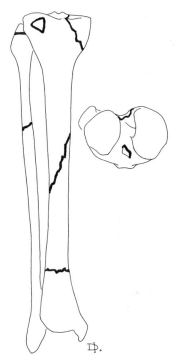

Figure 12–96 Tibial fractures.

the shaft of the tibia is reduced in the Emergency Room and the patient is hospitalized to assure that elevation is maintained and swelling is not excessive, and to allow early weight-bearing under the direction of a physical therapist.

To obtain the reduction the supine patient is moved toward the end of the cart far enough to allow 90 degrees of knee flexion. The knee is allowed to flex over the end of the cart with the foot hanging free. The patient is given IV Valium and Demerol. After the fracture is reduced by traction on the foot, gravity maintains the reduction while the operator wraps the plaster dressing over two layers of sheet wadding. The ankle is maintained in a neutral position for most fractures. An equinus position of the foot helps prevent posterior angulation in the skier's boottop fracture. While the plaster sets, anterior and posterior pressure is applied to the plaster just below the knee, molding and narrowing it around the proximal portion of the tibia. This accomplished, the knee is extended to a straight position, avoiding hyperextension. The thigh and knee portions of the long leg plaster are then applied, molding carefully in the anterior posterior direction just below the patella. A walking heel is applied. There may be up to one-half of an inch of shortening, which is acceptable. However, angulation must be corrected by wedging the plaster. During the first few days the patient experiences intermittent dependent pain as he begins partial weight-bearing with crutches, which are usually discarded during the third week. This long leg walking plaster is usually replaced in about two months by a short leg walking plaster. Most adults are removed from plaster after approximately three months.

Ankle

LATERAL MALLEOLUS (Fig. 12–97). Our most common lower extremity fracture is an isolated oblique distal fibula fracture. The fracture line is below the ankle anteriorly, then proceeds obliquely proximally and posteriorly. Lateral x-rays demonstrate the degree of displacement. There may be an associated medial ankle ligament injury. Reduction is accomplished with the patient sitting or lying on the edge of the cart. The involved leg hangs free in front of the operator with the knee flexed to 90 degrees. Reduction is accomplished by inverting the foot to tighten the lateral ligament and displace the distal fibular fragment distally. The operator's fingertips are then placed behind the distal fibula fragment and it is pulled forward and internally rotated to its former position. The forefoot is rested upon a support to prevent inversion and equinus when plaster is applied. The operator then has two free hands with which to apply the plaster and maintain the fibular reduction. A short leg plaster dressing is applied with a walking

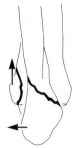

Figure 12–97   Lateral malleolus fractures.

heel. A postreduction film is obtained and walking is encouraged as early as possible. The plaster is left on for six weeks. Nonunion is rare.

POSTERIOR MALLEOLUS. Vertical fracture of the posterior lip of the tibia is seen alone or in combination with other ankle fractures. The articular cartilage does not reach the posterior edge of the tibia and therefore, a large fragment must be present before the fracture line extends into the ankle mortise. Displacement can frequently be improved by local pressure or by carrying the great toe into extreme dorsiflexion. When there is upward displacement of the fragment which includes more than one-third of the articular surface, open reduction is recommended.

MEDIAL MALLEOLUS (Fig. 12–98). Medial malleolus fractures which enter the ankle joint at the shoulder of the mortise remove the medial stability of the joint and create

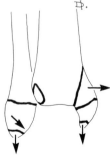

Figure 12–98   Medial malleolus fractures.

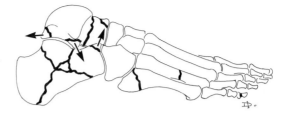

Figure 12–99 Fractures of the foot.

an irregular cartilage surface if they are not anatomically reduced. The infolded periosteum prevents an anatomical closed reduction. The anterior opening of the fracture line can often be improved by holding the foot in dorsiflexion before plaster application, and therefore open reduction and internal fixation are given favorable consideration in all displaced medial malleolus fractures that cannot be reduced anatomically.

Foot

CALCANEAL FRACTURES (Fig. 12–99). A calcaneal fracture most often follows a fall from a height. The bone has a thin cortex not suitable for internal fixation. I routinely apply a short leg walking plaster and begin weight-bearing as soon as tolerated. Weight-bearing will allow the remainder of the tissues in the leg and foot to maintain function and reduce atrophy while the fracture heals. The involvement of the subtalar joint often precipitates degenerative arthritis and fusion may be required. Also, following these fractures the normal lever arm of the tendo Achillis is altered and the patient has a persistent limp.

These patients must also be checked for an associated compression fracture of the spine.

TALUS. Most fractures of the talus follow dorsiflexion or plantar flexion injuries. After traumatic plantar flexion of the ankle, the posterior tubercle of the talus is fractured from the body. Simple walking plaster is applied and no reduction is necessary. The neck of the talus is frequently fractured in dorsiflexion injuries. The subtalar joint is

disrupted with displacement of the neck. A closed reduction may bring about the necessary anatomical reduction by bringing the foot into extreme equinus. After a dorsiflexion injury the lateral process may be fractured. Other small chip fractures are frequently seen. A short leg, nonweight-bearing plaster is used in these cases until fracture union occurs. Occasionally, open reduction and internal fixation may be indicated to maintain an anatomical reduction. If the neck fracture is displaced and associated with dislocation of the body of the talus from the ankle joint, attempts at closed reduction are unsuccessful. Aseptic necrosis complicates the management of displaced fractures of the neck of the talus.

METATARSAL. Transverse fracture of the base of the fifth metatarsal is the most common fracture of the metatarsals. It follows an inversion injury and avulsion of the tip of the metatarsal by the peroneus brevis tendon. Adequate, comfortable treatment is achieved with a short leg walking plaster for four weeks. Painless nonunion frequently follows treatment.

REFERENCES

1. Blount, W. P.: Fractures in Children. Baltimore, Williams and Wilkins Co., 1955.
2. Charnley, J.: Closed Treatment of Common Fractures. Baltimore, Williams and Wilkins Co., 1967.
3. Hawkins, L. G., Pomerantz, M. and Eiseman, B.: Laparotomy at time of pelvic fracture. J. Trauma, 10:619–623, 1970.
4. Hawkins, L. G., Storey, S. D. and Wells, G. G.: Intravenous lidocaine anesthesia for upper extremity fractures and dislocations. J. Bone Joint Surg., 52A:1647–1650, 1970.
5. Miles, J. S.: Basic principles of fracture therapy. Surg. Clin. North Am., 41:1453–1462, 1961.

Orthopaedics 13

AUGUSTUS A. WHITE, III, M.D., D. Med. Sci.,
and PETER JOKL, M.D.

8. Fatigue fracture of the tibia or fibula
C. *Knee and upper leg*
   1. Dislocated fibula
   2. Bursitis of the knee
   3. Semimembranosus bursitis (Baker's cyst)
   4. Idiopathic osteoarthritis of the knee
   5. Rupture of the quadriceps mechanism
   6. Stress fracture of the distal femur
   7. Myalgia paresthetica
D. *Hip*
   1. Trochanteric bursitis
   2. Iliopectineal bursitis
   3. Ischial bursitis ("weaver's bottom")
   4. Fatigue fracture of the hip
   5. Arthritis of the hip
E. *Upper Limb*
   1. Bursitis of the shoulder
   2. Supraspinatus syndrome
   3. Rupture of the rotator cuff
   4. Fibrous ankylosis of the shoulder (frozen shoulder)
   5. Bicipital tendinitis
   6. Arthritis of the shoulder
   7. Recurrent shoulder disloca- tion
   8. Recurrent posterior dis- location of the shoulder
   9. Suprascapular nerve irritation
   10. Rupture of the proximal biceps tendon
   11. Rupture of the distal biceps tendon
F. *Elbow*
   1. Olecranon bursitis
   2. Lateral epicondylitis (tennis elbow)
   3. Medial epicondylitis (golfer's elbow)
   4. Total elbow prosthesis
G. *Wrist*
   1. Stenosing tenosynovitis (DeQuervain's disease)
   2. Arthritis of the wrist
   3. Carpal tunnel syndrome

4. Ganglion
5. Ulnar tunnel syndrome
6. Avascular necrosis of the lunate (Kienböck's disease)
7. Navicular fracture
H. *Soft tissue injuries*
I. *Spine*
   1. Problems of neck-shoulder- arm syndrome
   2. Cervical spondylosis
   3. Acute herniated cervical disk
   4. Cervicothoracic outlet syndromes
   5. Cervical ribs
   6. Scalenus anticus (anterior scalene) syndrome
   7. Costoclavicular syndrome
   8. Hyperabduction syndrome
   9. Reflex sympathetic dys- trophy
   10. Differential diagnosis of neck-shoulder-arm pain
   11. Whiplash
   12. Scoliosis
   13. Anklyosing spondylitis
   14. Low back pain with or without sciatica
      a. Group I. Acute low back pain (0–3 weeks) with or without radiation into the leg
      b. Group II. Subacute low back pain (3 weeks–6 months) with or without sciatica
      c. Group III. Chronic low back pain (6 months) with or without radia- tion into the leg
      d. Group IV. Chronic low back pain (6 months) with one or more lum- bar spinal operations
   15. Spondylolysis and Spondylolisthesis
   16. Coccydynia
   17. Camptocormia
   18. Spinal Orthoses
J. *Comment*

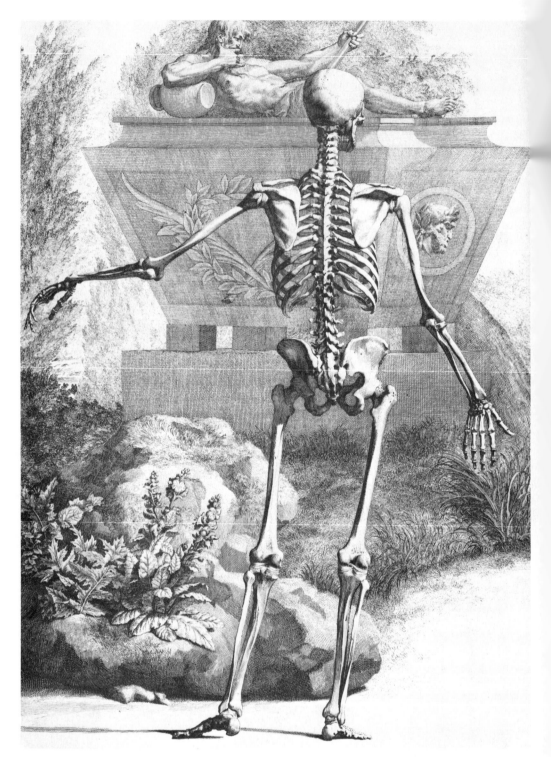

Figure 13–1   This eighteenth century art work by Albinus symbolizes the musculoskeletal system. Approximately one-third of patients who seek medical care have symptoms involving this system. (Bernhard Siegfried Albinus [1697–1770]. Tabulae Sceleti et Musculorum—Corporis Humani. Leiden, J & H Verbeek, 1747. Courtesy of The Francis A. Countway Library of Medicine.)

INTRODUCTION

In this chapter we will present an overview of the general management of some frequently encountered problems of the musculoskeletal system. The entities are selected from the perspective of orthopaedic specialists to provide information that will be useful for both the patient and the physician. Some are included because knowledge about them avoids trouble or decreases the likelihood of a missed diagnosis. Other entities are discussed because we have noted them to be mismanaged by nonorthopaedic surgeons.

In most instances the material is presented in the outline form shown in Table 13–1. The disease and a brief statement of the problem are given, followed by a section on clinical evaluation. A "typical" history is included whenever it is feasible. The most important physical findings and laboratory studies are included. The complete workup requires an assessment of the patient's general health from the clinical history, followed by an appropriate physical examination. Obviously, in some situations the routine laboratory studies will be either unnecessary or inadequate. Special diagnostic studies are discussed briefly where applicable. The clinical section is followed by a section on management. The advice given includes guidelines regarding important information to be communicated to patients about their problems. It is impossible, however, to indicate the specific information that should be given to a particular patient.

To review the use of some of these comments and guidelines: Provide a comprehensive but uncomplicated explanation of the disease process to the patient. Tell the patient what, if anything, he can do to help himself. Always search to find and communicate whatever realistic reassurance can

TABLE 13–1 Basic Outline of Presentation of Diseases

The Problem
Clinical Evaluation
    History
    Physical examination
    Routine laboratory studies
    Special studies
Management
    Advice to patient
    Medications and nonsurgical orthopaedics
    Surgery
Discussion

be offered. Anticipate patients' questions and anxieties. Remarks such as the following can sometimes be very important: "This problem is not due to cancer"... "Even though you are uncomfortable and in pain now, your condition is not caused by a serious disease"... "In due time you will be able to go back to your athletics, hobbies, work, etc."... "Even though you've had this problem before, it's not a chronic disease"... "Your back is giving you a lot of trouble, but it won't make you paralyzed"... "You have a type of arthritis, but it's not the kind that will put you in a wheelchair." Suggestions about specific medications and nonsurgical methods are followed by a brief discussion of surgical considerations. The final section includes a variety of miscellaneous items such as interesting facts about the disease, differential diagnosis and special factors.

We believe that this disease/problem-oriented type of presentation will be convenient and useful to the reader who is evaluating a particular patient. We will sometimes vary the format when the material can be better presented in another manner. This occurs in the sections on toeing-in, on neck-shoulder-arm pain and on low back pain. We hope that the reader will find all of the material useful and informative.

Childhood Problems

THE FOOT

Supernumerary Digits

The Problem

The obstetrician, pediatrician, mother or grandmother will usually have noticed the extra toe on one or both feet. The grandmother will usually be the person most concerned.

Clinical Evaluation

The deformity is congenital, and once discovered it may cause some anxiety in the patient's family. The extra toe may be anywhere in the foot. However, it is usually on the medial or lateral side (Fig. 13–2).

It is desirable to ascertain whether or not the extra toe has motor function by stimulating movement and by careful observation. One should also observe both the appearance and function of the foot to determine which extra toe is the least normal. X-rays will show which toes have the

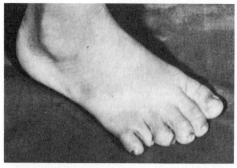

Figure 13–2 A supernumerary toe on the lateral side of the foot. Although it is most convenient to remove the lateral toe, one should make the appropriate observations to ensure that the least functional toe is the one that is removed.

most normal phalanges and articulations.

Management

The parents are advised that this condition will do no harm and will not upset the child's balance. However, it may cause difficulty with the fitting of shoes and with acceptance by the child's peers when he is barefoot. The parents may be told that it is normally a minor surgical procedure to amputate the extra toe. Surgery is usually recommended at 6 to 12 months of age. This gives ample time for growth and observation to determine which toe is least desirable functionally and cosmetically.

Hallux Valgus-Metatarsus Varus

This is not usually a clinical problem prior to adolescence. The detailed discussion in the adult section applies to the adolescent as well. The condition is often associated with a metatarsus adductus, which is discussed in the following section.

Metatarsus Adductus

The Problem

This is a condition in which the fore part of the foot is adducted in relation to the hind part.

Clinical Evaluation

Forefoot adduction is usually noted by a relative, a physician or a nurse practitioner. Often it is seen just after the child begins to walk when the feet are more closely observed. It may also be described as a child "toeing-in" or being "pigeon-toed."

PHYSICAL EXAMINATION. The limb should be checked for any evidence of neurological deficit. There are two key aspects. The first is that the only deformity is adduction of the forefoot in relation to the hind part. There should be no supination of the forefoot and no varus or equinus deformity of the ankle. The presence of any of these conditions implies that the patient may have a clubfoot deformity rather than simple forefoot adduction. The second clinical aspect is a determination of whether or not the deformity is fixed or readily correctable by manipulation of the foot.

The foot may be manipulated carefully by holding the heel with the toes pointing upward. The forefoot is then pushed at the point of the distal portion of the first metatarsal toward the fibular side of the foot. If the foot deformity corrects itself, the foot is supple; if it does not, one is dealing with a fixed deformity.

In the latter case, dorsal, plantar and lateral views of the foot should be taken. These provide a baseline and give some indication of the extent of the bony deformity. One should also look for any other possible anomalies of the foot.

Management

If the deformity is believed to be correctable in a child of three years or less, the parents are taught how to manipulate the foot to the corrected position and are advised to do this on some frequent schedule, such as with each diaper change. They may be reassured that the prognosis is excellent and that the deformity will probably be corrected completely with this treatment. However, even if there is some slight residual deformity, it is not likely to interfere with walking or athletic activity. Some of the greatest athletes in the world toe-in.

If the child is older or has a fixed deformity, a series of well-molded plaster casts are required. The casts should be changed every 7 to 14 days, depending on the severity of the deformity, the rate of correction desired and practicality. The technique for application of these casts is very important and, again, the same basic maneuver used to test the rigidity of deformity is important in the casting procedure. Ideally, the child should be relaxed and feeling comfortable at the time of the application. Gentle, firm management will generally help the child to remain relaxed and cooperative. We have applied benzoin or Ace adherent to the legs followed by two thicknesses of Webril. One to three rolls of two-inch or three-inch plaster, depending on the size of the child, are then applied.

Sometimes this deformity is seen in later life when it is truly fixed and not correctable after three or four months of vigorous, conscientious treatment with plaster. When this happens, surgical correction is indicated.

Usually in a child under two years of age this condition can be corrected by soft tissue releases of the tarsal-metatarsal joints. For the older child with significant deformity, the surgical treatment of choice is a laterally based wedge resection through the tarsal-metatarsal joints.

Discussion

In most cases the correctable metatarsus adductus is due to positioning *in utero*, and some think that when present in the very young child it will probably correct itself spontaneously. However it may not, and all concerned feel better when something is being done.

The key to the diagnosis and management of this problem is the correctability of the deformity. We believe that those deformities that are correctable can generally be managed by the nonspecialist on an outpatient basis.

Clubfoot (Talipes Equinovarus)

The Problem

There are three major components of this deformity, which are usually noted at birth: (1) abnormal forefoot adduction and supination, (2) varus deformity of the hind part of the foot and (3) equinus deformity. The magnitude and resistance of each of the three components may vary considerably. A severe deformity is not only unsightly but may also be the cause of considerable pain and disability. There are a large number of anatomical abnormalities that have been observed in the congenital clubfoot. The problem is to make the foot and ankle a functional structure. It is rarely possible to make the foot normal; however, certain major structural deformities may be improved and the foot placed in a functional position that will minimize pain and disability.

Clinical Evaluation

The deformity is usually recognized at birth or may be associated with some neurological or neuromuscular disease. The true clubfoot is an idiopathic condition that involves the foot and ankle and is present at birth. Talipes equinovarus deformity may also be seen with polio, Charcot-Marie-Tooth disease, lead poisoning, cerebral palsy, arthrogryposis and several other conditions.

PHYSICAL EXAMINATION. The patient should be studied carefully in order to rule out neurological diseases. Paralysis of the peroneal muscle group with muscle imbalance and spastic or hyperactive posterior tibial muscles can result in a clubfoot-like deformity.

The foot is then examined to determine the quality of the skin, the circulatory status and — most important — the relative severity of the three major components of this deformity. The extent to which these different components of the deformity are fixed or correctable is also noted.

LABORATORY STUDIES. X-rays of both ankles are obtained and the films evaluated for the presence of bony deformity and the relationship of the talus and calcaneus on both lateral and Kite angle views. The position of the navicular in relation to the talus is also observed.

If there is a problem in obtaining a clear history and if neuromuscular problems cannot be ruled out on clinical examination, electromyogram studies of specific anterior and posterior tibial muscles may be required. Usually it will be possible to make the correct neurological diagnosis with the help of a neurologist. Muscle biopsies are sometimes required for a definitive diagnosis.

Management

The advice to the patient and parents depends entirely upon the severity of the deformity. The degree of severity is a combination of the extent of the abnormality and its resistance to correction. A mild, supple deformity that is treated from birth will probably become a completely functional, almost normal foot with cast treatment and little or no surgery. It should be emphasized, however, that follow-up is required for the entire growth period in any patient with clubfoot. Parents and patients should be told something different in situations where there is a significant extent of fixed deformity with anatomical and radiographical evidence of gross anomalies. There is likely to be some disability associated with the foot and leg, and one or several surgical procedures will be needed to gain the maximum correction and function for the patient.

Both management and prognosis vary with the severity and fixation of the deformity and the age at which treatment is begun. If the diagnosis is made in the delivery room or nursery, plaster immobilization should be begun immediately in the position of maximum correction. Some of the less severe deformities in younger people may be treated by plaster fixation but should be managed by an experienced specialist.

The plaster technique is similar to that described for adduction; however, the molding and correcting forces applied in the cast are more complex. First, forefoot adduction and supination is corrected maximally, then the varus deformity of the hind part of the foot must be improved. In later serial cast applications the equinus deformity may be corrected. This cannot be done, however, if the Kite angle remains "locked" closed, as shown in Figure 13–3A.

Initial casts are usually applied at weekly or biweekly intervals. When the foot is brought into dorsiflexion, pressure must not be applied only to the forefoot, as a "rocker bottom" foot may result with the hind part of the foot remaining in an equinus position and the forefoot in dorsiflexion.

The majority of clubfeet can be treated by gradual manipulation therapy as outined. In some instances the equinus deformity of the heel persists in spite of the attempt at stretching. This may be due to medial insertion of the tendo calcaneus (heel cord). Lengthening or transplantation of the heel cord insertion may be necessary. Surgical treatment is not usually undertaken in the first six months of life.

Reverse last shoes are prescribed after successful plaster correction, attached to a Denis Browne night splint. Also, the mother is instructed in stretching exercises to be performed at diaper changes.

A

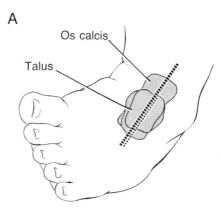

Os calcis

Talus

Uncorrected clubfoot deformity

B

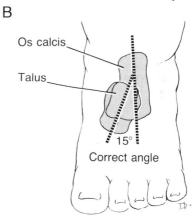

Os calcis

Talus

15°

Correct angle

Corrected clubfoot deformity

Figure 13–3 Correction for clubfoot deformity. *A.* Uncorrected clubfoot deformity. The axis of the talus and axis of os calcis are superimposed, as seen on x-ray. *B.* Corrected clubfoot deformity. The axis of talus and os calcis has been unwound to the normal angle of 15–20°. Difficulty in correction should be assessed by radiograph. Ordinarily the varus deformity is corrected first, followed by correction of equinus.

The status of the extremity is evaluated at follow-up visits during the first few years of life. Any indication of recurrence of the deformity is treated by resumption of plaster correction. In some instances additional surgical treatment is recommended for persistent muscle imbalance in the foot and ankle.

The more severe deformities in

older children are untreated deformities of two or more years' duration. These may be treated with soft tissue releases of the medial and posterior structures of the foot. In older individuals, the deformity will usually require a triple arthrodesis for correction. Sometimes some of the less severe deformities in older children can be corrected with a calcaneal osteotomy.

Discussion

This is one of the more difficult orthopaedic problems and should generally be in the care of the specialist. Rarely can the deformity be corrected completely, but under proper care, and especially when recognized early, the disability associated with the disease can be minimized.

Flat Feet

The Problem

The child is noted to have no arch, may be a bit clumsy and may wear shoes in an unsightly manner. A grandfather or a shoe salesman is often the one who has made the observation.

Clinical Evaluation

A family member or a shoe salesperson has observed the flat feet and has suggested that something be done. A child less than three years old may be a bit clumsy and fall occasionally. There is either no pain or simply an occasional complaint of pain following excessive activity.

PHYSICAL EXAMINATION. The goal of the physical examination is to rule out any serious disease process. The feet are observed standing and walking. If only one foot is flat, there may be some disease or deformity, especially if there is a pathological limp or a gait abnormality. The presence of a dorsal crease or a stiff foot with a tight ankle or spastic peroneal muscles suggests some other problem, namely, congenital vertical talus or peroneal spastic flat foot, respectively. The circulation should be checked and the foot examined for painful calluses. One usually finds nothing else but that the foot is indeed flat.

If the only finding is a flat foot, x-rays are not required. However, if they appear to be needed to convince the parents, or if there are any abnormalities in the examination, then x-rays are taken. Usually standing lateral and dorsoplantar views of both feet are adequate.

Management

The parents and the patient should be reassured that simple flat feet are not abnormal and do not represent any disease process. Moreover, some of the best athletes and fastest runners in the world have very flat feet. Clumsiness is normal among toddlers and others and not always attributable to flat feet. A flat foot — depending upon an individual's aesthetic taste — may or may not look as good as an arched foot, but it is just as functional. Special shoes are not necessary and will not "correct" the foot or create an arch, but they will not do any harm either, provided they are of the proper size. Surgery is contraindicated.

Discussion

In the absence of congenital vertical talus or other diseases, flat feet are not abnormal and need not be treated. Any foot may occasionally be painful, especially if it is overworked or placed in an inappropriately sized shoe.

Congenital Vertical Talus

The Problem

In this condition, the infant is born with a deformity characterized by a rigid foot with equinovalgus deformity of the hind part of the foot and a calcaneovalgus deformity of the forefoot, with dislocation at the talonavicular joint. This is differentiated from the other types of flat feet, which usually become apparent when weight-bearing is begun.

Clinical Evaluation

The deformity is characterized by a convexity of the sole (the "rocker bottom" foot) associated with tightness of the heel cord and prominence of the posterior portion of the os calcis.

Radiographs show a characteristic vertical position of the talus and a *horizontal position of the os calcis.*

Management

Treatment should be instituted early in infancy and usually requires operative measures.

Peroneal Spastic Flat Foot

The Problem

The patient presents with a painful foot and sometimes with a painful leg in the region of the peroneal muscles and tendons. The ankle is "stiff" and resists inversion. This is usually due to an abnormal talocalcaneal or calcaneonavicular coalition.

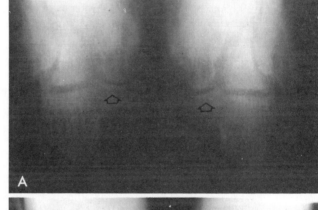
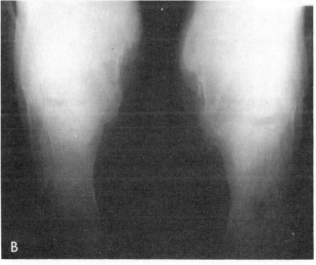

Figure 13–4 *A.* Normal 45-degree posteroanterior view of the talocalcaneal joint (Harris view). The joint between the talus and the os calcis at the point of the sustentaculum tali can be seen clearly. *B.* Tarsal coalition between the talus and the calcaneus totally eliminates the joint shown in *A.* (Reproduced with permission from Rankin, E. A., and Baker, G. I.: Rigid flatfoot in the young adult. Clin. Orthop., *104*: 244, 1974.)

Clinical Evaluation

There is usually a history of gradual onset of pain in the foot that will often have an intermittent course. The symptoms may be stimulated by activity. In the atypical case there may be a history of trauma, some systemic arthritis or infection. In most instances, however, the onset is spontaneous.

PHYSICAL EXAMINATION. The physical exam reveals severe flat feet on one or both sides associated with an antalgic or halting gait. Inversion of the foot and ankle is painful and either difficult or impossible. The spasm of the peroneal muscles may be seen or felt.

X-ray examination should include special 45-degree posterior-anterior views of the os calcis (to show a talocalcaneal bar) (Fig. 13–4) and an oblique projection of the hind part of the foot to show a calcaneonavicular bar. The x-rays shown in Figure 13–5 dem-

onstrate very well bilateral calcaneonavicular coalition. When there is a peroneal spastic flat foot in the absence of tarsal coalition, screening laboratory studies should be carried out to rule out systemic arthritis and infection. Osteoid osteoma has also been seen to cause the characteristic clinical findings of peroneal spastic flat foot.

Management

When a diagnosis other than tarsal coalition is made, the causative conditions are treated appropriately. When tarsal coalition is present, the patient who is having an early or an initial acute attack may be managed with plaster immobilization and analgesics. If these measures fail and the symptoms are intolerable, then surgical treatment is required. There are two types of procedures to be considered: excision of the abnormal bar, which

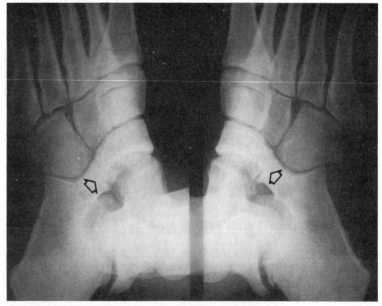

Figure 13–5 Oblique projection showing bilateral calcaneonavicular bars. An oblique projection may be obtained by placing the patient prone with the dorsolateral aspects of the feet next to the film cassette. The roentgen beam is then aimed perpendicular to the table. (Reproduced with permission from Rankin, E. A., and Baker, G. I.: Rigid flatfoot in the young adult. Clin. Orthop., *104*:244, 1974.)

may be purely bony or fibro-osseous, and triple arthrodesis of the ankle. The decision to fuse the tarsal and midtarsal joints is generally reserved for patients with a severe chronic condition or who have had previous operations for the condition. The prognosis for the appropriately selected surgical procedure is good.

Prehallux (Accessory Navicular)

The Problem

There are a number of bones in the foot that have secondary ossification centers. These normally fuse with the primary ossification centers to form an intact bone. Sometimes the fusion does not take place, and an accessory bone forms from the secondary center. This bone may be separated by fibrous tissue or synovial tissue. It is usually not symptomatic, but it may be.

Clinical Evaluation

The most commonly occurring accessory bone develops at the navicular. This bone is also probably the most frequently clinically significant one. It may be associated with flat feet and considerable pain.

Management

Initial treatment involves molded arch supports, analgesics and reduced activity. When this is not successful, moderate improvement may be expected with excision of the accessory ossicle and smoothing of the remaining navicular. The posterior tibial tendon frequently will have an anomalous insertion on the accessory navicular when the condition is present. Transfer of the anomalously inserted posterior tibial tendon to a more plantar portion of the foot has been recommended. We are not sure that this ma-

neuver has been justified either by rationale or clinical experience.

Calcaneovalgus Foot[2]

The Problem

In this deformity, which is recognized as the opposite of clubfoot, the ankle is quite mobile and the dorsum of the foot sometimes lies against the anterior aspect of the tibia. This condition is usually caused by intrauterine position, and almost always corrects itself spontaneously, unless associated with other neurological problems (e.g., myelomeningocele).

Management

Stretching exercises are shown to the mother, and the infant's foot and ankle are manipulated into the equinus and inverted positions at each diaper change.

Plaster treatment is indicated only for those feet in which the dorsal structures are tight, preventing manipulation of the ankle into the equinus position.

When weight-bearing is begun it is often necessary to employ shoes with medial heel wedges and medial Thomas heels, to prevent pronation of the hind part of the foot.

THE ANKLE AND LOWER LEG

Ankle Arthritis

The Problem

This is primarily a problem of diagnosis. The patient presents with a painful or swollen ankle, or both, which is presumably not related to trauma. The goal is to arrive at the correct diagnosis and then to determine the correct treatment.

Clinical Evaluation

The important consideration in the history is to rule out trauma, including the possibility of a puncture wound. Any history of other arthralgias, arthritis or skin rashes is important in evaluating the possibility of rheumatoid arthritis and rheumatic fever. Questions regarding fever, night sweats and furuncles are crucial to the evaluation of a possible infection. Bacterial infections, tuberculosis, fungal infections and brucellosis may all be considered. A history of weight loss or malnutrition may be associated with malignancy or scurvy, respectively.

PHYSICAL EXAMINATION. The important factors in addition to a thorough general physical examination relate to the examination of the ankle and other joints. Is the swelling truly in the ankle joint, as distinguished from the foot or the distal tibia? Is there local increased heat and redness? Is motion of the joint acutely and distinctly related to severe pain localized to the joint? These findings are suggestive of pyogenic arthritis or osteomyelitis of the distal tibia (see next section). Boggy, edematous swelling without erythema or increased warmth is more suggestive of chronic infections such as tuberculosis or a fungus infection. Modest swelling may be caused by a relatively rare condition called pigmented villonodular synovitis. Swelling that is localized to some region of the joint may be due to some benign or malignant neoplasm. Associated anterior and posterior muscle atrophy document to some extent the chronicity of the condition. The ankle should be checked for valgus and varus instability caused by some forgotten or unreported previous injury. The peroneal tendons should be palpated and given stress in an attempt to localize and identify any peroneal tendinitis.

LABORATORY STUDIES. The basic laboratory studies are a complete blood count, sedimentation rate, uric acid determination, rheumatoid factor test, ASO titer and routine x-rays of ankle and chest.

SPECIAL STUDIES. If the preceding evaluation did not document the diagnosis, skin tests for tuberculosis, fungus skin tests, aspiration of the joint[7] and gallium and technetium scans might be considered. If these are not successful in disclosing the diagnosis, biopsy should be obtained.

Management

The ankle joint may be entered with a needle for diagnostic or therapeutic purposes using the following technique: The skin may be anesthetized with an intradermal and subcutaneous injection of Novocain. The joint may be entered laterally between the fibula and the talus or medially between the talus and the medial malleolus of the tibia. For both approaches, the ankle is held in slight plantar flexion. The approach is about 1 cm above and anterior to the medial malleolus and just medial to the extensor hallucis longus tendon. The needle is then inserted posteriorly and about 30 degrees laterally into the ankle joint.

Most of the noninfectious forms of arthritis are treated with the appropriate medical therapy once a specific diagnosis is made. Salicylates (ASA), 650 mg q.i.d. while awake, provide satisfactory medical therapy in traumatic, degenerative and mild rheumatoid arthritis. In some instances a period of 3 to 6 weeks of rest and immobilization in a short leg cast is helpful in relieving symptoms of nonspecific arthritis. On rare occasions a patient may be given an intra-articular steroid injection for a painful ankle. This is not advisable for more than two or three times in any given joint because the liabilities of intra-articular cortisone are significant.

Discussion

This is a simplified work-up for arthritis in a child. We have not presented a detailed differential diagnosis. Many of the preceding suggestions can be carried out on an outpatient basis and will either lead to a diagnosis or have the evaluation well underway prior to hospitalization.

Osteomyelitis of the Distal Tibia

The Problem

This not uncommon clinical entity is important to diagnose as soon as possible.

Clinical Evaluation

A growing child will present with a very painful, swollen ankle, with or without an associated traumatic incident. There may not yet be a fever, but in most cases fever is present. The major complaint is very severe pain. Tenderness or pain is elicited by the slightest motion of the ankle or by very gentle touch.

PHYSICAL EXAMINATION. On examination there may be generalized swelling of the ankle joint and the distal tibia or simply a swelling about the distal tibia. The child absolutely refuses to walk on the leg in any fashion.

The initial x-rays may be normal or may show periosteal elevation and rarefaction of the bone characteristic of metaphyseal osteomyelitis. Needle aspiration of the joint or any fluctuant tender region of the distal tibia may produce pus for culture and Gram staining. If there is pus on aspiration, a technetium or gallium scan may show hyperactivity in the region.

Management

The patient should be treated initially with appropriate antibiotics as indicated by the results of the Gram stain while awaiting the results of the culture and sensitivity tests. When there is no aspirant or when the patient does not respond well to 48 hours of appropriate antibiotic treatment, then surgical incision, drainage, culture and curettage of the region should be considered.

Toeing-In

The Problem

Parent, relative, teacher or nurse notes that when the child walks, the toes "point in." The problem is to determine the severity and cause and to decide what, if anything, should be done about it. A child may toe-in because of forefoot adduction, clubfoot deformity, internal tibial torsion, femoral anteversion, and possibly from femoral torsion. Several disorders of neuromuscular function can also cause toeing-in. Such disorders are not considered in the following discussion.

Clinical Evaluation

The history is quite helpful. When the very young child up to one year or slightly older is presented, toeing-in may be due to intrauterine position or any combination of problems related to the forefoot, tibia or femur. From ages two to nine "habitual" patterns of sleeping and sitting may play an important role. Does the child sleep on his or her stomach with the hips, knees and feet in the internally rotated position? Is the child's habitual sitting pattern such that the hips and knees are flexed and the toes point towards each other with the dorsolateral portions of the feet touching the floor? The two feet are generally separated by some portion of the buttocks. A breech delivery will sometimes be associated with persistent femoral anteversion and consequently with toeing-in.

PHYSICAL EXAMINATION. Most of the characteristic causes of toeing-in can be ascertained on physical examination. Forefoot adduction and the clubfoot deformity were discussed earlier in this chapter.

Tibial torsion can be recognized by having the patient sit on the table, establishing the approximate major plane of motion of the knee joint and then the major plane of motion of the ankle joint. The ankle should be anywhere from neutral (zero degrees) to 20 degrees of external rotation in relation to the plane of motion of the knee joint. The lateral malleolus will be 15 to 20 degrees posterior to the medial malleolus. To the extent that the ankle is internally rotated, this is thought to represent an internal tibial torsion (Fig. 13–6). There may also be a moderate or excessive degree of genu varum (bowlegs). When the bowleg component of the deformity is excessive, one should be on the alert for Blount's disease or some form of rickets.

Femoral anteversion is recognized by testing the child in the sitting position and in the prone position. In the sitting position, the normal child can readily rotate one hip externally enough to rest the fibula of the ankle on the dorsum of the opposite distal femur and have the lower part of the rotated leg parallel to the floor. The internal rotation should be at least to a point at which the lower leg can form a 45-degree angle with the vertical. With femoral anteversion there is an excessive amount of internal rotation and limited external rotation. By placing the child in the previously described sitting and prone positions, the examiner can check that the previously described "habitual" pattern of sitting or sleeping is really the one that the patient is frequently in. The examiner can also detect whether the patient can assume the position with great ease. This tends to confirm the notion that the position is contributing to, if not causing, the deformity. Another important part of the examination is to have the child walk, run and sit, in order to get some appreciation of the severity of the deformity.

LABORATORY STUDIES. X-rays of the feet and knees are obtained if deformity is present. There are several radiographic techniques for discovering the magnitude of femoral anteversion. The following is a useful one. The patient lies supine with hips and knees flexed and the hips abducted 10 degrees. The x-ray beam is then directed perpendicularly downward onto the film, which is under the patient's pelvis. If there is any suggestion in the clinical presentation that some type of rickets may be involved, then serum calcium and phosphate determinations should be carried out.

Management

The basic advice to patients is that nature tends to correct the deformity spontaneously — to a considerable extent, if not fully. Moreover, except in the most severe deformity, a certain amount of toeing-in is compatible not only with normal function but with superior athletic performance. When the deformity is excessive or associated with significant proximal tibial epi-

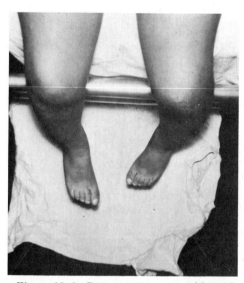

Figure 13–6 Patient sitting on a table with feet in the relaxed position shows considerable bilateral internal tibial torsion. The right leg shows a moderately severe amount of internal tibial torsion, while the left leg shows an extensive amount, approximately 50 to 60 degrees of internal tibial torsion.

physeal disease or with persistent femoral anteversion, then surgery may be considered. The decision to use some orthopaedic assistive device in addition to having the patient avoid habitual sitting and lying postures that contribute to the deformity is largely a matter of clinical judgment. The judgment considers parental anxiety, concern and understanding of the problem. Various devices, such as the Denis Browne splint or straps and strings that hold the heels together, may assist nature in the spontaneous correction or at least may help patients to avoid the contributing positions. These devices have not been proven to be effective, however, and it is quite doubtful that shoe wedges have any therapeutic effect whatsoever in these situations.

Forefoot adduction can be recognized by an abnormal alignment between the hind part of the foot, that is, the heel and the midtarsal joints, in relation to the metatarsal portion of the foot. Up to six months of age, if this is the only irregularity it can be treated by manipulation by the parent at each diaper change. After six months of age, the patient should be referred for consideration of casting to correct the deformity. Patients with clubfoot deformities should be referred immediately.

The Denis Browne bar or a Fillauer may be used to treat toeing-in that is due primarily to tibial torsion, but it is not helpful for forefoot adduction. It may be used for a child of any age who will tolerate it. Such children are probably somewhere between one and three years of age, depending upon the individual child's temperament. Usually the length of the bar is about the same as the child's shoulder width. The external rotation may be set anywhere between 45 to 65 degrees of external rotation, depending upon the deformity and the comfort of the patient.

Surgery is rarely necessary; however, when there is severe persistent femoral anteversion or proximal tibial epiphysitis (Blount's disease) then surgical correction is required. The procedures are generally proximal femoral or proximal tibial derotation and wedge resection osteotomies, respectively.

Blount's Disease

This is an idiopathic disease that occurs either in toddlers or in children between six and twelve years of age. The most striking deformity is that of bowed legs; however, in addition there may be severe internal tibial torsion. It is sometimes associated with obesity, but generally the patients are normal and healthy. The diagnosis is made radiographically. The x-rays of

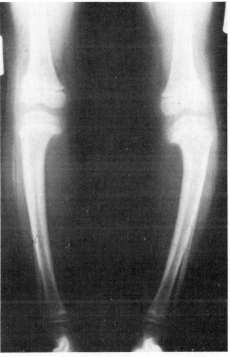

Figure 13-7 X-ray of proximal tibial epiphysitis, or Blount's disease. Note that in addition to the genu varum deformity there is considerable lipping of the proximal tibial metaphysis and disruption of normal epiphyseal line. Same patient's legs are shown in Figure 13-6.

the proximal tibial epiphysis show "breaking," a sharp prominence of the medial portion of the proximal tibial metaphyses. Either a widened or a narrowed and irregular medial portion of the epiphyseal line may also be seen on the anterior-posterior x-rays (Fig. 13–7).

This condition sometimes subsides and partially corrects itself after three or four years. However, in some instances, when the deformity is severe and there is no evidence of either partial correction or subsiding of the process, surgical correction is indicated.

Toe Walkers

The Problem

The child, age one and a half or older, is brought to the physician for advice because the patient consistently walks on his or her toes. The cause must be determined, or at least an evaluation should be made to detect serious and treatable conditions.

Clinical Evaluation

HISTORY. Usually there is no history of any particular disease. When the child starts walking, it is simply noted that he or she walks on the toes. It is important to check perinatal history, and any observations of spasticity or muscle weakness may be helpful in the diagnosis of cerebral palsy or muscular dystrophy. Any unusual bowel or bladder problems should be discussed.

PHYSICAL EXAMINATION. This should include a basic neurological evaluation, with special attention to spasticity. The patient is asked to recline on the floor and then to assume the erect position as rapidly as possible. If the patient has to extend the upper trunk by pushing the hands against the knees and upper thighs or demonstrates general weakness in the

process, this is suggestive of muscular dystrophy. Another important part of the examination is to determine perianal sensation and to examine motor function of the sacral plexus. Gastrocnemius and hamstring muscle weakness should be checked for, as should poorly developed calf muscles. Is there a tight heel cord, and can the ankle be dorsiflexed beyond 90 degrees with the knee either flexed or extended? There is a condition that is simply a congenitally tight Achilles tendon. Can the patient voluntarily walk without going up on the toes? Are there calluses over the metatarsal heads or any deformities of the foot?

LABORATORY STUDIES. The important laboratory studies are x-rays of the lumbosacral spine and of the feet. EMG studies may be considered if there is a significant possibility of lower motor neuron disease associated with spinal dysraphism or Charcot-Marie-Tooth disease.

SPECIAL STUDIES. On the rare occasion when muscular dystrophy is a serious consideration, muscle biopsy may be required.

Management

ADVICE. The parents may be told from the outset that toe walking is rarely associated with any serious disease, and once the unusual causes are eliminated they can be assured that the problem may disappear spontaneously or result in little or no disability. The most common situations found with toe walkers are a tight heel cord, with or without associated sacral or lumbosacral dysraphism, and simple habit. The dysraphism is usually recognizable by x-ray examination. The "habitual" toe walker usually will not have a tight heel cord but may develop one over a period of time. Thus, it can be difficult to separate the habitual from the idiopathic and from the occult spinal dysraphic toe walker. Obviously, the patient who can voluntarily walk normally is a habitual type. In some cases there may be associated psychological problems.

MEDICATIONS AND NONSURGICAL ORTHOPAEDICS. The most reasonable and most effective treatment for this condition is a regimen of plaster immobilization with progressive correction of any fixed equinus deformity. It may be necessary to start with long-leg casts if the equinus condition is contributed to by the gastrocnemius muscle. Up to six months of appropriate serial cast correction with long-leg and short-leg walking casts changed every two to four weeks seems like a reasonable attempt at correction. This treatment can also be helpful for the "habitual" toe walker.

SURGERY. In some situations in which the condition is causing the patient serious psychological problems, heel cord lengthening may be considered but is rarely a desirable solution.

THE KNEE AND UPPER LEG

Osgood-Schlatter Disease (Traumatic Epiphysitis of the Tibial Tubercle)

The Problem

Pain and localized tenderness directly over the insertion of the patellar tendon at the tibial tubercle.

Clinical Evaluation

Onset is commonly noted in adolescence associated with the "growth spurt" between the ages of 10 and 16 years. This is often concurrent with athletic activities or minor trauma to the tibial tubercle. Occasionally the symptoms become severe enough to restrict any active participation in sports.

PHYSICAL EXAMINATION. Pain is localized over the patellar tendon and is most acute at the insertion of the patellar tendon at the tibial tubercle. Soft tissue swelling is visible or palpable in this area. Unless the symptoms are severe, the range of motion of the knee is unrestricted, and the quadriceps muscle shows minimal, if any, atrophy.

LABORATORY STUDIES. Diagnosis is made most accurately from the history and physical examination. Roentgenograms of the knee joint show irregular ossification of the tibial apophysis and soft tissue swelling of the patellar tendon (Fig. 13–8). Rounded ossified fragments may be seen in the patellar tendon in more mature individuals.

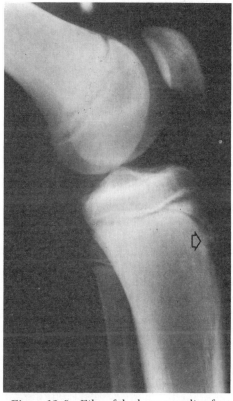

Figure 13–8 Film of the knee revealing fragmentation of the tibial tuberosity and swelling of the soft tissue over it. These findings are consistent with the diagnosis of Osgood-Schlatter disease.

Management

This type of epiphysitis is usually self-limiting but may, on occasion, persist for several years. Treatment should include a decrease in activity, the use of knee pads to protect the tibial tubercle from the trauma of everyday activities, and the avoidance of kneeling. If symptoms are incapacitating, cessation of all athletic activities and the use of oral anti-inflammatory agents such as aspirin for three or four weeks usually prove to be beneficial. Rarely, in extreme cases, complete immobilization in a cylinder cast is indicated.

Discussion

Parents and patients should be reminded that this is a self-limiting disease that usually ends with the cessation of growth.

Monoarticular Arthritis

The Problem

Parents usually note the gradual appearance of a limp and the inability to extend the involved knee fully in a child or adolescent.

Clinical Evaluation

Swelling, effusion and mild tenderness not associated with fever, rash or other major joint symptoms gradually develop over a period of weeks to months. There is no history of recent infection, sore throat or specific trauma.

PHYSICAL EXAMINATION. Unilateral synovial swelling, effusion and lack of full extension or flexion of the knee joint may be seen. Atrophy of the thigh musculature accompanies these symptoms.

LABORATORY STUDIES. Diagnostic studies should include x-ray of the in-volved joint to rule out the possibility of an unsuspected foreign body or of osteochondritis dissecans. Aspiration of the joint is imperative if effusion is present. Joint fluid should be evaluated for bacterial infection, and serum and joint fluid studies should be made to detect collagen diseases. It is most important to assess the possibility of a septic arthritis, including tuberculosis, and a tuberculin skin test should be performed.

Management

Once the presence of septic, tubercular and specific collagen disease arthritis has been excluded, treatment of monoarticular arthritis consists of rest for the involved joint and the use of oral anti-inflammatory medications. Treatment is often prolonged and may include an initial period of bed rest with traction in order to maintain the full range of motion in the knee. Once the synovitis appears to have stabilized, exercises for the lower extremity may be initiated. With stabilization of the initial acute synovitis, ambulation may be begun with crutches, avoiding any weight-bearing on the involved extremity.

Discussion

In view of the chronicity of this disease, it is often advisable to refer such a patient to an orthopaedic surgeon for extended treatment.

Septic Arthritis of the Knee

Clinical Evaluation

The patient complains of a rapid onset of knee pain, progressing to severe localized tenderness, swelling and inability to move the joint without excruciating pain. Often the history of a prior local furuncle (*Staphylococ-*

cus), sore throat (*Streptococcus*) or ear infection (*Hemophilus influenzae*) can be elicited, indicating the focus for the hemotogenous spread of this disease. Occasionally a local puncture wound is the source of infection. Gonococcal arthritis should be considered if the history warrants this possibility. It should be remembered that symptoms vary with the age of the patient involved. Be wary in evaluating the infant, since onset can vary from acute to gradual. Fever and localized symptoms may be minimal in this age group.

PHYSICAL EXAMINATION. Usually the child appears acutely ill with fever, flushing and shaking chills. Fixed positioning of the involved extremity is noted, with extreme pain elicited on attempted passive movement of the afflicted knee. There is localized erythema, effusion and synovial swelling of the joint. Other sources of infection should be looked for, including furuncles or an infected laceration. The skin surrounding the knee should be closely examined for any sign of recent trauma or puncture wound.

LABORATORY STUDIES. If infection is suspected, the knee joint should be aspirated immediately under sterile conditions, and the fluid should be evaluated as noted for monoarticular arthritis, including culture and sensitivity for bacteria under both aerobic and anaerobic conditions.[7] For all joint aspirations, the area should be carefully prepared and draped so as to maintain aseptic technique, and the physician should use a mask and gloves for the injection and aspiration process. The knee joint may be aspirated in the following manner: With the leg fully extended and the heel slightly elevated, an anteromedial approach is made. Since there is usually effusion, the patella can readily be made to ride up above the distal femur by pressing with the palm of the hand on the suprapatellar pouch. When this occurs, it is possible to grasp the patella between the thumb and forefinger and hold it

up away from the femur. The needle is simply inserted under the patella, going from the medial to the lateral direction in the coronal plane. One can generally perceive entrance into the joint prior to making contact with the cartilage on the medial facet of the patella. Should this occur, the needle is withdrawn slightly and then the joint is ready for aspiration.

Management

It is imperative to act with speed once a diagnosis of septic arthritis has been established. Any hesitation in treatment can allow irreversible damage to occur in the joint from the infective process. If the joint aspirate is clearly purulent, all attempts should be made at the time of aspiration to drain as much fluid from the knee joint as possible. Once an appropriate specimen has been obtained for culture and microscopic examination, the patient should be admitted to the hospital immediately for intravenous antibiotic therapy, and the involved limb should be immobilized in traction or splint. The joint should be closely observed and kept decompressed with repeated aspiration. Inability to keep the knee joint decompressed or poor response to antibiotic therapy warrants surgical débridement and irrigation of the infected joint.

Recurrent Dislocation of the Patella

The Problem

Occasionally dislocation of the patella is noted at birth, often associated with other congenital anomalies including abnormalities of the musculature of the thigh. This condition requires early specialized treatment. A much more common syndrome is seen predominantly in adolescent females. The patella either displaces laterally over the lateral femoral condyle and remains in this position or merely slips momentarily and returns to its original central position. The latter situation is more common and often occurs with activities such as walking or dancing.

Clinical Evaluation

The patient commonly complains of the knee "catching" or giving way, causing her to fall. The acute episode is usually followed by an effusion within the joint. There is on occasion a history of similar symptoms in other female family members.

PHYSICAL EXAMINATION. If a dislocation or subluxation has occurred recently, there is pain along the medial border of the patella. The patella will often feel quite mobile and may exhibit considerable retropatellar crepitus. A high-riding patella (patella alta) is often associated with this condition. Apprehension can be elicited from the patient if the patella is displaced laterally while the knee is extended and the quadriceps mechanism relaxed. The quadriceps muscles, especially the vastus medialis, exhibit atrophy. With the knee flexed, it is noticeable that the patella is laterally displaced and that the insertion of the patellar tendon is laterally placed on the proximal tibia. Fracture may be noted during acute dislocation.

LABORATORY STUDIES. Roentgenographic examination, including specialized tangential "sunrise" views of the patellofemoral articulation, shows lateral positioning of the patella in the femoral groove. Occasionally, an osteochondral fragment fractured during an acute dislocation may be noted.

Management

If symptoms are mild and of recent onset, the patient should be referred to a physical therapist for exercises to strengthen quadriceps and thigh musculature. If no improvement occurs with an active exercise program, or if

symptoms are chronic in nature, suggesting advanced chondromalacia (see page 540), surgical correction of the patellar alignment is indicated.

Patellar Tendinitis (Jumper's Knee)

The Problem

Pain over the patellar tendon in adolescents who are active in sports that require repeated jumping, such as basketball, volleyball or gymnastics, is the chief complaint.

Clinical Evaluation

Progressively severe pain over the patellar tendon occurs with jumping activities, decreases with rest and is exacerbated by activity.

PHYSICAL EXAMINATION. Pain and localized tissue swelling are observed over the patellar tendon. Occasionally, crepitation in the patellar tendon is noted on flexion and extension of the knee.

Management

These symptoms represent an overuse syndrome and usually occur early in the sports season. The patient should be advised to rest until the pain abates (seven to ten days) and may take an anti-inflammatory agent such as aspirin. Once the pain has resolved, athletic activities should be resumed at a gradual pace that does not exacerbate the pain. Often quadriceps exercises are beneficial to reduce atrophy of thigh musculature, which may accompany this injury.

Osteomyelitis of the Proximal Tibia and Distal Femur

Clinical Evaluation

The onset of severe incapacitating pain adjacent to the knee joint and associated with an acute febrile illness and shaking chills is the chief characteristic. This may be sudden or may be preceded by an episode of middle ear, skin or throat infection.

PHYSICAL EXAMINATION. Usually the child is acutely ill and irritable and complains of localized severe pain in the area of the knee. Infants will hold the affected extremity in a protected position and resist movement and examination. Palpation of the involved area often reveals localized erythema and hyperemia. There may be edema and occasional deep localized fluctuance.

LABORATORY STUDIES. Suspected acute osteomyelitis requires x-ray examination of the involved area, although results are rarely positive earlier than ten days after the onset of symptoms. In a suspected case of the disease, a complete blood count, sedimentation rate and blood culture should be made.

SPECIAL STUDIES. If the symptoms are poorly localized, a radioactive technetium bone scan should be considered in the face of negative x-ray examination.

Management

Once appropriate tests have been obtained and a high index of suspicion remains, intravenous antibiotic therapy should be initiated. Until positive identification and sensitivity tests of the infective organism are made, initial intravenous medication should consist of a penicillinase-resistant penicillin derivative. The involved extremity should be immobilized and closely observed. If symptoms do not subside over the next 24 hours, or if localized swelling, pain, fever and edema persist, surgical decompression of the involved area should be undertaken.

ADVICE. Osteomyelitis usually occurs in the metaphyseal region and does not involve the epiphysis (growth plate). However, in view of the prox-imity of these two structures, the parents and the patient should be warned of growth disturbance occurring subsequent to the infection and of associated damage to the epiphyseal plate.

Fatigue Fracture of the Proximal Tibia

The Problem

Localized pain over the proximal tibia associated with a new activity pattern, including running or jumping on hard surfaces, is the chief complaint.

Clinical Evaluation

A two- or three-week onset of localized pain associated with running or other athletic activities is noted. The pain increases in severity with activity and decreases with rest.

PHYSICAL EXAMINATION. Localized tenderness over the proximal tibia with an occasional periosteal elevation or mass that is palpable in the area of tenderness is found. Pain can be elicited by having the patient jump on the affected extremity or by manually bending the involved tibia.

LABORATORY STUDIES. Roentgenographic examination of the involved extremity will show some periosteal elevation or localized sclerosis if symptoms have been present for several weeks. Usually these studies will not be diagnostic initially. The technetium bone scan is an extremely sensitive test for this injury and can be positive within 24 hours of the onset of symptoms.

Management

This consists of decreased activity and immobilization in a protective long-leg walking cast for four to six weeks. There is a 20 to 30 per cent chance that a similar type of fracture will occur in the opposite extremity. Patients and parents should be advised that, following healing of the fracture, athletic activities should be resumed on a graduated schedule to allow both skeletal and muscular tissues to adjust to the increased stress of activity.

Chondromalacia of the Patella

The Problem

This disease is characterized pathologically by fibrillation of the articular surface of the patella. The onset may be traumatic, from direct blows to the patella, but more often it results from chronic attritional change. Predisposing factors are recurrent subluxation of the patella and genu valgum.

Clinical Evaluation

These symptoms are most commonly seen in adolescents and young adults who complain of diffuse knee pain associated with activities that are stressful to the knee joint, such as forced flexion of the knee, kneeling or walking down steep inclines. Occasionally there are recurrent effusions of the knee joint.

PHYSICAL EXAMINATION. Retropatellar crepitus and grating can be felt when the patella is manipulated within the femoral groove. There is, however, no correlation between the severity of retropatellar crepitus and grating and the severity of symptoms. Peripatellar tenderness and synovial swelling also are often noticed.

LABORATORY STUDIES. Routine radiographic views of the patella may not reveal any abnormalities. Occasionally, abnormalities of the patellar position in the femoral groove is noted on special tangential "sunrise" views, with narrowing of the patellofemoral joint space.

Management

In mild cases treatment should be directed at improving quadriceps strength through the use of isometric exercises. Bent leg exercises, knee bends, yoga positions and other types of flexed-knee exercises should be avoided. These forms of activity place increased stress on the patellofemoral articulation and may exacerbate symptoms. Rest from strenuous activity will often help to eliminate symptoms. Oral anti-inflammatory agents, specifically aspirin, may help to alleviate the symptoms if taken for a period of six to eight weeks while the conservative treatment regimen just discussed is undertaken. Resistant cases may require surgical treatment, but the patient should be advised that this mode of therapy has not proven to be uniformly successful.

Osteochondritis Dissecans

The Problem

Osteochondritis dissecans is a condition in which a segment of articular cartilage detaches from its bed with a small rim of subchondral bone, usually occurring from the posterior lateral portion of the medial femoral condyle. Occasionally the lesion is seen in the lateral condyle.

Clinical Evaluation

The most commonly affected joint is the knee, although this condition is also seen in the ankle, elbow and hip joints. It affects adolescent males more commonly than females. Occasionally there is an associated history of previous trauma, and rarely a family history of similar conditions can be elicited. Presenting complaints are those of diffuse joint pain, recurrent effusion and, if the fragment has detached from its base, episodic locking of the joint.

PHYSICAL EXAMINATION. There is atrophy of the surrounding joint musculature. Pain can be elicited on occasion by palpation in the area of the lesion. If the fragment has detached, a free mass may be felt within the knee joint.

LABORATORY STUDIES. Adequate roentgenograms of the joint are imperative. Special views, including a tunnel view of the knee joint, are necessary to visualize this lesion. An arthrogram and arthroscopic examination may be indicated to determine whether the articular fragment has detached itself from its subchondral base.

Management

If the articular surface has remained intact, cast immobilization for six to eight weeks is the treatment of choice to maintain the joint in such a position that no pressure is transmitted to the osteochondral fragment. If healing of the osteochondral fragment does not occur, or if it is noted that the fragment has detached from its base, operative fixation of the fragment is necessary.

Capsular, Ligamentous and Meniscal Injuries to the Knee

The Problem

The knee is a complex joint whose supporting and intra-articular structures are vulnerable to injury during vigorous physical activities.

Clinical Evaluation

The patient is usually seen following an acute injury involving the knee joint that occurred during some vigorous physical activity. Information about the mechanism of the injury, such as rotation or varus or valgus stress to the knee can be invaluable in directing attention to those structures that were injured. In chronic injuries of the knee, functional disability needs to be defined, and the occurrence of effusion, locking and episodic giving way may be indicative of intra-articular structural damage.

PHYSICAL EXAMINATION. A thorough visual examination of the knee, in which the presence of effusion and local ecchymosis is noted, should be completed prior to manual examination. An assessment of the integrity of the capsular, collateral and cruciate ligaments is made (see Figs. 13–9 to 13–12). Meniscal injury is often difficult to assess at the time of an acute injury and is of secondary importance initially. If the appropriate examination cannot be made because of patient discomfort, then the examination should be made under general anesthesia.

LABORATORY STUDIES. If the knee shows a tense effusion, arthrocentesis should be done under sterile conditions. The presence of fat globules in a sanguineous fluid points to the possibility of an intra-articular fracture. Roentgenograms of the injured joint (arthrograms) should be done routinely, looking for evidence of possible associated epiphyseal fractures or for radiographic signs of osteochondral fragments and ligamentous avulsion. Arthroscopic examination of acute injuries can define specific areas and degree of structural damage.

The previous discussion described the general evaluation of acute injuries. What follows is a brief description of the treatment for certain specific injuries to structures of the knee.

Medial Collateral Ligament

Injuries to the medial collateral ligament are seen most commonly. The knee is forced into an exaggerated valgus position, usually associated with twisting. In most severe injuries, complete loss of ligamentous continuity occurs, either as a result of avulsion of the ligament from its insertion or from its origin, or because of rupture of the ligament in the middle. Less severe forms of injury result from tearing of the fibers of the ligament, without evidence of instability. Examination of the knee should be performed as described previously, with the patient in the recumbent position. The knee is held in a slightly flexed position with one hand under the thigh and the other grasping the leg under the calf (Fig. 13–9). It is important to be certain that the patient relaxes the quadriceps muscles, because spasm or tension of this mechanism can stabilize the joint. A comparison should be made with the opposite knee to determine the presence or extent of instability.

PHYSICAL EXAMINATION. Minor sprains of the medial collateral ligament usually present with pain over the medial joint area. Tenderness can be localized, and little is seen in the way of tissue reaction. The pain is duplicated by acute flexion of the joint. No instability of the joint is noted. A padded dressing covered with an ACE bandage will often afford adequate symptomatic relief and should be used for ten days.

Moderate sprains will cause more intense pain. Weight-bearing is usually quite painful, but no instability is present. There is usually no effusion within the joint. A cylinder cast applied from the upper thigh to the lower leg will afford symptomatic relief and should be worn for a period of three weeks (Fig. 13–10). Weight-bearing is allowed, and the use of isometric exercises for the quadriceps is advised during the period of immobilization.

With a complete tear of the medial collateral ligament, instability is often

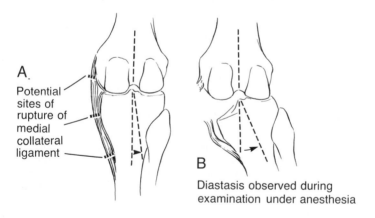

A. Potential sites of rupture of medial collateral ligament

B Diastasis observed during examination under anesthesia

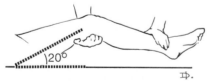

C Knee should be flexed 20° for examination to relax cruciate ligaments and allow diastasis to occur if medial collateral ligament is torn

Figure 13–9 Medial collateral ligament injury: technique of examination. *A.* Sites of rupture of the medial collateral ligament are indicated. Rupture occurs due to trauma from the lateral aspect of the knee. *B.* A diastasis is observed, as shown, during examination under anesthesia. *C.* The knee should be flexed approximately 20° during examination for medial collateral ligament injury, to relax the cruciate ligaments.

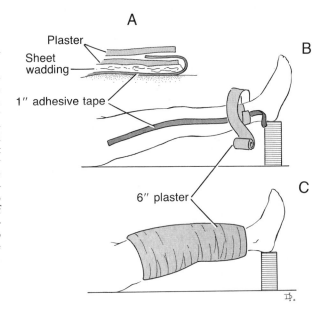

Figure 13–10 Cylinder cast for medial collateral ligament injury. A. A strip of 1 inch adhesive is applied to skin from the upper thigh to the ankle, after skin preparation with Ace adherent spray. An extra few inches of adhesive are left unattached, as shown, and later doubled back as illustrated in inset (B). Sheet wadding is applied next, followed by a circular roll of 6 inch plaster. The distal extra length of tape is incorporated into the plaster wrapping, to prevent downward displacement of the cast when the patient is ambulatory. The cast is molded snugly to conform to the natural contour of the leg (C), and the cast is not bivalved.

noted by the patient during attempted weight-bearing. The application of a valgus stress to the knee will show the presence of medial instability. Should there be any question regarding the presence of instability, the extremity should be examined under anesthesia with subsequent cast immobilization for four to six weeks if instability is verified.

Lateral Collateral Ligament

Injury to the lateral collateral ligament is less common. Often there is avulsion of the fragments from the head of the fibula, the site of insertion of the lateral collateral ligament. Occasionally, associated stretching injury to the common peroneal nerve is also present, causing a foot drop and anesthesia over the peroneal cutaneous distribution in the leg. Instability requires surgical treatment. Less severe injuries will respond to immobilization in a cylinder cast for a period of three to six weeks, as described for mild sprains of the medial collateral ligament.

Anterior Cruciate Ligament

Acute flexion injuries are the most common cause of injury to this structure. A bloody effusion within the knee joint associated with a positive drawer sign points to the diagnosis (Fig. 13–11). Operative treatment is most successful when the cruciate ligament is avulsed with a chondral fragment from its origin or insertion within the knee joint.

Posterior Cruciate Ligament

Isolated injury to the posterior ligament is extremely rare. This condition is recognized by a posterior "drawer sign" (Fig. 13–12). More often, the ligamentous injury is a component of other severe ligament damage in the knee joint that requires surgical treatment.

Meniscus

The menisci, or semilunar cartilages, are crescent-shaped segments of

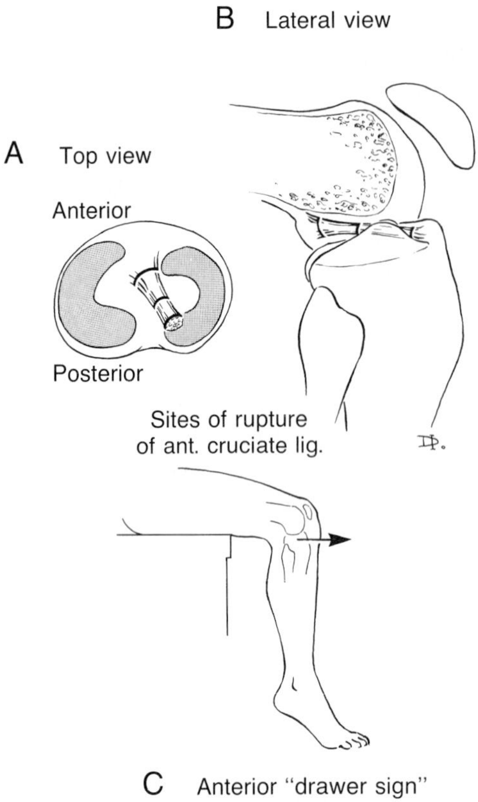

B   Lateral view

A   Top view

Anterior

Posterior

Sites of rupture
of ant. cruciate lig.

C   Anterior "drawer sign"

Figure 13–11   Anterior cruciate ligament injury (anterior "drawer sign"). *A* and *B*. Top view and lateral view of knee, showing the sites of rupture of the anterior cruciate ligament. *C*. Test for anterior cruciate ligament injury: the quadriceps is relaxed while the knee is flexed, by having the patient seated on a table. Increased mobility of the tibia on the femur is detected by grasping the calf and pulling the leg forward, toward the examiner. This motion simulates the opening of a drawer.

fibrocartilage attached to the tibia and are subject to damage from twisting injuries. The medial collateral ligament is contiguous with the medial periphery of the medial meniscus. The lateral meniscus is more mobile, and because of this it is less prone to injury.

CLINICAL EVALUATION

The patient usually mentions a rotatory injury, most often an inward twisting of the femur with the knee flexed. Pain is described as localized over the medial or lateral joint line. The patient may have felt a clicking or popping sensation in the area of pain and tenderness. The knee may have become incapable of extension after the initial episode or may have remained in the "locked" position.

PHYSICAL EXAMINATION. Examination of the joint after an acute injury will show the presence of effusion. The knee may be incapable of full extension. An inability to extend the knee fully may be due to intra-articular fluid rather than to trapping of the meniscus between the femorotibial joint surfaces. Tenderness is present in the joint line over the site of meniscal damage. Slight rotation of the tibia on the femur with the knee flexed will often reduplicate the discomfort.

LABORATORY STUDIES. After an x-ray film is taken to rule out the presence of other intra-articular conditions, the joint should be aspirated. If severe ligamentous injury can be ruled out and the findings point to a meniscal injury, decreased activity or immobilization on crutches for seven to ten days is indicated. Should there be evidence to suggest that the joint is locked, arthroscopic examination of the knee is

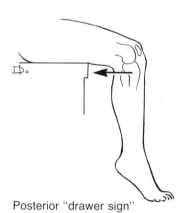

Posterior "drawer sign"

Figure 13–12   Posterior cruciate ligament injury (posterior "drawer sign"). The quadriceps is relaxed by flexing the knee while the patient is seated on a table. Increased posterior mobility of the tibia on the femur simulates closing a drawer, and indicates posterior cruciate ligament disruption.

indicated, with subsequent surgery if definitive mensical pathology is noted.

Chronic Meniscal Injuries

The symptoms described by the patient are usually less severe than those noted in the original injury. The patient may use terms such as "locking" and "giving way." In true locking the joint is caught in a position of flexion, usually of about 30 degrees, and requires manipulation by the patient or a companion for relief. The joint may be the site of recurrent effusions arising from a recurrent traumatic synovitis. Physical examination is the same as that for acute injury.

LABORATORY STUDIES. Routine x-rays of the knee joint should be taken. An arthrogram to evaluate the integrity of the menisci and arthroscopic examination of the knee joint should be routine.

MANAGEMENT

If a symptomatic meniscal tear is found, an arthrotomy for partial removal of the torn portion of the meniscus is indicated.

THE HIP

Congenital Hip Dysplasia

Congenital hip diseases include hip dysplasia, subluxation and dislocation (Fig. 13–13). The latter problem usually requires inpatient treatment, while the other two problems are commonly handled in the clinic.

The Problem

The child with the dysplastic hip is usually referred by a pediatrician. Limited abduction of the affected hip has been noted. With the thighs flexed 90 degrees, the affected extremity cannot be abducted. Occasionally the mother has noted difficulty in abducting the thighs while diapering the infant.

Clinical Evaluation

Occasionally the affected extremity will remain in a higher position than the opposite member owing to tightness of the abductor muscles and a pelvic tilt.

The condition is important in rela-

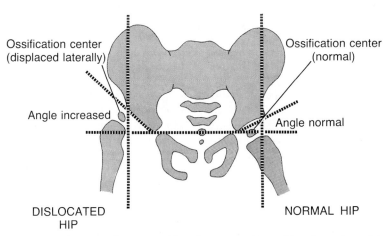

Figure 13–13 X-ray features of congenital hip disease. Dislocated hip shows lateral displacement of ossification center of femoral head and increased acetabular index angle. In dysplasia, the angle is increased, but the femur is not displaced laterally. In subluxation, the femur is malaligned with the acetabulum.

tion to differentiation from a true dislocation of the hip. On radiographs the
acetabulum is underdeveloped and
the acetabular index has an angle
greater than 30 to 40 degrees. There
does not appear to be lateral displacement of the femur. Delay in development of the ossification centers of the
femoral head may be noted in comparison with the opposite hip.

Management

Treatment consists of gradual correction of the abducted femur by the
mother. In severe cases a Frijka pillow
is employed for a period of several
months. In those instances when a
shallow acetabulum is seen on a radiograph but there are no physical findings, no treatment is necessary, as this
is probably a normal variant.

Subluxation

Clinical Evaluation

Subluxation of the hip is probably a
stage in the development of a true dislocation of the hip. Clinical and radiographic signs are similar to those seen
in hip dysplasia, with some exceptions. The abducted position of the
femur in relation to the pelvis is almost
always present. Asymmetrical thigh
folds are usually seen. The trochanter
on the affected side may appear more
prominent.

On x-ray films there is usually widening of the cartilage space of the hip
joint. With abduction of the hip there
appears to be malalignment of the
femur with the acetabulum.

Management

Initial treatment is directed at passive stretching of the tight abductor
muscles. Frijka pillow immobilization
of the hips is used. Observation of the
hip is indicated during the first year of
life to assure proper retention of the
acetabular-femoral head relationship.

Dislocation

Clinical Evaluation

Attention will be directed toward
recognition of the condition, as almost
all types of treatment include traction
supplemented by manipulation or operative procedures.

The hip dislocation is not always
present at birth but may develop in the
first months of infancy or even later.
Early recognition of the conditions and
prompt treatment are the important
factors in avoiding treatment failures.

In the preceding discussion, clinical
features were presented that aid the
practitioner in making the diagnosis of
hip dysplasia and subluxation. Most of
these clinical findings are also present
in the frank dislocation, i.e., limited
abduction at the hip joint, asymmetrical thigh folds and apparent tilting of
the pelvis. In addition, the normal fullness to palpation of the femoral head
distal to the inguinal ligament is absent. If the dislocation is bilateral the
perineum will appear widened. A
"clicking" sign may be felt when the
thigh, which is held in the flexed position, is abducted. The sign has been
described by Sharrard as a "visible or
palpable movement, often erroneously
described as a click." The femoral
head sliding over the acetabular rim
causes this sign.

In children who are walking, a gluteal limp is often present and is occasionally the presenting complaint.

Radiographic findings include those
features noted in dysplasia and subluxation, except that the femoral head is
laterally displaced. The acetabular
index is greater than 30 degrees.

Management

Treatment measures include reduction of the femoral head into the ace-

tabulum in an atraumatic fashion. The reduction, either by manipulative or operative means, is often preceded by a period of traction. Correction of the anteverted position of the femoral head is frequently necessary. In older children or after failures of other types of treatment, operative measures aimed at increasing the size, shape and direction of the acetabulum are often included.

Synovitis of the Hip

Clinical Evaluation

The clinical picture in this condition is one of acute onset, usually without antecedent trauma, in which the child complains of groin, thigh or knee pain. Typical findings are limited hip motion, especially internal rotation. As in coxa plana the age group affected is between five and ten years. A temperature elevation is often present, and the illness may follow an upper respiratory infection.

The intensity of the symptoms may cause concern about the possibility of a septic process. The absence of a peripheral leukocyte reaction and a minimal rise in the sedimentation rate will rule out the presence of this condition.

Management

Bed rest and traction will yield excellent pain relief. The restoration of free hip motion usually follows. Failure to regain full hip motion or recurrence of symptoms suggests that the youngster is suffering from the early stages of coxa plana.

Coxa Plana (Legg-Calvé-Perthes' Disease)

The Problem

This disease of uncertain etiology affects children between the ages of five and fifteen. It is characterized by changes in the femoral head very suggestive of an avascular necrosis and subsequent replacement.

There is a heavy male predilection (4:1, male to female). The disease is usually unilateral.

Clinical Evaluation

Characteristically the onset is noted with the appearance of a limp not related to previous trauma. Pain is often present in the inner aspect of the thigh and knee. Occasionally a youngster will present with a clinical picture within the hip joint associated with low grade fever, acute pain in the thigh and painful limitation of motion.

Usual findings on examination include a hip flexion contracture and limitation of internal rotation of the hip joint. A pelvic tilt associated with thigh atrophy is frequently seen.

X-ray films will usually show widening of the cartilage space and thickening of the capsular shadows. These findings, even though present after the initial symptoms have subsided, should suggest the diagnosis and are signals for institution of treatment.

Later x-ray films will show increased density of the femoral head. Rarefaction and sclerosis adjacent to the capital femoral epiphysis are frequently seen, accompanied by widening of the femoral neck.

Replacement of the femoral head is seen subsequently; lucent areas are present intermingled with radiodense segments. The outline of the femoral head may become enlarged and flattened, implying irreversible changes in the femoral head.

Management

In the early cases, when pain and spasm predominate, treatment by bed rest supplemented with mild traction may be indicated. Pain is not a dominant feature later in the course of the disease. The avoidance of weight-bearing is important in order to protect the femoral head during the replacement process; many methods have been used, but immobilization is difficult because the patients are in the active age group. The isolation of the child by such treatment measures as bed rest and spica immobilization seems unwarranted.

Use of a suspension sling and crutches is a popular method to prevent weight-bearing on the affected extremity and obviates the necessity of removing the youngster from social contacts. A Patten bottom, non–weight-bearing splint supplemented by a shoe lift on the opposite side will transfer much of the stress of weight-bearing to the ischium.

Protection from weight-bearing stresses should be continued until there is adequate replacement of the femoral head.

The best functional and radiographic results are obtained in those children who exhibit an early age of onset. There also seems to be a favorable correlation with promptness in instituting treatment.

Arthritis of the Hip

The Problem

In the differential diagnosis of hip pain in a child one must always consider the noninfectious forms of arthritis: rheumatoid arthritis, monoarticular rheumatoid arthritis, rheumatic fever and the group of vascular inflammatory diseases that may have an arthritic component. These include lupus erythematosus, scleroderma and Reiter's syndrome. The primary outpatient goal is to rule out bacterial infection, Perthes' disease and slipped epiphysis and to carry out the basic laboratory studies to make a diagnosis.

Clinical Evaluation

HISTORY. The pain is usually of gradual onset. It is important to remember that it may present as knee pain. There may be associated trauma. In most cases arthralgia or arthritis will be present in other joints. There is usually a history of antecedent pharyngitis and chest pain. The inflammatory vascular diseases may be associated with a rash or other skin changes. There is generally some history of a low grade temperature and there may be a family history of rheumatoid or vascular inflammatory disease.

PHYSICAL EXAMINATION. The patient is asked to walk, if possible, and the limp is observed. The patient is asked to stand on the affected leg and to flex the hip and knee on the opposite side (the Trendelenburg test). If the pelvis drops down and cannot be held level on the unaffected side, this is clearly indicative of organic pathology in the hip. This test may be positive due to severe pain or structural irregularities in and about the joint. The range of motion should be evaluated and may be also restricted or altered by pain and inflammation or by structural changes. The skin should be carefully examined for rashes, erythema or other conditions. There should be a careful check on lymphadenopathy.

LABORATORY STUDIES. The basic studies should include AP and lateral x-rays of both hips, a chest x-ray, complete blood count, sedimentation rate, urinalysis, rheumatoid factor test, L.E. cell preparation (if rash or multiple arthralgias are present), and EKG (if there is any question of rheumatic fever).

SPECIAL STUDIES. Joint aspiration culture and analysis and a technetium bone scan should be made.[7] For joint aspirations, the area should be carefully prepared and draped to maintain careful and thorough aseptic technique, and the physician should use a mask and gloves. The hip joint may be aspirated through an anterior or a lateral approach. The anterior approach is made after positioning the patient with the hip straight, in slight external rotation. The joint may be entered 2 to 3 cm below the anterior superior iliac spine, approximately 3 cm lateral to the femoral pulse. From the perpendicular position, the needle and syringe are then rotated about 60 degrees posteriorly, and then the joint is entered through fibrous capsule. At this point, if the diagnosis is not yet apparent, the consultation with a pediatrician, dermatologist or rheumatologist may be advisable.

Management

The advice and management will vary depending upon the diagnosis. The rheumatoid conditions are treated with salicylates and subsequently with steroids if severe enough. Surgery is considered in rare instances and generally is hip joint synovectomy, arthroplasty or fusion.

Septic Arthritis and Osteomyelitis of the Hip

The Problem

When there is a bacterial infection involving the hip joint, the goal is to make the diagnosis as soon as possible and then to make a judgment about the desirability of surgery.

Clinical Evaluation

HISTORY. The onset may be either acute or gradual, and it may sometimes appear to be associated with trauma. There may be either a low grade or a high temperature. In the acute phase, very severe pain is generally the most distinctive feature. The patient will often absolutely refuse even to touch the toe on the affected side to the ground. There may be referral of pain to the knee that is not usually of a sharp or severe nature.

PHYSICAL EXAMINATION. There is exquisite pain on motion or irritation of the joint capsule, sometimes even with the slightest manipulation of the hip joint. There may be swelling, tenderness and increased warmth at the joint region. If the situation is not acute and the patient will walk, he or she has an antalgic gait and a positive Trendelenburg test.

LABORATORY STUDIES. A complete blood count, sedimentation rate and AP and lateral x-rays of the hip should be taken. There is generally an elevated sedimentation rate and white blood cell count with a predominance of immature polymorphonuclear cells. The x-ray may show bulging of the joint as indicated by the configuration of the fat pad. There may also be mottled radiolucencies characteristic of osteomyelitis of the intra-articular portion of the proximal femur. When these tests and the clinical picture are not definitive, other tests may be required.

SPECIAL STUDIES. A technetium or gallium scan may be helpful in demonstrating an active infection process in the region.

A more important study, however, is that of aspiration of the joint in order to perform a culture, sensitivity tests and Gram staining of the aspirate. The aspiration is carried out as described in the preceding section. Blood cultures should also be carried out if the patient has a high temperature.

Management

ADVICE. Parents are informed that generally the prognosis of these infections is good when they are diagnosed and treated early. Sometimes treatment may require surgical drainage of the joint. When there is an old or resistant infection, cure may be a good deal more difficult, and there is a possibility of some residual disability that could require additional surgery.

MEDICATIONS AND NONSURGICAL ORTHOPAEDICS. If organisms appear upon Gram staining, then some combination of antibiotics should be started. The selection is based on whether the bacteria are gram-positive or gram-negative. The cultures in a small minority of cases of septic arthritis will not grow any organism. One has to make a decision about infection based on the entire clinical picture and start appropriate doses of antibiotics. If there is a positive culture, the antibiotic regimen should be adjusted to the sensitivity studies.

It is generally advisable to have both an evaluation of infectious disease and an orthopaedic evaluation of these patients because the damage and disability associated with septic arthritis of the hip are major. Difficult decisions must be made about open surgical drainage of the joint and about the type, efficacy and duration of antibiotic therapy.

Tuberculosis of the Hip

The Problem

This is a secondary type of tuberculosis infection that generally presents as a subacute or chronic problem. There is usually pain and stiffness with some wasting of regional muscles, and draining sinuses or associated trochanteric bursitis may also be present.

The diagnosis is made by complete blood count, sedimentation rate, skin tests, chest x-ray and hip x-rays and possibly by aspiration. When the biopsy is not characteristic and there are no acid-fast bacilli noted on acid-fast stain, the diagnosis may still be confirmed by guinea pig inoculation.

Management

Sometimes débridement, antituberculous therapy and immobilization of the hip will provide satisfactory results. However, it is frequently necessary to fuse the joint (arthrodesis) to achieve a pain-free, functional status.

Slipped Epiphysis

The Problem

The main problem also presents a great opportunity for the outpatient surgeon to make a most valuable contribution. The contribution can be the crucial one of early diagnosis of the condition and the prevention of additional slipping. The basic pathology is that of abnormal displacement (or gradual failure) between the head of the femur (the epiphysis) and the remainder of the bone. The displacement occurs in the third or fourth zone of the epiphysis, that is, the zone of hypertrophy or the zone of provisional calcification. The exact cause is not known; however, it appears to be associated with some imbalance of growth and sex hormones that results in an unusually large epiphyseal zone of hypertrophy, the third zone.

Clinical Evaluation

HISTORY. This is a disease that occurs in the first half of the second decade of life, more frequently in obese individuals but also in very slim hypogonadal types. The disease may present in a very subtle way, the most deceptive of which is that of mild pain and a limp in the *knee* area. Other cases may present with frank hip pain, and not infrequently there will be a history of trauma. Even when trauma is present, there may be an antedating history of a gradual onset of vague pain with a subtle limp.

PHYSICAL EXAMINATION. As mentioned, the disease seems to occur more frequently in the obese individual who is maturing slowly sexually, and it also occurs in the very tall, slim individual who has a relatively slow sexual maturity. The body habitus of the disease has suggested that it may represent some irregularity or imbalance between the production or activity of growth hormones and sex hormones.

In addition to the habitus described, the individual will have either an antalgic or a Trendelenburg gait and usually will show a positive Trendelenburg test.

The *toggle test* is a sign which is virtually pathognomonic and should alert the surgeon to the diagnosis. The key physical finding is that, with the individual supine, if one attempts to flex the affected hip in the neutral position, the leg will go very smoothly into abduction and external rotation as it is flexed. This pattern of motion is caused by the displacement that has occurred between the distal femur and the proximal capital epiphysis. When this is found, the individual must be considered to have a slipped epiphysis until proven otherwise (Fig. 13–14). Both sides should be checked in this manner very carefully. The opposite side may be normal and serve as

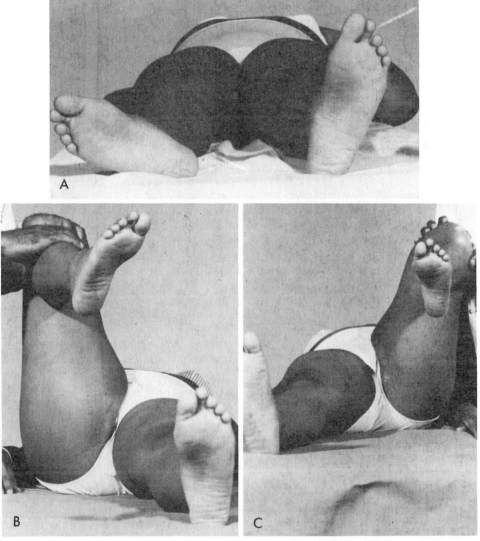

Figure 13–14 A. Typical slightly obese patient lying on a table with the right leg in external rotation. B. Right leg has been flexed and hip is flexed 90 degrees. Note that the lower leg and the foot point toward the midline, showing *external* rotation of the hip. This is a positive *toggle test* – a smooth motion with the hip moved to the flexed position is accompanied by external rotation and often abduction of the hip. C. On the left side when the hip is flexed there is no external rotation. Note that the tibia points straight ahead and not toward the midline, as was the case in the testing of the right hip shown in B. (Photos courtesy of Carleton West, M.D., Chicago, Ill.)

a control for the symptomatic side. There is, however, roughly a 50 per cent chance that a slip is present on this opposite side. If there are bilateral mild displacements, the abnormality will be subtle, noted only by the careful examiner. The involved hip will usually show limited abduction, flexion and internal rotation in comparison with the normal one.

LABORATORY STUDIES. The diagnosis is documented by x-rays, which should include an AP view of the pelvis to show both hips and frogleg lateral views of both hips (Fig. 13–15). The frogleg view is taken with the patient's hips placed in maximum abduction and external rotation, with the knees flexed and the plantar surfaces of the feet facing each other while their lateral surfaces rest on the x-ray table. Sometimes in the early stages of an epiphyseal slip the condition may not be recognized on a pure AP film, but if

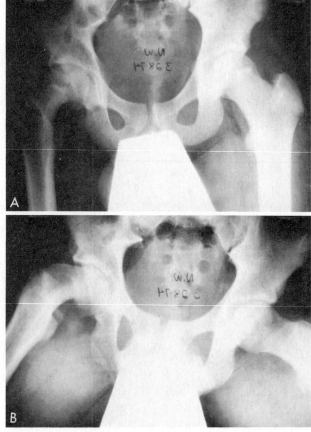

Figure 13–15 *A*. AP view of the pelvis showing a severe slip of the right femoral epiphysis. Note the shape of the proximal femur on the patient's right side. It is somewhat suggestive of an old pistol stock configuration. Note that on the left the head stands erect. On the right side the epiphysis has slipped medially and posteriorly. The physical finding of the positive *toggle test* described in Figure 13–14 would be present on the right side. *B*. Frogleg lateral view of both hips. In this view the posterior tilt can be seen. Again note on the right side the rounded pistol-stock deformity as compared with the left side, which is spherical and like a bulb at the end of a straight neck. It is important to note that, while the x-ray changes are obvious here, they can be more subtle, and when they are not obvious and diagnosis is suspected clinically and by physical examination it is important to obtain radiological consultation. It is crucial to diagnose this disease early, because the sooner the diagnosis is established, the more successful the treatment. (Photos courtesy of Lyle Micheli, M.D., Boston, Mass.)

frogleg lateral views are obtained one can see the slight relative slip of the femoral head on the involved side.

Management

ADVICE. The parents should be told that in many instances this can be a somewhat disabling disease. The outcome depends on the stage of the disease at the time of diagnosis and the course of the disease in a given patient. There may be complications such as avascular necrosis of the femoral head, idiopathic joint narrowing and arthritis in later life. The disease appears to be worse in blacks than in whites and in females than in males. The treatment, like the outcome, depends upon the stage at which the diagnosis is made and the individual characteristics of the disease. Treatment of any slipped epiphysis requires the participation of a specialist. In the acute situation these patients should be hospitalized and treated with traction with an internal rotation bar, and for 24 to 48 hours a very gentle attempt should be made to reduce the slip in traction. This can be very effective, especially in a slip of recent origin. When reduction is achieved, pins should be put across the epiphysis to maintain the reduction and stimulate fusion of the epiphysis. When a slip of large magnitude exists and cannot be reduced by gentle traction, then a Southwick biplane osteotomy should be considered.[6]

THE UPPER LIMB

Sprengel's Deformity

The Problem

Sprengel's deformity is a congenital malformation of the scapula with an elevated position of the shoulder associated with deformities of the cervical spine.

Clinical Evaluation

PHYSICAL EXAMINATION. Look for a unilateral elevation of the shoulder girdle with other developmental abnormalities of the associated musculature, spine and upper extremities (Fig. 13–16).

LABORATORY STUDIES. X-rays of the cervical spine and shoulder may reveal an osseous bridge (omovertebral bone) from the scapula to the cervical spine. In addition, an atrophied or deformed scapula will be noted on the AP view of the shoulder (Fig. 13–17).

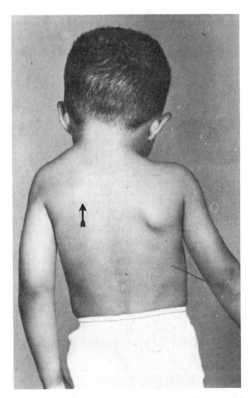

Figure 13–16 Three and one-half year old boy with Sprengel's deformity. Note high shoulder blade and fullness at base of neck on left side. Inferior angle of the scapula can be seen clearly on the right side. On the left side it is less prominent, but one can see the tip (arrow), which is significantly elevated above the level of the inferior angle of the scapula on the normal side.

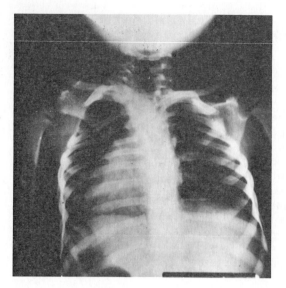

Figure 13-17 Note elevation of left scapula. Vertebral angle of scapula can be seen well above the clavicle on the left side. Note also the multiple anomalies of upper ribs of the left rib cage. X-ray anomalies of the cervical spine are also visible.

Management

Early management consists of stretching and exercising of the shoulder girdle. More definitive surgical correction should be considered when the patient is between three and seven years of age. Other associated congenital problems often require immediate care and treatment.

Erb-Duchenne Paralysis

The Problem

Traction injury of the brachial plexus at the time of birth, resulting in partial or complete paralysis of the involved extremity, is called Erb-Duchenne paralysis.

Clinical Evaluation

Often the injury is noted at birth and should be suspected with breech or difficult deliveries. The involved extremity may be flaccid or not actively used.

PHYSICAL EXAMINATION. A complete neurological examination of the involved extremity is needed to define the level of the lesion.

LABORATORY STUDIES. X-rays of the involved extremity and the shoulder girdle may at times reveal an associated fracture of the clavicle or involvement of the cervical spine.

Management

The initial treatment consists of prevention of muscle contracture using splints and passive motion. Depending on the severity of the initial injury, some regeneration of the nerve tissue may occur. At a later age (five to ten years), persistent muscle imbalances may be amenable to surgical correction.

Traumatic Subluxation of the Radial Head (Nursemaids' Elbow)

The Problem

Acute subluxation of the radial head occurs secondary to sudden traction on the extended elbow of a young child.

Clinical Evaluation

Acute onset of pain and discomfort is precipitated by a stumble or fall by a young child that was thwarted by the upward pull of an adult holding the child's hand. Occasionally at the time of injury a "click" may have been felt or heard by the adult.

PHYSICAL EXAMINATION. Following this injury, the elbow is held protectively by the child in a flexed and pronated position. Any movement causes extreme discomfort. A typical finding is an elbow that is acutely tender, especially to palpation in the area of the radial head.

LABORATORY STUDIES. X-rays of the involved area reveal a normal elbow joint because the dislocated portion of the articulation has not yet ossified, making it impossible to see the disruption on a routine roentgenographic view of the elbow.

Management

The injury is treated by gently flexing the elbow and supinating the forearm. Reduction is often felt or heard with an associated snap or click and immediate relief of discomfort. The involved extremity is placed in a sling and resumption of use of the arm is permitted as comfort allows. Parents should be warned of occasional recurrence.

THE SPINE

Atlanto-axial (C1-C2)
Subluxation and Dislocation

The Problem

The patient may present with pain and muscle spasm with the head in the so-called "cock robin" position. The head is rotated axially to one side and tilted or bent laterally to the opposite side. This may be associated with a variety of different pathological conditions of the upper cervical spine or the neck. This section will discuss some of the major conditions at the C1-C2 junction that may be associated with subluxations and dislocations in that area. The findings may be idiopathic, may present with Down's syndrome or may be related to trauma or to a large number of infectious processes.

Clinical Evaluation

The major considerations in C1-C2 subluxations and dislocations are given in Table 13–2.

HISTORY. There may be a history of trauma, pharyngitis or Down's syndrome or onset may be spontaneous with no previous signs or symptoms.

PHYSICAL EXAMINATION. The patient may show cervical muscle spasm. The sternomastoid muscle group should be examined carefully for fibrosis or tumor. The patient may be able to rotate the head actively to a normal position, or rotation may be possible only passively or not at all. The throat should be examined for evidence of pharyngitis, and regional lymph nodes should be evaluated.

LABORATORY STUDIES. The recommended x-ray studies are outlined in Table 13–2. A true lateral view of C1 may be obtained by taking a lateral x-ray of the skull with the cassette held next to the ear. Complete blood count, sedimentation rate and chest x-ray should be made, along with routine x-rays of the cervical spine and open-mouth views of the odontoid process.

Management

ADVICE. The management is based on the cause of the disruption and the response to conservative treatment. In nontraumatic situations, reduction should be attempted with axial traction or preferably with hyperextension of the head in the supine position using gravitational pull on the head as the

TABLE 13–2 Summary of C1-C2 Subluxations and Dislocations*

Type	Causes and Displacements	Physical Findings	Radiological Studies	Clinical Stability	Treatment
Bilateral Anterior	Dysplastic dens, trauma, infection, anterior displacement	Neutral or "cock robin" position of head	Lateral of C1, CT scan: anterior displacement of C1 on C2	Anterior displacement of 3 mm, neurological deficit—clinically unstable	Fusion or trial of conservative therapy
Bilateral Posterior (very rare)	Fractured, absent, or destroyed dens; posterior displacement	Patient may hold head in hands	Lateral of C1, CT scan: posterior displacement of C1 on C2	Clinically unstable	Fuse C1-C2
Unilateral Anterior (most common)	Arthritic conditions and infections; vertical axis rotation, IAR† at opposite joint	"Cock robin" position of head. Difficulty in rotating head away from direction in which it faces. No difficulty in moving further in that direction. Anterior tubercle of C1 may be shown to be displaced laterally by palpation of posterior pharynx.	Lateral of C1, CT scan: anterior displacement of C1 on C2. AP open-mouth laminograms C1-C2: lateral masses in different planes. Cineradiography or several radiographs of axial rotation: no motion of C1 or C2	With no neurological deficit, probably stable	Trial of reduction and conservative treatment. If symptoms require, fuse C1-C2.

Unilateral Posterior (rare)	Usually associated with a deficient or fractured dens; vertical axis rotation, IAR at opposite sides	"Cock robin" position of head	Lateral of C1, CT scan: *no* anterior displacement of C1 on C2. AP open-mouth laminograms, C1-C2: lateral masses in different positions. Cineradiography or serial radiographs of axial rotation: no motion of C1 or C2	With no neurological deficit, probably stable	Attempt reduction and, if symptoms require, fuse C1-C2.
Unilateral Combined Anterior and Posterior	Trauma; vertical axis rotation, IAR at dens	"Cock robin" position of head	Same as unilateral posterior	With no neurological deficit, may be clinically stable	Trial of reduction and conservative treatment; if not satisfactory, fuse C1-C2.

*From: White, A. A., and Panjabi, M. M.: Clinical Biomechanics of the Spine. Philadelphia, J. B. Lippincott, 1978. Reproduced with permission.

†IAR = Instantaneous Axes of Rotation

force for reduction. When a satisfactory reduction is achieved, the patient may be held in position by a halo apparatus — the second choice being a Minerva cast for 6 to 8 weeks. If reduction is not maintained, surgical treatment should be considered. The management of the specific types of subluxations is shown in Table 13–2.

Discussion

The major outpatient consideration for these patients is to distinguish muscle spasm and wryneck from a true subluxation or dislocation. This is achieved primarily by AP lateral x-rays of C1-C2 and a true lateral view of C1. If the diagnosis is made or is suspected the patient is best handled by someone with experience in the management of problems of the upper cervical spine.

Congenital Torticollis

The Problem

A young child has the head in the "cock robin" position owing to an idiopathic condition in which there is a tight or fibrotic sternocleidomastoid muscle. The position is cosmetically undesirable, and facial asymmetry will develop with growth.

Clinical Evaluation

There is sometimes a history of breech delivery or difficult labor. The problem is rarely noted at birth. It is usually noted within the first year, but not infrequently the child may be 3 or 4 years old.

There is a palpable tumor mass in the sternocleidomastoid muscle in about 20 per cent of cases or a taut muscle or fibrotic mass is palpable. Facial asymmetry may be present. If the head can be passively or — even better — actively moved to the erect neutral position, the prognosis is better.

When the condition is due to a tight sternocleidomastoid muscle, the cervical spine x-rays will be normal. X-rays should be checked carefully to rule out the possibility of C1–C2 disruptions, infection or tumor.

Management

If the child is very young (six months to two years) and there is no distinct tumor or fibrosis of the muscle, the parents are advised that nonsurgical corrective measures will suffice. If the child is older (three and a half to four years) or if there is muscle tumor or obvious fibrosis, surgery is likely to be required. Those situations in between these two extremes require careful weighing of the alternatives.

There is little to be lost by a three to six month trial of nonoperative therapy, which involves positioning the bed and turning the child's head in its sleep so that the sternocleidomastoid muscle on the involved side is stretched naturally. This means axially rotating the head to the side of the tight muscle and, whenever possible, tilting it to the side away from the tight muscle. Frequent passive and active manipulation of the head into the correct position is also helpful. A properly fitted cervical collar may be helpful in holding the neck in the corrected position.

If these measures are not successful, surgical release of the muscle is required. This should be done in the most cosmetically acceptable fashion. Release from the mastoid portion allows the scar to be covered by the hair.

Klippel-Feil Syndrome

The Problem

A great variety of developmental anomalies may occur in the development of the skull, cervical vertebrae, upper ribs and scapulae. Klippel-Feil syndrome is characterized by shortness of the neck owing to reduction in the number of cervical vertebrae or fusion of multiple hemivertebrae into one osseous mass. In addition, there may be congenital elevation (actually failure of descent) of the scapula (Sprengel's deformity), scoliosis, and associated mechanical, clinical, neurological or cosmetic problems. In most instances, however, this is not the case, and the situation is little more than a radiological curiosity.

Clinical Evaluation

HISTORY. There is usually no history other than a physical or radiological recognition of the deformity. Some patients may present because of limited motion of the neck or shoulder. The more severe cases present as cosmetic problems with short, webbed necks and low hairlines. There may also be an occasional abnormal tilt and rotation to the neck.

PHYSICAL EXAMINATION. Physical examination may show any of the previously mentioned anomalies. Range of motion of the shoulders should be checked to rule out limited scapular motion associated with Sprengel's deformity.

LABORATORY STUDIES. Routine AP and lateral views of the cervical spine and thoracic spine, including the scapulae, will generally demonstrate the mixture of deformities. Some of the extensive list of findings are partial or total occipitalization of C1, various anomalies of the odontoid process, failure of segmentation of all or part of two or more cervical vertebrae, hemivertebrae, cervical or thoracic spinal dysraphism, cervical or thoracic scoliosis, accessory ribs, fused or partially fused ribs, an omovertebral bone and elevation of one or both scapulae. A few of these findings are shown in Figures 13–18A and B.

Management

ADVICE. Unfortunately, there is little to be done of a cosmetic nature for these patients. Sprengel's deformity may be moderately improved. Pain or other neurological signs or symptoms that are associated with abnormal motion can be helped by arthrodesis of the appropraite segments in carefully selected patients. Excision of an omovertebral bone will generally improve function.

Scheuermann's Disease

The Problem

This is an idiopathic disease that involves the growing vertebral epiphyses and results in wedge deformity of the thoracic vertebrae, progressive kyphosis and sometimes pain.

Clinical Evaluation

HISTORY. There is nothing unique about the history with one possible exception. It has been observed that when young children perform hard work, heavy lifting or carrying they may have some predisposition to the disease.[8] Scheuermann's disease must be differentiated from poor posture as well as from physiological excessive sagittal plane curvature of the spine.

PHYSICAL EXAMINATION. The patient shows excessive posterior convex curvature of the dorsal spine. The compensatory lumbar curve may be supple, but thoracic kyphosis is fixed and cannot be altered actively or passively. This factor distinguishes habitual postural kyphosis from Scheuermann's disease. The deformity may show a sunken chest from the frontal view. The scapulae and shoulders tend to be rotated forward.

LABORATORY STUDIES. AP and lateral x-rays of the thoracic and lumbar

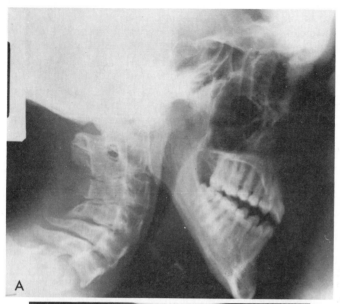

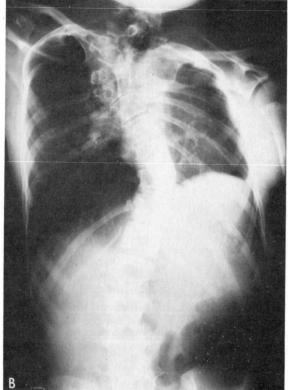

Figure 13–18 *A.* Congenital anomalies of the cervical spine in a patient with Klippel-Feil syndrome. Note the complete fusion of C1 and C2 and the unusual flattened abnormal lateral masses of the other cervical vertebrae. *B.* A much more severe case of Klippel-Feil syndrome with a number of other associated anomalies. Multiple congenital anomalies of the cervical and thoracic vertebrae, scoliosis of the thoracic vertebrae, numerous anomalies of the upper rib cage on the right side, and a prominent Sprengel's deformity of the left scapula can be seen. (Photos courtesy of Henry Sherk, M.D., Philadelphia, Pa.)

spine are required. The lateral view will show the excessive curves described previously. There may be extensive wedging of the upper and middle thoracic vertebrae and some scoliosis or irregularity in the vertebral ring epiphyses. Several Schmorl's nodes may also be seen in the involved vertebrae.

Measurement of the x-rays according to the Cobb method should not show a posterior sagittal plane thoracic curve of more than 40 degrees. The vertebrae should be examined to rule out osteoporosis, tumor and infection, especially tuberculosis. Osteoporosis is a generalized disease. Tumor is local, limited to one or two vertebrae. Tuberculosis may involve one to three vertebrae, usually includes the disk space and is associated with collapse and a perispinal soft tissue abscess. Other clinical considerations and additional laboratory studies will usually separate tuberculosis from tumor and, if not, a biopsy will.

Management

ADVICE. The parents may be advised that the pain can be controlled reasonably well with analgesics and reduced activity. As for the cosmetic effects of the deformity, a moderate correction may be achieved and maintained fairly well with a Milwaukee brace, which must be worn until shortly after the skeleton is mature. Exercises, although generally good for the health, cannot be expected to have any therapeutic effect on the deformity. Surgical correction involves major risks and should be considered only for severe deformities and with full appreciation of the risks involved.

The Milwaukee brace (Fig. 13–19) is worn 23½ hours per day. The patient may remove it for one half hour for swimming or bathing and may do anything he or she wishes while wearing the brace, except for participating in contact sports. Pelvic tilt and breathing exercises are used in conjunction with

the brace therapy. This orthosis is intended for the immature skeleton. It is not thought to have any correcting value in the mature skeleton.

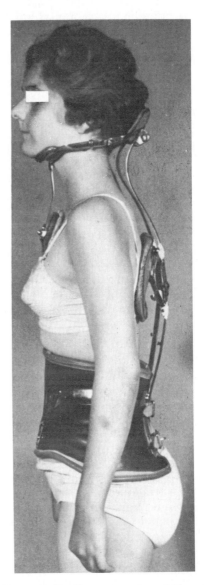

Figure 13–19 Patient wearing a Milwaukee brace for correction of Scheuermann's disease. The posterior thoracic pad is placed over the apex of the kyphos and the anterior pad just below the clavicle. The spine is relatively fixed and passively distracted by the occipital throat mold and by the pelvic girdle. (Reproduced with permission from White, A. A. and Panjabi, M. M., Clinical Biomechanics of the Spine. Philadelphia, J. B. Lippincott, 1978.)

Surgical correction involves extensive anterior and posterior exposure of the spine with release of anterior structures, correction of the deformity, posterior or anterior arthrodesis, or both, and Harrington instrumentation. Surgery is also sometimes indicated for progressive neurological deficit or compromise of cardiopulmonary function.

Scoliosis

The Problem

An adolescent develops an abnormal frontal plane curvature of the spine that is or may become an etiological factor in cardiopulmonary disease and is cosmetically displeasing or painful. The problem is to establish an effective screening system for early detection, to treat the early curves with orthotic devices and to carry out the appropriate surgical management in the selected patients who require it.

Clinical Evaluation

HISTORY. The deformity may be noted by a parent, friend, gym teacher or swimming coach. There are many diseases, most of which are listed in Table 13–3, that may be associated with scoliosis. Most of these conditions would be discovered in the history. The most common type of scoliosis, however, is idiopathic. There is a familial component to idiopathic scoliosis, and siblings of a patient should also be checked. The onset is usually in the early adolescence. A tailor or dressmaker may note some asymmetry while working on either the lower or upper part of a garment, for instance, when the hemline of a dress is askew or difficult to adjust. Patients may complain of pain in the spine or in the thoracoscapular region. When there are severe curves, patients may report some dyspnea with or without associated exertion.

TABLE 13–3   Classification of Scoliosis*

Alterations of intrinsic osseous structures
  Abnormalities of material properties of support structure
    Rickets (primary and secondary)
    Osteogenesis imperfecta
    Neurofibromatosis
    Infections or tumors
  Abnormalities of the geometry of the support structure
    Hemivertebrae
    Maldeveloped vertebrae
    Myelomeningocele
    Asymmetrical spina bifida
    Asymmetrical lumbosacral vertebral structure and articulation
    Fractures and dislocations
    Various surgical procedures
  Abnormal regional kinematics
    Congenital unilateral bars
    Partial failures of segmentation
    Asymmetrical sacralization of fifth lumbar vertebra
    Fractures and dislocations
    Surgery
Alterations of intrinsic ligamentous structures
  Marfan's disease
  Mucopolysaccharoidosis
  Myelomeningocele
  Surgery
Alterations in static or dynamic balance
  Neuromuscular static balance
    Polio
    Myelomeningocele
    Syringomyelia
  Neuromuscular dynamic balance
    Cerebral palsy
    Friedreich's ataxia
    Muscular dystrophy
  Postural dynamic balance
    Abnormalities of vestibular apparatus
    Visual disturbances
    Torticollis
    Leg-length discrepancies
  Thoracic static balance
    Rib removal (thoracoplasty); ipsilateral convexity
    Excessive thoracic scarring; contralateral convexity
Congenital scoliosis (deformity intrinsic to body)
  Infantile type
  Sprengel's deformity
  Klippel-Feil syndrome
  Multiple congenital anomalies
Miscellaneous forms of scoliosis
Idiopathic scoliosis

*From: White, A. A., and Panjabi, M. M.: Clinical Biochemics of the Spine. Philadelphia, J. B. Lippincott, 1978. Reproduced with permission.

PHYSICAL EXAMINATION. The patient should be viewed standing from the front, back and sides wearing no more clothes than a bikini swim suit (Fig. 13–20). The patient will show a frontal plane curve in one or more regions of the spine. There may be asymmetry of the pelvis or the shoulders, and a rib hump may be present on the convex side of a thoracic curve. In the lumbar spine there may be a paraspinous muscle prominence on the convex side of the curve. The tip of the spinous process may not be vertically over the intergluteal fold but may be shifted significantly to the right or the left, which is called decompensation. Viewed from the front, one side of the rib cage projects forward and the other backward. This is made obvious when the patient has well-developed breasts. When viewing the patient from each side, the examiner looks for thoracic kyphosis or lordosis and lumbar lordosis.

Neurological evaluation should include a check for long tract signs, abdominal reflexes, and general muscle strength on the lower extremity. Muscle wasting, fasciculations and spasticity should be checked.

LABORATORY STUDIES. Erect AP and lateral views of the involved regions of the spine will permit an adequate evaluation of the curve. From these films the Cobb angle can be measured and the deformity can be evaluated for congenital and structural anomalies (Fig. 13–21).

SPECIAL STUDIES. If the curve is 45 degrees or more, or if there are any cardiorespiratory symptoms, then cardiopulmonary function studies are recommended. Occasionally laminograms are ordered for an evaluation of unilateral failure of segmentation or to delineate other anatomical variations.

Management

ADVICE. Advice to the patient and parents is based largely on the severity

Figure 13–20 *A.* Patient with a mild to moderate right mid-thoracic scoliosis. Note that the *right* shoulder is carried slightly higher than the left. This degree of scoliosis is not likely to show with clothes, except that there may be difficulty with the hemline of a dress because of the asymmetry of the shoulders. *B.* Often a mild scoliosis can be made more prominent by having the patient bend forward. Here there is a rib hump on the *right* side. The rib hump is usually on the convex side of the curve, as shown here. Sometimes forward-bending will bring out very mild scoliosis and alert the physician to the need for following the patient closely or instituting brace treatment, depending upon the severity of the deformity. This maneuver is an important part of a scoliosis screening examination.

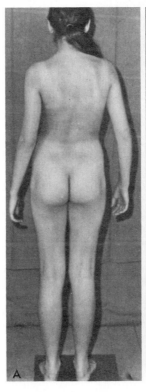
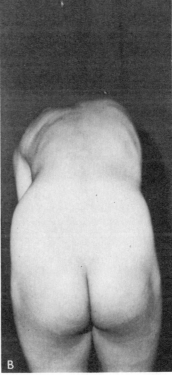

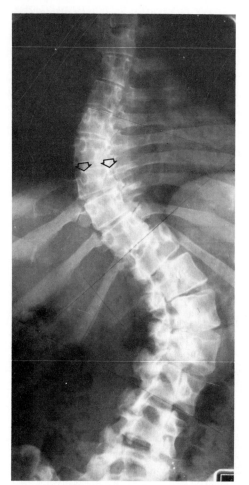

Figure 13–21 Severe double scoliotic curve. The primary curve is a 71-degree lumbar curve. Note the extensive structural changes in both the thoracic and lumbar curves. The lumbar curve shows excessive rotation, since the vertebrae are seen in almost complete lateral profile, even though the x-ray was taken as an AP view. The asymmetry of the pedicles in the thoracic region, as indicated by the arrows, is evidence of the abnormal rotation in that region.

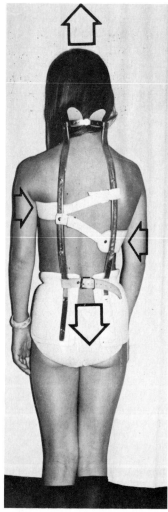

Figure 13–22 Simplified analysis of the forces active with the Milwaukee brace in the correction of scoliosis. The spine is subjected to axial stretching by equal forces, indicated by the arrows at the top of the head and on the hips. These forces are as follows: by way of the occipital pads and throat mold, there is an upward tensile force; the pelvic girdle exerts a downward tensile force. There is also a force exerted on the patient's left by the axillary pad and on the right at the apex of the curvature exerted by the thoracic pad. This serves as a counterforce in the horizontal direction. These various forces combine to correct the curve. This is *not* the same patient as shown in Figure 13–21.

of the curve. If the curve is mild (30 degrees or less) it can be watched and followed with x-rays every three, six or nine months depending upon whether or not it is progressing. The duration of follow-up is based on the patient's skeletal maturity as indicated by bone age and the condition of the vertebral and iliac apophyses. When the iliac apophyses are capped and fused, the rate of progression greatly diminishes.

A curve of greater than 30 degrees in an immature skeleton should be evaluated and followed by a physician who is experienced in the management of scoliosis. Some of the curves will need to be treated by a Milwaukee brace or some other appropriate orthosis (Fig. 13–22).

The decision to operate is a complex one based on several considerations. The major consideration is cardiopulmonary compromise. In severe cases this complication may be life-threatening. Pain and, to some extent, cosmetic considerations may be factors in the decision to operate. Curves of less than 45 degrees are rarely an indication for surgery. The most common procedure is instrumentation with Harrington rods and fusion of the vertebrae involved in the abnormal curve and adjacent to it.

Spondylolisthesis and Spondylolysis

These conditions are discussed in the adult section of this chapter under "Spine." In the child arthrodesis should be considered when a severely painful spondylolisthesis is documented to be progressive.

ARTHROGRYPOSIS

In this congenital condition the infant presents with contractures of major joints of the extremities. Abnormalities in the skeletal muscles have been described and are probably secondary to central nervous system changes. Bilateral dislocations of the hip are often seen along with ulnar club hands and club feet.

Treatment of the lower extremities is aimed at correcting the contractures to the greatest possible extent without compromising the circulation. The clubbed deformities of the foot and ankle can be helped by patient and prolonged plaster applications, but recurrence is frequent. Bilateral hip dislocations are quite refractory to treatment and perhaps should be left *in situ*, resulting in the formation of false acetabuli. Bracing of the lower extremities will often give stability, enabling the patient to be self-ambulatory. In the upper extremities continuing attempts to maintain the wrist and thumb in functional positions should be employed. Plaster splints and braces are employed. The muscles of the shoulder girdle are usually quite weak.

CEREBRAL PALSY

Cerebral palsy includes nonprogressive lesions of the central nervous system that interfere with the control of one or more limbs by paresis, incoordination or involuntary movement. Causes are numerous but the majority of cases today are the result of intrauterine or birth trauma, the incidence being one to two per thousand. Clinically, five types exist: spastic, athetoid, rigid, ataxic and mixed, of which the spastic type accounts for about 60 per cent.

Prognosis and rehabilitation potential are extremely variable, depending on the degree of both motor and intellectual involvement. Outpatient care must be directed at improving function and preventing deformity and complications such as scoliosis, contracture formation and hip dislocation.

Routine examination must be done to check range of motion, especially of hips, knees, ankles and hands. Hip abduction of less than 30 degrees in extension is a sign of impending dislocation. Progressive or persistent equinus sets the stage for permanent bony deformity.

Guided therapy programs can help the child immensely. Surgery such as adductor tenotomy and Achilles tendon lengthening can supplement therapy. The key to care is prevention of problems, not restoration of complications.

Adult Problems

In this section the authors have paid special attention to various aspects of outpatient orthopaedics that may be helpful or of interest to the reader involved in sports medicine.

THE FOOT

Athlete's Foot

The Problem

A relative increase in the flora of fungi in and about the foot results in infection of some portion of the foot, usually the region of the toes, causing scaling, redness, itching and blistering between the toes.

Clinical Evaluation

The feet usually have been allowed to become repeatedly sweaty or wet for an extended period of time, and the condition gradually develops and appears as just described.

Management

ADVICE. Patient education about prevention is important. Cotton and woolen athletic socks are generally preferable because they retain less moisture than socks of synthetic material. The feet should be dried carefully, and in humid conditions a nonirritating foot powder is recommended.

MEDICATIONS AND NONSURGICAL APPROACHES. When the weather permits, the wearing of sandals or open-toed shoes can be helpful. As direct treatment, aluminum acetate solution diluted 1 to 15 with water is recommended. The feet may be soaked in this for one half hour twice daily. The solution should be used only when the feet are in the noninflamed condition and not for more than five days if improvement is not evident. Tinactin, a recently developed over-the-counter medication, is also effective. Cases resistant to treatment should be referred to a dermatologist.

Blisters

The Problem

As a result of excessive pressure or friction on any part of the foot, there is irritation, inflammation and possibly secondary infection.

Clinical Evaluation

HISTORY. The patient generally has been overactive or has been normally active in improperly fitting shoes. The blister may be secondarily infected. With infection, the pain may have changed from a sharp surface pain — tender to the touch — to a deeper, more severe pain that (if on the plantar surface) may be more painful just when the foot is *unweighted*.

PHYSICAL EXAMINATION. When the foot is examined the blister may or may not still be intact. There will be considerable erythema and increased warmth, and if the blister is infected the presence of pus may be indicated by white skin about the margins of the blister. Popliteal, inguinal or femoral lymph nodes may be enlarged when there is an infection.

LABORATORY STUDIES. Sometimes a portion of the skin may be teased or carefully dissected away to confirm the presence of pus and to permit culture. This can also be achieved with needle puncture using local anesthesia if the blister is extremely tender.

Management

ADVICE. One important aspect of this situation is to discuss prevention with the patient. The patient may be advised to build up gradually to a particular level of stress to the foot. This allows the skin to adjust by developing protective hardening and calluses. If one knows ahead of time that an increased level of activity is to be anticipated, nature's preparation may be assisted by the application of tincture of benzoin compound (USP) once or twice a day for a couple of weeks ahead of time. The solution is applied over the bony prominences that are prone to blister formation. Another method is to apply a silicone-based ointment. This protects the skin in a different way by minimizing friction. There are two other very simple, practical measures to reduce friction. One is to wear two pairs of athletic socks, and the other is to be sure to wear properly fitting shoes.

MEDICATIONS AND NONSURGICAL ORTHOPAEDICS. In the early and noninfected phases, the important points

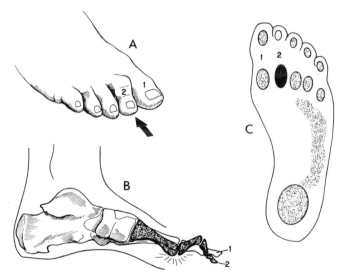

Figure 13–23 Mechanism through which a shoe that is too short can result in formation of a blister or painful callus over one of the metatarsal heads. In (A) the second toe is pushed in, causing it to curl or flex, as shown in the diagram. A short shoe might cause this pushing in. (B) shows a side view in which there is extension at the metatarsophalangeal joint and flexion at the interphalangeal joint that push the metatarsal head down deeper onto the sole of the shoe. In (C) the gray area represents the normal distribution of weight in a functional foot; that is, each toe and each of the metatarsal heads, the side of the foot, the heel, and sometimes even the medial border of the foot (as in flat feet) carry their fair portion of weight. When any one of these parts bears more than its share of weight (black area), stress is concentrated in that area, and pain and irritation followed by blisters and finally by chronic painful callus are the result. The toe indicated by the arrow has a hammer toe deformity.

are to eliminate or reduce the source of irritation and to keep the area clean as prophylaxis against secondary infection. When infection is suspected a culture of the organism should be made, followed by a course of tetracycline and any necessary changes when sensitivities are known.

DISCUSSION. Figure 13–23 shows some mechanisms through which one may develop a callus or a blister.

Calluses

The Problem

Due to a combination of an inner bony prominence and external pressure from footwear or weight-bearing or both, a callus develops over the bony prominence. The callus is frequently but not always painful.

Clinical Evaluation

The patient may complain of pain under the metatarsal heads on the plantar surface of the foot, under the tips of the toes, on the plantar surface over the interphalangeal joints, or on the dorsum of the toes. Painful calluses may also develop over various portions of the os calcis and about the first metatarsal head in the classic bunion, which is discussed later. Frequently there is a history of having worn shoes that are too short or with heels that are too high.

PHYSICAL EXAMINATION. The examination of the foot will usually show some imbalance of the type shown in Figure 13–23. Dorsal plantar and lateral standing x-rays of the feet can be helpful in the identification of osteophytes or other osseous anomalies that may be the irritating entity under the callus. Sometimes the problem may be only a normal bone that has come to be an irritant because of imbalance. The correct analysis of the source of the irritant and why it has developed is helpful if surgical correction becomes a consideration.

MEDICATIONS AND NONSURGICAL ORTHOPAEDICS. Calluses can be softened and reduced easily by applying salicylic acid colloidin (USP). The drug is applied after soaking the feet, and a callus pad is applied over the colloidin. Following this treatment a good deal of the callus may be safely scraped away with a relatively blunt instrument such as a wooden tongue blade.

In chronic situations or in cases where the salicylate therapy does not alleviate the pain, the "donut principle" may be employed. This principle is applied through the use of a pad that surrounds the callus but does not cover it directly. This technique moves the irritating portion of the shoe away from the tender hard apex of the callus to the surrounding normal skin. This is preferable to simply covering the callus, which may actually add to the forces and irritation that are applied to it. The appropriate "donut pads" may be readily obtained in a drug store as "Dr. Scholl's Pads," or they may be fashioned from felt or sponge rubber with a knife or scissors.

Painful calluses over the metatarsal heads may be helped by wearing a molded space shoe that has a transverse metatarsal bar. This bar is placed proximal to the metatarsal heads, shifting the weight away from them onto the more normal proximal tissue.

SURGERY. When conservative measures do not suffice, one must consider various types of surgical resection of the underlying bone or, in some instances, reconstructive procedures. The various surgical procedures are described in subsequent sections.

Paronychias

The Problem

Owing to the overgrowth of soft tissues at the sides of the toenail (usually on the big toe) or to the lateral growth of the toenail or to some combination of the two, the patient develops severe pain in the region. There may be an acute inflammation or an actual infection involved.

Clinical Evaluation

HISTORY. The patient has often worn shoes that are too tight or has cut the nails too close at their lateral edges. Occasionally this condition may occur without either of these antecedent situations. Pain may be present only upon irritation or pressure in the region or, when there is a closed-space infection, there may be pain even with the foot in a rested, elevated position.

PHYSICAL EXAMINATION. There may be moderate or severe swelling and inflammation over the lateral aspects of the nails. If infection is also present, there may be either drainage of pus or an abscess in the region.

LABORATORY STUDIES. If there is pus or an abscess, it is necessary to make a culture from the wound.

Management

ADVICE. The patient should be advised about adequately sized shoes and the proper cutting of the nails. The nails should be cut straight across, perpendicular to the long axis of the toe. The sharp edges of the toenails may be slightly rounded off with a nail file. The toes and feet should be kept as clean as the rest of the body.

MEDICATIONS AND NONSURGICAL TREATMENT. In most cases that are not infected, the acute situation may be resolved by proper footwear, soaking of the feet in tepid pHisoHex and tap water, and careful, gentle placement of cotton between the inflamed skin and the nail.

SURGERY. In chronic, resistant noninfected cases, resection is recommended for the lateral one-fourth to one-third of the nail and its nailbed, the overlying skin and scar tissue and a small (3 to 4 mm wide) strip of the adjacent skin at the side of the toenail. Hemostasis is achieved and the wound is allowed to heal by secondary intention. This results in a pain-free, epithelialized scar in the involved region.

If there is infection, the abscess must be released and cultured. The patient is treated initially with penicillin and subsequently treated according to the sensitivities of the organism cultured. When this is healed, the conservative treatment previously described may be employed. If that is unsuccessful surgery is indicated. The same steps are recommended for a wound that is already draining.

Hammer Toe

The Problem

Because of a relative fixed deformity of the toe, there is severe pain on the dorsum of the proximal interphalangeal joint. The deformity is that of hyperextension of the metatarsophalangeal joint and flexion of the proximal interphalangeal joint with its dorsal position much above the level of the other toes. Pain comes from chronic irritation of the tissues by the top of the shoe. There may be associated metatarsalgia and a painful callus over the corresponding metatarsal head.

Clinical Evaluation

HISTORY. There may be some distinct cause, such as neuromuscular disease or a lacerated flexor tendon, for this imbalance. However, there is usually no distinct associated disease. In most cases, the cause is footwear — a pathological result of shoes that are too tight (i.e., too short or too narrow) or those that have heels that are too high, or all of these.

PHYSICAL EXAMINATION. The deformity is shown in Figure 13–23. The painful area is located over the dorsum of the proximal interphalangeal joint. The joints of the toes should be checked for range of motion, crepitus, swelling, subluxation and dislocation.

LABORATORY STUDIES. It is generally a good idea to take standing dorsoplantar and lateral views of the foot. This will help rule out any unsuspected disease of the bones and joints and will permit a better appreciation of the structural anomalies of the forefoot. For example, is the metacarpophalangeal joint merely hyperextended? Is the pain caused by the callus over the joint or by some disease process within the joint?

Management

ADVICE. Here, as with most problems of the forefoot, the patient must be told tactfully that, although vanity may suffer, shoes that are too tight or not shaped to accommodate the human foot should not be worn. Moreover, human feet and ankles have not yet evolved to the point that we can walk in the equinus position without causing disease.

MEDICATIONS AND NONSURGICAL ORTHOPAEDICS. Some relief may be achieved with proper shoes and reduction of the callus by some of the techniques previously described. Sometimes the toe may be taped into alignment with the other toes. This may be done by having the tape pass (sticky side up) over the dorsal portion of the proximal phalanx of the involved toe and then sticking it onto the plantar aspects of the corresponding portion of the two adjacent toes. The sticky portion of the tape that remains exposed may be covered with another small piece of tape to prevent it from catching on stockings and from collecting dirt and lint.

SURGERY. Corrective surgery for this condition may be performed in an outpatient facility under local anesthesia and with the use of a tourniquet. The forefoot tourniquet is applied as follows: An Esmarch (rubber) tourniquet is laid on the dorsum of the foot so that the free end extends 8 to 10 cm beyond the tip of the toes and on to the dorsum of the foot to the base of the ankle. The remainder of the rolled tourniquet is then wrapped with moderate pressure, taking five to ten turns from the tips of the toes to the base of the ankle. The remaining roll can then be tucked under the final turn conveniently out of the way of the operative site. The free end of the Esmarch is then pulled in the direction that the toes are pointing until enough of the tourniquet is removed to expose the operative site for injection of local anesthesia and for surgery. The remainder of the tourniquet will maintain a bloodless field. If the patient is adequately sedated with morphine, this type of tourniquet can be tolerated for 60 to 90 minutes.

The procedure we recommend for the hammer toe that is resistant to conservative treatment is fusion of the proximal interphalangeal joint and resection of the proximal one third of the phalanx if there is persistent subluxation or dislocation at the metatarsophalangeal joint. The joint is exposed, denuded and fixed with a small stainless steel pin in the straight extended position. If the proximal phalanx was resected, the pin should also go into the metatarsal head with the toe aligned in the neutral position in relation to the metatarsal. This will allow healing with the toe in good alignment with its fellows. The wire may be removed in three to five weeks, closer to three weeks in the young (under 30 years) or healthy patient and closer to five weeks in the old (over 60) or unhealthy patient.

DISCUSSION. When fusion does not occur, the fibrous ankylosis is generally quite adequate for a satisfactory result.

Metatarsalgia

The Problem

The term *metatarsalgia* refers to pain in the forefoot that may be due to a variety of conditions. We shall treat these as a group and discuss several of the more common causes of forefoot pain. The specific problems to be discussed will be resistant plantar metatarsal calluses, Freiberg's disease, Morton's neuroma, march fracture (fatigue fracture) and splay foot.

Plantar Calluses

The Problem

Plantar calluses are discussed in detail on page 568. Here we deal with those for which conservative treatment was not successful or is not feasible.

Clinical Evaluation

HISTORY. The patient has not had relief and is either unwilling or unable to follow the previously described recommendations for conservative treatment.

PHYSICAL EXAMINATION. Examination demonstrates that the characteristic pain is produced with direct pressure. There may be two adjacent metatarsal heads involved.

LABORATORY STUDIES. The x-rays show a prominence over the plantar aspect of the metatarsal head or a "dropped" metatarsal head that corresponds with the location of the painful callus.

Management

Excision of the metatarsal heads is recommended under local anesthesia through a plantar incision at the base of the neck, using the tourniquet technique described in the section on "hammer toe." If two adjacent heads are involved, they may be resected through one longitudinal incision halfway between the two bones. If there is chronic dorsal subluxation of the metacarpophalangeal joints, it may also be desirable to divide the extensor tendons to the two associated toes.

Freiberg's Disease

The Problem

As a result of trauma or idiopathic epiphyseal dysplasia, a misshapen, sclerotic second or third metatarsal head develops, causing metatarsalgia or a painful plantar callus, or both, under the head of the metatarsal.

Clinical Evaluation

HISTORY. There may be a history of trauma, but the more usual situation is a history of moderate to severe pain in the region that may or may not be followed by the development of a painful callus. The symptoms are made worse by activities that apply additional stresses to the feet.

PHYSICAL EXAMINATION. A callus may be present, or there may be pain upon deep dorsal or plantar palpation. Pain may also be elicited by transversely squeezing the metatarsal heads together.

LABORATORY STUDIES. The x-rays may show increased radiopacity suggestive of decreased vascularity. There may also be a malshaped metatarsal head (Fig. 13–24).

Management

ADVICE. The patient may be told that the symptoms may be kept at a tolerable level by decreased activity and aspirin, 650 mg q.i.d. during the

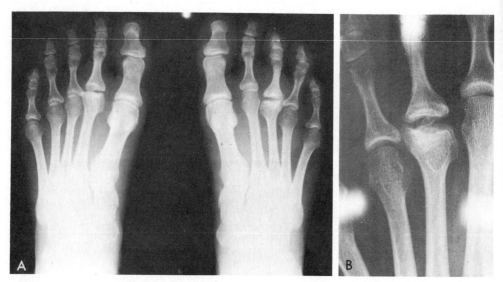

Figure 13–24 *A.* X-rays of a 22 year old female patient with bilateral Freiberg's disease. In the left foot the disease involves the second metatarsal head and in the right foot it involves the third metatarsal head. *B.* Close-up view of the disease in the right foot shows evidence of osteocartilaginous fragmentation into the joint. The right side was the most symptomatic and was successfully treated by resection of the metatarsal head.

day for seven days, followed by 650 mg p.r.n.

MEDICAL AND NONSURGICAL ORTHOPAEDICS. Shoe alterations may be tried, as previously described for metatarsal calluses.

SURGERY. When the above are not successful or cause too much of a hardship, surgical correction is an easy and effective alternative. Using the tourniquet technique described for hammer toe, the metatarsal head is transected at the base of the neck under local anesthesia, with an excellent prognosis for a satisfactory result.

Morton's Neuroma

The Problem

For reasons unknown, a neuroma develops in the region of the common digital nerve, usually between the third and fourth toe or sometimes between the second and third toes, causing severe pain (Fig. 13–25).

Clinical Evaluation

HISTORY. There is usually a gradual onset of discomfort in the region of the metatarsals in the middle or on the lateral side of the foot. It may be well localized between the third and fourth

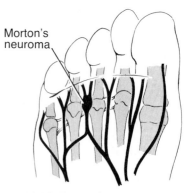

Figure 13–25 Morton's neuroma. Metatarsalgia may occur as a result of a painful condition caused by thickening of the sheath of the plantar nerves. Most commonly affected is the plantar nerve between the third and fourth toes, as illustrated here.

or the second and third toes. The symptoms may have a broad spectrum of intensity. Sometimes the patient may feel as if he has stepped on a small, sharp pebble, and the pain may be most severe. A dramatic example is that of the smug, well-dressed, sophisticated citizen who at one moment is strolling haughtily down the street and at the next moment is sitting on the curbside with one boot off, vigorously massaging the midportion of the metatarsal region. This patient has just stepped on his Morton's neuroma.

PHYSICAL EXAMINATION. The pain may be reproduced by squeezing the metatarsal heads together or by pressing on the dorsal and plantar surfaces between the third and fourth or second and third metatarsal heads. Another test is to manipulate two adjacent metatarsal heads in the region of the pain by pushing them together as they are moved up and down. This will sometimes catch the neuroma and further document the diagnosis. In some instances, one can demonstrate decreased sensation on the side of the toes that are adjacent to the space that separates them.

LABORATORY STUDIES. Standing dorsoplantar and lateral x-rays should be ordered to rule out other conditions such as Freiberg's disease. The x-rays should be normal when the correct diagnosis is interdigital neuroma.

Management

ADVICE. If the symptoms are severe, the diagnosis is reasonably certain, and the patient has had the problem for six to eight weeks, surgical excision has an excellent prognosis. The six to eight week period is a reasonable time to allow for spontaneous resolution of the condition. The patient may be advised about conservative treatment.

MEDICATIONS AND NONSURGICAL ORTHOPAEDICS. Aspirin, reduced activity and the use of thick, soft-sole shoes are recommended. A trial of one or more local cortisone injections in the region between the two appropriate metatarsal heads is also a reasonable treatment.

SURGERY. Using the Esmarch tourniquet technique described on page 570 and local anesthesia, the appropriate surgical procedure may be carried out. The neuroma and the branches of the nerves going to and from it are exposed through a dorsal or plantar incision. If a dorsal incision is used, the surgeon's assistant can help considerably by spreading the two toes with the fingers and pushing up from the plantar surface with the two thumbs. This maneuver generally delivers the neuroma right into the wound once the transverse metatarsal ligament has been cut. The dissection should be carried proximal and distal enough to the neuroma to define either a "Y" or an "X," as the case may be (Fig. 13–26A). At the center of either letter is the neuroma. Leading away from it towards the tips of the toes will be two nerves that are analogous to the top of the "Y" or the top of the "X." Leading into the neuroma on its proximal side will be either one common digital nerve at the bottom of the "Y" or two separate anastomosing branches analogous to the bottom of the "X." If whichever of the two letter-shaped areas that occurs is dissected free and excised, the patient is generally cured. Figure 13–26B shows a "Y" type of excised neuroma.

DISCUSSION. This condition is not infrequently bilateral, with the two sides presenting either simultaneously or in succession. When the patient has one side operated upon with success, the likelihood of the same diagnosis and a happy outcome on the other side is very good.

On occasion a patient may be encountered who has metatarsalgia that is only vaguely, if at all, characteristic of Morton's neuroma in terms of the history and physical examination described previously. If this patient is treated

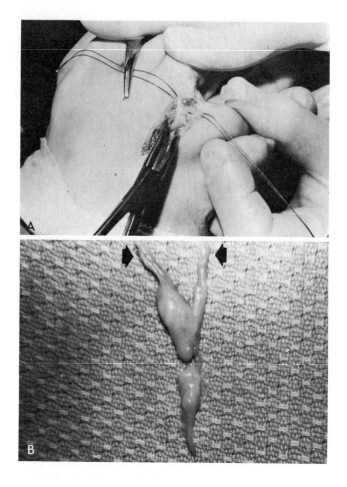

Figure 13–26 *A.* Surgical exposure of a Morton's neuroma through a dorsal incision between the third and fourth toes. The two sutures off to the side of the wound are placed near the two upper limbs of the "Y" figure of the neuroma. The hemostat is placed near the tail of the "Y." *B.* The excised neuroma. The arrows point to the location of the sutures shown in (*A*).

carefully with conservative measures, has a normal, stable personality well known to the physician, does not improve in four to six weeks and is carefully evaluated to rule out other causes of forefoot pain, the following may be considered. The patient may be offered a "Morton's exploratory procedure," which is done with the understanding that, although the physician is not sure of the diagnosis, given the clinical picture described, a neuroma may well be the cause. The minor procedure and the residual numbness between the toes is generally a small liability in the patient's judgment when compared with the chance of relief from the annoying and sometimes disabling pain. The outcome and the results have all

been good in the few patients we have operated upon under these circumstances. If we operate, we recommend removing the "Y" or the "X," whether it has a macroscopic neuroma or not.

Rheumatoid Arthritis with Metatarsalgia

The Problem

Metatarsalgia associated with rheumatoid arthritis is due to intrinsic synovial pathology as well as to major regional anatomical and biomechanical changes that are associated with the disease.

Clinical Evaluation

HISTORY. Usually the diagnosis will be obvious if the patient has a history of arthralgia and arthritis of these and other joints, particularly the metacarpophalangeal, elbow, knee, hip or neck joints.

PHYSICAL EXAMINATION. The patient may have thin, wasted limbs with fusiform swelling of the joints. In the earlier stages, more moderate swelling and erythema with increased warmth may be present. There may be the characteristic changes in the hand, with large, swollen or dislocated metacarpophalangeal joints and ulnar deviation of the fingers. The foot may show localized or generalized swelling of the metatarsophalangeal region. Warmth and erythema may or may not be present, depending upon the activity of the disease. Some or all of the metatarsophalangeal joints may be subluxated or dislocated and there are painful calluses over the metatarsal heads.

LABORATORY STUDIES. The basic laboratory studies should include a sedimentation rate, rheumatoid factor and uric acid tests and possibly a lupus erythematosus test.

SPECIAL STUDIES. If the diagnosis cannot otherwise be established, a skin or synovial biopsy might be considered.

Management

ADVICE. The patient may be told that the disease is chronic, with exacerbations and remissions. It can sometimes be progressive but may also arrest spontaneously. There are several types of treatment that will provide a significant increase in comfort and functional capacity.

MEDICATIONS AND NONSURGICAL ORTHOPAEDICS. Aspirin in therapeutic doses is the initial treatment of choice and is generally effective. Other drugs that may be helpful are indomethacin, phenylbutazone and gold compounds. The other important and effective therapeutic management involves decreasing the loads that are borne by the diseased foot. This is done by reducing activity and by shoe modifications. Materials such as crepe soles and sponge rubber inserts may be employed to dampen the forces that are transmitted to the metatarsal heads. The shoe can also be molded so that forces are taken up by other areas of the foot rather than by the region of the metatarsal heads. This result can also be achieved with the use of a transverse metatarsal bar worn proximal to the painful metatarsal head region. These measures, either separately or — preferably — in combination, can offer considerable therapeutic advantage. A good starting combination is aspirin, less time spent walking, sponge rubber inserts and a ⅜-inch wide transverse metatarsal bar. Other drugs, molded space shoes and more restriction of activity can also be tried. When nonsurgical therapy is unsuccessful, too inconvenient or impractical, then surgical intervention is indicated.

SURGERY. Resection of the four lateral metatarsal heads usually suffices. This may be done on an outpatient basis under a good intermetacarpal block through two longitudinal dorsal incisions. One incision is placed between the second and third metatarsal heads and the other is placed between the third and fourth. It is advisable to section the long extensor muscles to each of the four toes to prevent excessive dorsal displacement of the toes, which sometimes occurs following this procedure. The patient should be advised prior to surgery of the necessity of wearing some type of special shoes, such as the ones just described, even after the surgery.

DISCUSSION. There has been considerable discussion about the possible contraindications to surgery during some levels of activity of the disease. The indication for surgery is based on the magnitude of uncontrolled pain and disability and the possibility for correction with surgery, regardless of the activity of the disease.

Obviously, other surgically correctable conditions that may be noted in the forefoot should be scheduled for surgical correction at the same time.

March Fracture

The Problem

Like steel and other metals, bone demonstrates a type of fatigue failure. Repeated loadings, each of which as an isolated event would not be capable of causing a failure or a fracture, may with repetition over a period of time, result in a fatigue failure of the bone. Unlike metal, however, living bone demonstrates an active biological process in conjunction with the mechanical analysis just described.

Clinical Evaluation

HISTORY. The classic example is that of a previously sedentary young army recruit who, after a week or more of basic training, develops severe pain in the forefoot without a significant history of trauma. There may be pain in both feet. The patient may be anyone with a history of recent increase in an activity with repetitive loading, such as walking, jogging, running or dancing.

PHYSICAL EXAMINATION. This is generally normal. One must rule out other causes of forefoot pain such as interdigital neuroma, arthritis, gout, calluses and infection. There may be swelling and increased warmth in the region of the pain. Loads transmitted to the metatarsal directly in the swollen area or indirectly through deep palpation of the involved metatarsal may elicit severe pain. When no loads are applied to the forefoot, it is generally not painful. The temperature

should be normal, which helps to rule out acute osteomyelitis.

LABORATORY STUDIES. This should include complete blood count, sedimentation rate and x-rays. It is of interest to note that the x-ray may be perfectly normal for as long as 10 to 14 days after the onset of symptoms. However, one may see either a radiolucent or a radiopaque line across one or more of the metatarsals. Either of these findings virtually confirms the diagnosis. There may also be some radiopaque fusiform encapsulation callus of the metatarsal shaft in the region of the fracture. When the x-rays are normal within the first two weeks of symptoms, they should be repeated after a time interval that is appropriate to allow the changes to occur.

SPECIAL STUDIES. If for some reason it is crucial to evaluate more thoroughly a possible or impending fatigue fracture prior to the time that there is plain x-ray evidence of the lesion, one could obtain a technetium scan. This may demonstrate increased activity in the region of the impending fatigue fracture.

Management

ADVICE. The patient may be reassured that, with significantly decreased activity, there will be healing. It is interesting for the patient, especially in this situation, to have an uncomplicated explanation of the disease process. Although the condition may well heal by itself and the patient will be able to tolerate the pain associated with activity, he should be warned that the bone may break and displace completely. This can result in a longer course of disability and treatment.

MEDICATIONS AND NONSURGICAL TREATMENT. Aspirin in therapeutic doses is recommended supplemented with codeine in the acute phase, if needed. The patient's symptoms may reach tolerable level if he simply rests. The patient is generally more comfortable and more active in a short-leg weight-bearing cast with instructions to bear weight only as tolerated. Most fractures heal or require no further treatment after three to six weeks.

DISCUSSION. This is an easy diagnosis to make; however, it can also be easily missed if the history is atypical or not revealed and if the early x-ray examination is not followed by one taken two weeks after the onset of severe symptoms.

Hallux Valgus Metatarsus Varus (Bunions)

The Problem

There is abnormal medial angulation of the first digital ray of the foot. The first metatarsal points too much toward the midline of the body, and the first toe points too much away from the midline. The apex of the abnormal medial angulation is the articulation of the two bones. The prominent portion of the medial aspect of the head of the first metatarsal develops an exostosis and bursitis. The metatarsophalangeal joint may develop degenerative arthritis. There may be severe pain emanating from the bone, the bursa, the skin, an associated callus, the metatarsophalangeal joint or any combination of these structures.

Clinical Evaluation

HISTORY. The patient is usually a female, although the condition can exist in males who have a Morton's-type foot; that is, a foot with a shortened first metatarsal and a moderate congenital hallux valgus metatarsus varus. In any case, these patients complain of pain in the region of the exostosis. Initially, there is localized pain in the area of the bunion, and the development of osteoarthritis of the metatarsophalangeal joint is usually secondary. The patient complains of pain upon wearing shoes and pain with walking, with some relief obtained by removing the shoes. There may be a family history of bunions.

PHYSICAL EXAMINATION. The deformity, the callus and the bunion should be obvious (Fig. 13–27). One may be able to make some precise determination of the source and location of the pain through the examination. There may be erythema, swelling and tenderness to light touch suggestive of bursal inflammation. Tenderness to light touch in the absence of inflammation suggests callus pain. Pain from deep pressure on the exostosis may indicate that the bone itself is the source of the pain. Pain and crepitus evoked in association with manipulation of the big toe suggest the metatarsophalangeal joint as a source of the patient's discomfort. Obviously, there may be any combination of the various possible sources at any particular time. The foot should be evaluated carefully for tophi. The dorsalis pedis and the posterior tibial pulses are checked, as are color and warmth in and hair growth on the toes.

LABORATORY STUDIES. Standing dorsoplantar and lateral views of both feet are taken. The x-ray in Figure 13–28 shows a typical hallux valgus metatarsus varus with bunion formation. If the history or the examination is suggestive in any way of gout, a serum uric acid analysis should be made.

Management

ADVICE TO PATIENT. The basic principle is to avoid those mechanical factors that may be contributing to the irritation of the various components. If the patient wears high heels, have her eliminate them as one source of irritation. The equinus position maintained when walking in high heels applies tremendous forces to the foot. If the shoes also have tapered toes,

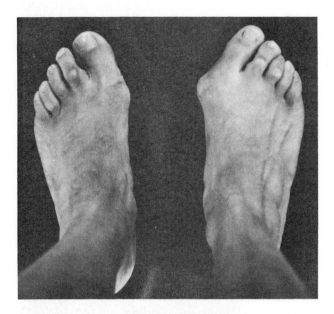

Figure 13-27 Note hallux valgus metatarsus varus and prominent bunions on the medial sides of both feet. (Photo courtesy of Marshall Holley, M.D., New Haven, Conn.)

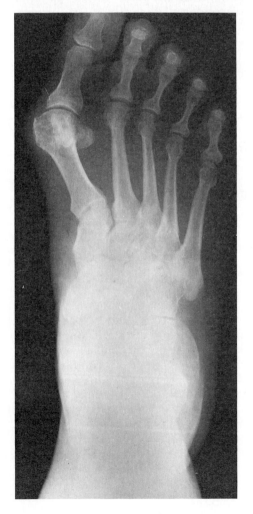

which is true of most high-heeled shoes, additional deformity as well as irritation over the painful bunion will often result. The patient should certainly not work in shoes that have anything other than flat heels. High heels and pointed toes should be eliminated, or their use should be kept to an absolute minimum.

MEDICATIONS AND NONSURGICAL ORTHOPAEDICS. The direct pressure of the shoe may be relieved by a donut-shaped pad; that is, one that can be placed around the exostosis to distribute the pressure of the shoe to other areas that are not painful or diseased. In addition, a so-called space shoe or broad shoe that has ample room may

Figure 13-28 X-ray view of bunion of great toe on right foot shown in Figure 13-27. Note varus position of first metatarsal ray and valgus position of phalanges. On the tibial side of the metatarsal head, prominent bone hypertrophy can also be seen. Overlying the hypertrophied area is a soft tissue shadow that represents the actual bunion. Note also the lateral subluxation of the sesamoid bones toward the fibular side of the first metatarsal head.

be employed to minimize the probability of irritation. To realign the toes, toe spacers placed between the first and second digits may also be employed. This is a temporary measure that may be helpful in the moderately symptomatic patient if used in conjunction with flat nonpointed shoes.

Therapeutic doses of aspirin, two 5-grain tablets every four hours while awake, will relieve pain and reduce inflammation involving the adventitious bursa overlying the bunion. Aspirin will also reduce arthritic pain, of course. When the pain is related to acute or subacute bursitis, local injections of cortisone with Novocaine may be employed as a temporary measure.

SURGERY. There is no bunion operation that will allow the patient to wear high-heeled or pointed shoes without pain and recurrence of deformity; however, there are a large number of operations for this condition.[2] The procedures may be grouped into three categories. One group of procedures corrects the deformity, removes the bunion and alters the joints. The second category includes the operations that remove the bunion and alter the joint, and a third category is simple excision of the bunion. Surgery is considered when the patient's pain and disability cannot be satisfactorily controlled by the previously described nonsurgical procedures.

When the pain is localized to the region of the exostosis and the patient is willing to wear the proper shoes, one may gain relief with a simple bunionectomy (Mayo procedure), which may be done as an outpatient operation.

If there is disease in the metatarsophalangeal joint, then a resection arthroplasty of the proximal portion of the proximal interphalangeal joint (Keller procedure) should be done in addition to removal of the bunion. This procedure may also be done on an outpatient basis.

When there is severe deformity, and especially in individuals younger than 25, one may consider some type of osteotomy to correct the metatarsus varus. Osteotomies involve a variety of techniques, including different procedures to remove or displace the bunion.[2] These operations are usually not elected in situations where there is metatarsophalangeal joint arthritis. The operation described by Mitchell is one of the more popular and effective procedures in this group.[4a]

Bunion of Lateral Aspect of Fifth Metatarsal Head (Tailor's Bunion)

This bunion is analogous to those described in the proceding section. It may be associated with varus deformity of the fifth metatarsal and of the fifth toe. The problem is aggravated by and may be caused by wearing high-heeled pointed-toed shoes. Removal of the exostosis under local anesthesia as an outpatient procedure is indicated if the analogous conservative measures suggested in the preceding sections do not suffice.

Both this problem and the common bunion may be associated with splayfoot.[2]

Gout

Gout is a disease of abnormal uric acid metabolism that results in high serum levels of uric acid, the development of tophi (chalky collections of sodium biurate crystals) and arthritis. The tophi may be seen in the bursae, the ears, the fingers or in various structures associated with the joint. Probably the most commonly affected area is the first metatarsophalangeal joint. The joint may be acutely painful, swollen and erythematous. There is often a family history of the disease, and the attacks may follow bacchanalian soirees. The suggested initial treatment is phenylbutazone, 200 mg two or three times per day. For interim control of uric acid levels, indomethacin or colchicine may be used, but it is recommended that such therapy be carried out under the supervision of a rheumatologist or an internist. Surgical removal of a painful, irritating tophus may be quite helpful. Any associated chronic arthritis should be treated with appropriate reconstructive surgery. A Keller-type arthroplasty for the metatarsophalangeal joint is likely to be a successful outpatient management of the symptomatic joint.

Painful Heels

The Problem

Either spontaneously or following trauma, a gradual or sudden onset of pain occurs in the plantar region of the heel. This may be due to a variety of conditions, the evaluation and management of which will be discussed as a group. There may be idiopathic, self-limiting inflammation of the skin and fat pad in the region of the heel. Inflammation may also occur in relation to isolated trauma (jumping onto the heels) or repetitive trauma (running). There may be a fatigue fracture or a plantar spur of the os calcis. The pain that we refer to in this section is deep under the skin and not associated with a blister or a callus. Unilateral heel pain can, of course, be caused by tumor or infection.

Clinical Evaluation

HISTORY. A history of running activity in a patient with relatively sedentary habits suggests fat pad inflammation or stress fracture. This is more likely to be associated with bilateral pain. A distinct history of trauma to the region makes the diagnosis easy. A chronic, gradually increasing pain is suggestive of a spur of the os calcis.

Any history of a puncture wound may implicate osteomyelitis or a deep inclusion cyst.

PHYSICAL EXAMINATION. Deep palpation to discover as accurately as possible the location of the pain is helpful in evaluating the x-rays. Calluses, if present, may be the source of pain and are more likely to be painful with light superficial palpation, as compared with deep pain elicited by greater pressures. Sometimes simultaneous pressure on both sides of the heel will also reproduce the pain.

LABORATORY STUDIES. The first study should be an x-ray, which will show or rule out reasonably well the presence of tumor or infection. A diagnosis of fatigue fracture cannot be eliminated by one set of x-rays. The initial set should be followed by another series taken at least 14 days after the onset of severe symptoms. If there is a spur of the os calcis, it is a probable source of the pain. If x-rays are normal, one should do a complete blood count and sedimentation rate to help rule out infection. If the clinical picture is suggestive of gout, rheumatoid arthritis or diabetes, then a serum uric acid test, a serum analysis for rheumatoid factor or a fasting blood sugar test is recommended.

Management

ADVICE TO PATIENT. This will depend on the diagnosis. In most cases there will not be a precise diagnosis, and the pain may be from pressure due to inflammation of the deep soft tissues and possibly of the periosteum. The patient can be assured that symptoms can be controlled and that recovery is likely without surgery, if this appears to be a concern.

MEDICATIONS AND NONSURGICAL ORTHOPAEDICS. A variety of conservation treatments have been used. Phenylbutazone, hydrocortisone injections, sponge rubber padding of the heel and reduced activity are all reasonable treatments to employ. Probably the best is the plastic heel cup.*

SURGERY. If nonsurgical treatment fails, several surgical procedures can be considered for this problem. In about half the patients there is no calcaneal spur to be removed. Chrisman and Snook[5] have suggested removal of the spur when present, but the major factor is excision of the medial inferior tuberosity of the os calcis.

Discussion

The covering of the heel is specially designed for the absorption and distribution of large loads. The os calcis is covered with thick skin and an abundance of subcutaneous fat. The fat is separated by rigid, somewhat radially orientated fibrous septa. The septa combine with the fat to form an effective cushioning or energy-absorbing mechanism. Pain may be caused by a local disruption of the structure and function of this organ with stress, concentration localizing pressure and pain in that particular area of the heel. The plastic heel cup may provide relief by rearranging the fat pad and septa, pushing and holding them so that the pressure is reduced. Removal of the medial tubercle may relieve pain by eliminating an area of stress concentration and allowing a broader base for weight-bearing.

Fatigue Fracture of Os Calcis

The Problem

Pain in the heel may be due to a fatigue fracture of the os calcis.

Clinical Evaluation

HISTORY. There is usually a history of vigorous, sustained activity that is

---

*Available through the M.F. Athletic Co., P.O. Box 6632, Providence, RI, 02904.

not habitual for the individual. The uninitiated jogger is a typical patient. The pain has a gradual onset and is greatly accentuated by running, jogging or even walking in some instances. This condition is analogous to march fracture and the various other types of fatigue fractures (see p. 576).

PHYSICAL EXAMINATION. On physical examination, one should try to demonstrate whether weight-bearing, jogging or standing aggravates the condition and causes the characteristic pain. When possible, the region of the heel should be carefully palpated. An area of exquisite, well-localized tenderness is suggestive of fatigue fracture of the bone.

LABORATORY STUDIES. Routine laboratory studies should include plain films of the os calcis region. Regular x-rays may be negative, however, for the first ten days to three weeks of symptoms (Fig. 13–29A and B).

SPECIAL STUDIES. If for some reason it is crucial to rule out or document the diagnosis prior to the ten-day to three-week waiting period, a technetium scan is necessary. This may show uptake (increased activity) in the region of the painful heel.

Management

The patient should be advised to stop running as long as the foot is painful. This is not good news for the average jogger. However, the foot should be rested until the reparative processes have a chance to work. The patient should be told that in all probability he or she will recover completely, with minimal residual symptoms or disability. The patient may be kept comfortable with salicylates or salicylates plus codeine.

Discussion

As mentioned previously, this condition has the same characteristics as fa-

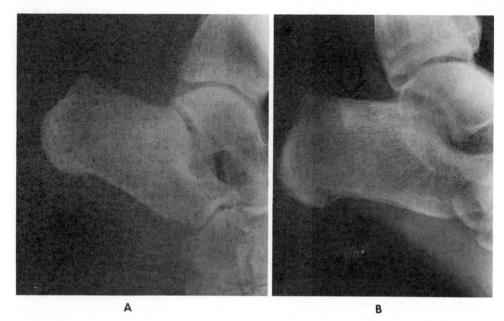

A   B

Figure 13–29   *A*. X-ray of feet of a healthy 23 year old nurse who complained of severe pain in both heels after having begun a daily jogging program 2½ weeks earlier. She had tenderness in the region of the os calcis bilaterally. *B*. X-ray of the same heel two weeks later. Using this film the previously suspected clinical diagnosis of fatigue failure or stress fracture of the os calcis can be confirmed.

tigue fractures in other regions of the body and may well be bilateral.

Flat Feet

The Problem

Some individuals do not have arches in their feet, and when these people develop foot pain, it is often attributed to the absence of arches. We take the somewhat controversial point of view that, unless an individual has congenital vertical talus or some other distinct, diagnosable anomaly associated with flat feet, the flat feet in and of themselves do not constitute a pathological condition and are not the cause of the individual's pain.

Clinical Evaluation

HISTORY.   An individual will present with pain in the plantar aspect of the foot, perhaps along the tibial margin of the foot or located centrally where the arch is in some feet or anterior or posterior to that area, or anywhere else in the midfoot, forefoot, or hind part of the foot. Either the patient or some other person has decided that this pain is caused by the patient's lack of an arch, and the patient comes demanding treatment for the flat foot. The patient may be wearing inappropriate shoes or may be using his feet excessively, either by increased activity on the feet on a less forgiving surface than he is used to or by additional weight-bearing. The history may reveal that the pain is due to strain or excessive use of the foot rather than to its flatness, or the pain may be attributable to any number of other conditions that may account for the flat foot. There may be failure of segmentation bars in the mid or hind part of the foot, rheumatoid or degenerative arthritis, Morton's neuroma, calluses, march fracture or other fatigue fracture, tendinitis, or another problem.

PHYSICAL EXAMINATION. The patient's foot should be examined carefully and the pain should be localized as much as possible. The examination may reveal some of the other conditions that have been described in this section of the chapter.

LABORATORY STUDIES. X-rays should be taken to determine if there is a peroneal spastic flat foot syndrome, which may be associated with failure of segmentation or abnormal bars connecting any of the midtarsal bones or the bones of the hind part of the foot. If this is suspected, tangential views should be taken to show the talocalcaneal joint, and various views rotating on the long axis of the foot to show possible calcaneal, cuboid and talonavicular joint bars should also be obtained. Sometimes a prehallux or an accessory navicular bone will be associated with flat feet, and this should be treated appropriately. The x-rays should be examined for any evidence of vertical talus, particularly if physical examination shows excessive flat feet or rocker-bottom feet with a dorsal crease.

Management

The patient should be managed according to the guidelines previously described for his particular condition. If the diagnosis is simply "flat feet," the patient should be reassured and encouraged. It may be helpful to diminish the burden on the foot by recommending either crepe-soled or ripple-soled shoes, which have an energy-absorbing capacity and so reduce the forces that are transmitted to the foot. Spongy inserts may also be used. A gently contoured molded arch support can be tried for the patient who insists upon having one.

Discussion

There is no convincing evidence that flat feet can be corrected or that flatness of the foot is associated with pain. Many millions of people in the world have absolutely flat feet and use them extensively without any complaint of pain or disability.

THE ANKLE AND LOWER LEG

Acute Sprains of the Medial Ankle

The Problem

Following eversion injury associated with some component of external rotation, dorsiflexion, or both, there is a variable amount of damage to the deltoid ligaments of the ankle. The ligaments may be stretched, partially torn or completely torn, as shown in Figure 13–30.

Clinical Evaluation

HISTORY. There may be a history of athletic injury in which the ankle and foot were twisted, or there may simply have been a fall. The patient usually complains of an acute onset of severe pain in the ankle. Sometimes an audible snap was noted at the moment

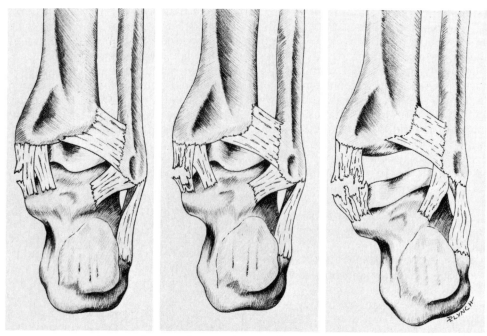

Figure 13–30   Schematic drawing of various degrees of ligamentous failure. The three figures show two stages of partial tearing and a complete disruption of the tibial collateral ligament of the ankle. The first level of injury, in which there is no gross anatomical disruption of the ligament, is not depicted here. The failure in that case occurs because the ligament has been deformed to the point that it has lost its normal elasticity.

of injury. Dramatic swelling may be observed by the patient soon after injury.

PHYSICAL EXAMINATION. The ankle may be grossly swollen and ecchymotic, depending upon how soon after injury the patient is seen. There may be only moderate swelling when the injury is relatively mild. If swelling and pain are not excessive, the ankle can be palpated carefully to demonstrate the exact location of the sprain or rupture. With sprain or rupture of the medial ligament, the area of greatest tenderness is on the medial portion of the ankle and the pain is accentuated by manipulating the ankle into the valgus position.

LABORATORY STUDIES. Anteroposterior, lateral and oblique x-rays of the ankle should be taken to rule out any fractures. If the injury is severe , one should consider giving an intra-

articular injection of Novocain and taking mortise views of the ankle, with the foot and ankle firmly manipulated into the valgus position. If this view shows abnormal tilting of the talus in the mortise, there is extensive rupture of the deltoid ligaments.

Management

ADVICE. The patient is told that some restriction of activity is required to allow the injury to heal. Generally, in mild and moderate sprains one can expect satisfactory healing within two to three weeks. More severe sprains may take four to six weeks. In the very active or athletic individual with gross rupture and instability, surgical repair may be considered.

MEDICATIONS AND NONSURGICAL ORTHOPAEDICS. Ice packs, elastic bandages and elevation are helpful in the first 48 hours. Aspirin, possibly plus codeine, may be used in the acute phase. Although elastic dressings, crutches and elevation may suffice with some therapists and patients, we do not consider this to be the treatment of choice. The tissues are rested and supported more securely by a short-leg cast worn for two to four weeks, followed by a graduated program of rehabilitation of the supporting muscles. The rehabilitation program is followed by some essentially pain-free jogging before a return to more vigorous activity is allowed. Premature stress may interfere with healing and produce a chronically unstable ankle.

SURGERY. When there is gross instability and the anticipated demands on the ankle are great, surgical exploration of the joints and direct repair of the ligament are advisable.

Discussion

Deltoid ligament injuries are less common than injuries to the lateral side of the joint. In both types of injury, the clinical considerations must allow for sufficient healing of the initial injury and proper rehabilitation after healing. These factors will reduce the incidence of re-injury and chronic instability of the ankle.

Acute Sprains of the Lateral Ankle

The Problem

With inversion in plantar flexion or internal rotation of the foot and ankle, there are associated injuries to the lateral ligaments of the ankle. These injuries are more common than medial ligament injuries, and the evaluation and treatment for both types of injury are the same.

Clinical Evaluation

HISTORY. The history is usually that of a twist and a pull of the ankle, with or without the factor of participation in athletics. There is immediate pain and swelling and sometimes an associated "snap" or "popping" sound.

PHYSICAL EXAMINATION. Pain and swelling generally occur, at least in the first few hours, on the lateral side of the ankle. Careful palpation just anterior and plantar to the fibular malleolus may elicit distinct tenderness. If tenderness is associated with an anterior "drawer" sign (the ability to pull the ankle and foot forward in the ankle mortise by an anteriorly directed force applied to the heel), then complete rupture of the anterior talotibial ligament is very likely.

LABORATORY STUDIES. Anteroposterior, lateral and oblique x-rays are needed to show the ankle mortise and the foot. If the injury is severe, and certainly if there is a positive "drawer" sign, the joint should be anesthetized with Novocain and stress views should be taken. Stress views are obtained by applying forces to the ankle and foot that place the ankle in the maximal varus position, then comparing these views with those of the uninjured ankle.

Management

The management is analogous to that described in the preceding section for acute medial ligament injuries.

Chronically Unstable Ankles

The Problem

Some patients will develop a syndrome in which they repeatedly stumble or fall, twisting their ankles. This results in pain and swelling on the medial or lateral aspect of the joint.

Clinical Evaluation

HISTORY. The patient has usually had one or more ankle injuries, and adequate healing of the previous injury or injuries has usually not occurred. This may be due to any combination of the following: the nature of the injury, the patient, the trainer, the coach and the doctor. The pattern of the episode of re-injury is quite variable among patients and even for a single patient. The injury may be minor or severe or may occur while walking on a nearly flat surface. The intervals between episodes may be days, weeks, months or as much as a year.

PHYSICAL EXAMINATION. Following re-injury of an unstable ankle, there is usually moderate or mild swelling. There may be mild, chronic, generalized swelling of the ankle. With lateral instability and minimal or no swelling, one can sometimes identify a sulcus in the area of the lateral tibial malleolar ligaments.

LABORATORY STUDIES. Stress views of the ankle of the type described for acute injuries may be helpful in establishing the extent of disruption of the ligaments.

Management

ADVICE TO PATIENT. There are two reasons for treating this condition. The first and most important is to provide for the patient's comfort and convenience. The second reason is that a very unstable and frequently irritated joint most probably presents a significant risk for the development of traumatic arthritis.

MEDICATION AND NONSURGICAL TREATMENT. Salicylates in therapeutic doses, wrapping with an Ace bandage, decreased activity and possibly the use of crutches and elevation will suffice in some instances. This is use-

ful for the acute "instability episode." In some situations where the instability is not of long standing (roughly, not more than a year), one might try a prolonged period of immobilization in a below-knee weight-bearing cast for six to eight weeks. This should be followed by a carefully supervised period of rehabilitation, including muscle redevelopment and jogging.

SURGERY. In more severe and recurrent conditions, surgical reconstruction of the medial or lateral ligaments may be desirable. These reconstructive procedures include repair of torn structures when possible. However, the major consideration is the restoration of medial or lateral stability using available expendable tendons tunneled through the malleoli and attached to the bone or soft tissues of the os calcis.

Discussion

In the evaluation of chronically unstable ankles one should consider the possibility of peroneal or posterior tibial tendinitis or subluxation.

Arthritis of the Ankle

The evaluation of an ankle arthritis in the adult is essentially the same as that recommended for a child. The adult is more likely to have degenerative arthritis, post-traumatic arthritis or an old, inactive inflammatory arthritis. Ankle fusion should be considered when the process is inactive, but the symptoms are too severe to be managed by conservative treatment.

Ankle Fusions

There are a number of different techniques for arthrodesis of the ankle. One particular technique that involves relatively less surgery than most procedures has been effective and is illustrated in Figure 13–31. Ankle fusion

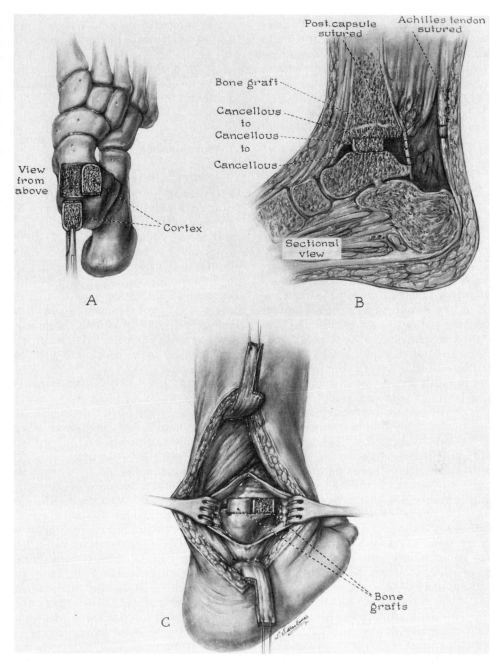

Figure 13-31 Diagrams of the basic surgical procedure for a relatively simple and atraumatic arthrodesis of the ankle. *A.* Positioning of the pieces of cortical calcaneus-iliac bone graft. *B.* Same positioning in a lateral section. *C.* Posterior view with the bone grafts in place. (Reproduced with permission from White, A. A.: A precision posterior ankle fusion. Clin. Orthop., 98:239–250, 1974.)

procedures generally eliminate pain and disrupt the normal gait only slightly. Studies have shown that, considering the prosthetic ankle joint replacements that are currently available, arthrodesis is generally the procedure of choice for treatment of intractable ankle joint pain.

Ruptured Achilles Tendon

This tendon sometimes ruptures, as a result of the strong forces applied to it in various athletic activities.

Clinical Evaluation

HISTORY. The patient is frequently a male aged 40 or older who played sports in the past but may be in somewhat less than optimum physical condition at the time of injury. In a typical case, the patient was participating vigorously in a basketball or tennis game. He jumped up or came down suddenly or made a sudden start, stop or cut. He and possibly others nearby may have heard a loud snap or "pop." The patient at this same moment may have had the sensation that he was kicked or hit on the back of the heel with the ball. He usually falls to the ground with great pain. Some patients will give a history of having had moderate pain in the region of the Achilles tendon for a period of time before the injury.

PHYSICAL EXAMINATION. There may be ecchymosis or mild to moderate swelling in the region of the heel, and the patient cannot walk on the toes. Weak plantar flexion may be present. The pathognomonic Simmonds' test for rupture of the tendon is performed as follows: With the patient in the prone position with both feet hanging off the end of the table (tibias supported by the table), each calf is squeezed firmly in the horizontal plane. On the normal side this maneuver will result in plantar flexion of the foot and ankle. On the injured side

there may possibly be a flicker of reaction but essentially no plantar flexion.[1] It may also be possible to see or palpate a sulcus in an area where a portion of the tendon should normally be.

LABORATORY STUDIES. It is desirable to take x-rays of the foot and ankle to rule out the presence of any bony injury.

Management

ADVICE. Once the diagnosis is certain, it is important to explain to the patient what has happened and to indicate that after healing occurs he will most likely be able to participate in sports again. However, it should be emphasized that this is a serious injury; there can be difficulty in healing and the whole process of treatment, healing and rehabilitation can take some time, namely four to six months or longer. We suggest that this injury be managed by a specialist who has had experience with it.

MEDICATION AND NONSURGICAL ORTHOPAEDICS. Elevation, elastic wraps and ice are desirable treatments in the acute phase of the disease. Their use may be followed by the application of a long-leg cast that holds the ankle in plantar flexion for four to six weeks, followed by six to eight weeks in a short-leg cast with the foot in the neutral position. This may seem a long time for treatment, but there appears to be a significant incidence of rerupture in patients who have only eight weeks of protected healing. Following removal of the cast, a heel lift may be worn for several weeks. A jogging program in which the patient works up to two or three miles of painless jogging per day is recommended before the patient goes back to vigorous running or competitive athletics.

SURGERY. Some specialists prefer to treat the initial injury with immediate direct suturing of the tendon. This technique should be followed by a program of protection and rehabilitation comparable to that described for the nonoperative treatment of the injury.

Discussion

The pain that some patients feel prior to rupture may serve as a warning. A preventive jogging program may be useful for males in the 40-plus age group who are not in condition and who feel heel pain. This will allow a partial injury to heal and permit some time for strengthening of the tendon before the patient participates in competition that might rupture the tendon. It can be difficult to choose between the surgical and nonsurgical treatment of this condition. However, it is accurate to state that in the hands of a competent clinician the patient can expect a satisfactory result.

Shin Splints and Anterior Tibial Compartment Syndrome

The Problem

Athletes involved in running, especially sprinters, will frequently complain of severe pain in the region of the shins or the anterior tibial compartment. This is usually a transient condition that resolves itself spontaneously. However, sometimes the pain may become intense and persist for weeks or months. When the condition becomes severe and progressive, it is referred to as anterior tibial compartment syndrome.

Clinical Evaluation

Most patients with shin splints never see a doctor. Sometimes, when pain is persistent, severe, progressive or associated with paralysis, patients do need medical and possibly orthopaedic attention. The history in less severe cases usually includes considerable sprinting, stopping and starting, possibly on a hard surface. The symptoms usually occur at the beginning of the athletic season and may be more severe shortly after running and at the beginning of running after 12 to 24 hours of rest. The diagnosis is likely to be anterior tibial compartment syndrome rather than shin splints when there is rapid progression of pain and paralysis or paresis of the anterior muscle, either spontaneously or associated with trauma to the shins.

In cases of shin splints there is usually tenderness to moderate or deep palpation in the anterior tibial compartment. Plantar flexion and inversion of the foot (stretching of the anterior tibial muscles) may also elicit the pain about which the patient is complaining. Anterior tibial compartment syndrome should be suspected when these findings are very acute and when, in addition, there is swelling, edema, engorgement or increased hardness of the anterior tibial muscles. The diagnosis is confirmed if paralysis or distinct weakness of the anterior tibial muscle group is present. X-rays of the tibia should be taken to rule out fatigue fracture. Recent studies have shown that pressure monitoring of the compartments may be helpful in the diagnosis and follow-up of patients with anterior tibial compartment syndrome.

Management

If diagnosed fairly early, shin splints can usually be managed by analgesia, elevation, massage and time. The athlete is generally opposed to reducing his or her activity temporarily and then gradually working back to the desired level; however, this is a desirable practice if it is at all feasible.

For the more severe and chronic cases the treatment is the same, except for two factors. These patients should be followed-up closely and warned about the possibility of anterior tibial compartment syndrome, and they may need to consider seriously a significant reduction of activity for several days.

Appropriate fasciotomy is indicated if the patient has acute anterior tibial compartment syndrome that does not improve rapidly with bed rest, elevation and ice in the hospital. Pressure monitoring of the compartment may be helpful in following the course of the disease and in evaluating the advisability of surgery.

Discussion

Although shin splints and anterior tibial compartment syndrome are discussed together and may represent stages of the same condition, there is no reliable evidence to support any such assumption. The etiology of shin splints and the initiating pathophysiology of anterior tibial compartment syndrome are not known.

Fatigue Fracture of the Tibia or Fibula

Fatigue fractures have been discussed on page 576. Uninitiated marchers, dancers and runners who have severe leg pain that is not simply from sore muscles should be suspected of having a fatigue fracture. This can be diagnosed from plain x-rays after 10 to 14 days and much sooner in some instances by technetium scan. The treatment is reduction of activity and protection of the bone by a cast or crutches, depending upon the severity of the symptoms and the extent and location of the structural failure of the bone.

THE KNEE AND UPPER LEG

Dislocated Fibula

The Problem

This is a relatively rare, isolated problem associated with rotatory injury involving the knee and ankle.

Clinical Evaluation

The injury is often associated with vigorous athletic activity in which the patient sustains a forceful rotatory displacement of the leg with the knee in the flexed position.

PHYSICAL EXAMINATION. The knee is held rigidly in the flexed position. There is acute pain localized over the lateral aspect of the knee joint, directly over the head of the fibula. The biceps tendon is noted to be in spasm. Comparison with the contralateral knee will show asymmetry in the area of the fibular head, with fibular prominence in the more common anterior dislocation and indentation in the rare posterior dislocation of the fibular head.

LABORATORY STUDIES. Comparison of lateral and anteroposterior roentgenograms of both knees will show malalignment of the involved proximal tibiofibular joint.

Management

Closed reduction is performed under anesthesia with the knee bent and the foot externally rotated, with posterior pressure on the anteriorly dislocated fibular head. Immobilization in a long-leg cast is required for three to four weeks following reduction.

Advice

This injury is secondary to severe rotatory stress on the involved extremity. The knee and ankle should be examined closely for ligamentous and osseous damage. The fibula should be palpated along its entire length for a possible fracture.

Bursitis of the Knee

The Problem

The knee is surrounded by several bursae, and inflammation of any of

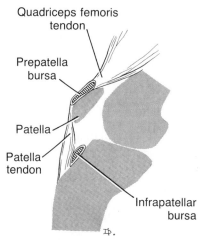

Quadriceps femoris
tendon

Prepatella
bursa

Patella

Patella
tendon

Infrapatellar
bursa

Figure 13–32 Bursae of the knee: prepatellar and infrapatellar. The prepatellar bursa is subcutaneous, and the infrapatellar bursa is located more deeply, posterior to the patellar tendon. Bursitis is treated by injection into the point of maximum tenderness.

these can mimic symptoms of meniscal and ligamentous injuries (Fig. 13–32).

Clinical Evaluation

A gradual onset of localized pain is often associated with the pursuit of a

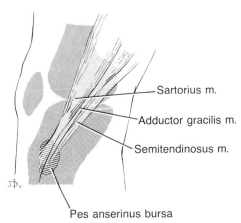

Sartorius m.

Adductor gracilis m.

Semitendinosus m.

Pes anserinus bursa

Figure 13–33 Pes anserinus bursa. The "goose's foot" bursa is located at the insertion of the sartorius, semitendinosus and adductor gracilis muscles in the medial tubercle of the tibia. The bursa presumably is named for the three separate tendons which insert at one point.

new physical activity. The pain is intensified following activities, and localized swelling occasionally appears. The most common bursitis of the knee is that of the prepatellar bursa; however, the infrapatellar, pes anserinus (Fig. 13–33) and popliteal bursae are also commonly afflicted. One should always search for a history of collagen disease, localized infection or gout that could be the cause of this pain.

PHYSICAL EXAMINATION. Acute localized tenderness is noted at the anatomical site of the bursa. Localized erythematous swelling may be palpable. The prepatellar bursa may occasionally show extreme swelling and fluid collection and may become septic owing to its subcutaneous location.

LABORATORY STUDIES. Aspiration of a fluctuant bursa should be carried out and appropriate examinations performed for crystals and inflammatory processes.

Management

In acute cases in which local infection can be ruled out, injection of a steroid compound can lead to dramatic relief of symptoms. In the case of septic bursitis, aspiration and oral antibiotic treatment is indicated once the organism is identified. With an infective process, elevation, splint immobilization and moist warm compresses are beneficial. In resistant cases associated with recurrent accumulation of septic fluid, open incision and drainage are indicated. Recurrent sterile fluid accumulation may occur in some patients with chronic septic and traumatic bursitis. Excision of the bursa should be considered in these cases if local compression does not alleviate the symptoms.

Semimembranosus Bursitis (Baker's Cyst)

The Problem

The popliteal cyst is an enlargement of the bursa that communicates with the knee joint just posterior to the medial head of the gastrocnemius muscle. When enlarged, the bursa presents between the gastrocnemius and semimembranosus muscles.

Clinical Evaluation

This condition is often seen in the preadolescent patient who has a painless mass in the medial portion of the popliteal space. The patient may describe recurrent swelling of the mass, and often there is an associated history of intra-articular disease in the knee joint. In older patients, the presence of the cyst may reflect synovitis of the joint secondary to rheumatoid or gouty arthritis or to another intra-articular derangement. The cyst may respond to treatment of these conditions.

PHYSICAL EXAMINATION. A firm, translucent mass in the popliteal space is palpable. Complete examination of the knee joint should be made to look for related intra-articular pathology. The popliteal mass should be palpated for pulsations and auscultated to rule out the possibility of a popliteal arterial aneurysm.

LABORATORY STUDIES. X-rays of the knee joint reveal a soft tissue mass in the popliteal area. These roentgenograms will also help to rule out a pathological process involving the osseous structures around the knee. An arthrogram and arthroscopy may be most helpful in evaluating the knee for any intra-articular disease.

Management

The popliteal mass usually resolves itself spontaneously once the intra-articular disease has been treated. On rare occasions, excision of the popliteal mass is indicated. In children, unless the cyst interferes with a neurovascular structure, no surgical treatment is indicated.

Idiopathic Osteoarthritis of the Knee

The Problem

A degenerative joint disease most often seen in elderly patients, this condition is occasionally due to a specific traumatic condition that has caused ligamentous instability and joint incongruity, leading to joint dysfunction.

Clinical Evaluation

There has been a gradual onset of pain and swelling in the knee over a period of several years. Often a related history of trauma or injury to the knee many years previously is given. Occasionally the onset cannot be ascribed to any particular episode. The pain usually increases with activity and intensifies with changes in the weather (usually cold or dampness). A history of gradually increasing deformity of the knee joint, represented by increasing valgus angulation, is noted by the patient.

PHYSICAL EXAMINATION. Depending on the severity of the degenerative changes, the knee may appear relatively normal or, in the more advanced cases, may be diffusely swollen. Gross crepitation of the patellofemoral and tibiofemoral articulations is often present on flexion and extension. In mild cases the only finding may be a minor effusion and some joint tenderness. Palpation may reveal the early formation of osteophytes along the joint margin. In the more advanced cases, examination should include measurement of valgus deformity of the involved knee joint and a search for effusion, synovial swelling and loose bodies in the knee joint and suprapatellar pouch. The degree of atrophy of the thigh muscles should be noted. A complete neurological examination should be made to rule out the possibility of a neurotrophic basis for the joint degeneration.

LABORATORY STUDIES. Roentgenograms of the knee are imperative to assess the degree of joint involvement (Fig. 13–34). These should be evaluated for the degree of osteophyte and cyst formation and narrowing of the joint space. VDRL and serum glucose level tests should be obtained.

Management

In the early stages, conservative therapy consists of weight loss and the use of oral anti-inflammatory drugs. A supervised exercise program is used to rehabilitate atrophied thigh musculature. If the examination reveals meniscal damage or the presence of intra-articular loose bodies, surgical repair or removal is recommended. In valgus deformity, joint débridement and synovectomy may prove to be beneficial when associated with a tibial osteotomy to realign the weight-bearing of the deformed joint. In advanced joint destruction none of these measures would prove beneficial. A total knee joint prosthesis or joint arthrodesis should be considered in that case.

Advice

Total joint prosthesis should also be considered in the elderly, relatively inactive individual. The patient's degree of discomfort and expected activity level should be assessed before one of the many available devices is rec-

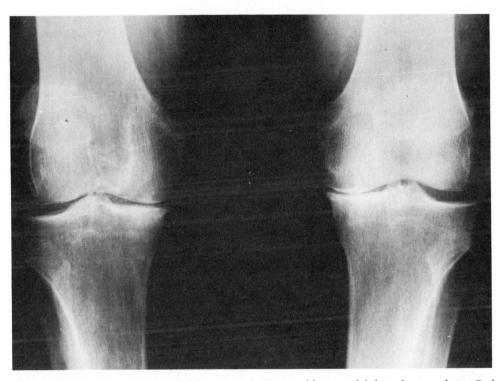

Figure 13–34 AP standing view of the knees of a 63 year old man with bilateral osteoarthritis. Both knees show narrowing of the medial joint compartment and spurring and lipping along the lateral and medial borders of the joint. This patient's main complaints were recurrent effusions and medial joint line pain when standing.

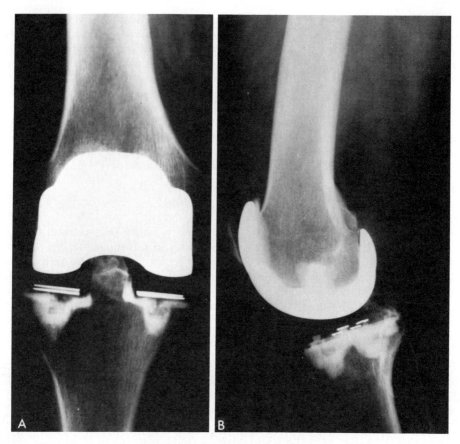

Figure 13–35 Anteroposterior (A) and lateral (B) views of a total knee joint replacement prosthesis. (Photos courtesy of Harris Yett, M.D., Boston, Mass.)

ommended. Figure 13–35 shows x-ray views of a patient with a total knee joint replacement.

Rupture of the Quadriceps Mechanism

The Problem

Rupture of the quadriceps mechanism may occur without fracture of the patella through the fibers of the quadriceps tendon or distally through the patellar tendon.

Clinical Evaluation

In younger individuals there is often a history of a forceful contraction of the quadriceps muscle when the body is thrust forward with the extremity forced into acute flexion. This is followed by the immediate onset of intense pain and inability to extend the knee actively against gravity. In some cases spontaneous rupture associated with chronic debilitating processes such as advanced renal and collagen diseases occurs.

PHYSICAL EXAMINATION. The diagnosis can be made from the presence of localized tenderness and a palpable gap in the quadriceps or patellar tendon with inability to extend the knee actively.

LABORATORY STUDIES. X-rays of the knee joint may localize the rupture. In cases involving the patellar tendon, the patella will be seen on the x-ray views to be in an unusually elevated position. In rupture of the quadriceps mechanism there is no change in the anatomical location of the patella.

Management

Surgical repair of the ruptured tendon is necessary.

Stress Fracture of the Distal Femur

The Problem

The basis for this injury is fatigue failure of the bone secondary to an unaccustomed activity level in untrained or inactive individuals.

Clinical Evaluation

Rapid onset of poorly localized pain associated with strenuous physical activity occurs over the distal femur or knee. The patient usually is a sedentary worker who, on the spur of the moment, participated in a long hike or a distance run. The pain occurs either during the activity or shortly thereafter.

PHYSICAL EXAMINATION. Pain and tenderness is noted over the distal tibia. The remainder of the examination is negative.

LABORATORY STUDIES. Roentgenographs are usually negative if done shortly after the onset of symptoms. However, they are necessary in order to rule out any local pathological process within the bone. Technetium bone scan may prove to be diagnostic in early cases.

Management

If a stress fracture of the femur is suspected, it is imperative that weight-bearing on the involved extremity be discontinued immediately. Disastrous displacement of untreated stress fractures has been documented. Treatment requires no weight-bearing and, if necessary, immobilization in a hip spica cast for a period of six to eight weeks. At this time, roentgenograms should show mature callus formation if adequate healing has taken place.

Advice

Activities should be resumed only after a period of supervised rehabilitation to obtain full motion and strength of the muscles and joints of the involved extremity.

Myalgia Paresthetica

The Problem

Compression injury of the lateral femoral cutaneous nerve (L2–3) causes numbness and dysesthesias over the lateral aspect of the thigh.

Clinical Evaluation

The patient usually gives a history of a gradual onset of numbness and dysesthesias over the lateral aspect of the thigh. Symptoms may be indistinct since the condition may occur insidiously, coming to the attention of the patient only when local trauma in this area produces less pain than that noted in the past. Dysesthesias include pain and a tingling sensation over the lateral thigh.

PHYSICAL EXAMINATION. Loss of two-point discrimination sensation or localization of dysesthesia over the cutaneous distribution of the lateral femoral cutaneous nerve is noted. Examination should include a complete neurological evaluation to rule out the possibility of nerve root compression, since the lateral femoral cutaneous nerve is only one of several nerves originating in the L2–3 area of the spine.

LABORATORY STUDIES. X-rays of the lumbosacral spine and the ilium on the involved side should be taken to rule out the possibility of an osseous or spinal abnormality impinging on the nerve.

Management

The patient should be advised that compression of the nerve by tight-fitting braces, corsets or belts in the region of the anterior superior iliac spine may result in injury to this nerve. Thus, all tight-fitting clothing should be avoided. Entrapment of the nerve as it exits beneath the inguinal ligament occasionally requires surgical decompression.

THE HIP

Trochanteric Bursitis

This condition is characterized by acute discomfort over the region of the greater trochanter owing to inflammation within the bursa (Fig. 13–36). Weight-bearing on the affected extremity increases the pain, and the patient usually presents with an antalgic gait.

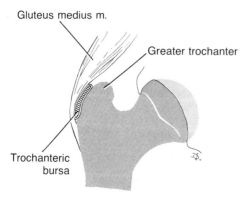

Figure 13–36   Anatomy of trochanteric bursa.

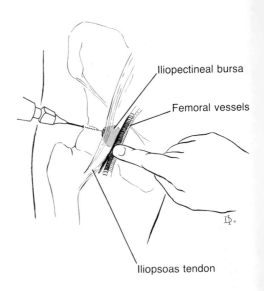

Figure 13–37 Iliopectineal bursa: anterior relationships and injection. The femoral pulse is identified. The needle is inserted as shown, lateral to the femoral pulsation. The tip of the needle is advanced until bone (the ilium) is encountered. This is usually at a depth of 2 inches or less in an average sized person. The needle is from a lateral angle, as illustrated.

The bursa may be a focus of tuberculous infection. In this condition, destructive changes are normally seen within the femur. In the usual nonspecific inflammatory involvement of the bursa, symptoms can be alleviated with the use of anti-inflammatory agents or by injection of steroids into the area.

Iliopectineal Bursitis

This bursa overlies the iliopectineal eminence and lies posterior to the psoas muscle (Fig. 13–37). It lies somewhat superior to the capsule of the hip joint with which it sometimes communicates. Inflammation or swelling within the bursa may compress the femoral nerve and cause pain referred into the thigh.

In the acute condition, the joint is held in the flexed position, and extension is painful from this position.

The presence of sepsis within the bursa needs to be differentiated from a psoas abscess and intra-articular hip disease.

Ischial Bursitis ("Weaver's Bottom")

Ischial bursitis is a common, painful condition due to inflammation in the ischial bursa. It may be relieved by injection of anti-inflammatory agents into the tender area overlying the ischial tuberosity. The relationship of the sciatic nerve is shown on the diagram (Fig. 13–38). One must take great care in injecting this region, in order to avoid damage to the sciatic nerve.

Fatigue Fracture of the Hip

As a result of repeated loading of the hip, usually in a patient who has been relatively inactive, the neck of the femur may undergo fatigue failure. The diagnosis should be entertained when unilateral or bilateral hip pain occurs in a relatively sedentary person who has recently begun a repetitive activity. If the plain x-rays do not show

the lesion, technetium scan should be considered. A crack in the superior femoral neck has the potential for complete separation and displacement.

The main consideration is to make the diagnosis as soon as possible, because once the diagnosis is known, bed rest with balanced suspension or internal surgical fixation should be considered.

Arthritis of the Hip

The Problem

Pain in the hip without a distinct history of trauma may be due to some type of arthritic condition.

Clinical Evaluation

The patient's age is a major factor in determining the etiology. Patients who are in the older age group when pain develops are likely to have osteoarthritis (Fig. 13–39). One should, of course, be on the lookout for tumor and infection in all age groups. Individuals in their twenties and thirties are more likely to have rheumatoid disease or

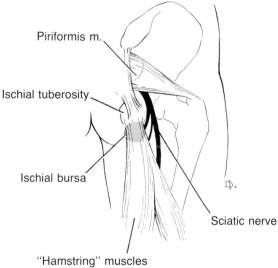

Figure 13–38 Ischial bursa: posterior view.

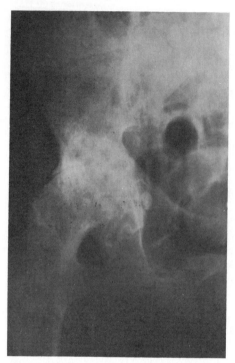

Figure 13-39 Severe osteoarthritis of the right hip. Note narrowing of the joint line and sclerosis. This patient has considerable cystic degeneration, more than is usually seen.

some of the other collagen vascular conditions such as lupus erythematosus or dermatomyositis. Patients in this age group may also have arthritis associated with avascular necrosis or a variety of the other conditions such as sickle cell disease, various clotting abnormalities and alcoholism or with steroid therapy.

Osteoarthritis is typically most symptomatic following periods of inactivity and, within limits, it tends to be less troublesome as activity increases. Most of the other conditions are made worse with activity, although the collagen vascular diseases, including rheumatoid arthritis, may have a spontaneous pattern of exacerbation and remission.

Osteoarthritis tends to involve the spine, hips, knees and the distal interphalangeal joints. Rheumatoid ar-

thritis may involve practically any joint. The elbows, wrists and metacarpophalangeal joints are more likely to be involved, however. Any of several joints may be actively symptomatic at any given time. There may be a family history of osteoarthritis or diseases in the collagen vascular group.

PHYSICAL EXAMINATION. The patient may walk with an antalgic gait or use crutches or a cane. The Trendelenburg test is generally positive, that is, if the patient stands on the symptomatic leg with the opposite hip flexed 90 degrees, the pelvis on the side of the flexed hip cannot be held horizontal and will drop down several inches. The patient with osteoarthritis will tend to hold the hip in slight flexion, abduction and external rotation. With rheumatoid disease there may be fusiform swelling of knees, fingers, wrist and elbow.

The patient should be examined for abnormal skin conditions (rash, discoloration). Subcutaneous nodules may be noted on the extensor surface of the forearm. Heberden's nodes may be found at the distal interphalangeal joints if the patient has osteoarthritis.

Examination of the hip may show limitation of motion in all parameters. Crepitus and pain may also be elicited as attempts are made to pass the joint through its range of motion.

LABORATORY STUDIES. If the diagnosis is not clear, the following laboratory studies are suggested: complete blood count, sedimentation rate, urinalysis, serum uric acid and rheumatoid factor tests and lateral x-rays of the hips.

Most patients with hip pain will have degenerative arthritis, avascular necrosis or rheumatoid arthritis. Usually the clinical information discussed up to this point will be adequate to make a diagnosis.

SPECIAL STUDIES. Some additional studies that may be needed to help with the diagnosis are: an L.E. preparation, joint aspiration for culture and synovial fluid analysis.[7] Joint aspiration technique is described on page 548. Guinea pig inoculation, skin tests and chest x-ray should be done if tuberculosis is suspected. A sickle cell test and hemoglobin electrophoresis may be helpful if avascular necrosis is a possibility. Technetium scan may also be helpful in that situation. In some instances the diagnosis can only be made after needle or open biopsy of bone or synovial tissue, or both.

Management

The treatment depends entirely upon the diagnosis. Nonsurgical treatment of collagen vascular disease is probably best given by a rheumatologist or an internist. Those patients to be treated orthopaedically may be managed as follows:

ADVICE. Considerable relief can probably be obtained with aspirin, crutches, physical therapy and reduced activity. This can be continued as long as it works satisfactorily.

MEDICAL AND NONSURGICAL ORTHOPAEDICS. The first approach is almost always aspirin, the use of a cane in the opposite hand, and physical therapy with a gentle active range of motion. This will sometimes suffice. More complex medical treatment for the collagen vascular group of diseases is also sometimes completely satisfactory.

SURGERY. Several surgical procedures are useful for various clinical situations involving arthritis of the hip. One is osteotomy of the hip. A wedge of bone is removed from the intertrochanteric region that permanently alters the orientation of the head of the femur in the acetabulum. This places different and probably healthier cartilage in juxtaposition across the joint. The procedure also alters the dynamics of fluid pressure in the head of the femur, which also may be therapeutic.

Surgical arthrodesis of the hip is another possibility. This is a fairly exten-sive surgical procedure that eliminates pain by eliminating the joint. An osseous fusion is established across the joint. Once the fusion is mature, the problem is solved forever. The procedure is fine for a heavy laborer but not for a sexually active female.

The third standard procedure is the implantation of a total prosthetic replacement for the joint (Fig. 13–40). The hip joint is most amenable to total joint arthroplasty, and the implants and procedures for it are very well developed. In a relatively young person (age 50 or younger), especially one who weighs 200 pounds or more or is extremely active, one can anticipate loosening or failure of the prosthesis

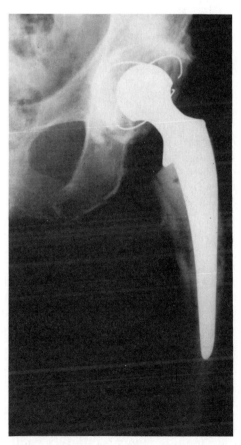

Figure 13–40 Total hip joint replacement. (Photo courtesy of Harris Yett, M.D., Boston, Mass.)

before the patient's death. In most cases there is an immediate happy result with this procedure, but other serious problems may develop when there are early or late complications. Nevertheless, this procedure is one of the most important advances in modern surgery.

Discussion

First, the correct diagnosis must be made. The main concern is to rule out infection or tumor. A thorough attempt should then be made to control the patient's symptoms with medication and nonsurgical therapy, if feasible. If this is not possible, the appropriate operation should be selected.

THE UPPER LIMB

Bursitis of the Shoulder

The Problem

The shoulder is surrounded by several bursae, all of which can be involved in a local inflammatory reaction. However, the subacromial bursa is the most common source of pain.

Clinical Evaluation

A rapid onset of acute, disabling pain in the shoulder is the chief complaint. Often a past history of mild shoulder discomfort associated with certain activities is elicited. The search for a specific cause of the pain, such as trauma or a particular activity, is often negative. The examiner should also look for a history of collagen disease of gout, since these may be the cause of the bursal inflammation.

PHYSICAL EXAMINATION. The patient presents with rigid splinting of the shoulder, which is diffusely tender to palpation. All motion, active or passive, is restricted because of pain.

Local erythema and increased temperature are noted in the area of the involved joint.

LABORATORY STUDIES. Roentgenograms occasionally show calcification of the rotator cuff, but this is not diagnostic, and the x-ray findings can be completely negative except for an elevation of the humeral head relative to the acromion due to surrounding muscle spasm. Occasionally the calcification in the rotator cuff erodes into the subacromial bursa, causing an acute and tender subacromial bursitis (Fig. 13–41).

Management

Complete immobilization in a sling provides significant relief. In most cases, infection of the subacromial bursa with a local anesthetic and an intra-articular steroid compound provides dramatic relief. Oral anti-inflammatory drugs such as phenylbutazone (Butazolidin) or indomethacin (Indocin), though slower-acting, are also effective in alleviating the inflammation.

ADVICE. The practitioner should be aware that subacromial bursitis is often secondary to other disorders about the shoulder, especially rotator cuff degeneration (see following section).

Supraspinatus Syndrome

The Problem

Pain develops because of degenerative changes in the rotator cuff. These changes are usually secondary to friction of the rotator cuff and of the subacromial bursa against the acromion. Initial fibrillation and fraying of this structure associated with calcaneous deposits in the tendon and the adjacent bursa occur. Eventually, tearing and occasionally complete rupture of the cuff occur. Pain emanating from

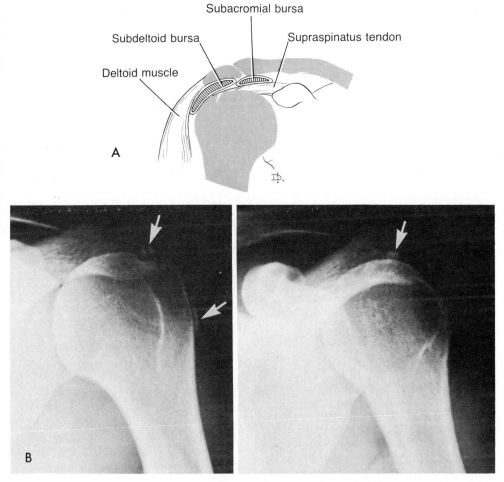

Subacromial bursa

Subdeltoid bursa

Deltoid muscle

Supraspinatus tendon

A

B

Figure 13–41 *A.* Diagrammatic representation of the relationship of shoulder bursae to the acromion and rotator cuff. *B.* X-rays of calcified tendinitis of the shoulder. Calcification in the subdeltoid bursa and supraspinatus tendon, as shown. The lesions are most apparent in the externally rotated view (*left*), and may be almost impossible to detect when the shoulder is internally rotated (*right*).

the rotator cuff is often difficult to differentiate clinically from that arising in the adjacent bursa.

Clinical Evaluation

The patient is usually 35 to 55 years of age and describes a gradual onset of pain of varying degrees of intensity that sometimes radiates into the lateral aspect of the arm. The pain is most severe with activities that demand extremes of motion. Often the patient volunteers the information that the pain occurs when donning a shirt or jacket or when reaching for an object above his head. A history of acute calcific tendinitis is often a precursor of the initial degenerative process of the rotator cuff.

PHYSICAL EXAMINATION. In degenerative changes of the rotator cuff, the range of motion of the shoulder is normal on passive examination. Active abduction between 80 and 120 degrees is often painful, and external rotation in the abducted position also causes symptoms. Some atrophy of the shoulder girdle musculature may be present in chronic cases.

LABORATORY STUDIES. X-rays of the shoulder in internal and external rotation and subacromial views may show calcific degeneration of the rotator cuff and the occurrence of subacromial spurs that may be aggravating the condition being considered.

Management

In mild cases, oral anti-inflammatory agents can be most helpful. In the young, active patient a short period of immobilization (four or five days) may be used to allow the inflammatory response to diminish. The physician should warn the patient that long periods of immobilization may lead to ankylosis (frozen shoulder). Oral anti-inflammatory agents should be tried in chronic conditions. In the more severe conditions, where pain is incapacitating, an injection of an intra-articular steroid may prove to be beneficial.

ADVICE. It is imperative, especially with older patients, to emphasize the importance of maintaining shoulder motion. Local injection of steroids should be limited to one or two times, since overexposure to steroid compounds may induce rupture of the rotator cuff.

Rupture of the Rotator Cuff

The Problem

Rupture of the rotator cuff occurs through an area of degeneration in the supraspinatus tendon.

Clinical Evaluation

The patient is usually more than 40 years old and describes the acute onset of severe shoulder pain accompanying a fall or stress to the shoulder. Often spontaneous pain and a "snapping" sound or sensation occur when an object is lifted or pushed. A previous history of shoulder discomfort similar to that of patients with supraspinatus syndrome can often be elicited.

PHYSICAL EXAMINATION. An acutely painful shoulder is noted with all active motion restricted because of pain and reflex inhibition. Palpation over the shoulder may reveal localized pain in the region of the rotator cuff, and in slender individuals a defect or step-off in this structure may occasionally be palpated. The erect patient cannot hold the straight abducted arm parallel to the floor without assistance. Clinically, differentiation between rupture of the rotator cuff and acute subacromial bursitis may be difficult.

LABORATORY STUDIES. In order to establish a diagnosis, the shoulder joint may be anesthetized by the injection of 1 per cent Xylocaine (5 cc given intra-articularly). Initiation of active abduction eliminates the possibility of complete rupture of the rotator cuff. Routine roentgenographs in both internal and external rotation should be taken to determine whether any associated calcific tendinitis is present. An arthrogram of the shoulder may help to diagnose a partial rupture of the rotator cuff.

Management

Partial ruptures can be treated by a short period of immobilization (eight to ten days). Complete ruptures in elderly or inactive patients can be treated similarly. Following the short period of immobilization, a supervised program of physical therapy that stresses range of motion and strengthening of the shoulder girdle musculature is instituted. Young, athletic patients with complete rupture of the rotator cuff benefit from surgical repair of the structure to maintain full strength and function of the upper extremity.

ADVICE. Patients treated nonoperatively do surprisingly well. Individuals to be treated surgically should be selected carefully. One criterion for this decision is the patient's active, vigorous and athletic use of the involved extremity. An active individual usually has the motivation for the active postoperative physical therapy that is required to regain full function of the shoulder joint.

Fibrous Ankylosis of the Shoulder (Frozen Shoulder)

The Problem

The origins of this condition are varied, but ankylosis arises most commonly from immobilization of the shoulder in the adducted position secondary to painful conditions within the joint. An inflammatory condition such as a bursitis, supraspinatus syndrome or bicipital tendinitis may result in ankylosis due to reflex restricted activity.

Clinical Evaluation

Often there is a history of humeral fracture, bursitis, supraspinatus syndrome or rotator cuff rupture, with the patient subsequently holding the shoulder in the adducted and immobilized position. Sometimes trauma to the elbow, wrist or forearm with associated shoulder immobilization initiates this condition.

PHYSICAL EXAMINATION. Examination reveals a limited range of active and passive motion of the shoulder.

LABORATORY STUDIES. Roentgenographic examination of the shoulder should be made to assess the degree of degenerative change within the glenohumeral articulation.

Management

The employment of gentle passive and active exercise by a skilled therapist will often suffice in the early stages of this disease. The importance of self-administered treatment at home must be stressed to the patient. On some occasions the use of ice pack prior to passive motion administered by the therapist will be more helpful than the usual applications of heat. Failure to show progress may require manipulative treatment under general anesthesia. During the procedure the joint is maneuvered through the full range of motion and maintained initially in the abducted, externally rotated position. Maintenance of the range of motion regained during manipulation depends on the passive and active exercises carried out following the treatment.

ADVICE. The saying, "an ounce of prevention is worth a pound of cure" is most applicable in this condition. Often the onset of ankylosis is insidious and rapid. With this in mind, the practitioner should stress to the patient the importance of maintaining some shoulder joint mobility in painful conditions involving the upper extremity, which must be rested to some extent.

Bicipital Tendinitis

The Problem

There are two distinct types of tenosynovitis of the bicipital tendon. The first is seen in athletes who present with an inflammatory reaction of the tendon due to overuse in activities such as baseball, gymnastics, bowling and swimming. The second type is seen in individuals over the age of 40 whose symptoms occur after trauma and strenuous exercise. Occasionally the onset is insidious, without any specific injury.

Clinical Evaluation

In young athletes there is a clear history of vigorous participation in one of the sports just named, often early in the season. Pain is exacerbated by practicing or competing in a specific activity that requires the use of the shoulder muscle complex. In older patients, some form of trauma, such as falling on the anterior aspect of the shoulder or jamming the humerus against the acromion in a fall on an outstretched hand, may be the initiating circumstance. Sometimes the onset is associated with a game of tennis or with shoveling snow. In older patients, this tendinitis can be part of a symptom complex involving other structures of the shoulder.

The pain is located in the anterior aspect of the joint. In severe conditions pain is sometimes described as radiating down the arm and into the posterior aspect of the scapula. It can be exacerbated by lying on the affected side. The patient should be asked whether the pain is associated with a snapping sensation in the shoulder joint. This may indicate that bicipital tendinitis is secondary to subluxation of the tendon from the humeral bicipital groove.

PHYSICAL EXAMINATION. Exquisite tenderness can be elicited by pressure over the tendon itself in the bicipital groove. The pain can be localized by placing the forearm into resisted supination with the forearm flexed. Abduction and external rotation of the arm is also painful. Snapping of the tendon indicates subluxation of the tendon in and out of the bicipital groove.

LABORATORY STUDIES. Roentgenographs of the shoulder help to rule out associated conditions such as calcific tendinitis. Axial views of the proximal humerus may show a bony spur within the bicipital groove. A shallow bicipital groove is further evidence for the diagnosis of a possible subluxating tendon.

Management

In the athlete four or five days of rest will usually alleviate all symptoms if treatment is started early. Often discussion with the coach and trainers can modify the patient's throwing, swimming or gymnastic style to avoid undue stress on this tendon. In older patients a brief period of rest followed by a supervised program of physical therapy, including heat and motion, should be tried. If conservative treatment is not beneficial, then a local injection of Xylocaine plus a steroid compound should be given into the bicipital tendon sheath. An effort should be made to *avoid* injecting the steroid into the bicipital tendon itself. Surgical intervention is necessary in chronic conditions that are refractory to other treatment and for subluxaating tendons.

Arthritis of the Shoulder

The Problem

Although the shoulder is not a weight-bearing joint, degenerative arthritis of this joint can be quite disabling. With a weight in the hand and the arm in the abducted position, because of the mechanics dictated by the long lever arm there is great force on the glenohumeral articulation, causing pain and discomfort in degenerative arthritis. A previous condition such as infection, fracture or collagen disease can cause degenerative changes; however, the cause for this condition in most cases is unknown.

Clinical Evaluation

The patient is invariably in the late fifties or older. A history of trauma, infection or other disease should be sought. Pain can usually be elicited with motion of the glenohumeral joint, gradually increasing and becoming more incapacitating over a period of many years. A history of hemoglobinopathy should be asked about, since aseptic necrosis of the humeral head occurs for the same reasons as noted for the femoral head.

PHYSICAL EXAMINATION. A limited range of motion involving the shoulder articulation is noted. Often crepitation and pain are elicited in moving the joint. Occasionally there is a history of locking, effusion and snapping secondary to the presence of loose bodies in this articulation. Atrophy of the shoulder girdle musculature often occurs secondary to reflex inhibition of muscle tone.

LABORATORY STUDIES. Roentgenographs of the shoulder will show the degree of loss of articular cartilage and other radiographic changes such as osteophyte formation associated with the degenerative disease process. Incongruity of the glenohumeral joint secondary to previous trauma may also be visualized.

Management

In the early phase of this condition conservative therapy, consisting of oral anti-inflammatory medications and a physical therapy regimen that emphasizes an active, supervised program of motion and strengthening exercises, should be tried. In more advanced, painful conditions, local injection of steroid into the shoulder articulation can be given once or twice. It should be remembered, however, that repeated injection of steroid compounds will hasten the already advancing degenerative process. If pain continues to be incapacitating, the patient should be evaluated in terms of his lifestyle and level of activity involving the use of the upper extremity. Fusion of the glenohumeral joint can give a functional and pain-free upper extremity. In addition, the insertion of a humeral head prosthesis or even a total joint replacement is possible and can dramatically reduce pain and restore some degree of lost motion. However, at the present level of technology, these joint substitutes cannot be ex-

pected to hold up under the stresses and activity level of an active young person.

ADVICE. The aim for individuals with chronic degenerative arthritis of the shoulder is to try to maintain an active and functional range of motion of the shoulder as long as possible. Once the degeneration has advanced, then surgical intervention should be advised.

Recurrent Shoulder Dislocation

The Problem

This is almost exclusively a malady of the young (16 to 30 year old) male. Usually there is a history of traumatic dislocation of the shoulder, followed by recurrent episodes of shoulder dislocation associated with minor stress on the glenohumeral articulation. Almost all of these individuals have joint instability secondary to laxity of the anterior or inferior joint capsule and insufficiency of the glenoid rim. Occasionally a traumatic osseous defect in the humeral head is present.

Clinical Evaluation

Usually the history includes recurrent anterior dislocation of the shoulder following an initial traumatic dislocation, which often was treated by a short, inadequate period of immobilization (less than three or four weeks). The patient states that the shoulder feels unstable and dislocates spontaneously when the arm is placed in an abducted and externally rotated position. The shoulder joint may become so lax that spontaneous dislocation can be induced by the patient. Specific information as to the site of the dislocation is important, since this condition must be differentiated from others such as subluxation or the possible but rare recurrent posterior dislocation.

PHYSICAL EXAMINATION. Apprehension can be elicited by abducting and externally rotating the suspected unstable shoulder. The patient often volunteers that he feels as if the shoulder will dislocate if abduction and external rotation are taken to the maximum degree. Following a recent dislocation, tenderness may be palpated in the anterior aspect of the joint capsule.

LABORATORY STUDIES. Roentgenographs of the involved shoulder in internal and external rotation will often show an osseous defect in the posterolateral area of the humeral head (Hill-Sachs lesion). Other findings include a fracture of the glenoid rim and an occasional loose body within the shoulder joint. Axillary views of the shoulder may show a shallow glenoid socket. An arthrogram of the shoulder shows a redundance and laxity of the anterior shoulder capsule. On occasion a true dislocation cannot be documented even though the history is compatible with joint laxity. Stability of the shoulder joint can be evaluated under general anesthesia with muscle relaxation. This examination can definitively assess the stability of the joint and substantiate the need for surgical repair. Examinations under anesthesia can be documented with the use of fluoroscopic cineradiography.

Management

The only effective method to treat this disorder is surgical repair to stabilize the shoulder joint. Many effective surgical procedures have been described in the literature.

ADVICE. It is important in this condition to document, by examination, history, past x-rays or a physician's statement, that dislocation has occurred. If this is not possible, the suggested laboratory examinations should be made before surgical intervention is attempted. The practitioner should be aware of the rare patient with diffuse joint laxity who can voluntarily dislocate or subluxate the shoulder joint. For these individuals effective treatment consists of exercise and advice to cease this maneuver. Surgery should be avoided in these patients because it is ineffective.

Recurrent Posterior Dislocation of the Shoulder

This is a rare entity and is usually associated with another condition such as seizure disorder, where dislocations occur secondary to involuntary muscle spasm. If this has caused chronic instability of the shoulder, repair of the posterior shoulder capsule can be attempted. Usually this should be done after the seizure pattern or the neurological condition is under control.

Suprascapular Nerve Irritation

The Problem

Entrapment of the suprascapular nerve occurs where it passes through the notch in the upper border of the scapula called the suprascapular foramen.

Clinical Evaluation

The patient describes vague pain over the posterolateral aspect of the shoulder. Often there is a history of trauma in which forceful adduction of the arm across the chest has caused a traction injury to the nerve.

PHYSICAL EXAMINATION. Pain is vaguely localized over the posterior aspect of the shoulder and can be elicited by forceful movement of the scapula forward and across the chest wall. Occasionally an acromioclavicular separation is associated with these findings, allowing for increased forward displacement of the scapula, thus exacerbating the traction injury to the nerve. Atrophy and weakness of the supraspinatus and infraspinatus muscles are present in injuries that are more than four weeks old.

LABORATORY STUDIES. X-rays should be taken to reveal a possible associated acromioclavicular separation. Electromyographic studies of the infraspinatus and supraspinatus muscles should be done to assess the degree of nerve damage and possible loss of innervation to these muscles. Infiltration of local anesthetic into the suprascapular notch should be attempted to see if this completely alleviates nerve pain secondary to neuritis.

Management

Electromyographic findings compatible with a traction injury should be treated expectantly, but nerve entrapment within the suprascapular notch requires surgical decompression.

Rupture of the Proximal Biceps Tendon

The Problem

Rupture is most common in the tendon of the long head of the biceps where it traverses the intertubercular groove. This dramatic and spontaneous injury usually occurs in middle-aged individuals.

Clinical Evaluation

Sudden and acute onset of pain in the shoulder, associated with a lifting maneuver is described. The patient often states that an audible snap occurred with the onset of pain. Most patients will notice a bunching of the biceps muscle in the distal aspect of the arm.

PHYSICAL EXAMINATION. In acute cases there is a dramatic bunching of the biceps in the distal end of the arm. Often ecchymosis is noted over the proximal end of the biceps and the anterior shoulder region (Fig. 13–42). Weakness, if present, is noted in active supination and flexion of the forearm.

LABORATORY STUDIES. None.

Management

In young, athletic patients, surgical reattachment of the biceps is indicated. In older patients, minimal functional disability occurs from this injury, so conservative treatment, which consists of a short period of immobilization until pain subsides, is used.

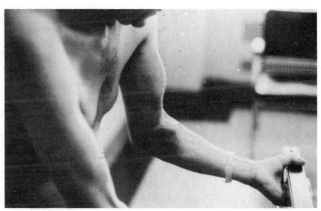

Figure 13–42   This patient has a rupture of the proximal (long head) biceps tendon. Note the "popeye" type of bulging of the biceps muscle in the lower part of the left arm. The bulging is accentuated by having the patient flex the elbow against resistance by attempting to lift the bed. The dark color on the inner arm is due to extensive extravasation of blood into the subcutaneous tissues.

Full functional use of the arm follows.

Rupture of the Distal Biceps Tendon

The Problem

This is a much less common injury that involves a tear of the distal musculotendinous junction of the biceps tendon at the elbow.

Clinical Evaluation

A sudden onset of pain over the anterior portion of the elbow during an episode of lifting or forced pronation is the presenting complaint.

PHYSICAL EXAMINATION. Ecchymosis may be present over the anterior region of the elbow. There is a bunching of the muscle in the proximal portion of the arm.

LABORATORY STUDIES. None.

Management

Surgical repair of the rupture is indicated, since this tear totally eliminates function of the biceps muscle at the elbow.

THE ELBOW

Olecranon Bursitis

The Problem

The bursal space between the insertion of the triceps on the olecranon and the skin can become distended with fluid secondary to irritation or trauma. This bursa is probably the one which is most commonly inflamed. Because of its superficial location, septic bursitis frequently occurs. A second olecranon bursa is found between the triceps tendon and the posterior ligament of the elbow, but this is rarely involved in bursitis.

Clinical Evaluation

Swelling is described directly over the olecranon prominence. It is occasionally painful but usually is asymptomatic. In acute conditions the occurrence is associated with trauma. In a chronic effusion work-related trauma, such as that of a traveling salesman who habitually rests his elbow on the door armrest while driving for long distances can often be elicited from the history. In septic arthritis, it is difficult to obtain any specific history. However, chronic asymptomatic bursitis often precedes it and, apparently secondarily, becomes infected because of a small puncture wound. A history of gout and collagen disease should be sought, since bursitis may be secondary to these conditions.

PHYSICAL EXAMINATION. In traumatic bursitis a fluctuant, tender swelling is noted over the proximal ulna. Surrounding ecchymosis may be present, and the fluid in the bursa may feel lobulated or lumpy owing to clot formation. This type of effusion is not translucent, while in chronic bursitis translucent fluid accumulations do occur. In a purulent olecranon bursitis, local erythema and acute tenderness may be present. Close examination of the skin may show a small localized puncture wound or a foreign body adjacent to the bursa.

LABORATORY STUDIES. Fluid aspiration should be done in chronic or possible purulent bursitis. The aspirate should be examined appropriately for infective processes or possible crystalline accumulation. Roentgenographic examination of the elbow and distal ulna should be made to assess the possible presence of a foreign body and to rule out an old fracture of the olecranon with associated loose bodies or nonunion.

Management

Treatment of traumatic bursitis should consist initially of a local compression wrap over a foam rubber sponge placed on the olecranon bursa to aid in the reabsorption of the accumulated fluid. In addition, this pad prevents recurrent trauma, which would contribute further to the formation of a chronic olecranon bursitis. This pad should be kept in place for a period of five to seven days. If no reabsorption of the hematoma has occurred and if the bursa is now filled with a free, clear, fluctuant fluid without clots, it should be given treatment similar to that used for chronic fluid accumulation.

Chronically accumulated fluid should be aspirated under sterile conditions. If the fluid is clear without sign of infection, one half cc of an intra-articular steroid solution may be instilled into the bursa. Following this treatment the bursa should be kept compressed with a sponge wrap just as described for a period of ten to fourteen days. The patient should be advised to avoid all trauma to the area of the olecranon bursa. After this time, if the effusion does not reaccumulate, a local protective pad (similar to the elbow pad used by basketball players) should be worn under the clothing for one month. If the fluid reaccumulates, the procedure may be repeated.

The fluid of septic bursitis should be aspirated and, following appropriate laboratory studies, the patient should be given an oral antibiotic. Initially this should consist of a broad-spectrum antistaphylococcal agent that is resistant to penicillinase. When definitive culture and sensitivity results have been obtained, other antibiotics may be prescribed accordingly. The bursa is examined in three days and, if the fluid has reaccumulated, aspiration is performed again. If purulent fluid continues to reaccumulate, incision and drainage of the bursa is indicated. On occasion, following infection or chronic recurrent olecranon bursitis, local therapy may be ineffective, and under these circumstances surgical excision of the bursa is beneficial.

ADVICE. Rheumatoid and gouty arthritis may be the primary cause of bursitis. Local treatment of the bursitis, however, would be the same as that described for chronic fluid accumulation.

Lateral Epicondylitis (Tennis Elbow)

The Problem

Pain over the lateral aspect of the elbow may be associated with any activity that demands repeated use of the forearm extensors. The symptoms have been attributed to pathological changes in the connective tissue of the extensor retinaculum, in the bursa and in the synovium and to compression of the radial nerve.

Clinical Evaluation

There is usually an occupational or athletic activity that is associated with the onset of pain over the lateral aspect of the elbow. Initially the pain is exacerbated by activity and relieved by rest. In more chronic conditions the pain can become continuous, often awakening the patient at night. A history of pain and dysesthesias radiating from the elbow to the dorsum of the hand should raise the suspicion of radial nerve entrapment. Inquiries about any previous history of neck or cervical spine injury should be made, for the answers may indicate that the primary etiology of the pain is cervical nerve irritation (see page 625).

PHYSICAL EXAMINATION. On palpation, pain is localized just distal to the lateral epicondyle. Dorsiflexion of the wrist against resistance reproduces the described pain. In patients with entrapment of the deep radial nerve, palpation over the nerve causes local tenderness with radiation into the dorsum of the wrist. Extension of the ring finger against resistance also causes pain in these patients. In patients with a history of chronic elbow pain, distinct atrophy of the forearm musculature can be noted. Neurological examination of the upper extremity should always be included to assess the cervical nerve root function.

LABORATORY STUDIES. X-rays of the elbow should be taken to assess the presence of calcification in the common extensor tendon. Often films of the cervical spine will be of value in assessing whether local pathology in this region is the cause of pain.

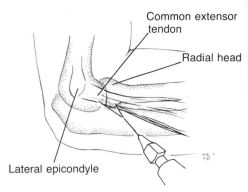

Figure 13–43 Injection for "tennis elbow." The area of maximum tenderness is palpated and injected. This is usually immediately adjacent to the origin of the common extensors from the lateral epicondyle of the humerus. The needle is carefully redirected into several points along the common extensors.

Management

In early acute cases, immobilization of the elbow for 10 to 14 days in a posterior splint and the use of oral anti-inflammatory drugs are effective measures for relieving symptoms. After this regimen, an exercise program should be initiated under the supervision of a qualified therapist to strengthen the forearm musculature before the offending activity is resumed. In cases that do not respond to this conservative treatment, local injection of steroids is often effective (Fig. 13–43). Following this injection, splinting and exercises are advised, using the pattern just described. This treatment regimen should be repeated several times if symptoms recur. A period of immobilization may be tried to alleviate pain in patients with deep radial nerve entrapment. If this is not curative, surgical decompression should be done. Steroid injection is contraindicated because of the danger of directly injecting the nerve. In the rare unresponsive patient, in whom several local injections of steroids have proven ineffective, one of several surgical procedures may be attempted.

ADVICE. The practitioner should keep in mind that elbow pain may be secondary to cervical nerve root entrapment, which could be the source of symptoms.

Medial Epicondylitis (Golfer's Elbow)

The Problem

This is a much less common problem than lateral epicondylitis. The symptoms of pain and history of injury are localized over the medial epicondyle of the elbow.

Clinical Evaluation

The onset of pain is associated with activities that stress the common flexor attachment at the medial aspect of the elbow.

PHYSICAL EXAMINATION. Pain is noted upon palpation over the medial epicondyle and somewhat distal to it. Volar flexion of the wrist against resistance reproduces the symptoms.

LABORATORY STUDIES. X-rays of the elbow are indicated to assess the possibility of any previous trauma to the medial epicondyle.

Management

Treatment is similar to that given for lateral epicondylitis, except that the injection is given medially (Fig. 13–44). Surgical intervention, however, is almost never required, since symptoms respond well to conservative local therapy. The exercise program should emphasize strengthening of the flexor musculature of the forearm.

Total Elbow Prosthesis

Advanced degenerative arthritis of the elbow joint is an indication for total prosthetic replacement of the elbow. Many different models are available for this surgical procedure. These joint replacements are successful only in selected individuals who suffer from extreme pain or discomfort from degenerative arthritis and who do not expect to use the arm in vigorous or demanding activities. Long-term studies con-

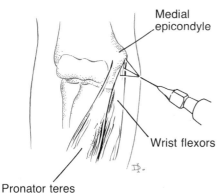

Figure 13–44 Injection for medial epicondylitis ("golfer's elbow"). The injection is performed at several points around the area of maximum tenderness. This is usually immediately distal to the medial epicondyle of the humerus, within the origins of the wrist flexors and the pronator teres muscle.

cerning the durability of the prosthesis are not available at present. Loosening and poor wear characteristics are major obstacles to its general use at this time. This procedure is indicated for elderly, relatively inactive patients.

THE WRIST

Stenosing Tenosynovitis (DeQuervain's Disease)

The Problem

The adductor pollicis longus and extensor pollicis brevis tendons share a synovium-lined sheath that is attached in the region of the styloid process of the radius. Inflammation of these tendons and their surrounding synovial sheath results in severe localized pain. In addition to the inflammatory process, congenital variation in the number of tendons sharing this common tendon sheath is thought to contribute to the syndrome.

Clinical Evaluation

Excessive occupational use of the wrist and thumb is a common cause of this condition. Pain over the radial aspect of the wrist is aggravated by grasping objects or clenching the fist. Often the pain is progressive, leading eventually to inability to do activities requiring the use of the thumb and hand.

PHYSICAL EXAMINATION. Cylindrical swelling is present over the radial aspect of the wrist. Pain can usually be elicited in the region of the swelling by forced ulnar deviation of the wrist with the thumb adducted and flexed toward the forearm (Finkelstein's test). In addition, local palpation may reveal pain or crepitation within the synovial sheath.

LABORATORY STUDIES. X-rays of the wrist are indicated to rule out possible local osseous abnormality.

Management

Splinting of the forearm with the wrist extended and in slight radial deviation often helps to alleviate the acute phase of this condition. When symptoms are long-standing, local injection of Xylocaine and steroids into the distal end of the tendon sheath will alleviate symptoms (Fig. 13–45). If no improvement occurs with steroids, then local surgical decompression of the synovial sheath is indicated.

Arthritis of the Wrist

The Problem

The wrist joint is subject to degenerative changes from previous traumatic conditions and is one of the joints most commonly involved in rheumatoid arthritis.

Clinical Evaluation

Pain in the wrist of gradually increasing severity is described, predated by a history of trauma or collagen disease. Depending on the degree of involvement, symptoms may be mild to severe.

PHYSICAL EXAMINATION. This includes an assessment of pain-free active and passive wrist motion. The examiner should be observant for signs of active rheumatoid arthritis, including the degree of synovial swelling and osseous deformity. Pronation and supination should be measured. The distal radioulnar joint should be examined for any degenerative changes. The extensor tendons should be observed for involvement and possible rupture at the point where they pass over the wrist joint.

LABORATORY STUDIES. Roentgenograms of the wrist should be made to assess the degree of degenerative change. Appropriate laboratory studies (CBC, sedimentation rate, rheumatoid factor and lupus erythematosus tests) should be carried out to evaluate for possible collagen disorders.

Management

In this complex joint, treatment must be individualized according to the type and severity of symptoms. Splinting may improve symptoms and may

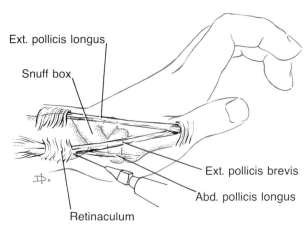

Figure 13–45 Injection for stenosing tenosynovitis (de Quervain's). Injection is performed at the site of maximum swelling and tenderness, which is usually the retinaculum of the extensor pollicis brevis and abductor pollicis longus. The needle is inserted tangentially along these two tendons, entering the retinaculum as shown.

be necessary to prevent the progression of deformity. However, in rheumatoid and advanced degenerative conditions, specific operative procedures such as synovectomy, arthrodesis or arthroplasty may be indicated.

Carpal Tunnel Syndrome

The Problem

This syndrome results from compression of the median nerve in the carpal tunnel. The median nerve and the flexor tendons of the fingers pass through this tunnel.

Clinical Evaluation

Symptoms of pain, numbness and tingling in the distribution of the median nerve are volunteered by the patient. Frequently there will be a history of pain that is most bothersome at night and that typically awakens the patient from sleep. The usual methods employed by the patient to alleviate symptoms are shaking the hand and running warm water over the fingers. Endocrine disorders that cause fluid accumulation, including diabetes and thyroid disease, may be initiating factors. Pregnancy and rheumatoid arthritis may be associated with this condition.

PHYSICAL EXAMINATION. On examination there may be visible swelling over the volar aspect of the wrist. The symptoms can usually be reproduced by holding the wrist in acute flexion for one minute. Hypesthesia is present over the distribution of the median nerve. In addition, two-point discrimination is diminished in the area innervated by the median nerve. Cervical nerve root involvement should be considered as a source of symptoms and must be ruled out by a thorough neurological examination. In advanced cases, atrophy of the thenar eminence will be noticeable.

LABORATORY STUDIES. Tangential x-rays of the wrist may show a bony abnormality within the carpal tunnel. Usually, however, the x-ray will be normal. Cervical spine x-rays should be made to rule out local nerve root compression. If endocrine disorders are suspected, appropriate tests should be obtained. Nerve conduction studies may help to localize the area of nerve root compression and to document the suspected condition.

Management

Splinting of the wrist and forearm with a volar appliance will often relieve the symptoms. If there is no medical contraindication, oral anti-inflammatory drugs may be employed in acute cases for three or four days. When the syndrome follows local trauma and is not progressive, this treatment is usually all that is needed. Under these circumstances the condition is self-limiting and will often subside spontaneously. In chronic cases surgical division of the transverse carpal ligament, with nerve decompression and neurolysis, is indicated.

Discussion

The most common pathological finding is a nonspecific inflammation and swelling of the synovial tissue. The syndrome commonly occurs in patients with rheumatoid arthritis and may follow a Colles' fracture. Local tissue swelling may be secondary to the fluid accumulation occurring in pregnancy, and the patient can be assured that this is a self-limiting circumstance.

Ganglion

The Problem

This is the most common tumor seen in the hand, occurring on the dorsal or

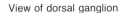

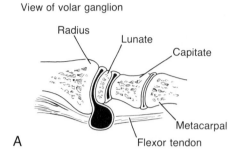

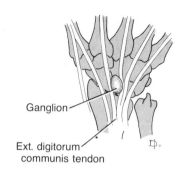

Figure 13–46 Ganglion. *A.* View of dorsal ganglion. The ganglion is shown in the most common location of ganglia of the wrist, presenting between the slips of the extensor digitorum communis, overlying the wrist joint. *B.* View of the volar ganglion. The most common location is on the radial aspect of the wrist, with the ganglion presenting just medial to the radial artery.

volar surface of the wrist (Fig. 13–46). The tumor can also evolve wherever there is a tendon sheath or joint capsule. This entity is rare in children and is most commonly seen in young women.

Clinical Evaluation

About one-half of the patients presenting with this mass will give a history of trauma, usually of a minor and repetitive nature, to the local tissues of the wrist. Often these masses are asymptomatic, but on occasion a ganglion can be painful. If the ganglion occurs adjacent to a vascular or neurological structure, compression will cause symptoms of ischemia or nerve irritation. Occasionally the mass will disappear spontaneously, only to recur after a period of time.

PHYSICAL EXAMINATION. A firm, translucent mass varying in size from a few millimeters to some centimeters in diameter is found. Often these masses are tender to palpation. Location of the ganglion in the region of a nerve or vascular structure should alert the physician to evaluate the competency of the structures in that region.

LABORATORY STUDIES. X-rays are helpful in confirming that the mass is a soft tissue structure.

Management

Rupture during manipulation leads to about a 60 per cent rate of permanent disappearance of the cystic mass. Some physicians advocate aspiration and the administration of steroids as effective treatment. The more definitive method is surgical excision of the tumor mass.

ADVICE. Regardless of the method of treatment chosen, the patient should be warned that the cystic mass may recur.

Ulnar Tunnel Syndrome

The Problem

Compression or injury of the ulnar nerve as it passes over the wrist and through Guyon's canal may produce symptoms of pain, weakness and dysesthesia over the distribution of the ulnar nerve in the hand.

Clinical Evaluation

Pain or dysesthesia in the little and ring fingers is described, associated with weakness of the intrinsic musculature of the hand. Occasionally there is a previous history of acute trauma or recurrent local contusion secondary to a specific occupational task.

PHYSICAL EXAMINATION. In chronic cases, atrophy and weakness will be noted in the intrinsic muscles of the hand. Dysesthesia and loss of sensory acuity are noted over the cutaneous distribution of the ulnar nerve. Palpation of the nerve along its pathway may localize an aneurysm of the ulnar artery or a small ganglion compressing the nerve within the canal. A careful neurological examination may identify the exact location of the compromised nerve.

LABORATORY STUDIES. Tangential x-rays of the volar side of the wrist and hand may indicate whether an osseous spur or fragment is intruding into Guyon's canal. Nerve conduction studies will show whether the nerve injury involves cervical or more distal nerves.

Management

A period of splinting and observation is indicated in acute traumatic conditions in which neurapraxia is the most likely diagnosis. If neurological degeneration progresses, or if a history of chronic progressive nerve dysfunction is elicited, surgical decompression and exploration of the ulnar nerve through its canal is indicated.

Discussion

Always eliminate the possibility of a more proximal lesion of the ulnar nerve occurring in the cervical plexus or elbow region.

Avascular Necrosis of the Lunate (Kienböck's Disease)

The Problem

Avascular necrosis of the lunate bone is most commonly seen in men between the ages of 20 and 40.

Clinical Evaluation

The patient often volunteers a history of trauma to the wrist such as a "sprain," followed by pain and swelling present for a period of several days to several weeks. There is then an asymptomatic period that is followed by a history of increasing pain in the wrist associated with manual activity. The pain becomes increasingly severe and progressive weakness of the wrist occurs.

PHYSICAL EXAMINATION. Local swelling and tenderness over the lunate is often noted on palpation. Dorsiflexion of the wrist is limited and painful.

LABORATORY STUDIES. Roentgenograms taken immediately after the initial trauma may be completely normal. With the onset of more chronic symptoms, repeat examination shows sclerosis of the lunate, and fragmentation and cystic degeneration of this bone later become evident. In advanced cases, secondary changes appear in the surrounding carpal bones.

Management

Initial treatment should consist of wrist immobilization in acute injuries with suspected lunate compromise. If avascular necrosis is discovered early, before fragmentation has occurred, immobilization of the wrist may prevent degenerative changes and breakdown while revascularization continues. Once fragmentation has occurred, local excision of the bone gives good results. If advanced degenerative changes involving the surrounding carpal bones and wrist joint have occurred, surgical intervention, including carpal bone excision or wrist fusion, may be indicated.

Navicular Fracture

The Problem

This fracture is known as the most commonly missed fracture in orthopaedics. Often the trauma and subsequent pain experienced by the patient are not severe enough to warrant medical attention. The navicular bone, having a tenuous blood supply, rapidly progresses to nonunion unless complete immobilization is accomplished.

Clinical Evaluation

Usually a history of wrist trauma or "sprain," followed by varying degrees of discomfort, is elicited. Wrist pain localized within the radial "snuffbox" is described. Occasionally the patient points specifically to the volar "snuffbox" as being the most acutely tender area.

PHYSICAL EXAMINATION. In relatively acute injuries, local swelling and tenderness is noted over the navicular. In more chronic injuries, pain may be produced by compression of the navicular within the volar "snuffbox."

LABORATORY STUDIES. On initial injury, x-rays may be negative for displacement or fracture line. Roentgenographic examination after two weeks often will clearly demonstrate the fracture line because of local bone resorption over the fracture site. Technetium bone scan, including local magnification views, represents an extremely sensitive technique for discovering this injury in suspected acute cases. (False positive results secondary to

local soft tissue hyperemia do occur with this method, however.)

Management

Treatment consists of rigid immobilization in a long arm cast with the elbow flexed at 90 degrees and the wrist in neutral position. The wrist should be placed in 15 to 20 degrees of dorsiflexion and the cast should include the thumb up to the interphalangeal joint. Even fractures due to untreated injuries up to six months old should be treated using this method. Immobilization of six to eight months may be necessary. In cases of nonunion of fractures that do not heal after an adequate period of immobilization, surgical intervention, including bone grafting, screw fixation or prosthetic replacement, may be indicated. Nonunion of fractures that is associated with degenerative changes of the wrist joint should be treated symptomatically. Painful wrist motion secondary to an old nonunited navicular fracture may be treated by one of several methods, depending on the circumstances. Excision of the navicular fragment, excision of the radial styloid, prosthetic replacement, proximal row carpectomy or wrist fusion represent some of the choices in this situation.

SOFT TISSUE INJURIES

In general, these injuries respond well to conservative, symptomatic treatment. Early effective management, however, especially in athletes, will significantly decrease the period of disability. In general, once skeletal injury has been ruled out, local treatment with ice packs placed over a compressive wrap and elevation for 24 hours will decrease the degree of soft tissue swelling and hematoma formation. Following this regimen, a period of controlled immobilization is most beneficial, maintaining the injured limb in a resting position for two or three days. This may require immobilization of the joint by using crutches or a sling in order to allow reabsorption of the local edema. After 48 to 72 hours of immobilization, local heat therapy may assist in further reabsorption of local swelling. Massage and the injection of absorptive enzymes into muscle and soft tissues that have been acutely injured have not proven to be beneficial.

The practitioner should remember that local reflex muscular atrophy may be rapid in onset following one of these injuries. In order to maintain full athletic and functional muscular activity, a specific exercise program to regain previous muscle strength should be instituted following recovery from the injury.

SPINE

Problems of Neck-Shoulder-Arm Syndrome

Patients will frequently present with pain in the neck, shoulder, arm and hand. The pain distribution may involve virtually any combination of the various regions and may vary somewhat in its location at different times. There are a number of conditions that may be the cause of the various pain syndromes. Once the physician is familiar with them it is usually not difficult to make an accurate diagnosis. Errors are made when a particular entity is not thought of and the wrong treatment is therefore initiated. In this section we will present the most common syndromes that cause neck, shoulder, arm and hand pain.

A few general comments should be made about these syndromes. They are presented in general order of progression from the most central to the most peripheral portion of the nervous system. Most of them involve some com-

bination of mechanical impingement or irritation on nerves or nerve roots and vascular impingement. However, the pain that the patient experiences may be either referred pain (e.g., cervical spondylosis causing interscapular or shoulder-arm pain) or pain from direct irritation or entrapment of the nerve (e.g., from an osteophyte in a neural foramen or from carpal tunnel syndrome). In addition, numbness, paresthesia and dysesthesia may be associated with nerve entrapment and inflammation. It is not always easy or even possible to identify exactly the type of pain involved or its precise mechanism.

Cervical Spondylosis

The Problem

In association with radiographic evidence of cervical spondylosis, some individuals will have considerable problems with neck, shoulder and arm pain.

Clinical Evaluation

HISTORY. The patient is usually over 30 years of age and likely to be female. There is sometimes a history of injury involving a fall, heavy lifting, twisting or a sudden stop (whiplash). These may or may not be significant. The pain may start in one or several sites, such as the neck, shoulder, arm or hand or any combination of these. Most typically it starts in the neck, or the area sometimes referred to as the interscapular region. The pain may be worse with activity and weather changes and improve with rest and analgesics. In some patients it is worse at night and in certain positions of the neck. There may be paresthesia and dysesthesia in the hand. The patient may also complain of weakness of the hand and arm and may drop things more frequently, presumably because of some combination of weakness and numbness, perhaps more often the latter. The pain is sometimes made worse by coughing and sneezing. The patient should be questioned about symptoms that might suggest an ischemic syndrome. Coldness, venous distention and discoloration in the hand are important observations. The patient may have had various treatments, such as a cervical collar, heat, massage, cervical traction or manipulation, with mixed or varied but generally unsatisfactory results.

PHYSICAL EXAMINATION. There may be some loss of motion in any combination of flexion, extension, lateral bending and axial rotation, but this is difficult to assess unless it is severe. Moreover, the prepain range of motion for the patient is rarely known. In some instances with acute pain there may be severe anterior or posterior muscle spasm or both, with or without an associated torticollis. The

head may be rotated and tilted, with a "cock robin" appearance.

The Spurling test (Fig. 13–47) may be positive. The patient is then tested for muscle strength, reflex activity and sensation. Table 13–4 describes the standard localization of neurological deficits. In addition, the lower extremities should be carefully examined neurologically to rule out the possibility of cord irritation, which can be be present with cervical spondylosis. Patients with this problem may have a pathological extensor reflex, loss of position sense, spasticity and unsteadiness of gait.

LABORATORY STUDIES. The patient should have anteroposterior, lateral and oblique x-rays of the cervical spine. The films are examined for localized or generalized cervical spondylosis. Anterior or posterior osteophytes as well as evidence of encroachment into the neural foramina may be seen on the oblique views.

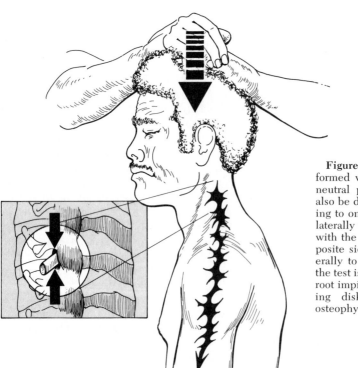

Figure 13–47 Spurling test performed with the patient's head in neutral position. The test should also be done with the patient looking to one side with the head bent laterally to that same side and then with the patient looking to the opposite side and the head bent laterally to the opposite side. When the test is positive it suggests nerve root impingement by either a bulging disk or a posterior-lateral osteophyte.

TABLE 13–4   Localization of Nerve Root Lesions by Physical Examination

Vertebral Interspace	Nerve Root	Weakness	Reflex Depressed	Sensation Decreased
C4–C5	C5	Deltoid and biceps	Biceps	Lateral aspect of humerus
C5–C6	C6	Biceps flexion and wrist extension	Brachioradialis	Radial aspect of forearm
C6–C7	C7	Finger and elbow extensions	Triceps	Middle finger
C7–T1	C8	Finger flexions	None	Ulnar aspect of forearm

One or more of the disk spaces may be narrowed, and on the AP view a more horizontal rather than a more vertical orientation of the uncinate processes may be seen. These films should be observed carefully to rule out any bony or soft tissue lesion that may be visible; one should also look for a cervical rib or a Pancoast tumor if the supraclavicular region can be seen.

SPECIAL STUDIES.   If the diagnosis is difficult and thought to be atypical of cervical spondylosis, other special studies may be indicated. EMG and nerve conduction studies may help to evaluate the possibility of nerve entrapment at the elbow or the wrist. EMG evidence of distinct peripheral nerve deficit may be helpful in a situation in which a possible emotional component is difficult to analyse. The Minnesota Multiphasic Personality Inventory (MMPI) and psychiatric interviews are also helpful in this situation. A myelogram is necessary if the clinical evaluation suggests cervical spondylosis severe enough to require surgery.

Management

The patient may be managed conservatively as long as he or she can tolerate the discomfort. After 9 to 12 months it is reasonable to consider surgery. In patients with clinical evidence of cervical myelopathy the time considerations are different, because surgery should be considered if there is no improvement with conservative therapy. In either case the patient should have a myelogram prior to surgery. Surgical results are much better when there is no myelopathy (evidence of long tract signs). The results with cervical spondylosis are best in patients who have unilevel radicular symptoms, who have had difficulty for over one year, and whose myelograms are positive and correlate with the level of their motor and sensory deficit. However, other patients who come close to having these criteria also enjoy good results. We can expect 80 to 95 per cent of carefully selected patients to have a good or excellent surgical result.

If the patient has not had adequate conservative treatment for 9 to 12 months then such a program should be commenced.

MEDICAL   AND   NONSURGICAL TREATMENT.   The analgesic and anti-inflammatory drugs should be used. Aspirin taken in therapeutic doses is always a good drug to employ unless there are contraindications. Indocin and Butazolidin can also be employed, and Darvon will sometimes suffice. When the pain is acute and severe, it seems reasonable on occasion to prescribe a short course of codeine with aspirin or Demerol. Cervical collars are sometimes helpful in symptomatic treatment even though they do not effectively immobilize the cervical spine (Fig. 13–48). Traction is also an appropriate technique that sometimes as-

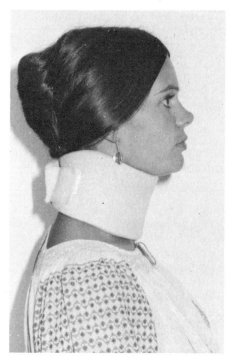

Figure 13–48   Model wearing a soft cervical collar. The collar is being worn in the standard position—in this case to prevent flexion more than extension. If the collar is rotated 180 degrees it can serve to diminish extension slightly more than flexion.

Discussion

Pain is a major factor in this disease and thus emotional and socioeconomic factors play a significant role in the presentation of the symptoms before and after treatment. It is difficult to select patients for surgery because many people have neck pain and many patients without neck pain have considerable degeneration in the cervical spine. However, an extended period of conservative treatment allows for improvement or for better understanding of the patient and his or her disease process. The differential diagnosis of neck pain is very important.

Acute Herniated Cervical Disk

The clinical characteristics of this condition may be thought of as more dramatic and accelerated versions of those seen in cervical spondylosis. Here the encroachment is made by the soft material of the anulus fibrosus rather than by combined osseous and ligamentous degenerative changes. There may also be evidence of myelopathy and muscle weakness. When the patient does not improve with rest and if the acute neurological changes per-

sists in symptomatic relief. Heat and massage are soothing and offer some temporary comfort. Practical suggestions for the comfort of an individual who has cervical spondylosis are given in Table 13–5.

SURGERY.   Depending upon the pathology, appropriately selected patients can enjoy a cure or considerable improvement from anterior diskectomy and arthrodesis of one or more vertebral interspaces. Some surgeons have suggested disk excision alone. We believe that the fusion technique opens up the neural foramen and immobilizes the segment that has diseased motion, and so provides two therapeutic benefits in addition to that of disk excision (Fig. 13–49).[9]

TABLE 13–5   Suggestions for Alleviation of Neck Pain

Avoid the tense "strain-or-stretch-the-neck" spectator position (chin projected forward and neck extended).

Avoid sleeping or reading while lying on the back with the neck flexed on a pillow.

Avoid holding the head and neck in any one position for prolonged periods.

Avoid excessive physical strain on the neck.

Avoid obviously tense and stressful situations.

Obtain adequate rest.

Keep the neck drawn back and chin tucked in when standing or sitting.

Use armrests when sitting.

Exercise gently but actively to maintain a full painless range of motion in the neck. Look up, down and to each side and try to touch the ear to the shoulder on each side.

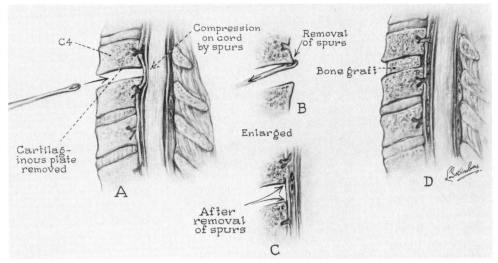

Figure 13–49 *A.* With light head traction, using rongeurs and small curettes, the disk space is cleared of all cartilage, gradually enlarged, and converted into a rectangular slot. *B.* A small curette is used to remove protruding spurs, especially in the posterolateral edges, always scraping from the edge away from the spinal cord and nerve root. *C.* It is not necessary or desirable to remove the posterior longitudinal ligament for degenerative disk disease. *D.* The rectangular graft must fit the rectangular slot accurately. If the posterior cartilage surfaces are not carefully removed, the graft may tend to extrude. The graft should be measured and fashioned so that it can be countersunk about one millimeter. (From White, A. A., et al.: Relief of pain by anterior cervical spine fusion for spondylosis. A report of 65 patients. J. Bone Joint Surg., 55:525–534, 1973.)

sist, then surgical removal should be considered immediately. This is in contrast to the prolonged period of conservative treatment used for cervical spondylosis. This approach protects the patient against a prolonged or increasing neurological deficit.

Cervicothoracic Outlet Syndromes

Several clinical syndromes that should be included in the evaluation of neck-shoulder-arm pain will be discussed under this heading. These conditions have been superbly illustrated elsewhere.[4]

Cervical Ribs

The Problem

The presence of a unilateral or bilateral rib or fibrous band at the C7 level of the spine is associated with some combination of neurovascular symptoms. These symptoms are presumably caused by encroachment of the rib on the brachial plexus and the infraclavicular vessels.

Clinical Evaluation

HISTORY. The patient is usually a female over 30 years of age. Neck pain is not a prominent symptom. The pain tends to be associated with numbness, paresthesia and dysesthesia and is located primarily in the ulnar side of the hand and forearm. There may be vascular changes such as discoloration, sweating or feelings of coldness.

PHYSICAL EXAMINATION. One or both hands may show atrophy and weakness of thenar muscles and intrinsic hand muscles. There may be cyanosis or increased sweating. A prominence may be palpable in the supraclavicular region. The subclavian artery may be relatively prominent or the rib itself may be palpable. It may be possible to irritate or aggravate the symptoms by palpation in the region.

LABORATORY STUDIES. Oblique x-rays of the C7–T1 region of the spine will show a well-ossified rib. A fibrous band running from C7 to the first thoracic rib can cause the same symptoms and will not show up on a regular x-ray.

SPECIAL STUDIES. If the clinical picture is such that differentiation from ulnar tunnel syndrome or carpal tunnel syndrome is difficult, then nerve conduction studies will be helpful. Arteriograms are also of use in the evaluation of a possible thoracic outlet compression syndrome or the presence of a fibrous band in place of a completely developed cervical rib.

Management

ADVICE. The patient is told that with conservative management there is a good possibility that the symptoms can be controlled at a satisfactory level. Surgery should be considered if there are progressive disabling neurovascular problems.

MEDICAL AND NONSURGICAL ORTHOPAEDIC CARE. The patient may be given salicylates that are supplemented occasionally with codeine. Individual patients should learn which activities and positions aggravate the symptoms and then avoid them. If the symptoms appear to be aggravated by droopy shoulders, muscle strengthening exercises to strengthen the shoulder elevators (trapezoids and rhomboids) would be beneficial. If obese arms and shoulders are thought to contribute to the drooping, then weight loss should be urged.

SURGERY. When surgery is indicated, resection of the cervical rib or fibrous band and transection of the scalene muscle should be performed. It has been suggested that when no distinct band or cervical rib is found at surgery, the middle portion of the first rib should be resected.

Discussion

The anatomical and pathophysiological mechanism of this cervical syndrome is interesting. In quadrupeds the neurovascular structures exit, for the most part, at right angles to their central sources. This causes essentially no traction or impingement on the neurovascular structure. However, in man, with his bipedal erect posture and loosely attached shoulder girdle, there is considerable drooping or caudad mobility of the upper limbs, which causes the neurovascular structures to take a sharp angular course as they exit from their source. The passageway for the brachial plexus and the subclavian artery is in the narrow triangle formed by the anterior and medial aspects of the scalene muscles and the first rib and has only a small margin of extra space. Thus a cervical rib, an extra band of fibrous tissue or even a somewhat fibrotic or tense scalenus anticus muscle could cause some degree of stenosis and symptoms in the upper limb. Any of several normal or abnormal anatomical structures in that region could cause stenosis. Other examples include (1) excessive hyperabduction of the shoulder, (2) a prominent transverse process of C7, (3) a fractured clavicle with gross malunion, excessive callus or pseudarthrosis, (4) exostosis of the first rib, (5) complete or partial congenital absence of the clavicle with excessive drooping of the shoulders, (6) excessive drooping of the shoulders for other reasons and (7) chronic or excessive carrying of weights that pull the shoulders down. Once the anatomy is thoroughly reviewed it is understandable that a sizeable number of conditions can affect the neurovascular structures in the area.[4] We suggest that the anatomical potential is present congenitally in many cases and that the symptoms present at age 30 because the shoulders tend to droop in adulthood at about that age, especially in the female.

Scalenus Anticus (Anterior Scalene) Syndrome

The Problem

This problem was mentioned in the preceding discussion. Subclavian artery and brachial plexus irritation is caused by passage through an anatomically or physiologically compromised interscalene triangle.

Clinical Evaluation

HISTORY. A patient, usually a female over 30, has progressive symptoms of some combination of pain, dysesthesia and numbness, usually in the ulnar side of the hand and forearm, although it may be anywhere in the hand or forearm. The symptoms may also be in the inner side of the upper arm. There may be coldness, increased sweating or color changes in the skin suggestive of vascular irritation. The neurovascular symptoms may be aggravated by hyperabduction of the shoulder.

PHYSICAL EXAMINATION. The limb is observed carefully for evidence of neurovascular compromise such as muscle wasting, cyanosis, excessive sweating or changes in the radial pulse. The radial pulse should also be checked by employing Adson's test. This is done by having the patient take a deep breath and hold it. The patient then extends the neck fully and turns the chin to the side of the arm symptoms. If the radial pulse is diminished or obliterated, this is strongly suggestive of interscalene triangle pathology. The test should be repeated as described but with the chin turned to the opposite side of the symptoms, because this sometimes obliterates the radial pulse on the painful side. This, too, is interpreted as a positive Adson's test.

LABORATORY STUDIES. The routine studies include standard x-rays of the cervical and upper thoracic region to observe for cervical spondylosis, Pancoast's tumor and cervical ribs. The status of the clavicle should also be examined on these films.

SPECIAL STUDIES. Arteriograms may be helpful in determining the extent of the subclavian artery constriction at the interscalene triangle or elsewhere. EMG and nerve conduction studies are useful if there is a question of nerve entrapment at the elbow or wrist.

Management

Surgical exploration is indicated, provided there is ample clinical evidence of neurovascular compromise when severe symptoms cannot be relieved by changing activity and other conservative measures described in the previous section. The anterior scalene muscle is resected; other structures, such as fibrous bands or the middle scalene muscle, should also be resected if the subclavian artery and brachial plexus are not sufficiently freed by the anterior scalenotomy.

Costoclavicular Syndrome

This syndrome is analogous to the cervical rib and scalenus anticus syndromes, except that the neurovascular compromise occurs between the clavicle and the first rib. The major difference is in the position of the shoulders associated with maximum reduction in the space between the clavicle and the first rib. In this syndrome the passageway is most compromised when the shoulders are thrust backward and downward, as when one carries a heavy backpack. When the shoulders are held in an exaggerated military position, the radial pulse may be diminished or eliminated if this condition is present. This may also occur in asymptomatic individuals.

There are several situations that may compromise the costoclavicular passageway. Irregularities of the clavicle include congenital anomalies of shape, partial absence, nonunion, malunion and fractures. Congenital anomalies of the subclavius muscle or the costocoracoid ligament as well as anomalies of the first rib can also be a cause of compromise of this space.

Diagnosis can be difficult. The symptoms and laboratory data to be evaluated are essentially the same as those described for cervical rib syndrome and scalenus anticus syndrome. In costoclavicular syndrome, the position of the shoulders that is associated with symptoms and radial pulse changes is different, however. Obvious clavicular and first rib abnormalities will help with diagnosis, as will the site of constriction seen on the arteriogram.

When surgical treatment is required, the procedure usually carried out is extraperiosteal resection of the clavicle, or it may be preferable to resect the first rib.

Hyperabduction Syndrome

The hyperabduction syndrome is related to sleeping with the arms held above the shoulders, elbows flexed and hands clasped behind the head. This position may be associated with the neurovascular thoracic outlet compression syndromes of the type described previously. The site of compression is thought to be either in the costoclavicular region or somewhat distal to it, underneath the pectoralis minor muscle just before it attaches to the coracoid process. In hyperabduction syndrome, in which abduction and external rotation of the shoulder with the hand above the head obliterates the pulse and reproduces the pa-

tient's symptoms, one may consider surgical intervention if the symptoms are severe enough. It is suggested that release of the pectoralis minor can be effective in relieving this condition.

Reflex Sympathetic Dystrophy

This condition probably involves, at least to some extent, a very long list of diseases. We discuss it here for several important reasons. The neurovascular conditions that are discussed here are likely to involve sympathetic nervous system symptoms. These include a cool extremity, vascular color changes, increased sweating, paresthesia and dysesthesia. Problems of reflex sympathetic dystrophy can cause pain in the neck, shoulder and hand. It is very important that these be recognized early so that vigorous treatment can be instituted.

The reflex sympathetic dystrophies are characterized by very severe pain associated with any combination of swelling, wasting, atrophy, excessive sweating, and slick, shiny, dry skin that may be either cyanotic or hyperemic. The disability is severe, the pain is excessive and there is usually significant associated psychiatric disease, along with great difficulty in treatment. The condition is poorly understood, and there are several diseases that we choose to think of as making up the group of reflex sympathetic dystrophies. These include shoulder-hand syndrome, Sudeck's atrophy, sclerodactylia, diffuse vasculitis and causalgia.

Treatment is very difficult and prolonged, but should be given with vigor and optimism. We suggest hospitalization in a place with an active physical therapy program, adequate facilities and psychiatric, orthopaedic and neurological specialists, including any other specialist who has experience in the management of this type of problem. Repeated sympathetic blocks and cervicothoracic sympathectomy in association with an active physical therapy progam is the basis of treatment.

Differential Diagnosis of Neck-Shoulder-Arm Pain

In the evaluation of neck and shoulder area pain, several other conditions should be considered in the differential diagnosis.

PANCOAST'S TUMOR. Palpate the supraclavicular fossa carefully. Observe a good x-ray of the apex of the lung on the side in question, looking for a superior pulmonary sulcus tumor. These patients usually have invasion of the first rib, which is eroded by tumor, and Horner's syndrome.

BURSITIS OF THE SHOULDER. There is usually localized tenderness in the supraspinatus or subdeltoid region. The pain is made worse by motion of the shoulder. A calcium deposit may be helpful in the differentiation process (see p. 600).

TENNIS ELBOW. Localized tenderness over the lateral epicondyle of the elbow that is made worse by shaking hands and by extension of the wrist or fingers against resistance may indicate "tennis elbow" (see p. 609).

DEQUERVAIN'S DISEASE. Localized tenderness and swelling in the region of the radial sheath that carries the extensor pollicis brevis and abductor pollicis longus tendons. Pain is made worse by Finkelstein's test: Make a fist with thumb in palm and deviate the wrist toward the ulnar side. This causes tremendous pain in the region of the tendon sheath (see p. 611).

CARPAL TUNNEL SYNDROME. Pain in distribution of the median nerve may be a helpful sign, but absence of typical distribution does not rule out carpal tunnel syndrome. Phalen's test and Tinel's sign near the wrist are helpful. Diagnosis may be confirmed with nerve conduction studies (see p. 613).

ULNAR TUNNEL SYNDROME. Pain and numbness in the distribution of the ulnar nerve, with possible hypothenar and intrinsic weakness or atrophy, may indicate ulnar tunnel syndrome. Diagnosis may be confirmed by nerve conduction studies (p. 614).

Through mechanisms that are not well understood, any of these syndromes may present with some combination of neck, shoulder and hand pain.

Whiplash

The Problem

Following a motor vehicle accident in which there is a hyperextension injury, the patient develops a variety of symptoms, including neck pain.

Clinical Evaluation

HISTORY. The individual typically is involved in an automobile accident, and problems develop either immediately or after several symptom-free days. In addition to neck pain, the patient may complain of headaches, numbness or weakness of both upper limbs, vertigo or tinnitus. There may be dysplasia or blurring vision and nystagmus. Any combination of these symptoms may have been present for days, weeks, months or years.

PHYSICAL EXAMINATION. There may be muscle spasm and limited range of motion in the neck, hyperalgesia over the posterior part of the neck and sensory loss either with or without a dermatome pattern.

LABORATORY STUDIES. The routine cervical spine x-rays may be normal. However, they may also show a number of changes that are not specific for this condition. These include loss of cervical lordosis, narrowing of disk spaces, formation of osteophytes, chip fractures or compression of the vertebral bodies.

SPECIAL STUDIES. Special x-ray studies should include views of the isthmus that may show fractures there or in the laminae. Fractures of the transverse process of C1 and of the joints of Luschka have been documented.

Management

ADVICE. Most patients with whiplash injury will improve almost completely with time. However, recovery can take a long time and unfortunately, not all patients do in fact recover. This is a situation in which empathy and reassurance are important. Although in some patients the potential financial compensation seems to affect the clinical presentation of the disease, in general whiplash patients should not be approached with any such bias. Patients with negative x-ray findings should be reassured and treated conservatively. Careful examination, understanding, accurate and empathetic communications and reassurance carry even more than their usual importance in the care of patients with whiplash injuries.

MEDICAL AND NONSURGICAL ORTHOPAEDICS. The initial treatment of patients with negative x-ray findings is analgesics, rest and gradual resumption of normal activities as tolerated. It is probably better to avoid the use of a cervical orthosis, but if this is not possible, a Thomas collar or a four-poster cervical orthosis may be used. Salicylates in therapeutic doses, supplemented with codeine when required, are suggested. Some patients will respond to cervical traction or to a program of cervical exercises that will gradually increase range of motion and muscle strength.

SURGERY. In a few patients after three to six months or more, clinical evidence of cervical spondylosis may develop at one or two levels. If the usual indications for surgery with cervical spondylosis are present, the patient should be offered the appropriate surgical treatment.

Discussion

This is one of the most difficult syndromes to manage, and many patients suffer extensively with this disease. A proper head rest in the motor vehicle is the most important consideration for the prevention of this injury.

Scoliosis

The Problem

Severe scoliosis (thoracic or lumbar) in the adult can be a significant problem, causing serious cardiorespiratory compromise, pain or significant deformity.

Clinical Evaluation

HISTORY. The patient usually has had untreated or unsuccessfully treated scoliosis since childhood. The most common form is idiopathic, but scoliosis can also be congenital, neuromuscular or another type. The patient should be questioned to determine, if possible, the etiology of his condition. It is important to get information about the patient's health, smoking habits and activity levels. Does the patient have dyspnea with normal activity? Is there incapacitating pain? To what extent can the pain be controlled with medication? To what extent is the cosmetic consideration significant?

PHYSICAL EXAMINATION. The finding of frontal plane curvature with axial rotation of the rib cage will be noted to varying degrees (Fig. 13–20A). The rib cage rotation (rib hump) can be seen more readily from behind with the patient bending forward at the hips and holding the knees straight (Fig. 13–20B). The patient may lean to one side, and there may be a real or functional change in leg length. Is pain associated with scapulothoracic motion or due to impingement from the lower ribs or the ilium? The patient should be carefully checked for any possible neurological defect.

LABORATORY STUDIES. Erect anteroposterior and lateral views of the involved portion of the spine are indicated. If there are cardiopulmonary symptoms, an EKG and pulmonary function studies should be carried out.

Management

ADVICE. The first decision to be made is whether the problem is mainly one of pain, cosmetic appearance or cardiorespiratory compromise. There may be some combination of these, and there may also be a problem of neurological compromise. The patient should be evaluated by a specialist and, in most instances, will be treated conservatively.

MEDICAL AND NONORTHOPAEDIC SURGICAL TREATMENT. The pain may be treated with appropriate analgesics. In some instances this may be supplemented with spinal orthosis, used for support and comfort but not for correction. When there is specific, well-localized pain in the spine, thoracic wall or ilium, it may be relieved with local injections of cortisone and Novocain.

The patient should be advised to stop smoking. Well-supervised exercises for breathing and range of motion are helpful in maintaining pulmonary function and residual spinal mobility.

SURGICAL TREATMENT. The indications for surgery in the adult scoliosis patient are relatively rare. In the younger adult up to age 35 or 40, the indications for surgery include improvement and prevention of further deterioration of cardiorespiratory compromise, neurological defect, pain or deformity or any combination of these. In the older age groups, the risk : benefit equilibrium changes, and surgery has more restricted indications. Clearly, any evidence of progressive neurological compromise should cause serious consideration of surgery, al-

though the prognosis of surgery is not good in an older patient with cardiorespiratory compromise.

Discussion

Good screening programs and appropriate management will reduce the number of adult scoliosis patients. In recent years, more of these patients have been operated upon successfully, but the risks are significant even when these patients are in the care of a specialist.

Ankylosing Spondylitis

The Problem

A disease somewhat akin to rheumatoid arthritis, ankylosing spondylitis occurs mainly in young men between the ages of 15 and 35 and causes severe pain and stiffness, primarily in the axial skeleton.

Clinical Evaluation

HISTORY. There may be a family history of the disease and associated iritis or arthralgias. The disease can present very much like an acute herniated anulus fibrosus. There may be chest pain, and stiffness in the spine and hips is a cardinal feature of the disease.

PHYSICAL EXAMINATION. The patient is often of asthenic build. One of the very early findings is limitation of chest expansion. Stiffness is also likely to be noted in the hip joints. A fixed loss of lumbar lordosis plus the rigidity of the entire spine accounts for the appelation "poker spine."

LABORATORY STUDIES. An elevated sedimentation rate and slight anemia may be present. HLA antigens may also be present. The earliest x-ray changes are usually seen in the sacroiliac joints. Increased radiopacity suggests sclerosis around the joints, although the joint itself becomes less distinct. This type of joint blurring may also occur in the manubriosternal joint and the symphysis pubis. The disk spaces calcify and the vertebral bodies change their structure so that the radiographic appearance of the spine comes to resemble a bamboo pole.

Management

ADVICE. The patient may be told that there is a chance that the disease will "burn itself out" before it progresses enough to cause great disability. However, the patient should know that a possibility exists that the disease will cause significant disability. There does not seem to be much that can be done to influence the course of the disease. Once the disease has stabilized, however, there are measures that can be taken.

MEDICAL AND NONSURGICAL ORTHOPAEDICS. Sleeping habits should be reviewed and changed as indicated to resist progression towards kyphotic deformity. The patient should avoid the flexed position as much as possible. Gentle, persistent exercises are important to preserve all available motion of the axial skeleton and other joints. Aspirin, or indomethacin (25 mg t.i.d.), or phenylbutazone (100 mg q.i.d.) are the drugs of choice for this disease.

SURGERY. Surgery should be considered in severe cases of kyphosis in which the patient cannot see the horizon. If the problem cannot be solved by surgical mobilization of the hip joints, then lumbar or cervical spinal osteotomy should be considered. Osteotomy is a high-risk procedure.

Low Back Pain With or Without Sciatica

Introduction

Our goal in this section is to present the information that is necessary in order to provide efficient, effective, risk-free care for patients with low back problems, with or without sciatica. This section will emphasize certain points in the history and physical examination. However, a full history and physical examination must be a part of the clinical evaluation of the patient.

When a patient complains of low back pain, with or without radiation into the legs, our goal is to be certain that we are not overlooking a diagnosable infection or tumor; we then must make the patient as comfortable as possible without subjecting him or her to unjustifiable risk. There are a number of different clinical techniques and skills that may be applied to achieve these ends. Four classes of patients with spine pain are shown in Table 13–6.

Idiopathic organic spine pain is the term we use to describe the clinical picture in which the patient, following evaluation, is thought not to have definite evidence of a herniated disk or any other specific organic diagnosis. Nevertheless, the clinical picture is compatible with organic disease and does not represent malingering or some type of functional ailment. A variety of terms are applied to this condition, including: acute low back strain, lumbar sprain or strain, mechanical low back pain, and mechanical derangement of the low back.

TABLE 13–6 Temporal Grouping of Patients With Low Back Pain

CLASSIFI-CATION	TYPE OF PAIN	DURATION
Group I	Acute	0–3 weeks
Group II	Subacute	3 weeks–6 months
Group III	Chronic	More than 6 months
Group IV	Chronic	More than 6 months and one or more operations

Group I. Acute Low Back Pain (0 to 3 Weeks) With or Without Radiation into the Leg

The Problem

Rule out tumor or infection and determine appropriate conservative treatment. Treat the tumor or infection if that is the diagnosis.

Clinical Evaluation

HISTORY. The patient may be of any age. The history is usually of low back pain that occurred following some form of physical stress (injury, lifting, jumping, wrestling, dancing or twisting). It is essential to learn whether or not the stress occurred on the job and whether or not litigation is likely to be involved. The symptoms may have started spontaneously or with minimal trauma.

It is important to know about any fever, malaise, weight loss, or pain in another area of the body. Have there been any urogenital or bowel symptoms? Have there been any arthralgias? Does the pain get worse with coughing, sneezing or straining at the stool? Is the pain alleviated with bed rest?

If the pain is relieved with bed rest and there is no fever, malaise or weight loss, and if the review of systems is otherwise normal, tumor or infection is less likely. When the pain becomes worse with activity, is relieved with rest and increases with coughing, sneezing and straining at the stool, the patient is likely to have an organic low back syndrome.

PHYSICAL EXAMINATION. Excessive, reliable, reproducible pain on percussion of one particular spinous process is suggestive of infection or tumor in that region. Other intrinsic spinal pathology, including disk disease, can also present this finding but it is generally not as dramatic or distinct.

There may be paraspinous muscle spasm with or without listing. Flexion, lateral bending and axial rotation are limited. One should look for a palpable step-off in the lower lumbar and lumbosacral region that may be indicative of spondylolisthesis. The patient's habitual relaxed standing posture should be carefully noted, especially when the patient stands with hip and knee slightly flexed on the painful side (Fig. 13–50). This is suggestive of nerve root irritation, presumably by the intervertebral disk.

A straight-leg-raising test may be positive. If there is sciatica (pain radiating below the knee) there may also be a positive crossed straight-

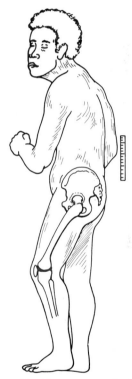

Figure 13–50 This stance is highly suggestive of the presence of a herniated disk or some other form of mechanical nerve root irritation in the lower lumbar spine. The patient sometimes stands in this position unconsciously, usually with a straight back, which reduces the posterior bulge of the disk, and flexed hips and knees, which minimize stretching of the sciatic nerve roots. (Reproduced with permission from White, A. A., and Panjabi, M. M.: Clinical Biomechanics of the Spine. Philadelphia, J. B. Lippincott, 1978.)

leg-raising sign or a positive Lasègue's sign. A positive straight-leg-raising sign is present when flexion of the hip with the leg straight and the patient supine elicits characteristic low back or leg pain at less than 80 to 90 degrees of flexion. The crossed straight-leg-raising test is positive when straight-leg-raising of the nonpainful leg causes pain to be elicited in the undisturbed, fully extended symptomatic leg at less than 85 to 90 degrees of flexion. Lasègue's test is given following a positive straight-leg-raising test of the involved leg. The test leg is extended to a point just below where the flexion elicited pain. The ankle of the test leg, which is flexed at the hip, is then dorsiflexed. If this last maneuver elicits sciatic pain in the leg, then Lasègue's test is positive. A positive result in the crossed straight-leg-raising test or in Lasègue's test, or both, is strongly indicative of nerve root irritation, presumably from a herniated intervertebral disk.[3]

The hips are maneuvered through their full range of motion. Any pain, crepitus or limitation of motion may indicate hip pathology that may be causing the patient's symptoms. The pulses should also be checked carefully because occlusive vascular disease can cause back, hip or leg pain.

The patient should then have each of the lumbar dermatomes and myotomes tested for sensory and motor function. The L3 and L4 nerve roots are likely to be normal if there is a symmetrical, active knee jerk and good quadriceps resistance on muscle testing. The L5 root is likely to be functioning well if the patient can walk on the heels and demonstrate good strength of the extensor hallucis longus on manual muscle testing. The S1 is likely to be functioning if there is no wasting of calf muscles, if the patient can walk on the toes and if the ankle jerks are active and symmetrical. Muscle weakness and sensory deficit that correspond to the same level are suggestive of nerve root involvement. (Table 13–6A).

LABORATORY STUDIES. If the clinical evaluation up to this point weighs convincingly against tumor or infection, no other laboratory studies are indicated in this acute phase, and the physician can proceed to consider the management of the condition. If this is not the case, these initial screening studies are suggested: anteroposterior and lateral x-rays of the lumbar and sacral spine. The AP view should be taken on a 14 by 17 inch film and should be centered so as to include the pelvis and hips. This is important because it permits the examiner to recognize a tumor or an infection in the hips or pelvis. Moreover, one may be able to recognize avascular necrosis of the hip or another unsuspected pathological condition that might cause low back pain with or without sciatica. The initial laboratory work should include a complete blood count, sedimentation rate, urinalysis and a chest x-ray if the patient has not had one within the preceding year. If there is still suspicion of tumor or infection after subsequent follow-up, then additional studies of the type suggested for Group II are indicated.

Management

ADVICE. Unless there is evidence of tumor or infection, the patient may be told that he or she is likely to be much better in a few days or several weeks. Moreover, some things can be done to help make the patient feel better.

MEDICATIONS AND NONSURGICAL ORTHOPAEDICS. The patient may be given salicylates, two 5-grain tablets every four hours while awake, with codeine added if the pain is severe. Bed rest, with the option of getting up to go to the bathroom, is suggested. This should be continued for one to two weeks. The patient is advised to get up as he or she feels better. The patient is re-evaluated in two to three weeks if improvement is unsatisfactory.

Discussion

Most patients will be either completely well or much improved by following this regimen. They can then be given some suggestions about how to avoid or minimize back pain (see Table 13–9).

Group II. Subacute Low Back Pain (3 Weeks to 6 Months) With or Without Sciatica

The Problem

Rule out tumor or infection and determine the appropriate conservative treatment. Surgery may be considered in select cases after three to four months of well-supervised conservative care. Tumor or infection must be adequately treated if that diagnosis is made.

Clinical Evaluation

HISTORY. The history may be the same as that in Group I, except that the problem has now been present for three weeks to six months. Usually some type of treatment has been attempted in addition to rest and analgesics. This may include physical therapy, traction, spinal orthosis, injections, manipulation, hospitalization for bed rest, or any combination of these. The patient should be questioned carefully about any history of fever, weight loss or change in gastric, intestinal, urogenital or respiratory function.

PHYSICAL EXAMINATION. The examination may also be similar to that described for Group I patients. There may be less muscle spasm and the pain may not be as sharp or acute with the various leg-raising tests. The patient's stance with hip and knee flexed on the involved side may be more pronounced. When sciatica is present, it may be more distinctive. Motor deficit and deep tendon reflex hypoactivity may be more obvious. There may be discernible muscle wasting. It should be emphasized, however, that patients are placed in Group II based on the duration of their symptoms, not on physical findings.

LABORATORY STUDIES. Complete blood count, sedimentation rate, urinalysis, and rheumatoid factor tests should be done. Anteroposterior x-rays on a 14 by 17 inch film, centered to include the pelvis and hips, and a lateral view should be taken. If there is any question of spondylolisthesis, oblique views of the lumbosacral region should also be included.

SPECIAL STUDIES. We suggest that a special study be done in patients over 60 years of age in Group II, in whom one is not reasonably certain about the etiology of their symptoms. We recommend that a technetium scan be done. This may permit discovery of an active lesion before it shows up by other radiographic techniques.

TABLE 13–6A   Localization of Nerve Root
Lesions by Physical Examination

NEUROLOGICAL LEVEL	WEAKNESS	REFLEX DEPRESSED	SENSATION DECREASED
L4	Anterior tibial muscles	Knee jerk	Medial foot
L5	Extensor hallucis longus	None	Mid-dorsum of foot
S1	Calf muscles	Ankle jerk	Lateral foot

A myelogram and EMG studies are indicated when the diagnosis of a herniated disk is almost certain and the clinical factors point towards surgery. Other special circumstances may require that a Minnesota Multiphasic Personality Inventory (MMPI) be administered.

Management

ADVICE.   If no other diagnosis is appropriate and the clinical picture fits with either herniated intervertebral disk or organic idiopathic low back pain, then the patient may be advised accordingly. Surgery should be considered if there is a distinct diagnosis of intervertebral disk disease and if symptoms are intolerable and not improved by any of the various forms of nonoperative therapy. Surgery should be preceded by a positive myelogram. If the picture is one of organic spine pain without clear-cut signs and symptoms of disk disease, the patient is encouraged to continue longer with nonoperative management.

Any other diagnosis that is made should be treated appropriately. Sometimes a patient will have a clinical picture compatible with severe lumbar osteoarthritis, spondylolisthesis or spinal stenosis. These may all be treated surgically when conservative treatment is inadequate and the symptoms demand relief.

MEDICATIONS AND NONSURGICAL TREATMENT.   We generally prefer to give patients in this group salicylates, Indocin and Darvon, with occasional codeine or phenylbutazone. We have not been enthusiastic about "muscle relaxants."

TABLE 13–7   Nonoperative Treatment of Low Back Pain — Category I

Rest, analgesics, anti-inflammatory drugs
Exercises
Heat and Massage
Axial traction
Orthotic devices
Local and regional injections

TABLE 13–8   Nonoperative Treatment of Low Back Pain — Category II

Isometric truncal exercises
Patient education and group therapy
Spinal manipulation

There appear to be two categories of nonoperative treatment for low back pain with or without sciatica. These are shown in Tables 13–7 and 13–8. Treatments in the first category give from 60 to 70 per cent satisfactory results, which is about the same as one can expect from a combination of placebo and spontaneous remission of symptoms. The other category of nonoperative therapy (shown in Table 13–8) may have a slightly higher success rate (70 to 80 per cent).

If one looks at Table 13–8 and considers the risk:benefit ratio, it appears that desirable nonoperative therapy is a program of isometric abdominal exercises and a patient education program. Although there are some risks associated with spinal manipulative therapy, in a carefully evaluated patient a manipulation technique shown in Figure 13–51 may be employed.

A nonisometric technique for developing abdominal tone is shown in Figure 13–52. The standard isometric abdominal exercises are done by vigorously contracting the abdominal muscles and holding them for two to three seconds, then relaxing. This should be done 10 to 15 times, two or three times a day. This exercise is *not* recommended for patients with cardiac disease.

A patient education program has been developed in Sweden. Slides and tapes for four lectures are available.* Table 13–9 shows some basic prophylactic and ergonomic suggestions of the type that the patient education program provides.

---

*Available from:
Mrs. Marianne Zachrisson-Forssell
AV-Producenterna
Lyckostigen 14
183 50 Täby
Sweden

Figure 13–51 This spinal manipulation is designed for the thoracic and lumbar areas of the spine. It appears to be one of the most frequently used techniques of medical scientists. The major thrust comes from the therapist's right hand rotating the pelvis forward and indirectly applying an axial torque to the thoracic and lumbar areas of the spine. The left hand is used to fix the thorax by taking up the reaction forces. (Reproduced with permission from White, A. A., and Panjabi, M. M.: Clinical Biomechanics of the Spine. Philadelphia, J. B. Lippincott, 1978.)

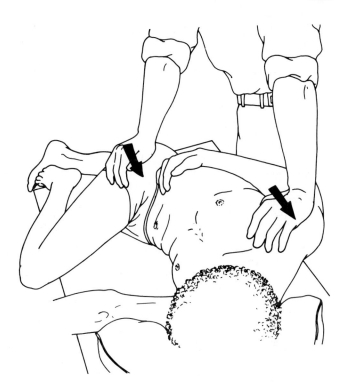

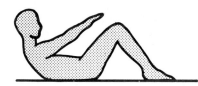

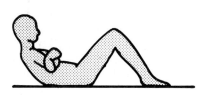

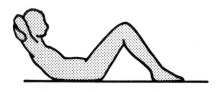

Figure 13–52 These exercises have been suggested as a method of strengthening the abdominal muscles. Note that the feet are always kept flat on the floor. The exercises increase in difficulty from top to bottom. Greater abdominal muscle forces are required in the bottom exercise as compared with the other two, because in this exercise the center of gravity of the upper body is farthest away from the axis of motion due to the rearward position of the arms. These exercises should be done slowly, with the head raised initially, followed by a curling-up movement of the upper trunk. (Reproduced with permission from White, A. A. and Panjabi, M. M.: Clinical Biomechanics of the Spine. Philadelphia, J. B. Lippincott, 1978.)

TABLE 13–9 Prophylactic and Ergonomic Suggestions For Patients With Spine Pain*

Exercise to maintain painless range of motion and muscle tone.

Avoid improper sit-ups and back extension exercises.

When sitting, use a lumbar support.

Use arm rests when possible.

Move around within the seat; also, get out of the seat occasionally.

Determine whether the flexed or extended lumbar position is more comfortable.

Use this position in walking, standing, sitting and lying down.

Avoid excessively high-heeled shoes.

When lying in bed during severe pain, flex hips 90 degrees.

Try sleeping on the floor on three blankets during severe pain.

Use a flat, firm bed otherwise.

Lift heavy objects using leg muscles and holding object close to you while doing a Valsalva maneuver.

Develop truncal muscles with isometric abdominal exercises.

Be careful about opening and closing windows.

Avoid sudden jerks or incremental loads when lifting or carrying.

Avoid heavy lifting and strenuous activity when the back is symptomatic.

Swimming is generally a good exercise.

Avoid obesity.

Sit on a bed or use a high table for changing diapers.

Avoid pain-related activities.

When standing for a long period of time, elevate one foot on a footrest.

*From White, A. A., and Panjabi, M. M.: Clinical Biomechanics of the Spine. Philadelphia. J. B. Lippincott Co., 1978.

We suggest that, in general, when surgery is not indicated there is an advantage to employing several of the low-risk nonsurgical treatment programs. This increases the chance for improvement and enhances the possibilities of placebo benefit.

SURGERY. For the highly symptomatic patient who cannot or will not wait longer it is reasonable to take a myelogram and, if the result is positive, to remove the disk at the appropriate interspace. The patient whose degenerative changes are mainly osseous and who has no sciatica should be encouraged to wait, if possible. However, if this is not feasible after a conscientious conservative effort, such patients may be helped by an appropriate spinal fusion.

Patients with well-documented spinal stenosis are encouraged to wait. When this is no longer possible they may be helped by removal of adequate portions of the posterior elements and by spinal fusion.

Discussion

Despite the discussion of surgery for Group II patients we recommend that *every* attempt be made to manage them nonsurgically. This is because many patients will be greatly improved after six months to one year and can function adequately without surgery. In this way the patient avoids the risk of surgery as well as the significantly decreased chance for relief of pain if the first surgical procedure is not successful. Moreover, the evidence suggests that delay of surgery does not compromise the benefit that it may offer later, even in the presence of documented disk disease. Lumbar neuromuscular deficit may return after disk surgery even when it has been present for 6 to 12 months prior to surgery.

On the other side of this issue, we should keep in mind a point that psychologists emphasize. They observe that when *pain* has been present for as long as a year, the mere removal of the organic cause of that pain is not enough to provide satisfactory relief. Some psychological treatment will be needed in addition to the surgical therapy. Thus the clinician must use good judgment in the recommendation of surgical or nonsurgical treatment for back and leg pain.

Group III. Chronic Low Back Pain (6 Months) With or Without Radiation Into the Leg

The Problem

These patients have had difficulty for a long period of time, and the diagnostic considerations are slightly different. When one can make a diagnosis that is surgically treatable and the patient has already had adequate nonsurgical management, surgical correction may be indicated.

Clinical Evaluation

The history is not different from that of the preceding group, except that the pain is more prolonged and the patient may have learned to live with it to some extent. However, it is not at an acceptable level. Usually the course of the pain is sporadic, with alterations in intensity. The patient has learned to avoid certain activities that may tend to aggravate it.

With this much time an infection will usually have presented itself clearly by fever, malaise or some other clinical manifestation. A tumor will usually have done the same, by weight loss, malaise and constant severe pain unrelieved by rest or analgesics. Some other evidence of tumor will also often be present. Gout, ankylosing spondylitis and other forms of arthritis will usually have developed into a more distinctive clinical picture by this time. Most patients with such a prolonged history will have a herniated disk, spinal stenosis, idiopathic organic spine pain or some other intrinsic spinal disease, such as spondylolisthesis or severe degenerative arthritis.

PHYSICAL EXAMINATION. If there is a profound neurological deficit with muscle wasting or bladder symptoms, one should consider a tumor of the neural elements. Otherwise the patient may show some of the findings suggestive of disk disease. Results of the various straight-leg-raising tests may not be as dramatic as in the more acute phases of the disease. There may be only subtle weakness or slightly diminished reflexes. Patients with disk disease that is resolving itself spontaneously may show improvement in muscle strength and loss of the hypoactive reflexes observed on previous examination.

LABORATORY STUDIES. These patients should have basic screening laboratory studies if they have not been done recently. Thus a CBC, sedimentation rate, urinalysis and rheumatoid factor tests are suggested. If there are no recent (within the last month) anteroposterior and lateral x-rays of the lumbar spine on 14 by 17 inch films, centered to include pelvis and hips, they too should be ordered.

SPECIAL STUDIES. If the patient is over 60 years of age and cancer is suspected, a technetium scan should be seriously considered. If the pain is severe enough for surgery and the clinical picture is suggestive of disk disease, a myelogram should be done. If there is any question of functional disease or psychogenic overlay, the MMPI should also be administered.

Management

ADVICE. If from the history and physical examination the patient appears to have a disk problem and the pain and disability is severe, the option of surgery should be offered. The patient should be told that the disk operation is likely to relieve leg pain more than back pain.

If there is some other specific diagnosis to account for the patient's back pain, such as spondylolisthesis or severe degenerative arthritis, that may be helped by arthrodesis, this procedure should be discussed with the patient. Arthrodesis provides greater relief for spondylolisthesis than for degenerative arthritis.

We do not think that patients with idiopathic organic spine pain in the lumbar region are good candidates for surgery. Many of these patients eventually have an arthrodesis with or without disk removal. Too many have no improvement and become members of the distressing Group IV, actually worse than they were prior to surgery. Group IV patients with idiopathic organic lumbar spine pain are best managed with a rigorous supportive program, exercises or other nonoperative treatment, patient education and a job change, if indicated.

MEDICATION AND NONSURGICAL ORTHOPAEDICS. The problems in this group are essentially the same as in Group II. When there is significant functional disability or obvious complications of the problem by the possibility of a lawsuit, these patients are best referred to a pain specialist. One should resist the tendency to try to help the patient by operating and should resist being manipulated into performing surgery. Such procedures rarely make the patient feel better and not infrequently make the condition worse.

SURGERY. Surgery may be helpful in cases of well-defined disk herniation and spondylolisthesis and occasionally in cases of spinal stenosis or severe degenerative joint disease.

Discussion

There is much we do not know about back pain. We can help patients with supportive therapy, and selected patients do benefit from surgical intervention. When we are not sure of the problem, there is a risk of making the situation worse with surgery. Patients who need a psychiatrist or a lawyer should be sent to one. Patients who cannot be helped should be sent to a pain specialist, and no surgery should be attempted.

Group IV. Chronic Low Back Pain (6 months) With One or More Lumbar Spinal Operations

The Problem

These patients are similar to those in Group III, except that their problems are more complex because they have had surgery but still have pain. If such patients have had more than one operation the problem is even more complex.

The problem is to identify those few patients in this group who may possibly be helped by surgery. The rest will need nonoperative supportive therapy, and perhaps a few will be best managed by a pain specialist.

Clinical Evaluation

HISTORY. These patients include a significant number of those involved in litigation. There may also be aspects of the history suggestive of a psychiatric disease. Some of these patients have had many other operations besides those on the spine. In many instances patients have also had a great number of spinal procedures.

There are several characteristic histories that deserve special mention here. One is the patient who has had one operation, namely, disk removal. This was followed by relief of leg pain and possibly by a return to work for a period of a year or more. The patient gradually develops back pain and may show narrowing and possibly degenerative changes at the interspace that was operated upon. The symptom aggravation pattern is compatible with mechanical irritation and a degenerative process. This patient may have a *good prognosis* with surgery.

Another patient is the type who has a spinal fusion and develops hypermotility and degenerative changes above the fused area or has a clinical picture of a herniated disk above it. This patient may also benefit from surgery.

Patients who have a fusion with clear clinical evidence of a pseudarthrosis have a moderately good prognosis for improvement after re-fusion across the pseudarthrosis. However, it is important to remember that the results of surgery for low back pain in patients who have had even one previous procedure on the low back have a significantly reduced probability of success, no matter what the clinical setting.

Many of these patients will complain of almost constant severe pain in the back, hips and legs, but pain may also be limited to the back. A large number of these patients will be addicted to some medication and are trapped in a rather depressing, disabled way of life.

PHYSICAL EXAMINATION. In addition to the findings described for Groups I to III, these patients will sometimes show other characteristics. They may move in a slow and deliberate manner, holding the spine very stiff and sometimes bent either slightly forwards or to one side. A tap with a rubber hammer or finger pressure in the lumbar region may elicit yelling, grimacing, jumping or falling that suggests excruciating pain. Pressure on the same area when the patient's attention is diverted may cause little or no such response. The back may be less rigid when the patient is reclining or sitting than when standing. A straight-leg-raising test may be positive in the supine position but not in the sitting position when the pulses are examined (Fig. 13–53).

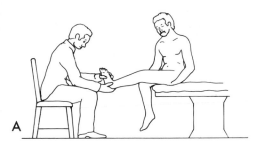

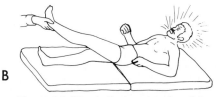

Figure 13–53 *A*. Patient is relaxed in a sitting position on the table while pulses are examined. Straight-leg-raising test here is greater than 90 degrees. *B*. When the patient is lying down, there is vigorous complaint even with less than 90 degrees of straight-leg-raising. This is inconsistent and suggestive of other than organic disease. (Reproduced with permission from White, A. A., and Panjabi, M. M.: Clinical Biomechanics of the Spine. Philadelphia, J. B. Lippincott, 1978.)

Although a patient may show a number of these traits it does not mean that he or she has no organic disease, but it does suggest that a cure, surgical or otherwise, is not a likely prospect.

LABORATORY STUDIES. The laboratory studies are the same as those given to Group III patients. One may wish to confirm the MMPI with a psychiatric interview.

SPECIAL STUDIES. A myelogram may be repeated if there is good evidence that a new or recurrent disk herniation has occurred. In some instances in which spinal stenosis is a possible diagnosis, a computerized axial tomogram of the lumbar region may confirm the diagnosis.

Management

ADVICE. When the cause of pain is not known or an organic basis cannot be found for it, it seems best simply to tell the patient that, even with the best knowledge, judgment and technology, it is not possible to say what the cause is. The patient may be sincerely reassured that the pain may lessen and that he or she does not have a lumbar spine infection or cancer. If it seems appropriate, one may refer the patient to a psychiatrist or to a pain specialist and possibly advise him or her to stay away from surgical treatment or any of the nonmedical so-called "magic cures."

If the evaluation points to some surgically correctable diagnosis, this can be discussed with the patient. If the physician feels that some additional nonsurgical therapy can be helpful, this too should be discussed.

MEDICATIONS AND NONSURGICAL THERAPY. Patients with chronic back pain should be treated with nonaddicting medications. Some of these patients may be helped by a patient education program combined with some type of group therapy. Any of the nonoperative programs that have not been tried with a particular patient deserve consideration.

SURGERY. The surgical procedures

have been discussed previously to some extent. The fusion procedure associated with disk removal for degenerative disease was presented. Refusion for distinctly discernible pseudarthrosis was mentioned. Surgery may be performed for a new or a recurrent disk herniation. Multiple laminectomies and foraminotomies followed by arthrodesis of involved joints have been suggested for spinal stenosis or as a salvage procedure for rare, carefully selected patients. This operation, which is relatively recent in spine surgery, has not been shown to be distinctly effective or ineffective.

Discussion

Be very careful about operating on patients in this group, especially if they have already had *more* than one procedure.

Spondylolysis and Spondylolisthesis

The Problem

There is pain and sometimes evidence of nerve root irritation associated with a defect in the pars interarticularis of a lower lumbar vertebra.

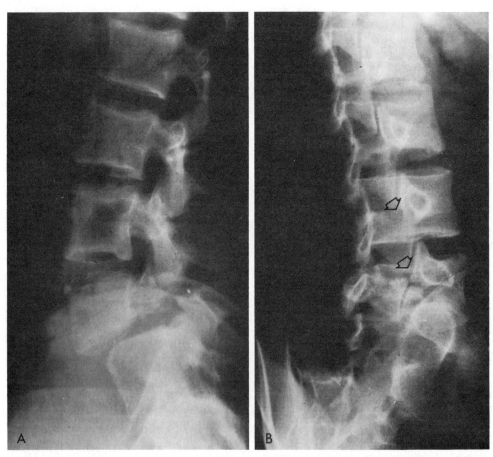

Figure 13–54   A. Lateral film of lumbar spine shows obvious spondylolisthesis with a 50 per cent slip or significant anterior displacement of L5 on S1. B. Oblique view of a patient with spondylolisthesis. Note the defect in the pars interarticularis. The upper arrow shows the neck in the "scotty dog" to be intact. The lower arrow shows a defect or fracture in the "neck" of the "scotty dog." The lower arrow indicates the defect in the pars interarticularis. This defect plus the anterior displacement constitute the diagnosis of spondylolisthesis.

Clinical Evaluation

HISTORY. Most characteristically, the history is of a gradual onset of moderate to severe lower back pain. The pain may be associated with vigorous activities or sometimes may occur after periods of sedentary posture followed by movement. There may sometimes be a history of participation in vigorous athletics, such as gymnastics, football, weight-lifting or wrestling. It is difficult to know whether or not these activities contribute to the cause, but it is not uncommon to find them as part of the history. In some instances, evidence of nerve root irritation, such as paresthesias, dysesthesias or deep pain in the distribution of the sciatic nerve, may be present. When this occurs, the symptoms may be aggravated by coughing, sneezing or straining at the stool. More often than not, however, the symptoms are those of chronic low back pain with some radiation into the hips and thighs.

PHYSICAL EXAMINATION. There may be muscle spasm, limitation of motion and accentuated lumbar lordosis, and often one can palpate a prominent spinous process in the region of the fourth or fifth lumbar vertebra, depending on the level of the disease. This is due to a combination of two factors. When spondylolisthesis occurs, that is, when one vertebral body slips forward onto the other, the whole upper portion of the spine above that level may be displaced anteriorly. Second, with the defect in the pars interarticularis the posterior elements of the vertebra below are moved posteriorly. These two factors result in the prominent palpable spinous process of the vertebra below the vertebrae which have shifted forward. This is an important physical finding.

In addition, depending on the extent of nerve root irritation or deficit, there may be a positive straight-leg-raising sign, Laségue sign or crossed straight-leg-raising sign. There may be reflex changes and muscle weakness also associated with nerve root deficits. Another finding that is sometimes present with spondylolisthesis is hamstring muscle tightness.

LABORATORY STUDIES. The diagnosis of spondylolysis or spondylolisthesis can sometimes be made using the plain AP and lateral films alone (Fig. 13–54A). When the diagnosis is not definite from these films but is suspected, oblique views usually will show the characteristic "scotty dog" sign, shown in Figure 13–54B.

When there is a question of nerve root irritation or neurological deficit, a myelogram is essential. This helps to confirm the diagnosis and to rule out a possible associated herniated anulus fibrosus. Electromyographic studies may be indicated if the presence or absence of neurological deficit is crucial in the evaluation process.

Management

ADVICE. When spondylolisthesis is associated with pain, the patient should be advised that, while the condition is a probable cause of pain, the pain that is being experienced may also be a transient spinal pain from which complete recovery may be expected. Moreover, even the pain that is associated with spondylolisthesis often will subside spontaneously, with or without conservative management.

MEDICAL AND NONSURGICAL ORTHOPAEDICS. Conservative management is a regimen of non-narcotic analgesics and possibly of anti-inflammatory drugs in conjunction with a lumbar orthosis which also gives abdominal support. This therapy should be carried out in conjunction with appropriate exercises for developing abdominal tone and proper instruction on ergonomics and basic activities of daily living that will help to alleviate the symptoms.

SURGICAL TREATMENT. When symptoms are prolonged and severe and are not relieved by the vigorous and carefully followed conservative treatment just discussed, it is appropriate to consider surgical intervention. This is rarely required for spondylolysis but not infrequently is needed for spondylolisthesis. The basic operation is a spinal fusion that prevents any subsequent abnormal displacement of the vertebrae and also is thought to alleviate pain that may be associated with excessive motion of degenerating joints. The fusion may be done either posteriorly or anteriorly.

Other considerations are whether or not the lumbar disk at the interspace involved should be removed and whether or not the detached portion of the posterior vertebral elements should be removed. These decisions are based on (1) the degree of spinal stenosis that is present, requiring decompression of the canal and (2) the presence or absence of a herniated intervertebral disk. When the latter is present the posterior vertebral elements are removed in order to expose the disk and remove it. In some instances there is a band of fibrous scar tissue that is thought to cause nerve root irritation. When that situation exists, it is advisable to remove the tissue.

Discussion

There are several interesting facts about this disease. The anatomical defect is present to different degrees in different racial groups. In the black American population, the incidence is about 2 per cent. In whites and Eskimos it is about 6 per cent and 60 per cent, respectively. One theory is that the defect is congenital, but this is not supported by anatomical observations. The disease appears to occur after age six or seven. The temptation is to assume that it has to do with the beginning of school and the significant additional amount of sitting. This seems to be rather a weak hypothesis. A number of people have the disease but do not have especially severe or an inordinate amount of back pain. It does seem to be the case, however, that in some patients with these defects there is an adequate organic problem, which can be relieved by appropriate surgical intervention when conservative treatment fails.

Coccydynia

Following an injury to the coccyx, such as a fall or blow, there is persistent pain in the region of the coccyx. Sometimes a distinct fracture can be seen on x-ray. When a displaced fracture is present, reduction should be attempted. This can be done by grasping the coccyx anteriorly with the index finger in the rectum and posteriorly with the thumb at the upper portion of the gluteal crease. The angulation may be corrected when there is acute pain, but reduction should be preceded by injections of Novocain into the region of the fracture.

Occasionally patients, usually females, will develop chronic, severe pain of months' to years' duration in the coccyx following a fall on the tip of the spine. This clinical syndrome is not well understood. The pain is constant but may be exacerbated by sitting or by moving the bowels. Injections of locally acting hydrocortisone and Novocain into the region of the sacrococcygeal joint are sometimes helpful. The symptoms may be alleviated somewhat by sitting on a round cushion with a hole in the center. These patients' diseases often have a significant functional component.

Surgical excision should be considered in some instances in which no evidence of compensation or functional overlay exists and the patient has had one year of conservative treatment without success.

Camptocormia

This syndrome has been described by several authors. It is rarely seen in civilian life, but when present the diagnosis can generally be confirmed readily. The patient is generally a modestly educated young male who complains of severe low back pain and is unable to stand erect. The individual is tilted forward and sometimes to one side or the other, often in a grotesque manner.

Endeavors to have the patient actively or passively assume an erect position while standing usually meet with total failure. The key, however, is that when he lies down on the examining table the "deformity" readily disappears. This classic type of hysterical disorder sometimes requires psychiatric care and considerable social support for improvement.

Spinal Orthoses

In this section a few brief comments are offered that will be helpful in the understanding and use of spinal orthoses. In most cases, the brace is employed to support (rest, assist), immobilize (protect) or correct the spine. In most instances the orthosis is employed to support the spine in order to provide symptomatic relief of pain.

There are many types of lumbar spine supports. Three of the basic types are shown in Figure 13–55. Mechanically, these braces generally are designed to provide increased abdominal support, which significantly reduces the forces on the spine. They usually create a less lordotic lumbar spine. In general, it is thought that a spine held in reduced lordosis is more comfortable. For symptomatic relief of most low back problems, the effectiveness of any of the three orthoses shown in Figure 13–55 will be about the same.

Cervical orthoses are used in the symptomatic treatment of cervical spine pain syndromes. The soft cervical collar does little to immobilize the cervical spine. It may have a place as a reminder or comforter and may offer some placebo effect. In order to provide any degree of immobilization a hard Thomas collar or a more extensive Philadelphia collar is required. For pain syndromes, we suggest that these devices be used as little as possible, consistent with the patient's ability to get along without them. Although there is no strong evidence, it is our clinical impression that when such collars are

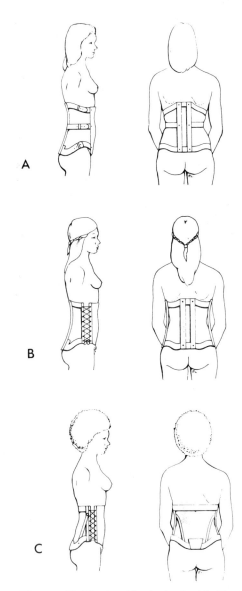

Figure 13–55 *A.* MacAusland (chairback) brace. This orthosis offers intermediate control for the upper lumbar spine in flexion and extension. It is less effective in lateral bending (no lateral uprights) and least effective in controlling axial rotation. *B.* Knight brace. This orthosis offers intermediate control for the upper lumbar spine in flexion-extension and lateral bending. (Note lateral uprights.) It is not an effective control of axial rotation. *C.* Williams brace. This orthosis exerts intermediate control against flexion-extension and lateral bending but not axial rotation. All three braces provide general support and stability through compression by the abdominal supports. (Reproduced with permission from White, A. A., and Panjabi, M. M.: Clinical Biomechanics of the Spine. Philadelphia, J. B. Lippincott, 1978.)

worn for a long time, strictly for symptomatic relief, dependency tends to develop.

COMMENT

We have briefly discussed a large number of topics. Our attempt has been to provide the most reliable, practical and accurate information on these topics. These capsule comments can never substitute for careful listening, history taking, thorough examination and sound clinical judgment. Our hope is that this chapter will complement those talents and therefore assist conscientious, though perhaps orthopaedically inexperienced, clinicians better to evaluate and manage their patients who have musculoskeletal problems.

Acknowledgment

Our special appreciation is given to Mrs. Carol Brunotte, Mrs. Mary Carroll, and the Beth Israel Hospital Department of Medical Photography for their assistance in the preparation of this chapter.

REFERENCES

1. Apley, A. G.: A System of Orthopaedics and Fractures. London, Butterworths, 1973.
2. Giannestras, N. J.: Foot Disorders: Medical and Surgical Management. Philadelphia, Lea & Febiger, 1976.
3. Hoppenfeld, S.: Physical Examination of the Spine and Extremities. New York, Appleton-Century-Crofts, 1976.
4. Lord, J. W., and Rosati, L. M.: Thoracic Outlet Syndromes. CIBA Clinical Symposia, 23(2):3–32, 1971.
4a. Mitchell, C. L., et al.: Osteotomy-bunionectomy for hallux valgus. J. Bone Joint Surg., 40A:41, 1958.
5. Snook, G. A., and Chrisman, O. D.: The management of subcalcaneal pain. Clin. Orthop., 82:163–168, 1972.
6. Southwick, W. O.: Osteotomy through the lesser trochanter for slipped capital femoral epiphysis. J. Bone Joint Surg., 49A:807–835, July, 1967.
7. Steinbrocker, O., and Neustadt, D. H.: Aspiration and Injection Therapy in Arthritis and Musculoskeletal Disorders. New York, Harper & Row, 1972.
8. White, A. A., and Panjabi, M. M.: Clinical Biomechanics of the Spine. Philadelphia, J. B. Lippincott, 1978.
9. White, A. A., Southwick, W. O., DePonte, R. J., et al.: Relief of pain by anterior cervical-spine fusion for spondylosis: a report of sixty-five patients. J. Bone Joint Surg., 55A:525–534, April, 1973.

14 The Hand

PAUL W. BROWN, M.D.

INTRODUCTION

The purpose of this chapter is to make clear what can and cannot be done properly and safely for injured and ailing hands in the Emergency Room and in the Outpatient Clinic. The attending physician should keep always in mind the first dictum of medical practice, "Primum non nocere." Unfortunately, too much is often attempted in the Emergency Room and more hands are harmed by too ambitious attempts at treatment than by too little. When faced with many of the poorer results of too much treatment administered in the interest of "saving time and money for the patient" or for "convenience," the hand surgeon is forced to conclude that the patient would have fared better if he had never seen a physician. When the capabilities and limitations of the Emergency Room and the Outpatient Clinic are honestly assessed, these environments can be properly used to relieve suffering and to treat or prepare the way for treatment of the injured hand. If ignorance or surgical arrogance is fostered in these places, the result will be a steady stream of complications referred to the hand surgeon or to the attorney.

THE ROLE OF THE EMERGENCY ROOM

Evaluation

An assessment of the damage to the hand can be made most thoroughly and adequately if the examining doctor is oriented toward diagnosis rather than therapy. Most injured hands are bleeding and the sight of blood seems to inspire the thought of surgery in many of us rather than an objective analysis of cause and effect. The Emergency Room certainly has great advantages in the treatment of minor trauma, but its highest value is in preparing the patient for proper treatment and in separating what is best handled on the spot from that which requires more extensive treatment.

Control of bleeding is seldom a great problem if one proceeds in a cool and organized manner. If bleeding obscures the wound the logical first step in the assessment of the wound is to stop the flow of blood. A fistful of surgical sponges covered with a mildly compressive elastic bandage will do the job in the majority of cases. I have not known exsanguination from a severed artery in the hand, wrist or forearm to occur, but occasionally it will be necessary to staunch the flow of blood by digital pressure or a tourniquet, a simple procedure which will then allow a full examination of the damage. Such an examination cannot be done well in the presence of a hovering parent or a distraught wife and they should be asked to remain in the waiting room, providing one does not forget to see them later and give them a report of one's findings.

The evaluation itself starts with the history of the injury or complaint. Not only is the nature of the accident or incident important, but also the nature of the environment, the exact time of the accident and the first aid treatment which has been given. The treatment for a laceration of a knuckle incurred by a knife is quite different from that for a laceration inflicted by someone's front teeth, since the contamination factors in the kitchen are quite different from those of the street. The patient's occupation and special requirements for the use of his hand as well as knowledge as to whether he is left-handed or right-handed are occasionally of importance in planning treatment.

The correct position for examination is to have the patient supine with arm outstretched on an armboard or table with a physician seated beside the hand. Good lighting is essential and need not include a glaring light directed into the patient's eyes. Many upright patients tend to faint when an injured hand is examined or manipulated; the

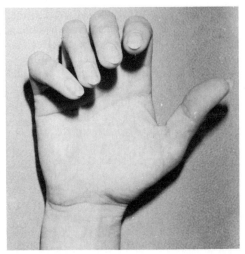

Figure 14–1 Position of examination. Note that the small finger is normally held in more flexion than the ring, the ring more than the middle and the middle more than the index. Also called the position of rest.

supine position obviates this possibility as well as reassuring the patient (Fig. 14–1).

Physical and visual examinations are next. Fear and anxiety are the greatest potentiators of pain and if the patient is supine and the physician proceeds in an orderly and confident manner, complaints of pain are seldom severe enough to interfere with the examination. Only rarely will narcotics or sedatives be required; if medication is indicated, diazepam (Valium) will act effectively and safely. An orderly inventory should be taken by tissue system: skin, vessels, nerve, bone and joint, tendon and muscle. Occasionally, the state of a particular structure will not be clear — e.g., the median nerve in a volar laceration of the wrist. In such cases one's curiosity must be curtailed by the admonition "do no further harm." Surgical exploration in the Emergency Room is out of order even in the search for the correct diagnosis. Generally, this will not be necessary and under ordinary circumstances, all damaged structures will be apparent without harming or hurting the patient.

What Can Be Done in the Emergency Room

Most dislocations and many fractures can be reduced in the Emergency Room. Some wounds can be closed. A spurting artery can be ligated or at least clamped. An occasional extensor tendon can be repaired and a burned hand may be immersed in ice water. Proper splints and dressings can be applied. Ideally, and with few exceptions, that is all! Unfortunately, the ideal is beset with necessary compromises of time, place, economics, bed availability and patient pressures, and we may be forced to extend the Emergency Room beyond its safe limits. For this we will pay a certain price of infection, wound breakdown, scarred-down tendons and other unhappy results. The greater our compromise, the greater the complications, and these will include such misfortunes as reflex sympathetic dystrophies, stiffened fingers and painful hands.

One very important thing the Emergency Room can do is to prepare for proper and prompt management of severe conditions beyond the capabilities of the Emergency Room. When time is important to results, and this is always true where débridement is necessary, the Emergency Room staff can save that time by notifying the attending physician and the operating room and taking care of preoperative and administrative details. The Emergency Room's task is not finished when the decision is reached to treat the patient further in the operating room.

Limitations of the Emergency Room

The limitations of the Emergency Room are implied in the foregoing. Nerves and tendons are not repaired, with certain obvious exceptions which will be dealt with later. Only the most simple skin grafts are undertaken and open reductions of fractures and dislocations are not done at all. Major débridements cannot be done well in the Emergency Room, and only the most obvious superficial burns can be assessed. The hand is terribly unforgiving of poor management and barely tolerant of the moderately good; most of these things can be done better in the operating room than in the Emergency Room and the damaged hand will insist on proving that time after time.

The Transition to Inpatient Status

The Emergency Room patient should become an inpatient when further care in the operating room is necessary within the next 24 hours or when the hand requires constant elevation, frequent observation, dressing changes or skilled nursing care. Cases not requiring immediate surgery but in which there is a reasonable risk of increasing edema should certainly be admitted: included in this category are wringer injuries in children and other crush injuries. Burns of undetermined extent should be admitted as should hand infections which show evidence of progression. Poor treatment in the first 24 hours may cause functional impairment that may take months or years of rehabilitation to correct.

The Outpatient Clinic

The results of treatment of the disabled hand can be facilitated or ruined by the follow-up care given that hand. Every hand surgeon is acutely aware that the postoperative management of the hand is just as important as the operation. Thus the Outpatient Clinic, like the Emergency Room, must have good facilities for examination of the hand. For most patients this is best accomplished with the patient sitting opposite the examiner with the hand resting on a small table of comfortable height. If sutures or wires are to be removed the examination may be painful and it is better to have the patient supine to remove the risk of fainting.

In the Outpatient Clinic dressings can be changed and splints made or adjusted, and a detailed record of the patient's progress in returning function to the hand can be made and kept. As future prescriptions may depend on the rate of progress, it is important that appearance, swelling, coloration, complaints of pain, strength and ranges of motion be carefully recorded. Consistency of nomenclature is necessary if records are to have value. The digits are not numbered, but are named: thumb, index, middle, ring and small. These may be abbreviated Th, I, M, R and S. The joints are metacarpophalangeal (MP), proximal interphalangeal (PIP) and distal interphalangeal (DIP); the thumb has only a single interphalangeal joint (IP). The joints are most commonly agreed to be at zero degrees when extended. If extended beyond this point, it can be recorded as a minus figure. Thus the MP joint of the right small finger which hyper-extends ten degrees and flexes to a right angle would be recorded as follows: RtSF MP — 10/90. A distinction may have to be made between active and passive ranges of motion (act. ROM and pass. ROM). The usual range of motion of the wrist would be recorded: 60/90; pro. 90, sup. 90.

In the case of nerve injuries careful motor and sensory examination is a necessary part of the record if the rate of regeneration of the nerve is to be assessed. Such recording may play an essential role in future decisions to re-explore a nerve or to intervene with secondary salvage procedures such as tendon transfers.

Most wounds of the hand, surgical and traumatic, are closed with synthetic sutures such as nylon. The simplest and most effective tools for suture removal are iris scissors with two sharp points and a mosquito type hemostat. Wire sutures may also be readily removed with these, although the scissors will not last indefinitely.

Kirschner wires used for internal splinting and for the fixation of frac-

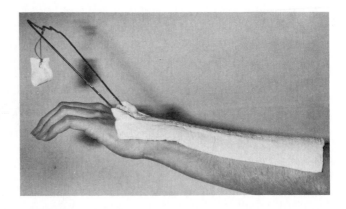

Figure 14–2 An improvised splint of plaster of paris, a bent coat hanger, rubber band and adhesive tape finger sling. When the plaster is set, it is affixed to the forearm with an ace bandage. This particular splint is designed to assist a finger in extension. Slings for each finger can be added.

tures and arthrodeses are generally buried just under the skin. Their removal is a simple outpatient procedure requiring the injection of a drop of local anesthetic, a nick in the skin and extraction of the wire with needlenose pliers whose jaws have been filed down to sharp points. Occasionally one cannot find the wire and if its removal is imperative a more effective anesthetic and a more extensive search and a tourniquet are required. Probing for elusive K-wires can be a painful experience for both physician and patient, and it is to be hoped that the former will not prolong the experience when simple measures are not enough.

Proper dressings can certainly be applied in the Outpatient Clinic and some simple splints can be fabricated out of plaster of paris, wire coathangers and rubber bands (Fig. 14–2). Some of the newer thermoplastics such as Orthoplast have some use in this regard. An understanding of what is needed in the way of a splint and some ingenuity are more important for most splints than fancy materials and elaborate equipment.

Equipment

The most essential equipment for dealing with impaired hands in the Emergency Room is an observant pair of eyes. Next most important is plenty of mild soap and water. Helpful but far less necessary are sutures and other surgical paraphernalia. With these priorities clearly in mind the type and extent of proper hand surgery in the Emergency Room can be better defined.

When dealing with wounds of the hand, the examiner or operator should wear a surgical mask. Surgical instruments needed are few and simple, but they should be small and reserved for delicate work. Necessary are a scalpel with expendable No. 15 blades, Adson or tissue fixation forceps, double pointed scissors, mosquito hemostats, a probe, a small bone rongeur, a Bunnell type hand drill and 0.045 inch Kirschner wires. A 4–0 plain catgut suture is adequate for tying off bleeders and 5–0 nylon or polyethylene swaged onto a small curved cutting needle is best for closing wounds of the hand and affixing skin grafts. Simple self-retaining retractors, skin hooks and small rake retractors complete the list. Anything more elaborate than this instrument inventory would indicate that work is being done in the Emergency Room that should best be done in the operating room.

A tourniquet has limited application in the Emergency Room and in the Outpatient Clinic. Simple débridement in the Emergency Room is generally best done without a tourniquet since recognition of devitalized tissue is easier when free bleeding can be seen. When a tourniquet is required, its level of application and duration of use may depend on the type of anesthesia used. A pneumatic blood pressure cuff should be used on the upper arm, a proper pressure for adults being 250 mm of mercury and for children 200 mm. Tourniquets used at wrist and forearm levels may cause nerve damage. A rubber band tourniquet around the base of the finger is dangerous except for procedures lasting only a few minutes. Since most patients can comfortably tolerate a tourniquet on the arm for about twenty minutes, this can be useful when carrying out small procedures on the hand under local anesthesia.

Anesthesia

This topic has been dealt with more thoroughly in Chapter 3, but reference should be made here to three types of anesthesia particularly useful to Emergency Room management of the injured hand. For all of these a solution of 1 per cent aqueous lidocaine is effective and safe. The first is local infiltration of the injured area. Producing an intradermal wheal, waiting a few seconds and then advancing the needle in various directions while injecting the solution should be a relatively painless procedure. A 1½ inch No. 22 hypodermic needle will suffice for this and the following methods. For effective use one should wait approximately ten minutes after injection before proceeding further. Solutions with epinephrine should not be used.

For work on one or two fingers a block of the digital or common digital nerve is often useful. The needle is introduced into the dorsal surface of the finger web, pointed volarward and toward the metacarpal head, and 2 milliliters of lidocaine are injected (Fig. 14–3). This is repeated for the other volar digital nerve, and if work is to be done on the dorsum of the proximal or middle segment of the finger a similar block of the dorsal nerves may be necessary.

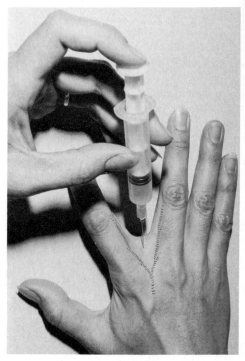

Figure 14–3 Common digital nerve block. The needle is directed toward the bifurcation of the nerve. If preceded by an intradermal wheal, the procedure should be almost painless.

Again it should be emphasized that no epinephrine should be used.

One of the most satisfactory types of anesthesia for Emergency Room work on the hand, wrist and forearm is the intravenous regional block or the so-called Bier block. This was described in Chapter 3, but it can be mentioned here that this type of anesthesia is easy and safe to use and is well accepted by children.

Related to methods of anesthesia are the safe, simple and analgesic properties of ice water. Ice water immersion of the painful burned hand is wonderfully effective in allaying pain and calming the patient, and is similarly useful for sprains, fractures and crush injuries. An ice water bath maintained for up to 15 minutes not only gives excellent relief of pain, but if used within an hour after the injury it may be very effective in preventing or decreasing the amount of edema that would otherwise develop.

Dressings and Splints

The hand dressing can be as important as the surgical treatment itself. Properly applied it can promote comfort, contribute to healing, and — most important — help to prevent or decrease edema. Improperly applied it can cause pain, contribute to stiffening and in fact irreparably damage a hand. The basic principle should be one of uniform mild compression — the dressing must be firm but not tight. Bunnell's concept of the position of function is still a very useful one in applying hand dressings even though some conditions may call for deviations from this position. These principles state that the hand is best maintained with the wrist in 30 degrees extension with moderate flexion of all MP and IP joints and with the thumb in moderate abduction. In this position both the transverse and longitudinal arches of the hand are preserved.

Wounds, whether sutured or left open, are best covered with fine mesh gauze. Somewhat better are plastic coated dressings such as Telfa or gauze impregnated with bismuth ointment such as Xeroform, since these allow blood to ooze through but do not stick to the wound when removed. Petrolatum fine mesh gauze is also good if the excess grease is scraped free — too much grease tends to cause maceration. Over the gauze are applied several flat gauze sponges; how much of the hand must be incorporated in the dressing is a question to be decided at this time. Any injury of the hand or of a digit causes edema of some degree. Whether this edema will be severe enough to interfere with healing or with return of the hand to normal function depends conjointly on the nature of the injury as well as on the postinjury management of that hand. Though one may hesitate to apply a complete hand dressing for a finger injury, it is safer to do so when there is a question of subsequent edema and pain.

For dressing an individual finger the various sizes of tubular stockinette known as Tubegauz are extremely convenient. Lacking this, a roller bandage gauze can be used, but this must be affixed with strips of adhesive tape. With such circumferential strips, care must be taken not to constrict venous return, and the patient must be cautioned to loosen the strips in the event of increasing swelling.

In dressing the entire hand the fingers should be separated by individual sponges, and the dorsal and volar surfaces of the entire hand, including the wrist, should be overlain with fluffed-up sponges in multiple layers. The dressings are then wrapped snugly with a slightly elastic roll of gauze such as Kling or Kerlex. The goal should be a firm dressing with evenly distributed compression; a compression dressing is definitely not a tight dressing. Material such as sponge rubber foam, polyurethane foam or mechanic's waste may be used in place of the gauze fluffs (Fig. 14–4).

A volar — and occasionally dorsal — plaster splint may sometimes be overlain on the compression dressing where immobilization is needed. A circular plaster cast seldom is needed for injury of the hand until the initial edema has subsided.

Equally important to the compression dressing is continuous elevation of the injured extremity. The duration of elevation is directly proportional to the damage done to the hand. Twenty-four hours will suffice for most injuries, but elevation may be indicated for several days when crushing has been a part of the injuring force. In the case of outpatient treatment, the patient should be instructed to suspend the hand in its dressing from the back of a chair moved next to his bed while he is sleeping. When he is up the forearm can be rested on top of the head or the hand rested on the opposite shoulder. Slings are generally inadvisable as they invite prolonged dependency of the hand and also tend to produce stiff elbows and shoulders.

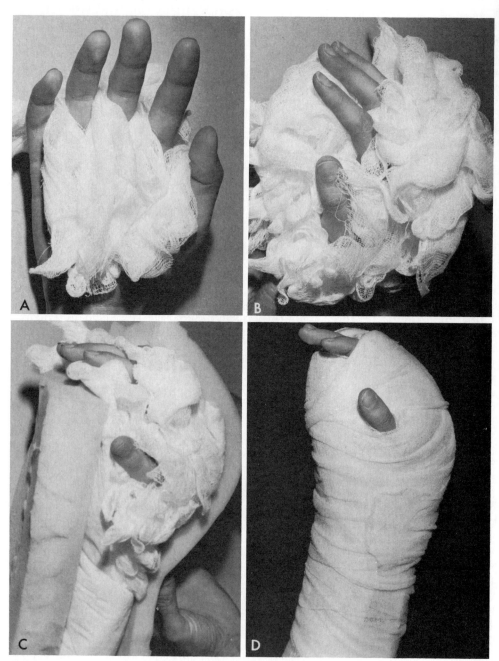

Figure 14–4 Applying the hand compression dressing. *A*. The fingers are lightly separated by surgical sponges. *B*. Many fluffed-up surgical sponges are applied to volar and dorsal surfaces. *C*. ABD pads or strips of polyurethane foam are applied from middle finger joints to just below the elbow. *D*. Firm, but not tight, compression is applied with Kerlix or Kling gauze. Ace bandage may be used but caution is necessary to avoid wrapping too tightly. Note "position of function." Elevation of the extremity should follow.

Static splints for digital fractures are illustrated in Chapter 12. Dynamic splints for uncomplicated problems can readily be fashioned from plaster splints, coathanger wire, rubber bands and safety pins. Such homemade splints may be definitive in some cases or may serve to start treatment until a more sophisticated brace or splint can be made by an orthotist.

TRAUMA

Open Wounds

An open wound represents a dual insult to the hand: first, a break in the integument with or without other tissue damage, and second, a factor of contamination. It is the latter which makes the open wound unique and potentially more dangerous than the closed injury. Lest this seem obvious to the point of being trite, let me point out that many of our complications and bad results stem from a lack of understanding of this fundamental. Pasteur's deathbed words are reputed to have been, "The organism is nothing, the environment is all." In dealing with the inherent dangers of wound contamination, two fundamentals must be understood: (1) as many of the contaminating organisms as possible must be removed from the wound without further damaging tissue, and (2) the tissue must be managed in such a way as to discourage multiplication of organisms. Anything which enhances such multiplication also enhances the transition from contamination, a nonpathological state, to infection, which definitely is pathological. The presence of devitalized tissue, hematoma, foreign material or edema tends to encourage infection. Translated into terms of practical action, our task is to remove as many bacteria as possible by irrigation, but since complete decontamination is not possible, we must improve the environment by débridement and by proper wound dressing and management.

DÉBRIDEMENT. Débridement is the key to wound healing. It may be as simple as the housewife holding her cut finger under running water before applying a Band-Aid, or it may be an exacting, time-consuming operation. It implies the removal of foreign bodies, devitalized or unsalvageable tissue and the removal of as many bacteria as possible. Foreign bodies such as splinters or lead shot may be easily removed, but the removal of foreign materials injected under pressure from a grease gun or paint gun may represent a formidable challenge. Organic material such as vegetable matter or bits of clothing must be removed, but the extraction of metallic bodies such as bullets or pieces thereof is rarely worth the surgical trauma required to find them.

Recognizing and removing devitalized tissue is the most difficult part of débridement. The hand has little expendable tissue, and the challenge is to save anything viable which is useful to future function, yet not to compromise healing and future function by leaving any dead or potentially dead tissue within the hand. Débridement is done without tourniquet, because bleeding of the tissues is often the best key to their viability. Skin which is obviously avascular should be removed; if in doubt as to its viability, leave the decision until two or three days have elapsed (Fig. 14–5). Subcutaneous fat that is dirty or badly traumatized should be removed. Muscle that bleeds freely should be retained; that which does not must be discarded. Bone fragments — even though completely detached from soft tissue — are never removed. If detached and dirty they should be washed off and returned to their place of origin. Nerves and tendons are rarely removed; even though frayed and dirty they may often be salvageable for future function, and therefore the physician should clean them off and leave them in place.

The best aid to the removal of bacteria is copious irrigation with sterile saline. This implies the use of a liter — or

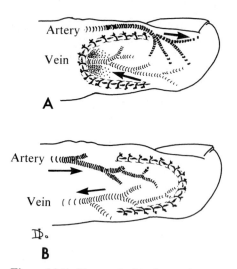

Figure 14–5 Traumatic skin flaps. The major problem and cause of necrosis in the distally based flap is inadequate venous drainage.

in severe cases many liters — of fluid and not a few squirts from a syringe. If the liquid is delivered by gravity through a narrow gauge nozzle the stream of fluid can be directed into nooks and crannies and with enough force to flush out bits of contaminants and devitalized tissue as well as a good proportion of the contaminating organisms.

CLOSURE AND NONCLOSURE. There are several conflicting approaches to the management of open wounds. Perhaps the most popular and certainly the most simplistic is to close them all. When this doctrine has been applied to all wounds, disasters such as wound breakdown, gas gangrene, amputation and death have been frequent. To go to the opposite extreme and leave all wounds open is certainly safer but hardly practical for many injuries. The challenge is to recognize those which may be safely closed — or better yet to recognize those wounds which would be benefited from early closure. This determination is often a difficult one: the factors to be considered are the nature and extent of the injury, the degree and type of contamination, the adequacy of decontamination and dé-

bridement and the length of time elapsed from the time of injury. To appraise all of these variables accurately and to apply them to a particular hand calls for objective analysis, knowledge and experience. If there is one simple rule, it must be: "If in doubt, don't close."

Wounds which generally can be safely closed are those which are cleanly incised, those which have been incurred in a relatively "clean" environment, those which have a small degree of soft tissue damage and those in which less than eight hours have elapsed from the time of injury until the time of closure. A useful distinction between the "tidy" and the "untidy" wound has been made by Rank and Wakefield,[7] but it should be noted that a seemingly tidy wound incurred the day previously does not permit safe closure, as it is no longer clean. Gunshot wounds, crush injuries, bites and wounds incurred in the barnyard are examples of wounds that should not be closed early.

Primary closure means suturing a wound within 24 hours of injury. This is probably the most common method used in the Emergency Room and despite the fact that most wounds so treated heal without complication, we must concern ourselves with those cases which are harmed by such treatment.

Delayed primary closure is done between the second and seventh day and is much safer for most wounds. Such wounds will still heal by primary intention and with fewer complications. The disadvantages for the physician and the patient are the time and inconvenience. A major advantage is that the "second look" at the time of redressing gives one the opportunity to find areas requiring redébridement, an opportunity that is denied by primary closure.

Closure after the sixth or seventh day is called secondary, and is used for more severe, untidy wounds, especially when there is some crushing of soft tissues. Secondary closure of wounds can sometimes be done by wound excision and suturing, but more commonly coverage is obtained with skin grafts or pedicle transfers, and these procedures will seldom be done in the Emergency Room.

With many wounds the doctrine of delayed closure may well be expanded to one of nonclosure. Some open wounds of the hand that are allowed to heal by secondary intention will give end results as good as the same types of wound that have been closed primarily. Transverse wounds of the volar aspect of the palm and fingers do particularly well when dressed properly with relative immobility of the adjoining joints, and will heal as well and as promptly as those that are sutured and with less likelihood of infection and wound breakdown. This doctrine is perhaps a difficult one for both physician and patient to accept, but once the former has seen a few wounds thus treated and has convinced himself of the usefulness of this technique, he will have little difficulty in convincing his patients (Fig. 14–6). For skin flaps which lift up or separate, adhesive tape strips may readily be used instead of sutures. The sterile adhesive Steri-Strips are quicker, cheaper and more comfortable to apply than sutures and they may be effectively used for skin closure as well as affixing skin grafts. Such tape sutures are very useful with a so-called trapdoor laceration, with lacerations of the fingers and on the dorsal surface of the hand.

Fractures and Joint Injuries

OPEN FRACTURES. It is widely written and accepted that open fractures of the hand must be closed and also that leaving an open fracture open invites infection. Neither of these dicta is true. If there is any question about the wound healing primarily because of contamination or the nature of the wound, the open fracture will heal better and with fewer complications if the wound is left open than if the wound does not accept closure and breaks down secondarily. The same is true of open joint injuries; contrary to popular teaching an open joint overlain by a dirty wound will do better left open, if active motion of the joint is encouraged. Such joints do not lose their

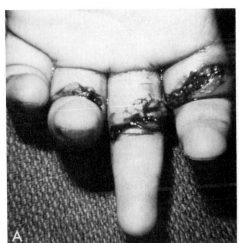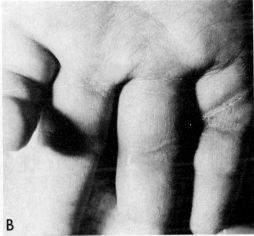

Figure 14–6 Nonclosure technique. Healing by secondary intention. *A*. Volar lacerations with an element of crushing. Underlying flexor tendons divided. Wounds were treated by débridement and copious irrigation, covered with fine mesh gauze and a mild compression hand dressing and suspension. No sutures were used. *B*. Same wounds 40 days later. No edema, no induration. Hand is now ready for reconstructive surgery for the tendons.

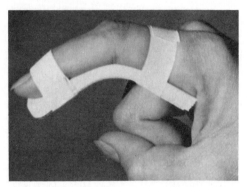

Figure 14–7 Splint for a fracture of the middle phalanx. Splint is aluminum and is padded with sponge rubber. The patient should be instructed to loosen the tape strips if swelling occurs.

articular cartilage nor do they tend to stiffen appreciably; on the contrary, the joint which becomes infected owing to premature closure often ends up with painful stiffness or ankylosis.

FRACTURES OF THE DISTAL PHALANX. These usually involve the distal tuft and may be remarkably comminuted, but no treatment other than a protective fingertip splint for comfort is necessary. This is a simple splint of aluminum placed on the volar side of the middle and distal phalanges with the DIP joint flexed 15 degrees. The end of the splint is curved up to cover the end of the finger to protect it from being painfully bumped.

FRACTURES OF THE MIDDLE PHALANX. Shaft fractures of this bone usually result from a crushing injury or from a blow by a heavy object. If undisplaced they should be immobilized for two to three weeks with an aluminum splint taped to all three phalanges with the interphalangeal joints in 15 degrees of flexion (Fig. 14–7). If angulated, the deformity should be corrected before splinting. If reduction cannot be retained by the splint, the fracture should be transfixed with a Kirschner wire drilled in from one side of the finger and left in place for three weeks. A fairly common injury combines a fracture of the volar portion of the phalanx with a dorsal dislocation of the remainder of the phalanx: i.e., a fracture-dislocation of the PIP joint. If not reduced accurately all useful function of this joint will be lost and an open reduction and internal fixation of two Kirschner wires as shown in the illustration is necessary (Fig. 14–8). This is generally a task for the operating room.

FRACTURES OF THE PROXIMAL PHALANX. The mechanism of injury of such fractures is usually the same as for the middle phalanx, and volar angulation of the fragments is common (Fig. 14–9). The proper treatment is reduction of the deformity followed by immobilization on a volar splint incor-

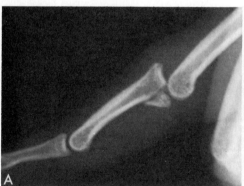
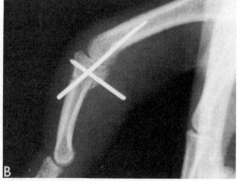

Figure 14–8 Fracture-dislocation of the PIP joint. *A.* Reduction of the dislocation cannot be maintained until the fracture is reduced and stabilized. *B.* This is best done with open reduction and K-wire fixation. The wires are removed in three weeks.

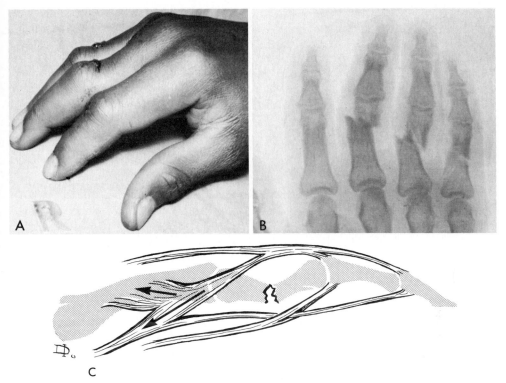

Figure 14–9 Fracture of the proximal phalanx. *A*. Typical deformity of volar angulation. *B*. Comminution, volar and lateral deformity are common. *C*. Volar angulation results from the deforming forces of the intrinsic muscles.

porated into a short arm plaster cast (Fig. 14–10). Placing traction on fingers is not only unnecessary but dangerous. Stiffened fingers may result from traction applied to straight fingers. Sloughs of volar skin and stuck-down flexor tendons may result from traction applied to fingers flexed over a splint. Unstable oblique fractures of the shaft of the proximal phalanx should be internally splinted with a transfixing Kirschner wire as with middle phalangeal fractures.

In reducing fractures of the phalanges or metacarpals care must be taken to correct rotatory as well as angulatory deformity. Careful inspection of both volar and dorsal surfaces is needed and the fingertips should be looked at end on (Fig. 14–11).

Fractures of the epiphysis of the base of the proximal phalanx in children and

Figure 14–10 Immobilization of the proximal phalanx fracture. A padded aluminum splint is shaped to conform to the moderately flexed finger and the slightly extended wrist and is incorporated into a plaster short arm cast. This splint and cast are also useful for metacarpal fractures.

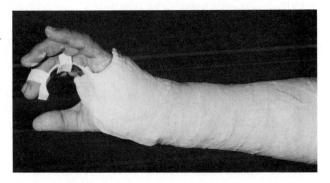

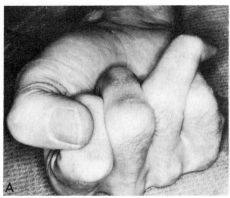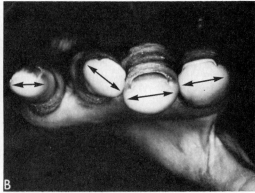

Figure 14–11 Malrotation of proximal phalanx fractures. *A.* This ring finger appeared fairly normal when the fingers were held extended. The deformity quickly became apparent when the fingers were flexed. *B.* Malrotation was apparent when the fingers were viewed end on.

adolescents may be corrected by manipulation, but if this is not possible and there are more than 10 or 15 degrees of angulation present, open reduction in the operating room may be necessary to avoid unsightly deformity. Such an injury is most common in the small finger.

METACARPAL FRACTURES. Most common of these is the neck fracture of the fourth or fifth metacarpals, the so-called boxer's fracture. If loose and easily reduced by manipulation, this fracture can be immobilized with a short arm cast extended over the dorsum of the hand and the involved finger with the finger flexed at the MP joint. Such a splint should leave the middle and distal phalanges free. Most often such fractures are impacted with the metacarpal head and neck flexed 30 to 60 degrees into the palm. In these cases manipulative reduction is usually impossible and they are best treated by accepting the deformity and allowing immediate active use of the hand as soon as symptoms allow, usually a few days. The patient with such an injury must be advised that the "knuckle" of the involved finger will forever remain obscure. The depression of the metacarpal head into the palm may be slightly uncomfortable when tightly grasping an unyielding object, but since metacarpals four and five are quite mobile

this will represent only a minor inconvenience for most people. If this is not acceptable to the patient, open reduction and K-wire fixation is the alternative (Fig. 14–12).

Less common but more serious are similar fractures of the neck of metacarpals two and three. As these metacarpals are relatively fixed, prominence of the head in the palm is a deterrent to strong and comfortable grasp. Therefore, if closed reduction is not possible, open reduction will be necessary. Two crossed K-wires introduced on either side of the MP joint will stabilize these fractures without the necessity for a cast or splint, and active motion of the MP joints can be allowed immediately. The wires should be removed after three weeks.

Oblique or transverse shaft fractures of the metacarpal which can be reduced can generally be adequately immobilized with a short arm cast that ends at the distal palmar crease, but this plaster dressing must be carefully molded to the transverse metacarpal arch and must be nonpadded. Oblique and unstable metacarpal shaft fractures which tend to telescope require K-wire fixation. Transverse shaft fractures which tend to angulate — and are fairly good risks for nonunion — require open reduction and fixation with crossed K-wires (Fig. 14–13). Intramedullary

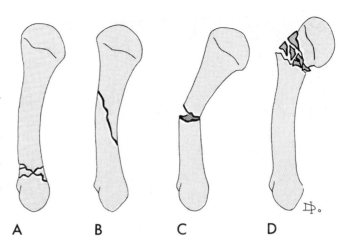

Figure 14–12 Metacarpal fractures. *A.* Comminuted fracture of the metacarpal base — generally stable and requires no splinting. *B.* Oblique fracture of shaft — usually treated with plaster splint or cast. *C.* Transverse fracture of shaft — usually angulates dorsally or displaces — generally best treated with internal fixation. *D.* Boxer's fracture of neck — reduction often impossible.

Kirschner wires introduced through the MP joint tend to give poor fixation and may jeopardize the joint. Fractures of the bases of the metacarpals are of little consequence and may be treated with active motion. Considerable pain and swelling may accompany these, and these symptoms are well handled by ice water immersion if seen within an hour or two of injury.

FRACTURES OF THE THUMB AND FIRST METACARPAL. Phalangeal fractures of the thumb are treated much the same as those of the fingers, though it is more difficult to shape an aluminum splint to conform to the thumb and thenar eminence, thereby immobilizing the MP joint. Shaft fractures of the first metacarpal are more often comminuted than are fractures of the other metacarpals. They can be readily immobilized by a plaster thumb spica, which is simply a short arm cast extended beyond the interphalangeal joint of the thumb. The thumb should be held

in the position of function, i.e., slight flexion and moderate abduction. (Fig. 14–14).

FRACTURES OF THE BASE OF THE FIRST METACARPAL. Fractures of the base of the thumb metacarpal are generally transverse, but they sometimes involve the carpometacarpal joint. The distal, larger segment is angulated in the position of flexion, which is quite compatible with good function. Since these are generally impacted and stable fractures, active motion will give a very acceptable result for most patients. If a patient requires a normal span, as with a pianist, an open reduction and K-wire fixation will be necessary. Base fractures with extension into the joint are often confused with Bennett's fractures, which, however, are really fracture-dislocations with proximal displacement of the distal fragment and the ulnar base or hook of the metacarpal remaining in place (Fig. 14–15). If the deformity is accepted, disability in the

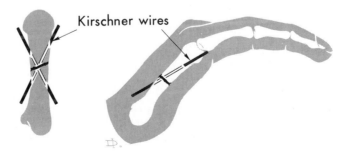

Kirschner wires

Figure 14–13 K-wire fixation of metacarpal fractures.

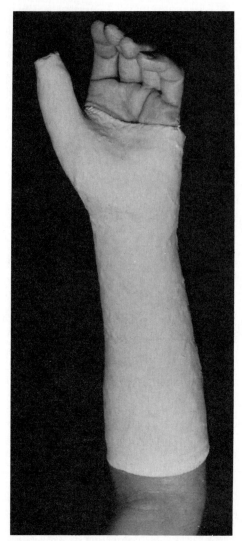

Figure 14-14 Plaster thumb spica. The plaster extends to the end of the thumb and the thumb is in a position of moderate abduction.

range of motion of the thumb will be moderate, but it is better to treat it by open reduction and Kirschner wire internal fixation. Treatment by skeletal traction is difficult, and often results in failure or complications.

JOINT INJURIES. Dislocations of the interphalangeal joints, like those of other joints, are emergencies because the functional result following such an injury is in direct proportion to the amount of time elapsed from injury until reduction. Reduction is generally a simple matter of pulling or manipulating the joint into normal position and is often accompanied by a palpable and sometimes audible snap. Ice water immersion for 10 or 15 minutes following reduction will result in decreased swelling and pain. Splinting with an aluminum splint for two weeks may then be followed by careful resumption of active motion.

MP dislocation of the thumb is caused by hyperextension of the proximal phalanx with rupture of the volar capsule and protrusion of the first metacarpal head through the two heads of the flexor pollicis brevis (Fig. 14–16). Reduction is accomplished by manual traction on the thumb while holding the MP joint in flexion to allow relaxation of the flexor pollicis brevis. Occasionally closed reduction will not be possible, in which case open reduction through a transverse incision in the proximal flexion crease of the MP joint is necessary. The same type of dislocation of the index finger MP joint may be

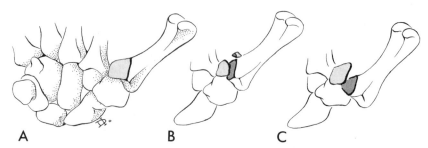

Figure 14-15 Fractures of base of first metacarpal. *A*. Stable — no displacement. *B*. Stable — slight displacement. *C*. Bennett's fracture–dislocation — reduction and fixation usually indicated.

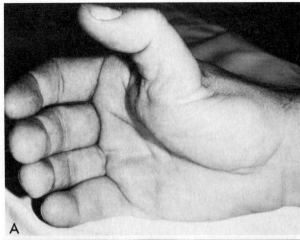

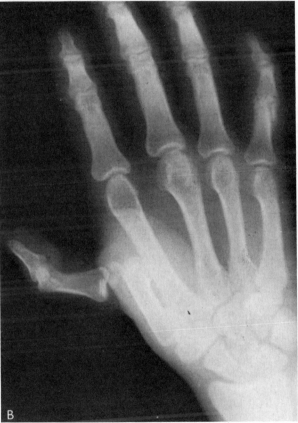

Figure 14–16 MP dislocation of the thumb. *A*. The metacarpal head is prominent on the volar surface. *B*. The proximal phalanx is displaced dorsally and proximally. Note the sesamoid bones.

seen and reduction is performed in the same manner. Following either open or closed reduction the digit should be immobilized with the MP joint flexed to 45 degrees for three weeks. If reduction is performed within several hours of injury, residual disability should be negligible.

Sprains of the PIP joints of the fingers represent a tear or stretching of the collateral ligaments and capsule. These injuries cause a surprising amount of

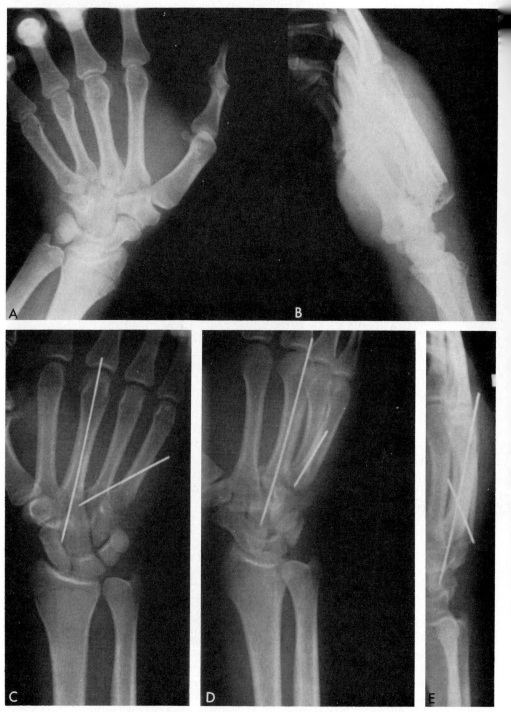

Figure 14–17 Carpometacarpal dislocation. *A*. Not recognized on AP x-ray. *B*. Readily apparent in lateral view. *C, D, E*. Manually reduced and transfixed with two K-wires.

persistent pain, swelling and stiffness of the joint. The joint should be immobilized for three weeks, and then active but protected motion may be started. Sprains or tears of the ulnar collateral ligament of the thumb MP joint are rarely successfully treated by splinting, and if recognized within two weeks of injury should be surgically repaired. Otherwise a condition of chronic instability called "gamekeeper's thumb" may result.

Carpometacarpal dislocations are uncommon and are difficult to recognize. Both physical deformity — difficult to recognize because of swelling — and a good lateral x-ray help in the diagnosis. They are easy to reduce but usually they promptly resume the position of dislocation when digital pressure is released (Fig. 14–17). They should be reduced manually and one or two K-wires drilled through the dorsum of the hand, transfixing the metacarpal base and the adjoining carpus. This wire should be left in place for three to four weeks.

Burns

THERMAL BURNS. The most difficult aspect of burn management is recognition of the depth of the burn or the degree of skin destruction. Many burns which at first seem devastating can be well managed on an outpatient basis. The most striking aspect is pain and this quite often is out of proportion to the depth of the burn. The burn cannot be objectively examined or analyzed until the patient is given relief from the pain and is quieted down, particularly children with burned hands. Ice water immersion is very effective for this and not only gives relief from pain but helps to control subsequent edema. Immersion for 10 minutes or so will soothe the patient and allow careful scrutiny of the burned area. The examiner will want to know the history of the burn and will wish to assess the depth of burn with close attention to the appearance of the

wound. Often it is not possible to be sure of either the area or depth of burn, and when in doubt it is important to hospitalize the patient. Superficial burns causing only partial skin loss and leaving adequate elements for normal skin regeneration are called first degree burns (Fig. 14–18). These can be managed in the Emergency Room, though the patient may have to return for regular follow-up examination and dressing changes. A light layer of mafenide acetate (Sulfamylon) cream covered with a regular compressive hand dressing will allow comfort, healing and some motion of the fingers. Dressings should be changed every three or four days until healing is well under way.

Deeper burns which involve the dermis heal slowly by the formation of granulation tissue. Though such granulations will eventually reepithelialize, the quality of this skin is relatively poor and areas greater than one centimeter in diameter are best covered with split thickness skin grafts. Such grafts can be laid on the raw areas and then overlaid with petrolatum or Xeroform gauze from which most of the

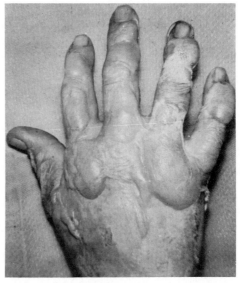

Figure 14–18 Superficial burn of the hand. The bullae are ominous in appearance but portend uneventful recovery with normal function.

grease has been scraped off. The gauze is then covered with the usual bulky dressing. Larger areas of dermal involvement (which some call second degree burns) should be treated on an inpatient basis, since more extensive grafting as well as daily attention to action motion of the fingers will be necessary.

Deep burns wherein all of the dermis is lost naturally require grafting usually preceded by débridement or escharotomy. Classically such a burned area is said to be anesthetic, but this is only relatively true and early classification of such a burn can be impossible. When in doubt, hospitalize. Electrical burns may appear at first to be small in area, but the apparent burn of the skin may only be the tip of the iceberg and extensive necrotizing damage may underlie it. Proper treatment cannot be planned until the extent of tissue damage is known.

CHEMICAL BURNS. Burns from caustic agents such as strong acids or alkalies are fairly common, and the immediate need is for removal or neutralization of the damaging agent. A copious amount of running water is the most effective means for this, but vinegar may be used to neutralize alkalies and chalk or lime water for acid burns. Solid phosphorus is more pernicious in that it is not easily washed free, although its oxidizing action will be halted by immersion of the hand in water. The phosphorus particles must be removed manually, and a 5 per cent solution of copper sulfate will neutralize any residual particles.

COLD INJURY. Frostbite, though common, is not benign as it represents local freezing of tissues. If extensive, permanent and irreversible damage results. Immediate warming by warm water immersion is the most effective first aid. Remember that frozen or near frozen tissues are damaged tissues and vulnerable to further injury, and thus the water should be warm (37° to 42° C), not hot. Pain may be intense with this type of injury and narcotics and sedatives may be necessary. The degree of damage may not be apparent for several or even many days, and it is often necessary to protect such hands with occlusive dressings. Sympathetic blocks are of little value in this type of injury.

Crush Injury

Crush injuries of the hand are often complex and may combine with fractures, joint damage, skin lacerations or tears, abrasions and injury to vascular structures, nerves and tendons. There is always an element of escape of extracellular fluid into the tissues. Formation of edema and its fixation in the tissues may cause more residual crippling than occurs from damage to any specific tissue or structure. Ice water immersion within an hour of injury will help considerably in preventing and controlling edema. This should be followed by immobilization of fractures, débridement of wounds and control or prevention of infection. A bulky compression dressing and constant elevation of the extremity are extremely important and may have to be continued for many days. The institution of active motion of the fingers within the dressing is also important to help prevent stiffening of joints.

Crush injuries can be deceptive, and the extent of damage may not be revealed until several days have elapsed. If any significant degree of crush has occurred, the patient should be hospitalized.

Wringer injuries of children are still fairly common and many are still mishandled. They may be superficial in degree or severe enough to compromise the entire extremity because of skin loss, severe swelling and the subsequent development of a Volkmann's ischemic contracture. The earlier the injured extremity is seen the more difficult it is to determine the severity of the crush. Even if there is only initial swelling, a few abrasions and moderate pain it is safer to assume the worst and to hospitalize the child, placing a firm compression dressing from fingertip to axilla and keeping the extremity elevated. The surgeon should be particularly attentive to any increasing complaints of pain. If there is obvious increasing swelling of severe proportions, prompt wide fasciotomy in the operating room may be required.

Foreign Bodies

Human beings are continually devising ingenious ways of introducing foreign objects through the skin of the hand. Wooden and bamboo slivers, pencil leads, pins and needles, broken knife points, steel filings and pieces of glass are commonplace. Bullets, often fragmented, shot pellets and the casings of detonating caps blown into the hand as the result of accident, altercation or experiment are also common. Most such objects should be removed, but this will depend on symptoms, size of the object and its location. Shotgun blast injuries at close range are devastating to a hand and a common mistake is to leave the felt or fiber shot shell wad in the depths of the hand because it is not apparent on x-ray films. Glass slivers of astounding size may be introduced through very small wounds. Most glass can be detected by careful scrutiny of x-rays. Children often sustain such injuries by a fall on the outstretched hand, introducing a sliver of broken glass into the palm in the region of the median nerve and its branches. After the bleeding has been stanched and the pain assuaged there may be no further symptoms. But careful palpation may elicit tenderness, indicating that a piece of glass which should be extracted is present in a dangerous area.

Removal of such foreign bodies in the Emergency Room is usually a practical course and can be done under local anesthesia and tourniquet ischemia when necessary. It is rarely necessary or advisable to close the incision.

The foreign body that has been deeply embedded for weeks or months before causing symptoms may not be as easy to locate or remove, and generally such removal should be done in the operating room. Foreign material long embedded may have caused the formation of an inclusion cyst or foreign body granuloma which will also have to be removed.

More important than the foreign body is the risk of infection it entails. After removal it is best to flush the wound thoroughly and to leave it wide open. Tetanus is an ever-present threat with any puncture or penetrating wound, and a booster dose is indicated for those previously immunized.

A barbed fishhook embedded in the finger should be cleansed with soap, the finger anesthetized, the hook passed through the finger, the point and barb clipped off, and the hook then backed out (see Fig. 4–6).

Fingertip Injuries and Amputations

These represent the most common type of hand injuries seen in the Emergency Room and the majority of them can be treated there. Power lawn mowers, automobile radiator fans, power saws, slicing machines and more mundane devices such as knives, handsaws and doors all take their toll of careless or inquisitive digits. As with most hand injuries the physician's goals are to relieve pain and to obtain healing with the best functional result, with appearance as nearly normal as possible. Unfortunately, it is not always possible to satisfy both the functional and cosmetic ideal. Female — and some male — patients frequently attribute more importance to the appearance of the hand than they will admit to and will therefore be unsatisfied with an excellent functional result if the appearance is unsightly. Despite some of our surgical pretensions, a cut off finger is a cut off finger, and both patient and physician must recognize that the state of the art is not yet such that the amputated part can be reimplanted and still consistently satisfy the criteria of use, appearance and comfort.

INJURIES TO THE FINGERNAIL AND NAILBED. Subungual hematomas, usually resulting from a misdirected hammer blow or a carelessly slammed car door, are painful, but prompt relief from pain is obtained by burning a hole through the nail directly over the accumulation of blood. This is simply done by straightening a paper clip and heating one end to a red hot temperature over a match or cigarette lighter. The hot end of the paper clip is touched to the nail and as the hematoma wells out, immediate relief from pain is obtained. This is a painless procedure but must be done before the hematoma has clotted.

Partially avulsed nails should be held in place as a temporary dressing by taping them in place with a Band-Aid. The loose nail will protect the underlying raw bed until it is sufficiently healed to require no protection. This takes two to three weeks, after which the nail generally is quite loose and can be easily removed. Often the base of the nail is avulsed, leaving one or both sides intact. In such a case the border of the avulsed portion should be trimmed and the nail then held in place with a Band-Aid. The base of the nail should not be forced back under the skin or infection may result.

When the nail has been completely avulsed, the bed should be protected by light petrolatum gauze and a dry dressing for about three weeks. Displaced or raised portions of the nailbed should be sutured in place to avoid distortions of the new nail.

If portions of the nailbed have been lost due to slicing or grinding injuries, the lost portion should be replaced by split thickness skin graft, but only after the denuded area has been fully debrided, gently scrubbed and irrigated. The graft should be a thin one and should be sutured in place leaving the ends of the sutures long so that they

may be tied over fine mesh gauze and several thicknesses of surgical sponge. If this stent dressing is then covered with Tubegauz, the finger can be returned to use promptly and the dressing cut free at the end of two weeks.

INJURY TO THE VOLAR PAD. Most injuries to the volar aspect of the fingertip are caused by lacerating or grinding agents. If reasonably clean or if further surgical cleaning can be done, they may be closed primarily by replacing flaps with sutures or Steri-Strips; if flaps are absent skin grafts may be used instead. Often such wounds have grease and dirt ground into them and cannot be cleaned satisfactorily. Such wounds should be fully and vigorously cleaned, but not closed. Closure or grafting can be done with more success and fewer complications a few days or even a week or two later. The concept of delayed primary closure is a sound one here and Iselin[4] refers to this as the "delayed emergency."

In those cases where skin has been lost it is often difficult to know if replacement is necessary. It will depend on the digit involved and the width or diameter and the location of the lost skin. Divots or strips of skin loss of approximately one centimeter or less in adult fingers will close satisfactorily by secondary intention. Pieces larger than this should be replaced by split thickness skin grafts, Wolfe grafts (see Fig. 14–21), or occasionally by cross finger flaps. If the loss is from the volar pulp of the thumb or index finger or in a child, the loss acceptable without grafting is smaller. Much larger areas of loss will of course heal but may result in hard, irregular or painful volar pads with some distortion or narrowing of the fingertip.

AMPUTATIONS. The basic rule in the Emergency Room is to save all viable tissue, but this may occasionally need modification. The Emergency Room is not the place for reconstructive surgery of the hand, but prompt action and good judgment here may often make any future reconstructive surgery unnecessary. This is often true in finger amputations because a good job by the first physician may often be the only surgical procedure needed. With any finger amputation the surgeon must satisfy two requirements: to preserve all length possible and to produce a functional digit. Function must take precedence over length unless cosmesis is more important to the patient than use, and it may thus be necessary to shorten the finger to make it more functional. Even more drastic is the injury requiring complete removal of a viable but useless finger in favor of obtaining better overall hand function (see Ring Injuries). Careful judgment is required and sometimes a compromise between the two requirements is necessary, but generally a short nontender finger with good sensation is better than a longer finger whose end is painful or numb. The patient's occupational requirement for the finger (or fingers) may well dictate the proper course.

The thumb is the most important digit for prehension, and preservation of length is most important. Nevertheless, comfort and sensation must also be considered and sometimes shortening is in order. The index finger is next in importance but will function fairly well if a functional portion of the middle segment is preserved. Such an index finger has a suitable key or lateral pinch, but the patient will substitute the middle finger for tip to tip pinch.

There is a distinction between complete and partial amputation (Fig. 14–19). Complete amputation means absolute severance, and reimplantation of severed fingers is still beyond the capabilities of the average surgeon, though many patients request that the severed member be "sewn back on." If the talent, facilities and indications all make the operation feasible, it is, of course, a task for the operating room. In partial amputation, there is some soft tissue connection; this is of value only when at least one neurovascular bundle is intact and in such cases careful fixation after cleansing is indicated. The more

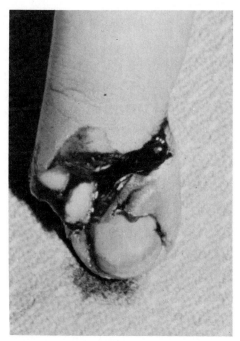

Figure 14–19 Incomplete amputation with comminuted fracture of distal phalanx. Replaced and held in place with a K-wire: no sutures. Excellent result.

distal a partial amputation and the younger the patient, the better the chance for survival. In questionable cases the decision should not be made in the Emergency Room; if only one or sometimes two fingers are involved, the repair should be done. If not successful, definitive amputation may be done later in the operating room. In any event, all attempts should be made to preserve the partially amputated finger, though the patient may have to be warned that survival of the finger is in doubt.

Closure of amputation stumps is obtained either by utilization of skin remaining on the stump or by skin graft or transfer. Skin flaps left by the wound should be utilized for closure after proper cleansing and removal of fat (Fig. 14–20). If the flap is too short to cover the stump, the phalanx may be shortened slightly, but if shortening is not desirable a combination of flap and graft can be used. Local sliding flaps

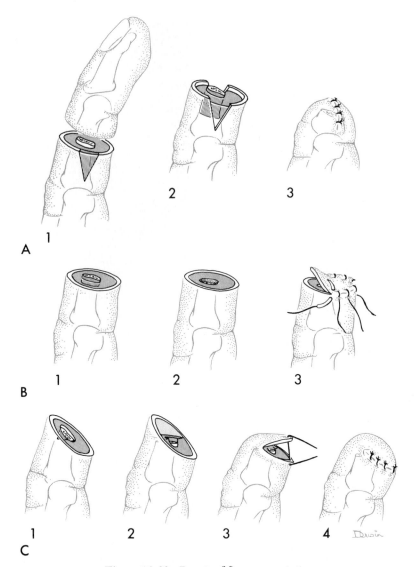

A 1   2   3

B 1   2   3

C 1   2   3   4

Figure 14–20   Repair of finger amputations.

should be used only by those experienced in their use — they are not generally a suitable method for the Emergency Room. The same is true for pedicle skin transfers, e.g., cross finger, thenar, palmar or thoracoabdominal flaps. These can be used by experts but others may find their disadvantages and complications will be more apparent than their advantages.

If skin must be transferred in the Emergency Room it should be in the form of a free graft and here there is a choice of split thickness or a thin full thickness (Wolfe) skin graft. The technique for these grafts is described in the following section and either of them is useful in closing amputations in the Emergency Room.

Split grafts grow or "take" more readily than full thickness grafts, but the latter result in tougher and more satisfactory coverage. Wolfe grafts are particularly suitable in children but their incidence of survival decreases with increasing age of the patient. Either type of graft should be sutured to the stump end under slight tension with interrupted 5–0 synthetic suture. It is best not to lay them directly on bone and therefore it may be necessary to nibble away enough of the exposed phalanx so that it lies 2 or 3 millimeters below the surrounding soft tissues. Three or four of the sutures should be left long enough to tie over several layers of gauze, forming a stent dressing. Tubegauz over this completes the dressing, which should be removed on day four or five and then replaced for about another week. If injuries to the hand are more extensive than a single finger amputation, a complete compression dressing and elevation of the extremity is required. Multiple amputations and mangled fingers are situations requiring a longer anesthesia and tourniquet time and better surgical conditions than are available in the Emergency Room.

Skin Loss

Loss of skin substance greater than approximately 1 square centimeter generally requires replacement by graft or transfer. This loss is not to be confused with wounds that are gaping but from which no skin has been removed; these will generally close very satisfactorily by suture, by tape or by spontaneous healing. Avulsions of skin are most common on the dorsum of the hand or fingers and can be replaced by split grafts after adequate cleansing. If in doubt about the degree of contamination or the adequacy of débridement, it is far safer to apply a dressing to the wound and to supply skin coverage as a secondary procedure some days later.

Split thickness skin grafts are most satisfactorily obtained with a dermatome, but since these are seldom available in the Emergency Room, grafts no larger than a postage stamp can be taken with a razor blade. The most convenient donor site is the proximal volar aspect of the forearm. The upper anterolateral thigh surface would serve even better, because the donor scar would be seen less frequently. For a graft 2 centimeters square a donor area of approximately 4 centimeters square should be anesthetized using subcutaneous infiltration of approximately 10 cc of 1 per cent aqueous lidocaine introduced with a 2 inch No. 22 needle. It would benefit both surgeon and patient to wait ten minutes after infiltration before cutting the graft, for this should be a painless procedure for both. The aim is to cut as uniform a graft as possible holding the razor blade almost parallel with the skin. The best thickness is 0.014 inch, but such a freehand graft will be quite irregular in both shape and thickness. The donor area of a graft this thick will show multiple punctate bleeding points and no fat. The graft should be transferred immediately to the recipient site and either sutured or taped in place with Steri-Strips. The donor site is covered with a single layer of fine mesh gauze and nothing more. The oozing blood will quickly clot and the patient should allow this gauze to fall off when it is ready to do so — generally in about ten days.

A simple technique is the use of a thin full thickness or Wolfe graft. Though the rate of take of this type of graft is somewhat less than that of split thickness grafts, it is preferable for areas requiring tougher skin, such as palmar surfaces and fingertips. Suitable donor areas are the volar aspect of the upper forearm, the antecubital region and the inguinal crease. The principle is to excise the graft as an ellipse after infiltration with the lidocaine and then to close the donor site as a straight line. After outlining the graft by a full thickness incision one tip of the ellipse is retracted with a skin hook and the graft reflected under constant tension; a scalpel is used to cleanly separate the graft from the underlying fat (Fig. 14–21). No fat should remain on the graft. As such grafts tend to curl up they are best sutured in place as with split thickness grafts. On examination after 10 to 12

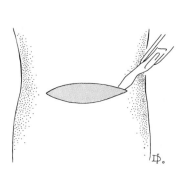

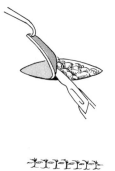

Figure 14–21   The Wolfe or thin full thickness skin graft.

days such a graft looks terrible, but after another week or two the blackened outer layers will peel off leaving good full thickness skin behind. The graft should be kept dressed until this healing has occurred.

The principal causes of skin graft loss are infection and hematoma. Infection is best prevented by very thorough débridement and irrigation of the recipient site and by a thorough surgical scrub of the donor site as well as careful aseptic technique. Hematoma is avoided by laying the graft on a surface which has ceased to bleed and by maintaining gentle but constant pressure on the graft with a proper dressing. Expressing any delayed hematoma formation from under the graft at three or four days will also help.

Tendon Injury

FLEXOR TENDONS. Hands with wounds on the volar aspect should be carefully examined for flexor tendon injury. Such injuries are easy to miss if the physician does not specifically watch for them. Sometimes the wound will gape enough to show severed ends of tendons, but frequently what appears to be a severed tendon is a portion of flexor pulley ligament or palmar fascia, and just as frequently a completely severed tendon will be retracted from the wound and not be apparent. The resting position of the hand and fingers is the best guide, especially in young children. A digit with lacerated flexors will demonstrate "hang out" as shown in Figures 14–22 and 14–23. Intact tendons can be checked by having the patient demonstrate functional flexor digitorum profundus by flexing the distal joint of each finger. The flexor digitorum sublimis is checked by the examiner by holding three fingers in full extension and having the patient actively flex the middle joint of the remaining finger. The flexor pollicis longus is checked by demonstrating active IP flexion of the thumb. Wrist flexors are easily demonstrated and palpated by active flexion of the wrist, as is the palmaris longus.[1]

The purpose of this examination is to inform the patient of the damage done so that arrangements can be made for

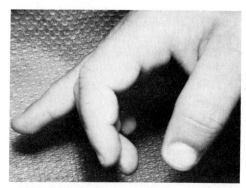

Figure 14–22   "Hangout" due to severed flexor digitorum profundus and sublimus in the middle finger of a child. This position is diagnostic and represents an alteration of the normal stance or position of the rest of the hand.

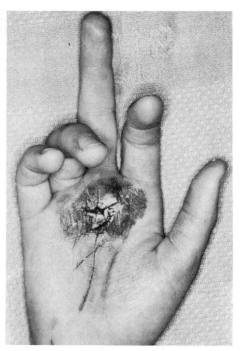

Figure 14–23 Same situation (in an adult) as in Figure 14–22. The palmar wound requires débridement, irrigation and no closure.

flexor tendon repair or grafting in the operating room when the wound is healed. Flexor tendons should not be repaired in the Emergency Room: unfortunately, many are and with uniformly poor results. Flexor tendon repair, either by direct anastomosis or free tendon graft or transfer, requires an experienced surgeon, the best of operating room environments and a sterile field. A transverse laceration of the volar aspect of the wrist may seem to invite primary repair of the underlying severed tendons in the Emergency Room. The temptation should be resisted, thereby avoiding the common complications of suturing the median nerve to severed palmaris or sublimis tendon, suturing tendons together with heavy silk, secondary wound breakdown, extra scar formation and a complete tenodesis of all the flexors to the digits.

EXTENSOR TENDONS. Though it is commonly recognized that primary flexor tendon repairs give poor results, many feel that repairs of extensor tendons are a much simpler matter. This is true for a few specific types and locations of injury, but most of the difficulties encountered in extensor tendon repair and the complications therefrom are so great that the Emergency Room is not the place for them. As with flexors, careful examination is imperative. The patient should demonstrate independent active extension of each of the MP joints and each of the IP joints. The extensor mechanism of the fingers is far more complex than the flexor: MP extension is by action of the extensor digitorum communis for the four fingers, plus the extensor indicis proprius for the index finger and the extensor digitiquinti for the small finger. The thumb MP joint is extended by the extensor pollicis brevis with an assist from the extensor pollicis longus. The thumb IP joint is extended by the extensor pollicis longus. The PIP joints of the fingers are extended mostly by the intrinsics — the interossei and lumbricals — but with an important contribution from the central slip of the extensor digitorum communis. Repairs of the extremely complex extensor mechanism over the dorsum of the fingers are difficult, and failures are more common than successes; they should be done under the best possible circumstances through a healed wound and in the operating room. With such injuries the proper approach is to thoroughly clean the wound, close it only if relatively clean and then splint the finger and wrist in full extension (i.e., 0 degrees) until wound healing is complete and definitive extensor tendon repair can be carried out.

Lacerations of the extensor hood overlying the MP joint may be repaired if the wound lends itself to primary closure. This very definitely does not include wounds inflicted by human teeth (see later discussion). End-to-end suture with 4–0 to 5–0 wire or synthetic suture can be done and the finger splinted in full extension for four weeks before active motion is allowed. The

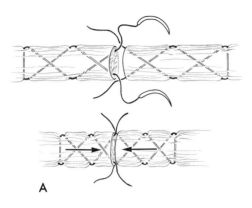

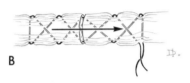

A

B

Figure 14-24 Tendon suture. A. Simpler method (preferred) — the two knots are buried at the anastomotic line. B. Classical Bunnell method — technique more difficult and with little real advantage over the simpler method.

single buried suture of Bunnell which is widely illustrated and looks very well in drawings is not so easy to use unless one has had considerable experience with it. A simpler technique is illustrated in which two sutures and therefore two knots are used. If the anastomosis is lightly rolled between the fingers the knots will disappear into

the anastomotic line and will cause no trouble (Fig. 14-24). With this type of suture the two ends of the tendon can be pulled tightly together with less likelihood of the surgeon breaking the suture and having to rethread it through the tendon, thereby further mangling the tendon ends.

Extensor tendons transected on the dorsum of the hand may be similarly repaired, but only if the wound lends itself to primary closure, and only if both tendon ends are readily accessible without extending the wound. Following such repair the usual bulky dressing is applied and the finger and wrist are to be immobilized at 0 degrees — i.e., in a straight line — with a short arm volar plaster splint extending to the finger tips for four weeks.

INCIPIENT BOUTONNIERE DEFORMITY. This deformity, a flexion contracture of the PIP joint with hyperextension of the DIP joint, is difficult and often impossible to correct once it has occurred (Fig. 14-25). Prevention is needed, requiring early recognition and treatment. The cause is severance of the central extensor slip over the PIP joint. Such an injury is not very impressive when first seen: usually there is a wound over the PIP joint and an inability to extend this joint actively for the last 20 to 30 degrees, though the joint will have full passive range of motion. Occasionally the wound on the

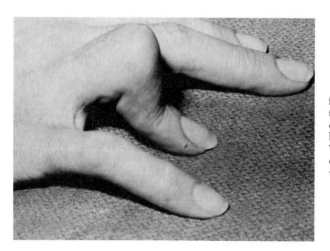

Figure 14-25 Boutonniere deformity. Late result of a rupture of the central slip of the extensor digitorum communis which was missed by the first examining physician. The finger was untreated and the deformity assumed this degree within three months.

dorsum of the joint will be in the form of a contusion and there will be no break in the skin. Caution is necessary here, for if the central slip is ruptured and the joint is allowed to assume a flexed position, the lateral bands of the extensor mechanism may migrate volarward, starting an insidious chain of events leading to the boutonniere deformity. Primary repair of the central slip is a job for the expert and should not be done in the Emergency Room. It is advisable to treat the wound only and to splint the finger and wrist at 0 degrees with a volar plaster splint for three to four weeks. If the splinting has been constant, satisfactory healing of the central slip will occur in many such cases. If the patient cannot extend the PIP joint fully after removal of the splint, it should be recognized that the tendon has healed with some lengthening, and surgical repair is indicated.

MALLET FINGER. Mallet or baseball finger is incurred by avulsion of the insertion of the extensor mechanism at the base of the distal phalanx or by severance of this tendon over the DIP joint. Frequently a fragment of bone will be pulled off the phalanx by the tendon. It is the most common tendon injury and is usually incurred by striking the end of the extended finger and forcing it into flexion against the resisting extensor mechanism. Following this the DIP joint lacks 20 degrees or more of active extension, though full passive extension is possible. It has been widely publicized that treatment must consist of immobilization of the PIP joint in flexion and the DIP joint in hyperextension, and many elaborate splints and modes of internal fixation have been devised for this. They are difficult to apply and more difficult to maintain and are really not necessary at all. If the injury is treated promptly — preferably within a few days of occurrence — by splinting the DIP joint in 5 to 10 degrees of hyperextension, the result will be good, and the patient will be far more comfortable than with more complicated splinting. Three methods

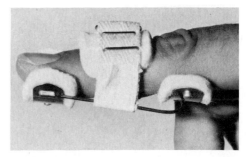

Figure 14–26 The safety-pin splint for mallet finger. When the central band is tightened, the DIP joint will be forced gently into slight hyperextension.

are available. The most satisfactory is a so-called safety-pin splint which is available as a stock item from most surgical supply houses (Fig. 14–26). This is a dynamic splint which, properly worn, applies a constant extension force to the DIP joint. It is imperative that it be worn constantly and without exception for a four week period. The patient must have this explained to him and he must cooperate if it is to work. The patient is also given an aluminum "ski tip" splint which he can substitute for the dynamic splint once or twice a day in order to wash his hands (Fig. 14–27). The patient must be cautioned against flexing the joint while changing splints. A second method is to use only the ski tip splint for the full four weeks. This does not give quite as good a result as the safety-pin splint, as it may leave

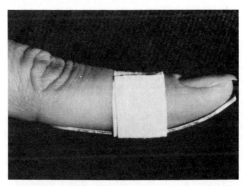

Figure 14–27 The aluminum ski tip splint for mallet finger.

the DIP joint with a deficit of 10 to 15 degrees of full extension. This deficit is somewhat unsightly but not significantly disabling. The ski tip splint, however, is much simpler and more convenient for the patient to maintain. The third method, which is suitable for children or patients who are unable to cooperate with splinting, is to drill a Kirschner wire the length of the distal phalanx and across the DIP joint while holding that joint in hyperextension. In placing the K-wire remember that the tuft of the phalanx lies directly beneath the nail and the wire should therefore enter the fingertip about 3 millimeters volar to the nail and not through the volar pad. The tip of the wire may be left protruding, covered with a Band-Aid and left in place for four weeks.

Nerve Injury

It is important to recognize nerve injuries in the Emergency Room, but they should be repaired in the operating room. Prompt recognition is important in planning treatment and in advising the patient on aftercare, and it has obvious medico-legal significance. Both motor and sensory examinations must be done before anesthetizing the extremity or any part of it. Obvious perhaps, but a common mistake is to wish one had checked fingertip sensation before the digital block had been done. An elaborate examination is not necessary: gross touch and pin-prick sensations are quickly checked and even in young children the latter should give some idea as to the presence or absence of sensation without the necessity of drawing blood with the examining pin.

It is far more accurate to ascertain the presence of two-point discrimination with a paper clip that has been straightened out and then bent into a horseshoe shape with the two ends approximately 1 centimeter apart. The patient who can tell (without looking) that he is being touched simultaneously with the two

points definitely has an intact nerve supply for that area.

Radial nerve sensation is of little importance, though easily checked over the dorsum of the hand and proximal segments of the thumb, index and middle fingers. Ulnar sensation should be looked for over the hypothenar eminence, the dorsum of the fifth metacarpal, the dorsal and volar aspects of the small finger, and the ulnar half of the ring finger. Not infrequently the ulnar nerve supplies sensation to all of the ring finger and the adjacent half of the middle finger. The median nerve supplies the rest: the volar aspect of the thumb, index and middle fingers and radial side of the ring finger, as well as the dorsum of the middle and distal segments of these digits.

Transection or damage to the median nerve will result in a thenar palsy with loss of opposition of the thumb. If the thenar eminences of both hands are palpated simultaneously and the patient is directed to abduct and oppose his thumbs the deficit on the injured side is readily apparent. Stab wounds of the proximal palm may transect the median recurrent (motor) branch, leaving the sensory digital branches intact.

Transection of the ulnar nerve gives a motor deficit which is easy to detect. Palpation of the first dorsal interosseous muscle while the patient is attempting to abduct the index finger, or asking the patient to abduct the small finger or to flex the small finger MP joint without bending the PIP or DIP joints will demonstrate paralysis of ulnar innervated intrinsic muscles. A stab wound in the palm may transect the deep ulnar or motor branch, leaving ulnar sensation intact.

In the case of an extremely clean, sharply incised wound occurring within the past hour or so, a primary neurorrhaphy may be indicated, but it should be done in the operating room by a trained and experienced team with proper instruments. In such a case it is the function of the Emergency Room to pave the way for the prompt transition to the operating room. Repair of the ulnar motor trunk or the median recurrent branch is feasible in the operating room. Severed digital nerves of the fingers and common digital nerves of the palm also lend themselves to successful repair when the repair is meticulously done under ideal circumstances, none of which exist in the Emergency Room. In dealing with the wound in the Emergency Room, there is nothing to be gained by the placement of marking or stay sutures in the nerve ends.

Arterial Injury

As with nerve injuries, the role of the Emergency Room is to recognize the injury and to initiate treatment. Transection of both radial and ulnar arteries may or may not cause a bloodless hand. Such an injury should certainly be suspected with a wrist laceration presenting with a blanched, cold hand even though there is little bleeding from the wound, as severed arteries are quick to close up and seldom present in the Emergency Room spouting blood. Such a situation requires a prompt end-to-end arterial anastomosis but it is rare that an Emergency Room will be adequately equipped or manned for such a procedure. If either artery is intact and the other severed, all that need be done is to ligate both ends of the severed artery and the other artery will more than suffice to supply the hand with blood. The same is true for digital arteries; one will do for a finger, but if both are transected the digit will be lost unless prompt repair of one or both is possible.

Intra-arterial injection of drugs such as barbiturates and others may cause complete arterial occlusion and destruction. The resulting avascularity plus the rapidly progressive edema are often severe enough to threaten the fate of the entire hand or any of its parts. The history is important in establishing the diagnosis but it is often not obtainable. Pain is very severe. Prompt surgical action in the form of wide fasciotomy is imperative if such a hand is to be salvaged. Here the primary role of the Emergency Room is to make the diagnosis and to expedite prompt treatment for the patient in the operating room. Suspicion of arterial injection of a drug is warranted in the patient presenting a white, tense, extremely painful hand without evidence of external injury.

The Mangled Hand

Industrial and farm accidents cause most of these, though automobiles, home power tools and shotguns make their contribution. The Emergency Room cannot deliver definitive treatment in most such cases, but it can play an absolutely essential role in setting the stage for and expediting such treatment. Assessment of the degree of injury, obtaining x-rays, cutting the red tape employed by hospital administrators, starting initial débridement, starting fluids, controlling shock and premedicating the patient will all serve to get the patient more quickly to the operating theater where complete débridement and repair can be undertaken. The golden period, though an old concept, is not an old-fashioned one, and it states simply that the more time elapsed from injury until proper treatment of the wound, the poorer the prognosis for uneventful healing of that wound.

Degloving and Ring Injuries

Circumferential degloving of a digit is typically incurred by the patient jumping off a truck or platform as the ring on the involved finger catches on an immovable object. The skin is circumcised at the level of the ring and stripped distally by the ring. Usually there is no fracture or dislocation and the extensor and flexor mechanisms are intact, and often the volar digital nerves and arteries as well. After cleansing the denuded digit and the reversed skin, the skin is peeled back onto the finger and the wound will then appear rather innocuous. Despite its good appearance, such a finger is usually fated to extreme functional loss because the subcutaneous veins and lymphatics have been disrupted and may be impossible to repair: during the ensuing days the finger becomes markedly swollen, painful and often gangrenous. When first seen in the Emergency Room it is best to warn the patient that he will probably end up with a useless, stiff or painful finger even if the finger does survive. Nevertheless, it is best to attempt to salvage it, and to debride or amputate later on when it is quite apparent to the patient that the finger is a detriment to overall hand function. After proper cleansing and thorough irrigation the skin edges should be approximated loosely with five or six sutures and a complete hand compression dressing applied, followed by continuous elevation for several days. If a microsurgical team is available, repair of the transsected vessels may save the finger.

Degloving of the dorsum of the hand usually results from the hand being jerked out of rollers or similar farm or industrial machines, creating a distally based flap of skin. Circulation to such a flap is often precarious, particularly as regards the venous and lymphatic drainage. Unless it is obvious that vascularity of such a flap is impaired, it should be debrided and lightly sutured in place as above. The patient should be advised that redébridement and possibly skin grafting may be necessary.

Grease and Paint Gun Injuries

Paint or lubricants forcibly injected into a finger from a pressure gun may dissect throughout the finger and hand and even up into the forearm. Such an injury may seem relatively benign for a few hours after the injection, but soon swelling, pain and stiffness become noticeable. Such injuries are surgical emergencies requiring detailed and prolonged dissection and débridement in the operating room under long-acting anesthesia. There are no effective first aid measures, and hot soaks are damaging: the only useful function of the Emergency Room in such an injury is to speed the patient to the operating room for proper and adequate débridement.

A similar injury may be caused by air or gas pressure guns, and the treatment for these is the same. Often the air or gas is a vehicle for abrasives or other foreign material which is forced throughout the tissues of the hand. Since the hand must be opened widely, such injuries carry a high infection risk.

Bites

A bite by human or animal teeth causes bruising and crushing of the skin and underlying tissue as well as laceration. It is an exceedingly dirty and potentially dangerous wound. The treatment consists of meticulous cleansing with soap under excision of any questionably viable tissue. Such wounds should very definitely not be sutured. Penicillin in heavy doses should be given until it is obvious that infection has not occurred. The open wound should be covered with light petrolatum fine mesh gauze and a dry dressing. Bites from animals of any species pose a risk of rabies, and it is important where possible to impound the animal that inflicted the bite. If there is the slightest possibility that the animal was rabid, immunization of the patient should be started despite the possible complications from this procedure.

Carnivores, particularly cats, carry virulent strains of pasteurella which cause nasty, indolent infections, and these are usually inoculated deep into the tissue of the hand bitten by these animals. Prompt treatment as outlined above followed by antibiotics will decrease the chances of such infection. Human bites are the most common and the most troublesome of all. They are most commonly incurred in fist fights in which the extensor surface of the MP joint is lacerated on the opponent's incisors. Contamination of the MP joint is common, and it is not rare to have such a joint or its extensor mechanism destroyed by the ensuing infection. Closing such a wound may endanger not only the joint but the entire hand or extremity. If the extensor tendon or hood has been severed, it should not be repaired and this should be left for a later procedure after the wound has healed. If the wound is presented several days after the bite, an infection, manifested by pain, erythema, induration and sometimes pus, is already present. The involved area must be widely opened, debrided and left open. Massive doses of an appropriate antibiotic should be used as well as a complete hand dressing, elevation and hospitalization. Such an infection is a serious matter and procrastination or halfway measures will cause serious complications.

Gunshot and High Explosive Wounds

The severity of these wounds depends on the type of structures damaged, the extensiveness of damage and the degree of contamination within the wounds. These factors in turn are dependent on the velocity and mass of the missile, the intensity of the blast and the environment of the hand when wounded. A knowledge of wound ballistics is helpful but not essential if a few basic concepts are understood. The greater the velocity of the missile and the greater its mass, the more energy will be expended in stopping its flight and the greater the mass of tissue that will be changed by the absorption of that energy. The role of the Emergency

Room physician is first to get the facts concerning the injury: the weapon or wounding agent, its caliber and load, the distance of the hand from the weapon, the time of the accident, whether gloves were being worn and what treatment has already been administered. The next task is an assessment of damage. A short but careful examination of the hand, including an x-ray film, should tell if the wound can be handled in the Emergency Room or must go to the operating room for more extensive treatment. In either case the same fundamentals apply: adequate débridement, copious irrigation, nonclosure of the wounds and a proper hand dressing and splinting followed by elevation and antibiotics and a tetanus booster.

Wounds inflicted by pistols of most calibers and by .22 caliber rifles are classified as low velocity wounds, and damage incurred by them is usually confined to the missile track. The wounds of entrance and exit should be debrided of any damaged tissue and the missile track irrigated generously. A roentgenogram may show that the bullet has fragmented within the hand, and it is usually best to leave these fragments undisturbed unless it is apparent that they are lodged against a vital structure, within a joint or are subcutaneous. Any bullet, particularly those of the larger caliber pistols, may cause a markedly comminuted fracture of a phalanx or metacarpal and occasionally of several bones. The bone fragments should never be removed even if completely detached from soft tissue and blood supply, as they will almost always be incorporated as part of the healing fracture and their removal may result in a serious deficit of bone. The size of the bullet is not a good criterion for the degree of damage: a .45 caliber pistol bullet is a very large missile, but it is quite possible for it to pass through a palm or even a finger with surprisingly little damage.

Far more important than size is the velocity of the bullet. The bullets from most high-powered sporting and military rifles are definitely high velocity. Even though they may pass completely through the hand with little apparent destruction, the energy they expend in the hand is transmitted throughout the entire extremity and may cause great damage a good distance from the missile track. This energy is dissipated in violent shock waves throughout the hand and may cause fractures, nerve damage and other injuries several centimeters away from the primary wound. Even if no specific structures seem to be harmed, the general disruption of the hand occurring in a few milliseconds may cause extensive edema and microhemorrhage which can permanently cripple the hand. Most such wounds require extensive débridement and intricate internal stabilization of fractures, and this, of course, should be done in the operating room. The complications and bad results obtained through inadequate débridement and by primary closure of such wounds are innumerable.

Shotgun blasts of the hand vary considerably, depending on the shot load and particularly the distance of the hand from the muzzle. Unfortunately, most such injuries are incurred with the hand directly against the muzzle and the damage sustained may be tremendous. It is not unusual to have several digits or even an entire hand carried away by such a blast. Not only is the force great at close range, but the mass of the shot pellets, wads and burning powder all contribute to blowing a large hole through the hand. Often such hands are gloved and bits of wool, leather and other contaminants are thus distributed throughout the wound. Though plastic wads are supplementing them, wads composed of animal and vegetable fiber and cardboard are still used in many shot shells and are serious sources of tissue destruction and contamination. These are particularly pernicious as they are usually not seen in a roentgenogram and may be easily missed in debriding the wound. The shot pellets themselves are of little consequence and need not be sought unless they are in a joint.

Explosive wounds of the hand in civilians are caused by detonating caps, dynamite, blasting powder, firecrackers, fireworks and (more *au courant*) tear gas grenades and homemade bombs. Even relatively small charges such as firecrackers may cause extensive wounding if the charge is enclosed within a container or within the grasping hand. Skin loss, multiple lacerations, fractures, amputations and extensive contamination by embedding of foreign material within the hand are seen with these wounds. The débridement and the recognition of salvageable tissue is a complex task and one for the operating room in most cases. Often there are burns associated with these injuries, and phosphorus and other powerful oxidizing agents from fireworks may be embedded in and under the skin.

It bears repeating that no wounds in the above categories should be closed. Delayed primary closure is feasible with many, and the advantages to this are that examination of the wound three or four days after injury offers the opportunity for a second débridement if the first has not proved extensive enough. Many of these wounds are closed secondarily, and in many cases the skin grafts and pedicle flaps are necessary.

INFECTION

Most serious infections of the hand start from small beginnings, and bad results stem from treatment that is inadequate or that is started too late. Prevention is best, of course, but once infection has started sharp observation and appropriate early treatment can prevent a progression of the infection into a crippling or loss of the digit or hand. Staphylococci are the most common causative agents, and antibiotics are far less useful than are prompt surgical measures.

Extent of nail removed

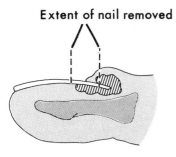

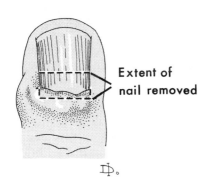

Extent of nail removed

Figure 14–28 Subungual abscess.

Paronychias

Paronychias are infections around the nail. Early in their development swelling, redness and pain occur at the side or the base of the nail. At this stage the infection may often be resolved by warm compresses, but if it has progressed to the point where pus has accumulated around the edge of the nail, the accumulation should be incised with a scalpel passed between the cuticle and the nail. If the infection has progressed to form a subungual abscess, pus will be apparent under the base of the nail, and the proximal half of the nail should be excised. Under digital nerve block the nail is transected

distal to the accumulation of pus and the proximal portion of the nail avulsed from its bed. The distal portion of the nail is left in place and the raw bed covered with petrolatum gauze and a small dressing (Fig. 14–28). A Band-Aid will suffice for the dressing and should be changed daily for about a week.

Felon

A felon is an infection in the volar pad of a digit which has progressed to abscess formation within the pulp space. Traversing this space are vertical septa running from the periosteum of the volar surface of the distal phalanx to the skin of the volar pad. Increasing pressure within these confined spaces causes severe pain, osteitis and sometimes necrosis of the phalanx. Once recognized, the proper treatment is surgical drainage and the goal is to cut through all the vertical septa and to allow free drainage of the entire pulp area. After digital nerve block a straight incision lateral to the nail may do the job, but it is often inadequately made and is therefore not recommended. It is better to extend this lateral incision hockey stick fashion around to the tip of the finger (Fig. 14–29). This distal portion should fall 3 or 4 millimeters volar to the nail bed and should not dip down into the volar skin which forms the tactile pad. Such an extension may result in a painful scar. After the incision is made the knife blade should be passed across the finger, breaking down all of the vertical septa. Pus and areas of necrotic pulp are removed and the wound lightly packed open with a wick of petrolatum gauze. This wick should not be

Figure 14–29 Incision for felon.

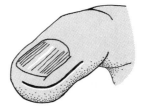

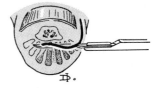

packed tightly into the wound. A fluffed dressing of the digit and hand is applied and the patient instructed to keep the hand higher than the head. Two days later the dressing should be changed and the gauze wick removed if the induration and erythema are markedly improved. If there is still some swelling and redness, leave the wick in for another two days. It is not necessary to close the incision and it will heal very well by itself as infection subsides.

With severe or neglected felons when the entire terminal digit is inflamed and swollen, a fishmouth incision which extends the above incision around to the other side of the finger is in order. This has been condemned by some, but if care is taken not to run the incision down onto the volar surface of the finger, the healed wound will be innocuous. After the incision has been made and the vertical septa transected, the end of the finger should gape open. No attempt should be made to close it, but a folded strip of Xeroform or petrolatum gauze can simply be laid in the wound and treatment proceeds as above.

Tenosynovitis

Infections of the flexor tendon sheaths of a digit usually start from a small puncture wound, but frequently this will be so small and obscure that the point of origin of the infection cannot be detected. These are dangerous infections and prompt recognition and treatment are necessary if a functional digit (or hand) is to be preserved. In a case that presents early, the patient has a painful finger which may be only slightly swollen but which feels tense to palpation. The finger is held slightly flexed, and active flexion of the digit by the patient causes pain along the flexor aspect. Passive straightening of the finger is even more painful. Many such cases will respond to appropriate antibiotics, bedrest, constant elevation of

the extremity and a warm, moist, bulky dressing. If, despite these measures, pain, swelling and redness increase and the pain progresses into the palm or wrist, the finger and flexor sheath should be opened through a midlateral incision along the so-called neutral line (Fig. 14–30). This incision should extend the length of the proximal and middle segments of the digit and should be left open, since it will heal spontaneously as the infection subsides. Pus in the sheath may or may not be encountered; if it is extensive, the sheath should also be opened in the palm and free drainage established. Whether to open the finger or to treat conservatively may be a difficult decision, but in the face of a worsening situation it is better not to procrastinate. An unnecessary incision is better than a finger that has lost function owing to sloughed or scarred flexor tendons.

Fascial Space Infections

Several potential fascial spaces exist in the hand. Any of them may be infected and become distended with pus. The treatment for all is prompt and adequate surgical drainage followed by treatment as described for tenosynovitis. The *middle palmar space* is most commonly infected. It lies dorsal to the flexor tendons and extends from the carpal tunnel to the distal palm and from the line of the third metacarpal to the hypothenar eminence. In opening this space care must be taken to protect the digital nerves and arteries as well as the flexor tendons and lumbrical muscles. *Thenar space infections* are characterized by marked swelling of the cleft between the first and second metacarpals. Drainage is best obtained through a transverse incision on the dorsum of the distal portion of the thumb web. The *hypothenar space* represents the third palmar space. This is rarely infected, but when it is it points dorsally. The *dorsal subcutaneous space* lies between the skin and the

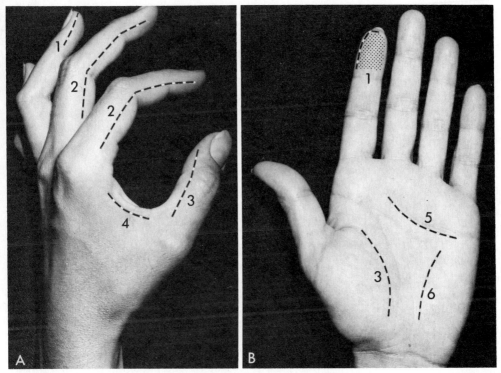

Figure 14–30 *A, B.* Incisions in the hand for drainage of infection.

1. Felon. This incision falls 3 or 4 millimeters volar to the tip of the nail. The dotted area represents the vertical fascial septa that must be transected by the knife blade. In severe cases this incision may be carried around to the opposite side of the finger forming the "fishmouth" incision.

2. Purulent tenosynovitis. This incision falls in the "neutral" line dorsal to the digital nerve and artery. The "neutral line" intersects the most dorsal portion of the flexion creases of the interphalangeal joints, which are easily determined by acutely flexing the finger.

3. Tenosynovitis of the thumb. The neutral line of the thumb is utilized in most cases, but in severe cases the ulnar border of the thenar eminence may also be opened.

4. Thenar space infection. A curved transverse incision through the dorsum of the thumb web allows direct access to the thenar space.

5. Middle palmar space infection. This incision is made 1 or 2 millimeters proximal to the distal palmar crease and extends from the third to the fifth metacarpal.

6. Hypothenar space infection. The ulnar bursa is approached through an incision on the radial side of the hypothenar eminence.

extensor tendons; it is rich in lymphatics and may become very swollen owing to infection in the palm and fingers. The space itself is not commonly infected, but when it is and pus is present, drainage by longitudinal incision is recommended. The same is true for the dorsal *aponeurotic space*, which lies between the extensor tendons and the metacarpals. *Web spaces* are three in number and exist between index and middle fingers, middle and ring fingers and ring and small fingers. When in-fected they point dorsally and are usually drained by means of a longitudinal incision through the dorsum of the finger web.

Lymphangitis

This generally starts from superficial injury, progresses rapidly and presents as pain, swelling and redness of the hand and sometimes of the forearm. The patient is febrile and toxic and the symptoms rapidly progress up the forearm to above the elbow. There are no findings of tendon sheath or fascial space infections. Subcutaneous abscesses may appear, but usually there are no localizing signs of infection. Surgical drainage is inadvisable except when there is definite localization of pus. The patient should be hospitalized and the entire extremity elevated and kept wrapped in warm, moist compression dressings to the axilla.

Cat Bite Infection

Pasteurella multocida infections from cat bites are treated with antibiotics, drainage where abscess formation has occurred, elevation and heat. These infections generally subside spontaneously in about two weeks.

Erysipeloid Infection

Erysipeloid infections are common in butchers, farmers and veterinarians. These are acute infections which subside spontaneously in about a month. Surgical intervention is inadvisable and penicillin is moderately effective. Wounds incurred while handling raw meat may be infected with Erysipelothrix and these should not be closed primarily, as they will frequently break down and result in more scarring than if left to heal secondarily.

CYSTS AND TUMORS

Ganglion

This is the most common of the extraneous growths of the hand other than warts. Most commonly located on the dorsal aspect of the wrist, ganglia may also be found on the volar side of the wrist and in the palm and fingers. Despite the various methods of injection and needling periodically report-

ed, the best method of treatment for symptomatic or unsightly ganglia is complete surgical excision in a controlled surgical environment. The more complete the excision, the less the incidence of recurrence. The same treatment is indicated for the small ganglia which are found on the proximal flexor pulleys over the metacarpal heads.

Giant Cell Tumor of Tendon Sheath Origin

These are also known as xanthomas and are the second most common tumors of the hand. They are benign but may cause local symptoms or bone erosion. They are usually located in the digits and present as firm, nontender, often irregular nodules. Their proper treatment is excision under tourniquet ischemia. They frequently have extensions around and under the flexor or extensor mechanisms and as their dissection may be complex should properly be done in the operating room.

Epidermoid Cysts

These are also called epithelial inclusion cysts. They develop following injury and are due to the implantation of epithelium into deeper tissues. They develop first as small nodules which are transiently tender and slowly grow to form subcutaneous cysts. Treatment is by surgical excision which can be done easily under digital block if the cyst is in a finger or under local infiltration if it is in the palm.

Mucous Cysts

These are the next most common tumor of the hand. They are present in older persons, usually with degenerative arthritis, and appear as painful cysts on the dorsum of the finger in the region of the DIP joint. Puncturing them produces a clear, gelatinous fluid and this relieves pain temporarily but results in either prompt recurrence or a bothersome ulcerative lesion. More satisfactory treatment is surgical excision of the entire lesion including the overlying skin, replacing the skin with a split thickness skin graft. This can usually be done adequately in either the Out-patient Clinic or the Emergency Room under digital nerve block and local lidocaine infiltration of a small donor site on the volar aspect of the forearm.

Pyogenic Granulomas and Foreign Body Granulomas

These are of inflammatory origin; the former are external and involve the skin and the latter are deep to the skin and form around a foreign body. The pyogenic granuloma is pedunculated, tender and ulcerated. It can be easily snipped off or excised and the base cauterized with silver nitrate. Foreign body granulomas require careful dissection in a bloodless field and most of them should be excised in the operating room.

Other Tumors of the Hand

Most tumors of the hand are benign and include lipomas, fibromas, enchondromas, hemangiomas, glomus tumors and warts. Warts will generally disappear as mysteriously as they occurred and within a few months. For extensive wart formation, dermatological consultation is generally indicated.

Squamous cell carcinoma is the most common of the malignancies in the hand. Malignant melanomas occur on the hand and have a particularly poor prognosis in subungual or palmar sites. Early excisional biopsy of palmar nevi is recommended to forestall malignant degeneration.

TENDON CONDITIONS

DeQuervain's Disease

This is also known as stenosing tenosynovitis and is manifested by pain over the radial styloid where crossed by the tendons of the abductor pollicis longus and extensor pollicis brevis. These two tendons share a common compartment covered by the extensor retinaculum. This condition is common in middle-aged females and can cause pain of disabling degree. Palpable tenderness can be demonstrated over the tendon compartment on the dorsal radial aspect of the distal radius. The pain is also produced or accentuated by forcible passive flexion of the thumb MP joint. Immobilization of the wrist and thumb in a plaster cast or splint may give relief of pain while immobilization persists, but the pain usually recurs when normal activity is resumed. Injections of the tendon sheath (not into the tendons themselves) with 2 ml of hydrocortisone gives prompt relief, but the pain usually recurs within a month or so. Repeated injection of the tendon compartment is inadvisable as degeneration and rupture of one or both tendons may occur. The only definitive treatment is surgical release of the compartment, which gives a definite cure in almost all cases. This procedure is best done in the operating room, but if the operator is experienced it may be done on an outpatient basis. Under tourniquet control a longitudinal incision is made directly over the affected tendon compartment. The retinaculum overlying the tendons is slit longitudinally, opening up the entire tunnel. Aberrant tendons and duplication of either of the tendons are common, but excision of these is not necessary. If there is a reactive tenosynovitis, the thickened synovium should be dissected free from the tendons. Some prefer to make a transverse incision, but the longitudinal incision gives almost as good a cosmetic result and has the added advantage that it is easier to avoid the sensory branch of the radial nerve which lies just radial to the tendons. Care should be taken to avoid traumatizing this nerve with either scalpel or retractors as it is often the source of troublesome neuromas. In making the longitudinal incision one should be careful to stop short of the transverse extension crease in the skin on the dorsum of the wrist.

Traumatic tenosynovitis can affect any of the flexor or extensor tendons, but is more common over the dorsum of the wrist. It is caused by excessive use of a particular tendon and is basically an inflammatory response of the tenosynovium to excessive motion. It is manifested by severe pain on motion and tenderness to palpation over the inflamed area. Palpable crepitation is often present when the tendon moves. Although it is similar to deQuervain's disease, surgical intervention is not needed. Splinting the tendon at rest for a couple of weeks will cause subsidence of the symptoms.

Trigger Thumb and Clutched Thumb

Snapping of the thumb when it is flexed is caused by thickening of the annular sheath of the flexor pollicis longus at the level of the MP joint, and it is a condition more common in infants than adults. Occasionally there is a concomitant nodule in the tendon itself. Cure is accomplished simply by longitudinal slitting and excision of the thickened portion of the sheath. This is done by a transverse incision through the flexor crease of the MP joint, care being taken to protect the digital nerves. Occasionally the thumb remains fixed in flexion and cannot be unlocked without surgical release. In the newborn whose thumbs are held tightly in the flexed position, the "clutched thumb" condition, the thumbs may sometimes be coaxed into the extended position by steady but gentle manual traction and held thus with plaster casts for several months. If the deformity is associated with congenital absence of the thumb extensors, reconstructive surgery is necessary.

Trigger Finger

Trigger or snapping finger is usually caused by a constriction in the proximal flexor pulley at the level of the metacarpal head. Often a corresponding nodule or thickening is present on the flexor digitorum profundus or at the bifurcation of the flexor digitorum sublimis. The treatment is release of the constriction by longitudinal slitting of the flexor pulley, which is exposed by a 2 centimeter longitudinal incision through the palmar skin overlying the metacarpal head. A transverse incision is recommended by some, but the longitudinal incision will heal almost as well and allows greater exposure with less danger to the digital nerves and arteries. A trigger finger will sometimes be the first sign of rheumatoid tenosynovitis, in which case a rheumatoid nodule and proliferative tenosynovitis may be found in one of the flexor tendons. An extensive tenosynovectomy may be necessary, and since this is difficult to forecast preoperatively, cases of trigger finger should be operated upon in the operating room.

Ruptured Tendons

Any of the flexor or extensor tendons may rupture as a result of trauma, rheumatoid involvement or other disease process such as tuberculosis. Finding the ruptured ends is not always an easy matter, and when found the severed ends can rarely be satisfactorily anastomosed. A segmental tendon graft or a tendon transfer is therefore frequently required. Such reparative surgery — and this includes avulsion of the flexor digitorum profundus from its insertion — should be done in the operating room.

Metacarpal Boss

The extensor carpi radialis longus and brevis insert on the dorsal bases of the second and third metacarpals respectively. The normal skeleton reveals dorsal bony prominences on each of the metacarpal bases, but in some patients, particularly those whose occupation requires repetitive, forceful wrist extension, a painful swelling and increase in size of this bony prominence may develop. The pain apparently is located in the fibers of insertion of the radial wrist extensors and is relieved by injection of the region with hydrocortisone. Occasionally immobilization of the wrist in extension for about three weeks will be necessary. Surgical shaving of the boss is indicated only when it is very large and persistently troublesome.

ARTHRITIS AND JOINT DISEASE

Rheumatoid Arthritis

Synovectomy, tenosynovectomy, repair of ruptured tendons and other reparative surgery for this disease should be done only in the operating room as well-planned procedures. Steroid injection of rheumatoid joints and tissues is commonly done and may give transient relief of symptoms, but repeated injection may cause such complications as tendon rupture and possibly cyst formation in the subcondylar bone.

Osteoarthritis

Degenerative arthritis of the hand will present in the Emergency Room and Outpatient Clinic either as painful arthritis of the thumb carpometacarpal joint or painful Heberden's nodes overlying the DIP joints of the fingers. The former is treated by arthrodesis or excision of the greater multangular in the operating room. When symptomatic, Heberden's nodes may be quieted by massage with an ice cube for a few minutes. They do not respond well to excision or injection.

Pyogenic Arthritis

Infections of the joints of the hand are usually caused by staphylococci introduced by trauma. Early joint infection is best treated by elevation and moist hot compresses, using antibiotics when appropriate. If these measures don't lead to regression of joint swelling and tenderness in two to three days, the joint should be opened and any debris or inflamed synovium excised. Contrary to some, I believe in leaving the joint wide open and starting active motion immediately. Such joints will heal very well. They will not lose their articular cartilage and will preserve normal or nearly normal ranges of motion.

Villonodular and Chronic Nonspecific Synovitis

A chronically swollen, thickened and moderately tender MP joint may have a hypertrophic proliferative synovitis due to repeated trauma or perhaps a low grade infection. Synovectomy is the prescribed treatment if one intra-articular injection of 25 milligrams of hydrocortisone does not cause subsidence of the findings and symptoms.

NEUROGENIC CONDITIONS

Carpal Tunnel Syndrome

Median nerve entrapment is common in the middle-aged, in the rheumatoid arthritic and following Colles' fracture. It is manifested by tingling and numbness in the median nerve sensory distribution in the hand, usually the thumb, index and middle fingers, but sometimes the tingling is present throughout the entire hand. Pain may be associated with this, and discomfort may involve the entire extremity. It is not rare for the presenting complaint to be pain in the forearm, or in the shoulder or even in the neck. The patient is often awakened by tingling in the fingers. He may resort to vigorous shaking of the hand or hands to obtain relief. Physical findings may be absent in the early cases but often there is a diminution in median sensation throughout the hand, manifested by a decrease in fine touch and two-point discrimination. There is occasionally thenar atrophy, and paresthesias may occur in the fingertips when the nerve is percussed on the volar aspect of the wrist. The main function of the Emergency Room or outpatient physician is to make a tentative initial diagnosis, so that follow-up studies and further testing can be done. If the diagnosis is confirmed early, surgical release can be done; surgery is very effective in reversing nerve changes. The longer these changes have been present and the older the patient is, the poorer the chance for regaining lost nerve function, particularly if there has been motor loss. An emergency situation exists with the elderly patient who has sustained a fracture of the distal radius which has been reduced and immobilized (usually in the flexed wrist position), and who then complains of pain or numbness in the fingertips. Such an extremity should be elevated and the plaster cast removed. A volar splint should be applied holding the wrist in neutral, even if this means losing the reduction of the fracture.

Reflex Sympathetic Dystrophy

In this category fall several complex conditions, such as causalgia, Sudek's post-traumatic atrophy, the shoulder-hand syndrome and others. Such past favorites as scalenus anticus syndrome and cervical rib have now been replaced by the thoracic outlet syndrome, but this too is related to this complicated group. In these there are apparently four components interacting in various combinations: a painful peripheral stimulus, spinal reflex arcs, sympathetic changes and finally interpretation and reaction to these peripheral phenomena by the higher levels of consciousness. Once such a condition is developed a vicious cycle is established and it tends to be self-perpetuating. Breaking the cycle at any one point is usually not effective and it must be attacked simultaneously at several points. Though it is true that the most "normal" individual may develop a reflex sympathetic dystrophy, more commonly it is seen in the inadequate personality type and in the outright neurotic. The approach then must be to relieve the painful stimulus as well as to deal with the patient's reaction to that stimulus. This is a time-consuming and patience-demanding process, but if the physician persists, often with the aid of a psychiatrist, most of such patients can be improved if not cured. Sympathetic block or stellate ganglionectomy is often tried, but these procedures are rarely effective unless done within the first few weeks of the development of the cycle. The most promising approach is the preventive one, which consists of dealing effectively with the painful lesion before a cycle can develop fully. Too often this depressing chain of events is fostered either by neglect of an injury or, even more commonly, by improper treatment, and one of the most common initial events is the tight plaster cast in which the patient's pain is treated by narcotics rather than by the relief of the pressure by bivalving the cast.

Self-Mutilation

Occasionally the Emergency Room or clinic physician will be faced with wounds of the hand which simply refuse to heal despite adequate treatment. These are usually on the dorsum of the hand and may be open or closed. Some patients who prefer to continue with compensation payments rather than return to work will deliberately or sometimes subconsciously keep an open wound of the hand from healing by picking at it or by traumatizing it in other ways.

A simple contusion of the dorsum of the hand may lead to persistent swelling and a painful hand edema which may last for many months. Known as Secretan's disease or peritendinous fibrosis, the condition is seen almost exclusively in insurance or compensation cases. The only treatment is to attempt to get the patient to use the hand as normally as possible and at the same time advise that all litigation be settled.

CONGENITAL DEFECTS

These range from mild syndactyly through innumerable combinations of defects to such severe conditions as congenital amputation of the hand or parts thereof. Few lend themselves to outpatient treatment. One exception to this is the infant who has a supernumerary digit on a small fleshy pedicle. Such a rudimentary finger can be easily snipped off and the small wound covered with a Band-Aid. If the pedicle is larger than about 3 millimeters in diameter, there may be a skeletal connection and more elaborate measures may be necessary. Attempts to repair syndactyly, congenital bands, bifid fingers and similar congenital anomalies should not be made on an outpatient basis, as the results obtained therefrom will be unsatisfactory.

DUPUYTREN'S CONTRACTURE

The only definitive treatment for Dupuytren's contracture is palmar fas-

ciectomy, an exacting operation which should be done only in the operating room. In cases where fingers are held contracted into the palm by a single longitudinal fascial band the operation may be simplified by percutaneous fasciotomy, which allows a partial release of the fingers. Severance of one or two fascial bands is simple to perform, but care must be taken not to cut too deep or to try for too great a release or the digital nerves, arteries and flexor tendons may be severed. Under local anesthesia a small bladed scalpel or tenotome is held flat on the palm and sloped transversely through the skin directly overlying the tight band. While applying traction to the contracted finger the knife blade is then turned perpendicular to the band and pushed down through the band. The knife pressure should be released as soon as the band is severed. This is a useful prelude to fasciectomy but is dangerous if one tries to accomplish too much. The small wound need not be sutured but will close spontaneously in about two weeks, after which the more complex operation can be done. During this time gentle but continuous extension splinting of the finger should be used to stretch out the skin and joint capsule.

SNAKE BITE

Time is of the essence in the case of snake bite, and simple first aid measures may greatly decrease the ensuing pain, edema, necrosis and systemic toxicity. If the patient is seen within 30 minutes, incision of the snake bite area and suction can remove a significant amount of venom. The incision should not be the commonly described cruciform type, as a single linear incision is preferable. Suction may be applied by mouth if there are no open lesions of the mouth, or by rubber bulb. Appropriate antivenom should be promptly administered, half in the area of the bite and the remainder intramuscularly. If the patient presents himself with a tourniquet on the arm this should be maintained until these immediate measures have been carried out. In no case should the tourniquet be left in place for more than two hours. Since much of the secondary damage may be caused by edema, dependency of the extremity should be avoided. Hypothermia of the hand and forearm with ice packs is quite effective in controlling pain and edema, but numerous cases of great damage from prolonged cold have occurred. Complications of cold injury have been severe enough to cause loss of the extremity above the elbow. Cold should not be used for longer than two or three hours and hospitalization is indicated in all cases.

Longitudinal fasciotomy is extremely effective in relieving pain and preventing muscle necrosis in severe bites in which massive swelling is obvious. The skin incision and fasciot-omy should be extensive and may extend from fingertip to elbow or higher. These wounds heal very well without closure or they may be subsequently covered with split thickness skin grafts.

REFERENCES

1. Brown, P. W.: Lacerations of the flexor tendons of the hand. Surg. Clin. N. Amer., *49*:1255–1268, 1969.
2. Boyes, J. H. (Ed.): Bunnell's Surgery of the Hand. Philadelphia, J. B. Lippincott Co., 1970.
3. Flatt, A. E.: The Care of Minor Hand Injuries. St. Louis, C. V. Mosby Co., 1963.
4. Iselin, M.: Delayed emergency in fresh wounds of the hand. Proc. R. Soc. Med., *51*:713–714, 1958.
5. Kanavel, A. B.: Infections of the Hand. Philadelphia, Lea & Febiger, 1939.
6. Milford, L.: The Hand. St. Louis, C. V. Mosby Co., 1971.
7. Rank, B. K., and Wakefield, A. R.: Surgery of Repair as Applied to Hand Injuries. Edinburgh, Livingstone, 1953.

15 The Breast

JOHN Q. GALLAGHER, M.D.

INTRODUCTION

The female breast has achieved a certain degree of attention from the present generation of the American public. The problems and diseases of this organ deserve an equal amount of attention from the physician — from house officer, family physician and surgeon. Cancer of the breast is the most common cause of death in women between the ages of 40 and 60. In fact, it is generally accepted that carcinoma of the breast is the most common cancer of women in the world today. Diseases of the breast therefore deserve a high degree of consideration in a text such as this which is devoted primarily to the care and treatment of patients not confined to the hospital bed.

During the past hundred years the sheer number of books and papers published on carcinoma of the breast stands in mute testimony to the confusion, controversy and apparent inability of doctors to establish a systematic approach to the treatment of this disease. A course of action that can withstand the vocal and written onslaught of our fellow investigators has yet to be found. The treatment of the patient with carcinoma of the breast extends over a long period of time. This, in many cases, may encompass a significant number of years in the life of the patient's attending physician. The actual time spent in hospital is relatively small compared with the years of follow-up care and hours spent plotting the best course of action for the individual patient whose free interval is past and who now presents with recurrent disease. The patient's total care should be a team effort involving close cooperation among the surgeon, physical therapist and, when indicated, the radiotherapist and chemotherapist.

There are problems other than cancer of the female breast, and these, though important to our patients, are proportionally far less complicated and controversial. These will be handled with little trepidation. The purpose of this short chapter, then, is to chart a course of action dealing with problems of the breast from benign to malignant. An attempt will be made to be concise and to summarize the voluminous

687

writings on the subject. The plastic and esthetic properties of the female breast will be avoided and left to those specifically interested in these problems.

THE EXAMINATION

Every doctor who as a matter of course in his daily practice examines the female patient would do well to establish a habit of spending three to four minutes teaching the patient to examine her own breasts. The doctor not only will have conducted a thorough examination, but hopefully will have encouraged the patient to check herself properly and routinely every month.[6, 9] In the premenopausal woman routine examination of the breast is best done several days after cessation of the menstrual period, because at this time breast enlargement is minimal and a mass is more easily detected. The history is important and

discomfort, swelling, skin changes, nipple discharge, as well as time of menopause, hormone therapy or family history of breast disorders all may prove significant to the patient's problem.

The actual examination should begin with inspection of size and symmetry of the breasts. Skin changes such as erythema or retraction, and any nipple ulceration or retraction are all significant (Fig. 15–1).

Gentle palpation of the entire breast in a systematic fashion should be demonstrated to the patient in both upright and supine positions. This will assure both doctor and patient future familiarity with the texture and consistency of her breasts. Areas of nodularity, old biopsy sites or abscesses should be accurately mapped out on the patient's chart. Careful palpation of axillary and supraclavicular areas completes the examination. Any change in the future detected by patient or doctor can then be more readily evaluated.

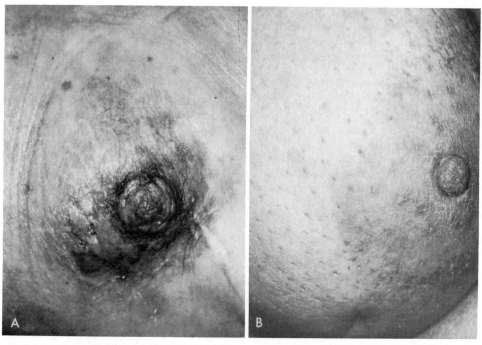

Figure 15–1 Carcinoma of the breast. *A.* Nipple ulceration and retraction in early subareolar carcinoma. *B.* Skin retraction ("peau d'orange") in advanced carcinoma.

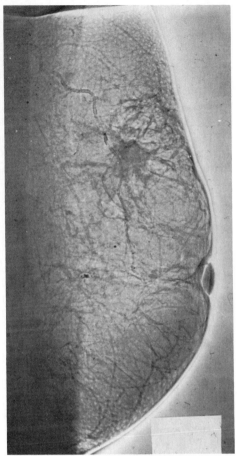

Figure 15–2 Xeromammogram of patient with carcinoma of the breast. Distortion and irregularity of ducts, increased density and flecks of calcification are the radiographic signs of malignancy in this patient with a mass deep in the breast.

The patient with large, pendulous breasts who is difficult to examine, as well as those patients with nodular and cystic breasts and particularly patients who have had a previous carcinoma all present distinct problems in accurate examination and routine follow-up care. The regular physical examination can be augmented with periodic xeromammograms (Fig. 15–2). This must be done judiciously, for much has been written recently about indiscriminate use of this technique as a screening procedure.[18] The patient with a strong family history of breast carcinoma or a woman with established cystic

disease in the dangerous age group should have xeromammograms every one to two years. This augments but does not replace the more frequent physical examination. This x-ray technique certainly is of great value in evaluating the remaining breast in the patient who has had a mastectomy, but it must be used carefully, with full knowledge of its dangers and limitations.

INFLAMMATORY CONDITIONS OF THE BREAST

Inflammatory lesions of the breast, though infrequent, cause considerable morbidity because of their chronic, indolent nature.[12] Engorged breasts in the neonate often become infected but usually respond readily to warm compresses and antibiotics. As always, suppuration is an indication for surgical incision and drainage. Pubertal enlargement is not really a true mastitis and should be handled conservatively with support and pain medication. The breast abscess as seen in adult women is a complex problem. Mammary duct ectasia, mammary fistulas and nonspecific inflammation may frequently be confused with carcinoma. The lactating breast is highly susceptible to infection. This condition usually responds quite readily to cessation of breast feeding, antibiotics and incision and drainage as indicated. Mammary duct ectasia is characterized by dilatation of the large ducts beneath the nipple and areola with periductal inflammation and fibrosis.[1] There may be associated nipple discharge with or without retraction. A painful tumor mass may form, making biopsy mandatory to rule out carcinoma. As the disease progresses, overt abscesses and fistulas may form. In our experience at the University of Colorado we have been singularly impressed by the fact that for many of the chronic inflammatory conditions of the breast — duct ectasia, abscesses or fistulas — simple

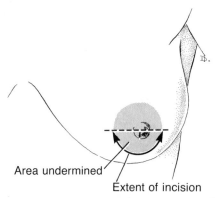

Figure 15–3 Circumareolar incision for wide excision of diseased duct system. The areola is elevated and the involved area is excised up to the nipple. Deep tissue is then closed, followed by delayed closure of skin in three to five days.

incision and drainage is not the definitive treatment. The average patient referred to the clinic with a chronic inlammatory condition has previously had one or two incision and drainage procedures. Our approach has been wide excision of the involved area with associated subterminal duct excision, including the entire area beneath the nipple and areola (Fig. 15–3). Because of the chronic infection, delayed primary closure of the skin is suggested. The underlying breast tissue is approximated with Vicryl or Dexon and three to five days later the skin edges can be pulled together with tape or previously laid sutures. With this approach recurrent disease has not been a problem.

CYSTIC DISEASE OF THE BREAST

In this age of enlightenment women are acutely aware of their susceptibility to carcinoma of the breast. No disease of the breast is more common or more confusing than lumpy, tender breasts, usually more pronounced just prior to menstruation. First of all, the patient must be reassured and the normal physiology of the cyclic changes of her breasts explained to her. If there

are dominant lumps that are mobile, well-circumscribed and appear fluctuant, the probability of cystic disease increases. Chronic cystic mastopathy (it is not truly a mastitis) is probably the most common breast ailment in premenopausal women. Because of high medical costs, as well as shortage of hospital beds, it appears unnecessary and meddlesome to admit women repeatedly to the hospital and perform partial mastectomies under general anesthetic.[4] The mental anguish associated with a hospital admission and the possibility of awakening with the loss of a breast is of great significance to the patient. If the patient, when first seen, presents with one or more discrete, fluctuant masses and is in the premenopausal age group, needle aspiration is in order.[16] With the fluid removed and the mass gone the patient can safely receive follow-up care.

Patients who have previously undergone biopsy and have an established diagnosis of fibrocystic mastopathy certainly should have needle aspiration when recurrent masses appear. In the event that no fluid is obtained or if a residual mass is present, the patient should be scheduled for breast biopsy under general or local anesthesia. Cysts that recur within two weeks or those that require multiple aspirations can also be scheduled for elective excision. A high degree of judgment must be used in following a regimen such as this, but it is a safe and conservative approach for the many women who present with this problem. The technique of needle aspiration is simple and relatively painless even without local anesthetic (Fig. 15–4). A syringe of appropriate size with a needle of 22 to 25 gauge is used after thorough cleansing and preparation of the breast. Light finger pressure assists in complete evacuation of the cyst. A common problem is the woman with multiple small cysts throughout both breasts who complains of considerable pain during the premenstrual period. Reassurance, pain medication, and

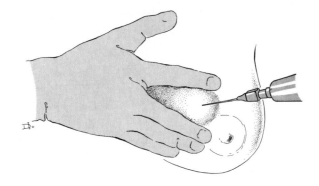

Figure 15-4 Aspiration of breast cyst. The cyst is identified, stabilized and evacuated by light finger pressure while syringe barrel is withdrawn.

support with a well-fitted bra will usually suffice. Small doses of diuretics given during the premenstrual period will often be of help. In extreme cases the use of an androgen such as methyltestosterone, 5 mg daily for the first three weeks of the cycle, may relieve the discomfort.

As estrogen function diminishes following menopause so do the problems with fibrocystic disease. On the other hand, if exogenous estrogen therapy is given postmenopausally, fibrocystic disease may often continue to present problems. This must be carefully and thoroughly explained to the patient. In carefully selected cases of young women with severe fibrocystic disease and particularly those with a strong family history of carcinoma of the breast, consideration may be given to a subcutaneous mastectomy with implantation of silastic prostheses. Many plastic surgeons have worked in conjunction with general surgeons in accomplishing this for the rare appropriate patient.

FIBROADENOMA

It is not an uncommon event for the physician to be confronted by a highly concerned young woman in her late teens or twenties who has just noted a firm mass in her breast and wants to be sure that it is not a cancer — right now! These young ladies, frequently accompanied by their distraught mothers, must immediately be assured and placed at ease. They must be told that their age places them in a relatively safe category.[5] The fibroadenoma that occurs in these young women usually is solitary, firm, mobile, painless and does not change in size or consistency during the course of her menstrual cycle. This is in opposition to the older patient with the multiple, painful masses of fibrocystic disease that usually will fluctuate with the menstrual cycle. For the young woman under 30 years of age who appears clinically to have a fibroadenoma we have, in the majority of cases, suggested excision under a local, or, in the patient who desires it, particularly if the lesion is large, under a general anesthetic. For those in this age group who do have a general anesthetic we assure them that they will awaken with their lump removed and both breasts intact. Permanent sections, consultations with a number of pathologists and thorough discussion with the patient and her family are in order before any radical surgery is embarked upon in a woman of this age group.

OUTPATIENT BREAST BIOPSY — INDICATIONS AND TECHNIQUES

There is nothing more certain to terrify a woman than the discovery of a lump in her breast. The lump is most often discovered by the woman herself or by her primary physician. The usual "All-American" technique has been to admit the patient to the hospital when the lump has been verified by her attending physician and to explain to her that she will be placed under a general anesthetic and if the mass is a cancer her breast will be removed and the situation resolved. In the United States today this is not always acceptable to the average American woman. She is quite familiar with the various women's magazines that discuss in detail the pros and cons of all the various modalities in the treatment of breast cancer. She is really much better informed and not ready to accept the didactic approach of the surgeon. The average knowledgeable American woman knows of the different operations and in many cases would like to thoroughly discuss these with her attending surgeon. There has never been any well documented evidence showing that biopsying a carcinoma and then following this with definitive surgical treatment two to five days later has altered the outcome of the surgery or the long-term course of the disease. Certainly not all patients are candidates for outpatient local breast biopsy, but the majority of women (more than 75 per cent) can receive this procedure and the physician can obtain a diagnosis (Fig. 15–5) without jeopardizing her eventual outcome. Little needs to be said about the time saved, compared with the long operation in which biopsy is followed by frozen section followed by possible definitive modified or radical mastectomy. As over 80 per cent of the biopsies done in this country prove to be benign, the hospital cost is certainly something to be considered, and the nation as a whole and the state medical societies in particular are concerned with hospital cost containment. The procedure of local outpatient breast biopsy costs about 10 per cent of the conventional admission for one to two days for the similar operation performed in the operating room under general anesthesia.

The technique of outpatient breast biopsy is relatively simple. A thorough

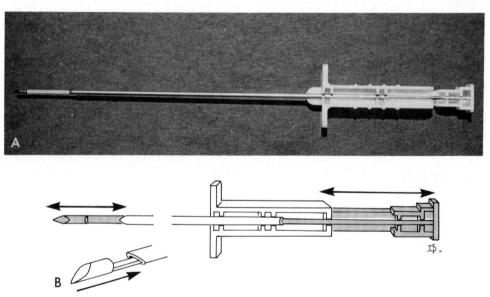

Figure 15–5 Disposal biopsy needle for breast biopsy. *A.* Needle assembled. *B.* Technique of biopsy. The hollow needle and obturator are inserted into the mass with the obturator (shaded portion) withdrawn. The obturator is then advanced by pressure on the plunger. The direction of the needle is then altered slightly, and the obturator is withdrawn, bringing with it a fragment of tissue. Needle and obturator are removed from patient, and tissue is extracted from obturator. (Travenol Laboratories, Inc.)

preoperative explanation in the physician's office is mandatory. The majority of women not only will accept this when it is explained but are quite happy that they do not have to go into the hospital and endure a general anesthetic with the possibility of waking up without a breast. Intravenous or IM Valium at the time of the outpatient breast biopsy is a very helpful adjunct to the procedure. This too must be explained to the patient and used on an individual basis. It is mandatory that the patient be brought to the outpatient department by a friend or relative who will return her to her home. When the patient knows that she will be admitted strictly to the outpatient department, placed under sedation with Valium and the breast lump removed in a manner probably less traumatic than having a tooth removed, she is generally very receptive to this approach.

This technique can generally be done in the outpatient department by the operating physician himself. In selected cases he may want to have a nurse available to help retract in addition to the circulating nurse. The IV Valium, if indicated, is given to the patient when she first lies supine on the operating table. The 10 mg syringe of IV Valium is inserted in the vein on the opposite arm and 5 to 7 mg are slowly injected. The syringe is then taped to the patient's arm and, if necessary, more Valium can be administered during the procedure This is highly selective; in many cases a simple injection of 5 mg or more may suffice and the syringe can be removed. The alternatives are to give the patient oral Valium preoperatively or an IM injection of up to 10 mg one half hour before the procedure. Some patients require no sedation whatsoever.

The technique varies with the individual patient and her lesion. The large, deep seated lesion in a pendulous breast might well not be amenable to this procedure and would warrant either needle biopsy or biopsy under general anesthesia. Generally

speaking, however, for the appropriate lesion with preoperative preparation this technique can be accomplished under local anesthesia. With intravenous Valium, by the time the patient's breast is prepared she also is well sedated for the biopsy. A transverse or circumareolar incision should be planned, which could easily conform with the possible planned modified or radical mastectomy should the mass prove malignant. In the average patient with no allergies or other reasons to avoid adrenalin we have found that 2 per cent Xylocaine with adrenalin in the conventional field block will provide sufficient anesthesia for removal of the breast mass. Generally, 10 cc of 2 per cent Xylocaine with adrenalin (if this is appropriate), drawn up in a No. 20 needle, then infiltrated with a No. 22 to 27 needle, will not only provide adequate anesthesia, but will minimize blood loss (Fig. 15–6). The patient is awake, and continuing conversation with her can not only reassure her but prepare her for every movement her physician might make.

Following the circumareolar or transverse incision (Fig. 15–7) bleeding should be minimal because of the 2 per cent Xylocaine with adrenalin; however, troublesome bleeders can be clamped and suture ligated with 3-0 Dexon. The disposable electrocautery unit, which is readily available, can also be used. The mass — which must have been carefully identified prior to injection of the local anesthetic — can then be grasped with an Allis or Leahy clamp and excised. Metzenbaum or other scissors, in addition to the judicious use of a scalpel, can facilitate this removal (Figs. 15–8 and 15–9). Following the removal of the mass a "bimanual" exam with the surgeon's fingers inside the wound and also outside the skin edges can locate any further masses that might be in the quadrant of the suspicious lesion. After the mass has been excised there is generally a significant defect present. This defect should be adequately closed, in layers

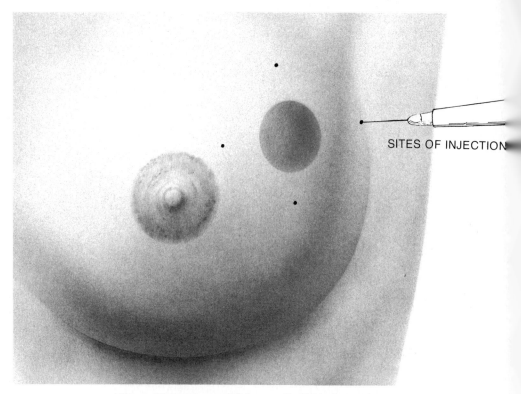

SITES OF INJECTION

Figure 15–6   Mass in left breast. Field block anesthesia.

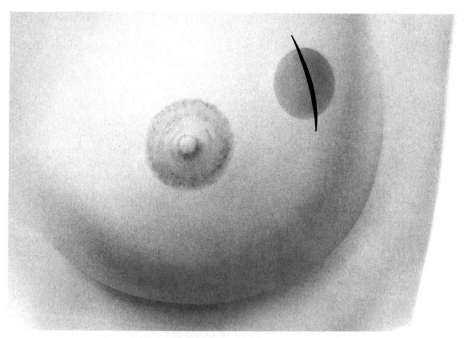

Figure 15–7   Incision.

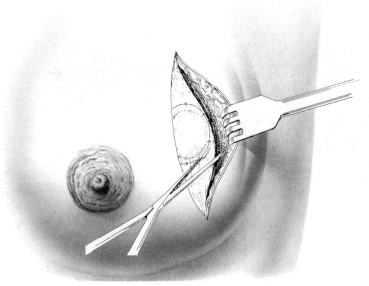

Figure 15–8 Dissection. The incision shown here and in the following illustrations has been enlarged to show details. In actual practice it should not be enlarged to this extent, in most cases. The smaller incision shown in Figure 15–7 will suffice.

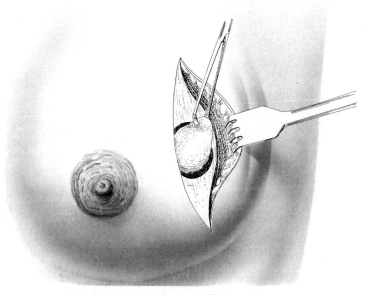

Figure 15–9 Removal of breast mass.

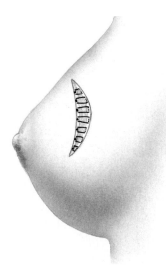

Figure 15–10   Closure in layers.

beginning from the very bottom of the defect, using atraumatic sutures of either Dexon or Vicryl (Fig. 15–10). This accomplishes two things: it closes the defect and at the same time obliterates all dead space and possible troublesome bleeders. A cosmetic closure is important and dimpling of the skin should be avoided. In a high percentage of cases a very good cosmetic result can be obtained. Utilizing either Dexon or Vicryl a subcuticular closure can assure a very good cosmetic result (Figs. 15–11 and 15–12). Following the procedure it is important that the patient, as well as her friend or relative, be thoroughly instructed in postoperative care. The wound should be dressed with a pressure dressing and the patient advised to wear a bra for the following 24 hours. After this period of time she can remove the

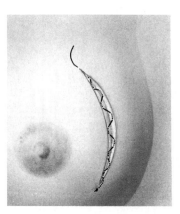

Figure 15–11   Subcuticular closure of skin.

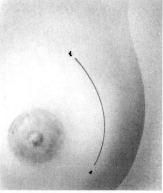

Figure 15–12   Finished closure. As noted in Figure 15–8, the actual incision would be smaller than that shown here.

dressing and shower or bathe. It is generally advisable to wear a bra night and day for the next three to four days.

The majority of breast biopsies that are done will prove to be benign, so the patient has undergone a relatively atraumatic incident in her life, compared with the hospitalization, general anesthetic and worry over possible loss of her breast. If the lesion does prove to be malignant, discussion with the operating physician, the patient and her family can discuss further steps that might be indicated in the treatment of her lesion.

In recent years there has been more interest shown in reconstructive breast surgery following mastectomy for carcinoma. The criteria for this surgery are very strict and only those patients who did not have a high grade carcinoma, multiple positive nodes or any indication for radiotherapy would be eligible. With a well established section revealing a positive diagnosis of carcinoma, possibly low grade, and hopefully a small lesion or lobular carcinoma, the problem might warrant discussion with the interested patient and an equally interested and motivated plastic surgeon for possible consideration of breast reconstruction following a complete and adequate extirpative cancer operation. These considerations are important prior to the definitive surgery. A transverse incision and, if indicated (as in the majority of breast carcinomas operated on today), a modified radical mastectomy retaining the pectoralis major will aid the plastic surgeon in the later reconstruction of the breast if she is a suitable candidate for this procedure.

NIPPLE DISCHARGE

The complaint of spontaneous discharge from the nipple is second in frequency only to finding an actual lump in the breast.[14] The resultant worry to the patient is understandable and she must immediately be reassured that this is not necessarily an outward sign of an underlying cancer. Only then should a systematic, logical plan for the approach to this problem be outlined to the patient. First of all, it should be made clear that a nonspontaneous, self-induced discharge is usually harmless and of no pathological significance. The puerperal discharge of lactation is, of course, a normal physiological process. The cloudy, purulent discharge associated with mammary duct ectasia and fistula has been dealt with above. The bloody or serosanguineous discharge which a generation ago was believed to be a sure sign of underlying cancer is of greatest concern to the patient. It is now established that though the underlying cause for this discharge must be determined, it is most likely due to a benign lesion, the most common of which is an intraductal papilloma.

Cytological study, a simple procedure and an additional diagnostic aid, depends wholly on the availability of an interested, diligent and well-trained cytologist. A negative cytological study means nothing. Though we have emphasized the benign nature of these discharges it must be made clear that in patients over the age of 50 years, cancer, not a benign lesion, is the most frequent cause of this discharge.[19] If an associated mass is present there is no problem, as it *must* be excised.

The patient presenting with a discharge and no mass must then be thoroughly examined in an effort to establish the quadrant containing the underlying pathology. This is done by palpating firmly in a radial fashion over the entire breast (Fig. 15–13). If the quadrant which is the source of discharge can be localized, the involved ductal system can then be surgically excised. In an older woman and in patients in whom no preoperative localization can be elicited it is then advisable to completely excise the

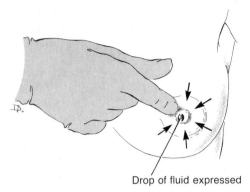

Drop of fluid expressed

Figure 15–13 Radial palpation of duct system to determine source of nipple discharge.

central duct system. This is done through a circumareolar incision extending no more than halfway around the areola, as described earlier (Fig. 15–3). The nipple and areola are elevated, the central duct system identified, and a generous underlying wedge of tissue removed, including the contents of the nipple, to assure excision of the entire major duct system. The defect is closed with buried catgut or Dexon and the nipple and areola replaced. The only possible occasion for simple mastectomy would be in the older patient presenting with a significant discharge, no mass and in whom the previously mentioned excision of the major duct system demonstrated no significant benign lesion to explain the discharge. This decision requires judgment, often aided by consultation with one's colleagues.

CARCINOMA OF THE BREAST

The definitive surgical treatment of carcinoma of the breast has no place in the subject encompassed by this book. The correct surgical approach is and has been under question for the past 80 years.[20] During this time we have seen treatment evolve from conventional radical mastectomy through extended radical mastectomy, and lately

to a modified conservative radical operation.[12] This latter approach has been generally accepted in England and is receiving considerable attention in this country. No absolute statement should be made, however, until there is clear-cut evidence from well-controlled studies comparing the various surgical procedures, such as those conducted by the National Adjuvant Breast Project.[7, 8, 11] In order to facilitate and plan the course of primary therapy, including the wishes and desires of the patient, we attempt to establish the exact diagnosis prior to the time of definitive surgery whenever possible. This can be done simply with the use of the disposable biopsy needle described earlier or possibly with needle aspiration biopsy as described by Kline.[13] This is often done for suspicious lesions seen in the office or clinic. A benign diagnosis necessitates performance of an open biopsy if the lesion is at all suspicious. With a diagnosis of carcinoma the situation is clear. When the results of the needle biopsy or possibly an open biopsy under local anesthesia are known, the course of action can be discussed with the patient and her relatives. Further tests, such as liver functions, bone survey and so on, may be indicated. It would also seem that there is less chance of tumor seeding with this approach compared to open excisional biopsy at the time of the radical surgery. The operative time saved is obvious.

Postoperative Care

Once the patient has been discharged she again enters that phase in her disease which is relegated to outpatient care. The immediate problems which vex the surgeon or surgical resident assigned to the outpatient clinic concern the skin flaps. Seromas under these flaps require needle aspiration. This must be done carefully under sterile conditions, and a pressure dressing should be applied. Strict instructions must be given to the patient regarding care of the dressing and the importance of returning promptly for a follow-up visit. If a significant amount of fluid reaccumulates after one or more aspirations, a small rubber drain should be inserted for two or three days.

Scattered areas of skin necrosis may be seen at or near the suture line on the first outpatient visit. These are usually due to faulty technique, such as skin flaps shaved unnecessarily thin or flaps approximated with undue tension, often with large retention sutures. Multiple closely placed skin sutures usually will prevent this problem. Prompt removal of sutures within 10 to 12 days, followed by application of basic principles of wound care should complete this phase. If necessary a skin graft can be performed at the appropriate time. When the wound is clean the graft can be performed on an outpatient basis under local anesthesia.

Physical rehabilitation is an important but frequently neglected factor following radical or modified radical breast surgery. Personal motivation should be stimulated by the surgeon with the help and expertise of the hospital physical therapist. Often this department, so readily available, is grossly neglected postoperatively in the care of the patient who has had a mastectomy. It should be made very clear to the premenopausal patient that she should, under no circumstances, take estrogens in any form, including oral contraceptives (the "pill"). The danger of stimulation of growth of any residual cancer is the reason for this injunction.[17]

Postoperative radiotherapy continues to be a controversial issue. A survey of the literature and the varied statistics leaves one in a state of doubt and confusion. The fact remains, however, that high voltage therapy can, under the proper circumstances, sterilize carcinoma.[10] We recommend postoperative radiotherapy for those patients with one or more positive nodes and for subareolar or medial quadrant lesions. There has been increasing interest shown among chemotherapists in placing the premenopausal postoperative patient with positive nodes on a regimen of drugs appropriate for this disease.[21] This will be dealt with specifically in another chapter of this book.

Is subsequent pregnancy a danger for the premenopausal patient who has undergone treatment for carcinoma of the breast? There is no absolute answer to this question. In the past, carcinoma of the breast in a pregnant woman was thought to be an indication for therapeutic abortion. We no longer believe that this is true. The young patient who has undergone primary treatment for carcinoma of the breast might well consider having a child if she is well apprised of the situation, and is free of disease after two or three years.[5] This question obviously must be carefully and thoughtfully considered according to the needs of the individual — necessitating extremely close rapport between the physician and his patient.

A routine of postoperative follow-up care is mandatory in tumor surgery. The postmastectomy patient should be seen at regular intervals for a thorough examination of the operative sites, areas of lymphatic drainage and particularly the remaining breast. Chest x-rays and xeromammographic examination of the remaining breast are suggested at yearly intervals. It is well established that at least 7 to 8 per cent of women develop carcinoma in the remaining breast.[19] Any complaints of bone pain, particularly in the back or hips, should be promptly investigated with an appropriate bone survey. These regular examinations reassure both the patient and her physician.

If recurrent disease is found in one of these periodic examinations, the so-called "free interval" is over. The patient then enters an entirely new phase in the management of her disease. The first and most important consideration is to explain to the patient and her immediate family the full meaning of the presence of recurrent disease. This is best discussed with the closest relatives first.

The explanation possibly may be modified in discussions with the patient on the basis of recommendations from the relatives. A positive approach offers reassurance to the patient. Emphasis should be placed on the many means of therapy at our disposal. The physician should then plan a sequential approach — not offering everything at once, but always having one more additional form of therapy available when the existing one fails. The patient with incurable cancer is often unbelievably optimistic, usually welcoming any form of therapy that may offer a glimmer of hope.

Management of Recurrent Breast Carcinoma

The first treatment of recurrent breast cancer generally lies in the realm of the radiotherapist. He has a success rate of up to 70 per cent in the palliative management of breast cancer. His role is particularly important when the disease involves portions of the bony skeleton within a field which can be treated practically and safely. He can often achieve remarkable results in superficial soft tissue metastasis and not only can alleviate pain but can also prevent pathological fractures by radiating weightbearing areas of the skeleton. There are limitations to this form of treatment. It is a local, not a systemic approach, and there is a distinct limit to the amount of radiation which can be given over any period of time. Radiation therapy offers little to the patient with visceral involvement such as metastasis to lung or liver. ^{32}P, a radioactive phosphorus substance, is taken up in areas of bone metastasis

and affords significant palliation for patients who have multiple areas of involvement. Pleural effusions due to metastases can be controlled in up to 50 per cent of cases by radioactive gold or colloidal ^{32}P. The skilled radiotherapist can offer much in the way of palliation to the patient with recurrent breast cancer.

The beneficial effects of castration in the female with carcinoma of the breast were first noted by Sir Astley Cooper in 1829. Even today the issue as to who should receive this treatment remains unsettled. From the voluminous writings on this subject it would appear that the patient most likely to respond to oophorectomy is a woman nearing menopause who has soft tissue or osseous metastases and who had a relatively long free interval. Prophylactic castration following mastectomy probably does not add anything when one considers the entire spectrum of the disease. The effect of castration in prolonging survival and the beneficial effects on metastases are likely to be the same whether oophorectomy is performed early or late. We therefore usually wait until the extent or location of metastases makes the need for it obvious. Objective response to oophorectomy then helps to direct the course of further therapy.

Certainly one of the most important advances in the treatment of carcinoma of the breast over the past few years has been the development of laboratories across the country to determine some prediction of hormonal dependency of mammary cancer.[3] Estrogen and progesterone binding assays are being done on an ever increasing basis. When these tests are positive they prove to be an invaluable aid to the therapeutic team in evaluating all parameters with the possibility of ablative hormonal therapy. The evaluation and interpretation of these tests by the pathologists performing them has widened the scientific approach to the problem of hormonal manipulation. Every physician performing breast surgery, be it primary mastectomy or excision of metastatic lesions, should be aware of the most convenient laboratory to which he might send these specimens. The individual laboratories vary as to their requirements, but generally a small fresh specimen packed in dry ice can be sent to them for a determination of estrogen and progesterone binding capacity.

As metastatic disease progresses there is usually some thoughtful consideration given to further ablative therapy such as adrenalectomy. There have been a number of reports from large referral centers suggesting that adrenalectomy can offer a distinct remission in up to 50 per cent of the cases.[15] This, however, is a procedure which must not be embarked upon lightly. It is an operation of some magnitude, one of the more difficult abdominal procedures. It is performed on a patient with a known fatal disease. Certainly operative mortality figures coming from a large center can be misleading and do not apply to the surgeon who rarely approaches this area.

There are no absolute criteria available to detect the patients who will benefit most from an adrenalectomy. It is generally believed that young patients who have responded to oophorectomy after first experiencing a significant free interval and who now present with primary bone or skin metastasis stand the best chance of receiving significant palliation. Hypophysectomy, too, can produce beneficial results in those patients who satisfy the same criteria as the candidates for adrenalectomy. As indicated earlier, the estrogen and progesterone binding assays can aid much in determining the appropriate patient for these ablative operations. Postoperative endocrine regulation is not too difficult in the patient of moderate intelligence. Oral cortisone acetate in doses of 50 mg per day and Fluorinef 0.1 mg every other day is generally all that is necessary to control the patient after adrenalectomy.

The beneficial effects of castration in premenopausal women with metastatic breast cancer are similar in many ways to the effects produced by administration of hormones. As experience broadens and data accumulates it is becoming increasingly clear that androgens or their synthetic equivalents have a palliative value in both premenopausal and postmenopausal women with metastatic disease. Androgens are particularly valuable to the younger, premenopausal woman with disseminated disease. Fortunately, it is no longer necessary to submit her to the indignity of visible and aggravating side effects. Fluoxymesterone (Halotestin) and testolactone (Teslac) are oral androgen preparations which are frequently effective with the absence of masculinizing side effects. Estrogens often can offer distinct help to the postmenopausal woman. Since breast cancer in young women can be stimulated by estrogens, they should be used only by postmenopausal women. There can be complications of hormone manipulation. Vaginal bleeding in postmenopausal women may require dilatation and curettage but will usually respond to cessation of therapy. Serum calcium must be followed closely, particularly in patients with osseous metastases. Nausea, vomiting and lethargy progressing to disorientation and coma are signs of hypercalcemia. Treatment includes cessation of hormones, increased fluids, steroids and phosphate.

Significant progression of disease after an adequate trial of hormone manipulation would prompt the physician to change to a new modality of treatment. Administration of corticosteroids offers a high degree of subjective improvement in the patient who is in the latter half of the course of metastatic carcinoma of the breast. There is no hard and fast rule regarding indications and dosages. Oral prednisone in doses of 10 to 30 mg per day is convenient and usually offers a degree of subjective improvement. Once therapy is begun it is generally continued indefinitely.

Chemotherapy continues to make rapid strides in the treatment of breast carcinoma. The oncologist is an important element in the team approach and in most centers oncology has evolved into a specialty. Multiple drug therapy in appropriate cases can produce significant palliation. This subject is covered in full detail in Chapter 25.

SUMMARY

The diseases of the breast have been outlined briefly. Absolute conclusions regarding treatment of breast cancer must be avoided. When we compare the results achieved during the past hundred years with the effort expended on clinical and laboratory research it is evident that the problem is far from solved. The investigators of the next generation can rest assured that this is a fertile field for their interest and efforts. Cancer of the breast is the most common cancer in women and our record in treating this condition is still unsatisfactory.

REFERENCES

1. Abramson, D. J.: Mammary duct ectasia, mammillary fistula and subareolar sinuses. Ann. Surg., *169*:217–226, 1969.
2. Auchincloss, H.: Modified radical mastectomy: Why not? Amer. J. Surg., *119*:506–509, 1970.
3. Block, G. E., et al: Prediction of hormonal dependency of mammary cancer, Ann. Surg., *182*:342–352, 1975.
4. Bolton, J. P.: The breast cyst and the hospital bed. Arch. Surg., *101*:382–383, 1970.
5. Earley, T. K., Gallagher, J. Q., and Chapman, K.: Carcinoma of the breast in women under thirty years of age. Amer. J. Surg., *118*:832–834, 1969.
6. Eckert, C.: How to evaluate and manage breast lumps. J.A.M.A., *234*:839–840, 1975.
7. Fisher, B.: The surgical dilemma in the primary therapy of invasive breast cancer: A critical appraisal. Curr. Probl. Surg., 1–53, Oct, 1970.
8. Fisher, B., et al: Ten year follow-up results of patients with carcinoma of the breast in a cooperative clinical trial evaluating surgical adjuvant chemotherapy. Surg. Gynecol. Obstet., *140*:528–534, 1975.
9. Gallager, H. S.: Early Breast Cancer Detection and Treatment. New York, John Wiley and Sons, 1975.
10. Gutman, R. J.: Role of supervoltage irradiation of regional lymph node bearing areas in breast cancer. Amer. J. Roentgenol. Radium Ther. Nucl. Med., *62*:722–724, 1969.
11. Haagensen, C. D.: Diseases of the Breast. Philadelphia, W. B. Saunders Co., 1974.
12. Handley, R. S.: Benign breast diseases: Surgical aspects. Proc. R. Soc. Med., *62*:722–724, 1969.
13. Kline, T. S., and Neal, H. S.: Role of needle aspiration biopsy in diagnosis of carcinoma of the breast. Obstet. Gynecol., *46*:89–92, 1975.
14. Leis, H. P., Jr., and Pilvich, S.: Nipple discharge. Hosp. Med., 29–53, November, 1970.
15. Moore, F. D.: Carcinoma of the Breast. Boston, Little, Brown and Co., 1968.
16. Rosemond, G. P., Maier, W. P. and Brobyn, T. J.: Needle aspiration of breast cysts. Surg. Gynecol. Obstet., *128*:351–354, 1969.
17. Schwartz, M. D.: An information and discussion program for women after a mastectomy. Arch. Surg., *112*:276–281, 1977.
18. Schwartz, H. M., and Reichling, B. A.: The risks of mammograms. J.A.M.A., *237*:965–966, 1977.
19. Seltzer, M. H., Perloff, L. J., Kelley, R. I., and Fitts, W. T.: The significance of age in patients with nipple discharge. Surg. Gynecol. Obstet., *131*:519–522, 1970.
20. Spratt, J. S., Jr., and Donegan, W. T.: Cancer of the Breast. Philadelphia, W. B. Saunders Co., 1967.
21. Tormey, D. C.: Combined chemotherapy and surgery in breast cancer: Review. Cancer, *36*:881–892, 1975.

16 The Heart and Lungs

BRUCE C. PATON, M.R.C.P. (Ed.),
F.R.C.S. (Ed.),
and MELVIN M. NEWMAN, M.D.

Heart and Great Vessels

Heart and Great Vessels

Bruce C. Paton, M.R.C.P. (Ed.), F.R.C.S. (Ed.)

Cardiac surgery might not, at first sight, seem a suitable topic for discussion in a text on outpatient surgery. The initial contact between surgeon and patient, however, is likely to be in the outpatient clinic or office, and post-operative visits to the clinic are an essential part of the patient's care. It is in the Outpatient Department, therefore, that the surgeon makes the first assessment of the problem, and it is again in this department that the results of the operation are evaluated, often for many years.

PREOPERATIVE EVALUATION

The classic approaches of history-taking and physical examination are as important in a complex problem such as the preoperative evaluation of a cardiac patient as in other fields. Even though objective data derived from cardiac catheterization, angiocardiography, pulmonary function tests, tests of coagulation, renal function and biochemistry combine to fill out and amplify the clinical picture, a surprisingly large proportion of relevant information can be obtained from the history and examination. In some instances, such as cases of uncomplicated patent ductus arteriosus or secundum atrial septal defect, a history, examination and EKG, chest x-ray or fluoroscopy are all that is needed to make the diagnosis and lay the foundation for advice about operation. Under these circumstances the decision is made neither easier nor more sure by embarking upon more complex and expensive forms of examination. The more complex the problem, however, the greater becomes the need for supporting data to ensure that the right operation is advised at the right time.

History

Questions should be directed toward the discovery of the defect, a determination of the present severity of illness and the course of progression between discovery and the time of examination. Each type of cardiac disease has a natural history. Where, in this natural history, is this patient? Critical points on such a life history curve are the start of disease, the inception of reversible symptoms, irreversible symptoms and death. If these points are mentally plotted along a time base the patient's position on the curve can be estimated, and the natural outlook that is faced can be determined.

Many types of congenital heart disease are operated upon before any symptoms have arisen; in most cases of acquired disease the best time for operation is after the development of reversible symptoms but before the start of irreversible symptoms.

Congenital Heart Disease

The following questions should be asked:

(1) Were there any predisposing illnesses during the mother's pregnancy, such as rubella or other virus diseases, or exposure to toxic drugs? Because the heart and cardiovascular system are completely formed by the tenth week of intrauterine life, most factors likely to cause defects should affect the fetus within this period. The rubella syndrome can develop in mothers exposed during the second trimester, but cardiac defects are not as common

as defects of other systems when exposure is that late.

(2) What was the condition of the child during and immediately after delivery? Was cyanosis present? Was a murmur heard? Was there respiratory difficulty?

(3) What has been the health of the child since birth? Specific questions should be asked about

    (a) rate of growth and development;
    (b) exercise tolerance;
    (c) frequency of respiratory infections;
    (d) changes in color of skin and mucous membranes with exercise or crying;
    (e) petechial hemorrhages or difficulties with coagulation;
    (f) fainting spells or blackouts;
    (g) feeding problems, especially dysphagia.

It is sometimes difficult to assess with accuracy the exercise tolerance of a child. Obviously, if the child is not yet crawling or walking this may be difficult, but general levels of activity may be an indication. In older children other factors may obscure the true state of affairs. Often the exhortations of parents, school authorities and doctors result in the child becoming relatively inactive and giving up sports which he previously played without difficulty. If the question is then asked, "Well, what do you do after school when no one is there to stop you?" a more honest appraisal may be reached. The child may say that he plays football, throws baskets or plays baseball without difficulty. How well does he keep up with his brothers or schoolmates? Don't just accept a protective mother's answer that "Oh no, Jimmy can't play baseball!" Jimmy may be able to do a lot of things that his mother never knew, and the mother may have to be out of the room before the doctor receives a truthful reply.

The differential diagnosis between congestive heart failure and pneumonia is difficult to make in small infants.

If, for instance, parents say that a six month old child was in the hospital on several occasions during the first three months of life with "pneumonia," the correct interpretation may be that the infant was in congestive failure. Dysphagia and respiratory problems within the first few weeks of life suggest a vascular ring. Many children with left-to-right shunts have an increased frequency of upper respiratory infections. This frequency, however, is not necessarily related to the severity of the lesion, the size of the shunt or the presence of pulmonary hypertension.

Cyanosis is an important sign indicating a right-to-left shunt, usually intracardiac. However, in a newborn infant, cyanosis is more likely to have a respiratory than a cardiac cause, and, therefore, a history of cyanosis apparent immediately after birth is not pathognomonic of cardiac disease. In many instances a history of cyanosis appearing weeks or even months after birth is more diagnostic. At that time, the ductus may close or changing intracardiac pressures may accentuate a right-to-left shunt.

Severe cyanosis of several years' duration may be associated with coagulation defects that must be diagnosed and treated before operation.

Syncope occurring during or immediately after exertion may be due to aortic stenosis; but other cardiovascular and neurological causes must be sought.

Acquired Heart Disease

Most patients with acquired heart disease are adults by the time symptoms become severe enough for operation to be considered. The origin of the disease, however, may have been in youth and questions about early health are appropriate. For instance:

(1) Were there obvious predisposing diseases? Rheumatic fever, acute pericarditis, or history of a murmur during childhood?

(2) At what time and under what circumstances was a diagnosis of cardiac disease first made? Was the diagnosis made because symptoms led to an examination; or was an examination made for routine purposes of insurance or employment and the diagnosis made then?

(3) If the patient was asymptomatic when the diagnosis was first made, when did symptoms first develop and what were the symptoms?

(4) What has been the progression of symptoms since they first developed?

(5) To what extent is the patient now functionally disabled? As with children, extensive and detailed questioning is often necessary to arrive at a true picture of disability. The reply to such a question as "How well do you manage stairs?" may be deceptive if it is then determined that in the normal course of daily life the patient never encounters stairs. A comparison of the patient's capabilities with that of his spouse may be useful. A patient may admit that his wife now seems to walk too fast, or that during the lunch interval his business associates walk too quickly. What was the patient able to do 12 or 6 months ago that he can no longer do?

All these questions are directed toward discovering the nature, severity and progression of symptoms. Merely to note in the chart that a patient has "two-block D.O.E." (dyspnea on exertion) seldom tells the whole story.

Dyspnea is the commonest symptom of cardiac disease and signifies pulmonary congestion. Although it is evidence of left-sided failure, it also occurs with pulmonary hypertension or increased pulmonary blood flow. Patients with pulmonary venous hypertension and incipient left-sided failure often start coughing with exertion, as well as becoming dyspneic.

Nocturnal dyspnea is a significant symptom when present. "Two-pillow orthopnea," however, is a meaningless description. Many normal people sleep with two pillows and patients with genuine nocturnal dyspnea find that two pillows provide insufficient elevation and support.

Medical purists have long taught that leading questions should not be asked, but if this principle is strictly adhered to, much useful historical information remains unacquired. If a patient is asked a straight question such as "Do you ever become so short of breath at night that you have to sit up on the side of the bed?" both patient and doctor are likely to have the same concept of the severity of the symptom. The answer is usually a plain "yes" or "no."

Of all symptoms of acquired disease none is more difficult to elucidate than pain. Ryle[10] described a sequence of questions to ask about pain which has not yet been improved upon:

(1) Character
(2) Severity
(3) Location — e.g., chest, abdomen, superficial or deep
(4) Extent — covered by a hand or a fingertip
(5) Radiation
(6) Time of onset of first attack
(7) Length of each attack
(8) Time between attacks
(9) Precipitating factors
(10) Relieving factors
(11) Associated symptoms — vomiting, sweating and faintness, among others

In most instances answers to these questions will provide a clear picture not only of the symptom but also of the etiological factors.

Pericardial pain is precordial and burning or pricking in nature. Because adjacent pleura may be involved, the pain is often accentuated by movement, respiratory effort or coughing. Pericardium is not a very sensitive membrane, and only the inferior portion, innervated by branches of the phrenic nerve, is pain sensitive. Post-operative pericardial pain is rare, although pericardial reaction is present in all patients after cardiac operations.

If pericarditis is anterior a friction rub may be audible, but posterior pericarditis may produce pain without a rub.

Myocardial pain is central, deep behind the sternum, and aching, crushing or squeezing in character. It may radiate to the jaws, arms or fingers, and radiation is frequently bilateral. Feelings of weakness, arm numbness, fear and impending death are not uncommon. Pain that is located in the left chest and is pricking, sharp or stabbing is seldom myocardial in origin, even though the patient may be convinced of having heart disease.

Angina is usually provoked by exercise but may be started by a fit of anger or emotional shock. A typical attack rises quickly to a plateau of severity sufficient to make the patient stop whatever he is doing, and then subsides after a few minutes. *Stable* angina is that which can be predicted by the patient to be associated with particular types of exertion. *Preinfarction*, *crescendo* and *unstable* angina describe a spectrum of pain of increasing severity and duration of attacks with diminishing provocative stimuli, often associated with temporary electrocardiographic changes of ischemia but not of infarction nor with enzyme changes.

The clinical diagnosis of angina is not always easy. Anxiety states, esophageal spasm, diaphragmatic hernia and extreme dyspnea from any cause may result in central chest pain not dissimilar to angina. Anxiety states are often associated with left inframammary pain that comes on after, rather than during, exercise. Pulmonary hypertension, both arterial and venous, which increases with exertion may cause pain very similar to typical angina.

Physical Examination

Inspection

A systematic approach to examination of the heart starts not with the application of a stethoscope to the chest but with general observation of the patient and an examination of the periphery. Examination begins as soon as the patient walks into the office. Is he young or old, fat or thin, emaciated or short of breath? Does he move around easily and with assurance or slowly and cautiously as though expecting the onset of pain, or is he incapacitated by shortness of breath? What is his color? Is there generalized cyanosis, or the cyanosis of peripheral stasis? And, perhaps the most important distinction of all, does he look ill or well?

The patient should be stripped to the waist, seated at about 45° elevation and in a good, slightly side-directed light. Note pulsations in the neck. Are they arterial or venous? If venous, estimate roughly the venous pressure and the presence and magnitude of an accentuated V-wave. If arterial pulsation is obvious is it normally located in the carotids or is it suprasternal, as is characteristic with coarctation of the aorta? Does the pulse pressure seem to be abnormally wide? Inspection of the precordium is directed toward determining the cardiac apex, any obvious asymmetry of the chest, pulsations and signs of cardiac activity. The weight, size and configuration of the patient must be taken into account in interpretation of all these findings.

Palpation

Palpation starts at the periphery with examination of the pulses. Are pulses present or absent? What is their volume, timing, rate and rhythm? What is the blood pressure and are there inequalities of pressure between limbs? Hepatomegaly and peripheral edema indicate congestive failure.

Feel over the precordium and neck for thrills, which should be timed against the cardiac cycle. When the ventricles become hypertrophied, their activity is transmitted to the precordium as distinctive impulses. Right ventricular hypertrophy is best felt along the left sternal border as a rather sharp tapping impulse, while left ventricular hypertrophy is transmitted as a strong rolling, heaving apical impulse. During systole the hypertrophied right ventricular outflow tract travels directly anteriorly during contraction, but the left ventricle, in contracting, pushes the whole heart forward in a somewhat rotatory manner, imparting a much broader, more widely distributed thrust to the precordium.

Percussion

In the classic sequence of physical examination, percussion follows palpation, but it contributes little to examination of the heart per se. It is very useful in detecting pleural effusions and large pneumothoraces. However, percussing out the cardiac apex is not of much help except perhaps when a pericardial effusion dampens the precordial manifestations of cardiac action.

Auscultation

Because auscultation is instinctively regarded as the most important facet of cardiac examination, it is worthwhile to reconsider the information that may already have been acquired by this stage of the examination before a stethoscope is used. The presence or absence of cyanosis of cardiac origin immediately separates patients with right-to-left shunts from all others. The peripheral pulse wave can be diagnostic of coarctation, aortic stenosis and insufficiency and suggestive of a patent ductus. Atrial fibrillation points to mitral disease, especially stenosis, arteriosclerotic disease or thyrotoxicosis.

Tricuspid insufficiency may be diagnosed from the venous pulsation. Visible wide arterial pulses reconfirm an impression of aortic insufficiency. The precordial impulse indicates left or right ventricular hypertrophy and, if pulmonary valve closure is palpable, pulmonary hypertension. The presence, location and timing of thrills are pointers to a diagnosis of patent ductus, valvular stenosis or insufficiency, ventricular septal defects, tetralogy of Fallot and unusual shunts such as rupture of a sinus of Valsalva. By the time, therefore, that auscultation is started the diagnosis has often been made and the stethoscope merely confirms what has already been found.

For the finer points of auscultatory diagnosis any standard textbook of cardiology should be consulted. It is important, however, that the surgeon have a system for listening to the heart. Each area — aortic, pulmonary, tricuspid and mitral — should be listened to in order. By timing against the pulse or precordial impulse the first and second sounds can be confirmed. Then listen to the sounds individually. Are two or more sounds present? Are they of normal volume? If they are split is this a constant finding during all phases of respiration? Next listen to the systolic and diastolic intervals. Murmurs are usually graded in intensity on a basis of I to VI, I being the softest and VI so loud that it can be heard without direct application of the stethoscope to the skin. Murmurs should be analyzed for the location of maximum intensity and radiation, magnitude, character, precise timing within systole or diastole and impingement upon the opening and closing sounds.

Aortic murmurs are accentuated by making the patient sit up, lean forward and exhale. Similarly, low-intensity mitral diastolic rumbles are best heard when the patient is tilted over to the left side. If the patient is made to sit up and down in bed a couple of times and then listened to while lying on his left side, some hard-to-hear murmurs of mitral stenosis may become audible.

Not all murmurs signify cardiac disease, and it is obviously important to try to distinguish as simply as possible between significant and insignificant murmurs. This problem arises most often in children, and the commonest insignificant or "functional" murmurs are: (a) a low-frequency musical or grunting murmur best heard between the left sternal border and the apex; (b) a soft, blowing early systolic murmur heard over the pulmonary area, associated with normal splitting of the second pulmonary sound. The chest x-ray and EKG should also be normal. (c) Venous hum: this high-pitched hum is usually heard on the right side over the superior cava but occasionally may be heard in the left intraclavicular region and confused with the continuous murmur of a patent ductus arteriosus. The hum changes with alterations in the position of the neck and may be obliterated by compressing the jugular veins.

Most innocent murmurs are of low-grade intensity, and they are never associated with other abnormalities such as thrills or cardiomegaly or with changes in the chest x-ray or EKG.

If there is any doubt about the patient's functional capacity have him walk up the hallway or some stairs or "mark time" in the office and observe for yourself the effects of exercise.

When the history and physical examination are completed, an anatomical diagnosis has usually been reached. The functional capacity of the patient has been assessed from both history and examination. In most cases, therefore, ancillary tests such as radiography and cardiac catheterization are used to confirm a diagnosis already made and to provide objective data of its severity.

Radiography

A full "cardiac series" should be taken on all patients at the first visit.

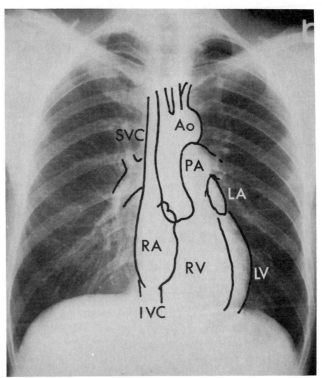

Figure 16–1 Normal AP chest film, with cardiac chambers outlined. SVC, superior vena cava. RA, right atrium. IVC, inferior vena cava. AO, aorta. PA, pulmonary artery. RV, right ventricle. LA, left atrium. LV, left ventricle.

This includes PA and lateral views of the chest, and PA, right and left oblique views after a barium swallow. Oblique views are not worth taking in children under two years of age. At subsequent visits a PA view may be all that is necessary to determine if the size of the heart has changed and to view both lung fields.

In order to interpret the cardiac findings in a chest x-ray, knowledge of normal anatomy is required (Fig. 16–1). Alteration in configuration of the cardiac shadow can then be interpreted with knowledge of the chamber involved. Some principles that influence the enlargement of cardiac chambers and the great vessels are important.

Cardiac Chambers

(1) Enlargement is more likely to be caused by increased intracavitary volume than by increased pressure. Increase in volume may be due to additional flow derived from an in-tracardiac shunt, retrograde flow secondary to valvular insufficiency or dilatation due to myocardial disease or failure.

(2) Myocardial hypertrophy may be considerable before the external dimensions of the heart are noticeably enlarged. Stenotic lesions, therefore, are not associated with great cardiac enlargement until failure induces ventricular dilatation.

(3) When valvular insufficiency is present the chamber immediately upstream is enlarged the most. If the insufficiency is of an atrioventricular valve, both upstream and downstream chambers are enlarged.

(4) When an intracardiac shunt is present, enlargement involves the downstream chamber and great vessel.

Great Vessels

The pulmonary vessels and aorta increase in size for three reasons: (1) increased intravascular volume (flow or congestion), (2) poststenotic dilatation and (3) intrinsic disease of the vessel walls. Pulmonary vessels may also be increased in number.

The size of a vessel is closely related to the flow within it. Because increased flow usually affects one or another of the cardiac chambers, isolated enlargement of the pulmonary artery or aorta is more likely to be due to poststenotic dilatation or localized disease than to increased flow. An increase in flow also enlarges distal vessels, such as the peripheral pulmonary vasculature.

Looking at a Chest Film

A good working system for looking at chest films is the assessment of the following factors in the order listed:[3]

(1) Check that the film is correctly viewed. Left stomach bubble and left cardiac apex — normal; right stomach bubble and right cardiac apex — situs inversus (dextrocardia); left stomach bubble and right cardiac apex — dextroversion.

(2) Survey the bony structure, looking for defects due to noncardiac disease as well as those associated with cardiovascular disease such as rib-notching.

(3) The overall size and localized enlargements of the cardiac shadow should be noted and interpreted according to their anatomical sites. A knowledge of the best view for evaluating enlargement of each chamber is important, because enlargement apparent in one view may be confirmed or refuted by appearances in another view (Table 16–1).

(4) The lung fields. Examine lung parenchyma, vascular patterns and extrapulmonary lesions such as effusions. The lung fields are best divided into upper, middle and lower thirds for comparison between both sides.

Evaluation of the pulmonary vessels should distinguish between vascular-

TABLE 16–1 Optimum Views for Cardiac X-ray

TARGET	BEST VIEWING ANGLE
Right Auricle	AP
Right Ventricle	RAO
	Lateral
Pulmonary Artery	AP
	Lateral
Left Auricle	AP (with barium)
	LAO (with Ba)
	Lateral (with Ba)
Left Ventricle	LAO
Aorta	
ascending	AP; LAO
arch	LAO
descending	LAO

LAO — left anterior oblique
RAO — right anterior oblique
AP — anteroposterior

ity (the number of vessels), perfusion (increased or decreased flow) and congestion (with associated signs of decompensation). Differences between central and peripheral vascular patterns are also important. Severe pulmonary hypertension, for instance, may be associated with large hilar vascular shadows but with attenuated, sparse peripheral shadows. In high flow, left-to-right shunts, however, enlargement of the vessels extends to the periphery.

Some changes are more obvious in upper than lower zones or vice versa. The "upturned mustache" effect, in which hilar vessels turn toward the upper lobes, is characteristic of mitral stenosis, but a large main pulmonary artery without peripheral enlargement suggests pulmonary valve stenosis.

Engorged lymphatics in the basal lobes are the basis for the so-called Kerley lines associated with pulmonary venous hypertension and failure.

Serial observations are essential. In the long-term follow-up of cardiac patients changes in the x-ray appearances may tell a story more graphically than the patient's words.

Electrocardiography

Few surgeons become expert at electrocardiographic interpretation and in most instances this is not necessary.

In the diagnosis and follow-up of operable heart disease features of the electrocardiogram most important to the surgeon are: (1) rhythm, (2) heart rate, (3) major defects in conduction, (4) evidence of ventricular hypertrophy, (5) evidence of acute ischemia, (6) changes associated with drugs such as digitalis and (7) evidence of electrolyte imbalance (Fig. 16–2).

Especially in congenital defects specific electrocardiographic changes are associated with certain lesions. Because left axis deviation is so unusual in young children, it is a finding of great significance. A severely cyanosed infant with left axis deviation almost certainly has tricuspid atresia. A child with left axis deviation and evidence of a left-to-right shunt at the atrial level has an endocardial cushion defect of some variety unless other evidence proves differently.

Evidence of ventricular hypertrophy confirms clinical evidence often obtained by other means. Postoperatively, diminution or disappearance of changes of ventricular or atrial hypertrophy is good evidence of a favorable result. If EKG changes do not fit with other clinical data, or re-evaluation of the situation is necessary, in patients with multiple valvular lesions the EKG may provide important evidence of ventricular preponderance.

Cardiac Catheterization: Angiocardiography

It is important that the cardiac surgeon be familiar with normal values obtained by cardiac catheterization, with methods for calculating cardiac output and vascular resistances, and with interpretation of data (Tables 16–2 and 16–3).

Catheterization

The following information is obtainable by cardiac catheterization:
(1) The presence, anatomical location, magnitude and direction of shunts.
(2) The presence, location and severity of valvular obstructive lesions.
(3) The presence, location and severity of valvular regurgitation.
(4) Cardiac output, vascular resistances and responses to stimuli such as exercise, hypoxia or drugs.

Angiocardiography

Cardiac catheterization determines changes in physiology, but angiocardiography outlines changes in anatomy, and it is the anatomy that the surgeon has to change in order to alter the physiology. Angiocardiography provides the following information:

(1) Evidence of the exact site of intraventricular obstructive lesions. Although catheterization may accurately locate an infundibular obstruction in the outflow tract of the right ventricle, only angiocardiography delineates the exact location, length and severity of the obstruction. It is from angiocardiographic appearances and not from pressure data that the surgeon can determine the technical difficulties involved in the operation.

(2) Evidence of valvular insufficiency. The assessment of mitral and tricuspid insufficiency from pressure tracings alone is not very accurate. A left or right ventricular injection of dye, however, may indicate the severity of the lesion.

Aortic insufficiency can similarly be evaluated, but because measurement of aortic diastolic pressure is such a good test for determining the degree of insufficiency, angiocardiography is not essential merely to diagnose this lesion.

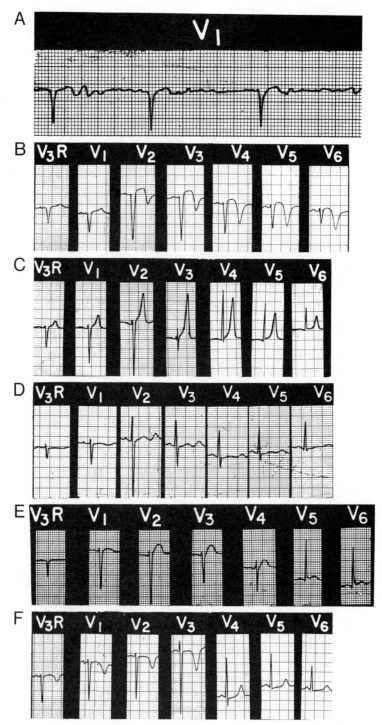

Figure 16-2   Examples of ST and T wave changes due to several causes. *A.* Digitalis effect with atrial fibrillation. *B.* Acute ischemia and infarction. *C.* Hyperkalemia. *D.* Hypokalemia. *E.* Hypercalcemia. *F.* Hypocalcemia.

TABLE 16–2   Normal Values for Intracardiac Pressures

| | Pressure (mmHg) | | |
	Systolic	Diastolic	Mean
Right atrium	3–7	−2 to +2	2–7
Right ventricle	15–30	0–7	
Pulmonary artery	15–30	5–15	10–20
Pulmonary wedge			5–12
Left atrium			4–12
Left ventricle	100–140	4–12	
Aorta	100–140	65–90	70–90

(3) Ventricular function and contractility can be accurately assessed from cineangiocardiograms. Knowledge of ventricular function is of great importance in cases of valvular disease, and when dyskinetic or akinetic areas are suspected in patients with coronary disease and postinfarction scars.

(4) Coronary arteriograms should probably be made in all patients in the "coronary age group," i.e., males above 35 and females above 45, regardless of the lesion for which they are being investigated. In patients being evaluated for coronary disease, good biplane cineangiograms are a *sine qua non*. In other patients, however, it may be of great importance to know whether the coronary vessels are normal. If a patient with severe aortic valvular stenosis has angina he may also have coronary disease and might be better off with both valve replacement and coronary bypass than with valve replacement alone. Before the advent of successful direct operations upon coronary arteries, knowledge of the state of the coronary vessels was important only in assessing the risks involved in an operation. But indications for coronary angiography in patients with primarily noncoronary lesions have now been widened, because if coronary lesions are discovered it may be possible to incorporate their treatment into the overall management of the patient.

Laboratory Examinations

The following tests should be made routinely on all cardiac patients: CBC, electrolytes, BUN, creatinine and urinalysis. Liver function tests are indi-

TABLE 16–3   Formulae for Calculating Common Parameters

Cardiac output (Fick method): $CO = \dfrac{O_2 \text{ consumption (ml/min)}}{\text{Systemic A–V } O_2 \text{ difference (vols. \%)}}$

Vascular resistance $(R) = \dfrac{\text{Pressure gradient}}{\text{Flow}}$

Pulmonary vascular resistance $= \dfrac{\text{Mean PA pressure–Mean LA pressure} \times 80}{\text{Pulmonary blood flow}}$

(Normal: under 3 units, or 240 dynes-sec/cm^5)

Systemic vascular resistance $= \dfrac{\text{Mean arterial pressure (mmHg)}}{\text{Cardiac output (L/min)}}$

(Normal: under 20 units, or 1600 dynes-sec/cm^5)

cated if there has been clinical suspicion of abnormal hepatic function.

Tests of coagulation are not normally necessary unless the patient has been receiving anticoagulants or if there has been a history of abnormal bleeding. Patients with severe cyanotic heart disease commonly have a variety of coagulation defects and should be appropriately investigated. The older the patient and the more severe the cyanosis, the greater the likelihood of a severe defect of coagulation[16]. If left uncorrected these defects may lead to severe and uncontrollable small vessel hemorrhage during operation and excessive and even fatal hemorrhage in the postoperative phase.

Medications

Medications most commonly received by patients before operation are digitalis, diuretics, potassium, propranolol, coronary vasodilators and anticoagulants.

Digitalis administration is stopped 48 hours before operation. If the patient has been receiving digoxin most will have been excreted within 48 hours. Digitoxin is a long-acting preparation and should be stopped three to four days before operation. Withdrawal of digitalis is important to avoid digitalis intoxication secondary to potassium fluxes that occur during extracorporeal bypass.

There is some uncertainty about the need to stop propranolol before operation. The hemodynamic effects of propranolol continue for about 36 hours after serum levels are negligible,[8] and, therefore, it may be advisable to withdraw propranolol about 48 hours before operation. However, several studies also indicate that, in coronary patients, continuation of propranolol up to and through operation can be carried out safely. The depressant hemodynamic effects seem to be more prolonged and more accentuated in children than in adults. Therefore, in

children propranolol should be stopped at least 48 hours, and preferably one week, before operation.

Anticoagulants are often given to patients with atrial fibrillation who may or may not have already suffered from peripheral emboli. There is no need to restore the prothrombin level to normal before operation, and too sudden a cessation of Coumadin anticoagulation may induce rebound hypercoagulability. Arrange the dosage so that the patient is admitted to hospital with a prothrombin time of 30 to 40 per cent of normal. Bleeding complications are rare if the prothrombin time is at this level.

There is no need to start antibiotic treatment before the patient is admitted to the hospital. Note any allergy to antibiotics so that agents can be chosen that will not induce reactions.

If the patient has focal infections of the urinary tract or oropharynx, time is saved by treating these on an outpatient basis before admission.

ASSESSING THE RISK

One of the most important decisions the cardiac surgeon has to make is the determination of the point reached by the patient on the natural history curve of his defect. Diagnosis is often simple. No unique skill is required to diagnose aortic insufficiency, but great judgment may be necessary to decide the correct time for operation. Numerous factors must be taken into account in assessing the risk in each case.

Congenital Heart Disease

Different factors are important at different stages of childhood. In general, children either require operation in infancy because the severity of the defect is causing crippling and life-threatening hemodynamic difficulty, or operation can be safely delayed for several years until the child is older.

In small infants, the following factors increase the risk of operation: pulmonary hypertension, severe cyanosis, prematurity, superimposed respiratory complications and additional severe congenital defects.

Obviously the risk is greater with a severe than with a less severe defect, but even patients with severe defects can be operated upon with an acceptable risk if operation results in a radical improvement in hemodynamics. An infant in congestive failure with a large patent ductus arteriosus may be transformed almost immediately by closing the ductus. The operation, in this instance, results in rapid, total hemodynamic cure. On the other hand, a child with severe but reversible pulmonary hypertension may have a stormy postoperative course and prolonged convalescence until the pulmonary vascular changes recede.

During the past few years, great improvements have occurred in results of definitive operations on infants. The use of profound hypothermia and circulatory arrest permits a precision of operative technique not previously obtainable. Improvements in postoperative care, especially respiratory support, have decreased postoperative mortality and morbidity.

There is an increasing tendency toward early definitive repair of most defects. It used to be thought that an early palliative operation, for complicated defects, followed by later total repair was the optimal course of action. This is no longer thought to be so. Many defects can be safely repaired at an early age.

Tetralogy of Fallot has been repaired with a mortality rate under 10 per cent, under the age of one year. Ventricular septal defects that are symptomatic can also be repaired with a low mortality rate after six months of age. There may still be a place for pulmonary artery banding in infants under six months of age.

The presence of pulmonary hypertension adversely affects the outlook in many defects. Severe, fixed pulmonary hypertension, unresponsive to oxygen or Priscoline and in excess of 10 units, is almost always an absolute contraindication to surgery. The greater the pulmonary hypertension, and the less reactive the pulmonary bed, the greater the risk of operation. In transposition of the great vessels, fixed pulmonary hypertension is almost always present by two years of age, and corrective operations for this lesion should always be done before this age.

Reactive pulmonary hypertension may not always revert to normal after operation.

Congestive failure is not necessarily a bad prognostic factor, provided that failure is not due to myocarditis, endocardial fibrosis or irreversible pulmonary hypertension. When failure is secondary to a mechanical problem such as a stenotic valve that can be restored to normal function by an operation, the outlook is good. In young patients with multiple rheumatic valvular lesions, assessment of the relative importance of myocardial and mechanical valvular factors is very difficult. Measurement of pressures such as the left ventricular end-diastolic indicates at best only the current functional capacity of the left ventricle. These measurements do not indicate the ability of the ventricle to recover once the valvular lesion has been repaired. In young patients, fortunately, if a severe valvular lesion exists some improvement can be expected after repair even if myocardial disease also exists.

Congenital heart disease is occasionally encountered in adults, either because the diagnosis has been missed earlier or because a palliative operation was done in early life. The commonest exception to these examples is the middle-aged patient with calcific aortic stenosis discovered at operation to have a bicuspid aortic valve. In general, the risks of correcting congenital lesions in adults are not high, unless there are fixed pulmonary changes or there has been severe impairment of ventricular function.[1]

Down's syndrome and other forms of mental deficiency are commonly associated with congenital heart disease. The decision whether or not operation should be carried out in such children involves an assessment of the incapacity due to the mental deficiency, the severity of the cardiac defect, the risks involved and the overall improvement anticipated in the child's condition and ability to look after himself, enjoy life and benefit from remedial training. The wishes of the parents are paramount. The author's personal opinion is that few children with mental deficiency should be denied operation, especially if the risks involved are reasonably low. If the quality of the child's life might be improved by increasing his physical capabilities, then operation would seem to be entirely justified.

Acquired Heart Disease

Several factors are common to the assessment of patients with acquired heart disease, among them the relative importance of valvular malfunction and myocardial disease. If the primary problem is a mechanically poor valve and the myocardium seems to be strong, then a good result can be anticipated and the mortality rate should not be high (Table 16–4). If several valves are involved the risk increases, mainly because of associated myocardial disease with chronic congestive failure, complicated drug therapy and coexisting pulmonary problems.

Patients with stenotic lesions are often more improved by operation than those with valvular insufficiency. The reasons for this are not entirely clear. The heart is usually smaller in patients with valvular stenosis than in those with regurgitation. Increased volume loads due to regurgitation may

TABLE 16–4 Mortality After Operation*

Aortic valve replacement	3–8%
Mitral valve replacement	3–8%
Multiple valve replacement	8–25%
Open mitral commissurotomy	1–2%
Coronary bypass:	
Good LV function	<5%
Bad LV function	5–30%

*Rates based upon published figures.

result in greater myocardial stretching and subsequent fibrosis than do pressure loads. Regardless of the causes, heart size in patients with regurgitation will decrease neither as rapidly nor as completely as in those with valvular stenosis.

The New York Heart Association classification of functional severity is a useful index by which to classify patients to be operated upon, but it is not necessarily a prognostic indication of how patients will fare after operation. Patients in Class I should probably never be operated upon. Patients in Class II may be operated upon under some circumstances and those in Classes III and IV are almost by definition candidates for operation. Some of the most dramatic results are obtained in patients in Class IV, perhaps because they have the greatest reasons for improvement.

Very few patients should now be regarded as inoperable. Severe congestive failure per se is not a contraindication. Massive cardiomegaly with clearcut evidence of mild valvular disease but severe myocardial dysfunction or very severe renal, hepatic or pulmonary disease may suggest that the lesion is inoperable. Every surgeon can nevertheless point to individual patients in whom these conditions existed and who were helped by operation. The prospect for such patients without operation is universally grim.

Renal function should always be assessed preoperatively. If the BUN is normal and urinalysis does not indicate infection or proteinuria, no further investigation is necessary. If the BUN and creatinine are elevated and creatinine clearance is depressed, the risk of renal dysfunction postoperatively is increased. If these changes seem to be on the basis of chronic congestion rather than primary renal parenchymal disease, the prospect for improvement after operation is good. Primary renal disease cannot be expected to improve and may impose a significant risk during the immediate postoperative phase. Once the initial recovery phase has been reached the period of risk has usually passed.

Hepatic function is sometimes depressed by chronic congestive failure. Improvement of congestive failure after operation may result in a similar improvement in hepatic function. During the postoperative period, when the products of hemolysis secondary to perfusion must be effectively handled by the reticuloendothelial system, pre-existing diminution of hepatic function may contribute to temporary postoperative jaundice.

In patients with suspected hepatic dysfunction, defects of coagulation should be sought and corrected if found.

Respiratory disease often accompanies cardiac disease and in most cases is secondary to it. Patients with independent chronic obstructive respiratory disease must be very carefully evaluated by pulmonary function tests. Even severe respiratory disease may be tolerated during the postoperative phase with the aid of respirators; and correction of cardiac defects, especially those contributing to pulmonary congestion or hypertension, may greatly improve the overall respiratory state. However, severe obstructive respiratory disease considerably increases the risks of operation.

Previous embolic episodes may be both an indication for operation and a source of added risk. About 50 per cent of patients with previous emboli are found at operation to have an intra-atrial clot that can be the origin of intraoperative emboli or, if inadequately removed, the propagating point for later emboli. Recognition of this danger also decreases it, because intraoperative techniques should prevent dissemination of emboli.

If a patient is hemiplegic there is a slightly increased risk of postoperative pulmonary complications because the cough of these patients is not as strong as is normal. Aphasia may present some nursing problems and details of pre- and postoperative care should be explained in great detail to aphasic patients, since their disability isolates them from those who attend them.

Neurological problems should be carefully noted before operation because neurological complications of open cardiac surgery are not unknown, and if the preoperative state is not noted, postoperative problems may be difficult to evaluate.

Other associated diseases are occasionally encountered. Diabetes of moderate severity does not impose any great problem. Severe diabetes associated with diminished renal function obviously adds to the risks, but under these circumstances the real question is whether cardiac disease or diabetes poses the greater threat to the patient's life.

Gout is not uncommon in association with valvular disease. The commonest complication of this association is an acute flare-up after operation, and the patient should be warned that this may occur.

Marie-Strümpell's ankylosing spondylitis is sometimes associated with valvular disease. The patient with a rigid spinal column and no movement of the thoracic cage is particularly liable to pulmonary complications. The ribs, however, can be retracted without difficulty through a midline sternotomy.

Hematological diseases such as

thrombocytopenia or chronic leukemia present special problems. Any hematological disease that might affect coagulation must be fully investigated and, if possible, corrected before a cardiac operation is contemplated. Chronic leukemia is not a contraindication to operation, but platelet dysfunction is common in these patients and their ability to clot properly must be assured.

TRICUSPID DISEASE. Of all valvular lesions this is perhaps the most difficult to assess. Clinical examination is helpful if there is obvious venous pulsation in the neck, distinct murmurs, hepatomegaly and peripheral edema. In approximately one-third of patients who require tricuspid valve replacement there is no preoperative evidence of significant disease.

Hemodynamic measurements made at cardiac catheterization are often undiagnostic. Cardioangiography with injection of dye into the right ventricle will confirm the presence of tricuspid regurgitation. But because the catheter must pass through the tricuspid valve, false positives are not uncommon. Isolated tricuspid disease is uncommon and the overwhelming clinical picture may be that of the associated aortic or mitral disease. The surgeon's finger at the time of operation probably remains the best means for evaluating tricuspid function.

Severe tricuspid disease may cause persistent hepatic dysfunction, ascites and peripheral edema. If the operation is postponed until these have been fully compensated, there may be unnecessary delay. A reasonable period of bedrest and preoperative therapy is advisable, but as soon as improvement has reached a recognizable plateau, operation should be carried out.

Tricuspid valves seldom need to be replaced, as either the annuloplasty of deVega or the ring annuloplasty of Carpentier appear to be superior operations.[2, 5] The necessity for tricuspid repair, in addition to prosthetic replacement of either aortic or mitral

valve, adds considerably to the rate of mortality. This is not because tricuspid repair is so dangerous but is a reflection of overall cardiac decompensation if tricuspid repair is necessary.

MITRAL DISEASE. More surgical experience has been gained with the treatment of mitral stenosis than with any other valvular disease. During the past decade there have been changes both in the surgical approach to this problem and in the nature of the problem itself. Whereas the early experience with mitral stenosis was with closed commissurotomy in young patients, present experience is with open operations on older patients.

Patients in Class I do not require operation. They will usually live for many years without disability. As soon as symptoms develop and the patient moves into Class II, operation should be seriously considered. One of the genuine tragedies of medicine is the young woman with mitral stenosis who suddenly develops atrial fibrillation, cerebral embolism and hemiplegia. Recognition, therefore, is necessary not only of the diagnosis but of the phases of danger. As the patient approaches 40, atrial fibrillation with attendant dangers of embolism becomes more likely. Once atrial fibrillation is established, embolism is a constant danger that can be ameliorated by relief of the stenosis.

In most instances mitral stenosis can be treated by open mitral commissurotomy. But even if the valve is flexible and a good result is obtained, the operation should be regarded as palliative. Continued abnormal flow and turbulence result in slowly progressive re-stenosis, and the process is not due to continuing rheumatic activity.

Valve replacement is reserved for patients with accompanying insufficiency, calcified valves or extreme degrees of fibrosis and subvalvular contraction of chordae and papillary muscles. The choice of valve is still a matter for individual preference because no single technique has been shown to be unequivocally superior to all others. Operative mortality for isolated mitral replacement is about 5 per cent in most centers, although higher and lower figures are also quoted. The postoperative embolic rate has been reduced to less than 5 per cent with recent prosthetic valves. This major reduction in embolic rates in the past few years has been due to changes in valve design. Because embolic episodes are no longer such a major complication, the real issue in the choice between a synthetic prosthetic valve and a tissue valve now revolves around the relative stability and longevity of the different types of valve.

Valvuloplasty for mitral insufficiency can be a very effective operation when the valve is not calcified and is still mobile. Valve replacement is necessary in all other cases of mitral insufficiency.

Although functional results as measured by improvement in symptoms are good after mitral valve replacement, objective data obtained at postoperative catheterization often show residual gradients across prosthetic valves which increase with exercise. Pulmonary hypertension and vascular resistance decrease so that at rest they are at approximately the upper limit of normal, but with exercise both pressure and resistance increase. There is often no correlation between improvement in symptoms and objective data, and patients with persistent severe pulmonary hypertension are sometimes dramatically improved and able to resume activities long since given up. The scientist worries about the objective data, but let us not forget that the patient is more concerned with his symptoms.

AORTIC VALVE DISEASE. Of all acquired valvular defects aortic stenosis is perhaps the most satisfactory to treat. Patients with severe symptoms and congestive failure preoperatively improve rapidly after operation: heart size comes down even before the patient leaves the hospital and exercise capabilities are restored even to patients in their late sixties and seventies.

How severe should aortic stenosis be before operation is warranted? Several factors must be considered: symptoms such as angina or syncope make operation a fairly urgent necessity. Operation should be advised if the gradient is greater than 50 mmHg at rest and rises with exercise. If the cardiac index is much below normal a lesser gradient may be significant. But in most instances valves with a gradient of about 30 mmHg have remarkably few pathological changes except for some thickening of the cusps and a few millimeters of fusion at the commissures. Although this fusion can be relieved it is not worth subjecting a patient to a major operation to do so little. If this grade of aortic stenosis coexists with another valvular lesion that demands operation it is worthwhile to look at the aortic valve at the same time and relieve whatever stenosis exists.

Left ventricular end diastolic pressure (LVEDP) is an important index of ventricular function and suggests myocardial dysfunction if elevated above 15 mmHg. If the LVEDP is very high, the cardiac index low and the gradient moderate, myocardial fibrosis may be severe. The risk of operation is increased and the final result may be poor. Electrocardiographic evidence of left ventricular strain or periinfarction block is also a bad prognostic sign. The presence of these electrocardiographic changes has been held to be a contraindication to operation because of the high mortality rate that is associated. This has not been our experience, but postoperative difficulties, arrhythmias and failure may be expected more frequently in these patients than in those with more normal electrocardiograms.

After a patient with aortic stenosis becomes symptomatic, death ensues in three to five years. Therefore, the onset of symptoms is an indication that operation should be carried out with reasonable urgency. Although sudden death has often been thought to be a major feature of aortic stenosis, congestive failure is more commonly the terminal event.

All patients with aortic stenosis should have selective coronary arteriograms before operation to distinguish between angina due to the valvular disease and that due to coronary arterial disease. If both diseases are present they may both be treated at the same operation with valve replacement and saphenous vein bypass of the stenotic coronary artery.

Patients with aortic insufficiency have a different natural history pattern from those with aortic stenosis. Whereas those with stenosis are usually in their fifties before symptoms develop, patients with insufficiency are commonly in their thirties when dyspnea on exertion, nocturnal dyspnea and congestive failure become manifest.

The optimal moment for operation is more difficult to decide in patients with aortic insufficiency than in those with stenosis. Some patients with aortic insufficiency and huge hearts with a wide-open valve are capable of considerable physical exertion, to an extent quite beyond the usual expectation. After symptoms develop, about five to seven years elapse before death.[14] Therefore, although the development of symptoms is an ominous sign, there is no extreme urgency in advising operation. It is presumed that ventricular fibrosis is likely to develop progressively in patients with large hearts and, since it is irreversible, it diminishes the result of the operation. For this reason operation is usually advised soon after patients become symptomatic. Age should be taken into consideration, for an asymptomatic patient in his twenties with free insufficiency probably has almost a decade before him without symptoms. A man in his early forties is likely to develop

symptoms within a short span of time.

Diastolic pressure measured by a sphygmomanometer is as good an indication as any of the severity of insufficiency. If the diastolic pressure is greater than 60 mmHg, insufficiency is mild; between 50 and 60 mmHg it is moderate; and below 50 mmHg it is severe. It is important to notice the heart rate when diastolic pressure is measured. If the rate is rapid, the diastolic pressure will not be as low as when the rate is slow, and the functional severity of the insufficiency may be underestimated.

Heart size, left ventricular end diastolic pressure, cardiac index, evidence of pulmonary congestion and severity of symptoms must be taken into consideration in deciding about operation.

CORONARY ARTERY DISEASE. There are four results of coronary atherosclerosis for which operation may be necessary: (a) occlusion, partial or total, of one or more coronary vessels; (b) postinfarction scars and left ventricular aneurysm; (c) postinfarction intracardiac defects such as ventricular septal defect or papillary muscle dysfunction and mitral insufficiency; and (d) conduction defects requiring insertion of a pacemaker.

It is now accepted that coronary bypass surgery is an effective palliative technique for the relief of angina and also increases longevity. The prime indication for operation is severe angina unresponsive to energetic medical management. Nonoperative management should include treatment with nitroglycerine, long-acting nitrates, and Inderal. "Risk factors" should be controlled both before and after operation; dietary modification, cessation of smoking, control of hypertension and weight reduction are all part of a complete medical regimen. Only control of hypertension is likely to have an immediate effect on angina.

A definition of severe angina obviously varies from patient to patient, depending upon age, functional aspirations and occupation. Assuming acknowledgement of these factors, everyone with incapacitating angina should have coronary angiography. It is from the combination of history and clinical findings and results of angiography that the final decision is made.

Lesions that demand surgery are (1) obstructions involving the left main coronary artery, (2) severe (>70 per cent) left anterior descending lesions, (3) lesions separately involving LAD and circumflex systems, (4) multiple lesions of all vessels, with satisfactory distal arteries suitable for grafting and (5) good left ventricular function in combination with the indications listed above.

Lesions for which the results of operation are not so good and for which the indications are therefore, weaker are (1) diffuse multiple lesions with poor "run-off" and inadequate sites for grafting, (2) diffusely poor akinetic left ventricle and (3) diffuse disease in diabetic females.

Isolated obstruction of the right coronary system rarely, if ever, warrants operation, unless angina is very severe and the right arterial obstruction is the only visible cause of the problem.

Left ventricular function, more than any other single factor, influences operative mortality and final outcome.[4] With good left ventricular function operative mortality is around 3 per cent, even if many vessels have to be grafted.[15] The worse the function of the left ventricle, the higher the mortality rate, even as high as 25 to 30 per cent. With improved techniques for intraoperative myocardial preservation, including deep hypothermia and hyperkalemic, hypothermic arrest — as opposed to normothermic ischemic arrest or induced fibrillation — the results of operation on these high-risk patients have improved. The simplest index of left ventricular function is ejection fraction (EF). If the ejection fraction is >40 per cent mortality will be low; if EF <20 per cent mortality will be high. (A similar correlation also obtains in valvular disease.)

Risks must always be assessed against potential results. Total relief of angina can be expected in 70 to 80 per cent of patients, partial relief in 10 to 15 per cent and no change or worsening in the remainder. Prolonged graft patency occurs in 75 per cent of vein grafts and 95 per cent of internal mammary grafts. Grafts that are patent one year after operation are likely to remain open for several years.

Evidence is now available from several sources that patients live longer after bypass operations than do patients with similar disease without operation. Isom[17] reported 88 per cent survival (including operative deaths) five years after operation, compared with 65 per cent survival without operation in patients with two-vessel disease, and only 45 per cent survival in those with triple-vessel disease. After five years 80 per cent of those operated on remained free of further infarction.

In patients with postinfarction scars and ventricular aneurysm the most important indication for operation is congestive failure. Cardiac catheterization and left ventricular angiography should be used to confirm the diagnosis and to demonstrate the extent of dynamic impairment. Failure of an aneurysm to fill with dye may be due to clot. A large area of paradoxical expansion is always associated with reduced cardiac output. Coronary angiograms should be made because vein bypass may be necessary to improve function of the healing left ventricle. An occasional patient may require operation because of repeated peripheral embolism arising from clot within an aneurysm.

Similar indications obtain in patients with postinfarction ventricular septal defects or papillary muscle dysfunction. The extent of failure and all other hemodynamic data must be fully assessed. Operation is indicated solely to cure the physiological disability and not to deal with the anatomical lesion alone.

Talking to the Patient

It is essential both morally and legally that the surgeon talk with the patient and explain what is advised, why it is advised and what may be expected. Many cardiac operations on children are prophylactic — closure of a secundum atrial septal defect or a small ventricular septal defect, for example — and parents are entitled to a frank discussion of the need for an operation. It would be easy to tell a parent that the child has a "hole in the heart" and *must* have an operation. In many instances a defect may be present, but there is no urgency about operation, and operation should be arranged when financial, social and other factors are convenient.

Questions that patients ask fall into several categories. First, they want to know what is wrong with them, why an operation is necessary and what the risks are. The answers should be forthright and as complete as the background of the patient will permit. Second, they want to know what to expect, where the incision will be, how long the operation will take, how long they will be in hospital, how long the convalescence will be and the details of postoperative diet, drugs and activities. Some patients have strange ideas about the technical aspects of cardiac surgery, and it is surprising how many patients believe that the heart is totally removed from the body, repaired and returned to its original site. Third, the patient will want to know about the financial cost. Crippled Children's Services and other agencies pay for the care of many patients, but it is advisable to have someone in the admissions office who is conversant with the costs of cardiac surgery and the helping agencies available to plan with the patient how best to deal with these problems.

Except for details of postoperative convalescent care all these questions should be answered before the patient is admitted. For several years, all cardiac surgical patients admitted to the University of Colorado Medical Center have received an explanatory booklet which also serves as notice of admission. Similar explanatory booklets or sheets are easily made up to answer local needs.

Before the patient leaves the hospital, detailed explanations of expected progress, diet to be followed and drug regimens should be given. This may best be done by a suitably trained nurse. If the patient is to receive anticoagulants, very specific and perhaps even written instructions should be provided, emphasizing the dangers of excessive and inadequate therapy and the need for laboratory control.

POSTOPERATIVE EVALUATION

Details of postoperative follow-up vary with each patient and each lesion, but certain principles can be followed in assessing how well a patient is recovering from the operation.

Functional Progress

By the time the patient leaves hospital he is on his feet most of the day and capable of looking after all personal needs. Thereafter, progress depends upon his own efforts as well as physiological recovery. It is impossible to detail exactly what every patient may or may not do. Recovery from a cardiac operation is similar to retraining an athlete — progressive, acceptable and tolerable activity is desirable. Whatever the patient can do without undue tiredness, pain or shortness of breath is acceptable. Between four to six weeks after operation the patient should be back to full activity. Patients with prosthetic valves should be warned against undue activity for three months in order that complete healing and fixation of the valve may take place before it is subjected to the tachycardia and increased blood pressure of exertion.

Few patients discuss the resumption of sexual activity, but provided that reasonable exercise capability has been achieved there is no reason why sex should not be resumed.

The patient's achievement in resuming and improving upon preoperative exercise tolerance is probably the best single sign of satisfactory progress. If the patient has been asymptomatic before operation total resumption of activity must be aimed at. The greater the disablement before operation the greater the possible improvement. Questioning of patients must be detailed and as objective as possible to evaluate improvement in exercise tolerance. Patients sometimes feel that they should always report improvement so as not to disappoint their doctor. This otherwise praiseworthy attitude should not deceive the physician. Return of symptoms and a decrease in exercise tolerance after a period of improvement should always be regarded as an ominous sign. If operation has involved closure of a shunt, it should be determined whether the shunt has reopened; if a prosthetic valve has been used, other signs of valve dysfunction should be looked for.*

Physical Findings

During routine postoperative examination the following points should be noted:

Wound

The wound should be well healed, without infection or keloid formation, and painless. The midline sternotomy

---

*See page 739, Syndromes of prosthetic valve failure.

wound is notorious for poor healing with a broad scar or the development of keloids. Midline epigastric herniae occasionally develop at the lower end of a midline sternotomy where the linea alba has been divided. Wire sutures may become prominent and painful, especially in thin patients. If sufficient time has elapsed for the sternum to heal and a wire suture causes discomfort, it should be removed.

Cardiovascular System

Examination is carried out in the routine manner and is a comparison between pre- and postoperative features. After a successful operation, congestive failure should have disappeared or diminished, cardiac action should be quieter and palpable evidence of ventricular hypertrophy should decrease. Changes in murmurs must be correlated with what is anticipated. After relief of pulmonary valvular stenosis, for instance, the murmur is always still present, although often of a more vibratory character. Patients with prosthetic aortic valves all have a short systolic murmur. However, in addition to listening for the expected, listen also for the unexpected, the signs that tell of trouble. Redevelopment of murmurs that had previously disappeared, the appearance of new murmurs or changes in character or intensity of murmurs that have been long present should always arouse suspicion. The disappearance of a murmur caused by a surgically induced shunt is equally ominous. If fever is present the important question is whether or not the patient has endocarditis. Malaise, anemia, petechial hemorrhages, splenomegaly, changing murmurs and newly developed congestive failure point to infectious endocarditis. A sense of reasonable well-being in spite of the fever, pericardial rub or pleural effusion, lymphocytosis and splenomegaly suggest that the patient has a postcardiotomy syndrome.

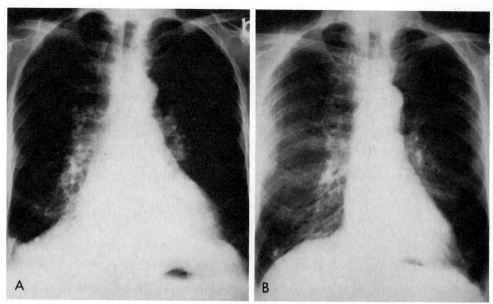

Figure 16–3 Preoperative (*A*) and postoperative (*B*) chest x-rays of a patient with aortic stenosis. A gradient of 167 mmHg was present across the aortic valve before replacement by a ball valve. Film *B* was taken four months after operation.

Radiologic Evidence

Heart Size

Reduction in heart size may be anticipated after most operations (Fig. 16–3). The few exceptions include cases in which heart size has been normal to start with, and in a few lesions such as tetralogy of Fallot in which heart size increases after operation. After operation for stenotic lesions heart size tends to come down more rapidly and completely than after operation upon regurgitant lesions.

After a left-to-right shunt has been closed, heart size should decrease within a few weeks. Persistence of cardiomegaly suggests that closure of the defect has been incomplete.

Pulmonary Vascularity

When pulmonary vascularity has been increased before operation and the cause has been completely eliminated by operation, vascular patterns return to normal within three months.

Although flow through the lungs is acutely restored to normal by the operation the vessels still remain large and it takes time for them to respond to the diminished flow by a decrease in size. Persistently increased vascularity for more than three months after operation may be regarded as evidence of incomplete closure or reopening of the defect. If vascularity increases after a period of diminution, reopening of the defect must be suspected.

In those defects in which diminished pulmonary vascularity is present preoperatively, an increase in vascular patterns is apparent immediately after operation and remains unchanged. An excessive increase in vascularity raises the suspicion that a right-to-left shunt has been converted into a left-to-right shunt by breakdown of the repair.

Electrocardiographic Evidence

Electrocardiographic evidence of ventricular hypertrophy recedes after a successful operation (Fig. 16–4). The interval during which recession may

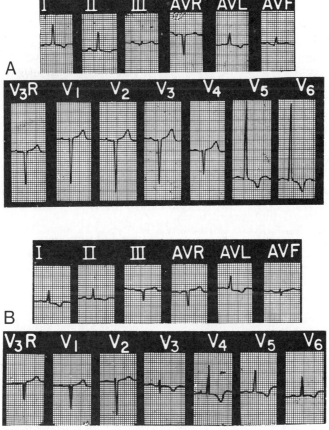

Figure 16–4 Electrocardiographic evidence of regression of left ventricular hypertrophy within eight months of replacement of a stenotic aortic valve. *A*. Before operation. *B*. Eight months after operation.

be anticipated varies with the degree of hypertrophy, but signs of left ventricular hypertrophy may begin to diminish within two weeks after successful replacement of the aortic valve for aortic stenosis.

Conduction defects of the right bundle are constantly present after right ventriculotomy and are related to incision of the anterior wall of the right ventricle. This abnormality does not alter the prognosis.

Other arrhythmias and conduction defects commonly seen are atrial fibrillation and flutter, nodal rhythms, premature ventricular contractions and, occasionally, complete heart block.

The arrhythmia is most often related to the underlying pathology. But elec-

trolyte abnormalities or digitalis toxicity should be sought.

Complete heart block is almost invariably iatrogenic and is present from the moment of operation. In rare cases, complete heart block can revert to normal sinus rhythm many years after operation. This is a happy exception to the rule that if complete heart block is present when the patient leaves hospital it must be regarded as permanent and treated accordingly.

Laboratory Examinations

Blood Counts

Routine blood counts are made at the first two or three postoperative visits and thereafter if there are indications such as fever or anemia.

During the first week to ten days after an operation involving extracorporeal circulation the hematocrit falls to 30 to 32 per cent because the generation of cells circulated through the pump has a shorter life span than normal. Within a month after operation the hematocrit should be back to normal. If the hematocrit is not normal by this time a source of bleeding or hemolysis is sought.

The development of anemia months or years after operation is always a source of concern. If the patient has a prosthetic valve, hemolysis must be suspected (see page 739). A combination of fever with anemia raises the possibility of bacterial endocarditis. An iron deficiency anemia is probably due to chronic blood loss; therefore, it should be remembered that patients with prosthetic cardiac valves are not immune to peptic ulcer or carcinoma of the colon. Look for the usual causes of anemia.

Biochemical Tests

Routine electrolyte examinations are rarely necessary as part of the follow-up examination. By the time a patient leaves the hospital he should be in electrolyte balance. If prolonged treatment with digitalis and diuretics is necessary, periodic measurement of serum potassium is important to ensure that potassium supplementation is adequate.

In some patients with preoperative impaired renal function the BUN becomes elevated after operation. Renal function may take several weeks to return completely to normal and an elevation of BUN a month after operation is not necessarily a sign of permanent renal damage.

If liver function has been depressed before or after operation, standard tests of function are necessary to confirm that improvement has occurred.

Hemolysis

Hemolysis is a possibility in several situations after cardiac surgery. Any situation in which a leak may occur around or through a valve or intracardiac patch may give rise to hemolysis. Mild jaundice and anemia are the clues. A falling hematocrit not responding to iron or transfusion and an elevated bilirubin provide objective data. Plasma hemoglobin and haptoglobin levels, an elevated reticulocyte count and a shortened red cell life confirm the clinical diagnosis.

Drug Therapy

Cardiac Drugs

DIGITALIS GLYCOSIDES. The most important function of these is their positive inotropic action. Systolic contractile force and cardiac output are increased and the Starling curve relating left ventricular stroke work to left atrial filling pressure moves upwards and to the left (Fig. 16–5). Stroke volume is increased and elevated ventricular end-diastolic pressure is restored

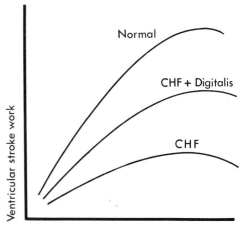

Figure 16–5 The effect of digitalis on the Starling curve is shown. Cardiac function, depressed in congestive failure, is improved by digitalis, but is not restored to normal.

to normal. The heart rate is slowed, especially in patients with congestive failure. This slowing in rate may be not so much a primary action of the drug as a secondary effect of the increase in cardiac output. If there is atrial fibrillation, the frequency of signals from the atrium to the A-V node is so great that many impulses are extinguished within the node. The frequency of ventricular response depends upon the refractory period of the A-V node. Digitalis prolongs the refractory period so that a greater number of atrial signals fail to pass through the A-V node, and the ventricular response becomes slower. Vagal activity is increased, slowing ventricular response.

Digitalis also has important peripheral actions. In normal subjects digitalis induces arteriolar and venous constriction. In patients with congestive failure the opposite occurs and there is an indirect vasodilator action. There is also a shift in pooled blood from the portal to the systemic venous bed.

Salutary effects are produced by digitalis in patients with heart disease but without failure. The stress of a chronic pressure load is withstood better by a digitalized myocardium, and with improvement in contractile force the necessity for increased sympathetic tone is reduced. Systemic and pulmonary venous pressures are reduced and symptoms are proportionately alleviated.

The effect of digitalis is in proportion to the dosage. A small effect is achieved by a small dose, and maximal effect is obtained by the maximum tolerable dose.

The effects of digitalis are influenced by several factors, including electrolyte levels (especially potassium), endocrine hormonal actions and other drugs. High serum potassium levels diminish the inotropic effect of digitalis but also reduce the incidence of toxic arrhythmias. Low potassium levels do not affect the inotropism of digitalis, but a low serum potassium, by itself, increases myocardial contractile force.

The electrocardiographic effects of digitalis are characteristic. The earliest effect is a sagging depression of the S–T segment. As digitalis action increases, S–T depression becomes more marked, heart rate slows and the P–R interval is prolonged. If toxicity develops, multiple ventricular extrasystoles, pulsus bigeminus and various degrees of heart block may appear.

The cardiac glycosides are all toxic and the margin between therapeutic effect and toxicity is quite narrow. If a rapidly metabolized agent such as digoxin is used, toxic manifestations should disappear within 12 hours of the last administration of the drug, but if a long-acting agent such as digitoxin is used, toxic effects will persist.

The common symptoms of toxicity are:

Gastrointestinal — anorexia, nausea, vomiting, abdominal discomfort, diarrhea. Anorexia and nausea usually appear first, and early digitalis toxicity should be suspected in any patient receiving a maintenance dosage who suddenly loses appetite and becomes nauseated.

Cardiac — changes in rate, rhythm and conduction. Ventricular extrasystoles, pulsus bigeminus, paroxysmal tachycardia, bradycardia and, in extreme cases, ventricular tachycardia and fibrillation. Any of these changes should be taken as an indication of toxicity and treated accordingly.

Miscellaneous systemic effects — headache, visual disturbances, skin rashes and eosinophilia have all been reported. With the exception of headache these symptoms are uncommon.

When a patient develops signs and symptoms of digitalis toxicity four steps must be taken: (a) stop all further doses, (b) measure serum electrolytes, (c) obtain a new EKG trace and (d) measure the serum level of digitalis. If the potassium concentration is low, supplementary potassium should be given. If the primary manifestation of toxicity is a cardiac arrhythmia, extra potassium may have to be given intravenously. A dose of 3.0–5.0 mEq given slowly IV may immediately stop a bigeminal rhythm or multiple extrasystoles. Even if the serum potassium concentration seems to be within normal limits, intracellular levels may be low, and a small dose of potassium given intravenously may be very beneficial without changing the plasma concentration to a measurable extent.

Antiarrhythmic drugs, quinidine, procaine amide, lidocaine and propranolol may be used when severe digitalis toxicity leads to dangerous supraventricular and ventricular arrhythmias. Great care must be taken in their use because of their propensity to lower cardiac output. Phenytoin is useful in the conversion of digitalis-induced supraventricular and ventricular arrhythmias to normal sinus rhythm with very little concomitant reduction in cardiac output.

Patients treated chronically with digitalis and diuretics should receive oral potassium supplements (15 mEq one to three times a day). Potassium should not be given to patients with seriously impaired renal function.

DIGITALIS PREPARATIONS. There are many different preparations available. The commonest in use are:

Digoxin for oral, IM or IV use. Loading dose is 1.0–1.5 mg in divided doses over 24 hours; maintenance dose by mouth is 0.25–0.50 mg per day. Digoxin begins to act within one hour of intravenous administration and within a few hours of an oral dose. Excretion is quite rapid and most of its effectiveness disappears within 48 hours of stopping administration.

Digitoxin (U.S.P.). This is a very potent, slow-acting preparation. The dose is 0.6 mg IV, followed by 0.2–0.4 mg every 4 to 6 hours for a total dose of 1.2 mg. Oral dosage is 0.6 mg twice at 12-hour intervals, then 0.1–0.2 mg per day. After intravenous administration 6 to 10 hours are necessary before its

effect begins. After stopping chronic usage, 2 to 3 weeks may elapse before complete regression of action and disappearance of blood levels.

ANTIARRHYTHMIC DRUGS. Several drugs are used specifically for their antiarrhythmic actions. Other drugs such as potassium have isolated usefulness in the treatment of specialized arrhythmias. The most commonly used antiarrhythmic drugs are described below.

Quinidine. Like many antiarrhythmic drugs, quinidine increases the refractory period of cardiac muscle, decreases excitability and slows conduction. The drug is absorbed rapidly by mouth. About 15 per cent is excreted and the rest is metabolized. Use of quinidine is indicated for the conversion of atrial fibrillation or flutter and ventricular and nodal tachycardias to normal rhythm. It is useful in the suppression of frequent premature beats. A test dose of 100–200 mgm should be given before starting doses of 200 mgm every four to six hours. The dose is increased daily to 400 mgm and then to 600 mgm every six hours, to a maximum of 600 mgm every two hours for five doses. Toxic effects (cinchonism) include vertigo, headache and tinnitus. Hypotension with widening of the QRS complex occurs sometimes and typical drug rashes are not uncommon.

Lidocaine. Although lidocaine is absorbed after intramuscular administration it is given intravenously in the treatment of arrhythmias. The usefulness of lidocaine is greatest in the emergency treatment of ventricular arrhythmias. Onset of action is almost immediate, and it has an effective half-life of 15 to 20 minutes. Metabolism takes place almost entirely within the liver. The initial dose is 1 mg per kg, which can be repeated after five minutes, or a continuous microdrip infusion can be used in a dose of 1 to 2 mg per minute. A convenient preparation is 1.0 gm in 500 ml, which is prepared by mixing 50 ml of 2 per cent lidocaine with 450 ml of saline. This solution contains 2 mg per ml and can be utilized in a therapeutic trial at a rate of 1 ml per minute for 30 minutes for a 60 kg patient. Toxic side effects are primarily related to the central nervous system. Large doses may cause drowsiness, convulsions or collapse. One of the advantages of this drug is that doses up to 5 mg per kg do not depress myocardial contractility.

Procaine amide. Absorption of procaine amide from the gastrointestinal tract is effective within 60 to 90 minutes of oral administration. The effect of a single dose lasts 5 to 10 hours. Procaine amide is eliminated unchanged via the kidneys.

Although procaine amide is most effective in the treatment of ventricular arrhythmias it is also useful in the treatment of atrial premature contractions and atrial tachycardia, and is moderately successful in the prevention of recurrent atrial fibrillation. About 90 per cent of patients with ventricular premature contractions respond to this drug.

Daily divided doses of 1.0 to 6.0 gm are used to start treatment. A stable therapeutic level should be obtained within three days. More even levels are obtained by smaller doses every four hours than by larger doses every six hours. Procaine amide can be given intravenously, 100 mg every five minutes, for emergency treatment. Blood pressure should be carefully monitored during such treatment.

Toxic effects, especially after intravenous use, include hypotension, widening of the QRS complex and myocardial depression. Nausea, vomiting and skin rashes may occur. A syndrome similar to systemic lupus erythematosus has also been reported after prolonged oral administration. If the drug is stopped the symptoms slowly disappear.

Propranolol hydrochloride. Propranolol is a specific blocker of beta-adrenergic receptor sites, and therefore prevents the chronotropic, inotropic and vasodilator effects of beta-adrenergic stimulating agents. In large doses the drug also depresses cardiac action and acts as an antiarrhythmic drug. Propranolol therapy is a balance between adequate beta-adrenergic blockage and maintenance of adequate cardiac function. By blocking adrenergic stimuli, propranolol diminishes myocardial oxygen requirement and is therefore beneficial in the treatment of angina.

Propranolol is almost completely absorbed from the gastrointestinal tract and achieves a peak effect within one to one and one-half hours of administration. Its effectiveness lasts two to four hours. There is little correlation between serum levels of the drug and therapeutic effects, and correct dosage has to be achieved by clinical titration.[8]

The indications for propranolol are (1) the control of angina (in conjunction with other measures), (2) the control of tachyarrhythmias, both atrial and ventricular and (3) suppression of myocardial outflow tract spasm, as in tetralogy of Fallot or idiopathic hypertrophic subaortic stenosis.

Treatment with propranolol should, if possible, be stopped 48 hours before operation in adults, and one to two weeks before operation in children.

ANTICOAGULANTS. Anticoagulants are given preoperatively to patients with valvular disease, especially mitral disease, atrial fibrillation and a history of peripheral embolism. Some patients may have been receiving anticoagulants for a long time before being seen by the surgeon. It is not necessary to stop therapy completely before operation. If the prothrombin time is greater than 30 per cent of normal at the time of operation unusual bleeding is not usually encountered.

In many such patients anticoagulation is restarted again after operation even if a prosthetic valve has not been inserted. It is difficult to know how long anticoagulation should continue. There is some evidence that stopping anticoagulation leads to a rebound phenomenon with hypercoagulability and an increased likelihood of embolism. It is also clear that the incidence of embolism after, for instance, a good mitral commissurotomy is much less than that before operation and that the increased flow rate through the valve diminishes the chances of subsequent episodes. No hard and fast rules can be given.

After insertion of a prosthetic valve, anticoagulation is usually started as soon as chest tubes are removed. In spite of conflicting evidence and the hope that a prosthetic valve might be designed that is without embolic complications, most surgeons still anticoagulate patients with prosthetic valves. Patients with porcine valves, especially mitral, should be on anticoagulants for three months.[9] Most embolic episodes occur within the first year after operation, but there is no period beyond which immunity from embolism is assured. If contraindications to anticoagulation (such as peptic ulceration) develop more than a year after insertion of a prosthesis, it is probably safe to stop treatment slowly.

The anticoagulants most commonly used are heparin, bishydroxycoumarin (dicumarol) and sodium warfarin (Coumadin).

Heparin. Heparin inhibits the clotting of blood and acts on all three stages of coagulation. The clotting time is prolonged in proportion to dosage. It is not effective when given by mouth, but is effective after subcutaneous, intramuscular or intravenous injection. Heparin is metabolized by the liver and has a relatively short half-life; some is excreted in the urine.

Administration for immediate effect is by intermittent intravenous injection. A dose of 100 units (formerly termed 1.0 mg) per kg is therapeutically effective and prolongs the clotting time two to two and a half times normal for four to eight hours. When treatment is being initiated, clotting time should be measured prior to injection of the dose and approximately 30 minutes later. This enables the physician to assess the peak and troughs of therapeutic effectiveness.

Continuous IV administration of 200 mg (20,000 units) heparin in 500 ml of 5 per cent dextrose in water gives a more continuous therapeutic benefit but is more difficult to control.

For long-term use the subcutaneous route is necessary. A very fine needle (No. 25 or 27) should be used and injections should not be given repeatedly in the same site. An initial dose of 30,000 to 40,000 units is given and, thereafter, about 20,000 units every 12 to 24 hours. The clotting time should be measured a few times about midway between each dose to try to establish a satisfactory therapeutic level.

Heparin is counteracted by protamine sulfate in an intravenous dose of one to one and a half times the dose of heparin. Antagonistic effects are rapid and clotting time should be normal within seven to ten minutes of administration.

Protamine can itself act as an anticoagulant if given in too large a dose. It can also result in temporary pulmonary hypertension and a reduction in cardiac output if given too rapidly. For these reasons the appropriate dose of protamine should be diluted in 100 to 150 ml of 5 per cent dextrose and given over a 10 to 20 minute period.

Bishydroxycoumarin (dicumarol). The effects of this agent are very similar to those of warfarin sodium (Coumadin). The most important action of these drugs is to depress the prothrombin complex, but other clotting factors are also affected. Administration is oral and there is a latent period of 12 to 24 hours before an effect is obtained. It is important that this latent period be taken into account when treatment is being started and when the dosage schedule is being worked out. If the drug is taken in the afternoon the effect of that dose will not be measureable until the following day. (The latent period is longer with warfarin sodium.)

Numerous factors affect the action of this and similar drugs; among them are the following (1) Diet: a change in fat intake by changing vitamin K absorption may influence the response. (2) Liver function: depression of hepatic function, from whatever cause, increases the patient's susceptibility to the drug. The development of postoperative serum hepatitis, for instance, is an immediate indication for a drastic reduction in the dosage. (3) Intercurrent diseases: during minor intercurrent diseases such as flu, the dosage should be reviewed and prothrombin times measured more frequently than usual to make sure that desirable therapeutic levels are maintained. (4) Drugs: sulfonamides, quinine, quinidine steroids and salicylates in excess of 1.0 gm per day increase sensitivity to these drugs. These drugs must either be avoided or increased vigilance should be maintained if their use is essential.

The most important complication of anticoagulant treatment is hemorrhage. If the prothrombin time is kept between two to two and a half times the control time or 20 to 25 per cent of normal, hemorrhagic complication should be rare. If the prothrombin time falls below 15 per cent of normal, spontaneous hemorrhage — retroperitoneal, intracranial, nasopharyngeal, gastrointestinal or into the urinary tract — is increasingly likely. Some hemorrhagic complications such as bleeding gums may be relatively trivial, but severe gastrointestinal or intracerebral bleeding may be catastrophic. When bleeding occurs treatment with the drug should be stopped. If hemorrhage is not severe this alone may be adequate. But vitamin K (2.5 to 5.0 mg by mouth) may have to be given. In severe cases the dose of vitamin K may have to be increased to 10 mg parenterally. For immediate effect transfusions of fresh blood or fresh frozen plasma will restore coagulation to normal.

Warfarin sodium (Coumadin). The initial dose is 20 to 30 mg by mouth followed by a daily maintenance dose of 2.5 to 10 mg depending upon sensitivity of the patient to the drug. The latent period between ingestion and response is 24 to 36 hours and the effect of a single dose may last for four to five days. This delayed action is extremely important in calculating doses and in determining why a dose may seem to be too small or too great. The prothrombin time you measure today reflects the dose of the day before yesterday. The complications and antidotes necessary are the same as with dicumarol therapy.

Platelet Inhibitors. The initiating feature in the development of a thrombus is the aggregation of platelets. If this process is prevented the subsequent deposition of thrombus may be avoided. Three functions of platelets can be measured: (1) platelet aggregation, which is the tendency of platelets to stick to each other, (2) platelet adhesiveness, which is the tendency of platelets to adhere to foreign surfaces, and (3) platelet survival time. A reduction in platelet adhesiveness or aggregation may be beneficial in preventing platelet adherence to foreign surfaces. A shortened platelet survival time is, however, evidence of deleterious platelet dysfunction, and there is strong correlation between shortening of platelet survival time and tendency to clot formation and postoperative thromboembolism.

Several nonsteroidal anti-inflammatory agents such as aspirin, sodium salicylate and sulfinpyrazone have been found to inhibit ADP-induced platelet aggregation and to prolong platelet life. This both explains some of the complications of treatment with these drugs and also raises the possibility of preventing thrombus formation by the administration of these or similar drugs. Patients who are known "clotters," with a history of several thromboembolic episodes, should have their platelet survival time measured and, if it is shortened, restored to nor-

mal by the administration of sulfinpyrazone.

DIURETICS. *Thiazides.* These drugs
are effective orally and are useful in
the treatment of congestive failure and
hypertension. They induce loss of both
sodium and potassium, and dietary supplementation with potassium, 1.0 gm
three to four times per day, is necessary
during prolonged administration. Thia-
zide drugs are contraindicated if there
is renal failure. Eight or nine different
drugs in this group are available, all of
roughly equal potency. Dosage depends upon the drug used. Toxic effects include skin rashes, gastrointestinal disturbances, hyperglycemia and
even diabetes. In susceptible patients a
flare-up of gout may occur.

Ethacrynic acid: Furosemide. These
are very potent agents which induce a
profound diuresis within 30 to 60 minutes of ingestion. Diuresis of both sodium and potassium is greater than with
thiazides. Because of the potency of
these agents they should not be used
unless congestive failure is severe, and
even then should be given in small
doses, 20 to 50 mg, to see what effect is
obtained. These drugs can be given
safely when renal function has been
impaired.

ANTIBIOTICS. The general principles that govern the use of antibiotics
obtain in cardiac surgery. Most surgeons give antibiotics prophylactically
to cover the period of operation, and the
evidence is that infections are thereby
reduced. By the time a patient leaves
the hospital antibiotic administration
has usually been stopped.

Antibiotic coverage should be given
to all patients with congenital or valvular disease, after prosthetic replacement during dental work, urological
manipulations, operations for noncardiac disease or intercurrent infections
that are more than trivial. Young patients with rheumatic heart disease
should continue to take penicillin prophylactically until the age of 35.

Special Techniques

Phonocardiography

Phonocardiograms are not made routinely in the follow-up of all types of
cardiac patient but may be useful when
following patients with prosthetic heart
valves. The first sound of a normally
functioning aortic prosthesis is louder
than the second, and the magnitude of
aortic opening sound to aortic closing
sound (AO/AC) should be greater than
0.7 — a ratio of 0.5 to 0.7 is borderline
and a ratio smaller than 0.5 is presumptive evidence of aortic ball variance.

Ultrasound

Echocardiography has been developed more rapidly during the past few
years than any other cardiovascular
diagnostic technique. A textbook on the
subject should be consulted for detailed descriptions of echocardiogra-
phic techniques and findings.

Some of the many advantages of the
technique are that it is noninvasive,
repeatable at frequent intervals and
precise.

The surgeon should be aware that the
technique can be used to demonstrate:

(1) valve movements, both natural
    and prosthetic;
(2) anatomical relationships between
    valves;
(3) ventricular cavitary size;
(4) ventricular wall movement;
(5) aortic diameter; and
(6) pericardial effusions or pericar-
    dial thickening.

From the tracings measurements can
be made of:

(1) stroke volume;
(2) valve annulus diameter (aortic);
(3) LV outflow dimensions; and
(4) mitral valve cusp velocity.

Because of the large amount of
information obtainable the technique
is extremely useful in diagnosis of
congenital heart disease, especially

complicated defects in small infants; estimation of valve stenosis, especially mitral, pulmonary and aortic; and follow-up of patients with prosthetic valves. Characteristic echoes are produced from each type of valve, and poppet movement can be measured with great accuracy.

Newer multi-crystal methods now make real-time observations of cardiac movement possible. These techniques, when perfected, may to some extent supercede angiocardiography.

COMPLICATIONS

Complications Common to All Operations

1. Postcardiotomy Syndromes[7]

The various syndromes have been comprehensively reviewed by Kirsh (1970). Three have been recognized, but as the etiological factors of none are known the relationship between them is also obscure.

The *postpericardiotomy syndrome* is characterized by pericarditis and pleuropericardial involvement with fever, chest pain and friction rubs. It usually develops two to three weeks after operation. A fever of 101° to 104° F. is common. The patient feels generally unwell with sweats, chills and myalgia. The white cell count is elevated with a normal lymphocyte count. Improvement takes one to four weeks. Activities should be restricted; aspirin, 10 gr q.i.d., may be sufficient to alleviate symptoms. Steroids are rarely necessary. If the patient is receiving anticoagulants and salicylates are contraindicated, acetaminophen is a useful substitute.

The *postperfusion syndrome* is not as common as the postpericardiotomy syndrome and occurs in only about 5 per cent of patients after operations in which extracorporeal circulation has been used. Fever, lymphocytosis and splenomegaly are the distinguishing features. Atypical lymphocytes, constituting 25 to 80 per cent of the white count, appear in the blood soon after the development of fever and persist for as long as three months. The syndrome usually starts within the first six weeks after operation and lasts for two to four weeks. The course is benign. Pleuropericardial complications are not a feature. Treatment consists of aspirin or other antipyretics. There is strongly suggestive evidence that this syndrome may be caused by a cytomegalic virus transmitted by blood transfusion.

A *biphasic postcardiotomy syndrome* has also been described. The first phase starts a few days after operation with fever, tachycardia and a vesicular periorbital rash. The second phase starts three to six weeks later with similar fever, perioral lesions and pleuropericardial manifestations. Atypical lymphocytes are found in the blood smear but not in such high proportion as in the postperfusion syndrome.

2. Infection

Infection may appear in the late postoperative period in two ways: (a) as a wound infection or (b) as bacterial endocarditis or septicemia.

Wound infection becomes apparent with all the classic local signs of calor, dolor, rubor and tumor. If an infected stitch is the source of trouble it must be removed. If infection involves the sternal stitches a decision must be made about the stability of the sternum, the possibility of deep mediastinal infection and even the possibility of sternal osteomyelitis. A superficial wound incision may be a minor complication, but a mediastinal infection with sternal dehiscence is potentially catastrophic. If a sinus grows along the tract of an infected suture the patient may have to be readmitted to hospital for curettage of the tract.

Bacterial endocarditis is a potential

hazard in all patients with intracardiac defects before or after operation. After valve replacement infection develops in a small percentage of patients, with perhaps slightly greater frequency after graft replacement than after prosthetic replacement.

The patient with infection presents with some signs and symptoms similar to those of the postcardiotomy syndromes. Fever, elevated white count and splenomegaly are found. Perhaps the most important, immediately distinguishing feature is the obvious illness of the patient with septicemia and endocarditis, whereas most patients with postcardiotomy syndromes maintain a good appetite and feel reasonably well in spite of fever. Changing murmurs, petechiae, emboli and splinter hemorrhages may be found. Numerous blood cultures must be made as soon as the diagnosis is suspected and before antibiotic treatment is started. Although the prognosis is grave if infection develops on a replaced valve, recovery is possible, sometimes after prolonged antibiotic treatment and sometimes after removal of the infected valve.

3. Congestive Failure

Congestive failure must not be taken as a satisfactory diagnosis, per se. The physician must always look beyond the immediate situation to determine the underlying cause. Postoperatively, congestive failure may be due to a continuation of the cardiac problem for which the operation was performed or it may be due to the development of a new complication.

If the patient was in chronic failure before operation, weeks or months may elapse before failure disappears in spite of a hemodynamically excellent result. Severe myocardial fibrosis or coronary disease may slow down or prevent total recovery.

Congestive failure occurs after operations for congenital as well as acquired disease. After total correction of the tetralogy of Fallot many patients are left with persistent right ventricular hypertension, a closed interventricular septum and a right ventricle recovering from a large incision. Congestive failure is common, but almost always responds satisfactorily to standard management with digitalis and diuretics.

The most ominous onset of failure is that which occurs after a period, perhaps a long period, of well-being. The first suspicion must always be that something has gone awry with the technical result of the operation.[6] A patch on a septal defect may partially dehisce, a previously opened valve may have slowly restenosed or a prosthetic valve may no longer be functioning adequately. Technical problems are usually fairly easy to pinpoint. Recatheterization may be necessary to confirm and measure a reopened shunt, the development of a new murmur being the warning clue. Only after it is certain that the result of the operation is still technically intact should other sources of trouble be invoked. Myocardial disease, coronary disease, or systemic hypertension may be responsible. Myocardial factors are most difficult to diagnose and are often established only by elimination of other causes.

The treatment of congestive failure in the postoperative patient is no different from that prescribed in other circumstances. Immediate recourse to increased diuretics and salt restriction is not always necessary. The patient's activities, diet and habits should be reviewed; he may have been indulging, soon after operation, in activities that are too strenuous, and sometimes a short period of bedrest is all that is necessary to restore compensation. If failure is severe and a technical problem exists, the patient must first be admitted to hospital; failure is then treated and the hemodynamic situation and the necessity for reoperation are reassessed after failure has abated.

4. Wound Problems

DISRUPTION. If a thoracotomy wound disrupts at all, it almost always does so before the patient leaves hospital. Infection is the commonest cause of late disruption and must be treated accordingly. Not all disruptions of sternotomy wounds must undergo reoperation. If there is no infection, the skin is intact and the wound is stable from a ventilatory point of view, the final endpoint may be firm fibrous union. Minor degrees of sternal movement and clicking may be annoying to the patient but may be preferable to another operation and the risk of introducing infection where none already exists.

The midline sternotomy is the most frequently used incision for cardiac operations. Cosmetically it leaves much to be desired. It protrudes above a fashionable level in girls and often heals as a wide scar, occasionally as a true keloid or hypertrophic scar. Painful keloidal healing is difficult to deal with. Excision and resuture may result in an acceptable scar, and local injections of hydrocortisone may also relieve symptoms and diminish scar formation.

In children a pigeon-breast deformity may develop after midline sternotomy. This can, in part, be avoided by taking good periosteal sutures as part of the closure. These stitches tend to prevent eversion of the sternal edges in the flexible juvenile chest.

5. Rhythm Problems

Arrhythmias and conduction problems are common. Some begin during the operation and persist; others start postoperatively and may be intermittent or permanent.

ATRIAL FIBRILLATION. This is probably the most frequent arrhythmia. Provided the rate of ventricular response is adequately controlled with digitalis, the patient will probably tolerate the irregularity. Cardiac output can, however, be increased by restoring normal sinus rhythm. If an attempt is made at electrical conversion within the first two weeks after operation normal rhythm may be achieved but seldom persists. If there is a delay of four to six weeks the likelihood of permanent conversion is greater. At the time of electrical conversion the patient should be fully digitalized and should receive quinidine after conversion. Patients with atrial fibrillation also tend to have a slightly higher incidence of peripheral emboli after valve replacement than patients in sinus rhythm.

ATRIAL FLUTTER. Atrial flutter sometimes develops after operations which involve the right atrium, such as closure of an atrial septal defect. The arrhythmia is sometimes resistant to therapy and sinus rhythm cannot be restored. The usual treatment is full digitalization followed by a course of quinidine. Electrical conversion is rarely of value in restoring sinus rhythm.

NODAL RHYTHM. Nodal rhythms do not seem to be as persistent as atrial arrhythmias. A nodal rhythm is quite common at the end of operation but usually disappears within a few days. An occasional patient develops chronic nodal bradycardia. This may reduce cardiac output to the point of disability; if the rate constantly remains below 55 per minute, thought should be given to the need for a permanent transvenous pacemaker.

HEART BLOCK. Most instances of complete heart block after cardiac operations are iatrogenic. Patients with endocardial cushion defects, large ventricular septal defects and tetralogy of Fallot run a small (5 per cent) risk of induced heart block. With detailed anatomical knowledge of the course of the conduction bundle and satisfactory surgical techniques for placing sutures without injuring the bundle, the risk should be small. Complete block may develop during aortic valve replacement and, very rarely, with mitral valve replacement. In some cases, the block is temporary, but if block persists for four weeks after inception a permanent pacemaker should be inserted. Two drugs are of some usefulness in complete block — isoproterenol hydrochloride and ephedrine. Steroids appear to be of benefit in patients with postinfarction block.

Isoproterenol may be used intravenously in an emergency — 0.05 to 0.1 mg, or 1 to 2 mg in 500 ml of 5 per cent dextrose in water. Sublingual absorption (10 to 15 mg) is sometimes helpful. Ephedrine 15 to 60 mg by mouth, has a beneficial effect in some patients. Prednisone 10 to 15 mg per day may be tried if there are no other contraindications and especially if myocardial ischemia rather than direct mechanical damage to the bundle is suspected.

There is some evidence that prolonged iatrogenic heart block in children may not have as serious a prognosis as was once thought. However, with increasing reliability of pacemakers the risks of a fatal standstill would not seem to be worth taking, and insertion of a pacemaker is advisable.

6. Respiratory Complications

By the time the patient leaves the hospital most complications have been successfully treated. A few complications may become chronic and require continued management.

TRACHEAL OR SUBGLOTTIC STENOSIS. After prolonged ventilation by a respirator with a cuffed endotracheal tube, there is some mucosal damage in almost every patient. Minor degrees of noncritical stenosis may occur unnoticed in many patients. If severe stenosis occurs it may not become manifest for several weeks until the patient returns with respiratory distress and stridor.

If ventilation has been through an oro-or nasotracheal tube the commonest site for stenosis is subglottic. On laryngoscopy subglottic swelling with a slit-like orifice can be seen. If ventilation has been via a tracheostomy the site of obstruction may be at the healed tracheostoma or lower down, at the level of the cuff or tip of the endotracheal tube.

When the patient is first seen he may be in acute and potentially lethal respiratory distress. If the obstruction is subglottic a tracheostomy below the obstruction will afford relief, or it may be possible to pass an endotracheal tube through the narrow passage. If the obstruction is secondary to a previous tracheostomy, obtaining a good airway may be difficult. In the case of stenosis at an old tracheostomy, reopening the wound may permit the passage of a tube into the distal trachea.

Stenotic areas lower down pose the greatest problem. It is difficult to dilate these areas via the larynx through a bronchoscope, but bronchoscopy may be necessary initially in order to determine the site of obstruction. Reopening the tracheostomy provides better and closer access to the stenosis. Depending upon the site of obstruction, an uncuffed tracheostomy tube or a longer endotracheal tube may be passed through the narrow part.

Subglottic obstruction is due to granulation tissue and swelling. Radiotherapy has been used successfully in reducing the size of these masses. Most of the more distal obstructions are due to contracting scar tissue although there may be superimposed edema. Tracheograms should be made to delineate the problem.

There are two long-term solutions — first, repeated dilatation; second, resection and repair. Through a tracheostomy the distal areas of obstruction can be dilated with Hegar dilators. Topical anesthesia is necessary. At first dilatation may be necessary every 48 hours. Eventually a permanent lumen of adequate caliber may be achieved. If dilatation is not successful, definitive repair is the only solution.

PLEURAL EFFUSION: HEMOTHORAX. Small effusions may collect because of congestive failure, and in most instances there is no need to tap them. If respiratory distress is due to excessive accumulation of fluid, thoracentesis (Fig. 16–10) may be necessary.

The management of hemothorax is a source of discussion. If a patient acquires a sizeable hemothorax, should or should it not be evacuated surgically and a decortication carried out? Much of the information about the management of these cases comes from military sources and from observing the course of events in traumatic cases. This information may not be directly applicable.

If the hemothorax is small and does not contribute to respiratory distress, and if there is no evidence of infection within it, it should be left alone. Aspiration is not necessary, may introduce infection and is inadvisable if the patient is receiving anticoagulants. Hemothoraces of this magnitude will be absorbed quickly without residual constrictive fibrothorax. In children even quite large collections will be absorbed if given time. If the hemothorax is large or seems to be infected, tube thoracotomy (Fig. 16–11), followed possibly by decortication, may be necessary.

7. Complications of Valve Replacement

EMBOLISM. Peripheral embolism as a major complication of valve replacement became apparent soon after the first prosthetic valves were inserted. During the first few years of experience with valve replacement, the incidence of embolism was very high — 10 to 15 per cent after aortic replacement and 30 to 50 per cent after mitral valve replacement. Research indicated that the emboli arise from junctional areas between cloth and metal. Fibrin and pseudoendothelium adhere to the cloth but break away from the metal. By covering metallic parts with cloth this problem was significantly reduced. With most valves used in the past decade the incidence of embolism after valve replacement of all sorts has been reduced to 3 to 5 per cent.

Embolism after homograft or xenograft replacement is not unknown, although it is less common than that after prosthetic replacement. An embolism rate of 0–2.5 per cent has been reported by various authors.

It is important to realize that only a small proportion (about 1.5 per cent) of embolic episodes are fatal, and about an equal percentage result in residual damage. Most episodes are transient and without sequelae.

HEMOLYSIS. After valve replacement, hemolysis is usually an indication of valve malfunction. Hemolysis has been reported in patients with a Beall disk mitral valve without mechanical malfunction. Perivalvular leaks, ball variance, and clots on the suture ring causing leakage through the valve can hemolyze cells.

If hemolysis is mild the hematocrit can be maintained with iron therapy. If, however, the hematocrit continues to fall, blood transfusion may be necessary. When hemolysis is severe, even transfusion at regular intervals is inadequate, and reoperation is then mandatory.

Other factors must be considered. Prosthetic valves with silastic poppets may develop ball variance, and the hemolysis is then a sign of variance. If other evidence of variance coexists, reoperation becomes a matter of some urgency. If the prosthetic valve is of a type (e.g., metal ball) in which variance is not possible, other causes for hemolysis must be considered.

SYNDROMES OF PROSTHETIC VALVE FAILURE.[6] Increasing long-term experience with valve replacement has made it abundantly clear that no type of valve — prosthetic, homograft or heterograft — is devoid of problems. Although some of these difficulties have been referred to elsewhere in this chapter the subject is of such importance that the various syndromes should be collectively described. Although the clinical manifestations are those of congestive failure, embolism, hemolysis and arrhythmias, it is perhaps easiest to look separately at the difficulties with aortic and mitral valves.

Aortic valve failure. When faced by a patient with probable valve failure it is very important to know precisely what type of valve has been used. Ball variance, for instance, has only been reported in valves with silastic balls. Not all valves with silastic poppets have a high incidence of variance, whereas some, such as the Starr-Edwards model 1000 aortic valve (no longer used), had a high incidence of variance. Disk valves (Kay-Shiley), free-floating valves or tilting valves (Bjork-Shiley, Wada) are subject to cocking and fixed tilting of the disk. Homografts and heterografts are liable to cusp rupture and retraction and, occasionally, massive calcification.

Loss of opening valve sound is pathognomonic of ball variance, but this sign is found in only about 25 per cent of patients with variance. If still present, but diminished in intensity so that the opening sound is less than half the intensity of the closing sound, variance is likely.

The late appearance of hemolysis, failure, emboli, arrhythmias and new murmurs should all be taken as evidence of a mechanical problem. Palpitation, dizzy spells, syncope and angina may also be warning signs. When these symptoms are associated with jaundice or anemia the diagnosis should be assumed unless there is overwhelming evidence to the contrary. Prosthetic aortic stenosis is due to a clot that prevents normal movement of the poppet, either as a collar on the suture ring or a thickening around the struts or apex of the cage. Aortic insufficiency, however, is most likely to be due to uneven accumulation of a clot, permitting leakage around the poppet; or a leak around the fixation ring.

Aortic insufficiency, ranging between minor and severe, is a common complication of homograft valve replacement, but does not seem to be as common with porcine xenografts. The late appearance of an aortic diastolic murmur may signify development of a tear in a cusp and the patient's progress must be watched very carefully in case insufficiency increases to produce hemodynamic difficulty. A diastolic murmur without a change in diastolic pressure is not of hemodynamic importance, but may presage impending difficulties.

Mitral valve failure. As with aortic valves the single most important warning indication is the development of symptoms after a good result.

Mechanical problems with mitral prostheses are most frequently associated with clinical evidence of pulmonary congestion and left-sided failure. If the signs and symptoms are persistent, a "steady-state" problem such as a valve leak is probably the cause. If paroxysmal episodes predominate, an intermittent cause such as acute tilting or sticking of a ball or disk is probably present. Progressive evidence of mitral stenosis indicates a buildup of clot on the valve that restricts motion but preserves competence, whereas evidence of insufficiency indicates that some process is preventing proper closure of the poppet or that there is perivalvular leakage.

Variance has been uncommonly found in mitral ball valves. Disk valves may wear at the edges and become notched. When this happens free movement is impaired. Usually the initiating force is an accumulation of fibrin between the disk and the ventricular wall which pushes the disk against the opposing struts. A metal disk may prevent notching but does not prevent cocking and tilting. As soon as one of these syndromes is suspected every possible means must be used to confirm or deny the diagnosis. Auscultation, phonocardiography, ultrasound, radiology (including fluoroscopy and angiocardiography) and laboratory data should all be used in evaluation.

If the evidence points definitively or strongly to a diagnosis of mechanical malfunction, whether of the aortic or the mitral valve, reoperation should be planned for an early date. The mortality rate for emergency reoperation is 60 to 80 per cent, but for a semi-elective reoperation the mortality rate is only 10 to 15 per cent.

8. Congestive Failure

If a patient develops left ventricular failure after valve replacement, two questions must be answered. Is there some problem with the replaced valve? Is failure due to myocardial or coronary disease? Clinical examination may or may not provide the answer. If there is a new murmur or a louder murmur than before, or if valve sounds have changed, a valve defect must be suspected. If failure supervenes without these changes endocardial or myocardial fibrosis may be the cause. When failure begins soon after operation it may be due to too early activity, inadequate digitalization or improper adjustment of diet or diuretics. When, however, failure starts after a period of improvement and well-being, other causes must be sought. Assessment must first be made of valve function, using radiological, ultrasound, phonocardiographic and other necessary methods. Cardiac catheterization and angiocardiography may be necessary to demonstrate perivalvular leaks because not all of these are clinically audible.

Management depends upon the findings. Late left ventricular endocardial fibrosis has been described after replacement of the mitral valve. The lesion is a response to turbulence and the impingement of ventricular filling jets on the endocardium. Clinically, patients with this problem present with congestive failure; management is difficult because a precise diagnosis is not possible, nor is there specific treatment.

Coronary disease should be treated according to the usual indications. Coronary ostial stenosis due to a jet lesion from an aortic prosthesis has been successfully treated, and this lesion and more distal occlusions could be treated by saphenous vein bypass.

PACEMAKERS[12]

The necessity for a pacemaker may be either temporary or permanent (Table 16–5). Pacemakers may be classified as *fixed rate*, in which the rate is pre-set at the factory; *variable fixed rate*, in which there is a possibility of changing the rate but which always delivers a regular signal to the heart, regardless of intrinsic cardiac rhythm; *synchronous* in which the atrial impulse is picked up by a special electrode and used to trigger delivery of an impulse to the ventricle and *demand*, in which the R-wave is used either to stimulate or to inhibit the impulse generated by the power source.

Insertion of Endocardial Leads

TEMPORARY. Temporary pacemaker leads are inserted using a technique

---

TABLE 16–5 Indications for Use of Pacemakers

ATRIOVENTRICULAR BLOCK
(a) With slow idioventricular rate (P)
(b) With Stokes-Adams attacks (P)
(c) With congestive failure (P)
(d) After myocardial infarction (T) → (P)

TACHY/BRADY ARRHYTHMIAS (SICK SINUS SYNDROME)
(a) To prevent (T) → (P)
(b) Overcome (T) → (P)

AFTER CARDIAC SURGERY
(a) To increase postop heart rate (T)
(b) Management of iatrogenic A-V block (T) → (P)
(c) Control of postop arrhythmias (T)

SINOAURICULAR BLOCK WITH VERY SLOW HEART RATE

CONGENITAL COMPLETE HEART BLOCK

(P) = Permanent; (T) = Temporary.

similar to that for subclavian vein cannulation (see page 100). Under local anesthesia in the fluoroscopy room a No. 14g needle is inserted into the subclavian vein. A No. 5 temporary pacing electrode is passed through this and the needle withdrawn. Positioning of the electrode in the right ventricle is done under fluoroscopic control. The lead is firmly attached to the skin by a stitch and connected to an external battery-operated power source.

PERMANENT. Permanent pacemakers may have transvenous or epicardial leads. Transvenous leads are inserted under local anesthesia and with fluoroscopical control via a cephalic, external jugular, internal jugular, axillary or subclavian vein. The cephalic vein route is easiest and may be approached through a 3-inch incision inferior to the lateral one third of the clavicle. After the vein is isolated in the deltopectoral groove the lead is inserted into the vein and positioned in the apex of the tight ventricle. The lead should lie in a gentle curve, without intracardiac loops. The power source is buried subcutaneously through the same incision. In thin patients the generator may be buried beneath the muscle for greater protection (Fig. 16–6).

Epicardial lead placement requires a thoracotomy, unless a spiral tipped lead is used that may be inserted through the bed of the 4th left costal cartilage or through a subxiphoid, transdiaphragmatic approach.

Changing of Pacemaker Generator

For elective changing of a pacemaker battery the patient is admitted to hospital one day before the operation and can usually be discharged 24 hours following operation after satisfactory function of the new battery has been confirmed.

The patient is positioned on the table with the battery location suitably exposed. Electrocardiogram leads are at-

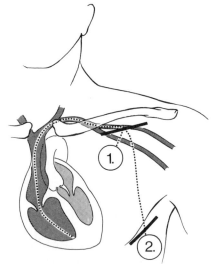

Figure 16–6 Transvenous pacemaking. The lead is advanced into the right ventricle via the cephalic vein, exposed beneath the clavicle. The generator may be buried in the infraclavicular area (1), or beneath the pectoral fold (2).

tached for continuous monitoring. Under local anesthesia (1 per cent Xylocaine without epinephrine) an incision is made over the battery, reopening the old wound. The smooth endothelialized pocket around the battery is opened widely enough to permit exteriorization of the battery. Depending upon the system for attachment of the endocardial leads to the battery, the appropriate connections are loosened. An alligator clip lead is made ready and led off the table to an external battery source. With a minimum of delay the battery is detached from the leads and the alligator clips immediately fastened to the bare ends of the endocardial leads. Cessation of pacing can thereby be reduced to a few seconds.

The external power source should be provided with a variable input so that the threshold required to pace the heart can be measured and noted for future reference. The new battery is brought into proximity to the lead ends, the alligator clips are removed and the connection made between leads and new battery with minimal delay. If any problems of manipulation arise, the leads are immediately withdrawn and reconnected to the external power source, which should not be turned off until reconnection to the new battery has been safely accomplished.

The battery is replaced in its pocket, which is liberally irrigated with bacitracin before resuturing of the wound in layers. Stitches may be removed after seven days.

Assessment of Pacemaker Failure

The causes of failure to pace are (1) battery failure, (2) breakage of lead, (3) dislodgement of endocardial lead, (4) failure of electrical component other than battery, (5) perforation of endocardial lead through myocardium into pericardium and (6) fibrosis around lead resulting in increased electrical resistance.

With these causes in mind the following tests should be made when a patient presents with pacemaker failure:

(1) Is the pacemaker pacing but the patient not picking up the impulse? Examine the EKG. The pacemaker spikes should be visible if the batteries are still working.

(2) Is the impulse strong enough to cause pacing? Measurement of the pacemaker artifact on the EKG is deceptive, but it may be of help if the measurement can be compared with a similar previous tracing. X-ray examination of the batteries can determine if they have become seriously rundown. The time since implantation of the batteries will also be a valuable clue. Mercury-zinc batteries should last 24 to 30 months, but lithium batteries are expected to last four to twelve years.

(3) Is the impulse getting to the heart? Take x-rays to examine for fractured leads. Several views should be taken from different angles. X-rays will also demonstrate a change in position of a lead or apparent perforation of the myocardium. If a specific cause such as a lead fracture or worn-out batteries can

be determined, appropriate steps can be taken to remedy the situation. If a cause cannot be determined, exteriorize the battery under local anesthesia, remove the leads from the battery and attach them by jumper cable to an external power source. The threshold for pacing can then be determined. If the threshold is normal, the power source should be renewed, but if it is excessive, the old lead may have to be removed and replaced by another. If no pacing can be achieved, the electrode is probably fractured and must be replaced.

Transvenous leads may become fixed by fibrosis to the tricuspid valve or the right ventricular endocardium. Attempting to pull out such a fixed lead by force is hazardous. If the lead does not come out easily the safest course is to insert a second lead by an alternative route.

PERICARDIAL PROBLEMS

Pericardial Effusion

The clinical manifestations of pericardial effusion depend upon the nature of the underlying disease and the hemodynamic changes due to the effusion. Trauma, uremia, infections, neoplasms and collagen diseases are among the many possible causes. In some instances the primary cause is obvious, in others a detailed search must be made for the cause, and open pericardial and myocardial biopsy may be a necessary part of the investigation.

Fatigue, dyspnea, orthopnea, abdominal swelling and peripheral edema are the presenting features. Venous pressure is elevated and engorged neck veins are easily seen. Precordial activity is diminished, but there is evidence by palpation and percussion of an enlarged heart. Radiologically a large globular heart shadow is seen, with elimination of the usual indentations along the cardiac borders.

Special diagnostic investigations include cardiac catheterization with angiography, scanning with radioactive isotopes and echocardiography. The diagnostic intracardiac pressures are a raised venous pressure and elevated end-diastolic pressure in both ventricles. Systemic pressure and cardiac output are both reduced. If the right atrium is filled with radiopaque dye the distance between the atrial wall and the edge of the cardiac shadow can be measured and represents the depth of effusion. When severe tamponade supervenes, the patient is clinically in shock. He is cool, peripherally cyanosed, with a small, thready, rapid pulse; cardiac output is diminished acutely in spite of high venous pressure.

The intrapericardial volume necessary to induce tamponade is variable and depends, in part, upon the rapidity of accumulation of fluid. Pericardium does not stretch acutely and, therefore, even 150 ml of effusion accumulated rapidly in a previously normal sac may elevate intrapericardial pressure sufficiently to reduce venous return and impede diastolic filling. If, however, the development of effusion is slower, the pericardium may have time to stretch and several hundred ml may accumulate without tamponade.

In either circumstance removal of a relatively small (25 to 50 ml) volume may reduce intrapericardial pressure sufficiently to improve cardiac function.

Never decide, therefore, that there cannot be tamponade because the volume of pericardial fluid seems to be too small. Nor should a conclusion be reached that a large effusion should automatically result in tamponade.

Pericardiocentesis

Before embarking upon elective pericardiocentesis examine the scanning and radiological evidence carefully to determine if the effusion is loculated and to assess the size of effusion.

There are three routes of entrance into the pericardium: (a) through the angle between the xiphoid process and the left costal margin, (b) at the cardiac apex and (c) through the left fourth or fifth interspace just lateral to the sternum. The preferred route is (a) because there is the least chance of damaging neighboring structures — lung, internal mammary artery, left anterior descending coronary artery — via this route.

The patient is positioned in a sitting position elevated to about 45°, and the lower chest and upper abdomen are thoroughly prepared and draped (Fig. 16–7). Under local anesthesia a long 20g needle is inserted in the angle between the left costal margin and the xiphoid process in an upward and posterior direction. The needle is inserted with a 20 ml syringe attached and the operator aspirates while advancing the needle. An alligator clip lead attached to the needle acts as one lead of an EKG which is monitored continuously while the needle is inserted. A change is noted if the myocardium is entered.

It is usually possible to feel the needle puncture the central tendon of the diaphragm and pericardium and immediately thereafter fluid may be aspirated into the syringe. If movement of the heart is felt against the needle tip, the needle is withdrawn slightly. If a large volume of chronic effusion must be drained, a small plastic tube can be introduced into the pericardial sac through the lumen of a large-bore needle and left in position, draining into a container.

Pericardial Drainage

If pericardiocentesis is not successful a simple method of pericardial drainage has been described by Schlein[13]. Under local anesthesia a five inch vertical incision is made in the

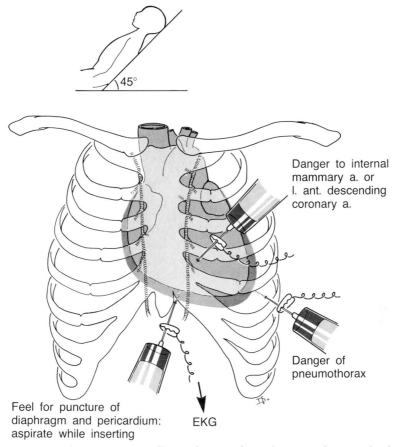

45°

Danger to internal
mammary a. or
l. ant. descending
coronary a.

Danger of
pneumothorax

Feel for puncture of
diaphragm and pericardium:
aspirate while inserting

EKG

Figure 16–7 Pericardiocentesis. A needle may be passed into the pericardium via the three routes indicated. Each route has some disadvantages. An EKG lead is clipped to the needle to monitor contact between needle and myocardium.

midline over the xiphoid process. Dissection is carried down through the linea alba to the diaphragm. The xiphoid process is raised superiorly, the fibers of the diaphragm are divided and the pericardium exposed and entered. Ample drainage is obtained and, if necessary, a tube can be left within the pericardial sac for prolonged drainage.

Constrictive Pericarditis

In constrictive pericarditis the heart becomes entrapped by a thick encircling fibrous scar that obliterates the pericardial sac and may become cal-

cified. Venous return is reduced by contracted scars around the caval orifices, and diastolic filling is impeded by constricting pericardial scar.

Venous congestion, hepatic enlargement, ascites and peripheral edema highlight the clinical picture. Peripheral cyanosis and cool extremities reflect a low cardiac output.

The techniques of radiology, scanning and ultrasound used to demonstrate a pericardial effusion can also be used to determine the presence and thickness of pericardium. Pericardial calcification is sometimes easily seen on a plain film, but the mere presence of calcification does not by itself denote constriction.

The treatment of constrictive pericarditis is widespread pericardiectomy, from phrenic nerve to phrenic nerve, with release of scar around the caval openings.

CARDIAC TRAUMA

Closed Injury

Evaluation of the integrity of heart and great vessels should be part of the investigation of every patient who has sustained a crushing or deceleration injury of the thorax. Attention should be directed along two lines.

(1) Is there damage to the heart? There may be myocardial contusion of every degree from a mild bruise to infarction readily discernible by electrocardiography. Atrial and ventricular walls, including the septum, may rupture, giving rise to a hemopericardium or a large intracardiac shunt. Disruption of the papillary muscles can cause mitral insufficiency.

Accumulation of a pericardial effusion may result in tamponade, and development of a shunt or valvular dysfunction may cause congestive cardiac failure.

Myocardial contusion may cause the symptoms and effects of myocardial infarction and is probably commoner than most statistics would indicate.

(2) Have the great vessels been damaged? Severe deceleration injuries may rupture the aorta. The commonest site for this is at the ligamentum arteriosum, but it may also occur in the ascending aorta, intra- or extrapericardially and at the roots of the main branches of the aortic arch. A widened mediastinum, seen on x-ray, should immediately arouse suspicion of aortic injury. If the first film was a "portable," widening should be confirmed by taking a 6 foot A/P film. Aortography is necessary for a definitive diagnosis.

Immediate mortality of traumatic aortic rupture is about 80 per cent. Among the 20 per cent who reach the hospital and in whom the diagnosis is made, mortality is about 25 per cent. Immediate operation is essential and should precede, or be included in, exploration for other problems. The *treatment* of closed injuries depends upon their nature. Contusions should be treated like myocardial infarctions of comparable severity. Rupture of a chamber into the pericardium may first require pericardiocentesis for relief of tamponade before definitive repair. Intracardiac shunts require open operation, but if congestive failure can first be controlled medically risks may be decreased.

Penetrating Injuries

Stab and gunshot wounds in and around the heart demand rapid evaluation and action if lives are to be saved. Two questions have to be answered immediately:

(1) Is the patient bleeding to death?

(2) Is there acute tamponade, and an equal but different threat to life?

Massive free bleeding into pleura and pericardium leads to acute hypovolemic shock. The most important distinguishing feature between hemorrhage and tamponade is the presence of high venous pressure in the latter. If, however, there is a combination of massive hemorrhage and tamponade the intrapericardial pressure necessary to induce tamponade is not as great as in a patient with a normal blood volume. Venous pressure may not then be elevated.

Penetrating thoracic wounds that injure the heart alone are uncommon, except after stab wounds. Gunshot wounds are likely to involve lung, esophagus, trachea and great vessels, and these possibilities must be constantly kept in mind.

Cardiac tamponade is more likely after stab than gunshot wounds. Out of 547 patients with thoracic gunshot wounds treated in Vietnam only 7 presented with tamponade.

The outcome after cardiac injuries depends upon the size of the wound and the interval between injury and treatment. Small wounds, less than 1 cm in length, may seal themselves quite rapidly, especially if the wound is a clean stab of a ventricle. Atrial wounds are less likely to seal spontaneously. Large wounds may cause death due to blood loss before treatment can be started. If the patient reaches the Emergency Room alive, he has, by definition, demonstrated that the wound is temporarily compatible with life.

Treatment

Immediate evaluation includes (1) assessment of shock, (2) search for signs of tamponade, (3) examination of entrance and exit wounds and a determination of organs that may have been injured and (4) chest x-ray for signs of hemopericardium, hemo- and pneumothorax.

Immediate treatment includes (1) assurance of airway and ventilation, (2) insertion of catheters for measurement of venous pressure and infusion of blood and fluids, (3) insertion of chest tubes for drainage of hemothorax and pneumothorax and (4) pericardiocentesis, if there is direct evidence of, or strong suspicion of, tamponade.

Indications for immediate operation are (1) a moribund patient. Resuscitation should be started in the Emergency Room, with transfer of the patient to the operating room as soon as possible. There should be no hesitation in opening the chest in the Emergency Room, provided endotracheal intubation and support of ventilation are possible. A 3 minute ride to the operating room may be fatal. (2) Immediate evacuation of 1000 ml to 1500 ml of blood by chest tube, followed by 500 ml in the next hour. (3) Redevelopment of tamponade after one suc-cessful pericardiocentesis. (4) Evidence of injury to the great vessels.

THE FUGITIVE CATHETER[11]

The use of plastic catheters for intravenous infusions has become so widespread in the past few years that needles have become almost passé. An unpleasant dividend of this technique is the loss of a catheter into the cardiovascular system. There are two common causes of this complication. Either the catheter is improperly secured to the skin, so that it becomes disconnected and slips intravenously, or the end of the needle previously inserted into the vein for passage of the catheter severs the catheter, and the free segment is carried away by the circulation.

If loss of the catheter is recognized at the moment of occurrence, rapid application of circumferential pressure high and proximal on the same limb may catch the catheter. Palpation is extremely deceptive, especially around the elbow. Don't cut down on what is presumed to be a catheter without radiological proof of its presence.

Take x-rays of the limb and thorax. If the catheter is radiopaque it will be spotted in the limb, right side of the heart or pulmonary artery. Because radiopaque catheters are now available, catheters that are not radiopaque should be avoided. Searching for a nonopaque catheter is frustrating and unfruitful.

If the catheter is lodged in the limb, a tourniquet is applied to prevent migration and it is removed under local anesthesia. Special instruments such as the Dormia basket catheter and the Ross snare are needed for removal of a catheter from the heart.

There is still some controversy over the best therapeutic approach to this problem.[11] Many patients are now walking around harboring within them a piece of plastic catheter without any symptoms. In most instances there are no sequelae. There have been reports of septic emboli and hemorrhage, and removal of all fugitive catheters has been advised.

A middle-of-the-road course seems acceptable. All catheters still in the limb should be removed. An attempt should be made to extract, by cardiac catheterization, all catheters within the heart. If the catheter is in the distal pulmonary arteries, leave it alone.

Antibiotics should be given for about one week after the incident. Anticoagulants do not seem warranted (any more than with endocardial pacemaker electrodes). At any sign of further complications, the catheter should be surgically removed.

REFERENCES

1. Beach, P. M., Bowman, F. O., Kaiser, G. A. and Malm, J. R.: Total correction of tetralogy of Fallot in adolescents and adults. Circulation, *43*: Suppl. I, 37–43, 1971.
2. Carpentier, A., Delouche, A., Dauptain, J., Blondeaur, P., Pinnica, A. and Dubost, C.: A new reconstructive operation for correction of mitral and tricuspid insufficiency. J. Thor. Cardiovasc. Surg., *61*:1–13, 1971.
3. Daves, M. L.: Skiagraphing the mediastinal moguls. New Physician, *19*:48–54, 1970.
4. Fox, H. E., May, I. A. and Ecker, R. R.: Long-term functional results of surgery for coronary artery disease in patients with poor ventricular function. J. Thor. Cardiovasc. Surg., *70*:1064–1072, 1975.
5. Grondin, P., Meere, C., Limet, R., Lopez-Besoc, L., Delcan, J. L. and Rivera, R.: Carpentier's annulus and DeVega's annuloplasty. J. Thor. Cardiovasc. Surg., *70*:852–61, 1975.
6. Hylen, J. C., Kloster, F. E., Starr, A. and Griswold, H. E.: Aortic ball variance: diagnosis and treatment. Ann. Intern. Med., *72*:1–8, 1970.
7. Kirsch, M. M., McIntosh, K., Kahn, D. R. and Sloan, H.: Postcardiotomy syndromes. Ann. Thorac. Surg., *9*:158–179, 1970.
8. Leaman, D. M., Levenson, L. W., Shiroff, R. A., Babb, J. D., DeJoseph, R. L., Hayes, A. H. and Zeus, R.: Persistence of biologic activity after disappearance of propanolol from the serum. J. Thor. Cardiovasc. Surg., *72*:67–72, 1976.
9. Pipkin, R. D., Buch, W. S. and Fogarty, T. J.: Evaluation of aortic valve replacement with a porcine xenograft without long-term anticoagulation. J. Thor. Cardiovasc. Surg., *71*:179-186, 1976.
10. Ryle, J. A.: The clinical study of pain: with special reference to the pains of visceral disease. Br. Med. J., *1*:537–540, 1928.
11. Richardson, J. D., Grover, F. L. and Trinkle, J. K.: Intravenous catheter emboli. Experience with 20 cases and collective review. Am. J. Surg., *128*:722–730, 1974.
12. Schaldach, M. and Furman, S.: Advances in Pacemaker Technology. New York, Springer-Verlag, 1975.
13. Schlein, E. M., Bartley, T. D., Spooner, G. R. and Cade, R.: A simplified approach to therapy of uremic pericarditis with tamponade. Ann. Thorac. Surg., *10*:548-551, 1970.
14. Segal, J., Harvey, W. P. and Hufnagel, C.: A clinical study of one hundred cases of severe aortic insufficiency. Am. J. Med., *21*:200–210, 1956.
15. Ullyot, D. J., Wisneski, J., Sullivan, R. W., Gertz, E. W. and Roe, B. B.: Improved survival after coronary artery surgery in patients with extensive coronary artery disease. J. Thor. Cardiovasc. Surg., *70*:405–413, 1975.
16. von Kaulla, K. N., Paton, B. C., Rosenkrantz, J. G., von Kaulla, E. and Wasantapruek, S.: Preoperative correction of coagulation in tetralogy of Fallot. Arch. Surg., *94*:107–111, 1967.
17. Isom, O. W., Spencer, F. C., Glassman, E., et al.: Does coronary bypass increase longevity? J. Thor. Cardiovasc. Surg., *75*:28–37, 1978.

Thorax: Lungs and Esophagus

Melvin M. Newman, M.D.

INTRODUCTION — OUTPATIENT EVALUATION AND TREATMENT

The office practice of the thoracic surgeon revolves around questions of diagnosis of tumors, infections or minor trauma. In this age of exponential cost increases, the skillful physician is able to complete essential diagnostic studies and plan appropriate treatment strategies for the ambulatory patient and to reserve expensive hospital time for more complicated tests and definitive treatment. The Emergency Room experience deals with more immediate threats to life that impose urgency upon diagnosis and decision.

History

The office practice of thoracic surgery depends more upon details of the history than do many other specialties. Many patients have had chronic respiratory complaints but the first important question is: Why does the patient present himself *at this time*? Does he have pain, cough, hemoptysis, dyspnea, fatigue or weight loss? How rapidly have symptoms developed?

Physical Examination

Rubin[85] has listed 15 frequently neglected physical findings in four groups:

(1) Pulmonary periostopathy and clubbing of digits
   a. Rest pain but no pain on joint motion
   b. Floating or sponginess of nail bed
(2) Signs of bronchial obstruction
   a. Bagpipe sign of a partially obstructed bronchus
   b. Pendular motion of trachea toward the side of obstruction or pneumothorax or inspiration and away from the affected side on expiration
   c. The palpable but inaudible rhonchus
(3) Specific tracheal signs
   a. Absence of upward laryngeal movement on swallowing (fixation by mediastinal mass)
   b. Deviation of trachea toward right or left sternomastoid muscle
   c. Increased depth of jugular notch (anterior mediastinal tumor)
   d. Fluctuation of trachea on palpation (distension of cervical esophagus)
   e. Respiratory fremitus in tracheal obstruction
   f. Anterior d'Espine's sign (loud tracheal sounds on auscultation over sternum indicate a large anterior mediastinal tumor)
(4) Specific signs in the neck
   a. Auscultatory crepitus above the clavicles (mediastinal emphysema)
   b. Ecchymosis at root of neck and over upper thorax (mediastinal hemorrhage)
   c. Supraclavicular lymph nodes may become palpable when patient coughs or strains
   d. Unilateral loss of bulging on Valsalva maneuver and retraction on Mueller maneuver (carcinoma at apex of lung)

X-ray

The interpretation of roentgenograms is aided by an organized inspection routine.[103] The mnemonic C-H-E-S-T (*C*avity, *H*eart, *E*dges, *S*oft tissue,

Thorax, bony) has been suggested by Fordham.[36] One first looks at the chest wall for symmetry, contraction of interspaces, rib erosion and extrathoracic soft tissue swelling. Next scan the pleura from apex to base for thickening, fluid or air collections and changes in the leaves of the diaphragm. Next, scan the mediastinum and cardiac shadow for shifts to right or left and abnormal contour. Then look at the lung parenchyma for masses, infiltrates, radiolucencies, or changes in radiodensities between the right and left side or the upper and lower portions of the lung. Compare the vascular patterns right and left. Finally, if infiltrates are present, try to determine if they are alveolar or if they are interstitial (interstitial fibrosis versus Kerley's lines).

Special Techniques

Single posterior, anterior and lateral chest films are useful for initial screening. More information about a suspicious area can be obtained by a variety of simple techniques: the apical lordotic projection, oblique projections and the use of coning down and focused grid to decrease tissue scatter. Since image-intensifying equipment has come into general use, fluoroscopy again has become more popular as a supplement to roentgenograms for assessing mobility of the right and left leaves of the diaphragm, equal ventilation of the right and left lungs and normal versus abnormal motion of cardiac silhouette. When supplemented with a few swallows of barium, fluoroscopy may add several dimensions to our understanding of the x-ray shadows.

Body section radiography, or tomography, is invaluable for separating contiguous areas of similar density and for demonstrating small metastatic lesions. Two new developments, xerotomography[66] and computerized axial tomography (computer-assisted tomography, CAT) may give even more infor-

mation in selected patients but at the expense of increased radiation exposure. The greatest utility of CAT scanning at present appears to be in the study of mediastinal masses and pleural metastases. Unfortunately, a very old examination, the stereoscopic posterior-anterior chest film, is rarely used anymore, even though it may sometimes give as much three-dimensional spatial information as the CAT scan.

Finally, there will always be special situations where angiocardiography will be essential for evaluation of superior vena caval obstruction or abnormalities of the heart and the aorta and its branches.

Endoscopy

Bronchoscopy and esophagoscopy can be done in a well-equipped office that has all the facilities to cope with emergencies, including untoward drug reactions, hypoxia or cardiac arrest. Bronchograms also can be done advantageously at the same sitting as bronchoscopy if x-ray facilities are available. These techniques will be discussed in more detail later.

Sputum Examination

Sputum studies are useful in proportion to the effort made in securing deep cough specimens. Bacteriological specimens should be cultured for pyogenic bacteria, mycobacteria and fungi as quickly as possible to avoid overgrowth of saprophytic bacteria. Cytology depends upon rapid fixation to stop autolysis of the desquamated cells. Some cytologists prefer to examine smears fixed in ether-alcohol or 95 per cent ethanol and others supplement this with study of sections of centrifuged and formalin-fixed sputum. Many cytologists have reported a success rate of 90 per cent in diagnosing bronchogenic cancer from three consecutive sputum smears. The three or four days after bronchoscopy are likely to provide the best sputum specimens for cytology and for culture of bacteria and mycobacteria. When sputum smears must be mailed to the laboratory, they can be fixed by spraying the slides with a polyvinylpyrrolidone solution.[110]

Skin Tests

Skin tests for tuberculosis, histoplasmosis and coccidioidomycosis are used now with greater discrimination, since they merely indicate previous infection and give little help in assessing activity of current disease. If active histoplasmosis or coccidioidomycosis is suspected, it is important to draw blood for precipitin and complement fixation tests before the skin tests are done to avoid an anamnestic response and falsely high values. We no longer use the blastomycin skin test, which lacks specificity. Although Silzbach and other investigators believe the Kveim test is specific for sarcoidosis, Israel and colleagues think the test may be of historical interest only, since the antigen may be specific not for sarcoidosis but for proliferating lymphoid cells.[50]

Lung Biopsy

In many cases the cause of pulmonary infiltration can be determined only from lung biopsy. Diagnoses of carcinoma, tuberculosis, sarcoidosis, pyogenic infection, *Pneumocystis carinii* infection and fungus infection have been made in this way. Biopsies have been done transbronchially with a biopsy forceps or brush passed through the fiberoptic bronchoscope,[32] guided by fluoroscopy; percutaneously with the Vim-Silverman needle; by aspiration through size 22 to 18 needles positioned fluoroscopically,[25] and by percutaneous use of a high-speed turbine-driven hollow drill.[116] There has been a high incidence of pneumo-

thorax with all the percutaneous procedures and occasional hemorrhage with all types of biopsy. Chest tube drainage is frequently, and thoractomy rarely, needed; therefore, lung biopsy by percutaneous or by thoractomy approaches remains a hospital procedure.

Node Biopsy

When there is palpable lymphadenopathy, node biopsy or cervical fat pad biopsy under local anesthesia is perfectly feasible as an outpatient procedure.

Mediastinoscopy

When no nodes are palpable, it is preferable to hospitalize the patient for general endotracheal anesthesia and to do a formal mediastinoscopy (Fig. 16–8). Mediastinoscopy and bronchoscopy are frequently combined under one general anesthetic and, in good risk patients, could be done as outpatient procedures.

Indications for Thoracotomy

After preliminary diagnostic studies have been completed, exploratory thoracotomy may be indicated for diagnosis or definitive treatment. Pulmonary resection must have clear justification. The most important question one should ask about any surgical or medical procedure is: What are we trying to accomplish for *this* patient?

Tuberculosis

Tuberculosis today tends to be an illness of youth and old age. As in most other infections, effective treatment rests upon (1) isolation of the mycobacteria in culture and in characterization of their antibiotic sensitivities; (2) adequate doses of two to four ap-

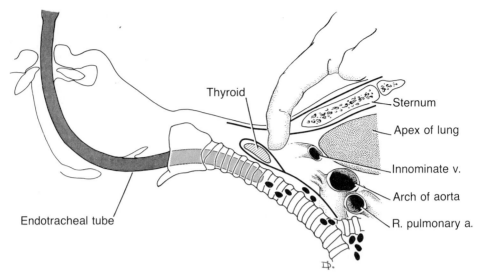

Figure 16–8   Mediastinoscopy. The neck is entered by a low collar incision which follows the skin creases. Blunt dissection can be carried down along the pretracheal fascia to the bifurcation of the trachea. Nodes can then be selected by inspection through the mediastinoscope and biopsies can be made of them.

propriate antibiotics given in combination for an adequate period of time; and (3) continuous observation and repeated reculture to insure continuing efficacy of treatment.[5] The evidence is increasingly convincing that intensive treatment with isoniazid, streptomycin and rifampicin for six months may be just as effective as the former treatment courses of one and a half to two years with combinations of streptomycin, isoniazid and paraminosalicylic acid.[37] An often overlooked responsibility is examination and skin testing of household contacts; although there is still some controversy, many believe that prophylactic therapy with isoniazid for one year may prevent the development of clinical tuberculosis in patients who have recently converted their PPD skin tests to positive.[4]

Today, surgery for tuberculosis is reserved for mechanical problems that antibiotics cannot repair. These include

(1) an area of destroyed lung tissue of limited resistance to secondary infection;

(2) the bronchial problems: bronchostenosis, bronchiectasis, bronchopleural fistula;

(3) the diagnostic problem of the small solid lesion ("coin lesion"); and

(4) chronic empyema, which frequently is a mixed infection with *Mycobacterium tuberculosis* and pyogenic organisms such as *Staphylococcus aureus*.

The atypical mycobacteria can also produce lung disease that in every way resembles classical tuberculosis except for a slower time course. *M. kansasii* responds to chemotherapy moderately well; however, *M. intracellularis* (Avian-Battey group) responds poorly and incompletely to chemotherapy, and in these patients a localized, persistent thick-walled cavity or a solid necrotic residual may be an indication for segmental resection or lobectomy.[29] There are rarely indications today for pulmonary resection in children with pulmonary tuberculosis.

Fungal Infection

Treatment of pulmonary fungal infections parallels that of tuberculosis. Agents available for chemotherapy are fewer.[7] Amphotericin B is effective against the widest number of fungi. Penicillin is effective against susceptible strains of actinomyces and sulfadiazine has been effective against many strains of nocardia. The compound 5-fluorocytosine has been especially promising in cryptococcal infections and against some strains of Candida (Monilia). Again, the role of surgery is to remove mechanical problems in order to make chemotherapy more effective.

Cancer

Lung cancer is the most common lethal neoplasm in men older than age 45 in the United States today. The incidence has increased more than 1000 per cent in cases proven at autopsy since 1900. In 1978, 92,000 people died of lung cancer in the United States alone. Surgery still offers almost the only chance for cure.

The best results in the treatment of lung cancer have been obtained in patients with small asymptomatic lesions discovered by routine roentgenograms. However, in the prospective study of 6027 volunteers by Boucot and Weiss,[111] 121 developed lung cancer during a ten-year period, and, despite chest x-rays every six months, only 8 per cent of the group survived five years after discovery of the tumor. Fontana and colleagues at the Mayo Clinic are conducting a prospective ongoing study of 4042 men over the age of 45 who smoke one or more packs of cigarettes daily.[35] Ninety per cent of the group have adhered to the routine of a chest film and three-day pooled sputum cytology every four months. Suspicious cytological findings are followed up with fiberoptic bronchoscopy and brushing. Chest x-rays were abnormal in only 24 of 33 patients with cytologically demonstrated cancer. The rate of cancer detected was six per 1000 man-years of surveillance.

Screening methods other than sputum cytology have been disappointing. Although about two-thirds of patients with far advanced lung cancer have elevated serum levels for carcinoembryonic antigen (CEA), the test is of little value in minimal disease. There is still hope that specific tumor-associated antigens can be isolated for use in early diagnosis.[48]

Saccomano[92] has demonstrated the synergistic carcinogenic effects of cigarette smoking and radon inhalation in uranium miners in Colorado and Utah. Cessation of smoking tends to restore the bronchial cytological findings toward normal after a period of years. Arnold Reif, a pathologist, estimates that 81 per cent of lung cancer is caused by smoking and that 20 per cent of *all* cancer in the United States results from smoking.[92] The Lahey Clinic statistics from 1956 to 1972[8] show that the rate of lung cancer in women who smoke has doubled in that time and that now women constitute 29 per cent of lung cancer patients. Originally, the report of Wynder and Graham[112] showed a strong correlation only between epidermoid (squamous) carcinoma and smoking; however, more recent studies show significant increases in oat cell and adenocarcinoma in heavy smokers as well. If one also considers the high incidence of coronary arterial disease in heavy smokers,[1] smoking can be described in no other way than as irrational behavior; there is no way to rationalize irrational behavior.

There are certain rules-of-thumb concerning operability in lung cancer. Weight loss still tends to be an ominous sign; it may not preclude resectability of a lesion but it decreases the likelihood for surgical cure. Phrenic or recurrent nerve paralysis does not always preclude resection but again argues against possible cure.

Accumulation of pleural fluid does not necessarily rule out curative resection, provided that the fluid is a result of pulmonary suppuration distal to an area of bronchial obstruction and is not due to seeding of the visceral and parietal pleura by tumor nodules. If the pleural fluid is free of tumor cells, one should not rule out exploratory thoracotomy.

The introduction of mediastinoscopy by Eric Carlens in 1959 was a major advance (Fig. 16–8). Its increased utilization followed the demonstration that patients with mediastinal node involvement, especially of the "perinodal" type, were not likely to benefit from pulmonary resection.[52, 80] However, a more recent study has shown a five-year survival rate of 25 per cent in patients who had squamous cell carcinoma with ipsilateral mediastinal metastases who were treated by resection and postoperative radiation to the mediastinum.[57] Peripheral lesions less than 2 cm in diameter are infrequently associated with mediastinal metastases except for small undifferentiated (oat cell) carcinoma.[49]

RESULTS. Once the patient has developed symptoms, most clinics report a survival of only 6 to 8 per cent for the entire group with brochogenic cancer. Attempts to improve survival with preoperative supervoltage irradiation were received enthusiastically when it was found that a large number of tumors were made resectable. However, two carefully randomized series have failed to show any improvement in survival.[65]

PALLIATION. Palliation must be considered in terms of both quality and length of life. Palliative resection is sometimes justified to stop distressing hemoptysis or to remove foci of suppuration that cannot be controlled by antibiotics. Comfort is increased but not length of survival.

X-ray therapy may be useful in relieving pain in bone metastases or pain resulting from invasion of the chest wall. Sometimes an obstructed bronchus can be opened to relieve dyspnea or infection. In the British Medical Research Council series, overall survival was longer in patients with oat cell carcinoma treated with radiation than in those treated surgically;[69] however, many thoracic surgeons can point to a few five-year survivors who had lobectomies for small peripheral oat cell cancers.

Initial studies of chemotherapy failed to show any benefits in series of patients from Veterans Administration hospitals or in a combined university hospital series. Currently, treatment with combinations of two to four drugs is under study. The median survival of patients with small cell undifferentiated (oat cell) carcinoma is four to six months from time of discovery, and median survival with chemotherapy is about one year. Benefits are much less with epidermoid and adenocarcinoma. Side effects with intensive chemotherapy are sometimes severe and the quality of life must be balanced against the number of days of increased survival.[98]

THE PROBLEM OF THE SOLITARY PULMONARY NODULE. The extensive chest x-ray surveys done by the U.S. armed forces during and after World War II seemed to indicate that, in men over the age of 40, the solitary uncalcified pulmonary nodule might have as high as a 35 per cent chance of being malignant, whether primary or metastatic. By contrast, in surveys in civilian populations, only 2.4 to 3 per cent of all nodules showed malignancy. However, in males over the age of 44 who had nodules more than 39 mm in greatest diameter, the probability of malignancy was one in three.[47]

There is general agreement that the nodule that shows massive or laminar calcification is probably caused by a granuloma (tuberculosis, atypical mycobacterial infection or fungus infection), whereas scattered flecks of calcium in a nodule are still compatible with cancer. Hamartomas usually have a characteristic pattern of patchy calcification that is readily recognized on tomography so that the patient can avoid thoracotomy. Rigler[88] feels that a notch in the edge of a nodule is strongly suggestive of malignancy. Lillington sums up current thinking well: "In patients over the age of 35 with an uncalcified nodule of unknown stability, the possibility of primary malignant tumor is sufficiently great that such a lesion must be considered malignant until proven otherwise, and managed accordingly. . . . An attempt to obtain a tissue diagnosis by needle aspiration biopsy or brush biopsy is advisable in most cases. . . . If no diagnosis is obtainable, exploratory thoracotomy is advisable in most instances."[61]

Functional Criteria for Surgery

PULMONARY. One must always ask the question: Is the patient able to afford the loss of any more functioning pulmonary tissue? Many years ago Max Pinner asked the question in a different way: What shall it avail the patient to be "cured" of his tuberculosis if he never again will be able to leave his bed to do a few hours' work or climb one flight of stairs?[82] Often one can gain a useful estimate of the patient's ability to withstand a lobectomy or pneumonectomy by a detailed study of his daily activities. How many flights of steps can he climb? How far can he walk on level ground without distress in either legs or chest? Does he wheeze or become blue with exertion? Can he blow out a match at a distance of two feet with unpursed lips? It is tempting to estimate pulmonary function from the x-ray film, but this is always inferior to actual studies of ventilation and of blood gases. The detailed laboratory values are available in Physiology of Respiration by Comroe[23] and in other textbooks. In general a patient of average size who has at least 2 liters of total vital capacity and who can expel 65 per cent of that in the first second of forceful expiration and who has disease localized to a lobe can probably be tided over an operation. He may have severe diffi-

culty after operation and may require prolonged assistance of ventilation.[10]

CARDIAC. Cardiac catheterization has been useful in borderline cases. The normal individual can increase ventilation at least tenfold and can triple his cardiac output with strenuous exercise. Under these circumstances pulmonary artery pressure may rise slightly in the normal individual or may actually fall, whereas the person who has lost more than half of the perfusable pulmonary vascular space will almost always show a rise of 15 to 20 mm of mercury or more in mean pulmonary artery pressure. Temporary occlusion of the right or left branch of the pulmonary artery with a fluid-filled balloon was first introduced in Sweden by Carlens (1951) and in this country by Paul Nemir (1953); it serves as a "functional pneumonectomy."[19] Arterial blood gas studies at rest and after breathing 100 per cent oxygen for 20 minutes will also tell much about intrapulmonary mixing and the ventilation/perfusion ratios ($\dot{V}/\dot{Q}$).

Endocrine Abnormalities

Various types of endocrine abnormalities have been associated with malignant tumors of the thymus, of the lung, of the pleura and of the retroperitoneal tissues. These have included paradoxical antidiuretic hormone production, secretion of insulin or insulin-like materials, hypercalcemia from parathormonelike materials, Cushing's syndrome from anomalous ACTH secretion and secretion of norepinephrine and epinephrine by extra-adrenal pheochromocytomas.[73]

Mediastinal Tumors

Mediastinal tumors are less common than tumors of the lung. Often one clue to the type of tumor involved is its position.[64] In the upper anterior mediastinum the substernal goiter can usually be identified easily by fluoroscopy — it is adherent to the trachea and moves upward on swallowing. A little lower in the anterior mediastinum the two most common tumors are thymoma and enlarged lymph nodes involved by lymphoma or Hodgkin's disease. The teratomas, dermoids and embryonal cell carcinomas are all rare. Lymph nodes in the midmediastinum may simulate tumor when they are affected by various granulomas such as tuberculosis, atypical mycobacterial infections, fungal infections or by involvement by metastatic tumor from lung or esophagus. Posteriorly, the neurofibroma is almost unique.

Thymic tumors have been of special interest because of the association of the thymus with myasthenia gravis, first noted in 1901 by the German pathologist Carl Weigert. On May 26, 1936, Alfred Blalock did the first thymectomy specifically for treatment of myasthenia gravis. His patient, a 19 year old woman who had had symptoms for four years, was well 25 years later. After a lapse from grace for nearly two decades, thymectomy is making a comeback as treatment for what is now considered as an autoimmune disease. Studies by Osserman and associates[81] indicate that thymectomy works as well in men with myasthenia gravis as in women. Duration of symptoms had little prognostic value in their series. Since most patients have either a normal or hyperplastic thymus, it is a waste of time to attempt to demonstrate a tumor in every patient as a justification for thymectomy.

Idiopathic Pleural Effusion

Idiopathic pleural effusion is ominous. All effusions should be aspirated for diagnosis (Figs. 16–9 and 16–10). Smears and cultures should be done for pyogenic bacteria, acid-fast bacteria and fungi. Transudates (e.g., from heart failure) almost always contain

less than 3.0 gm of protein per 100 ml, while exudates from infarct, cancer, empyema or tuberculosis almost always contain more than 3.0 gm per cent.[16] Potts and associates have shown that pH measurements are quite useful: pH was above 7.30 in benign effusions and below 7.30 in empyema.[60]

Malignant cells sometimes can be shown on direct smears stained by the Papanicolaou or hematoxylin-eosin method, but results may be better after mixing the fluid with an equal amount of 10 per cent formalin, centrifuging and then embedding and sectioning the "button" of cellular debris at the bottom of the tube. Tissue culture has been helpful in the diagnosis of mesothelioma and metastatic adenocarcinoma in effusions.[76]

Spontaneous Pneumothorax

Spontaneous pneumothorax used to be considered pathognomonic of pulmonary tuberculosis. Today it usually results from rupture of focal areas of obstructive emphysema which are often in portions of the lung adherent

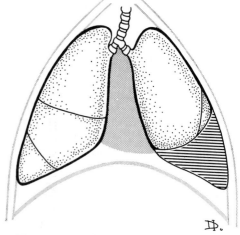

Figure 16–9 Pleural effusion. In pleural effusion, the fluid level curves up along the chest wall. If hydropneumothorax exists, there is an obvious, straight airfluid interface. Hydropneumothorax implies a connection with the bronchial tree.

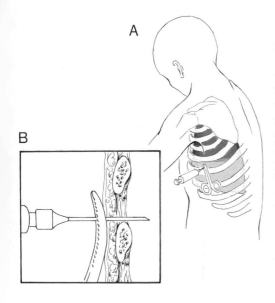

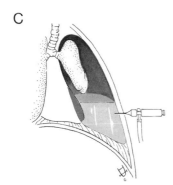

Figure 16–10 Thoracentesis. A. Thoracentesis is best done with the patient seated and leaning forward slightly. B. An 18 gauge needle with a 45° bevel is introduced just above the top of the rib. A plastic cannula (e.g., Intracath, Longdwel, or Angiocath) works well and is less likely to lacerate the underlying lung than a metal needle. C. When large volumes of fluid must be removed, a three-way stopcock between the needle and a 30 to 50 ml syringe permits drainage through a length of rubber or plastic tubing into a collecting bottle.

to the apex of the chest from an old infectious process. My own policy is to treat the first or even second episode (Fig. 16–11 A, B, C) of spontaneous pneumothorax with catheter drainage (size 16F) of the affected pleural space. However, in individuals who have had episodes on both sides of the chest or

more than two episodes on the same side of the chest, the recommendation is for a thoracotomy to excise or oversew areas of blebs (on the surface of the lung) or bullae (originating below the surface of the visceral pleura) and to strip off the parietal pleura to insure a firm symphysis between the surface of the lung and the chest wall. This latter procedure does not completely prevent blowouts from the surface of the lung, but it means any such blowout will form a very localized pneumothorax and not be life-threatening.

The former enthusiasm for treatment of emphysema by extensive excision of emphysematous blebs or bullae has been tempered by the increasing evidence that patients with airway obstructive disease have a generalized process affecting the whole lung and that any surgical intervention is likely to have extremely short-term benefits. There are a few individuals who have localized giant bullae and minimal evidence of generalized airway obstruction who may still be benefited by judicious local excisions.

Empyema — Resection and Open Drainage

Empyema is still with us despite antibiotics and increased awareness. The diagnosis sometimes can be made by a direct smear of pleural exudate, even though growth of bacteria has been suppressed by antibiotics given prior to consultation. Tube drainage is the first maneuver using a large (24–32 F) catheter placed by closed thoracostomy (Fig. 16–11) on water seal drainage. If the fluid is very thick or the empyema wall quite dense, then we do not hesitate to revert to the old maneuver of rib resection and open drainage.

Each new generation of surgeons (and physicians) must relearn the dictum arrived at by the Empyema Commission of the U.S. Army after World War I: "Empyema is cured only by

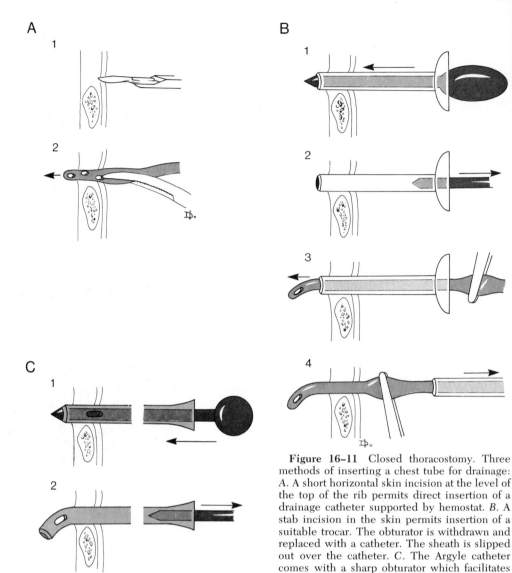

Figure 16–11 Closed thoracostomy. Three methods of inserting a chest tube for drainage: *A.* A short horizontal skin incision at the level of the top of the rib permits direct insertion of a drainage catheter supported by hemostat. *B.* A stab incision in the skin permits insertion of a suitable trocar. The obturator is withdrawn and replaced with a catheter. The sheath is slipped out over the catheter. *C.* The Argyle catheter comes with a sharp obturator which facilitates insertion through a small skin incision.

eliminating the space, either by bringing the lung out to meet the chest wall, or failing this, by bringing the chest wall down to meet the lung (thoracoplasty)."

Postpneumonectomy empyema is the exception to the rule. It is often possible to sterilize the space after open drainage, to close the bronchial fistula, if present, and to close the chest wall again.[54]

Chronic Constriction–Decortication

Chronic constriction of the lung by a layer ("peel") of granulation tissue and fibrin is best treated by decortication.[24] There are a few patients with extensive fibrosis of the underlying lung who are not candidates for decortication but who can be treated by chronic open drainage or marsupialization of the empyema cavity to the outside and who remain relatively symptom-free for many years, until they finally succumb to their pulmonary insufficiency. We have not hesitated doing localized Schede full-thickness excisions of the chest wall in order to marsupialize chronic empyema cavities, and the patients have been grateful for relief which has often extended for over a decade or more. Fortunately, since few patients are being treated by artificial pneumothorax any more for tuberculosis, the chronic "mixed" empyema (tuberculosis plus pyogens) is almost a museum piece.[31]

Postoperative Problems

Pain

Postoperative care after thoracotomy must not be neglected. Persistent intercostal neuralgia is often troublesome. Light percussion on the chest wall often will locate a "trigger zone." Direct block of this or a block of two intercostal nerves above and below the segment, repeated two or three times, may be all that is needed. Claggett[22] has suggested division of the intercostal nerve above the line of incision prior to opening the rib spreader, since he feels that many cases of intercostal neuralgia in the older patient are the result of excessive traction upon posterior sensory roots in the patient who has already developed considerable stiffening of the thoracic cage. One per cent lidocaine has been an effective blocking agent, as discussed later under rib fracture.

Persistent Air Space

The problem of the persistent air space in the patient who has had recent pneumonia or in the postoperative patient always comes up. One of the most common problems is the pneumatocele which may persist for weeks or months after an episode of pneumonia or pulmonary trauma. This is not a surgical problem. If the patient is asymptomatic and has had adequate antibiotic treatment for his pneumonia, we prefer merely to watch such spaces until they disappear. If there is a fluid level or if the patient has cough, fever or leukocytosis, then we consider this a lung abscess and start with treatment of appropriate antibiotics, based on cultures of sputum or pleural fluid, and this course of antibiotics is usually four to six weeks in duration. Postpneumonia pneumatocele is most common after staphylococcal pneumonia, but a subsequent lung abscess may be due to other microorganisms. Persistent air spaces have also been described in children after pertussis and usually need only careful observation until they disappear.

THE EMERGENCY ROOM

"Chance favors the mind that is prepared."

These words of Louis Pasteur's have been quoted thousands of times but never in a better context than that of the Emergency Room.

Priorities

An ordered system of priorities is essential (a) to save life, (b) to preserve function as far as possible and (c) to minimize disfigurement.[42] The priorities are
(1) Maintain ventilation;
(2) Stop obvious external bleeding;
(3) Replenish the blood volume and insure adequate circulation;
(4) Treat cardiac wounds;
(5) Evaluate and treat central nervous system damage;
(6) Repair the ruptured viscus;

(7) Stabilize and later reduce and fix fractures.

Ventilation

The importance of ventilation can be illustrated by simply holding one's breath. Only a trained athlete such as an experienced underwater swimmer can hold his breath voluntarily for more than 40 to 60 seconds. The accident victim is fortunate if he reaches the Emergency Room within 30 minutes after the catastrophe. Fractures and lacerations about the face with bleeding into the upper airway cause obvious airway obstructions. However, fracture of the larynx must always be suspected when there is laryngeal tenderness, crepitus or stridor, and it may be overlooked until the patient is in serious difficulty. This is one of the few instances when emergency tracheostomy is justified; otherwise it is safer to insert a bronchoscope or endotracheal tube for ventilation and perform a formal tracheostomy sometime in the next 24 hours (see Chapter 11). Tracheostomy is best done over an endotracheal tube in the operating room with adequate equipment, light and assistance.[75]

Cricothyroidotomy was uniformly condemned in the older surgical literature because of an allegedly high rate of subsequent subglottic stenosis; however, Brantigan and Grow have demonstrated in more than 650 patients that cricothroidotomy through a short transverse incision is safe for both emergency and elective use.[11]

Several points cannot be emphasized too often. Instead of "stop, look and listen," the command should be "strip completely, look, feel and listen." Ventilation can often be observed better by looking at the patient's chest movements from the foot of the bed. Inequality of movement of the right versus the left thorax can often be evaluated by palpation with the fingers on the rib margins and the thumbs laid along the spine. If the patient is awake and cooperative and has an intact glottis, pneumothorax can be detected more quickly by palpation of vocal fremitus than by percussion or auscultation.

Physical Signs and Emergency Treatment

Some physical signs may give clues as to the severity of injury: "splinting" of movements of chest or abdo-

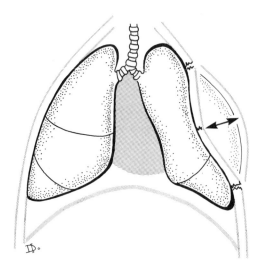

Figure 16–12 Paradoxical motion — flail chest. *Parodoxical motion* of the chest wall results from multiple fractures of contiguous ribs. Each rib or costal cartilage must be fractured anteriorly and posteriorly to cause the chest wall to be pulled in on inspiration and pushed out on expiration. This can markedly decrease alveolar ventilation. Immediate treatment with an endotracheal tube connected to volume-cycled respirator will improve ventilation and bring arterial Po_2 and Pco_2 back toward normal. An elective tracheostomy can safely be done in the operating room at any convenient time in the next 48 hours.

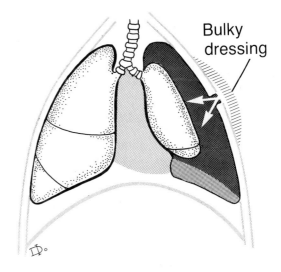

Figure 16–13 Sucking chest wound. A *sucking chest wound* can be occluded by petrolatum (Vaseline) gauze covered by a bulky dressing. If the lung is also lacerated, application of an occlusive dressing will produce a tension pneumothorax. Therefore, if the patient has any evidence of respiratory distress, a thoracostomy tube is inserted in the fifth or sixth interspace in the midaxillary line to remove air and blood and expand the lung.

men, *flail chest* with paradoxical chest wall motion (Fig. 16–12), respiratory distress, ecchymoses at the base of the neck, subcutaneous emphysema, difference in breath sounds between the right and left sides, absence of a point of maximal impulse at the cardiac apex and a change in the percussible liver dullness. *Sucking chest wounds* (Fig. 16–13) can be closed with Vaseline gauze and a bulky dressing held in place by tape. If there is suspicion of a *tension pneumothorax* (Fig. 16–14) do not wait for the x-ray but confirm by thoracentesis (Fig. 16–10) and then insert a thoracostomy tube (Fig. 16–11). Although many textbooks still show insertion of chest tubes in the second interspace in the midclavicular line and the seventh interspace posteriorly, I have come to believe that the patient is much more comfortable if tubes are inserted in the midaxillary line and that they work just as well in this position with less restriction of the patient's movements. As shown in Figure 16–11, the demonstration of free air or blood in the pleural space is followed immediately by insertion of a trocar and a tube. At one time there was enthusiasm for inserting the largest possible chest tube, but again experience has shown that a size 16 catheter is usual-

ly more than adequate for the upper tube to remove air.

One may want to insert a size 24-36 plastic tube by means of direct incision into the pleural space because of intrapleural bleeding. The quickest

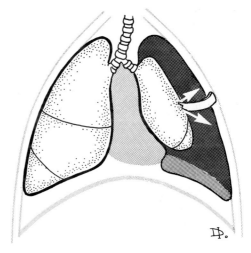

Figure 16–14 Tension pneumothorax. *Tension pneumothorax* results from a laceration of the lung which produces a one-way valve effect. During straining or coughing, air is forced into the pleural space under high enough pressure to displace the mediastinum, interfere with ventilation of the other lung and with venous return to the right atrium. Immediate insertion of a chest tube can be lifesaving. Occasionally, tension pneumothorax can result from bronchiolitis, rupture of an emphysematous bulla, or even a necrotizing pneumonia.

way in general to stop bleeding in the pleural space is to expand the lung expeditiously. This usually requires at least two chest tubes with suction of minus 15 to minus 25 cm of water. If the patient continues to bleed more than 500 ml during the second hour after the tubes have been inserted, this is taken as an indication for immediate thoracotomy. In the military experience in Viet Nam, 94 per cent of hemothorax problems were controlled with tube drainage alone and only 6 per cent of patients required thoracotomy.[109]

If there is an unremitting flow of air from the chest tubes, one has to suspect either a ruptured bronchus or deep lacerations of the lung surface by spicules from fractured ribs, both of which require immediate operation.

Eijgelaar and van der Heide[28] found that x-ray demonstration of air in the deep cervical fascial planes along the trachea and along the large vessels enclosed by the middle cervical fascia was a very strong indication of a ruptured bronchus or trachea.

Subcutaneous emphysema may be annoying but in itself is rarely serious. It can occur from a laceration of the nasopharynx when air is forced beneath the skin, or from mediastinal emphysema from a tracheal laceration, or it may simply represent the end of an involuntary Valsalva maneuver with rupture of alveoli at the periphery of the lung and dissection of the air back along the vascular sheath, as originally described by C. C. Macklin in 1936. When subcutaneous emphysema produces severe discomfort, excess air can often be massaged into a few pockets where it can be aspirated aseptically with an 18 gauge needle.

Stabilization of the Chest

By simple inspection, one can see whether or not there is paradoxical motion of the chest. This implies fractures of several ribs in at least two places (Fig. 16–12), making an unsupported flap of chest wall which is pulled in with inspiration and pushed out with expiration, thus diminishing pulmonary ventilation. Despite recurrent articles in the surgical literature advocating stabilization of the chest wall with towel clips, pericostal stainless steel wire traction sutures and even Kirschner wire fixation of rib fragments, I remain convinced that internal splinting by artificial ventilation is superior. Blood gases can be maintained in the normal range and the patient requires less narcotics. The original contribution of Moerch and Avery represents the best approach: insert a cuffed endotracheal tube immediately and start artificial ventilation with a volume-cycled respirator. Within 24 to 48 hours the endotracheal tube can be replaced by a cuffed tracheostomy tube. Positive pressure ventilation is then maintained for ten to twenty days, until the chest wall has been stabilized by fibrosis at the fracture sites.[3]

Trinkle and associates feel that too much emphasis has been placed on the flail segment of thoracic wall and that the basic problem in closed chest injuries is the underlying pulmonary contusion. With close attention to treatment of the damaged lung, many of their patients did not need tracheostomy and prolonged positive pressure ventilation.[106]

Monitoring of Blood Gases

Cyanosis can be seen only when the patient has more than 5 gm of reduced hemoglobin per 100 ml of blood, and the hypovolemic patient may die before this level is reached. Inadequate ventilation can quickly be demonstrated from an arterial blood sample by a saturation below 90 per cent and a PCO_2 above 50 mm of mercury. Repeated arterial samples are the best guide to the adequacy of ventilation.

Probably the single greatest advance in the treatment of patients with all types of acute pulmonary insufficiency has been monitoring of arterial blood samples. Arterial puncture is easily done by puncture of radial, brachial or femoral arteries with a 20 gauge needle. Currently available equipment for determining arterial oxygen saturation, pH, Po_2 and Pco_2 can give rapid, accurate values as guides to therapy.

Bleeding

External

External bleeding can generally be controlled with finger pressure or pressure dressings initially. Definitive vascular repair or ligation should be done under aseptic conditions in the operating room. More difficult problems arise from lacerations of intercostal arteries or the internal mammary artery and these may require emergency thoracotomy for control.

Internal

Evaluation of internal bleeding is more difficult. It is important to check pulses and blood pressures in both upper and lower extremities repeatedly for symmetry; this is often a clue to aortic laceration or false aneurysm after blunt trauma. Fractures of the first rib are very frequently associated with injuries to innominate or subclavian arteries, aortic arch and brachial plexus.[87] As soon as ventilation and circulating blood volume have been restored to normal, plans should be made for definitive repair (see page 746 for assessment and treatment of heart wounds).

Treatment of Hypovolemia and Shock

While all the above measures are being taken, other members of the team have begun treatment for hypovolemia and shock. A central venous pressure cannula should be inserted by a convenient route: antecubital vein, jugular vein or subclavian vein (see Chapter 4). At least two plastic cannulas or cutdowns should be inserted. As soon as central venous pressure has been measured accurately, fluid infusion should be begun with lactated Ringer's solution to increase circulating blood volume. Plasmanate can be added as soon as blood has been drawn for typing and cross-match. Up to one liter of low-molecular weight dextran (dextran 40) can be given without interfering with the coagulation mechanism.

Associated Injuries (Diaphragm, Spleen, Liver, Kidney, Brain)

A Foley catheter is inserted in the bladder to monitor urinary output. Cross-match enough blood: most patients subjected to massive injury should have at least six units of blood cross-matched initially. Plan the logical approach to stop any continuing bleeding. Even the least experienced surgeon soon learns that lower thoracic injuries on the left carry a high suspicion of rupture of the spleen and sometimes laceration of diaphragm, and low thoracic injuries on the right may be combined with lacerations of the liver and of the right kidney. Traumatic rupture of the diaphragm (Fig. 16–15) frequently follows a massive, sudden compression of the abdomen and demands immediate surgical repair. Stab wounds of the lower chest and upper abdomen have had a high incidence of diaphragmatic laceration with appearance of a diaphragmatic hernia later;

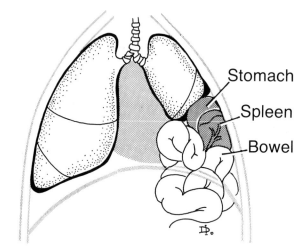

Figure 16–15 Traumatic rupture of diaphragm. Massive blunt trauma to the abdomen can split the diaphragm (usually the left leaf) in the direction of its fibers. The spleen, stomach, splenic flexure of colon, and small bowel may be forced into the pleural space and may markedly interfere with ventilation. Immediate operation is essential. A similar but more slowly developing situation has followed stab wounds (in the left lower chest or left upper abdomen) that lacerate the diaphragm.

all should be explored in the operating room.

The problem of central nervous system damage is always with us. Few patients subjected to massive injury to the torso and extremities have escaped without a concussion at the minimum. The problem of differentiation between cerebral concussion, contusion and laceration on the one hand and between acute extradural or subdural hematoma on the other is often difficult and calls for neurosurgical consultation as early as possible.

Rib Fractures

Uncomplicated rib fractures can cause much discomfort. Analgesics will relieve most patients, but if there are multiple fractures, much more relief can be achieved by intercostal nerve block (Fig. 16–16). Blocks may have to be repeated every six to eight hours for the first few days after injury. The patient is then able to ventilate more effectively and to clear the bronchial tree by coughing. In general, strapping of the chest is much less effective in reducing pain and is likely to cause blistering of the skin. In a few instances, when one or two lower ribs have been fractured, circumferential restriction of the en-

tire chest by a belt or by tape may give some comfort.

Transportation

Finally, the reader may wonder why the acutely injured patient has not been taken for x-ray studies up to this point. Experience again has shown that the least amount of moving around that need be done in order to accomplish treatment is to the patient's advantage. Plan the evaluation and emergency treatment in a logical fashion so that the patient needs only one trip to the x-ray department, either on the way to the intensive care area or to the operating room. If extremity fractures are splinted before he makes this trip, further blood loss around the fracture sites will be minimized and it will be easier to maneuver the splinted extremity into the best position for x-ray studies.

Summary

In summary, the patient who comes to the Emergency Room after massive trauma must be considered in imminent danger of death. Chest injuries may be involved in more than half of

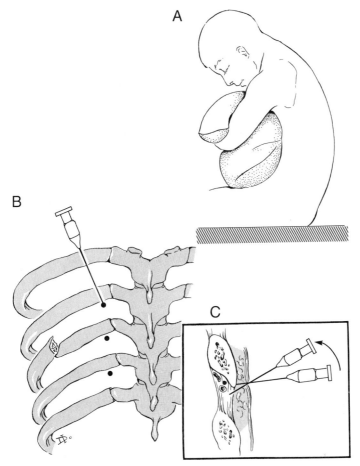

Figure 16–16 Relief of pain from fractured ribs. *A*. The patient is usually more comfortable sitting up with the arms grasping a pillow, thus throwing the scapulae forward. *B*. The sensory fields of the intercostal nerves overlap. In order to relieve the pain of fractured ribs, one must block one nerve above and one below the fractured rib, as well as the nerve adjacent to the fracture. *C*. A 22 gauge needle is inserted through a skin wheal of 1% lidocaine until it touches the lower border of the rib; then it is angled downward to pass just beneath the edge of the rib. It is not necessary to produce paresthesias by contact with the nerve. Five ml of 1% lidocaine injected within a few millimeters of the nerve will diffuse to produce an adequate block. Always get a chest x-ray after the block to be sure no pneumothorax has resulted from inadvertent laceration of the lung during the block.

the cases. A logical, preformed plan for diagnosis and decision will save more lives than misguided enthusiasm and technical virtuosity.

ESOPHAGUS

History

Just as with pulmonary disease, it is important to learn why the patient presents with his symptoms at this time. Is there incoordination of swallowing with regurgitation of fluid through the nose, suggestive of neurological disease? Is there pain in the throat or substernally with swallowing (odynophagia)? Is there difficulty in swallowing (dysphagia), manifested by a vague sensation of soreness or something sticking in the esophagus? Are there symptoms to suggest gastroesophageal reflux, such as "heart burn," regurgitation when bending over to put on shoes, regurgitation of gastric contents or staining of the pillow during sleep?

Physical Examination

A fairly good index of severity of symptoms is the degree of weight loss. Physical examination begins with a careful evaluation of the mouth and teeth, since symptoms may be related to swallowing large masses of unchewed food. Inspection of the posterior pharynx and base of the tongue with a mirror takes only a few minutes and is often helpful. Only a limited physical examination of the cervical portion of the esophagus is possible and therefore roentgenography and endoscopy provide much of the relevant information.

X-RAY

Many radiologists prefer to start the examination with thick barium, the consistency of toothpaste, to study motility in the pharynx and upper esophagus. Thinner barium is more useful for study of the lower esophagus and for evaluation of reflux. The image-intensifying fluoroscope has reduced radiation dosage to the patient and has facilitated recording on film or video tape. The repeated playback of cine records of swallowing and peristalsis gives more information than can be obtained by the skilled observer from a single observation of the screen. Spot films complement the motion studies.

Special tricks are helpful. In the case of foreign bodies, which today are often radiolucent plastic, the patient can swallow a piece of soft bread or absorbent cotton saturated with barium sulfate suspension and this will often be arrested by the foreign body. Sometimes esophageal spasm or stricture can be assessed

better by observation of the passage of a marshmallow coated with barium sulfate. Some maneuvers may help to demonstrate reflux from stomach into lower esophagus: the Trendelenburg position, having the patient stand sideways to the screen and bend forward from the waist, the Mueller and Valsalva maneuvers and external pressure on the abdomen.

A concise account of esophageal morphology and movement is given by Zboralske and Freedland[117] and by Templeton.[101] A more extensive monograph by Stein and Finkelstein[96] outlines a helpful checklist of diagnostic features: (1) caliber; (2) intraluminal radiolucencies; (3) marginal contour; (4) mucosal pattern; (5) peristalsis; (6) position and displacement; and (7) food residue or detritus.

Endoscopy

Bronchoscopy and Esophagoscopy

Bronchoscopy and esophagoscopy are often done at the same sitting and will be discussed together here. The history of endoscopy has been concisely reviewed by Richard Meade.[68] The contributions of Chevalier Jackson were remarkable and were largely responsible for the popularization of bronchoscopy and esophagoscopy in this country in the early part of the century. The classic text of Jackson and Jackson[51] is still worth study.

Fiberoptic endoscopes (Figs. 16–17 through 16–19) have increased the ease, range and versatility of visual examination of the bronchi, esophagus, stomach and duodenum. The major advantages of fiberoptic bronchoscopy have been greater comfort for the patient, access to segmental and subsegmental bronchi, better examination of the upper lobes and facilitation of transbronchial biopsy and brush biopsy in the periphery of the lung. The major complications have been hypoxia and arrhythmias with

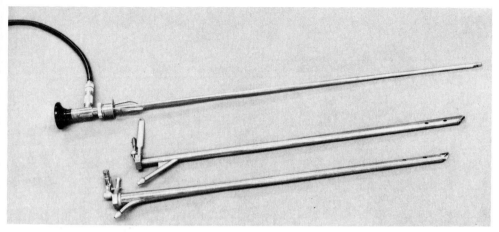

Figure 16–17 Bronchoscopes. *Top.* Right angle telescope with fiberoptic light carrier. *Middle.* Classic Chevalier Jackson tubular design. *Bottom.* Modern conical tube found in the Broyles, Holinger and C. L. Jackson instruments.

bronchoscopy[99] and perforation during esophagoscopy.

The fiberoptic bronchoscope can easily be passed through an endotracheal tube or tracheostomy stoma to remove secretions. The major disadvantages of fiberoptic endoscopes are expense, susceptibility to damage that requires return to the factory for expensive repairs and limitations in effective sterilization by chemical means.

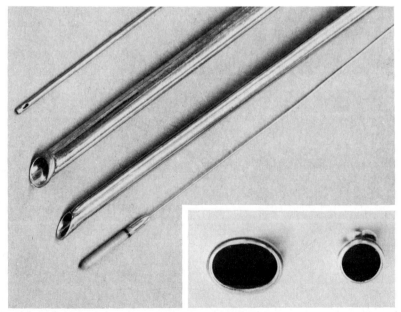

Figure 16–18 Rigid esophagoscopes. *Left upper to right lower.* Suction tube with solid rounded end and side holes; oval esophagoscope of Robertson or Jessberg type; cylindrical esophagoscope of Chevalier Jackson; soft rubber bougie — "lumen finder." *Inset.* End-on views of Robertson (*left*) and Jackson (*right*) esophagoscopes to show the marked improvement in working space available with the oval cross section as compared with the cylindrical tube with the same anteroposterior diameter.

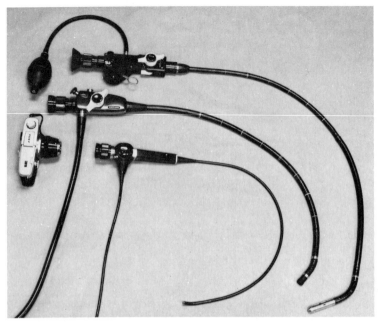

Figure 16–19   Flexible endoscopes. *Top.* Gastroscope. *Middle.* Esophagoscope. *Bottom.* Broncho-scope. The camera at left can be adapted for use with all three instruments.

There are situations in which the open, rigid bronchoscope or esopha-goscope is superior: when there is a need for large biopsy forceps or for large bore suction tubes to remove blood clots, inspissated secretions or crusts; during manipulation of large foreign bodies; and for dilation of strictures under visual control. The rigid and flexible scopes serve com-plementary functions and the endo-scopist must be skilled in the use of both.[115]

In conjunction with the endo-

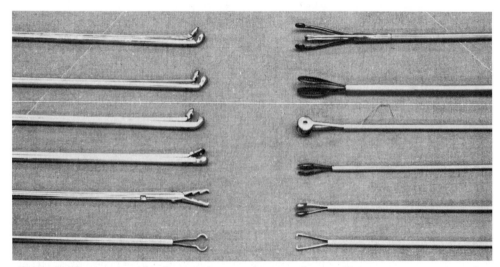

Figure 16–20   A variety of endoscopic biting and grasping forceps. The instrument at upper right is a Clerf safety pin closer.

scopes, a complete set of suction tips, biopsy forceps and forceps for removal of foreign bodies is essential (Fig. 16–20).

Pediatric Problems

Infants present special problems because the small airway permits passage of only a 3.0 or 3.5 mm open tube. Visibility has been likened to observing the far wall of a ballroom through a very small keyhole. A size 14 F urological panendoscope has been used with ventilation maintained through the cystoscope sheath. The Storz Company has brought out a size 7 F telescope based on the Hopkins cylindrical lens system that can be used both for cystoscopy and bronchoscopy.

The Endoscopist

The most important factor in bronchoscopy or esophagoscopy is the endoscopist. An experienced, obviously knowledgeable physician who moves gently but deliberately gives an enormous amount of nonverbal reassurance to the patient.

Premedication

We feel that premedication is essential. Formerly, a short-acting barbiturate such as seconal or amytal was used together with 0.4 to 0.6 mg atropine and a narcotic by intramuscular injection. For several years, I have found that diazepam (Valium), 5 to 15 mg orally one hour before the examination, has been superior to a barbiturate in relieving anxiety and producing muscular relaxation. Atropine 0.4 mg is given intramuscularly 30 minutes before the examination to decrease salivation. Depending upon the size of the patient and his previous reaction to narcotics, I have used 5 to 10 mg of methadone orally one

hour before the examination, 50 to 100 mg of Demerol (meperidine) intramuscularly or intravenously 5 to 30 minutes before the examination or 5 to 10 mg of morphine intramuscularly. In most patients the combination of diazepam 10 mg and methadone 5 mg by mouth one hour before the examination has been effective for endoscopy and for most minor surgical procedures with local anesthesia.*

An occasional patient may come to the examination quite tense and anxious. Five to 10 mg of Valium given slowly intravenously to the point of mild dysarthria will produce tranquility, muscular relaxation and amnesia for the procedure.

General Anesthesia

General anesthesia has been used routinely for babies, children and extremely apprehensive adults. Modern techniques for general anesthesia have removed any justification for immobilizing the helpless little patient for endoscopy without premedication or anesthesia, as formerly practiced by Jackson and Jackson and their pupils. Ventilation during anesthesia seems most efficient by the Sanders Venturi attachment, which eliminates the need for the cuirasse respirator or other complicated gear.[70] General anesthesia is used routinely in some clinics for esophagoscopy, but our experience has been that most patients tolerate esophagoscopy under topical anesthesia quite well.

---

*Roche Laboratories, the manufacturer of Valium, has the following sentence in the package insert: "Valium (diazepam) is not recommended for bronchoscopy and laryngoscopy because increased cough reflex and laryngospasm have been reported." The manufacturer inserted this because "In early trials with Valium, one investigator reported laryngospasm and coughing in his patient." My personal experience has been that diazepam is an excellent agent for premedication before endoscopy and is not accompanied by any increased incidence of laryngospasm.

Topical Anesthesia

Topical anesthesia was formerly a ritual that involved the use of concentrations of cocaine of from 4 to 10 per cent. Some patients have had severe and even fatal reactions to cocaine, and consequently this was supplanted in many centers by the use of 1 per cent Pontocaine, but reactions continued to occur. Lidocaine as a spray (2 per cent) and as viscous Xylocaine (4 per cent) has been very widely used with a low incidence of side effects. In recent years, dyclonine hydrochloride (Dyclone) has been used almost exclusively as our topical anesthetic agent. Our routine is to measure out a total of 20 ml of 0.5 per cent Dyclone in a medicine glass and not to exceed this amount. The pharynx and tongue are sprayed slowly and systematically to eliminate the gag reflex. Since Dyclone has a slower onset of action than Pontocaine or cocaine, this takes about five minutes. We have the patient breathe slowly while a mist of Dyclone is sprayed over the glottis. This is followed by three intratracheal instillations of 2 to 3 ml each. The trick here is to have the patient expire completely just before the anesthetic solution is delivered into the glottis through a malleable laryngeal cannula. The patient must take a deep breath and cough and, as a result of the cough reflex, he aspirates the material deep into the bronchial tree. Our patients have had no toxic reactions from Dyclone used in this fashion.

Dyclone shares with Pontocaine and some other topical anesthetic agents the property of inhibiting growth of bacteria, mycobacteria, and fungi. When cultures are of critical importance, lidocaine or even 4 per cent cocaine for topical anesthesia might be preferred. As mentioned previously, positive cultures and positive specimens by cytology are most likely to be obtained from sputum coughed up during the two or three days following bronchoscopy, and these will no longer be affected by the topical anesthetic agent.

In preparation for endotracheal intubation, the anesthesia staff often prefers to use 3 to 5 ml of Xylocaine (lidocaine) injected percutaneously into the trachea. For prolonged endotracheal intubation, percutaneous superior laryngeal nerve blocks with 1 per cent lidocaine have been used, but I feel this technique adds very little to topical anesthesia for a routine bronchoscopy.

An ingenious method for topical anesthesia has been devised by Christoforidis et al.,[20] who have used an ultrasonic nebulizer and cascade impactor to produce a mist of particles of which 80 per cent are less than 10 microns in diameter. Adequate anesthesia can be produced in seven to ten minutes with 4 to 7 ml of 4 per cent lidocaine with no stimulation of cough and virtually no discomfort for the patient. As ultrasonic nebulizers become more available, this method of self-administered topical anesthesia will undoubtedly become increasingly important.

In preparation for esophagoscopy the pharynx and tongue are sprayed with 0.5 per cent Dyclone as for bronchoscopy and in addition, the patient swallows 10 to 15 ml of viscous Xylocaine in small sips, a procedure which gives excellent topical anesthesia of mouth, pharynx and cricopharyngeal area.

Some endoscopists insist upon general anesthesia for all esophagoscopy; however, this does not seem necessary except in children too young to cooperate. There is no good evidence that routine use of general anesthesia will result in a lowered incidence of esophageal perforation.

Position of Patient

In the classic method of Chevalier Jackson the patient was supine for all

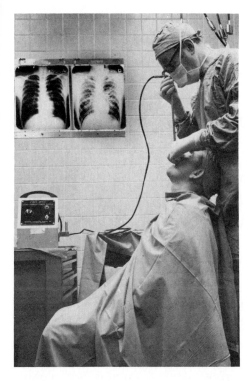
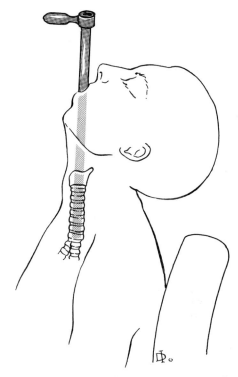

Figure 16–21   Bronchoscopy in the sitting position. *Bronchoscopy in the sitting position* is often more comfortable for the patient. The x-rays are available for continual comparison with the endoscopic findings.

endoscopy and his head was securely controlled by an assistant. This is still useful when bronchoscopy is performed under general anesthesia, when the assistance of gravity is needed for manipulation and extraction of foreign bodies, and for almost all esophagoscopy. Bronchoscopies at this center are often performed with the patient sitting in a straight backed chair (Fig. 16–21), or reclining slightly on the operating table or in bed.[13] Patients in this position can breathe more comfortably and have less fear of suffocating. A special assistant is not needed to hold the head.

Foreign Bodies – Technique of Removal with Physiotherapy

Foreign bodies in the air passages may threaten life because of glottic obstruction, and this tends to be a problem more often in elderly or alcoholic patients. The foreign bodies in the lower respiratory tract occur most commonly in children under school age. Jackson and Jackson[51] have presented one of the widest experiences with endoscopic removal of foreign bodies from the bronchi and esophagus. Burrington and Cotton[15] have described a method that uses a bronchodilator by aerosol and postural drainage and coughing, assisted by the physiotherapist. They have been able to recover more than 80 per cent of foreign bodies inhaled by children by this method. If the foreign body cannot be coughed up, endoscopy is an important technique that prevents bronchial obstruction and secondary suppuration, which is especially common when vegetable foreign bodies such as peanuts have been aspirated. In the case of the esophagus, the oval cross section of the Jessberg, Robertson, Moersch type of esophagoscope (Fig. 16–18) is especially useful in manipulating and removing foreign bodies.

Congenital Lesions— *Tracheoesophageal Fistula and Atresia of the Esophagus*

In *Surgery of the Esophagus* by Sealy and Postlethwait[83] one can find an excellent discussion of congenital anomalies of the esophagus. Commonest is atresia of the midesophagus with tracheoesophageal fistula, which seems to occur about once in 3000 live births. The experienced nurse often makes the diagnosis in the newborn nursery; the clue is excessive production of frothy mucus. Attempts to pass a size 10 to 12 F soft rubber catheter into the stomach will meet obstruction about 10 cm from the mouth. Occasionally the diagnosis may be missed until the baby has developed considerable respiratory embarrassment from aspiration.

Diagnostic Techniques

Anteroposterior and lateral chest films in the upright postion will show the configuration of the heart and whether or not there is air in the stomach and small bowel; sometimes they will show the gap between the tip of the catheter in the upper segment and the air column in the lower esophageal segment. The severest problem in these babies is aspiration pneumonia; therefore, barium is used sparingly to outline the upper esophageal pouch. Formerly, instillation of 1 or 1.5 ml of Gastrografin or other water-soluble contrast material was used to outline the upper pouch, the contrast material being aspirated through the inlying soft rubber catheter immediately after exposures have been made. Many radiologists

feel that the hypertonic Gastrografin produces more pneumonitis than barium sulfate; however, barium sulfate can cause granulomas when retained in the lung. Swenson[100] has used a size 8 F soft rubber catheter with three holes at the tip which is passed through the nostril into the upper esophageal pouch, on which constant suction is maintained to remove saliva and minimize further aspiration.

Surgical Repair and Results

T. M. Holder et al.[45] collected 1058 cases from 84 pediatric surgeons. Eighty-six percent of the patients fell into group C with a blind upper esophageal pouch and fistula between trachea and lower esophageal segment. About half had associated congenital anomalies of heart, gastrointestinal tract, genitourinary system, musculoskeletal system or central nervous system. Imperforate anus was noted 99 times. Gastrostomy before or after repair did not appear to reduce complications or mortality. The overall survival rate in 431 full term infants with type C malformation who weighed more than 5 pounds was 72 per cent.

Most authors have advised primary repair of the esophagus when the ends of the esophagus can be joined without undue tension. If tension appears excessive at the proposed suture line, then division of the fistula, cervical esophagostomy, gastrostomy, and later reconstruction with transposed colon, will decrease mortality.

Holder, McDonald, and Woolley[46] advocated primary repair except in the critically ill baby or the infant weighing less than 5½ pounds. Various authors have reported that 25 to 40 per cent of infants with tracheoesophageal fistula have been premature. In this group results were remarkably improved by doing a Stamm gastrostomy under local anesthesia as soon as the diagnosis was made to minimize reflux into the trachea. The tracheal fistula was divided by a retropleural approach through the right thorax 18 to 36 hours later. Repair of the esophagus was done one to six months later, when the infant's condition appeared favorable. By this method they were able to salvage 9 out of 15 patients in a very high risk group.

Carcinoma of Esophagus

Diagnosis

Nearly sixty-five years have elapsed since Franz Torek of New York City successfully resected a carcinoma of the esophagus transthoracically,[105] yet our salvage rate for patients with this disease has improved but little since esophagectomy with primary esophagogastrostomy was introduced to the western world by W. E. Adams and Dallas Phemister in 1938. Symptoms of mild substernal distress may evolve very gradually into high grade obstruction. Gradual weight loss and nutritional anemia may be ignored initially by patients and physicians. Cancer of the esophagus has often extended considerable distances through the submucosal lympatics before the patient has disabling symptoms which take him to the physician. Fluoroscopic studies[58] and endoscopy will usually make the diagnosis. However, some patients may be unsuitable even for fiberoptic esophagoscopy, especially those who have marked stricture or angulation of the esophagus, patients who have severe cardiovascular disease or airway obstructive disease or those with severe arthritis of the cervical spine. For patients such as this Fennessy et al.[33] have suggested inserting a catheter down to the level of the lesion under fluoroscopic control and then brushing the surface with nylon and steel brushes to obtain cells and shreds of tissue for microscopic examination.

Treatment

Once the diagnosis has been established, the goal is to restore swallowing function as quickly and safely as possible. Cancer of the esophagus tends to spread long distances through the submucosal lymphatics even before symptoms are significant, so cure is unusual.[39] Esophagectomy with esophagogastrostomy in a single operation is now most widely accepted; even if it does not cure, it can restore function. More complicated, multistaged procedures involving jejunal or colon interposition have higher mortality and no better results.[40]

There is general agreement that simple gastrostomy does not prolong life or comfort. X-ray therapy by multiple port or rotational techniques, supplemented by bouginage when necessary, has given relief to many patients[91] and has produced a few long-term cures of lower esophageal tumors. Intraluminal plastic tubes have been used to restore a channel for swallowing in patients too debilitated to withstand esophagogastrostomy; in carefully chosen patients this has made the remaining few months of life more comfortable.[78] Chemotherapy has had little to offer so far. There is one report of restoration of a lumen through the tumor by the local escharotic effect of cyclophosphamide and 5-fluorouracil injected directly into the tumor via esophagoscopy.[74]

Hemorrhage and Trauma

Hemorrhage is not a common accompaniment of esophageal disease except for rare catastrophes, such as erosion of an aortic aneurysm into the esophagus. The commonest causes of hematemesis are gastric or duodenal ulcer and erosive gastritis. The next commonest is esophageal varices.[18] Finally, there is the Mallory-Weiss syndrome in all its variations, ranging from a simple split of the mucosa of the lower esophagus to intramural hematoma of the esophagus to a full thickness tear into the pleural space, usually on the left. There is almost always a history of excessive food and alcohol intake and an episode of vomiting immediately preceding the episode of bleeding. Although there is no universal agreement on early use of esophagoscopy, numerous reports indicate that early endoscopy can be valuable in differential diagnosis of bleeding. Endoscopic electrocoagulation has successfully stopped hemorrhage in some cases of Mallory-Weiss syndrome; otherwise open operation and suture ligation of the bleeding points are needed.[108] If frank rupture of the esophagus has occurred, then immediate thoracotomy is indicated.[89]

In addition to Boerhaave's syndrome, esophageal injury can result from sharp and blunt trauma, both internal and external, and from burns. Jones and Samson and Nemir, Wallace and Fallahnejad have done extensive reviews.[53] The key to successful treatment of all esophageal injuries is early diagnosis, surgical closure and adequate drainage.[94]

The special problem of esophageal varices will be discussed in Chapter 18 on liver disease.

Corrosive Injuries

Chemical Burns — Types

Chemical burns of the esophagus continue to pose some of the most difficult technical problems. Acid burns tend to produce superficial coagulation while alkali burns produce a rapid hydrolytic destruction of protein which may progress through the full thickness of the esophageal wall within a few minutes. Eighty-six per cent of the lye burns in the series of Sealy and Postlethwait[83] occurred in children under the age of five years. The series reported by Yudin[114] consisted largely of sulfuric acid burns, because sulfuric acid is commonly used as a desiccant to prevent frosting of storm windows in Russia. By the time the patient reaches the Emergency Room with an alkali burn, attempts at neutralization are of no value, a conclusion borne out by Leape et al.,[59] who in a study of sodium hydroxide burns in animals found that much of the damage was done within the first few seconds after contact. Liquid caustic was worse than granular in their clinical series.

Burrington has described a characteristic full thickness circumferential burn of the esophagus that results from ingestion of Clinitest tablets. The strictures are usually extremely dense, resistant to dilation and require local excision and reanastomosis of the esophagus.[14]

Treatment

ESOPHAGOSCOPY AND STEROIDS. Previous treatment regimens, such as that published by Salzer in 1920, emphasized avoidance of esophagoscopy for several weeks after the burn. Bouginage was begun three to seven days after the burn and was continued for at least six months. It has been estimated that at least half of the patients did not require this period of extended and uncomfortable treatment. The current approach, as reviewed by Egan,[27] calls for esophagoscopy under general anesthesia within 24 hours after the patient has been admitted to the hospital, since pharyngeal burns are not always accompanied by esophageal damage. If esophagoscopy is stopped at the level of the first evidence of burn of the esophagus, the incidence of perforation will be kept low. If no burns are found in the esophagus or cardia, the patient is kept overnight for observation and then sent home with careful instructions to the parents to watch for any symptoms of interference with swallowing. If there is an esophageal burn, the patient is started on cortisone and an antibiotic. The work of Rosenberg et al.[90] demonstrated the advantages of cortisone in delaying maturation of fibroblasts and inhibiting collagen formation so that the epithelium could regenerate over the burned surface. The addition of antibiotics was especially important in patients who were on cortisone. Yarington and Heatly[113] at the University of Rochester used methylprednisolone sodium succinate (Medrol) intramuscularly in doses of 20 mg every eight hours for children under the age of two and 40 mg every eight hours for older patients. The University of Oregon routine[27] with 60 patients was to use parenteral dexameth-asone 1 mg daily or oral prednisone 60 mg daily for three or four days and then a maintenance dose of from 5 to 10 mg of prednisone daily together with ampicillin. The steroids are continued until esophagoscopy, performed at intervals of two to three weeks, demonstrates that the mucosa has healed. Fluoroscopic studies are made six months after steroids are discontinued. Strictures are dilated either with woven dilators (silk or nylon) or with the Hurst type of mercury-filled bougie (Fig. 16–22). More complicated or multiple strictures require a gastrostomy and retrograde dilatation. Ashcraft and Holder found that direct injection of prednisolone into short experimental strictures has aided in their dilation and resolution.[2]

DILATATION. Dilatation therapy can be carried on successfully for many years, as Salzer and many others have demonstrated. When dilatations

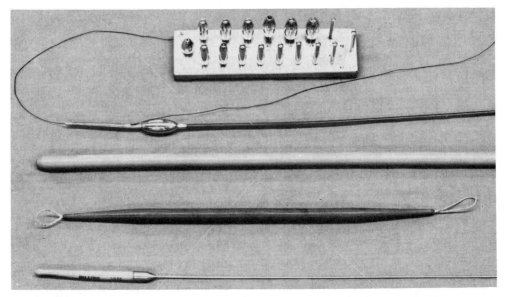

Figure 16–22 Esophageal bougies. *Top* to *Bottom:* The Plummer dilator has a flexible coil spring tip which follows a previously swallowed silk thread. The shaft unscrews and a series of metal olives can be positioned just behind the flexible tip. Next, the Hurst mercury-filled, flexible dilator is probably the easiest for the patient to use at home. The torpedo-shaped Tucker bougies have loops at both ends to facilitate their being drawn antegrade or retrograde in patients with established gastrostomies. The woven nylon Jackson dilators have olive-shaped tips to reduce the likelihood of perforation. Holinger has developed miniature dilators on the same pattern for use in infants with esophageal strictures.

are done over a previously swallowed string or are carried out over a looped string through a gastrostomy, the incidence of perforation is not great. It is important not to try to proceed too rapidly; Chevalier Jackson's old rule of not increasing the diameter by more than three gradations of bougies at any one sitting is still a good one. Dilatations must be kept up two or three times a week for a prolonged period and then from once a week to once a month indefinitely. Some patients learn to swallow a Hurst dilator at home with little difficulty. If a lumen of at least size 30 French through the esophagus can be maintained, the patient can manage baby food. If a dilator larger than 42 F can be passed, then a normal diet, well chewed, can be swallowed. With extensive, long, multiple strictures, either dilatation eventually becomes laborious as maturing collagen continues to contract, or the patient becomes dissatisfied with the multiple dilatations. In such cases esophageal substitution with colon has been helpful. A common technical problem is stenosis of the anastomosis at the level of the cricopharyngeus, since scarring in the area just below the cricopharyngeus is usually very extensive after a lye burn. Some surgeons have felt that a second operation for total esophagectomy should be done once the esophagocolostomy has been successfully accomplished, since the incidence of carcinoma in old lye strictures of the esophagus is quite high.

Disorders of Esophageal Motility

It has been said that 90 per cent of clinical problems with the esophagus are related to disordered tone or motility.[41] The consequences range from dysphagia to gastroesophageal reflux. By combining the results of cineroentgen studies with manometric studies at various levels in the esophagus, we now have a much clearer understanding of normal and disordered physiology.[21] Esophageal motor disorders can be reflections of systemic disease.[71]

Differential Diagnosis

Lindsay[63] has classified these under the headings of muscular disturbances (diffuse scleroderma or generalized systemic sclerosis, dermatomyositis, myasthenia gravis, secondary myasthenia and senility); innervation disturbances (peripheral neuritis, the jugular foramen syndrome, central nervous system lesions of amyotrophic lateral sclerosis, syringomyelia, multiple sclerosis or poliomyelitis, lesions of the medulla from tumor, inflammation or trauma); and psychic disturbances producing the familiar globus hystericus. Some authors have included the pulsion diverticulum, which almost always occurs posteriorly between the leaves of the upper and lower portions of the cricopharyngeus sphincter, as the result of a postulated asynchrony of the upper and lower constrictor fibers. The Plummer-Vinson syndrome of iron deficiency anemia and cricopharyngeal dysphagia is well recognized, but the pathogenesis is still unexplained.[74]

Spasm

Spasm of the esophagus can occur alone or may be associated with disordered peristaltic activity of the esophagus. Milder degrees of spasm cause the appearance of the corkscrew esophagus. Diffuse spasm with muscular hypertrophy has also caused dysphagia and in some patients has been associated with pulsion diverticula and hiatal hernia.[55] A long myotomy will relieve symptoms in a majority of patients.[34]

Achalasia

Our knowledge of the lower esophageal sphincter has been increased by the study of patients with reflux and especially by study of patients in whom the sphincter fails to relax, a condition commonly called achalasia. The excellent monograph on achalasia by F. H. Ellis and A. M. Olsen[30] brings together the clinical background and experimental studies. In man there is degeneration of ganglion cells in the lower esophageal segment. In cats failure of the lower esophagus to relax is produced by bilateral cervical vagotomy or destructive lesions in the dorsal motor nucleus of the vagus nerve. The syndrome of achalasia was first described in 1674 by Thomas Willis, who described palliation by bouginage. Plummer in 1906 reintroduced bouginage, and forcible dilatation with a hydrostatic bag remained the method of choice at the Mayo Clinic for many years; however, the even better results following longitudinal myotomy of the lower esophagus (Heller procedure) have tended to displace dilatation in recent years. In the Mayo Clinic experience there was one operative death in 300 cases. Three patients had a postoperative empyema. Ninety-four per cent of 256 patients who could be followed from 1 to 17½ years experienced definite improvement and 83 per cent reported good to excellent results. Eleven per cent had only a fair result, but were still symptomatically improved.

Complications — Esophagitis and Carcinoma

When peptic esophagitis has occurred, it has usually been due to carrying the Heller myotomy too far down on the stomach and completely disrupting the lower esophageal sphincter mechanism or to deranging the phrenicoesophageal support mechanism with subsequent hiatal hernia and gastric reflux. In addition, persistence of dysphagia after a Heller procedure demands further investigation by fluoroscopy and esophagoscopy,

since there appears to be a markedly increased incidence of carcinoma of the esophagus in patients with achalasia.

Hiatal Hernia and Reflux Esophagitis

Diagnosis

Hiatal hernia and gastroesophageal reflux are not necessarily coexistent. By special maneuvers, up to 60 per cent of adults can be shown to have some degree of herniation of the esophageal hiatus. Contrary to earlier studies, the incidence does not increase with age.[67] Stilson et al.[97] examined 1027 patients aged 9 to 90 and found that the Trendelenburg maneuver and straight leg raising were insensitive tests for herniation. A prone or right oblique position detected about 25 per cent of the cases. A block of balsa wood interposed between the abdomen of the prone patient and the examining table revealed approximately 98 per cent of the total hernias discovered and in their hands the water syphon test revealed 93 per cent of the total. Sixty-nine per cent of the patients who had a positive water syphon test had a demonstrable hiatal hernia, and 54.5 per cent of the total patients with hiatal hernia had a positive water syphon test. The combination of manometric studies with pH studies in the lower esophagus has been more dependable in diagnosing reflux.[21] This helps to explain some of the failures in preventing reflux after what appeared to be adequate anatomic repair of the hernia.

Sphincter Mechanism — Chalasia and Achalasia

There is a functional sphincter in the lower esophageal segment that relaxes in response to peristaltic waves initiated by swallowing. The sphincter works more efficiently when situated below the diaphragm where it is exposed to the positive pressure of the abdomen, than above the diaphragm where it is influenced by the negative intrapleural pressure. The tone of the lower esophageal segment is increased slightly in normal individuals by administration of pentagastrin, but gastrin causes no increase in tone in patients with reflux.[56] The acute angle of entry into the fundus of the stomach appears to aid in prevention of reflux. Reflux can occur in the absence of hiatal hernia, as in the series of Hiebert and Belsey,[43] and most patients with hiatal hernia do not have symptoms of regurgitation or esophagitis. The term "chalasia" (excessive relaxation) has been proposed for the hypotonic cardiac sphincter as the antonym to "achalasia" (failure to relax).

Treatment

When there are mild symptoms of gastroesophageal reflux without evidence of dysphagia, bleeding or aspiration, then a regimen of six small meals, antacids and sleeping with the head of the bed elevated about 15 to 20 cm can be tried. In children below the age of two, this treatment is likely to be successful, even though the hiatal hernia can be demonstrated twenty years later.[17] In adults, however, once there is evidence of esophagitis by endoscopy, only a small minority will improve without surgical correction of the reflux.[9] Lilly and Randolph have used the following as their indications for surgical repair in children: persistent vomiting, inadequate nutrition (failure to thrive), recurrent aspiration pneumonitis and bleeding.[62]

Baue and Belsey[6] have emphasized several points in the surgical treatment: (1) adequate mobilization of the lower esophagus and cardia, (2) inversion of the lower esophagus into the fundus of the stomach to maintain the acute angle of entry of the cardia,

(3) some type of gastropexy to maintain an appreciable length of esophagus within the abdomen and (4) adequate approximation of the crurae of the diaphragm to prevent recurrence of the hernia. The operations of Hill[44] and Nissen[77] differ in details but have similar objectives to the Belsey procedure. Urschel and Paulson[107] have reported excellent success with the Belsey repair. Their experience has included a larger number of patients with pulmonary disease secondary to aspiration (50 per cent) than in most other series.

Several authors have reported treating stenosis secondary to peptic esophagitis by effective repair of the hernia followed by bouginage.[104] More severe cases require interposition of a segment of colon or jejunum. Thal[102] has devised an ingenious method for splitting the full thickness of the stricture and filling the defect with a portion of the fundus of the stomach, which then becomes covered by esophageal epithelium. There are still some unsettled problems in the treatment of long-standing peptic esophagitis. Some workers have argued for vagotomy and a drainage operation of the stomach, such as pyloroplasty, while others have felt that vagotomy might predispose to achalasia of the cardia.

Mucosal Injury and Repair

The consensus now is that the so-called Barrett's esophagus probably represents areas of peptic esophagitis where the squamous epithelium has been replaced by glandular epithelium from the fundus of the stomach.[12] It is important to keep in mind the high incidence of carcinoma of the esophagus in patients with the Barrett esophagus, achalasia and old lye strictures. Patients who have had dysphagia and substernal burning for many years may fail to recognize that a slow crescendo of symptoms may mean cancer.[72]

Food Impaction

In older people a large bolus of meat may occasionally become wedged in the esophagus. This may result from a combination of inadequate dentition and some impairment of esophageal motility. An x-ray should first be taken to determine whether or not the piece of meat contains bone. If bone is present, endoscopical removal is mandatory. If no bone shadow can be seen, one can try a proteolytic enzyme such as papain (Adolph's Meat Tenderizer), either sipped by the patient over several hours or dripped in via a Levin tube passed down to the obstruction.[18]

Benign Tumors

Benign tumors of the esophagus are much rarer than carcinoma. The leiomyoma is commoner than the lipoma. Both can usually be enucleated without opening the mucosa.[93]

Webs and Rings

Webs or rings in the mid or upper esophagus probably represent congenital anomalies resulting from a failure of the formerly solid cord of cells of the embryonic esophagus to canalize completely. The so-called Schatzki ring seems to occur almost always in association with hiatal hernia and seems most of the time to mark the junction of gastric mucosa with esophageal squamous epithelium.[84]

Summary

In this short space it has been impossible to cover all aspects of pulmonary and esophageal disease. That work is reserved for textbooks. Whenever possible, attempts have been made to include references to the literature of the past five years, to points of controversy and to recent reviews in depth. The discipline of thoracic surgery continues to advance rapidly and repeated trips to the current literature will be needed to keep pace with its progress.

REFERENCES

1. Aronow, W. S.: Effect of cigarette smoking and of carbon monoxide on coronary heart disease — critical review. Chest, 70:514–515, 1976.
2. Ashcraft, K. W. and Holder, T. M.: The experimental treatment of esophageal strictures by intralesional steroid injection. J. Thorac. Cardiovasc. Surg., 58:685–691, passim 1969.
3. (a) Avery, E. E., Mörch, E. T. and Benson, D. W.: Critically crushed chest. J. Thorac. Cardiovasc. Surg., 32:291–309, 1956.
   (b) Blair, E. and Mills, E.: Rationale of stabilization of the flail chest with intermittent positive pressure breathing. Am. Surg., 34:860–868, 1968.
4. Barlow, P. B. et al.: Preventive treatment of tuberculous infection. Am. Rev. Resp. Dis., 110:371–374, 1974.
5. (a) Bates, J. H.: Treatment of tuberculosis. Adv. Int. Med., 20:1–21, 1975.
   (b) Barlow, P. B.: Treatment of tuberculosis. Basics of RD (American Lung Association), 5:18–23, 1976.
   (c) Lester, T. W.: Chemotherapy for tuberculosis. Postgrad. Med., 60:112–117, 1976.
   (d) Bailey, W. C., Raleigh, J. W. and Turner, J. A. P.: Treatment of mycobacterial disease. Official statement of the American Thoracic Society. Am. Rev. Resp. Dis., 115:185–187, 1977.
6. Baue, A. E. and Belsey, R. H. R.: The treatment of sliding hiatus hernia and reflux esophagitis by the Mark IV technique. Surgery, 62:396–404, 1967.
7. (a) Baum, G. L. and Schwarz, J.: Diagnosis and treatment of systemic mycoses. Med. Clin. North Am., 58:661–681, 1974.
   (b) Abernathy, R. S.: Treatment of systemic mycoses. Medicine, 2:385–394, 1973.
   (c) Utz, J. P., Becker, A., Buechner, H. A. et al.: The pulmonary mycoses: Diagnostic and therapeutic guidelines with self-assessment, 1976. American College of Chest Physicians, 911 Busse Highway, Park Ridge, IL 60068.
8. Beamis, J. F., Stein, A. and Andrews, J. L.: Changing epidemiology of lung cancer.

Med. Clin. North Am., 59:315–325, 1975.

9. Behar, J. et al.: Medical and surgical management of reflux esophagitis. A 38-month report on a prospective clinical trial. N. Engl. J. Med., 293:263–268, 1975.

10. Boushy, S. F., Billig, D. M., North, L. B. et al.: Clinical course related to preoperative and postoperative pulmonary function in patients with bronchogenic carcinoma. Chest, 59:383–391, 1971.

11. Brantigan, C. O. and Grow, J. B., Sr.: Cricothyroidotomy: Elective use in respiratory problems requiring tracheotomy. J. Thorac. Cardiovasc. Surg., 71:72–80, 1976.

12. Bremner, G. G., Lynch, V. P. and Ellis, F. H., Jr.: Barrett's esophagus: congenital or acquired? An experimental study of esophageal mucosal regeneration in the dog. Surgery, 68:209–216, 1970.

13. Brown, R. K. and Kovarik, J. L.: Bronchoscopy in the sitting position. Surg. Clin. North Am., 49:1421–1424, 1969.

14. Burrington, J. D.: Clinitest burns of the esophagus. Ann. Thorac. Surg., 20:400–404, 1975.

15. Burrington, J. D. and Cotton, E. K.: Removal of foreign bodies from the tracheobronchial tree. J. Ped. Surg., 7:119–122, 1972.

16. Carr, D. T. and Power, M. H.: Clinical value of measurements of concentrations of protein in pleural fluid. New Engl. J. Med., 259:926, 1958.

17. Carre, I. et al.: A 20-year follow-up of children with a partial thoracic stomach (hiatal hernia). Aust. Paediatr. J., 12:92–94, 1976.

18. Cavo, J. W. et al.: Use of enzymes for meat impaction in the esophagus. Laryngoscope, 87:630–634, 1977.

19. Charms, B. L.: Unilateral pulmonary artery occlusion. *In* Zimmerman, H. A. (Ed.): Intravascular Catheterization. Springfield, Charles C Thomas, 1966.

20. Christoforidis, A. J.: Use of ultrasonic nebulizer for the application of oropharyngeal, laryngeal and tracheobronchial anesthesia. Chest, 59:629–633, 1971.

21. Clark, J., Moosa, A. R. and Skinner, D. B.: Pitfalls in the interpretation of esophageal function tests. Surg. Clin. North Am., 56:29–37, 1976.

22. Claggett, O. T.: Personal communication, 1971.

23. Comroe, J. H. et al.: Physiology of respiration. Second Edition. Chicago, Year Book Medical Publishers, 1974.

24. Coon, J. L. and Shuck, J. M. Failure of tube thoracostomy for empyema: An indication for early decortication. J. Trauma, 15:588–594, 1975.

25. (a) Dahlgren, S. and Nordenstrom, B.: Transthoracic needle biopsy. Stockholm, Almqvist & Wiksell, 1966.
    (b) Nordenstrom, B.: Transthoracic needle biopsy. New Engl. J. Med., 276:1081–1082, 1967.
    (c) Nordenstrom, B. and Bjork, V. O.: Dissemination of cancer cells by needle biopsy of lung. J. Thorac. Cardiovasc. Surg., 65:671, 1973.
    (d) McCartney, L.: Further observations on the lung patch technique. Am. J. Roentgenol. Radium Ther. Nucl. Med., 124:397–403, 1973.

26. Dodds, W. F.: Current concepts of esophageal motor function: Clinical implications for radiology. Am. J. Roentgenol., 128: 549–561, 1977.

27. Egan, R. S.: Corrosive esophagitis — a review of therapy. Northwest Med., 68:1007–1009, 1969.

28. Eijgelaar, A. and Homan van der Heide, J. N.: A reliable early symptom of bronchial or tracheal rupture. Thorax, 25:120–125, 1970.

29. Elkadi, A., Salas, R. and Almond, C.: Surgical treatment of atypical pulmonary tuberculosis. J. Thorac. Cardiovasc. Surg. 72:435–440, 1976.

30. Ellis, F. H. and Olsen, A. M.: Achalasia of the Esophagus. Philadelphia, W. B. Saunders Co., 1969.

31. Eloesser, L.: Of an operation for tuberculous empyema. Ann. Thorac. Surg., 8:355–357, 1969; S. G. & O., 60:1096–1097, 1935.

32. (a) Fennessy, J. J.: Transbronchial biopsy of peripheral lung lesions. Radiolgy, 88:878–882, 1967.
    (b) Fennessy, J. J., Fry, W. A., Manalo–Estrella, P. and Frias Hidvegi, D. V. S.: The bronchial brushing technique for obtaining cytologic specimens from peripheral lung lesions. Acta Cytol., 14:25–30, 1970.
    (c) Willson, J. K. V. and Eskridge, M.: Bronchial brush biopsy with a controllable brush. Am. J. Roentgenol. Radium Ther. Nucl. Med., 109:471–477, 1970.
    (d) Ellis, J. H., Jr.: Transbronchial lung biopsy via the fiberoptic bronchoscope: Experience with 107 consecutive cases and comparison with bronchial brushing. Chest, 68:524–532, 1975.

33. Fennessy, J. J., Frias Hidvegi, D. V. S. and VariaKojis, D.: Transcatheter biopsy of esophageal lesions. Radiology, 96:123–126, 1970.

34. Ferguson, T. B. et al.: Giant muscular hypertrophy of the esophagus. Ann. Thorac. Surg., 8:209–218, 1969.

35. Fontana, R. S., Sanderson, D. R., Woolner, L. B. et al.: Mayo Lung Cancer Project: Status report. Chest, 67:511–522, 1975.

36. Fordham, S. D.: Quick tips on evaluating x-rays. Res. Staff Phys., May 1976, pp. 77–83.

37. Fox, W. and Mitchison, D. A.: Short course chemotherapy for pulmonary tuberculosis. Am. Rev. Resp. Dis., 111:325–333, 1975.

38. Graham, E. A.: Some fundamental considerations in the treatment of empyema thoracis. St. Louis, C. V. Mosby Co., 1925.

39. Gunnlaugsson, G. H. et al.: Analysis of the records of 1657 patients with carcinoma of the esophagus and cardia of the stomach. Surg. Gynecol. Obstet., 130:997–1005, 1970.

40. (a) Hankins, J. R. et al.: Carcinoma of the esophagus. The philosophy for palliation. Ann. Thorac. Surg., 14:189–195, 1972.
    (b) Dillon, M. L., Jr. et al.: What is the rational treatment for carcinoma of the esophagus and cardia? J. Thorac. Cardiovasc. Surg., 68:321–327, 1974.

41. Henderson, R. D.: Motor Disorders of the Esophagus. Baltimore, Williams and Wilkins Co., 1976.

42. (a) Hewlett, T. H.: Sheft's initial management of thoracic and thoraco-abdominal trauma. Springfield, Charles C Thomas, 1968.
    (b) Hood, R. M.: Management of thoracic injury. Springfield, Charles C Thomas, 1969.
    (c) Martin, J. D., Jr., Haynes, C. D., Hatcher, C. R. et al.: Trauma to the thorax and abdomen. Springfield, Charles C Thomas, 1969.
    (d) Baker, R. J., Boyd, D. R. and Condon, R. E.: Priority of management of patients with multiple injuries. Surg. Clin. North Am., 50:3–11, 1970.

43. Hiebert, C. A. and Belsey, R. H. R.: Incompetency of the gastric cardia without radiological evidence of hiatal hernia. The diagnosis and management of 71 cases. J. Thorac. Cardiovasc. Surg., 42:352–359, 1961.

44. Hill, L. D.: An effective operation for hiatal hernia. Ann. Surg., 166:681–692, 1967.

45. Holder, T. M. et al.: Esophageal atresia and tracheoesophageal fistula. A survey of the surgical section of the American Academy of Pediatrics. Pediatrics, 34:542–549, 1964; Ann. Thorac. Surg., 9:445–467, 1970.

46. Holder, T. M., McDonald, V. G. and Wooley, M. M.: The premature or critically ill infant with esophageal atresia: Increased success with a staged approach. J. Thorac. Cardiovasc. Surg., 44:344–355, 1962.

47. (a) Holin, S. M., Dwork, R. E., Glaser, S., Rikli, A. E. and Stocklen, J. B.: Solitary pulmonary nodules found in a community-wide chest roentgenographic survey. Am. Rev. Resp. Dis., 79:427–439, 1959.
    (b) McClure, C. D., Boucot, K. R., Shipman, G. A. et al.: The solitary pulmonary nodule and primary lung malignancy. Arch. Environ. Health, 3:127–139, 1961.
    (c) Overholt, R. H., Bougas, J. A. and Woods, F. M.: Surgical treatment of lung cancer found on x-ray survey. New Engl. J. Med., 252:429–432, 1955.
    (d) Wilkins, E. W.: The asymptomatic isolated pulmonary nodule. New Engl. J. Med., 252:515–520, 1955.
    (e) Davis, E. W., Peabody, J. W. and Katz, S.: The solitary pulmonary nodule. A ten-year study based on 215 cases. J. Thorac. Cardiovasc. Surg., 32:728–770, 1956.
    (f) Steele, J. D. and Buell, P.: Survival in bronchogenic carcinomas resected as solitary pulmonary nodules. Proc. Natl. Cancer Conf., 6:835–839, 1970.
    (g) Higgins, G. A., Shields, T. W. and Keehn, R. W.: The solitary pulmonary nodule: Ten-year follow-up of Veterans Administration —Armed Forces cooperative study. Arch. Surg., 110:570–575, 1975.

48. (a) Hollinshead, A. C., Stewart, T. H. M. and Herberham, R. B.: Delayed hypersensitivity reactions to soluble membrane antigens of human malignant lung cells. J. Natl. Cancer Inst., 52:327–338, 1974.
    (b) Veltri, R. W. et al.: Isolation and identification of human lung tumor-associated antigens. Cancer Res., 37:1313–1322, 1977.

49. Hutchinson, C. M. and Mills, M. L.: The selection of patients with bronchogenic carcinoma for mediastinoscopy. J. Thorac. Cardiovasc. Surg., 71:768–773, 1976.

50. Israel, H. L. and Goldstein, R. A.: Relation of Kveim-antigen reaction to lymphadenopathy. Study of sarcoidosis and other diseases. New Engl. J. Med., 284:345–349, 1971.

51. Jackson, C. and Jackson, C. L.: Bronchoesophagology. Philadelphia, W. B. Saunders Co., 1950.

52. Jepsen, O.: Mediastinoscopy. Copenhagen, Munksgaard, 1966.

53. (a) Jones, R. J. and Samson, P. C.: Collec-

tive review: Esophageal injury. Ann. Thorac. Surg., *19*:216–230, 1975.

(b) Nemir, P., Jr., Wallace, H. W. and Fallahnjehad, M.: Diagnosis and management of benign disease of the esophagus. Curr. Probl. Surg., *13*:1–74, 1976.

54. Karkola, P., Kairalvoma, M. I. and Larmi, T. K. I.: Postpneumonectomy empyema in pulmonary carcinoma patients. J. Thorac. Cardiovasc. Surg., 72:319–322, 1976.

55. Kaye, M. D.: Oesophageal motor dysfunction in patients with diverticula of the mid-thoracic esophagus. Thorax, 29:666–672, 1974.

56. Kaye, M. D. et al.: Responses of the competent and incompetent lower esophageal sphincter to pentagastrin and abdominal compression. Gut, *17*:933–939, 1976.

57. Kirsh, M. M. et al.: The effect of cell type on the prognosis of patients with bronchogenic carcinoma. Ann. Thorac. Surg., 13:303–310, 1972.

58. Koehler, R. E., Moss, A. A. and Margulis, A. R.: Early radiographic changes in carcinoma of the esophagus. Radiology, *119*:1–5, 1976.

59. Leape, L. L. et al.: Hazard to health — liquid lye. N. Engl. J. Med., *284*:578–581, 1971.

60. (a) Light, R. W., Moller, D. J. and George, R. B.: Low pleural fluid pH in parapneumonic effusion. Chest, 68:273–274, 1975.

(b) Potts, D. E., Levin, D. C. and Sahn, S. S.: Chest, *70*:328–331, 1976.

61. Lillington, G. A.: The solitary pulmonary nodule. Am. Rev. Resp. Dis., *110*:699–707, 1974.

62. (a) Lilly, J. R. and Randolph, J. G.: Hiatal hernia and gastroesophageal reflux in infants and children. J. Thorac. Cardiovasc. Surg., 55:42–53, 1968.

(b) Johnson, D. G. et al.: Evaluation of gastroesophageal reflux surgery in children. Pediatrics, 59:62–68, 1977.

63. Lindsay, J. R.: Functional disturbances of the upper swallowing mechanism. Ann. Otol. Rhinol. Laryngol., 64:766–776, 1955.

64. Lyons, H. A.: Mediastinal tumors. *In* Spain, D. M. (Ed.): Diagnosis and Treatment of Tumors of the Chest. New York, Grune and Stratton, 1960.

65. (a) MacMahon, B. et al.: Preoperative irradiation of cancer of the lung. Preliminary report of a therapeutic trial, a collaborative study. Cancer, 23:419–430, 1969.

(b) Shields, T. W., Higgins, G. A. Jr., Lawton, R., Heilbrunn, A. and Keehn, R. J.: Preoperative x-ray therapy as an adjuvant in the treatment of

bronchogenic carcinoma. J. Cardiovasc. Thorac. Surg., 59:49–59, 1970.

66. (a) Maklad, M. F., Ting, Y. M. and Ravikrishman, K. P.: Xerotomography of peripheral lung lesions. Chest, *64*:516–518, 1976.

(b) Muhm, J. R., Brown, L. R. and Crowe, J. K.: Use of computed tomography in the detection of pulmonary nodules. Mayo Clinic Proc., *52*:345–348, 1977.

67. Mandelstam, P. and Lieber, A.: Cineradiographic studies of the esophagus in normal adults. A study of 146 subjects ranging in age from 21 to 90 years. Gastroenterology, 58:32–39, 1970.

68. Meade, R. H.: A History of Thoracic Surgery. Springfield, Charles C Thomas, 1961.

69. Miller, A. B., Fox, W. and Tall, R.: Five-year follow-up of the Medical Research Council comparative trial of surgery and radiotherapy for the primary treatment of small-celled or oat-celled carcinoma of the bronchus. Lancet, 2:501–505, 1969.

70. Morales, G. A. et al.: Ventilation under general anesthesia for bronchosopy. J. Thorac. Cardiovasc. Surg., 57:873–878, 1969.

71. Mukhopadhyay, A. K. and Graham, D. Y.: Esophageal motor dysfunction in systemic diseases. Arch. Int. Med., *136*:583–588, 1976.

72. (a) Naef, A. P. et al.: Columnar-lined esophagus: An acquired lesion with malignant predisposition. Report on 140 cases of Barrett's esophagus with 12 adenocarcinomas. J. Thorac. Cardiovasc. Surg., 70:826–834, 1975.

(b) Borrie, J. and Goldwater, L.: Columnar- cell-lined esophagus: Assessment of etiology and treatment. A 22 year experience. J. Thorac. Cardiovasc. Surg., *71*:825–834, 1976.

73. Nathanson, L. and Hall, T. C.: Lung tumors: How they produce their syndromes. Ann. N.Y. Acad. Sci., 230:367–377, 1974.

74. Nelson, C. S.: Chemotherapy as the definitive form of therapy in esophageal carcinoma. J. Thorac. Cardiovasc. Surg., 63:827–837, 1972.

75. Newman, M. M.: Tracheostomy. Surg. Clin. North Am. 49:1365–1372, 1969.

76. (a) Newman, M. M., Trapani, I. T. and Riley, E. A.: Unusual tissue culture findings in a case of pleural mesothelioma with prolonged clinical course. Am J. Ther. Clin. Rep., 1:115–139, 1975.

(b) Monif, G. R. G., Stewart, B. N. and Block, A. J.: Living cytology. A new diagnostic technique for malignant pleural effusions. Chest, 69:626–629, 1976.

77. Nissen, R.: Gastropexy and "fundoplication" in surgical treatment of hiatal hernia. Am. J. Dig. Dis., 6:954–961, 1961.

78. (a) Palmer, E. D.: Peroral prosthesis for the management of incurable esophageal carcinoma. Am. J. Gastroenterol. 59:487–498, 1973.

    (b) Thomas, A. N.: Treatment of malignant esophageal obstruction by endoesophageal intubation. Am. J. Surg., 128:306–312, 1974.

79. Palmer, E. D.: Disorders of the cricopharyngeus muscle: A review. Gastroenterology, 71:510–519, 1976.

80. (a) Palva, T., Viikari, S. and Ingberg, M.: Pulmonary carcinoma. Mediastinoscopic criteria for curative resections. Dis. Chest, 56:156–158, 1969.

    (b) Shields, T. W. et al.: Relation of cell type and lymph node metastases to survival after resection of bronchial carcinoma. Ann. Thorac. Surg., 20:501–510, 1975.

    (c) Stanford, W. et al.: Results of treatment of primary carcinoma of the lung — analysis of 3000 cases. J. Thorac. Cardiovasc. Surg., 72:441–449, 1976.

81. (a) Papatestas, A. E., Alpert, L. I., Osserman, K. E. et al.: Studies in myasthenia gravis: Effects of thymectomy. Am. J. Med., 50:465–474, 1971.

    (b) Sambrook, M. A., Reid, H., Mohr, P. D. et al.: Myasthenia gravis: Clinical and histological features in relation to thymectomy. J. Neurol. Neurosurg. Psychiatry, 39:38–43, 1976.

82. Pinner, M.: Collapse therapy. *In* Pulmonary Tuberculosis in the Adult. Springfield, Charles C Thomas, 1945.

83. Postlethwait, R. W. and Sealy, W. C.: Surgery of the Esophagus. Springfield, Charles C Thomas, 1961.

84. Postlethwait, R. W. and Sealy, W. C.: Experiences with treatment of 59 patients with lower esophageal web. Ann. Surg., 165:786–796, 1968.

85. Rabin, C. B.: New or neglected physical signs in diagnosis of chest disease. J.A.M.A. 194:546–550, 1965.

86. Reif, A. E.: Editorial. J. Natl. Cancer Inst., 57:1207–1210, 1976.

87. Richardson, J. D., McElvein, R. B. and Trinkle, J. K.: First rib fracture: A hallmark of severe trauma. Ann. Surg., 181:251–254, 1975.

88. Rigler, L. G., and Heitzman, E. R.: Planigraphy in the differential diagnosis of the pulmonary nodule; with particular refer-

89. (a) Rogers, L. F. et al.: Diagnostic considerations in mediastinal emphysema: A pathologic-roentgenologic approach to Boerhaave's syndrome. Am. J. Roetgenol., 115:495–511, 1972.

    (b) Curci, J. J. and Horman, M. J.: Boerhaave's syndrome: The importance of early diagnosis and treatment. Ann. Surg., 183:401–408, 1976.

90. Rosenberg, N. et al.: Prevention of experimental lye strictures of the esophagus by cortisone. Arch. Surg., 63:147–151, 1951. Ibid. 66:593–598, 1953.

91. Rubin, P., Goodner, J. T., Nakayama, K., Pearson, J. G., Rider, W. D.: Cancer of the Gastrointestinal Tract. II. Esophagus: Treatment — localized and advanced, J.A.M.A., 227:175–185, 1974.

92. Saccomano, G., Archer, V. E. and Auerbach, O.: Development of carcinoma of the lung as reflected in exfoliated cells. Cancer, 33:256–270, 1974; 34:2056–2060, 1974.

93. Seremetis, M. G. et al.: Leiomyomata of the esophagus. An analysis of 838 cases. Cancer, 38:2166–2177, 1976.

94. Sheely, C. H. et al.: Penetrating wounds of the cervical esophagus. Am. J. Surg., 130:707–711, 1975.

95. Shields, T. W.: The fate of patients after incomplete resection of bronchial carcinoma. S.G. & O., 139:569–572, 1974.

96. Stein, G. N. and Finkelstein, A. K.: Tumor Atlas of the Gastrointestinal Tract. The Esophagus and Stomach. Chicago, American College of Radiology — Year Book Medical Publishers, 1973.

97. Stilson, W. L. et al.: Hiatal hernia and gastroesophageal reflux. A clinicoradiological analysis of more than 1000 cases. Radiology, 93:1323–1327, 1969.

98. (a) Strauss, M. J.: Combination chemotherapy in advanced lung cancer with increased survival. Cancer, 38:2232–2241, 1976.

    (b) Einhorn, L. H. and Hornback, N. B.: Treatment of oat cell carcinoma of the lung. J.A.M.A., 237:2177–2178, 1977.

    (c) Holoye, P. Y. et al.: Combination chemotherapy and radiation therapy for small cell carcinoma. J.A.M.A., 237:1221–1224, 1977.

99. Suratt, P. M., Smiddy, J. F. and Gruber, B.: Fiberoptic bronchoscopy complications. Chest, 69:747–751, 1976.

100. Swenson, O. et al.: Repair and complications of esophageal atresia and tracheoesophageal fistula. N Engl. J. Med., 267:960–963, 1962.

101. Templeton, F. E.: X-ray Examination of the

Stomach. Chicago, University of Chicago Press, 1964.

102. Thal, A. P. et al.: New operation for distal esophageal obstruction. Arch. Surg., 90:464–471, 1965.

103. There are many excellent textbooks of roentgenology, and not all can be listed here. Four useful texts are:
    (a) Felson, B.: Fundamentals of Chest Roentgenology. Philadelphia, W. B. Saunders Co., 1960.
    (b) Fraser, R. G. and Pare, J. A. P.: Diagnosis of Diseases of the Chest, 2nd ed. Philadelphia, W. B. Saunders Co., 1977.
    (c) Medelman, J. P.: Normal Roentgen Anatomy. *In* Rabin, C. B. (ed.): Roentgenology of the Chest. Springfield, Charles C Thomas, 1958.
    (d) Rigler, L.: Pleura, Mediastinum and Lungs. Vol. IV, Part 2: Roentgen Diagnosis. New York, Grune and Stratton, 1975.

104. (a) Toledo-Pereyra, L. H. et al.: Management of acid-peptic esophageal strictures. J. Thorac. Cardiovasc. Surg., 72:518–521, 1976.
    (b) Woodward, E. R.: Surgical treatment of reflux esophagitis and stricture. Postgrad. Med., 61:143–150, 1977.

105. Torek, F.: The first successful case of resection of the thoracic portion of the esophagus for carcinoma. Surg. Gynecol. Obstet., 16:614–617, 1913.

106. Trinkle, J. K. et al.: Management of flail chest without mechanical ventilation. Ann. Thorac. Surg., 19:355–363, 1975.

107. Urschel, H. C., Jr. and Paulson, D. L.: Gastroesophageal reflux and hiatal hernia. Complications and therapy. J. Thorac. Cardiovasc. Surg., 53:21–32, 1967.

108. Villar, H. V. et al.: Emergency diagnosis of upper gastrointestinal bleeding by fiber optic endoscopy. Ann. Surg., 185:367–374, 1977.

109. Virgilio, R. W.: Intrathoracic wounds in battle casualties. Surg. Gynecol. Obstet., 130:609–615, 1970.

110. Water-soluble Fixative Spray. Richard Allen Medical Industries, 1335 Dodge Avenue, Evanston, IL 60204.

111. Weiss, W., Seidman, H. and Boucot, K. R.: The Philadelphia Pulmonary Neoplasm Research Project. Thwarting factors in periodic screening for lung cancer. Am. Rev. Resp. Dis., 111:289–297, 1975.

112. Wynder, E. L. and Graham, E. A.: Tobacco smoking as a possible etiologic factor in bronchogenic carcinoma — A study of 684 proven cases. J.A.M.A., 143:329–336, 1950.

113. Yarington, C. T., Jr. and Heatly, C. A.: Steroids, antibiotics and early esophagoscopy in caustic esophageal trauma. N.Y. State J. Med., 63:2960–2963, 1963.

114. Yudin, S. S.: The surgical construction of 80 cases of artificial esophagus. Surg. Gynecol. Obstet., 78:561–583, 1944.

115. (a) Zavala, D. C.: Diagnostic fiberoptic bronchoscopy: Techniques and results in 600 patients. Chest, 68:12–19, 1975.
    (b) Zavala, D. C. et al.: Fiberoptic and rigid bronchoscopy: The state of the art. Chest, 65:605–606, 1974.

116. Zavala, D. C.: Pulmonary biopsy. Adv. Int. Med., 21:21–45, 1976.

117. Zboralske, F. F. and Friedland, G. W.: Diseases of the esophagus. Present concepts. Calif. Med., 112:33–51, 1970.

118. Zollinger, R. M. and Nick, W. V.: Upper gastrointestinal tract hemorrhage. J.A.M.A., 212:2251–2254, 1970.

17 Peripheral Blood Vessels

J. CUTHBERT OWENS, M.D., and
ROBERT B. RUTHERFORD, M.D.

a. Origin of emboli
b. Diagnosis
c. Objectives of treatment
C. *Arterial injuries*
1. Initial blood loss
2. Diagnosis
3. Treatment
D. *Chronic occlusive arterial disease*
1. Diagnosis
2. Pathology
3. The lower extremities
4. Location of the occlusion
5. Symptoms
6. Signs
7. Ancillary diagnostic studies
a. Invasive diagnosis
b. Noninvasive diagnosis
(1) Doppler examination
(2) Segmental limb systolic pressures
(3) Ankle pressure response to provoked hyperemia
(4) Plethysmography
(5) Velocity wave form analysis
8. Treatment
a. Natural history
b. Risk of operative procedure
c. Preoperative in-hospital evaluation
d. Nonoperative (medical) management
e. Instructions to patients with arterial insufficiency
E. *Arteritis*
1. Thromboangiitis obliterans
2. Collagen diseases
3. Other forms of arteritis
F. *Aneurysms*
1. Abdominal aortic aneurysm
2. Iliac artery aneurysm
3. Lower extremity aneurysm
4. Visceral arterial aneurysm
5. Mycotic aneurysm
G. *Extracranial and aortic arch occlusive disease*
1. Transient ischemic attacks
a. Diagnosis
b. Noninvasive diagnostic studies
c. Treatment
2. Aortic arch syndrome
a. Diagnosis
b. Treatment
3. Vertebral basilar arterial insufficiency
4. Fibromuscular hyperplasia
5. Kinked internal carotid artery
6. Emergency carotid artery surgery

7. Asymptomatic stenosis of extracranial carotid artery
IV. **CELIAC AXIS AND MESENTERIC VASCULAR DISEASE (ARTERIAL AND VENOUS)**
A. *Etiology and pathogenesis*
B. *Acute mesenteric ischemia*
1. Acute mesenteric artery thrombosis
2. Acute embolic occlusion
3. Acute mesenteric nonocclusive ischemia
4. Acute inferior mesenteric artery occlusion
5. Acute mesenteric venous thrombosis
C. *Chronic intestinal ischemia*

V. **ARTERIOVENOUS FISTULAS**
A. *Physiological changes*
B. *Closure of the fistula*
C. *Etiology*
D. *Sites of arteriovenous fistulas*
1. Extremities
2. Aorto-inferior vena caval fistulas
3. Pulmonary arteriovenous fistulas
4. Renal arteriovenous fistulas
5. Portal circulation arteriovenous fistulas
6. Arteriovenous fistulas of neck and face
7. Pelvic arteriovenous fistulas
E. *Diagnosis*

VI. **LYMPHEDEMA**
A. *Etiology*
B. *Classification*
C. *Primary lymphedema*
1. Congenital lymphedema
2. Lymphedema praecox
3. Lymphedema tarda
4. Differential diagnosis
5. Diagnostic studies
6. Complications
D. *Secondary lymphedema*
E. *Treatment for primary and secondary lymphedema*
F. *Lymph collection in wounds*

VII. **MISCELLANEOUS PROBLEMS**
A. *Cold Injuries*
1. Chilblain
2. Immersion or trench foot
3. Frostbite
a. Predicting outcome
b. Freezing process
c. Classification
d. Predisposing factors
e. Environmental factors
f. Early treatment

INTRODUCTION

This chapter is devoted to the identification and treatment of peripheral vascular problems as they are seen in an outpatient setting, whether it be a private office, clinic or emergency department. Less than 20 percent of patients with peripheral vascular disease require hospital admission and even fewer require operation. While the indications for hospitalization and operation will be discussed, the major emphasis here will naturally be on those conditions that ordinarily can be managed entirely on an ambulatory basis.

The examining clinician must be constantly aware of the interrelationships between the peripheral vascular system and all other body systems, for a vascular problem may be either caused or influenced by associated disease entities; for example, Raynaud's phenomenon and collagen diseases, leg ulcers and metabolic diseases and recurrent venous thrombosis and coagulopathies. Further, many conditions causing pain or swelling in an extremity are assumed to be of vascular origin by the primary physician, who will frequently request a consultation with a vascular specialist. It is important, therefore, to be familiar with the distinguishing diagnostic features of such nonvascular conditions. In fact, it is because of this familiarity that the vascular surgeon often treats these cases. For this reason, some of these conditions have been included in this chapter, for example, causalgia, thoracic outlet compression syndrome, neurotrophic ulcers and cold injuries.

HISTORY

CODE: 0 = absent
        1+ = mild, < normal
        2+ = moderate, norma
        3+ = severe, > normal

Name _____ Date _____

PAST HISTORY

allergies _____ operations _____

injuries _____ major illnesses _____

pregnancies _____ phlebitis _____

pulmonary embolism _____ serious infections _____

cardiac: angina _____ CHF _____ MI _____

      arrhythmia _____ DOE _____ orthopnea _____

respiratory _____

diabetes _____

hypertension _____

renal _____

neurological: cerebrovascular _____

            peripheral _____

venereal disease _____

arthritis, collagen vascular _____

other _____

FAMILY HISTORY

same condition _____ other vascular _____

diabetes _____ hypertension _____ CVA _____ cardiac _____

clotting abnormalities _____

PERSONAL AND SOCIAL

alcohol _____ tobacco _____

education _____ psychological _____

occupations _____

travel _____

drug use: past _____

         present _____

Figure 17–1   Peripheral vascular worksheet.

Illustration continued on the opposite page

Initial Clinical Evaluation

The initial clinical evaluation of a vascular condition involves reaching a presumptive diagnosis on clinical grounds; using noninvasive diagnostic measures to confirm the diagnosis; weighing the degree of disability and the natural course of the underlying disease against the risk and success rate of the various operative and nonoperative therapeutic alternatives; and, when necessary, confirming the diagnosis and the extent and degree of involvement by angiography. Finally, no decision can be made without combining the sociological, pathological, anatomical and physiological findings in the individual patient. Even though one's experience and judgment can make this all-important process of patient identification and selection straightforward in most cases, there will always be some patients in which

I. COMPLAINTS   RANK   SEVERITY   DESCRIPTIVE COMMENTS

pain _____

weakness _____

hot/cold _____

numb/sensitive _____

discoloration _____

swelling _____

ulceration _____

varicose veins _____

II. LOCATION: r/l, medial/lateral, dorsal/ventral

    toes _____ foot _____ ankle _____ leg _____ knee _____

    fingers   hand   wrist   forearm   elbow

    thigh _____ hip _____ back _____ other _____

    arm   shoulder   neck   _____

III. ONSET: sudden/gradual

IV. DURATION: _____ days/weeks/months/years

V. FREQUENCY: _____ times/day/week/month/year

VI. TEMPORAL PATTERN: continuous/intermittent/day/night/none

VII. COURSE: static/better/worse/fluctuates

VIII. INTERFERES WITH: sleep/work/exercise/other

IX. INFLUENCING FACTORS (A = aggravates, R = relieves, O = no effect)

    elevation _____ dependency _____ exercise _____ rest _____ heat _____

    cold _____ weather change _____ menses _____ emotions _____ vibration _____

    pressure _____ position _____

    activity _____

    other (including Rx) _____

Figure 17–1 *Continued*

the disease process or its management is neither obvious nor definitive.

There are few areas in medicine in which the conditions encountered lend themselves so readily to diagnosis solely on the basis of thoughtful history and careful physical examination as vascular diseases. Specialists in this field are often surprised at their colleagues' difficulties in assessing peripheral vascular problems. The vast majority of these problems are caused by one of two basic disease processes (arteriosclerosis and thrombophlebitis), which predominantly affect the lower rather than the upper extremity or visceral circulations and present with pain, a change in appearance or

sensation (swelling, discoloration or temperature change) or some form of tissue loss (ulceration or gangrene). By applying a systematic, problem-oriented approach to these complaints, the clinician will often be able to predict the status of peripheral circulation even before the examination, to understand the reason for pain by its character and location, to predict the cause of lower extremity swelling by its distribution and associated skin changes and to tell the cause of leg or foot ulcerations by their location and appearance.

Unfortunately, there is a tendency, as one becomes adept at this, to turn the anticipated one-hour consultation

PHYSICAL EXAMINATION

Name _____ Date _____

Ht. _____ Wt. _____ Pulse _____ Temperature _____ B.P. _____

General _____ Head and Neck _____

Heart _____

Lungs _____ Abdomen _____

		UPPER		LOWER	
EXTREMITIES		right	left	right	left
SKIN	warm/cool				
	atrophied/thickened				
	cyanosis/mottling				
	pallor/rubor				
	capillary filling				
	hair growth				
	nails				
EDEMA	brawny/pitting/spongy				
	degree				
	extent				
MUSCULOSKELETAL	subcutaneous: atrophy/fibrosis				
	ulceration/tissue loss				
	discoloration/pigmentation				
	erythema/cellulitis/lymphangitis				
	symmetry/atrophy/hypertrophy				
	joint enlargement/swelling				
	range of motion				
	reflexes				
	sensory				
	motor				

Figure 17–2   Peripheral vascular worksheet.

Illustration continued on the opposite page

with a new patient into a five-minute interview and spot diagnosis, or to handle a clinic full of chronic but familiar problems single-handedly in an hour or two, bypassing the systematic approach with increasing frequency and abbreviating consultation notes and clinical records. Eventually the ability to transmit this knowledge to other clinicians in an organized fashion becomes attenuated. It may be useful, therefore, for the experienced as well as the inexperienced clinician to maintain a formal framework upon which these diagnostic skills can be superimposed. This need may be filled by a diagnostic check list or evaluation form such as the one presented in Figure 17–1. This approach not only avoids embarrassing oversights but also can preserve the details of the initial evaluation for later dictation and function as a temporary record until the transcribed note reaches the files. Parts may be filled in by auxiliary personnel. In a larger clinic devices such as tabular check lists, particularly if modified for each of the major disease entities or operations encountered, can provide the background for clinical investigation. The forms shown here (Figs. 17–1 and 17–2) are only intended to be examples. Obviously this will not suit everyone, and each physician

ARTERIAL SURVEY

	RIGHT			LEFT		
	pulse	bruit	aneu-rysm	pulse	bruit	aneu-rysm
carotid						
subclavian						
brachial						
radial						
ulnar						
abdominal aorta						
iliac						
femoral						
popliteal						
dorsalis pedis						
posterior tibial						

VENOUS SURVEY   CODE: N = normal; P = prominent, tense; V = varicose;
T = thrombosed

	RIGHT	LEFT
greater saphenous		
lesser saphenous		
anterolateral thigh		
posteromedial thigh		
anterior tibial		
posterior arch		
perforators		
intracutaneous venules		
tourniquet test		

DEMOGRAPHIC DATA

Name _____ Date _____ History no. _____

Address _____ Occupation _____

Age _____ Sex _____ Nationality/Race _____

Referring physician _____ Telephone no. _____

Address _____

Figure 17–2 *Continued*

should develop his or her own version.

History and Physical Examination

The history of patients with vascular diseases usually centers around key complaints that often can be developed by pointed questioning into a reasonable presumptive diagnosis even before a physical examination has been started. It is not our intention to discuss the major diagnostic considerations of all forms of vascular disease. These will be covered later in the appropriate sections of this chapter. Rather, an attempt will be made, mainly by using the lower extremity as an example, to demonstrate the value of knowing which questions to ask and which physical signs to seek. This problem-oriented approach is preferred to the common practice of describing an uncorrelated list of vascular signs and symptoms.

The Painful Extremity

The most common presenting symptom in lower extremity vascular disease is pain. *Acute arterial occlusion* does not always produce the well-known five P's — pain, pallor, pulselessness, paresthesia and paralysis. In fact, if the pain is not severe and sustained or if the patient does not experience motor or sensory loss, he may not seek immediate medical help, and the missing pulses may not be detected until later, when the patient presents with intermittent claudication or is examined for other reasons. Nevertheless, the initial pain of acute arterial occlusion is usually fairly characteristic. It begins suddenly and rapidly reaches a crescendo. The patient will commonly describe a sensation of the leg being "struck" by a severe, shocking pain that renders it weak. If standing at the time, he may be forced to sit down immediately or even crumple to the ground as the extremity gives way. The pain may quickly subside in intensity, and, depending on the severity of the ischemia that remains after the initial wave of vasospasm has passed and collateral channels are recruited, it may either subside completely or settle into one of the typical pain patterns of chronic ischemia described later.

Chronic arterial insufficiency of the lower extremity produces two very reproducible pain syndromes, intermittent claudication and ischemic neuritis. Other pain patterns, such as night cramps, gout or causalgic-type pain, may be accompanying complaints but are not necessarily indicative of ischemia.

Intermittent claudication, though derived from the Latin word for *limp*, has by usage come to mean a discomfort or disability associated with exercise. Depending on the level and extent of the arterial occlusive disease, the patient may present with buttock and thigh claudication, calf claudication or foot claudication, either singly or in contiguous combination. The most common type, *calf claudication*, is easily recognized as a cramping pain in the calf that can be reproduced consistently by a certain amount of exercise and completely relieved by a minute or so of rest.

Intermittent claudication is not always a symptom in arterial occlusion. Frequently, elderly patients will experience no symptoms from superficial femoral artery occlusion because the occlusive process is gradual enough to allow concomitant development of collateral circulation and because their sedentary existence protects them from claudication.

Patients with a more proximal (aortoiliac) distribution to their arterial occlusive disease will usually suffer from *buttock and thigh claudication*, although a significant number will complain mainly of calf claudication. Buttock and thigh claudication commonly does not produce the severe, cramping, muscular pain experienced in the calf. The sensation is more of an aching discomfort associated with weakness. These patients may even deny the existence of pain per se, complaining only that their hip or thigh "gives out" or "tires" after they have walked a certain distance. Patients with osteoarthritis of the hip or knee may complain of a similar extremity discomfort that is also brought on by exercise, but, important in the differentiation of the two is the fact that the amount of exercise causing symptoms in osteoarthritis is variable, and the symptoms do not disappear as promptly with rest, vary in severity from day to day and are frequently associated with changing weather conditions. Also, low neurospinal pain may simulate claudication secondary to aortoiliac occlusive disease, especially with standing, as the associated lordosis further narrows the neurospinal canal. Since older patients sometimes have diminished femoral pulses and proximal bruits reflecting some degree of aortoiliac artery stenosis, it is not unusual for these other painful conditions to be wrongly ascribed to vascular disease. This is a classic example of the importance of matching symptoms and signs in terms of severity and distribution. It is unusual to have significant hip or buttock pain from iliac artery stenosis without associated thigh or calf claudication. Furthermore, aortic or complete iliac artery occlusion with absent femoral pulses on at least one side is usually necessary for such proximally distributed symptoms.

Finally, aortoiliac occlusive disease severe enough to produce disabling claudication will nearly always be associated with impotence in males. The absence of impotence in a male with bilateral hip or thigh pain should make one suspect that the pain may not be due to aortoiliac occlusive disease. Occasionally, a patient with true buttock and thigh claudication will complain that this discomfort, or numbness and weakness, is also brought on by sitting. This is presumably because sitting on the buttocks significantly impedes flow through collateral pathways passing through these areas.

Foot claudication with a vascular basis is very rare. It may exist independent of calf claudication if the occlusive lesions diffusely involve all the infrapopliteal arteries, but it is just as commonly associated with more proximal occlusions and calf pain. Foot claudication has a greater relative frequency in vasculitis, such as thromboangiitis obliterans, than in arteriosclerosis obliterans because of the typically more distal distribution of occlusive lesions in vasculitis. The complaint is usually that of a painful ache, a "drawing" pain or cramp in the forefoot associated only with walking. Such a patient will usually also complain of a "wooden" or "burning" sensation or numbness, or both, in the same distribution and of his foot always being cold at night. He will frequently have been diagnosed as having "flat feet" and have visited several podiatrists or tried a variety of arch supports or "orthopedic" shoes. This

rarest form of lower extremity claudication usually occurs only with advanced degrees of arterial insufficiency and therefore is commonly associated with ischemic "rest pain" of the foot.

Ischemic neuritis is typically a nocturnal deep "rest pain" of disturbing severity, which diffusely involves the entire leg, foot or only the area distal to the metatarsals, although it may be localized to the vicinity of an ischemic ulcer of a pregangrenous toe. Frequently, it may be so severe that it requires hospitalization and is not relieved even by substantial doses of narcotics. The horizontally sleeping patient is typically awakened by this pain and forced to get up and do something about it. He may sit up and rub or hold the painful foot, get up and pace the floor or walk to the medicine cabinet to take an analgesic. Any of these responses will relieve the pain fairly promptly, but only by unwittingly recruiting the help of gravity in improving the perfusion pressure to the distal tissues. Although the patient may at first wrongly attribute the relief to rubbing the foot, walking or even to an amazingly fast-acting analgesic, eventually he learns to sleep with his foot dependent, either by dangling it over the side of the bed and resting it on a chair or by sleeping out the night in a lounge chair. This deep pain pattern is too characteristic to be missed by the careful interrogator. Episodes of *gouty arthritis* may accompany this type of pain or may be a separate entity that needs to be excluded.

Causalgic-type pain, which is a discomfort most severe at night, is best characterized as a superficial burning pain with hyperesthesia. It may also accompany the pain of ischemic neuritis or be a separate entity. The combined pains are incorrectly identified as a single entity, namely "rest pain." As will be discussed later, the treatment and prognosis of these two pain patterns are often dissimilar.

Night cramps localized to the calf at

bed rest have no known vascular origin; rather, they are thought to result from an exaggerated neuromuscular response to stretch. However, they are so common in older patients, some of whom may even have pulse deficits or other signs of arterial occlusive disease, that the complaint should alert the examining physician to rule out limb ischemia. Night cramps are also prevalent in those patients who permit themselves to experience multiple episodes of intermittent claudication while ambulatory.

Pain associated with *venous disease* of the lower extremity is not as characteristic as the arterial pain syndromes. Fortunately, these conditions are usually easily recognized by their associated physical findings. Significant pain is not a common complaint of patients with primary *varicose veins*. In fact, excluding those women who localize their pain only to the long saphenous vein just prior to a menstrual period, one must be suspicious of patients with varicose veins who present with pain, particularly if the varicosities are of long standing and were not previously painful. Such patients may be suffering from extremity pain of another, more obscure etiology and have blamed it on the visible varicosities. Occasionally, varicose veins will produce a "pulling," "pricking," "burning" or "tingling" discomfort that is well localized to the varicose veins themselves, unlike the diffuse sensation of fatigue or heaviness that more commonly predominates. Although these symptoms are relieved by elevation, as is typical of venous discomfort, the tingling and burning sensation often worsens before it subsides during the initial period of elevation.

Venous thrombosis in the lower extremity may cause little or no pain until the associated inflammatory reaction (phlebitis) is significant, in which case there will be localized tenderness along the course of the involved vein. Swelling, either early or later in the postphlebitic period, is often associated with a moderate aching discomfort and a tight or heavy sensation, but severe, "bursting" pain is rare, unless the patient is spending too much time in the upright position and still has significant residual obstruction to venous outflow. It is clear that while the symptoms associated with venous obstruction, in the absence of associated inflammation, are extremely variable, their aggravation by standing and relief by elevation is consistent, and this relationship should always be explored.

Patients with *other forms of extremity pain* are often referred to the surgeon under the false presumption that their complaints are circulatory in origin. Therefore, it is important to recognize the nonvascular extremity pain syndromes, or at least the common ones associated with nerve or musculoskeletal derangements. As previously noted, the pain of arthritis or sciatica is usually fairly characteristic and easily distinguishable from that due to vascular disease. However, there are three other extremity pain conditions that can masquerade as vascular disease because of the associated vascular signs. Painful *peripheral neuritis* is often seen in patients with diabetes mellitus or chronic alcoholism. The alcoholic with peripheral neuritis often has ruborous skin changes, while the diabetic patient with peripheral neuritis is frequently noted to have not only rubor and trophic skin changes but absent peripheral pulses as well. In these patients the examiner may mistake the problem for arterial insufficiency rather than for the early stage of diabetic or alcoholic neuropathy. The neurological signs may be subtle, often no more than a patchy loss of light touch, vibratory sense and two-point discrimination. However, peripheral nerves are tender to palpation on both upper and lower extremities.

The second misleading type of extremity pain is *reflex sympathetic dystrophy* or *minor causalgia*. As in neuritis, the pain produced is usually burning in character. Major causalgia, associated with incomplete nerve injury, is usually easily recognized, but the minor variety, which may follow relatively minimal trauma or acute circulatory problems such as venous or arterial occlusion, must always be kept in mind by the vascular surgeon. A common case is the patient who has residual discomfort following back surgery (disk operations. lumbar fusions), which is often labeled as "arachnoiditis." Typically, the signs of autonomic imbalance that originally attracted the attention of the referring physician will be present. The causalgic extremity may be warm and dry initially but later becomes cool, mottled or cyanotic. Eventually, trophic changes develop that are similar to those of arterial insufficiency. The pain is not always classically superficial, burning and localized to the distribution of a somatic nerve, as originally described. If there are reasonable grounds for suspicion after initial evaluation, relief of the pain by a proximal arterial injection of 25 mg of tolazoline HCl (Priscoline), confirmed later by a documented paravertebral sympathetic block, will establish the diagnosis.

The third and most subtle of these misleading extremity pain conditions appears in the female patient who complains chiefly of aching or painful legs identified as *"restless" or "crazy" legs*. The patient is most likely an aggressive individual with a high level of anxiety in a stressful environment. Owing to repeated episodes of muscle tension during these stressful periods, the extremities become uncomfortable. Examination reveals tenderness in all muscles of both upper and lower extremities, and often variable color changes may be noted in the hands and feet, which are also more moist than expected.

Physical Examination

The painful extremity is usually examined by a prejudiced clinician if a careful history has been taken, for the reasons given above, and it is difficult to be systematic when physical findings confirming one's suspicions immediately catch the eye. However, a complete and thorough initial examination should be carried out. A previously undetected diastolic hypertension, carotid bruit, fibrillating heart or abdominal aortic aneurysm can be the dividend of such thoroughness. Furthermore, documentation of the state of the peripheral pulses may well have future value. Examination of the abdomen should consist of more than a brief palpation for an occult aneurysm. For example, lower abdominal bruits may provide the only physical clue of aortoiliac occlusive disease in a patient with buttock and thigh claudication, since there may be no signs of chronic ischemia, and peripheral pulses may be palpated readily. Iliac artery obstruction will often produce not only a bruit but a diminution of the femoral pulse, but since a hemodynamically significant stenosis may produce as little as 10 mm Hg pressure gradient across the iliac artery at rest, the absence of the latter finding does not rule out this possibility.

If such a patient is exercised to the point of claudication, he will usually "lose" temporarily his previously palpable pedal pulses because of the marked decrease in vascular resistance that occurs in exercising muscle distal to an obstruction and the increased distribution of flow to muscle beds proximal to the obstruction. This is the basis for the practice of monitoring ankle pressure following lower limb exercise.

Femoral pulses may be difficult to palpate in muscular or obese patients unless the hips are externally rotated and the vessels are palpated lateral to the pubic tubercle, where they are covered by a smaller amount of fat. The popliteal pulses are often difficult to palpate even for the experienced examiner, so difficult in fact that the knowledgeable surgeon who feels them too easily will usually suspect the presence of a fusiform popliteal aneurysm. Holding the knee partially flexed, with the patient in the supine position, and allowing it to fall gently back into the examiner's hand, which is positioned so that the proximal interphalangeal joints hook the tendons while the fingertips sink gently just lateral to the midline of the popliteal space, is an effective means of palpating for a popliteal pulse. Many clinicians routinely sit down and have the patient turn to the prone position, flex the knee and have the foot rest on the examiner's shoulder while examining for the pulse within the popliteal space as well as above and below the area. The locations of the posterior tibial pulses in the hollow behind the medical malleolus and of the dorsalis pedis pulse along the dorsum of the foot between the first and second metatarsal bones are well known. Less well appreciated is the fact that the dorsalis pedis pulse will not be palpable in almost 10 per cent of normal individuals. Routinely, and especially in such cases, the lateral tibial artery, which is the terminal branch of the peroneal artery, should be sought just anterior to the lateral malleolus. A warm room and a light touch is the best combination for the most accurate detection of peripheral pulses. When there is a suspicion that the examiner is feeling his or her own pulse, someone should monitor the patient's radial pulse while the patient's pulse rate is identified.

Severe claudication may be associated with atrophy of the calf muscles, but unless this is unilateral and produces asymmetry it may escape detection. Loss of hair growth over the dorsum of the toes and foot is another relatively common sign of arterial insufficiency and may be accompanied by thickening of the toenails secondary to slowness of nail growth. However, more advanced ischemic changes (such as atrophy of the skin and its appendages and the subcutaneous tis-

sue, which causes the foot to become shiny, scaly and "skeletonized") usually do not appear in the absence of ischemic "rest pain." Delayed return of the capillary blush after pressure on the pulp of the digit or slow venous filling after the elevated extremity is dropped back into the dependent position are also signs of advanced ischemia. Buerger's sign, that is, cadaveric pallor on elevation and rubor on dependency, occurs with very restricted arterial inflow and chronic dilation of the peripheral vascular bed beyond, particularly of the postcapillary venules. The dependent toes may appear so red and refill so rapidly after pressure application that the uninitiated may mistakenly consider this to be evidence of hyperemia rather than an expression of severe ischemia. Localized pallor or cyanosis associated with poor capillary filling is usually a prelude to ischemic gangrene or ulceration. At this advanced stage of ischemia, the foot may be edematous from being maintained continually in the dependent position in an attempt to relieve the ischemic pain.

As previously stated, lower extremity pain secondary to venous disease is inconstant. In addition, the discomfort caused by venous distention from whatever cause is similar in its character, as is its relief by elevation. Therefore, the physical findings associated with these venous problems may be extremely helpful in differentiating among them. For example, *varicose veins* may be the result of primary saphenofemoral incompetence or may be secondary to deep venous and perforator incompetence. In the untreated state, the latter condition produces brawny edema, stasis dermatitis and ulceration. By contrast, the edema associated with primary uncomplicated varicose veins is mild and rarely appears early in the day; dermatitis with pigmentation is restricted to the skin immediately overlying prominent varicosities; and ulceration does *not* occur. Furthermore, primary varicose veins typically involve the main saphenous vein rather than scattered tributaries, and they do not refill quickly upon standing after a tourniquet has been applied to the upper thigh (positive tourniquet test).

An acutely thrombosed superficial vein will feel like a tender cord and may be surrounded by erythema, warmth, swelling, induration and other localized signs of inflammation. Even an acutely thrombosed deep vein, if associated with a sufficient inflammatory reaction, may result in tenderness along its course. However, it will usually produce a more generalized edema distally. If the deep calf veins are thrombosed, there may be pain on dorsiflexion (Homans' sign), tenderness on anterior-posterior but not on lateral compression of the calf (Bancroft's sign) and prompt pain in the calf if a sphygmomanometer cuff is inflated around it to 80 mm Hg pressure (Lowenberg's sign). However, these signs are said to be present in less than half the patients with acute deep venous thrombosis. The oft-quoted rate of one third false positive and one third false negative diagnoses of thrombophlebitis when made on clinical grounds alone applies more to an inpatient population, in whom occult thrombosis is more likely to occur, and swelling is more likely to be absent in patients receiving bedrest. On the other hand, outpatients with this condition usually present *because* of signs or symptoms, and therefore a higher rate of diagnostic accuracy may be expected in this setting. Nevertheless, it should be remembered that this diagnosis can be made confidently on clinical grounds only in cases with extensive major venous thrombosis (for example, in phlegmasia cerulea dolens or phlegmasia alba dolens) or when associated with a marked inflammatory reaction. As discussed later, it is far better both for diagnostic and follow-up purposes to examine the patient anatomically for changes in normalcy

than to use a gross test identified by eponyms.

The Swollen Leg

After the painful leg, limb swelling is the most common problem about which the surgeon is consulted. In examining the swollen lower limb, the consultant should remember another 5 P's: pressure, protein, permeability, paresis and 'pendency. Plasma constituents move into the tissues and return to the vascular space during circulation, according to Starling's law. The balance of factors influencing this process is a delicate one, particularly in the lower extremity, where gravity provides an additional complicating factor. The valved venomotor pump mechanism is presumably an evolutionary adaptation to man's assumption of the upright position, for if a normal person were to stand motionless long enough, venous pressures at the ankle would stabilize in the range of 80 to 100 mm Hg, and swelling and petechial hemorrhages would appear. However, with a competent venomotor pump mechanism, even modest activity of the calf muscles, such as occurs in intermittently shifting one's weight, will reduce this pressure to 20 to 30 mm Hg, and what little swelling accumulates during the day will usually disappear overnight when the body is horizontal. Patients who do not take advantage of this respite, for example, patients who sleep night after night with their feet dependent to relieve ischemic pain, will develop chronic swelling, as will patients with a peroneal palsy or an arthritis or fused ankle, who cannot activate the leg's venomotor pump.

Increased permeability secondary to inflammation will result in swelling if the extremity is not kept elevated. Similarly, swelling is seen in secondary aldosteronism. The lymphatic system is the route by which extravasated protein is returned to the central circulation. If the clearance capacity of this system is restricted because it is congenitally hypoplastic or obliterated by episodes of lymphangitis, or if its outflow is obstructed or interrupted by surgery or malignant lesions, or if it has been influenced by radiation, protein-rich lymph will accumulate in the tissues. A similar mechanism, in reverse, applies in hypoproteinemia, and this occasional cause of swelling should be considered in obscure cases. Other than in compartment syndromes, lower limb swelling is confined to the skin or subcutaneous tissue, or both, external to the deep fascia.

High venous pressure is the most common cause of extremity swelling. This increased peripheral venous pressure may be cardiac in origin, as in right-sided heart failure of tricuspid valvular disease, or may be due to intrinsic venous obstruction, as in peripheral venous thrombosis, or to extrinsic compression, as may occur to the left iliac vein by the right iliac artery. Most commonly, however, it is due to the unrelenting and unopposed transmission, in the upright position, of gravitational pressure through in-

competent valves of the deep and communicating veins of the postphlebitic leg to the superficial tissues. Venous hypertension secondary to arteriovenous fistulas is rarer but causes similar though more localized changes.

Clinically, the differential diagnosis of swelling may be difficult when it is of brief duration, but in the chronic state characteristic physical findings appear that greatly simplify matters. When a patient presents with a chronically swollen leg, the experienced examiner may make the correct diagnosis in over 95 per cent of cases simply by noting its distribution, its response to elevation and the associated discomfort and skin changes. These and other diagnostic considerations pertinent to chronically swollen lower extremities are listed in Table 17–1.

If there are no obvious associated skin changes and the edema "pits" readily on pressure, its cause is usually central or systemic, that is, cardiac in origin or due to hypoproteinemia or secondary aldosteronism. The distribution of this type of swelling, sometimes called orthostatic edema, is diffuse but greatest peripherally, always involving the foot. The edema asso-

TABLE 17–1   Differential Diagnosis of Chronic Leg Swelling

Characteristic	Venous	Lymphatic	Cardiac (Orthostatic)	Lipedema
Consistency of swelling	Brawny	Spongy	Pitting	Noncompressive (fat)
Relief by elevation	Complete	Mild	Complete	Minimal
Distribution of swelling	Maximal in ankles and legs Feet spared	Diffuse, greatest distally	Diffuse, greatest distally	Maximal in ankles and legs Feet spared
Associated skin changes	Atrophic and pigmented, subcutaneous fibrosis	Hypertrophied, lichenified skin	Shiny, mild pigmentation, no trophic changes	None
Pain	Heavy ache, tight or bursting feeling	None or heavy ache	Little or none	Dull ache, cutaneous sensitivity
Bilaterality	Occasionally, but usually unequal and left predominant	As often as not, but left predominant when unilateral	Always, but may be unequal	Always

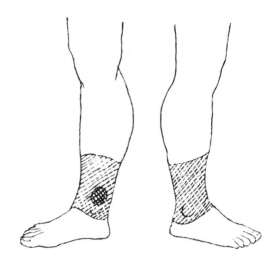

Figure 17–3 The "gaiter" zone (shaded), the area of predilection for postphlebitic (stasis) ulcers. (From: Rutherford, R. B.: The nonoperative management of chronic venous insufficiency. *In*: Rutherford, R. B. (ed.): Vascular Surgery. Philadelphia, W. B. Saunders Co., 1977, p. 1238.)

ciated with peripheral venous disease, even in the acute stage, does not "pit" readily. In the chronic stage it is frankly "brawny" and is associated with characteristic skin changes caused by chronic venous hypertension. The breakdown of extravasated red cells causes the characteristic pigmentation and, along with increased protein in the interstitial fluid, leads to inflammation and fibrosis in the subcutaneous tissues. Later, the skin becomes atrophic and breaks down with minor trauma. These components of so-called stasis, or postphlebitic, dermatitis have a "gaiter" distribution, as shown in Figure 17–3, and even in earlier stages when edema predominates, the feet are often relatively mildly affected compared with the ankles and lower half of the legs. This occurs because the venous hypertension is transmitted to the superficial veins by incompetent perforator veins located in this "gaiter" area. Eventually, progression of these chronic changes converts the skin and subcutaneous tissues of the leg from a diffusely edematous process to a pigmented, atrophic, tightly scarred zone that, when viewed in contrast to the proximal edema, leads to the descriptive term, "the inverted champagne bottle leg."

The distribution of lymphedema is diffuse but is always greater distally,

beginning with the toes and moving upward. This swelling is neither pitting nor brawny but "spongy" in character, in that while it does not significantly resist deformation by pressure, the skin and subcutaneous tissues immediately return to their original position as the pressure is withdrawn. Skin pigmentation and ulceration are rare. If anything, the skin eventually becomes hypertrophic. The end stage of chronic lymphatic insufficiency, elephantiasis, with its folds of thickened, lichenous skin hanging over the ankle, is too characteristic to be missed.

Occasionally women will present with chronically "swollen" legs that have none of the above characteristics. Although often reluctant to admit it, they will usually confess that they have always had "thick" ankles. These patients, and often other female members of their family, have maldistribution of fat characterized by excessive peripheral deposition. For unknown reasons, such patients are prone to superimposed orthostatic edema and complain of a dull ache and sensitivity of the overlying skin. However, this swelling, sometimes referred to as *lipedema*, never completely subsides after elevation or the use of diuretics. Furthermore, it is symmetrical with a relative *sparing* of the feet.

Occasionally a patient may state that

his legs swell immediately on arising, but during detailed questioning it becomes obvious that he is merely describing venous filling.

Finally, complaints of swelling that always feels greater to the patient than it appears to the examiner may represent a form of dysesthesia. If such patients also complain of superficial burning discomfort and show signs of autonomic imbalance, one should suspect a minor form of causalgia or reflex sympathetic dystrophy.

The Ulcerated Leg

The third most common problem for which consultation is requested is leg ulcers. There are only three common types of chronic ulceration likely to be encountered in the lower extremities — ischemic, stasis and neurotrophic ulcers — and they are readily distinguished one from the other, as outlined in Table 17–2. *Ischemic ulcers* are usually quite painful, and typical ischemic "rest pain" in the distal forefoot with nocturnal occurrence and relief by dependency is likely. These ulcers may have irregular edges at first, but when they become chronic they are more likely to be "punched

out." They are commonly located distally over the dorsum of the foot or toes but may occasionally be pretibial. The ulcer base usually consists of poorly developed grayish granulation tissue. The surrounding skin may be pale or mottled, and the previously described signs of chronic ischemia are invariably present. Probing or debriding the ulcer causes little bleeding.

Neurotrophic ulcers, on the other hand, are completely painless but bleed with manipulation. They are deep and indolent, often surrounded by a chronic inflammatory reaction and callus. Their location is typically over pressure points or calluses, for example, the planter surface of the 1st and 5th metatarsal-phalangeal joint, the base of the distal phalanx of the great toe, the dorsum of the interphalangeal joints of the toes with flexion contractures, the callused posterior rim of the heel pad or bony prominences on the leg or the ankle. The patient is usually a long-standing diabetic with a neuropathy characterized by patchy hypesthesia and diminished positional sense, two-point discrimination and vibratory perception.

The *stasis or postphlebitic ulcer* is located within the "gaiter" area shown in Figure 17–3, most commonly near

TABLE 17–2 Differential Diagnosis of Common Leg Ulcers

Type	Usual Location	Pain	Bleeding With Manipulation	Characteristics	Associated Findings
Ischemic	Distally, on dorsum of foot or toes	Severe, particularly at night Relieved by dependency	Little or none	Irregular edge, poor granulation tissue	Trophic changes of chronic ischemia
Postphlebitic (stasis)	Lower third of leg (gaiter area)	Mild, relieved by elevation	Venous ooze	Shallow, irregular shape Granulating base Rounded edges	Stasis dermatitis
Neurotrophic	Under calluses, pressure points (plantar aspect of 1st or 5th m-p joint), bony prominences of leg or ankle	None	Brisk	Punched out, with deep sinus	Demonstrable neuropathy

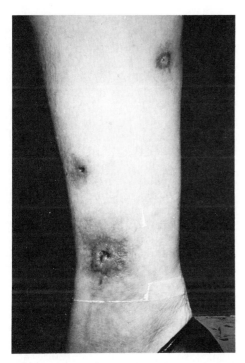

Figure 17–4 Chronic leg ulcers resulting from vasculitis. Often mistaken for postphlebitic ulcerations.

the medial malleolus. It is usually larger than the other types of ulcers, irregular in outline but also shallower and with a moist, granulating base. It is always surrounded by a zone of stasis dermatitis, as previously described.

Over 95 per cent of all chronic leg or foot ulcers fall into one of these three recognizable types. The remainder are hard to distinguish except that they are not typical of the other three types. Vasculitis, hypertension and syphilis all may produce leg ulcers. Vasculitis often produces multiple punched out holes and an inflamed indurated base that, when biopsied, suggests fat necrosis or chronic panniculitis (Fig. 17–4). Hypertensive ulcers represent focal infarcts and are very painful. They may be located around the malleoli, particularly laterally. Luetic ulcers are uncommon today, but in any atypical ulcer, this or other systemic causes of ulceration such as chronic ulcerative

colitis with pyoderma gangrenosum or tuberculosis should be suspected. Long-standing ulcers that are refractory to treatment may represent an underlying osteomyelitis, cancer (usually melanoma or squamous carcinoma) or a secondary malignancy.

Finally, although most patients with ulcers of one of the specific etiologies just discussed will blame trauma as the initiating agent, trauma may occasionally be the primary etiological factor, with the chronicity of the ulcer being related either to the slow healing that is characteristic of the lower one third of the leg or possibly to a degree of arterial insufficiency that would otherwise be subclinical. Such ulcers will often heal with nonspecific therapy such as intermittent elevation and the application of Unna's boots.

In summary, the identification and treatment of peripheral vascular problems is exemplified by the approach to the painful, swollen or ulcerated leg in order to stress the value of a problem-oriented approach, careful interrogation and thoughtful examination, all guided by an experienced index of suspicion. Having completed this initial assessment at the bedside or in the office, the clinician must next consider the need to proceed further diagnostically, either for the sake of diagnosis itself or to provide further objective information upon which to base therapeutic decisions. Whether the basic diagnosis is obvious or not, the location and extent of the vascular disease and the degree of circulatory impairment can often be documented by noninvasive methods of study, as described later in the chapter. Angiographic confirmation is usually obtained only if necessary to make major therapeutic decisions, including the feasibility of reconstructive vascular surgery. Since these procedures are not without significant risk and expense, the choice between operative and nonoperative treatment should often be made before proceeding with angiographic studies.

VENOUS DISEASE

Thromboembolic Disease

Venous thrombosis and its complications are among the most common diseases seen on an outpatient basis. These diseases occur both as acute processes and as chronic conditions.

Definition and Classification

Venous thrombosis may be defined as a partial or complete occlusion of a vein by a thrombus. An antecedent or secondary inflammatory reaction is present in the wall of the vein. Its importance lies in its frequent occurrence and its serious, sometimes fatal, sequelae.

Venous inflammatory processes are associated with local thromboses that invariably evoke a secondary inflammatory reaction. The two processes of thrombosis and inflammation cannot be separated from each other. Variation in the degree of inflammatory reaction has led to a classic division of venous thrombolic disease into two categories, phlebothrombosis and thrombophlebitis. This categorization is not universally accepted, since there is always some inflammatory reaction present, and therefore all cases should be included under the one term, *thrombophlebitis.*[5]

All states of thrombus formation are directly related to the time elapsed and to the clinical signs present. The clot may vary from an initial sludging and adherence to the intima of the "backwash" of a valve cusp to the formation of an organized clot. Thrombophlebitis theoretically leads to an organized clot and phlebothrombosis to an unorganized clot. *Phlebothrombosis* as a specific diagnostic term should be assigned only after objective histopathological examination of the specimen. *Thrombophlebitis* is the more appropriate term to use clinically.

The common sites of involvement by thrombophlebitis are the veins of the extremities — the femoral, popliteal and tibial veins, the subclavian, axillary and iliac veins, and the superior and inferior vena cava. Venous thrombosis may be localized or confluent, involve several venous tributaries, occur in a patchy or scattered fashion and be either fulminating or insidious in onset. Although thrombophlebitis characteristically presents in one lower extremity, phlebography and autopsy studies may also demonstrate similar lesions in the asymptomatic limb. Since numerous nonthrombotic disorders may present similar clinical features, it is common to question the reliability of signs and symptoms of venous thrombosis when they are based primarily on a clinical impression. However, in the majority of patients in whom there are distinct inflammatory signs (swelling, pain and tenderness limited to the venous anatomical site), the manifestations of the disease process are clear-cut and diagnosis is ordinarily simple. In some patients the manifestations may be so bizarre and erratic that a diagnosis can be made only by exclusion.

Etiology and Pathogenesis

Intravascular thrombosis is not yet completely understood. The common denominators leading to the development of thrombosis, irrespective of the primary disease or operative procedure, are: (1) primary endothelial lesions of the vein wall with subsequent inflammation and thrombosis, (2) slowing and eddying of the blood flow with sludging and inflammatory reaction in the wall of the vein, and (3) physical and chemical changes in the blood itself, producing hypercoagulability (Virchow's triad). Thrombophlebitis is the end result of an imbalance in the physiochemical forces that maintain the vein endothelium undisrupted and the blood in a fluid state.

When blood coagulates, the final result is the formation of fibrin, which is the stroma of the clot. This white fibrin matrix produces the network that catches the thrombocytes, leukocytes and erythrocytes. This process may be normal, decreased (hemorrhagic diathesis) or increased (abnormal thrombosis).

When the clotting process is enhanced, the contributing or triggering factor may be localized and result in a thrombosis. A thrombus may produce an embolus or it may be diffuse, causing obstruction of small as well as large vessels and interfering with venous outflow and even arterial inflow. When the diffuse process is extensive, a marked consumption of clotting factors occurs that is termed *consumption coagulopathy.* A more detailed discussion of the clotting process is presented later.

Thrombophlebitis

Clinical Features

The cardinal findings in thrombophlebitis are those of inflammation: Celsus' classic quartet of dolor, calor, tumor and rubor. Redness may be present disproportionately and may occur concurrently with other symptoms and signs. The following clinical patterns refer mainly to thrombophlebitis of the lower extremity, but analogous manifestations can be expected elsewhere.

LOCAL MANIFESTATIONS. 1. *Subjective pain* in varying degrees is often sensed as "soreness" or "pins and needles" in the involved or distant area, or both, and the extremity may feel heavy. Pain is accentuated by motion or dependency, and relief is obtained by inactivity and elevation. Muscle cramps often indicate deep vein thrombophlebitis but may easily be misinterpreted when not accompanied by additional signs and symptoms. Severe low back or groin pain may ac-

company iliofemoral thrombophlebitis. Causalgia, a burning type of pain, or ischemic neuritis (deep pain), is sometimes present on or within the foot when there is evidence of decreased arterial supply following massive venous thrombosis to the limb, that is, phlegmasia cerulea dolens. A common complaint in superficial veins is the burning pain localized to the course of the greater or lesser saphenous vein.

2. *Objective pain,* not to be confused with direct tenderness, may be elicited by indirect compression on the vein. This maneuver is recommended only as a rapid screening method. The well-known Homans' sign is deep pain evoked in the upper posterior calf on dorsiflexion of the foot with the knee extended. Grasping the entire muscle mass of the calf also causes pain. The misleading aspect of Homans' sign is that it is positive in a large number of nonthrombotic disorders, particularly those that involve the muscles or nerves of the calf.

Another misleading test is Lowenberg's sign, which elicits pain in the calf when a blood pressure cuff is applied to the region of the knee and inflated to 100 to 120 mm of mercury. A modification of this test is the Ramirez sign, in which the blood pressure cuff is placed on the leg and inflated to 40 mm of mercury. Pain may be produced in the region of the thrombotic calf vein and should disappear promptly with release of the pressure. The Perthes test is positive if the patient develops pain upon walking with a tight elastic bandage on the leg or a tourniquet on the thigh. This test was popularized as a method to determine deep vein obstruction in patients having varicose veins. However, when the Perthes test is positive, treatment is required for venous thrombosis, not varicose veins. These tests are often misleading when specific nonthrombotic disorders are present.

Tenderness of a mild, moderate or marked nature is provoked by direct digital pressure along the course of the involved pain. This simple test is probably the most accurate method of diagnosing thrombophlebitis, for it locates the most inflamed site. This method of examination is *strongly recommended,* not only to rule out nonthrombotic disorders but also to localize the extent of the tenderness and to follow its response to therapy. Since this requires detailed anatomical examination of the extremity, it provides a means of differentiating between deep vein thrombosis and such common entities as superficial thrombophlebitis, gastrocnemius or plantaris muscle rupture, sciatic nerve neuritis or entrapment syndromes, as well as less common nonthrombotic leg disorders. Tenderness of the deep veins is diffuse or radiates over the course of the vessel and is usually confined to sections where the veins can be easily delineated, as in the inguinal region, Scarpa's (femoral) triangle, Hunter's (adductor) canal or the popliteal fossa. A positive Bancroft's sign is tenderness induced by firm, steady pressure in the midportion of the calf posteriorly toward the tibia, but not on lateral compression. This is a far better method of examination than Homans', Lowenberg's, Ramirez' or Perthes' tests. Tenderness may also be elicited by pressure over the malleoli or plantar surfaces.

3. *Color changes* usually present as red linear streaks corresponding to the path of the superficial vein, and the involved extremity has an inflamed appearance. Dusky cyanosis may occur distal to the occlusion of a large vein. Occasionally, a pale blue or white appearance of the extremity may follow spasm of an artery that rests against an inflamed vein. The red lines are warm to the touch; the pale areas are cool or cold. When a significant amount of deep vein obstruction results in a bluish foot and leg, elevation of the extremity does not produce much of a decrease in the blue color. The same results are noted when subclavian or axillary vein thrombosis obstructs the venous outflow of the upper extremity.

4. *Local swelling* or *induration* of the red streaks and tissues immediately adjacent to either of the saphenous veins or their tributaries produces cordlike prominences that may remain for several weeks after anti-inflammatory therapy has eliminated the red streaks and pain.

5. *Edema* results from congestion of the venous, lymphatic and capillary beds beyond the thrombophlebitic obstruction. Gross edema from distal blockage of larger veins causes disproportion and a doughy feel to the limb. Swelling of the leg is not characteristic of superficial thrombophlebitis, since the saphenous systems conveys no more than 10 per cent of the venous circulation from a normal limb. Ambulatory patients are more likely to have edema than bed patients, since gravity influences the location of swelling. This is why the clinical diagnosis is more accurately made in outpatients than inpatients: 75 per cent vs. 50 per cent. The more cephalad the venous occlusion, the more likely it is that the patient will have discomfort from the swelling and the higher the incidence of venous thrombosis as verified by phlebography. Edema and a waxy, pale discoloration account for the typical appearance of *phlegmasia alba dolens* (milk leg). In the early stages the skin may be cool. Later, when reflex vasospasm is relieved by the inflammatory reaction, the leg becomes warm. Occasionally, there may be marbleization (cutis marmorata) or "cobweb" mottling of the skin (harlequin skin).

6. *Enlarged or dilated veins* may appear and be diagnostic of the presence of a deep vein obstruction because of the increased load of venous return through venous collaterals. The veins of the involved foot and leg may become quite prominent. As many as three sentinel veins may appear over the tibia on the upper third of the leg (veins of Pratt). The superficial venous tributaries in the groin may become

prominent with iliac vein thrombosis or with bilateral prominence of these vessels when the inferior vena cava is involved. With subclavian, innominate or superior vena cava venous occlusions, prominent veins are noted in the shoulder area.

SYSTEMIC MANIFESTATIONS. 1. *Fever* may be slight or absent, depending on the amount of perivenous inflammatory reaction and the presence or absence of infection. Fever is usually limited to the early stages of the disease and subsides within a few days. An unaccountable, transient subnormal temperature is sometimes one of the earliest signs of thrombophlebitis (Michaelis' sign).

2. The *pulse rate* increases in stepladder fashion. Tachycardia may occur when a significant amount of inflammation and edema cause an attendant sequestration and reduction in intravascular volume.

3. The *erythrocyte-sedimentation rate* tends to parallel the degree of fever. Although it is nonspecific, this test is used as an index of resolution or progression of the disease.

These systemic signs become extremely important when thrombophlebitis is being considered in patients with paralysis of the lower extremities. The legs are invariably swollen in these patients, and incapable of feeling pain.

Typical Clinical Patterns

The general clinical patterns are fairly consistent in thrombophlebitis, but the symptoms and signs may vary. The atypical or rare forms are less easily identified and the condition may be recognized only at autopsy.

Deep Thrombophlebitis (Thrombophlebitis of the Femoral Vein and Veins of the Muscles of the Calf)

The most common location of thrombophlebitis is in the veins of the calf or in the superficial, deep and common femoral vein, or in both. The symptoms and signs are variable and may include none or all of the clinical manifestations described in the preceding section. Common presenting symptoms include:

(1) Calf pain, especially with contraction of gastrocnemius and soleus muscles

(2) Pain in the thigh

(3) Edema in calf or thigh

(4) Pulmonary embolus from a silent thrombosis of calf or femoral veins

A very rare presenting symptom is a paradoxical embolus to the arterial system in a patient with a patent atrial or ventricular septal defect.

Superficial thrombophlebitis, which occurs in the saphenous system, may progress into deep thrombophlebitis by extension of the thrombus through perforating veins or by extension across the saphenofemoral junction at the fossa ovalis. Deep thrombophlebitis of the common femoral vein may progress to involve the iliac vein and the inferior vena cava. When iliofemoral thrombophlebitis occurs, the thigh almost invariably becomes swollen. Deep thrombophlebitis may later subside completely or may produce a postphlebitic syndrome, characterized by chronic edema, pain and late-appearing ulcerations of the lower third of the legs, particularly in the area of the malleoli.

Superficial Thrombophlebitis (Thrombophlebitis of the Saphenous Veins)

Although this is a common condition occuring with or without varicose veins, it may be associated with more serious problems. Its symptoms are pain, local tenderness, reddish-blue discoloration and usually the formation of a palpable cord localized to the lesser or greater saphenous veins or to their tributaries. Since deep venous thrombosis may also be present, the outcome may depend on its detection and the type of therapy instituted. The saphenous vein carries only a small amount of the venous return from the extremity. Therefore, generalized swelling of the leg and foot should not occur unless deep vein thrombophlebitis is present or unless the patient has a history of postphlebitic syndrome as previously stated. Propagation of the thrombus to the saphenofemoral junction may be the source for a pulmonary embolus. Therefore, it is essential that patients with superficial thrombophlebitis have frequent examinations to evaluate the extent of the local tenderness and vein changes from the thrombosis.

Silent Thrombosis (Unorganized Clot)

The presence of a silent thrombosis should be considered in questionable thromboembolic states, especially when predisposing factors are present. Silent thrombosis is the term used to identify an unorganized clot; it may be unsuspected until a pulmonary embolus has occurred and death is imminent, or in other cases there may be varying degrees of apprehension, malaise, chest pain, cough, fever, tachycardia, cyanosis, dyspnea, pallor, hypotension and sweating. In pulmonary embolization, a pleural rub or rales may lead the observer to conclude that an embolus is the cause of shock, and a thorough search for the source of the embolus in the lower extremities or pelvic veins is sometimes rewarding. Hemoptysis is absent or is a late manifestation. Electrocardiographic tracings are equivocal or may be mistaken for coronary occlusion, and the roentgenographic opaque triangle of pulmonary infarction is rarely seen. A small primary embolus that has been overlooked may be followed in a week or ten days by a fatal secondary embolization. When the histories of a majority of patients with fatal emboli are carefully reviewed, a primary embolism is usually noted in retrospect. This impression has been supported by re-

ports regarding patients who have undergone a pulmonary embolectomy. Roentgenological changes that are seen on a routine chest film or a pleural rub usually do not become evident until two or three days after embolization has occurred.

The commonly recognized stage of thrombophlebitis is not the extreme of silent or of massive venous occlusion but that which has previously been described under Deep and Superficial Thrombophlebitis.

Massive Venous Occlusion

This uncommon disease of the limb is actually an accentuation of iliofemoral thrombophlebitis. It can be classified into three venous thrombotic entities according to the severity of signs and symptoms. Iliofemoral thrombophlebitis per se is the mildest of the three (see earlier discussion of deep thrombophlebitis). The two severe forms are *phlegmasia alba dolens* (milk leg) and *phlegmasia cerulea dolens* (blue phlebitis).

PHLEGMASIA ALBA DOLENS. This is a syndrome caused by severe iliofemoral thrombophlebitis. Historically it is called "milk leg" because of its occurrence during the postpartum period. In the majority of patients it occurs on the left side, supposedly owing to inherent abnormalities of the iliac vein such as an intimal web or compression from the right iliac artery as it crosses over the left common iliac vein. Clinical findings are caused by severe venous thrombosis as well as by some degree of lymphatic obstruction. The onset of edema is sudden and is often accompanied by severe pain. Swelling of the thigh is a characteristic feature and local tenderness can be elicited in the groin over the femoral triangle and possibly above, in the iliac fossa. The superficial collateral veins in the inguinal area become dilated and are usually prominent. The foot is cool early and later becomes warm.

Pedal pulses are palpable, although difficult to feel when foot and ankle edema is marked. However, capillary flow is good and ischemia is not a problem. Fluid loss into the extremity may be significant and hypovolemia may become a concern.

PHLEGMASIA CERULEA DOLENS. This syndrome is the most severe of those associated with iliofemoral thrombophlebitis (Fig. 17–5). Gangrene of the leg is a probable complication. The onset is usually violent, with agonizing pain. The extremity is cold, tender, cyanotic, sometimes swollen and suffused with a violescent discoloration. It finally becomes shiny, livid and markedly edematous and develops blisters on the toes and foot. Vasospasm is severe and gangrene may ensue because of the marked venous congestion accompanied by the resultant arterial deficiency. To differentiate this entity from acute arterial occlusion, one should remember that arterial occlusion alone never results in edema. Also, the absence of a history of intermittent claudication should exclude chronic arterial disease as a contributing factor. If arteriospasm is complete or sustained, the gangrene is "dry" and well demarcated; otherwise, the gangrene is also accompanied by compartment swelling and is the "wet" or venous type. The progression is usually swift and the outcome may be death from shock or pulmonary embolization. In almost all cases it is associated with an underlying condition. Arterial deficiency in deep-vein thrombosis ranges from no decrease to complete absence of the arterial flow.[90] Since a large amount of blood and fluid is sequestered in the thrombotic limb,[1] hypovolemia is a potential hazard and may require treatment.

Thrombophlebitis of the Subclavian or Axillary Vein

This is a relatively benign variety of thrombophlebitis. The manifestations are indistinguishable from thrombophlebitis in other veins. The arm is swollen due to venous obstruction, and prominent veins are usually noted over the pectoral area. Raising the arm during examination fails to relieve the blueness or venous engorgement of the extremity. Because this condition often follows unusual or excessive use of the arm or unusual posturing, it has been called "effort thrombosis" or "straphanger arm." The patient may have a history of thoracic outlet com-

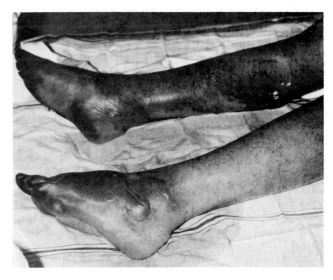

Figure 17–5 Massive venous thrombosis of iliofemoral and calf veins resulting in gangrene of the feet. Note edema, cyanosis and blister formation. Patient had multiple pulmonary emboli initially that masked radiological evidence of carcinoma of the lung.

pression syndrome in which the subclavian vein is trapped between the
clavicle and the first rib. Details of this
syndrome will be discussed later in
the chapter.

Migratory Thrombophlebitis

This condition appears as isolated,
red, painful areas, usually involving
superficial veins in separate parts of
the body. It has been associated with
cancer, thromboangiitis obliterans,
nonbacterial endocarditis, collagen
disease, drugs and familial traits toward clotting. Underlying disorders
should be searched for and the patient's clotting profile should be studied. Treatment should consist of an anti-inflammatory agent, subcutaneous
heparin on an ambulatory basis, or
both.

Pelvic Thrombophlebitis

Pelvic vein thrombosis may be difficult to diagnose unless evidence of the
predisposing gynecological and obstetrical conditions are noted on pelvic
examination. Systemic manifestations
may raise suspicion of venous thrombosis in the pelvis. Occasionally, when
the hypogastric vein is thrombosed,
perivenous inflammation may involve
the obturator nerve which passes beneath the vessel. Discomfort may then
be referred to the adductor muscles of
the thigh or to the knee.

Inferior Vena Cava Thrombosis

Occlusion of the inferior vena cava
by an isolated thrombus is rare because of the large volume of blood
flowing through the vessel, but it may
occur following caval interruption procedures. Occasionally vena caval occlusion occurs from extension of iliac
vein thrombophlebitis. When a spontaneous thrombosis does occur, associated disorders causing the condition include tumors such as lymphoma or
hepatoma, trauma, retroperitoneal fibrosis, scleral obstruction of the hepatic vein and massive infection in children who develop severe dehydration
and blood dyscrasias. Swelling and
congestion may appear in the lower
extremities and dilation may appear in
the superficial veins on the anterior abdominal wall. Venous flow occurs from
the groin toward the umbilicus in the
superficial or the deep epigastric
veins, or both (Fig. 17–6) instead of in
the opposite direction as is normal. A
directional Doppler (flowmeter) may
be used to confirm this flow pattern.
Other than the occurrence of pulmonary emboli, the most serious complication is extension of the venous thrombosis into the renal veins, causing the
nephrotic syndrome.

Superior Vena Cava Thrombosis

Many diseases may cause this disorder, such as tumors, aortic aneurysms, mediastinitis and histoplasmosis. The head — particularly the
conjunctiva — becomes   edematous
and cyanotic; the arms and chest swell
and dilated veins appear in the neck,
arms and upper trunk. The patient may
develop vertigo and syncope with exercise (Fig. 17–7).

Septic Thrombophlebitis

Most cases are sequelae of infected
sites of venous catheters or are seen in
conjunction with burns of the extremities or following obstetrical and gynecological manipulations. There are the
usual local manifestations of thrombophlebitis, plus cellulitis, abscess formation and accentuated systemic reactions. Cavernous sinus thrombosis
from jugular venous dissemination
may appear long after chronic mastoiditis has subsided. Neonatal omphali-
tis may give rise to portal venous
thrombosis several months later. Other
types of septic thrombophlebitis in-

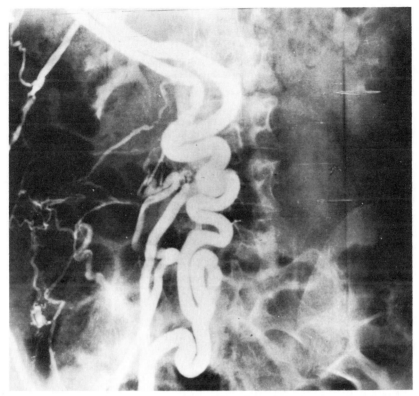

Figure 17–6 Venogram demonstrating collateral flow through deep epigastric vein one year following ligation of inferior vena cava in a patient with congenital hypercoagulopathy.

Figure 17–7 Superior vena caval occlusion from histoplasmosis. Note dilated veins over neck, arms, shoulders and thorax.

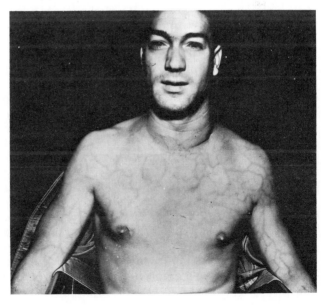

clude pylephlebitis, renal vein thrombosis, vena caval thrombophlebitis, mesenteric vein thrombosis, acute cor pulmonale due to thrombotic occlusion of the pulmonary arteries, and pelvic thrombophlebitis.

Differential Diagnosis

The diagnosis of thrombosis of the *superficial* veins of the lower extremity is usually quite easy. The swelling and inflammatory signs are localized along the course of the saphenous veins or along one of their major tributaries, and one can often feel the cord-like thrombosed vein.

In contrast, the diagnosis of acute deep venous thrombosis (DVT) may be extremely difficult on clinical grounds alone. Approximately half of patients with *clinical* signs compatible with DVT have a normal venogram, and conversely, more than half of DVT cases are not detected clinically. There is no significant difference in the incidence of the commonly accepted clinical signs and symptoms of phlebitis between cases in which venograms confirm the presence of DVT and those in which they are normal.[16, 30] However, there is a significant difference between an inpatient and outpatient population in regard to the presentation of DVT. In high-risk hospitalized patients, the incidence of DVT detected by either routine radioactive fibrinogen scans or venograms may exceed 50 per cent with as many as 85 to 90 per cent being clinically occult. On the other hand, outpatients rarely present unless they have signs and symptoms, so that a correct diagnosis may be arrived at on clinical grounds in up to 75 per cent of patients.

The more common disease entities that may be confused with peripheral thrombophlebitis are listed in Table 17–3.

The superficial veins of the lower extremities are frequently a source of "false phlebitis." Many women, partic-

TABLE 17–3 Differential Diagnosis of Deep Thrombophlebitis

"False phlebitis" ("hormonal phlebitis") — pain in saphenous veins immediately prior to menstrual periods and during pregnancy
"Epidemic phlebodynia" — painful cords in the legs during cyclical periods of water retention in women
Cellulitis
Lymphangitis
Superficial (saphenous) thrombophlebitis
Muscle strain
Muscle rupture — gastrocnemius or plantaris
Sciatic neuritis
Posterior tibial neuritis
Entrapment neuritis
Spontaneous night cramps
Arterial insufficiency
"Restless" or "crazy" legs
Lymphedema, congenital and acquired

ularly those with varicose veins, develop pain and tenderness on the medial aspect of one or both limbs just prior to menstrual periods. The pain is frequently described as burning in nature, and the complaint is localized to the saphenous veins and is termed "hormonal phlebitis." When the extremity is elevated, the vein collapses (an event that does not occur in thrombophlebitis). Pain subsides following menstrual flow. During pregnancy and when anovulatory hormones are used, a similar discomfort may occur, and the patient also notices fluid retention and increased prominence of the limbs. A detailed history and examination plus elevation of the limbs and Doppler studies should exclude venous occlusion. Discontinence of the anovulatory hormones usually relieves symptoms. Another entity known as "epidemic phlebodynia" has been described in young women who develop palpable cordlike structures in the legs. This is thought to be a variant of water retention. Elevation of the limbs allows the superficial veins to collapse. Ballottement, percussion or Doppler studies of the saphenous system should demonstrate venous patency. No specific treatment is of benefit because the condition eventually subsides spontaneously.

Congenital and acquired lymphedema may simulate the chronic postphlebitic syndrome but can be distinguished in most patients by history and physical examination. The differential diagnosis of the swollen leg has been discussed in the introduction to this chapter. Pelvic venography is now utilized to identify patients with iliac vein entrapment by the common iliac artery, since this appears to be a contributory cause of unilateral lymphedema of the left lower limb in some patients (Fig. 17–8).

Cellulitis, with or without lymphangitis, may also be difficult to differentiate from venous thrombosis. However, in most instances of cellulitis the fever is high, which is unlikely in thrombophlebitis unless it is septic.

Leukocytosis or a shaking chill also differentiates cellulitis from thrombophlebitis. Antibiotics would exclude the possibility of differentiation.

Superficial thrombophlebitis of the saphenous veins in the thigh or calf presents a disturbing problem, since these veins overlie the course of the deep venous system in these two areas. Palpation of a tender cordlike structure, erythema localized to the saphenous vein, or establishment of patency of the vein by elevation, ballottement, percussion or a Doppler ultrasound probe over the vein and comparison of the measurement of each extremity's circumference will assist in establishing the diagnosis. When in doubt, the patient should be assumed to have deep vein thrombosis also and should be treated accordingly.

Muscular complaints in the leg may easily simulate deep vein thrombophlebitis. Mention has been made previously of the signs that may mimic the presence of thrombophlebitis. These are positive Homans', Lowenberg's or Ramirez' signs, which may be elicited in numerous muscular as well as sciatic nerve disorders. Moreover, all of these conditions may coexist. Muscle strain or rupture of the gastrocnemius or plantaris muscle after direct trauma or following unaccustomed sudden or strenuous exercise in middle-aged men or women can cause severe discomfort in the calf of the leg, with swelling, tenderness and a "diagnostic" dorsiflexion sign. A history of diffuse tenderness located medial or lateral to the midline of the calf, swelling over the muscle rupture area and the presence of ecchymosis at the ankle or lower third of the leg establishes the diagnosis of a gastrocnemius muscle rupture. Plantaris muscle rupture may be present, with tenderness that is usually high in the calf in the popliteal space but occasionally in the midcalf. Leg soreness may occur following spontaneous night cramps. Treatment with quinine, benadryl or chloroquine

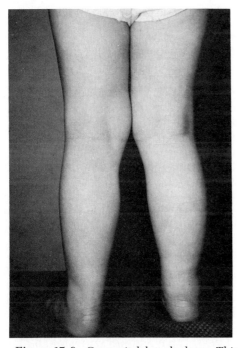

Figure 17–8 Congenital lymphedema. This child with bilateral mild edema was treated with the Jobst pneumatic pressure machine at weekly intervals. Her condition was stable and did not require surgery. Pelvic venography is utilized in such patients to look for entrapment of the iliac vein.

should result in relief for the majority of patients and thus establish the diagnosis of night cramps alone.

Included in the differential diagnosis is a strange syndrome identified as "restless" or "crazy" legs. The history of its presence periodically during or after a stressful situation, fatigue or hormonal changes, and the presence of minimal physical findings other than tender muscles in the extremities should help establish this diagnosis.

When swelling is painless and bland and develops with ambulation, the diagnosis is lymphedema. Following femoral-popliteal bypass, swelling of the thigh and leg may occur, owing to disturbance of lymphatic channels and increased flow of arterial blood. If calf discomfort occurs, this is strongly indicative of thrombophlebitis. Most often, this complaint occurs in an extremity that was severely ischemic from recent acute arterial occlusion. The leg pain develops within 48 hours after reconstruction, and tenderness is usually localized to each of the compartments; namely the lateral, posterior or anterior areas of the leg. These findings usually exclude venous thrombosis unless it is demonstrated on phlebography.

Another difficult diagnostic problem is the differentiation of thrombophlebitis from sciatic nerve irritation due to entrapment neuritis. Tenderness over the sciatic nerve on the posterior aspect of the thigh and absence of adductor canal tenderness or tenderness in the calf and the posterior aspect of the thigh will exclude the diagnosis of thrombophlebitis. The possibility of both conditions being present may need to be considered. Peripheral neuritis may be localized to one extremity but usually is bilateral and more generalized, as discussed earlier in this chapter.

Diagnostic Methods

The many clinical observations that can be utilized to establish the diagnosis of acute venous thrombosis have been discussed. However, since it is difficult to make the diagnosis accurately on clinical grounds alone, and because thrombophlebitis may have serious and often fatal complications, supplemental diagnostic methods may be necessary. Ancillary diagnostic measures are employed chiefly in three types of patients with suspected venous disease: those with *silent thrombosis,* when thrombophlebitis is suspected but signs and symptoms are minimal or nonexistent; those in whom *pulmonary embolism* is suspected or established but in whom no peripheral evidence of thrombophlebitis is displayed on examination; and those who are believed to have diseases that are considered in the *differential diagnosis* of thrombophlebitis. The following diagnostic procedures have been proposed in a group of disorders that have a high incidence of deep vein thrombosis.

Noninvasive Approach

Currently, there are only two approaches to the noninvasive diagnosis of deep venous thrombosis that help bridge the gap between the uncertainty of clinical diagnosis and the accuracy of phlebography. One involves the monitoring of venous "flow" with a Doppler probe, and the other employs plethysmographical measurement of provoked venous volume shifts. Both are relatively easy to perform at the bedside and therefore will be described in detail.

DETECTION OF DVT BY DOPPLER VELOCITY DETECTOR. Ultrasonic instruments that take advantage of the Doppler effect in monitoring the "flow" of blood in accessible peripheral vessels have found widespread clinical application in this decade. In principle, sound reflecting from a moving object will change in frequency in direct proportion to the velocity of the object. In practice, taking advantage of the fact that the only significantly moving "objects" in the tissues of a resting extremity are red blood cells, a 5 to 10 MHz ultrasound beam is directed from a transmitting piezo crystal at the selected vessel, using known anatomical landmarks. The adjacent receiving crystal in this same probe receives the reflected sound and passes it through a differential amplifier that amplifies only those frequencies that are more than 50 to 60 cycles per second different from the transmitted frequency. The resulting signal falls into the audible range, producing arterial and venous sounds so characteristic normally that the abnormalities produced by luminal obstruction are easily recognized.

The common term "Doppler *flow-meter*" is actually a misnomer because it detects velocity rather than flow. This differentiation is important in studying arterial disease but has no practical significance in the study of peripheral veins, so continued reference to venous "flow" is justifiable. Whereas the arterial sound is synchronous with heartbeat, the venous sound rises and falls with respiration and can be likened to a high wind rhythmically rushing through the trees. The details of this test and its physiological basis have been well described by Sumner.[83]

In the legs of a supine individual the sound decreases with inspiration, as the diaphragm descends and causes increased intra-abdominal pressure, and increases with expiration, as the diaphragm rises and intra-abdominal pressure falls. Ordinarily, these phasic changes can be detected in all the major veins of the lower extremities down to and including the posterior tibial and greater saphenous veins at the ankle. Finding such a phasic signal virtually assures the observer that all the venous channels proximal to the position of the Doppler probe are patent, or at least functionally patent. In contrast, continuous, nonphasic flow, although indicating that the vein immediately below the probe is patent, suggests that there is obstruction of the vein channel cephalad to the probe and that blood is flowing continuously into collateral veins bypassing that obstruction. Respiratory variation is much less noticeable in females. The opposite effect of sound increasing on inspiration and decreasing on expiration occurs in the veins of the upper extremities of subjects who breathe thoracically or who are examined in the upright position. As shown in Figure 17–9, proximal compression of the vein manually, or by forced expiration

Figure 17–9 Venous flow responses to augmentation maneuvers. *A* and *B* show normal responses; *C* and *D* show abnormal responses typical of venous vascular incompetence. (From: Sumner, D. S.: Evaluation of the venous circulation using the ultrasonic Doppler velocity detector. *In*: Rutherford, R. B. (ed.): Vascular Surgery. Philadelphia, W. B. Saunders Co., 1977, p. 181.)

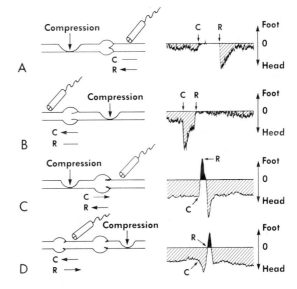

in the case of iliac veins, should stop forward venous flow without producing retrograde flow. Compression of the veins distal to the monitoring position should produce augmenation of flow, which will be weak or absent if the vein at the point of compression is thrombosed. Major deep venous occlusion will often produce enough increase in flow through the parallel, superficial (saphenous) vein that the difference is noticeable when compared with the opposite side. Thus, by detecting the presence or absence of deep venous flow and by determining (1) if it is phasic with respiration or continuous, (2) whether or not it is augmented following the application of distal compression or the release of proximal compression and (4) whether or not ipsilateral saphenous flow is increased, one can diagnose proximal DVT with an accuracy of greater than 85 per cent.[83]

The major weakness of this approach is that thromboses below the knee are hard to detect if they do not involve the posterior tibial vein. Examination of the anterior tibial vein is less satisfactory and the thrombi in the peroneal vein and gastrocnemius and soleal sinusoids are impossible to detect. Previous thrombophlebitis leaves a residue of occluded and recanalized veins, dilated collaterals and incompetent valves that make recognition of superimposed acute venous thrombosis extremely difficult. Also, since the Doppler probe accurately detects only the presence or absence of venous "flow" and only roughly assesses its quantity, a long propagated clot originating in a venous valvular sinus could escape detection. Unlike calf vein thrombi, these clots are particularly dangerous, and failure to recognize their existence is one of the most serious weaknesses of the Doppler venous examination. However, reports of such a diagnostic error have not been presented, and abnormalities in venous flow pattern produced by nonadherent thrombi usually allow their detection. Finally, it should be realized that sound transmission through excessive fat, hematoma and scar tissue is poor and may create false impressions.

PLETHYSMOGRAPHIC DETECTION OF DVT. Major changes in venous volume can be produced by intermittently damming up and releasing venous outflow. The basis for this approach is that these changes can be indirectly measured by plethysmographic techniques and are significantly reduced by deep venous thrombosis (Fig. 17–10). Stated simply, an obstructing deep venous thrombus will dam up venous outflow so much that an additional superimposed obstruction will produce a *relatively* lesser increase and, when subsequently released, a relatively slower rate of decrease in venous volume than is normally observed. The plethysmographic methods that can be employed to measure these changes in venous volume indirectly are the monitoring of (1) changes in calf circumference with a strain gauge,[6] (2) changes in segmental calf volume by an emcompassing air-displacement cuff,[73] and (3) changes in electrical impedance.[60] Although these methods vary in technical detail, they all employ the same principle and appear to be relatively comparable in accuracy. Because it is currently the most popular technique, impedance plethysmography (IPG) will be described in greater detail here.

The impedance of a segment of an extremity depends primarily on its blood volume. Although small changes in blood volume occur with each cardiac cycle, much greater changes in volume occur with each respiratory cycle, probably because the venous system holds more than 80 per cent of the blood volume. In this technique a weak high-frequency alternating current is passed by circumferential electrodes through a segment of calf, and the resulting changes in voltage are detected by additional monitoring

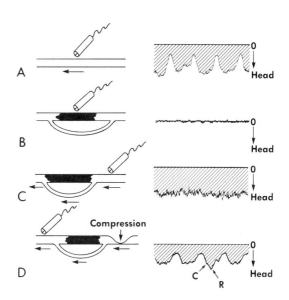

Figure 17–10 Changes in venous flow pattern produced by an obstructing thrombus. *A.* No obstruction, normal flow pattern. *B.* Probe over obstruction. *C.* Probe distal to obstruction. *D.* Lack of augmentation when vein is obstructed distal to the probe. (From: Sumner, D. S.: Evaluation of the venous circulation using the ultrasonic Doppler velocity detector. *In*: Rutherford, R. B. (ed.): Vascular Surgery. Philadelphia, W. B. Saunders Co., 1977, p. 182.)

electrodes, accurately reflecting changes in resistance, which in turn accurately reflect changes in venous volume.

Originally, the diagnosis of DVT by IPG was based only on the recognition of a dampening of the phasic volume shifts associated with respiration. Normally a change greater than 20 per cent should be seen. Comparison with the contralateral limb was often confirmatory. Subsequently, the practice of measuring the initial or maximum rate of venous outflow (VO) produced following obstruction of flow by deep inspiration was introduced.[60] The variability of patient effort during this maneuver limits its reproducibility and produces too wide a range of normal values. To overcome this, a 45-second inflation of a thigh cuff to 50 to 60 mm Hg is used.[89] The leg is slightly elevated (to eliminate variations in pooling) and externally rotated (to encourage muscle relaxation). The knee is lightly flexed to avoid the extrinsic popliteal vein compression associated with complete extension. The cuff is rapidly inflated and the increase in venous volume or capacitance (VC) after 45 seconds is measured. The cuff is then rapidly deflated and the slope of

the initial rapid venous outflow (VO) is monitored. The inclination of the initial downslope is a measure of maximum venous outflow but, rather than measure this slope, the decrease over the first one to three seconds is usually used. Although the major emphasis has been on VO or MVO, it has been shown by Hull and associates[42] that, because of some variability in the degree of venous pooling, it is advisable to plot the VO against VC, as shown in Figure 17–11. Using discriminant analysis they established the slope of a VC-VO line that separated abnormal from normal cases with 98 per cent accuracy. Impedance plethysmography had a specificity of 97 per cent and a sensitivity of 93 per cent for proximal deep venous thrombosis (that is, of the popliteal, femoral and iliac veins). However, its false negative diagnosis rate with venographically documented distal (calf) venous thrombosis was 83 per cent. Its sensitivity was 83 per cent in asymptomatic proximal vein thrombosis and 78 per cent in nonobstructing proximal vein thrombosis. There is an increasing rate of false negative diagnoses with the passage of time following the onset of thrombosis. False positive findings also occur in conges-

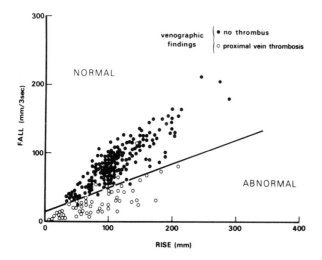

Figure 17–11 This graph shows how well plotting venous capacitance (rise) against venous outflow (fall) separates venographically documented cases of proximal DVT from normal cases. (From: Hull, R., Van Aken, W. G., Hirsh, J., et al.: Impedance plethysmography using the occlusive cuff technique in the diagnosis of venous thrombosis. Circulation, 53:696–700, 1976.)

tive heart failure, arterial insufficiency and previous phlebitis. Nevertheless, these studies demonstrate the degree of accuracy that can be achieved with IPG in experienced hands. Even under less rigorous conditions, its accuracy is probably equal to a careful venous Doppler examination (that is, in the range of 85 per cent), with both tests sharing the failing of inability to diagnose minor calf vein thrombosis. Combined, their accuracy probably approaches that of venography for deep vein thrombosis at or proximal to the popliteal vein, that is, those cases in which treatment with heparin and complete bedrest is necessary to prevent pulmonary embolism. Currently most clinicians are willing to embark on heparin therapy for DVT on the basis of these studies alone, saving phlebography for those cases in which there is a discrepancy between these tests and the clinical impression.

THERMOGRAPHY. The clinical use of thermography or infrared photography has had limited acceptance as a screening device for venous disorders. This is probably because of the high cost of the apparatus and the availability of other simpler methods that record information of more importance than temperature alone.

Invasive Approach

PHLEBOGRAPHY. Faced with a 30 to 50 per cent false positive-false negative diagnosis rate for the clinical diagnosis of DVT, many clinicians formerly resorted to phlebography before making any therapeutic decisions. This practice was also encouraged by the fact that the implications of a diagnosis of DVT are often serious and may dictate the need for extended anticoagulant therapy and strict adherence to a regimen of intermittent leg elevation and elastic support. Even a single, uncomplicated instance of phlebitis may greatly affect insurability and employment. However, phlebography is an uncomfortable, invasive study that cannot be performed at the bedside or in iodine-allergic patients, and, even in competent hands, it is associated with a small but definite rate of diagnostic error and morbidity. In some clinical settings, the expense and the unavailability of proper equipment or trained personnel may pose limitations. Therefore, while phlebography still must be considered the definitive method for diagnosing deep venous thrombosis, it is impractical for screening or serially monitoring patients. When indicated, two methods of phlebography study may be used: (1) ascending phlebography from the foot, in which the superficial and deep veins of the extremity are studied and (2) direct femoral vein puncture, in which venous pressure and the iliac portion of the venous system are investigated. Osseous phlebography, which has been used when venipuncture could not be performed, has essentially been abandoned.

VENOUS PRESSURE. Venous pressure, which was once used to evaluate varicose veins and chronic deep vein obstruction or insufficiency, is now usually taken only when phlebograms are being performed. In both iliac thrombophlebitis and lymphedema, comparison of pressures in the femoral veins may reveal the source of the disorder. Iliac thrombophlebitis is four times more common on the left than on the right because of external compression by the right iliac artery or the presence of an intraluminal web. A difference of 2 mm Hg between the two sides indicates iliac vein obstruction. Confirmation is made by exercise when there is an increase of 3 mm Hg or more in venous pressure.

RADIONUCLIDE PHLEBOGRAPHY. Radionuclide phlebography, usually performed with ^{125}I or other radionuclide-labeled albumin microspheres, avoids some of the problems of contrast phlebography and has the additional advantage of providing a concomitant lung scan, but it is associated with a significant rate of false positive diagnoses and does not eliminate the need for expensive equipment and specially trained personnel.

RADIOACTIVE FIBRINOGEN SCANNING. This is another radionuclide method for detecting DVT. It has proven to be extremely sensitive, even for small calf vein thromboses. In fact, it is not infrequently positive when a concomitant venogram detects no abnormality, in which instance it is impossible to determine if this is a false positive test or if a small early thrombus is present in a valve cusp not visualized by venography. This test is less accurate in detecting more proximal thrombi and is not reliable in detecting iliac vein thrombosis. Finally, although FDA restrictions on the use of homologous, as opposed to autologous, albumin have now been lifted, its widespread clinical application is still limited by the fact that it has to be injected prior to the development of deep venous thrombosis. Its main value is as a prospective clinical research tool, as in the evaluation of anticoagulants and of other methods of preventing DVT.

Treatment of Thrombophlebitis

When treating thrombophlebitis, it is important to do no harm. No single therapeutic agent or specific is known at present that will either prevent or cure all types of thrombophlebitis. A disease with such a varied pathogenesis and clinical course as thrombophlebitis can be expected to respond capriciously to therapy. It is essential that a working plan be followed that is based on the appreciation of both the pathophysiology and the natural course of the disease.

Objectives of Therapy

The objectives of therapy are:

(1) to eliminate all etiological factors (congenital or acquired coagulopathy);

(2) to eliminate all secondary contributions (infection, respiratory depressant, polycythemia, sludging, etc.);

(3) to improve venous outflow and retard swelling (elevation of lower limbs and elastic support);

(4) to decrease established phlebitis (anti-inflammatory agent);

(5) to prevent clot propagation and speed resolution (anticoagulation therapy — heparin);

(6) to prevent recurrence (anticoag-

ulation therapy – heparin, or pro-thrombin depressant therapy – Cou-madin);

(7) to avoid late sequelae – anti-coagulation therapy, progressive am-bulation, elevation and elastic support; and

(8) to support the patient's own re-sources for mitigating the disease and its complications.

Prophylaxis

Prevention begins with history-taking and identification of the factors that predispose to thrombophlebitis. The patient is asked about occupation-al and other environmental conditions, drugs utilized, allergies and tenden-cies to bruise or bleed easily; he should also be questioned about quick clotting and erythematous reactions in superficial veins adjoining the site of an injury. A history of previous throm-bophlebitis may be elicited by dis-cussing varicosities. The presence of polycythemia, arteriosclerosis or con-gestive heart failure will indicate a predilection to thrombophlebitis. A re-cent history of weight loss, abdominal pain or cough may suggest the possi-bility of cancer. The family history should be explored to uncover possi-ble hereditary clotting traits.

The physical examination is often contributory. Obesity, cardiac dys-rhythmias or impingement on the veins caused by pregnancy, garters, girdles or fractures should be noted. Multiple old scars and bruises, especi-ally of the ankles and legs, should lead to careful evaluation of the venous sys-tem. Deep venous incompetence, which is particularly significant in geriatric patients, may be identified by a few simple maneuvers. Probably the best determining factor of deep vein incompetence is a history of swelling in one extremity before noon every day.

To aid the physician in detecting pa-tients most susceptible to thrombo-phlebitis, a clotting profile should be obtained for those patients who have a history of venous thrombosis. Clotting profiles should also be obtained for pa-tients who are presently taking, or have recently used, medication that has a known incidence of thromboem-bolic complications and for patients who have specific disorders that may predispose to thrombophlebitis (see section on the clotting process). A sim-ple approach is the use of a clinical scoring table like that shown in Table 17–4, which is a modification of a table devised by Farmer and Smithwick.[22] Any patient whose total score reaches 6 during hospitalization is considered susceptible to thrombophlebitis.

Other criteria, such as the presence of ulcerative colitis, soft tissue trauma,

TABLE 17–4   Scoring System for Risk of Thromboembolism*

Factor	Points
Age 50 or more	3
Major abdominal or pelvic surgery	3
Presence of cancer	2
Serious postoperative complications	2
Prolonged operation (three hours or more)	2
Obesity	1
Varicose veins	1
Abdominal distension	1
Infection, particularly intra-abdominal or retroperitoneal	1
Prolonged immobilization (ten days or more)	1
Heart disease	1
Shock during or after operation – sys-tolic pressure below 80, with pallor and tachycardia for 30 minutes or more	1
Blood dyscrasia or anemia (Hb. 10 gm or less)	1
Previous thromboembolic disease	1
Dehydration	1

*A total score of 6 or more indicates suscepti-bility to thrombophlebitis.

thoracic injuries and fractures, may be added.

The reversal of some conditions that predispose to thrombophlebitis may be impossible at short notice in surgical patients. Nevertheless, useful prophylactic measures can be instituted at the time of hospital admission. When surgery is elective and one can temporize, the risk of thrombophlebitis may be lessened in several ways:

(1) Overweight individuals are placed on dietary control.

(2) Smoking is forbidden.

(3) Varicosities are treated when possible.

(4) Physiological imbalances are rectified as much as possible.

(5) Dermatological disorders such as eczema and epidermophytosis are treated.

(6) Chronic infections, such as those occurring in the bronchi or urinary tract, are noted. Antibiotics and anti-inflammatory agents are used as indicated.

(7) Knee-length elastic stockings should be used routinely both pre- and postoperatively.

(8) Constricting bandages and pressure points on the lower extremities are avoided.

(9) Common sense and proper surgical technique are the best precautions against postoperative complications. Proper positioning of the patient on the operating table is vital.

(10) "Risk" patients are optimal candidates for prophylactic low dose heparin as described in the following section.

Some of the programs instituted preoperatively may need to be continued during and immediately after surgery. Some surgeons recommend that all patients who were ambulatory before surgery receive dorsiflexion of both feet several times at the termination of the operative procedure to increase the flow within an already lethargic venous circulation. Active and passive use of leg muscles is beneficial immediately after operation unless contraindicated. Early ambulation must be individualized. Venous catheters should be inspected frequently and discontinued as soon as possible. Cutdowns should be confined to the upper extremity unless they are life-saving.

If immobilization is prolonged, passive and active exercises should be started early with the help of a trained physiotherapist. Stasis may be the precursor of sludging and clotting of the blood, but active exercise must be limited by the patient's endurance. (The clotting process and prophylactic anticoagulation are discussed in detail later in this chapter.)

Initial Management

The clinician following up any surgical or nonsurgical patient shortly after hospital discharge should recognize that thromboembolism may still be a hazardous complication. Such instances occur far more frequently when prophylactic measures were not emphasized constantly prior to and during hospitalization. Whether or not a patient has recently been discharged from the hospital, it is obviously essential for the surgeon to be aware of which cases of acute thrombophlebitis require admission and which can be treated on an outpatient basis.

Excluding those patients who require prophylactic heparin or Coumadin or antiplatelet therapy (see later section on prophylactic anticoagulation), the only patients who should be treated as outpatients are those who have acute thrombophlebitis of the superficial veins with no symptoms or signs of deep vein involvement. Usually a five-day regimen of a strong anti-inflammatory agent, such as phenylbutazone (Butazolidin), will relieve the patient's complaints and abort the inflammatory process. Any failure of response or recurrence of complaints in such patients should indicate the same hospital admission and full heparin therapy as in patients with deep vein thrombophlebitis.

Complications and Sequelae

The outcome of thrombophlebitis in any particular case is unpredictable, since the course of the disease does not always appear to be governed by the usual natural history. It is often controlled with little or no treatment, only to recur weeks, months or years later in the same vein or in another one. Sometimes it shows a stubborn progression, cannot be contained and leads to death or chronic incapacitation.

Complications begin when the thrombus extends by continuity; it then shrinks and becomes firmer or more adherent, and finally it may fill the entire lumen or float beyond its site of attachment and block other veins. A severe perivenous inflammation may occur, with constitutional symptoms present. Suppuration of the affected vein may ensue and remain localized or result in bacteremia and septic emboli. Even when infection does not occur, the thrombus may detach and become a pulmonary embolus and infarction, which sometimes is fatal. Restoration of vein function, recanalization with incompetent valves or contraction and permanent obliteration of the vein may develop.

The fate of the thrombus depends upon the degree of derangement of the vessel or the blood. If the involvement is minimal, the entire process can undergo rapid resolution. Significant inflammation or disease prolongs the abnormality. Disturbances in circulation or changes in coagulation aggravate the condition. Gangrene may occur from thrombosis of large venous trunks and collateral veins and from marked spasm of the distal arterial tree. The gangrene of thrombosis is like frostbite — it is rarely deep.

The main pathophysiological manifestation of acute thrombophlebitis is obstruction of venous blood flow. The degree of venous impairment varies according to the vessels involved, the extent of the process, the presence of aggravating factors and the availability of collateral circulation.

As mentioned before, any chest complaint, no matter how minor, from a recently discharged surgical patient should alert the examining physician to the possibility of a pulmonary embolus. This is especially true when the patient has or has had lower extremity pain, swelling, or both, postoperatively. The chest complaint or the lower extremity signs and symptoms, or both, provide the "golden" period for preventing a fatal pulmonary embolus, since studies have verified repeatedly that a primary embolus precedes the majority of fatal emboli by several days. Recognition is therefore essential.

Pulmonary Embolism

The diagnosis of pulmonary embolism can be very difficult to make. Most competent clinicians lean toward diagnosis and treatment of pulmonary emboli on suspicion alone because of the difficulties in establishing a firm diagnosis and because of the risk of death and disability when it goes undiagnosed.

Any major hospital should recognize the importance of immediate procedures to establish the diagnosis of a pulmonary embolus. Sudden death is admittedly uncommon in patients who die as the result of pulmonary embolism. However, these patients are often in precarious condition, and further delay in establishing diagnosis may result in a fatal outcome. Errors in diagnosis are reduced when an expert team is available to perform the necessary diagnostic procedures. Centralization of equipment, personnel and facilities is therefore essential. Pulmonary emboli may arbitrarily be divided into categories: massive, moderate and minor; or, massive pulmonary embolism, branch embolism and peripheral embolism. Variables relating to pre-existing pulmonary or cardiac disease, acute right heart failure, tachypnea and cyanosis are the hallmarks of massive or critical embolus.

A plain chest film, electrocardiogram and blood gas measurements (especially for PaO_2) are initially taken to differentiate embolism from other diseases such as pneumothorax, aneurysm of the aorta and acute cardiac conditions. Decreased vascular markings lead to the suspicion of an embolism or pulmonary infarction. A normal film does not exclude a pulmonary embolus. Angiography is essential if embolism is suspected.

Radioactive lung-scanning should precede angiography, since a normal scan excludes a massive or branch embolus. Lung-scanning is currently performed with ^{131}I-labeled albumin administered intravenously or after inhalation of radioactive xenon.

Chronic Venous Insufficiency

This condition is usually the result of damage caused by thrombophlebitis and is thus called the "postphlebitic syndrome." The management and treatment of chronic deep venous insufficiency is aimed primarily at preventing disfigurement from chronic leg edema, pigmentation and ulceration, eliminating pain resulting from the complications of venous congestion, and halting the recurrence of venous thrombosis. Until the aggressive use of anticoagulant (heparin) and specific anti-inflammatory therapy for thrombophlebitis became widely accepted, few patients escaped these sequelae. Therefore, the occurrence and severity of these sequelae are minimized and are far less common when treatment for thrombophlebitis is prompt and adequate.

ETIOLOGY. The term "postphlebitic" implies that there is a previous history of deep venous occlusion, yet approximately 20 per cent of patients have no prior history of thrombophlebitis. Some may have had cardiac disease, extremity injury, a previous operation, or may have been pregnant —the common conditions in which venous thrombosis may have developed silently. Further, the development and severity of the syndrome depend on the extent to which the deep venous valves are destroyed by the thrombosis, the amount of inflammation of the vein wall and the surrounding tissues, and the adequacy of treatment of the acute episode of thrombophlebitis. The thrombosis may occlude the venous tube totally or partially. Collateral veins compensate for the localized occlusion, even without heparin or anti-inflammatory therapy. However, when the venous thombosis is extensive and involves more than the calf veins, the femoral veins or the iliac veins, the extent to which the deep vein valves are demolished becomes the critical factor. When this occurs, neither recanalization nor collateral venous channels will be capable of handling the load of venous return efficiently.

The delicate valves that are found throughout the venous system in the extremities are apparently an evolutionary adaptation to the erect posture. They break up a column of blood from ankle to atrium that, if unopposed, would exert a potential gravitational force of 110 to 120 mm Hg. Thus, if one were to stand completely relaxed and motionless for several minutes, venous pressures in this range would develop in the ankles. However, even modest motion, such as shifting one's weight, will contract the calf muscles around these valved venous segments and force the blood upward. Regular, rhythmic motion such as walking will "pump" the venous blood upward and reduce the ankle venous pressure to the 0 to 30 mm Hg range. Without a competent venomuscular pumping mechanism, we would all have swollen legs and petechial hemorrhages by day's end. In fact, in patients with paralytic afflictions, severe arthritis or fusion of the ankles, these problems can exist even in the absence of deep venous thrombophlebitis.

As previously stated, the edema that immediately follows deep venous thrombosis is purely obstructive in origin and quickly subsides as collateral veins develop and the patient is kept in bed with legs elevated. Typically, the patient receiving anticoagulants is discharged after 10 days and given a regimen of external elastic support (either Ace bandages or elastic stockings) and progressive ambulation, short of edema. At 6 to 12 weeks, when anticoagulant therapy normally is discontinued, the patient and his physician may not see the necessity of continued elastic support, since the legs appear normal or nearly so. However, although the deep venous system eventually becomes recanalized, the delicate valves remain imprisoned in organized thrombus, the result being a patent but valveless deep venous system that now transmits the gravitational pressure of the blood unimpeded from the heart to the ankles. The deep venous valvular incompetence alone is not enough to produce serious stasis sequelae.

The final common pathway that leads to stasis dermatitis and ulceration is a transmission of the high pressures that normally occur in the deep venous system in the ambulatory state to the superficial tissues through incompetent perforator or communicating veins. It is the anatomy of these perforating veins, shown in Figure 17–12, that determines localization of these stasis changes and ulcers in the previously mentioned "gaiter" area (Figure 17–3) — that is, the lower half of the leg, extending upward from the malleoli. These perforator veins may be involved by the initial thrombosis and may therefore also become incompetent, or they may simply dilate because of back pressure from the valveless deep venous system until their valves, too, become incompetent.

Although the aftermath of thrombophlebitis is the cause of 90 to 95 per cent of all cases of chronic venous insufficiency, two other rarer causes may be seen. One is a congenital or hereditary incompetence of one or more of the perforator or deep veins, similar to the inherited saphenofemoral incompetence that causes varicose veins. A second and more common cause is long-standing primary saphenous vari-

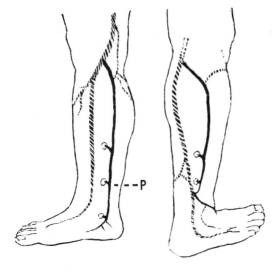

Figure 17–12 The usual location of the medial and lateral perforator veins and their relationship to the greater and lesser saphenous, respectively. (From: Rutherford, R. B.: The nonoperative management of chronic venous insufficiency. *In*: Rutherford, R. B. (ed.): Vascular Surgery. Philadelphia, W. B. Saunders Co., 1977, p. 1238.)

TABLE 17–5 Venous Pressure Changes With Exercise (Erect Posture)

Condition	Resting Pressure	Pressure After Exercise	Time to Return to Normal
Normal veins	90 mm Hg	0–30 mm Hg	31 seconds
Primary varicose veins	90 mm Hg	45–60 mm Hg	3 seconds
Postphlebitic syndrome	90 mm Hg	75–90 mm Hg	Immediately

cose veins in which, although the original defect is only saphenofemoral incompetence, the continued recircuiting of venous blood in the upright position down the saphenous system and back through the perforator veins eventually dilates the latter until their valves become incompetent. Here also the deep veins may be incompetent on a congenital or hereditary basis. It is only in this rare circumstance that stasis ulcers can be truly called "varicose ulcers." This lesion will be discussed in detail later in the section on leg ulcers.

As seen in Table 17–5, the patient with postphlebitic syndrome, unlike the normal person, will produce little if any venous pressure drop during exercise. In fact, the pressure will occasionally increase. Those who decrease their venous pressure during exercise will rarely sustain this drop, whereas the normal person will quickly decrease this pressure with exercise, and it will take several minutes for the pressure to build up again after the exercise has been discontinued. Patients with primary varicose veins fall in an intermediate position in such tests.

Thus, the final common pathway in chronic venous insufficiency is the transmission of deep venous hypertension into the superficial veins and the superficial tissues. When this occurs, sometimes weeks or months after the initial episode of thrombophlebitis, edema recurs when the patient is upright for any significant period of time. Plasma fluid constituents are forced into the interstitial spaces, and

extravasation of plasma proteins and red cells also occurs. This causes a low-grade inflammatory reaction, and a bluish-brown pigmentation develops as the red cells disintegrate. The end result of prolonged periods of this type of damage is stasis dermatitis, with brawny edema, subcutaneous fibrosis, pigmentation and cutaneous atrophy (Figure 17–13).

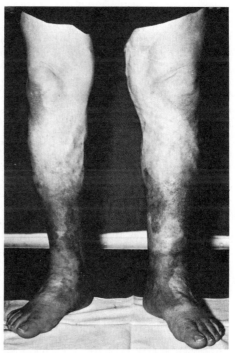

Figure 17–13 Brawny edema, subcutaneous fibrosis, pigmentation and superficial veins secondary to chronic deep thrombophlebitis. Ligation and excision of varicose veins is contraindicated initially. Treatment consists of the standard therapy for the postphlebitic syndrome, as described in the text.

In the natural history of untreated thrombophlebitis, the frequency of stasis dermatitis and ulceration increases with time. After ten years, three-fourths of these patients will have advanced stasis changes, and half will have had stasis ulcers.[9] Ulcers generally occur within seven years on the average, but may occur as late as several decades after the initial episode of thrombophlebitis. Seldom does an ulcer appear earlier than two years after the acute episode.[66] Unfortunately, stasis changes are subtle and gradual at first, and the patient comes to accept a degree of swelling, discoloration and aching in the involved leg. It is often not until some minor trauma leads to a skin break that develops into an actual postphlebitic ulcer that he again returns to the physician.

Others, particularly orthopedic patients, may develop a silent deep venous thrombosis, and when the leg swells after the cast is removed, they are often told that such swelling is due to poor muscle tone and will disappear in time. However, it appears that over 50 per cent of patients with major fractures of the lower extremity develop deep venous thrombosis.

DIAGNOSIS. Diagnosis of the postphlebitic syndrome is based on a history of deep vein thrombophlebitis followed by edema and any combination of skin pigmentation, dermatitis, subcutaneous fibrosis, chronic ulceration, varicose veins, recurrent infection or disabling subjective complaints such as heaviness, fatigue or pain. When there is no history of thrombophlebitis and no other cause such as cardiac disease, primary lymphatic obstruction, collagen disease, recurrent trauma, simple varicose veins or paralysis can be elicited, this syndrome is considered as nonthrombotic.

Females outnumber male patients possibly because of their higher incidence of obesity, menstrual cycles producing intermittent water retention, use of oral contraceptive drugs or infrequent participation in exercise programs.

Of the 10 per cent of patients who require hospital admission, the most common reasons are: recurrent thrombophlebitis, cardiac failure, extensive cellulitis of the limb, large resistant ulcers, varicose veins requiring excision and ligation and ulcers necessitating excision and grafting or subfacial ligation of venous perforators, or both.

The diagnosis requires the presence of unilateral or bilateral lower extremity edema. Swelling almost invariably appears in the morning hours but is seldom the major complaint. Trauma often is a contributory cause of the

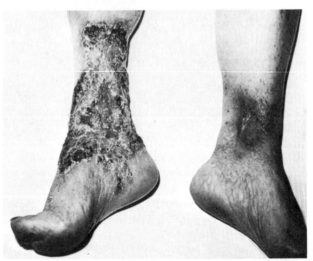

Figure 17–14 Squamous carcinoma arising in chronic postphlebitic ulcer. Ulceration present for many years at the ankle; finally underwent malignant degeneration.

ulcer and may be the major reason for reappearance of the syndrome. Rarely do the leg ulcers develop into malignant lesions unless they have remained unhealed for 15 years or more (Fig. 17–14). Achilles tendon fibrosis may occur when a nearby ulcer has been untreated for a significant period. Varicose veins are a very common factor and may precede the syndrome or develop after its onset.[66]

Other disorders are present in the majority of patients and may cause the reappearance of the syndrome or limit the therapeutic response. The disorders most often present are obesity; cardiovascular conditions including cardiac failure, cor pulmonale, hypertensive cardiovascular disease and arteriosclerosis obliterans; psychiatric conditions; metastatic cancer; and recurrent thrombophlebitis attributed to a hypercoagulable state. Multiple disorders are not uncommon. Additional conditions or situations that may cause or contribute to the postphlebitic syndrome are: oral contraceptive drugs, sclerosing therapy for varicose veins, surgery of varicose veins while the extremity is not free of morning edema, "hardware" present from open reduction of a fracture, and interruption of the inferior vena cava during an episode of deep vein thrombophlebitis, in which ineffective therapy has been given in the postoperative period.

Venography may be necessary to establish a diagnosis. The iliac veins and inferior vena cava should be studied with bilateral pressure readings. Since there is a higher incidence of left lower extremity involvement, the initiating or contributory factor may be from iliac vein pathology. The possibility that a major vein was injured during pelvic or groin surgery such as inguinal hernia repair should also be considered, especially when prominent superficial veins are noted in the groin area. Coagulation studies are essential for all patients having recurrent episodes of thrombophlebitis. Use of a Doppler flowmeter, impedance plethysmography, venous pressure tests or labeled isotopes may be beneficial in screening certain patients.

TREATMENT. Treatment is planned principally on an outpatient basis, following a complete general medical examination that includes a total evaluation of the extremity involved and of the patient's overall problem. The clinician first initiates a conservative treatment program consisting of (1) patient cooperation, (2) treatment of allied disorders, (3) control of infection and (4) compression and exercise of the extremity.

Patient cooperation is strongly emphasized, for thorough education is necessary in the physiopathology of the condition, both for immediate care and for continuing prophylaxis. Mimeographed instruction sheets are issued and the patient is repeatedly "quizzed" on this material. Cooperation implies both compliance with instructions for limb care and willingness to assist in caring for allied disorders.

Allied disorders are so frequently present that "total" treatment is essential. Patients with cardiac failure may require digitalization, diuretics and salt-poor diets. Obesity necessitates weight reduction. Thrombophlebitis, when still clinically active or recurrent, requires admission to the hospital and treatment with heparin until the patient is asymptomatic. However, superficial thrombophlebitis can be managed with an anti-inflammatory agent such as Butazolidin (phenylbutazone) prescribed orally for three to five days (100 mg, t.i.d., p.c.). Successful treatment of the allied disorder is a prerequisite to optimal primary treatment of the postphlebitic syndrome.

Infections, whether dermatitis, epidermophytosis or infected ulcers, are treated with the knowledge that the majority are superinfected with fungi (Fig. 17–15). Therefore, treatment is begun by means of warm soaks for the leg, including the foot, of potassium permanganate, 300 mg in two quarts of

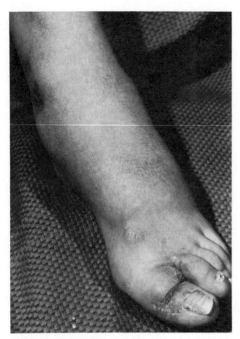

Figure 17–15 Lymphedema, cellulitis and fungal infection of the foot superimposed on chronic thrombophlebitis. Treatment is given as in the postphlebitic syndrome, and in addition potassium permanganate immersion is prescribed for 30 minutes, three times per day for three days. The potassium permanganate solution is 1:1000 (120 mg in 1 quart of water.) Systemic antibiotics are also administered.

water, three times daily for 30-minute periods for three days. This controls the fungus and tends to dry the ulcer and also tests the patient's interest in his treatment, for the toenails will become black when instructions are properly followed. If there is significant cellulitis surrounding the ulcer, a broad-spectrum antibiotic (e.g., ampicillin or erythromycin) is administered, or an antibiotic is applied topically in a water-soluble base (e.g., polyethylene glycol) to the ulcer twice a day. When parenteral antibiotics are necessary for a widespread cellulitis, admission to the hospital may be advisable. However, antibiotic therapy is seldom necessary when fungicidal therapy, periodic elevation, diuretics and anti-inflammatory drugs are used. Enzymatic debriding preparations

have been found to be relatively ineffective and unnecessarily expensive.

After this initial "cleaning up" period, an Unna's paste boot (Fig. 17–16) is used for periods of one to three weeks until the ulcer is completely healed. Unna's boot has been used for leg ulcers since the nineteenth century. It consists essentially of a gauze dressing impregnated with gelatin, zinc oxide and Caladryl. An Ace bandage is applied over this moist cast-like dressing from the base of the toes to just below the knee. This combination provides, in essence, a medicated support dressing that the patient cannot readily remove. No other medication, gauze or other material should ever be applied to the ulcer beneath the boot. The paste impregnated in the gauze of the boot must be in direct contact with the bed of the ulcer. If the ulcer is too deep, an attempt should be made first to stimulate granulation and to fill in the defect before a series of Unna's boot applications are begun. Often, these ulcers will be much shallower after the surrounding edema and inflammation are reduced by elevation, diuretics and an anti-inflammatory agent. Initially, the Unna's paste boot is reapplied on a weekly basis if drainage or odor dictates. Otherwise the boot is changed every three weeks. Often it is reapplied one or two times after the ulcer heals to allow the new skin to mature.

Edema usually clears by elevation overnight, but some patients require a longer period of continuous elevation to reach the edema-free state. A daily diuretic is prescribed for most patients. Active and passive exercise are recommended during elevation, especially when edema is slow in subsiding. Progressive ambulation is begun, using elastic compression support, only after the edema has disappeared or lessened significantly on arising or when the patient is wearing an Unna's paste boot.

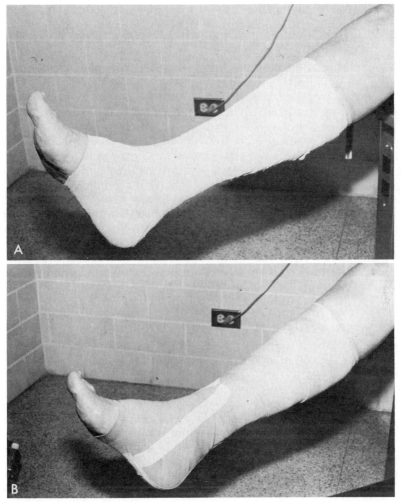

Figure 17–16 Application of Unna's paste boot to leg with postphlebitic ulcer. *A.* Medicated paste (gelatin, zinc oxide and Caladryl) impregnated gauze roll shown after being wrapped on leg from toes to upper third of leg. *B.* Cloth-rubber (Ace) bandage applied over boot with tape at ankle to maintain its position. Dry gauze roll may be used to separate paste boot from Ace bandage. No daily care necessary from one to three weeks. Patient required prior treatment for fungus infection, inflammation and edema of leg.

Three types of *elastic compression* may be used for support. If the leg is markedly swollen and edema returns on dependency in less than one hour, or if previous therapy with cloth-rubber bandage support has failed, pure rubber (Esmarch) bandages are advised. A cotton stocking may be worn beneath this bandage to avoid skin reaction to the rubber. Most cases, however, require only elastic stockings or cloth-rubber compression bandages from the beginning. Elastic stockings are substituted for the cloth-rubber or pure rubber bandages as soon as practical, especially following an increase to two or more hours of edema-free ambulation. The stockings should be tailored or well-fitted for the patient's edema problem. Unlike pneumatic compression, elastic stockings do not force fluid from the limb; they only delay the progress of the edema. This delay time is directly related to the quality of the compression or elasticity provided by the stocking. Therefore, thin or sheer "elastic" stockings are not recommended. No patient is instructed to wear an elastic support above the knee. Objections to the use of full-length elastic hose or tights are: (1) they produce a garter effect at the knee or groin, or both, during flexion, (2) thigh edema cannot be optimally controlled by compression, (3) they are costly to replace every four months or less, and (4) patients do not regularly use them, since they are difficult and time-consuming to apply. Seldom does thigh edema remain after recognized therapy. Therefore, swelling below the knee becomes the most significant problem. Occasionally, Unna's boots are utilized permanently with changes made monthly for patients who develop recurrent ulcers in spite of adequate preventive measures. Patients who may need this approach are: (1) those who are aged and prone to sitting most of the day, (2) those whose employment requires prolonged periods of standing or sitting, (3) those who are uncooperative even after a thorough educational program and (4) those who are unable to utilize the "venous heart" leg muscles of the involved limb because of a fixed ankle or knee joint.

The time permitted for standing, sitting or active ambulation is limited to 30 minutes prior to the appearance of fullness, heaviness, fatigue or edema in the extremity. The patient then returns to extremity elevation above the heart level for at least a 15-minute period. Each week the period of ambulation is increased short of the identified appearance of the fullness or edema, after a trial period demonstrates a lengthening of the previous symptom index. The patient should be informed that these time periods may fluctuate with the type of activity. Improvement should be seen each week. Otherwise the patient's habits and daily activities are reviewed and discussed to find the rea-

son for failure. When a two-hour edema-free period has been reached (frequently within two weeks), the patient is permitted to return to work, provided he elevates the extremity above the heart level for 15 minutes every two hours. This period is extended to four hours if no edema appears, then to six, and finally is left to the patient's discretion. During waking hours the patient faithfully wears an elastic stocking until the limb is edema-free. Elastic compression is usually necessary thereafter only when the lower extremities will be dependent with little or no movement for a prolonged period.

The patient is repeatedly instructed not to ambulate when fullness or swelling is present or without his elastic support. Each case must be individualized throughout the treatment. Foot care is emphasized and prophylactic medications are ordered: talcum and antifungal powder for the "sweating" foot or leg utilizing an elastic stocking, and lanolin or an ointment with a water-soluble base for the dry, scaly, scarred or indurated limb. Corns, calluses and thickened toenails are included in the therapy as well as repeatedly stressing the importance of foot hygiene by quoting the adage: "Never wash your face without washing your feet."

Operable conditions should be corrected early in the program to bring about a successful outcome. Grafting may be recommended for the indolent ulcer that necessitates immediate healing for economic, environmental or other practical reasons. However, these reasons seldom create a problem, since most ulcers heal within six weeks to three months when Unna's boots are utilized, provided the invading fungus infection is cleared and the edema is controlled. Wide excision and grafting of an ulcer is advised only when healing is unduly delayed or when the ulcer has been present for several years and there is a possibility that malignant changes have occurred within the lesion. An ulcer that has undergone malignant degeneration is not only extremely rare but also is probably the only occasion where an amputation is indicated.

A *large brawny ulcer* that fails to respond to nonoperative management may be considered for a subfascial vein ligation, radical excision of the ulcer and skin grafting. When one is tempted to perform a modified Kondoleon or Linton procedure on these patients it should first be recognized that such a radical approach is not a definitive operation. Furthermore, the patient must still follow a rigid postphlebitic syndrome program. Invariably, when this policy is not enforced the patient's previous problems recur within a few years.

We have rarely found it necessary to excise and graft postphlebitic ulcers. This position has been influenced by our own past experience and that of others who had a high incidence of surgical failures or recurrent ulcers after previous "successful" excision and grafting. The morbidity and cost to these patients becomes prohibitive. Several of our referred patients have experienced as many as 10 unsuccessful attempts to excise and graft their leg ulcers, and one such patient had 16 procedures! Adherence to the nonoperative regime described here resulted in healing of their ulcers within a few months. The later patient's ulcer site has remained healed for 15 years.

An *equinus* (equinovarus) *deformity* resulting from the shortening of the Achilles tendon is a complication that should be avoided by preventive measures. Its presence is noted in women with a large ulcer partially overlying the tendon who walk with the heel off the ground or who wear high-heeled shoes for relief of pain. Immediate grafting and a later tenoplasty may be required for those patients who do not demonstrate improvement during an ambulatory nonoperative program. Patients are advised to sleep with a posterior ankle splint on the involved limb.

Any patient with a cold, sweating, cyanotic or pale foot who complains of intolerable pain with hyperesthesia about the leg ulcer should be identified as having *causalgic-type pain*. The methods of establishing diagnosis and treatment for this type of pain are described later in this chapter. Rarely is a sympathectomy indicated since pharmacological sympathetic denervation is almost always successful. These patients universally resist the application of any type of topical medications, especially an Unna's paste boot. Therefore, relief is an essential factor in their therapy. The deep discomfort about the ulcer site is *somatic pain*, which is controlled by means of an antiinflammatory agent with or without a mild sedative.

Surgery for *varicose veins* should not be considered lightly in patients with a postphlebitic syndrome. The procedure is contraindicated in any patient until the morning and afternoon edema of the leg has been controlled. This requires three to six months of conservative therapy. When indicated, the major benefits derived by the patient are both prophylactic and therapeutic. Prophylactically, the operation greatly reduces the possibility of recurrent superficial thrombophlebitis and eliminates the painful chronically inflamed subcutaneous veins. These veins are a potential hazard and their removal is often very rewarding. Therapeutically, the afternoon swelling that may have been present before surgery usually disappears. To achieve this improvement it is essential for the patient to walk a few minutes out of every waking hour for several days following operation, with elastic support to the knee, and to follow the postphlebitic syndrome routine rigidly. If no swelling appears during the day after several months of this regimen, the patient may ambulate without support. However, he is warned that extremity trauma or infection or prolonged sitting or standing may cause the syndrome to recur, necessitating reinstitution of the elevation-exercise regimen, including the daily use of an elastic support. Such trauma includes sclerosing therapy by injection to residual veins.

The *nonoperative management* of chronic venous insufficiency takes much time and patience on the part of the physician. The reward is that it obviates the expense of inpatient care, and the two-hour edema-free rule for return to work decreases the number of employee hours lost to industry. Fitting the therapy into the patient's daily routine is essential. The type of elastic compression is carefully chosen and its function thoroughly explained. Additional emphasis is placed on the utilization of the American custom of coffee breaks and the lunch hour. These allow the patient to have two-hour intervals between the beginning of the work day, coffee break, lunch hour, coffee break and the end of the day; each can be interspersed with 15-minute periods of elevation of the extremity above the heart level.

Insistence that the extremity be edema-free prior to beginning ambulation is a sound and established principle, for it allows collateral veins to develop without hindrance. Most major veins recanalize and all establish collaterals. Until the changes occur there will be a delay in the initial phase of the recovery period. Much of this delay may be due to the additional harm created by the recanalization when collaterals have not been protected during and after development. Compression of these vessels beneath the integument by the surrounding edematous tissue can only cause harm in this process.

There is general agreement regarding the initial treatment of acute thrombophlebitis and its early complications; it must be aggressive and thorough. The postphlebitic syndrome should likewise be treated with the same broad viewpoint.

The physician's motivation to attempt nonoperative management of chronic venous insufficiency, even though it is a time-consuming process,

is provided by confidence in the ultimate success of this regimen and the knowledge that every "convert" is one less patient who will require periodic applications of Unna's boots. A trained nurse or other assistant can be invaluable in this task. In some clinics, particularly those in Europe, the physician sees the patient only twice, barring complications: first at the time of the initial evaluation and later for an educational session after the ulcer is healed. The routine management in the interim is carried out by properly trained and supervised nurses or physician's assistants.

The program described herein gives 85 per cent excellent to good results.[66] It follows to a degree what Luke identified in 1949 as the "new way of life" concept, but the restrictions should not necessitate any radical change in the patient's activity for the future.[53] Admittedly, an occasional case will be more complicated than average, and such a patient should not be assigned to a trained nurse or physician's assistant. Fortunately there are very few patients who find it necessary to change their occupations, restrict their daily activities, or receive ambulatory anticoagulant (subcutaneous heparin) therapy. Unsatisfactory results that occur are due to the failure or inability of the patient to adhere to an established program. These include patients with incurable diseases (such as malignancies), pulmonary or cardiac failure, cirrhosis, ankylosed lower extremity joints, mental diseases, hypercoagulable states and obesity that is resistant to treatment.

INSTRUCTIONS FOR PATIENTS WITH POSTPHLEBITIC SYNDROME. Education of patients is an important part of the treatment for postphlebitic syndrome. The following instructions can be given to each patient:

Your condition is known as the postphlebitic syndrome. It is important that you thoroughly understand this plan of treatment. The condition that you have may lead to complications which will be severely incapacitating, but *with your cooperation* we may control your present disability and gradually restore you to comfort and useful activity.

WHAT IS THE POSTPHLEBITIC SYNDROME?

The postphlebitic syndrome refers to the condition that frequently follows inflammation of the deep veins of the lower extremity. It may range in severity from mild painless swelling of the feet and legs to tremendous enlargement of the entire extremity, accompanied by varicose veins, deep leg ulcers and even *dangerous* infection. Either one or both legs may be involved.

The process begins with inflammation and clotting of the blood in the veins of the feet and legs. At this stage, there is tenderness in the calf muscles, usually accompanied by swelling of the legs and fever; this is called "phlebitis." Most cases of phlebitis subside without further trouble. However, two things may occur during the phlebitis which lead to the postphlebitic syndrome:

First, the tubes or vessels that carry blood from the legs back to the heart (called veins) become plugged. This blocks the drainage of blood from the legs, and the resulting back pressure may cause swelling.

Second, another network of smaller vessels that accompany the veins carries tissue juices from the legs back to the heart; these are called lymphatic vessels. They, too, may become inflamed and obstructed, particularly if there is any infection in the foot or leg. This blocks the lymph (tissue juice) drainage from the legs and will also cause swelling of the legs and feet, which your doctor calls *edema*.

Both the veins and the lymphatic vessels contain one-way valves, which assist in the return of fluid to the heart with movement of the muscles. These valves act the same as the handle of a water-pump, which removes water from a well. When these valves are damaged, the fluid may move in both directions when the vessels are compressed by the muscles. This, plus plugging of these damaged vessels, results in increased back pressure and a more sluggish circulation. Therefore, any smaller vessels that are able to take over by detouring around the obstruction are also blocked by the swelling.

Now a vicious circle has developed, in which swelling of the legs and obstruction of the damaged vessels with the loss of the valves aggravate one another.

This last point is extremely important, for the plan of treatment aims to break up the vicious circle by removing a key link in the cycle, namely, by *keeping the swelling out of your legs*. In addition, infection that is present should be cleared by your doctor, and good foot care should be instituted to prevent any future occurrence or recurrence of infection.

No matter how advanced your postphlebitic syndrome may be, proper treatment will result in marked and encouraging improvement, but your full cooperation is absolutely essential. From the beginning, your attention should be directed toward keeping the swelling out of your legs. This will prevent further damage to the remaining drainage vessels and allow new ones to develop and take over the work of those that have been damaged. Special problems, such as varicose veins and leg ulcers, will be handled at the proper time — AFTER THE LEG SWELLING IS UNDER CONTROL.

PLAN OF TREATMENT

Two methods are used to remove and prevent a recurrence of swelling in your legs:

(1) Elevation of the legs on at least two pillows;

(2) Elastic stockings, applied whenever you are erect, and occasionally necessary in some patients when the legs are elevated.

Elevation removes the fluid from the legs by means of gravity. When the legs hang down, gravity works against the drainage vessels, and swelling prevails.

The elastic stocking gives the drainage vessels support and delays the time at which additional leg swelling will appear. Seldom is an elastic stocking necessary above the knee, since it is more difficult to put on and to keep in place, does not compress the thigh as well as the leg and may produce a garter effect at the knee and intermittently prevent drainage from the leg.

Powder the legs before applying the stocking, especially during the summer. In most cases, the stocking may be left off the extremity while it is elevated in bed — but be sure to put the stocking back on before arising in the morning.

The Postphlebitic Routine

(1) The first step in your treatment is to get *all* of the swelling out of your legs by means of elevation. This may be accomplished during one night's rest. However, in a few cases it may take days. Your doctor may prescribe "water pills" to assist the removal of the excess fluid in your legs.

(2) Once you have removed *all* of the swelling, you are ready to start a gradual increase in walking. Remember that you regulate your walking so that you *never allow swelling to return in your legs*. Observe that a full feeling beneath the stockings warns you that swelling has just begun to appear. Stop walking and do not allow your legs to be down when this fullness appears. They need to be elevated above the level of your body immediately. This fullness may develop in 15 minutes, 2 hours or even more or less. Don't be discouraged, for improvement will soon begin.

When the time this fullness appears has been noted, your next period of walking will be just short of this time. For example, if the fullness appears in 90 minutes, elevate your legs for 15 minutes at ninety minutes after arising, then walk or have them dependent for only 60 minutes (30 minutes less than the fullness period) and elevate them again above the level of your body. This time routine is continued for the remainder of the day. The same routine is continued for a few days and then the dependency period increased to the previous time of fullness. If no fullness occurs, then walk or have the legs dependent until fullness does occur. When it does reappear then repeat the routine of elevation, starting again 30 minutes prior to the new noted time of fullness. Now you are walking more than before. In this manner, you will increase the time you are up, in accordance with your findings. Some people will quickly increase their walking and in a few weeks return to full activity, without swelling in their legs; others will have to go very slowly, being up for only short intervals each day for a week or more, until new drainage vessels develop that will allow longer walking periods without swelling of the legs.

During the period of increasing activity, there are three rules to follow:

(1) Always reapply your elastic stockings *before lowering your legs from bed in the morning or during the day.*

(2) When you are up, *walk*, for walking helps pump fluid from the leg by muscular milking action on the vessels. When you are not actually walking, elevate your legs, either in bed or on a chair. Be an executive; put your feet on the desk!

(3) (a) Do not *sit* with your legs hanging down.

(b) Do not *stand* in one position when you could be sitting with your legs elevated.

If it is imperative that you return to work, you may do so if the swelling does not occur for at least two hours after standing. However, frequent rest periods should be taken at work, and if possible the legs should be elevated on a chair so that progress will continue. When you are able to be on your feet the entire morning without swelling, the time is approaching when you will be free of swelling the entire day with elastic stockings.

Three things retard this program:

(1) Failure to cooperate — routine has not been followed.

(2) Obesity — reduction in weight will be ordered by your doctor, and will be most helpful.

(3) Infection — failure to remove this hinders your efforts in the program. In addition, poor foot care delays the possibility of a successful outcome.

Keep your feet as clean as your face!

Even though you have returned to normal activity and no swelling appears in your legs with or without elastic stockings during the entire day, there is always the possibility that at some future date you may have a return of this swelling, and it will be necessary for you to repeat the routine. If you discontinue the use of elastic stockings when you are free of swelling it is suggested that you wear them when you are required to sit or stand for long periods.

Conclusion

You must remember that no matter how slow your progress may seem to you now, the *quickest* way for you to return to useful and normal activity is to follow this postphlebitic routine religiously. So when you feel your legs getting heavy and tight under the elastic stocking – take warning, and *elevate your legs.*

Remember – KEEP THE SWELLING OUT OF YOUR LEGS!!![66]

Varicose Veins

Abnormally enlarged veins are termed varices or varicose veins. Varicosities usually occur in the lower extremities. They are important clinically because they predispose to venous thrombosis and venous insufficiency. Generally they are dilated, elongated and tortuous. However, a significant number of patients have a long saphenous vein that is straight, thick-walled and apparently normal in appearance but that shows free reflux of blood into tributaries that are obviously varicose. Despite their normal appearance, these veins show a saphenofemoral valvular incompetence with a positive tourniquet test. A normal variant that may be misleading is *venous ectasia*. This condition usually occurs in men whose leg veins are prominent but neither tortuous nor thick-walled. These patients usually have similarly enlarged veins in their upper extremities. The valves in these veins are competent and give a negative tourniquet test, and the condition is asymptomatic.

Varicose veins may be classified as *primary* when they are the result of congenital or acquired incompetence of valves or weakness of the wall of the veins. *Secondary* varicose veins are the superficial collateral tributaries that develop following venous occlusion from thrombosis or arteriovenous fistula. The differentiation can be very difficult unless an adequate history is obtained and the state of the patient's venous return is carefully evaluated.

Etiology

Varicosities are caused by the presence of one or more of the following: increased intraluminal pressure, destruction or absence of the venous valves, deterioration of the vein wall or a lack of support of the veins by the surrounding tissues. Once varices occur they usually become self-perpetuating, with increasing dilation and incompetence. The examining physician frequently finds it difficult to determine whether the varicosities are congenital, familial or acquired. Congenital or familial origin is generally considered a factor in at least 65 per cent of the cases. Acquired varicosities are caused by repeated trauma to the lower extremities, by pregnancy, by thrombosis in the deep veins, by occupations requiring long periods of standing, by obesity, by undergarments that constrict the thighs and by chronic infections requiring prolonged rest. Each of these factors should be carefully scrutinized in taking the history, for the cause of the disorder often has a bearing on the type of treatment.

Congenital varicose veins are seen in patients who present with venous insufficiency soon after puberty. These patients often develop small arteriovenous fistulas with or without cutaneous hemangiomas. They usually have a hereditary history of varicosities and form large varicosities during pregnancy. They frequently present markedly incompetent superficial veins without a history of trauma, deep vein thrombosis or infection.

Varicosities that develop after *trauma* are not uncommon, although a history of superficial or deep vein thrombophlebitis occuring after injury may be difficult to obtain. Incompetent veins do not develop until weeks or months after the trauma and do not necessarily show enlargement of the entire saphenous system. Physical findings demonstrate that the varicosities are due to incompetent valves in the perforating veins that connect the superficial veins with the deep veins below the saphenofemoral area. Uncomplicated, primary varicose veins per se do not produce morning swelling of the leg or ankle. Therefore, any patient presenting with a history of past or present leg edema should be carefully studied, since the lower extremity complaints may not be due to the obvious varicose veins (Table 17–1). Cardiac, hepatic or renal disease may be the cause of edema. No patient should have surgery for varicose veins when leg edema is present. If there is a past history of leg edema in the morning, the cause should be treated and under control before surgery is undertaken. Varicose veins that develop in the postphlebitic syndrome should not be ligated or removed until the syndrome is under control, since they constitute a small but important pathway for venous return and will often recur.

Another intriguing aspect of congenital varices is the presence of macroscopic arteriovenous connections. These can be noted at surgery by opening the saphenous vein and viewing the minute arterial connections under magnification.[28] These A-V connections become prominent during pregnancy and in cirrhotic patients.

Pregnancy is probably the most common acquired cause of varicose veins. Varices do not usually form until the second or third pregnancy. Increased abdominal pressure is a major factor, but hormonal factors are also believed to play a large part in the etiology. Treatment is preferred in the first trimester and no later than the seventh month. Most patients should avoid surgery for varicosities that develop during pregnancy, since the majority lessen in severity or disappear following delivery. Surgery can be scheduled in the immediate postpartum period or as an elective procedure. Labial varices are seldom treated unless they fail to regress after delivery. Labial varices suggest the presence of pelvic varices, especially in the broad ligament. Many obstetricians fear the possibility of hemorrhage from labial varices during an episiotomy and may therefore advise a cesarean section. If noted during pregnancy, labial varices should be operated upon on a prophylactic basis between pregnancies if delay is warranted. When surgery must be performed for labial varices during pregnancy, it should be performed as early as possible to lessen the possibility of infection of the labia occurring as a complication and creating a serious problem during and after delivery. Surgery is definitely not advised during the third trimester.

One entity not relieved by varicose vein surgery is the *restless leg syndrome*. This complaint is most common in women in whom there is stress produced by career commitments or the seemingly endless responsibilities of caring for a number of aggressive children. Owing to the tension of her environment the patient experiences fatigue in her legs and finds they are uncomfortable during the evening. She frequently describes them as "crazy legs" and finds comfort only in rest, sedation or walking on a cold floor.

A word is in order regarding the commonly used term, *varicose ulcers*. This term should be abandoned, for it implies that the ulcer is due to varicose veins. There is no such entity unless a significant arteriovenous fistula is present. Incompetent veins feeding the area may be a contributory factor, but the main source of the disability is disorder in the deep venous system. These patients should not be informed that excision of the incompetent superficial veins can cure the ulcer. On occasion the ulcer may heal but the "cure" is short-lived, since the problem involves the deep venous system. Ninety per cent of the lower extremity blood returns to the systemic circulation via the deep venous sytem.

Anatomy

The lower extremity has two systems of venous outflow, the deep and the superficial. The deep system is represented by the posterior tibial, the anterior tibial and the peroneal veins which drain to the popliteal vein and then into the superficial femoral vein at the adductor canal. The superficial vein forms the common femoral vein after receiving the profunda femoris vein at the inferior portion of the fossa ovalis in Scarpa's triangle. This is just below the saphenofemoral junction. The superficial venous system, represented by the long (greater) and short (lesser) saphenous veins, is the site of varicose veins. The two systems are connected by communicating veins that pierce the deep fascia of the extremity. There are usually two or three communicating or perforating veins in the thigh and approximately six in the leg. The long saphenous vein drains the medial aspect of the foot, crosses anterior to the medial malleolus and continues up the inner aspect of the leg, going behind the condyles of the tibia and femur. It progresses in an oblique line to the fossa ovalis, where it enters the common femoral vein just inferior to the inguinal ligament. Besides the numerous perforators that join the long saphenous vein with the deep system, there is occasionally a communication with the short saphenous vein, which drains into the popliteal vein. In many instances, two long saphenous veins pass the medial area of the knee and join at the lower third of the thigh or continue to the saphenofemoral junction. Three to five tributaries are present near the saphenofemoral junction. Some of these may join the common femoral rather than the long saphenous vein. As mentioned earlier, an accessory saphenous vein may be noted at the saphenofemoral junction joining directly with the femoral vein or connecting with the saphenous vein just below the saphenofemoral junction. Valves are present in both the long saphenous and the perforator veins. Those in the long saphenous vein open superiorly, while the perforator valves open toward the deep system. The saphenous nerve closely accompanies the vein from the medial malleolus to the lower third of the thigh, where it enters the adductor canal and continues cephalad as the femoral nerve.

The short saphenous vein begins on the lateral aspect of the foot and runs 1 cm posterior to the external malleolus. It drains the lateral aspect of the leg. It usually ascends to the tendon of Achilles and then progresses up the posterior midportion of the calf to enter the popliteal space. In some cases it penetrates the deep fascia and joins the popliteal vein, usually at the mid-upper third of the leg between the heads of the gas-

trocnemius muscle. This vein also has several perforators connecting with the deep veins of the leg. The short saphenous vein is accompanied by the sural nerve from the lateral malleolus to the midportion of the calf, where the nerve penetrates the fascia and continues to join the sciatic nerve in the area of the popliteal fossa.

Anomalies of both the long and short saphenous veins are common and should be searched for during the examination and at operation. Failure to recognize anomalies is the most common cause of so-called "recurrences." A better descriptive term, which should not be considered uncomplimentary to the surgeon, is "missed" varices. Every surgeon has on occasion "missed" removing all obvious varicosities. Preoperatively, this possibility should be explained to the patient.

Symptoms

Symptoms of varicosities vary among patients. However, careful questioning almost always reveals some symptomatology when prominent veins are evident. In every case, the physician should examine the lower extremity completely, including the arterial system, to exclude any other basis for the patient's complaints. Disfigurement of the extremities is obviously an indication for operation but it is very much overemphasized. The true reason for evaluating the patient for surgery is frequently not listed.

There may be an increased tendency to fatigue of the muscles of the leg and a sensation of fullness, congestion and soreness in the region of the veins after standing for a variable period of time. The actual course of the long or short saphenous veins may be traced by the patient as the bothersome site for his or her complaints, especially by female patients during the period of two or three days just prior to menstrual flow, at which time the veins appear larger. There may be burning pain and itching in the area overlying the varices. Muscular cramps occasionally occur, particularly at night. The patient's symptoms often seem disproportionate to the amount of actual pathology observed; nevertheless, they almost invariably clear up on removal or obliteration of the involved veins. Swelling, when present, is minimal and localized around the ankle after the patient has been on his feet all day. Swelling occurs in the evening and disappears during the night.

Primary varicosities seldom show skin changes. Secondary varicosities frequently show skin changes and symptoms that pertain both to the varicosities and to the underlying venous disorder. Itching, dermatitis, morning edema, fibrosis and ulceration in the region of the ankle are usually the result of deep vein incompetency or trauma.

Treatment is rarely indicated for intracutaneous *spider-like* or telangiectatic venules, which are fairly common on the thighs of women. Although sclerosing therapy may be used for cosmetic reasons, the resultant skin pigmentation and the reappearance of these minute varicosities does not justify the effort, unless bleeding occurs following minor trauma.

A few minor varices should not be blamed for all of the patient's leg symptoms.

Examination

Inspection of the lower extremities is conducted with the patient standing on a footstool. Distended veins may be related to the long or short saphenous system. Spiderlike intracutaneous venules may be separate or related to obvious large vein varicosities. Similar small venular dilatations occurring at the ankle or foot suggest deep venous insufficiency, long-standing varicosities along with a history of repeated pregnancies or a strong history for congenital varices. This third small group of patients, termed "vein formers," are

the patients who may develop recurrent varicosities following adequate varicose vein surgery.

A number of tests are available for examination of varicosities. Some should be abandoned and others used only when indicated, and a few should be conducted regularly on all patients. Varicosities below the knee are almost always plainly visible to the examiner; however, frequently the long saphenous vein in the thigh with its connecting tributaries from the leg, and occasionally the short saphenous vein, are not obvious owing to a large amount of subcutaneous fat. This prevents proper mapping of the venous pattern. Accurate determination of the size of the vein being examined is difficult to assess, and areas where incompetent perforators are present may be obscure. Tourniquet tests are usually valueless in these patients, for the flow pattern seldom can be demonstrated. This problem is far more evident in females than in males. The following tests are advised:

PERCUSSION OR BALLOTTEMENT (SCHWARTZ-HEYERDALE) AND DOPPLER TESTS. These tests are utilized to identify the course of the long and short saphenous veins and augment the information obtained from visualization and simple palpation. They also demonstrate variables such as the presence of more than one long saphenous vein or a variable course of the short saphenous vein. The short saphenous vein should be traced into the popliteal vein or into the long saphenous vein below the knee or in the thigh. It may also have connections to the popliteal and long saphenous veins. In addition, when there is a marked localized enlargement of the long saphenous vein in the thigh, an incompetent perforator may be looked for. To orient patients as to the source of their disorder, they are permitted to feel the size of the enlarged incompetent main vein in the thigh during percussion. The percussion is extended around the medial aspect of the thigh to determine if additional accessory saphenous veins are present and to determine where a tributary enters the saphenous system. Percussion may also demonstrate that a soft bulge on the leg is actually muscle herniating through a small fascial defect. This can be confirmed by its appearance and disappearance during dorsiflexion and extension of the foot. No pulse wave is transmitted from one of these bulging areas.

To perform the percussion or ballottement test, the examiner's hand is placed at the level of the lower third of the medial aspect of the thigh with the fingertips on the area where the vein is expected to be present. The other hand is used for percussion or ballottement of the vein below this level. By moving both hands along the vein, it is possible to map the vessel and its branches completely. Experience with this method allows the examiner to determine the size of the vessels, their course, the amount of scarring in the vein wall and the number of incompetent perforators. These last may be observed at points of bulging of the vein at the thigh or along the leg medial to the tibia. The percussion test does not establish competence of the venous channel or the direction of flow.

However, the cough test with palpation over the saphenofemoral junction will aid in establishing competence. These tests can be performed more easily if a Doppler flowmeter rather than the fingertip is used to demonstrate reflux.[23]

TOURNIQUET TESTS (BRODIE-TRENDELENBURG). These tests are used mainly for patients who have questionable varices or to rule out any connection between the short and long saphenous vein in the thigh. It is difficult to determine the vein causing reflux in the short saphenous vein — that is, whether the reflux comes from the popliteal vein, the long saphenous vein or a perforating vein.

The tests are performed by having the patient lie supine on the examining table with the lower extremity raised above the level of the body until all superficial veins are collapsed. Thumb pressure is applied over the fossa ovalis, or a tourniquet is applied lightly at midthigh or on the upper leg. Specific sites may be controlled by thumb pressure in the calf during the time the tourniquet is in place. The patient is then allowed to stand erect and the following occurrences may be observed: (1) retrograde filling of an incompetent vein to the tourniquet, with the vein below this area remaining empty; (2) rapid filling of the saphenous vein from the deep system below the tourniquet, demonstrating perforator incompetence; (3) sudden retrograde filling of the vein approximately 15 seconds after the tourniquet is released, denoting total vein incompetence; and (4) sudden filling of the vein below the tourniquet before it is released, demonstrating incompetence of the short saphenous vein or the perforating veins. The tourniquet may be applied at any point along the lower extremity.

These methods of examination determine the incompetence of the long or short saphenous vein or both, and allow the examiner to recommend the type of surgery necessary to remove the veins. These tests have limited usefulness, since most patients with varicose veins are women, generally with moderately obese thighs, in whom the long saphenous vein flow pattern cannot be determined with these test maneuvers.

TOURNIQUET WALKING TEST (PERTHES' TEST). This test was once popular as a means for demonstrating deep vein incompetency. It involves placing a tourniquet on the thigh and instructing the patient to walk. If the veins empty below the tourniquet it is concluded that the deep veins are competent. A modification of the test is the use of an elastic support to the knee. In this case, if discomfort develops shortly after ambulation, the deep venous system is considered occluded. The presence of edema during the morning or early afternoon hours is a more reliable means of evaluating the efficiency of the deep venous system. Until proved otherwise, the deep venous system is considered functionally adequate if morning or early afternoon edema does not occur. Venography or supplemental procedures may be performed to confirm the adequacy of the deep venous system, but they are not essential when an adequate history and physical examination do not disclose the presence of edema.

Treatment – Outpatient

Surgeons vary widely in their initial treatment of varicose veins. A thorough understanding of normal and abnormal anatomy, pathology and physiology of these vascular channels is necessary. Without such an understanding, various complications such as deep vein thrombosis, nonhealing ulcers, uncontrolled edema, lymphorrhea, causalgia and even loss of the leg are possible following surgery.

When the benefits that may be obtained from surgery are uncertain because the patient's complaints are indecisive or the varicosities are borderline, nonoperative treatment is advisable. Elastic stockings from toe to knee are prescribed and supplemented with intermittent elevation of the lower extremities above body level for short periods daily. Long periods of sitting or standing are to be avoided, especially in women prior to their menstrual periods. Panty girdles and other constricting garments and the varied use of high-heeled and flat-soled shoes are inadvisable. Mild exercise is suggested on a regular basis. Anxiety caused by the stress of career or home life is investigated, for such stress may cause muscle tension resulting in fatigue in extremities, called "restless" or "crazy" legs (see previous discussion). Frequently this entity is misdiagnosed as being due to varicose vein, even when the veins are not significant in appearance and unlikely to be the cause of the patient's discomfort.

Operative Treatment

Indications for surgery are (1) symptoms localized to superficial veins or to the entire extremity; (2) progression of either symptomatic or asymptomatic varicosities; (3) location of varices: the more proximal the varices are to the saphenofemoral junction, the stronger the indication; (4) superficial thrombophlebitis of less than 24 hours' duration, with no evidence of deep vein involvement; (5) severe associated inflammatory reaction, such as eczema or septic thrombophlebitis, overlying the vein or within its lumen following appropriate antibiotic and antiinflammatory therapy; (6) improvement of appearance; (7) prophylaxis against deep venous thrombosis and its complications; and (8) "recurrent" varicosities.

Contraindications for surgery are: (1) constitutional disease with poor prognosis; (2) uncorrected arterial occlusive disease; (3) advanced age with asymptomatic varicosities; (4) severe deep vein insufficiency with persistent edema; (5) pregnancy, especially after first trimester; (6) excessive obesity; and (7) Klippel-Trenaunay syndrome (congenital dysplastic angiectasis). Unnecessary surgery should be avoided; when in doubt, nonoperative measures should be instituted at least for a trial period.

Surgery for varicose veins does not always necessitate hospital admission. The following procedures can be performed on an outpatient basis in the operating room with no more risk than occurs with inpatient surgery.

1. HIGH LIGATION OF THE LONG SAPHENOUS VEIN WITH EXCISION OF A SEGMENT. This procedure alone may be all that older patients require. Dissection and partial excision of tributaries are absolutely necessary because

of anatomical variation that may be present at or near the saphenofemoral junction. Frequently the segment below is not obliterated owing to incompetent perforators.

2. HIGH AND LOW LIGATION OF THE LONG SAPHENOUS VEIN AND ITS PROXIMAL TRIBUTARIES WITH EXCISION OF A SEGMENT AT EACH SITE. Since this method does not remove the varicose segment, recurrences occur owing to a bifid or dual saphenous vein. In addition, a communicating vessel may develop as a result of an incompetent perforator.

3. HIGH AND/OR LOW LIGATION FOLLOWED BY RETROGRADE SCLEROSING THERAPY. This procedure has been almost universally abandoned because of the high incidence of complications from the sclerosing therapy, i.e., deep vein thrombosis and marked inflammatory response.

4. HIGH LIGATION AND EXCISION OF THE LONG SAPHENOUS VEIN AND ITS TRIBUTARIES FOLLOWED BY SEGMENTAL LIGATIONS AND PARTIAL EXCISION OF THE VEIN. Even with an extremely thorough examination before operation, perforators and communicating veins can easily be missed. This procedure is designed to locate and ligate the perforators and communicating veins.

5. HIGH LIGATION OF THE LONG SAPHENOUS VEIN AND ITS TRIBUTARIES FOLLOWED BY STRIPPING OF THE ENTIRE LONG SAPHENOUS VEIN UTILIZING AN INTRALUMINAL OR EXTRALUMINAL STRIPPER. By performing this procedure segmentally, especially in the thigh, the vein can be inspected in its entirety, and any variables present may be observed and surgically excised. One modification of this technique is to make two incisions, one at the groin and the second at the ankle, and to strip between the two points. This latter procedure is probably the most common method currently performed in most hospitals. However, since it is a crude, blind technique it misses variables and allows "recurrences." It also necessitates use of a full-length elastic bandage, which is objectionable because it limits knee flexion postoperatively and causes discomfort at the knee. The potential of deep vein thrombosis in the extremity is increased as a result of the trauma of surgery combined with subsequent postoperative splinting.

6. HIGH LIGATION OF THE LONG SAPHENOUS VEIN AND ITS TRIBUTARIES WITH EXCISION AND/OR STRIPPING BETWEEN MULTIPLE INCISIONS. This procedure is more radical than is usually required, especially when complete excision of the lower segment along with its surrounding scar tissue and underlying fascia is included.

A few patients may not be completely cured during the initial operation. They may have to return for further treatment, at which time an isolated segment may be ligated and excised. Some surgeons may prefer to use sclerotherapy for "mopping up" these isolated vein segments. Too often these isolated varices are connected and are the result of an incompetent major system (the long or short saphenous). Sclerosing therapy should be used in this case only when the major component has been ligated and excised.

Prior to surgery all patients should be informed that a major segment of the saphenous vein may be missed. Even though enough operating time has been allowed to clear a patient's varicosities there is still a chance, though minimal, of recurrent or "missed" varices. Admittedly, Procedure No. 6 is more lengthy than other approaches, but it assures the patient of complete extirpation of the offending veins with few exceptions. Only one extremity is operated upon at a time.

We recommend Technique No. 5 or 6 and, when indicated, the short saphenous vein is treated similarly either at the same time or at a later date. The extensive procedure as described in No. 6 is not usually recommended for older patients. Furthermore, it is important to advise a female patient to have surgery when it is indicated during the course of the disease rather than to tell her to "wait until you've finished having all your family."

Many vascular surgeons have suggested saving untortuous main channel saphenous veins, since they may be needed for arterial reconstruction later in life.

Anesthesia

The anesthetic should allow ambulation as soon as possible following surgery. Epidural anesthesia is preferable, although a light general or local may be employed. Spinal anesthesia is not desirable because of the possibility of lengthy motor paralysis and spinal headache. Epidural anesthesia may occasionally produce spinal headache when the dura has been entered. Properly applied local anesthesia can be very satisfactory.

Virtually all patients are ambulatory within two or four hours after operation and are instructed to walk a few steps or more every hour during the day. Ambulation is gradually increased until the patient is able to walk well. If general or spinal anesthesia is used, passive exercises should be carried out immediately after operation and for several minutes of every hour until the patient is capable of voluntary ambulation.

Local or epidural anesthesia has been used in all but 8 of 156 cases in which the senior author has performed the excision and stripping technique. Excluding those eight, the patients were discharged after a few hours under observation without being admitted to the hospital. This does not mean to imply that excision and stripping of varicose veins is a simple operation or that it could be an office procedure. The operations were closely supervised, and in no instance has either the patient or the surgeon felt that postoperative care was neglected. The operation was performed only on one extremity to lessen the patient's discomfort at home and to increase the

likelihood of compliance with the aforementioned instruction relative to ambulation. The few possible complications could easily have developed even if the patient had been admitted to the hospital. All patients received medication for sleep and for pain plus thorough instructions before leaving the hospital.

Reasons for discharging these patients immediately after surgery are: (1) the number of vacant beds in hospitals is often limited, and they should be kept available for patients who need admission; (2) postoperative therapy in the hospital offers very little that cannot be provided at home; and (3) financial saving to the patient and to third party insurance programs is considerable.

The procedure most often performed in this country is high ligation and excision at the saphenofemoral junction followed by complete stripping of the long and sometimes of the short saphenous veins. When this method of extirpation of the saphenous vein is performed, it is probably hazardous to discharge the patient immediately, especially if a pressure dressing is applied to the entire extremity. To avoid this and also to perform a more complete operation, it is better to advocate stripping only below the knee following complete ligation and excision of the varicosities in the thigh.

Preoperative Preparation

Morning swelling and ulcers are allowed to clear before surgery is performed; treatment of the sequelae of the postphlebitic syndrome has been discussed earlier in this chapter. Occasionally varices are marked on the skin before surgery, although the surgical procedure excises the incompetent segments causing the varices. Marking of varices is done the day before surgery on veins that do not follow the usual course or that have a bizarre pattern. An ordinary pen is used. The areas are scratched with a needle beside the marking before skin preparation is started and while anesthesia is being instituted.

Operation (Fig. 17–17)

We prefer a high longitudinal or slightly oblique incision from 3 to 5 inches long. This incision has specific advantages: (1) The incision is in line with the vessel that has been percussed and palpated and also with the femoral vein and artery so that it allows better visualization of these vessels should control be necessary. (2) Transverse incisions have a greater probability of cutting lymphatic vessels and traumatizing lymph nodes, sometimes resulting in lymphedema and lymphorrhea. We believe that the ankle swelling that may appear after operation is not necessarily an indication of deep vein thrombosis but is more characteristic of lymphedema. (3) Excision of a large segment under direct vision is readily possible by this type of incision. In addition, more of the wound is utilized since it is in line with and not transverse to the axis of the vessel.

The remainder of the incisions are also longitudinal along the course of the vessel, except the one used in the popliteal space for the short saphenous vein. We have found that this incision has a better cosmetic appearance on the extremity, particularly in females, since the lines of a woman's stocking run longitudinally rather than transversely.

CARE AND METHOD OF LIGATION. After the incision has been made up to the inguinal crease, the long saphenous vein is dissected to the sphenofemoral junction, with careful ligation of all tributaries, dissection of each tributary back as far as possible, and wide excision of each segment. From three to five tributaries may be expected. Because there may be a direct connection between the femoral vein and one of these tributaries or an accessory saphenous vein, the femoral vein is gently exposed and inspected on both the medial and lateral aspects to obviate recurrent varicosities originating from this area. Any blunt dissection against the axis of the vein is avoided to obviate puncture of the vessel. The saphenofemoral junction is then doubly ligated flush with the femoral vein, with the distal ligature being a transfixion suture. Dissection should be cautious because of the presence of the small external pudendal artery, which traverses the inferior portion of the fossa ovale. This artery may have its course over or beneath the long saphenous vein at this point. If it is damaged, it should be carefully ligated, since it is notorious as a site of postoperative bleeding.

METHOD OF SEGMENTAL STRIPPING. The inferior segment of the saphenous vein is dissected under direct vision and an attempt is made to localize the highest perforator or tributary, which is usually just inferior to the groin incision. Any communicating or perforating vessel is directly visualized, clamped and ligated. The superior dissection, which may include opening the sheath, also locates any accessory saphenous vein that may be present. The inferior segment of the long saphenous is utilized to locate the midthigh point of incision. A large majority of the incompetent perforators occur at this site. The superior wound is not closed until the segment between the two incisions has been dissected or stripped out. Here one end of the vessel is converted into the other wound and the perforator is ligated when present. In most cases the entire segment is removed under direct vision by gently pulling up (rather than back) on retractors. After the segment has been removed, the first incision is closed with interrupted sutures, carefully obliterating any pockets where serum may collect. The operation is then continued inferiorly in the same manner, with the third incision approximately four inches above the knee, avoiding the flexion crease. This third incision is

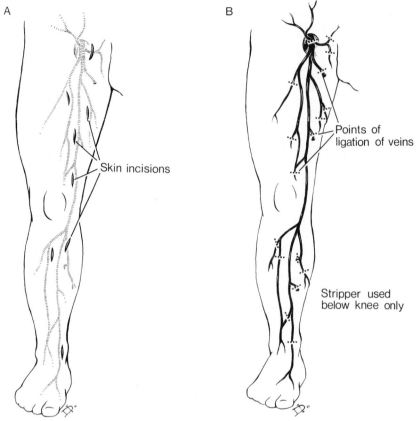

Figure 17–17 Surgery for varicose veins. High ligation and stripping of the greater saphenous vein is performed as described in the text. This operation can be performed on an outpatient basis when suitable anesthesia and postoperative recovery facilities are available.

Illustration continued on the opposite page

important in looking for a perforator or a bifid saphenous vein; when the latter is present both segments are stripped to the ankle. The next incision is just below the knee. When two saphenous veins are present in this area the incision is made at a point midway between the two vessels. The dissection of the saphenous vein in the thigh is done under direct vision to minimize the possibility of recurrences and the incidence of postoperative hematoma. Close observation is made for a communication with the short saphenous vein at any point along the long saphenous vein in the thigh, even though none was found on preoperative examination. In such cases the short saphenous

vein is excised or stripped at the same operation.

Occasionally no incision is made below the knee if the operator is confident that the long saphenous is a single segment that goes directly to the ankle. In such a case, the next incision is made over the internal malleolus in a longitudinal direction, and the stripper is placed into the lumen of the vein at this site. However, the procedure is much easier to perform if a fourth incision is made inferior to the knee. When the stripper is passed, care is taken that the first attempt allows easy passage of the stripper, since occasionally the vessel may go into spasm and make the second passage difficult. Perforation of

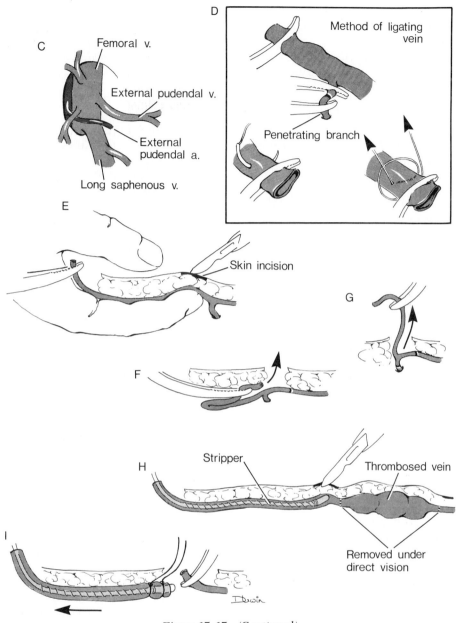

Figure 17–17 *(Continued)*

the vein wall may occur. When the operator is not sure of the specific course taken by one of the vessels observed, it can easily be traced by passage of the instrument.

Many types of intraluminal strippers are available — some have filiform tips, others have olive or acorn ends and some allow injection of saline to distend the vessel so that the stripper may be passed through a tortuous vein. The only type of stripper necessary is one that is sufficiently flexible and has small olive or acorn tips that are interchangeable.

The short saphenous vein is stripped and excised in approximately one out of ten cases. A transverse incision is made only at the popliteal space, and longitudinal incisions are placed at the midcalf and 1 cm posterior to the external malleolus. Special care should be taken to avoid damaging the sural nerve, which accompanies the vein inferiorly.

Four anatomical variations of the short saphenous vein are possible: (1) the short saphenous vein goes directly into the popliteal vein through the popliteal space; (2) the same connection with the popliteal vein is present but a tributary is evident coursing up the posterior aspect of the thigh and going into the deep system at a higher point; (3) the short saphenous vein does not enter the popliteal vein but connects with the long saphenous vein near the saphenofemoral junction; (4) the saphenous vein enters the deep fascia below the popliteal space, coursing between the two heads of the gastrocnemius muscle to join up with the popliteal vein. The stripper is introduced from the ankle to aid in identifying variables.

Only one lower extremity is operated upon at a time.

The incidence of recurrence has been less than 5 per cent, and half of these were vessels that had been missed at operation and therefore should not be considered recurrences.

Postoperative Care

The extremity is wrapped with an elastic bandage from the toe to the knee. Instructions are given to walk a few minutes of every waking hour and to elevate the extremity between ambulatory periods and at night. Mild sedation is given for pain and discomfort. Antibiotics are not indicated. Most patients return to their occupations within five or six days. On the seventh day, the wounds are inspected and the sutures generally removed.

Sclerosing Therapy

Sclerosing therapy enjoyed a vogue as the preferred method of controlling varicose veins in the 1930s and 1940s, replacing in popularity a number of surgical approaches peripherally directed at the varicose veins themselves but ignoring their underlying cause, saphenofemoral incompetence. When high ligation of the saphenous vein was combined with stripping or excision of its varicose branches, the pendulum swung back in favor of surgery and, in the United States at least, sclerosing therapy was almost abandoned. The relatively recent rekindling of interest in sclerosing therapy may have been stimulated by difficulties in mustering sufficient surgical resources (surgeons, operative time and surgical beds) to meet adequately the therapeutic demands posed by varicose veins, particularly in European countries that have socialized medicine.

Considerable uniformity has developed regarding the choice of a sclerosing agent, for 3 per cent tetradecyl sulfate (Sotradecol) has been found to be almost as active as but much less toxic than previous agents. It is a stable and soluble chemical of low enough viscosity that it can be injected through fine needles and, although its thrombogenic activity is less than that of some other agents, so is the associated perivascular inflammatory response.

The combination of improved injection technique and improved sclerosing agent has caused some surgeons to re-evaluate the role of sclerosing therapy in controlling varicose veins. In a randomized six-year clinical trial, Hobbs[39] has shown that, while sclerosing therapy produced better initial (first year) results than surgery, the tendency for recurrence with time was so great that by the fourth to sixth years surgery had re-established its superiority. Further analysis of this experience indicated that, while the advantage of sclerosing therapy persisted for "dilated superficial veins" and "incompetent perforators." the superiority of surgery for cases of primary saphenous varicosities was apparent early and increased with time. The senior author had the same experience and findings more than two decades ago.

Thus, it would appear that while blind enthusiasm for sclerosing therapy is certainly unwarranted, it does have a place in the management of varicose veins. When a proper high ligation of the saphenous vein has been carried out and the main channel stripped, sclerosing therapy can be effectively used to obliterate those small, tortuous varicose tributaries that are impossible to strip and difficult to excise. In addition, residual or recurrent varicose veins following surgery may be controlled by sclerosing therapy. Finally, gratifying results may occasionally be obtained by using sclerosing therapy to obliterate those spider-like clusters of subcutaneous venules, which are such a cosmetic problem to self-conscious women.

TECHNIQUE. Sclerosing therapy involves the injection of small volumes of sclerosing agent into the main lumen of the vein, which then is carefully compressed to *avoid* thrombus formation. This compression must be maintained until fibrosis has permanently obliterated the lumen. The veins are first explored by palpation and by a sliding finger, with the patient in the upright position, to determine "points of control" or major points of back filling. These are circled with a felt-tip pen, and then the patient is placed in the supine position. The veins are then injected at the marked sites with 3 per cent sodium tetradecyl sulfate, using disposable 2 ml syringes and 25 gauge needles. The usual injection is 0.5 ml, although 0.23 to 0.75 ml may be used, depending on the size of the varicose

segment. Immediately after each injection, a moist cotton ball is taped over the injection site. Afterwards the entire leg is wrapped with an Ace or other elastic bandage. Intermittent elevation of the legs above heart level (15 minutes q.i.d.) and continuous elastic compression are maintained for at least three weeks. Spider-like veins are injected with a 27 or 30 gauge needle using 0.1 ml of the same sclerosing agent foamed with air to a volume of 1 ml.

Until recently, sclerosing therapy had not been used at our institution for over twenty years because recanalization was found to be common following this method of treatment. When varicosities do recanalize (usually within two years) they are worse than when originally seen. Bizarre patterns of varicose veins develop when repeated sclerosing therapy is substituted for surgical removal of incompetent veins or is given to patients with a postphlebitic syndrome. Surgery, when undertaken at a later date, is time-consuming and difficult. Furthermore, extravasation of the sclerosing agent may result in ulceration and a peculiar type type of chronic edema, which is both disfiguring and disabling, localized to the skin. Improperly injected material, including the injection of too large a quantity, may initiate significant thrombophlebitis, both superficial and deep, and result in the postphlebitic syndrome.[66] The risk of complications may outweigh the benefits that can be derived from sclerosing therapy. It is strongly recommended that sclerosing therapy be contraindicated as a primary therapeutic method in patients with varicose veins and in patients with chronic deep vein incompetency.

Causes of Recurrences

Excluding recurrences that follow other procedures, the majority of recurrences are the result of missing or subsequent opening of incompetent veins connecting the saphenous and deep venous circulation. ·Three explanations for missed varicosities are (1) failure to ligate and excise points of communication with the deep penetrator; (2) failure to ligate and excise all tributaries at the saphenofemoral junction, including an accessory saphenous vein; (3) failure to make sure that both sides of the femoral vein are under direct vision; (4) failure to recognize the occasional long saphenous vein that is bifid just above the knee; and (5) selection of patients with varicosities secondary to deep or perforator vein incompetence.

Incompetency of the saphenous vein from the saphenofemoral junction is the same as incompetency from a deep penetrator connecting the saphenous vein at the superficial femoral vein.

Varicose Veins with the Postphlebitic Syndrome

Varicosities occur in two out of three patients with the postphlebitic syndrome. They invariably have morning swelling, whereas the patient with varicose veins alone has ankle swelling only late in the afternoon. Treatment of varicosities in the presence of the postphlebitic syndrome is not undertaken until a minimum of six months' therapy has been successfully accomplished. The swelling should be controlled until it occurs only late in the afternoon. Surgery is rarely indicated, but when performed it should include subfascial ligation of the perforator veins. Therapy regarding postphlebitic syndrome has been discussed earlier.

Varicose Veins with Acute Superficial Thrombophlebitis

Extremities of patients with acute superficial thrombophlebitis are closely examined for deep vein involvement. If no such evidence exists, they may receive high ligation and excision with stripping regardless of the presence or absence of varicose veins. This procedure was very frequently performed a decade ago but owing to the successful use of anti-inflammatory drugs, few now require surgery. Indications for performing the procedure are: (1) progressing thrombophlebitis, (2) thrombophlebitis approaching or present at the saphenofemoral vein junction, (3) septic or suppurative thrombophlebitis and (4) varicose vein surgery indicated anyway in the future.

ARTERIAL DISEASES

Peripheral arterial diseases are manifested most frequently in the lower extremities, but they are not clinically limited to these areas. Any acute or insidious pathological change occurring in an arterial vessel distal to the heart is considered as peripheral arterial disease.

Vasospastic Disorders

The three most common vasospastic disorders are Raynaud's phenomenon, acrocyanosis and livedo reticularis. Each of these conditions may occur as a primary disorder, as a secondary condition due to an underlying systemic disease, or as an entity resulting from some mechanical irritation to a major artery proximal to the symptomatic area.

Raynaud's Phenomenon

Raynaud's phenomenon is the most common vasospastic condition. A typical case involves first the tip of one or more fingers and later may progress to include the entire digit and even the hand. Usually the disorder begins unilaterally and later becomes bilateral. The toes and feet may be included in the symptomatology but never without the presence of upper extremity findings. Symptoms and signs are characterized first by intermittent pallor, a cyanosis, or both, and finally by reactive hyperemia. In an occasional patient, one or two of these color changes may be less prominent or absent. Numbness initially occurs in the digit(s), and "burning" paresthesias may develop later during the erythematous phase. Swelling of the involved fingers often occurs. Even though gangrene of the part is frequently feared by the patient, nutritional lesions are absent or limited to the skin, usually of the fingertips alone. These lesions vary from petechial spots and spontaneous subungual hematomas to frank ulceration. The condition is initiated by exposure to cold, trauma or emotional stress.

Any patient with Raynaud's phenomenon needs further study to determine the underlying basis for the condition. Three possibilities are currently considered: (1) The primary group, termed "Raynaud's disease," includes patients who have intermittent attacks with a symmetrical bilateral distribution, an absence of gangrene or cutaneous trophic changes and in whom an underlying cause is not established within two years. These patients most often are young females. (2) The secondary group includes Raynaud's phenomenon due to associated conditions such as collagen diseases, metabolic occlusive arterial disease, neurogenic lesions, drug and heavy metal intoxication and blood dyscrasias, including the rare entities of cryoglobulinemia, macroglobulinemia and cold agglutinins in the blood. (3) The third is Raynaud's phenomenon related to repeated mechanical trauma to the shoulders, hands and fingers. Occasionally these patients present clinical evidence of the thoracic outlet compression syndrome. In this group of patients there is continuous or intermittent irritation of the subclavian artery or vein or brachial plexus.

The studies required to determine the underlying basis for Raynaud's phenomenon begin with a blood clotting profile, a sedimentation rate and digital capillary examination. Digital plethysmography and Doppler studies are most useful for documenting the extent or absence of digital artery thrombosis and for assessing drug therapy. Immunological screening tests should be ordered when the history and clinical findings suggest the need to detect an associated disease. These tests include determination of antinuclear antibody and the rheumatoid factor, immunoglobulin electrophoresis, complement C3 test, antinative DNA antibody determination, Coomb's test and attempts to identify lupus erythematosus (LE) cells. Serum protein electrophoresis should also be included because of the possible association of serum protein abnormalities. Screening for cryoglobulins, macroglobulins and cold agglutinins is rarely productive yet is indicated in some patients. On occasion, nerve conduction velocity testing may provide documentation of the presence of nerve injury, compression or entrapment in the areas of the thoracic outlet, elbow and wrist. Skin and muscle biopsy that includes a small artery is a valid means of establishing the presence of an associated collagen disease.[72] Finally, digital arteriography may be of assistance in certain patients.

Laboratory procedures should be ordered cautiously when the only complaint is that of color changes in the extremity. Elaborate studies costing the patient hundreds of dollars are unjustly ordered when no other sign or symptom is evident from the history or physical examination. "Artful procrastination" is advised when considering these studies, yet close attention is paid toward treatment of the symptoms.

Treatment of Raynaud's phenomenon is generally concentrated on protection from exposure to cold, trauma and emotional stress.

MEDICAL TREATMENT. 1. The patient is thoroughly educated as to the nature of the condition and reassured that extensive gangrene will not occur. Known factors that precipitate vasoconstrictive episodes and occasional ischemic changes on the fingertips, such as cold, emotional upset, trauma, cigarette smoking and infection, are included in the discussion. The use of tobacco is strongly discouraged. Evidence of its effect is easily identifiable by finger symptomatology, gross evidence of sweating or vasoconstrictive activity demonstrated by plethysmography during a period of smoking. During winter weather, warm clothing is advised, including heavy stockings and gloves and protection of the head. Special heating devices for hands and feet may be suggested. Summer weather does not exclude additional protection, for it may be necessary in drafts, in low evening temperatures or in the presence of air conditioners. A change of climate may be advised, though it is rarely necessary.

2. Psychiatric evaluation is suggested only when it is needed to prevent or reduce significant manifestations of emotional instability.

3. Prophylactic care of hands and feet is mandatory. Any surgical procedure on digits is ill-advised and should be discouraged, since minor trauma may precipitate vasospasm and ischemia. When digital surgery is necessary, local anesthesia to the digit should never be used. Many of these patients are excellent candidates for causalgic pain syndromes. They are therefore warned of the hyperesthesia that may follow trauma or infection to their hands or feet and informed that pain can be treated by medical or surgical sympathetic denervation.

4. Underlying diseases or physical causes are constantly considered concurrently with treatment of Raynaud's phenomenon. The most prevalent of these are collagen diseases, especially scleroderma, which may be the earliest symptom or may not be clinically identified until several years later.

5. Several approaches to therapy may be initiated.

a. Mechanical entrapment causing arterial or neurological irritation in the shoulder area from a thoracic outlet compression syndrome may require some method of medical sympathetic denervation. Irritation may occur when shoulder exercises are advised before considering surgery, or following excision of the first rib in which an upper thoracic sympathectomy has not been performed (Fig. 17–18). A similar approach, medical or surgical, or both, should be considered when there is a contributory nerve injury, or entrapment of the ulnar nerve at the elbow or of the medial nerve in carpal tunnel syndrome.

b. If an underlying systemic disease, such as one of the collagen diseases

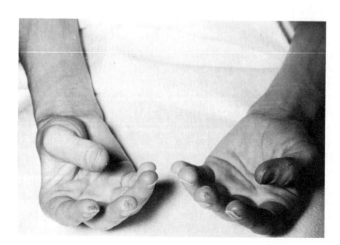

Figure 17–18 Raynaud's phenomenon due to entrapment in thoracic outlet. Note fingertip necrosis. Treatment: first rib resection and simultaneous extrapleural thoracic sympathectomy.

(especially scleroderma), is present and if ulcerations are present, the use of subcutaneous heparin is prescribed on a long-term basis. Sympatholytic drugs are also used to relieve superficial pain and to attempt to maintain a more normal digital color pattern. A third approach to drug therapy is the use of specific drugs to deplete catecholamines.

None of the treatments for Raynaud's disease and Raynaud's phenomenon is entirely satisfactory. Oral administration of sympatholytic drugs, sublingual use of nitroglycerine and intramuscular injection of estrogens have been used with varying results. These drugs have not produced sustained changes in signs and symptoms. The role of sympathectomy is also inconsistent. Almost all patients will show improvement for the first six months following operation, but half of the patients will subsequently develop a recurrence of symptoms and signs. The greatest improvement occurs in patients with digital-artery thrombosis and in those individuals who have been classified as having primary Raynaud's phenomenon. The outcome is poor in patients with scleroderma and other connective tissue diseases in which sympathectomy is contraindicated. These disorders are difficult to diagnose in their early stages, and the prognosis with any treatment may therefore be difficult to determine. Those patients who need therapy the most seem to respond least well. It is apparently worthwhile in these patients to help them through any exacerbation of their symptoms.

c. The following therapy is advised in patients with Raynaud's phenomenon:

The most promising drug now being used is reserpine, a drug with a potentially dangerous central depressant action. This effect is seen with oral therapy, in which doses should be about 0.25 mg daily. The preferred method of administration is intra-arterial, slowly infusing 0.25 to 0.5 mg or reserpine in 5 ml of saline solution into the brachial artery. On the first visit tolazoline hydrochloride (Priscoline) 25 mg may be added to the intra-arterial reserpine to judge the potential of the intra-arterial route. Some reports maintain that relief of pain and ulceration may be present for as long as six months. Our experience has shown clinical improvement for no more than three weeks. Some patients may again become responsive to therapy with sympatholytic drugs, to which they had become resistant.

Oral or intramuscular injections of reserpine are prescribed as tolerated from 0.25 to 1 mg. The blood pressure is regularly monitored on each visit to avoid the discomforts and hazards that may occur if it is significantly lowered. The side effects of reserpine are described in the instructions given to the patient. Reserpine administration has been reported to deplete catecholamines with or without depletion in serotonin. Response to reserpine has been gratifying in some patients with Raynaud's phenomenon, but it has been used less frequently when there is a need for repeated intra-arterial injections. The oral drug most often prescribed by us is guanethidine, 10 to 30 mg daily. Porter has found that the oral administration of norepinephrine-depleting drugs and alpha receptor–blocking drugs produces improvement in 80 to 90 per cent of patients.[72]

Sympatholytic drugs are prescribed separately for a few days to one week at a time to determine their effects on pain, temperature, skin color and the function of involved digits. These drugs are dihydro ergot alkaloids (Hydergine), 0.5 to 1 mg orally or sublingually; phenoxybenzamine hydrochloride (Dibenzyline), 15 mg; tolazoline hydrochloride (Priscoline), 25 to 50 mg; nylidrin hydrochloride (Arlidin), 6 to 12 mg; or cyclandelate (Cyclospasmal), 100 to 200 mg when necessary three times a day and at bedtime. Since the response to each of these drugs may vary, a record of the benefits and side effects observed will determine which drug or combination of drugs will be most beneficial. At present phenoxybenzamine hydrochloride is preferred and has been combined with guanethidine, with additional benefits. Medication should be used when symptoms are expected. Medication is therefore taken prior to exposure to an adverse environment, rather than on a specified time schedule. However, when vasospasm, pain or ischemic ulceration is continuously present, regular administration of medication is indicated. Because of recent success obtained by guanethidine and, in some patients, by reserpine therapy, sympatholytic drugs have lost much of their popularity. Their use is now reserved to cases in which these other drugs produce little if any benefit or are contraindicated. Sympatholytic drugs are also indicated when sympathectomy is being considered. When sympatholytic drugs produce a good response, relief of symptoms should be expected following sympathectomy.

SURGICAL TREATMENT. Surgical measures may be indicated when medical therapy fails to control digital complications such as pain, subungual hematoma, recurrent ulcerations, paronychia, atrophy of soft tissue and osteoporosis. The strongest indication for surgery is the presence of the thoracic outlet compression syndrome and the traumatization of subclavian vessels. This is rarely seen. We treat the thoracic outlet compression syndrome by shoulder exercises for at least three months prior to determining whether the removal of the first rib via the axilla or the posterior thoracic area is indicated. (A more detailed discussion of this subject will be given in the section on thoracic outlet compression syndrome.)

An upper thoracic sympathectomy is almost always performed when the first rib is removed for Raynaud's phenomenon. When thoracic sympathectomy is indicated, excision of the second and third ganglia is essential for ablation of sympathetic activity from the upper extremity. However, to lessen the possibility of an inadequate sympathetic

denervation because of the possible presence of anatomic variables. T_4, T_3, T_2 and the inferior half of T_1 are excised. The preganglionic fibers entering T_1 (which fuses with the inferior cervical ganglion) are avoided so that Horner's syndrome will not develop. When sympathectomy alone is performed, benefit is frequently less than optimum, although most patients do obtain some relief. Lumbar sympathectomy for lower extremity involvement requires ablation of L_2 and L_3, but a wider excision including L_1, L_2, L_3 and L_4 is usually performed. In males, L_1 is not included in the excision on one side to avoid possible impotence postoperatively. Good results should be expected from the procedure in most patients. When Raynaud's phenomenon is present in all four extremities, sympathectomy is performed at six-month intervals or only three extremities are denervated, to avoid the hazard of orthostatic hypotension and the nuisance of excessive perspiration in the undenervated areas of the trunk. Spacing the procedures allows time for readjustment of sympathetic tone in the proximal areas of each involved extremity. There is no indication for sympathectomy when scleroderma is accompanied by Raynaud's phenomenon, for the results have not been found to be worthwhile. Treatment for this condition is directed toward the underlying disease.

Acrocyanosis

Acrocyanosis is a benign vasospastic disorder in which bluish color, coldness and moistness of the hands and feet are usually *persistent rather than transient*. The cyanotic appearance becomes more intense in a cold and stressful environment. These changes are not accompanied by pain, and complications rarely occur. Patients obviously appear to have a dysfunction of the sympathetic nervous system and are classified as "sympathetic reactors." Other patients with similar problems include those in whom color changes are not predominant but whose hands and feet are constantly cold and clammy: the "wet fish" hand. In acrocyanosis, the volar aspect of the hands and feet is very moist, while the dorsal aspect is usually dry. Interestingly, the cyanotic appearance disappears on elevation and during sleep. The underlying cause for this disorder may be some circulating hormonal agent or a high intrinsic tone in the muscular media of the vessels.

The only therapy that is usually required is assurance of the patient that the cause of the intense blueness of the hands is merely the patient's embarrassment in public. All patients should also be warned to avoid an extremely cold environment, trauma and infection, for they are excellent candidates for the bizarre sympathetic disorders that occur in patients who are "sympathetic reactors."

Sympatholytic drugs may occasionally be prescribed. Sympathectomy is unwarranted, for the disease is almost always uncomplicated except for the signs previously described. These signs usually are less evident in later life.

Livedo Reticularis

Livedo reticularis, unlike acrocyanosis and Raynaud's phenomenon, is not localized to the digits, hands and feet but characterized by a purplish "fish net" mottling of the skin of the legs, thighs, forearms, arms or trunk. Superficial ulcerations, when present, are situated proximal to the hands and feet. Treatment is symptomatic. Rarely is a sympathectomy justified unless the ulcerations become progressively larger and fail to heal in spite of appropriate débridement, antifungal drugs and antibiotics. Sympatholytic drugs, reserpine or guanethidine may be tried. A search for an underlying collagen disease or blood dyscrasia is advisable. As

with Raynaud's phenomenon and acrocyanosis, education of the patient is essential. The patient should particularly avoid cold temperatures and emotional stresses.

Acute Arterial Spasm

Acute arterial spasm has often been blamed but never proved as the primary cause of ischemia of tissue. Therefore, it should be considered, diagnosed and treated as a contributory but not causative factor in the ischemic findings. Such concern frequently occurs in patients who have iliofemoral thrombophlebitis or phlegmasia cerulea dolens and arterial injury. In addition, certain patients during examination and at surgery demonstrate a marked tendency toward arterial spasm, which often cannot be satisfactorily explained. Other conditions, such as vasculitis, hypercoagulability, high levels of circulatory catecholamines, hypovolemia, hypertensive disorders and other physiopathological states, should be considered. These patients usually have a rapid progression of their disease and frequently are poor candidates for surgery.

Acute Peripheral Arterial Occlusion

Acute occlusions of peripheral arteries necessitate early and accurate diagnosis followed by emergency medical and surgical procedures. Signs and symptoms relate to the occluded site, the extent to which the vessel(s) is occluded, the extension of the associated embolus or thrombus and the promptness with which appropriate therapy is instituted. Embolization is the most likely cause when pallor, pain and a decrease or loss of sensation and function occur with a decrease in or absence of distal pulse(s). Thrombosis, although often acute with similar findings, is usually insidious in its development and preceded by prodromal complaints.

Embolism, thrombosis or trauma with or without laceration may cause arterial occlusion. Embolectomy provides a much higher success rate than a thrombectomy, since an occluding thrombus encompasses a longer segment of an artery, which almost always has extensive vascular disease.

Extremities and Aortic Bifurcation

Aortic, femoral and popliteal artery bifurcations are the usual sites of lodgement of arterial emboli, since the vessel narrows at the point of its division. The axillary and brachial artery bifurcations are the usual sites for occlusion of the upper extremity arteries. Seldom do occlusions of upper extremity arteries cause a loss of the part, even without treatment. However, the hazard of losing the extremity does exist and the possibility of morbid changes such as contracture, pain and forearm claudication is significantly high; therefore, an embolectomy is indicated to assure maximum restoration of function in the great majority of cases. Aortic, iliac and lower extremity embolectomies are always indicated, especially when the embolus is lodged at the aortic bifurcation, for the patient may lose not only both lower extremities but also his life when surgery is inordinately delayed. When any degree of abdominal pain accompanies the signs and symptoms of an aortic bifurcation embolus, a mesenteric artery occlusion should be considered until proved otherwise. The presence of multiple emboli should be considered as a common occurrence.

ORIGIN OF THE EMBOLI. Most emboli originate in the heart from an auricular thrombus due to fibrillation, vegetative disease of the aortic or mitral valve or from a mural thrombosis following myocardial infarction. Other sources are atherosclerotic plaques from the wall of the aorta or other major

artery, platelet aggregate material in an atherosclerotic ulcer ("blue toe syndrome"), a clot within an aneurysm, pulmonary vein thrombosis or a thrombus in an injured artery. Other causes for embolization include missiles, tumor particles, paradoxical emboli through a right to left shunt in the heart, air, amniotic fluid and fat. However, all except fat are so rare that unless the history is reinforced by clinical findings, they are not considered. Fat emboli are fairly common following trauma.

Fewer large arterial emboli are noted today owing to improved therapy for cardiac lesions. Cardiac and peripheral vascular surgeons routinely check for unexpected emboli peripherally following surgery.

DIAGNOSIS. The classic signs and symptoms of acute arterial occlusion of an extremity usually result in the proper diagnosis. However, the classic signs and symptoms are not present in all patients. Therefore, the examining physician needs an "index of suspicion" to lessen the hazard of mortality or an increase of morbidity. Accompanying the suspicion of the presence of an acute arterial occlusion must be an aggressive attempt to utilize supplemental diagnostic procedures.

Arterial occlusion should be considered in a patient who presents with sudden or insidious complaints referrable to an extremity that, without injury or infection, demonstrates pallor when it is in a horizontal position and becomes worse on elevation. Pain per se is not important initially in more than half of the cases. However, when the discomfort of paresthesia or numbness is listed as pain the percentage is much greater. Decrease in or loss of sensation and function is related to the site and extent of the occlusive segment in addition to previously present vascular disease. On the skin the lines of demarcation of sensation and temperature changes seldom coincide, and the occlusive site is frequently proximal to the area of symptomatic changes. A decrease in distal pulse amplitude is synonymous with an absent pulse in a patient with a blood pressure that is normal or above normal.

Supplemental diagnostic aids such as arteriograms, the use of a Doppler flowmeter, oscillometric readings or plethysmography may confirm the suspicion of arterial occlusion. Arteriogram studies are beneficial not only to confirm the site of occlusion but also to determine the patency of the distal arterial system. Owing to the potential of multiple sites of occlusion in one or both lower extremities, arteriograms should be performed preoperatively and also following removal of the embolus or thrombus or repair of the injured vessel.

Left atrial enlargement, atrial fibrillation, recent myocardial infarction or a history of intermittent claudication are clinical findings that may indicate the presence of an embolus or thrombus in the extremity. In approximately 10 per cent of patients no source of embolus is demonstrated. Calf or forearm tenderness is usually present in more than one compartment in patients with arterial embolism. In patients with venous thrombosis, however, only the posterior compartment of the leg is tender, and this usually occurs only in the midline of the calf.

OBJECTIVES OF TREATMENT. (1) Relieve arterial spasm and pain by intra-arterial tolazoline hydrochloride (Priscoline) 25 mg, paravertebral sympathetic blocks, continuous epidural or spinal anesthesia or sciatic or median nerve infiltration. However, as previously mentioned, this approach treats only the contributory and not the causative factors for the ischemic findings. Caution must be exercised in diagnosis and treatment if the patient is in shock or has a lowered blood volume. (2) Do not allow extremes of temperature to the ischemic part. (3) Protect extremity from trauma with cotton wadding or foam rubber and board to the foot of the bed. The extremity is placed in a dependent position. (4) Administer heparin immediately, 7500 to 10,000 units intravenously. Heparin therapy lessens the likelihood of further emboli, slows the progression of a pre-existing arterial thrombus and retards development of venous thrombosis and sludging in the distal arterial tree. Its use may save the patient from arterial occlusion elsewhere and may also save the occluded part when surgery is delayed or not undertaken. When surgery is not performed, heparin is administered subcutaneously, 15,000 to 20,000 units every 12 hours.

Surgery may have to be postponed if acute arterial occlusion occurs in a community that does not have personnel or facilities to perform definitive vascular surgery, if operating room space or specialized personnel are unavailable, or for other reasons including the patient's condition. Regardless of the reason for postponement, the aforementioned procedures plus the administration of antibiotics should be instituted prior to transfer to another hospital or to surgery. Acute arterial occlusion is an urgent-emergent condition; it is not critical except when acute mesenteric vascular occlusion is suspected.

The optimal period for surgery is within ten hours of occurrence for an extremity arterial occlusion but immediately for a major mesenteric vascular occlusion. Later exploration is justified for the extremity only if patency of the distal major vessel can be clinically demonstrated. An arteriogram is warranted in most cases. Operation is definitely indicated for patients with an embolus to the bifurcation of the aorta or the common iliac artery. Unless contraindicated, patients with arterial emboli or thrombi are continued on half of the prescribed therapeutic dosage of heparin and 5 gr of aspirin orally twice daily after operation to minimize the danger of a second embolus or thrombus. If the patient is being given heparin during hospitalization he is usually converted to oral Coumadin or aspirin for long-standing prophylactic therapy. Some patients may need fasciotomies, especially if there has been an inordinate delay in the procedure. Fasciotomies are not performed unless definitive arterial surgery has also been attempted.

In either medical or surgical treatment, consider the cause. In arterial injury, occlusion is due to local factors alone; return of circulation is highly possible and should always be sought regardless of the time required. However, in embolus or thrombosis, inherent diseases are already present and time is of the essence. Before undertaking any procedure, the body as a whole should be considered.

Arterial Injuries

The conservative or nonoperative approach to arterial injuries is no longer an acceptable means of treatment.[64, 85] To prevent crippling, loss of limb or organ or loss of life, an aggressive and confident application of current surgical procedures is mandatory. Injury to a major artery is not unusual in a hospital emergency department, nor is overt trauma the chief cause of the injury. There is a significant incidence of vascular injuries that occur during diagnostic procedures, at operation and during therapeutic cardiopulmonary bypass. Occasionally these occur as late occlusions and do not present for diagnosis until the patient returns for a follow-up examination with symptoms of vascular insufficiency.

Initial Blood Loss

When a vascular injury occurs it is essential that emergency medical personnel both inside and outside the hospital recognize not only the presence of blood loss but also the need to estimate the amount lost. Blood volume following hemorrhage from a vascular injury may be roughly estimated by a few simple questions, maneuvers and calculations. (1) Ask the ambulance attendant what he observed regarding the patient at the accident scene and en route to the hospital. "Was the accident severe or minor?" "How much blood did the patient lose at the scene and en route?" (2) When the patient arrives at the hospital and shows no signs or symptoms of shock, ask or note if the arm veins were or are prominent after applying a tourniquet prior to beginning intravenous fluids. If so, then blood loss has not been excessive. (3) Elevate the lower limbs. If the pulse decreases and the blood pressure rises the patient is in relative hypovolemia. This is known as the *tilt test*. These signs reverse if the head and thorax are elevated; therefore, it is advisable to check both the patient's blood pressure and pulse before and after any movement. (4) To calculate roughly the body's blood volume deficit, we recognize that the body's volume of blood in parts is equal to approximately one-fifteenth of body weight. Therefore, the average male weighing from 150 to 180 lb will have from 5000 to 6000 ml of blood. Loss of 1000 ml, or 16 to 25 per cent of this blood volume, results in a moderate state of shock. This amount or more can be lost in the tissues of the thigh following a femoral shaft fracture. A loss of 30 per cent causes a severe state of shock, endangering the patient's survival. If the bleeding is uncontrolled, the body plunges deeper and deeper into shock and death may result in a matter of minutes. A significant number of these patients' lives can be saved and shock can be prevented by initiating the diagnosis and care of both the vascular injury and the blood loss at the scene and by continuing this process within the entire emergency medical services system. All of the variable situations are well known to every physician but need to be identified and discussed with ambulance technicians.

Diagnosis

Diagnosis of an arterial injury is not always obvious. The classic sign is a significant bright red bleeding with the ischemic extremity appearing pale, cadaverous or mottled, cold to the touch, with collapsed veins and absence of pulses. Recognition of arterial injury is usually not difficult in a nonobtunded patient who complains of pain in a nonbleeding extremity with characteristic diagnostic signs. However, the signs may be misleading in the presence of arteriosclerosis, shock or arterial spasm. It is not necessary to confirm diagnosis by the absence of a peripheral pulse. The conclusion that a decreased distal pulse is due to spasm should not be entertained for a prolonged period, for spasm alone does not cause loss of tissue. As stated previously, a decreased distal pulse should be considered synonymous to an absent distal pulse until proved otherwise. With a normal or even a decreased distal pulse, a definitive diagnosis sometimes cannot be made until débridement of the wound reveals a vascular injury. All injuries above the wrist or ankle should be explored if a peripheral pulse is diminished or absent, provided the patient is not in shock. This aggressive approach should be taken to increase the possibility of a successful outcome and to combat the high incidence of vascular injuries without laceration following blunt trauma. In blunt trauma there may be no penetration of the skin, but the distal arterial pulse is decreased or absent due to an intimal tear, perivascular hematoma, soft tissue edema or entrapment of the artery between fragments of bone.

Following fracture, dislocation of a joint, snake bite or prolonged use of an improperly placed tourniquet, a sign of major vascular injury is the presence of "fracture blisters" in the distal portion of the extremity. In these patients, compartment fasciotomies are performed routinely after the injured artery is repaired. The deep fascia is unable to expand under pressure of muscle edema that may occur preoperatively from a snake bite (usually only one compartment is involved) or shortly after repair of the artery when diapede-

sis occurs. An expanding hematoma may be present in only one compartment. Both the muscle edema and the expanding hematoma may thereby further occlude the arterial circulation when arterial injury is present or they may obstruct the artery by their resultant pressure. Readings of pressure may be obtained in one or more of the compartments to confirm the diagnosis.

Penetrating wounds are frequently an indication of vascular injury and may constitute an immediate threat to life from exsanguination. Late sequelae such as secondary hemorrhage, false aneurysm and arteriovenous fistula may be equally hazardous and are further reasons for an aggressive operative policy. Additional criteria demanding operation are: a pulsating or expanding hematoma and a penetrating wound over the course of a large vascular bundle such as the neck, axilla, brachium, antecubital space, femoral-inguinal area, popliteal space and the forearm and leg areas. A patient presenting with a penetrating wound in these areas should be admitted to the hospital either for exploration of the involved compartment(s) or for observation in an intensive care unit for a decrease in muscle or nerve function or in arterial supply to the distal part. These patients are observed for a minimum of 24 hours. Wounds that penetrate the fascia in these areas should not be considered minor, because the potential of an avoidable amputation is too great. Occasionally a fasciotomy may be required following muscle rupture below the elbow or knee when the rupture is accompanied by bleeding and no major artery is involved.

Treatment

Treatment must follow certain guidelines both at the emergency site and en route to the hospital via ambulance as well as within the hospital Emergency Department. The following protocol is not intended to suggest that the techniques and concepts are original but to identify procedures that are expected to give satisfactory results for ambulance attendants trained as emergency medical technicians, for Emergency Department personnel and for surgeons who perform the definitive arterial repair.

Emergency care begins by applying pressure directly to the wound to control bleeding. When this is unsuccessful in stopping hemorrhage a tourniquet may be employed, though it is rarely necessary. When a tourniquet is necessary it should not be loosened until a pressure dressing has been applied and blood or plasma expanders are available to treat or prevent shock. If hemorrhage is excessive when the tourniquet is released, bleeding may be controlled by pressure over the major artery proximal to the site of injury. Clamping a vessel blindly with hemostats must be avoided, since this may lead to damage of veins and nerves and may crush a portion of the artery. Airway obstruction, cardiac arrest and monitoring of shock have priority over hemorrhage. Sterile technique should be utilized at the hospital to prevent infection. Arteriography, although not always essential, may be necessary to determine the presence of a pre-existing arterial lesion, the type of vascular injury that has occurred, or a more exact localization of the site of arterial injury.

Definitive treatment of arterial injuries requires special facilities. Every general surgeon has been trained to do definitive vascular surgery, but the equipment necessary for quality care of a patient with an arterial injury may not be available. When these prerequisites are not present, immediate treatment of the injury should be limited to hemostasis, wound care and stabilization of the patient so he can be safely transferred to a hospital having the required special facilities. Details are essential for successful arterial surgery. Eighty per cent of all arterial injuries should have a successful outcome. Compromise does not serve the patient's in-terest and increases the possibility of an unsuccessful result.

Measures taken preoperatively or prior to transfer to another institution should include continuation of emergency procedures plus the following: (1) A central venous pressure catheter is placed through the brachial or jugular vein or directly into the subclavian vein. Every attempt is made to stabilize the patient with Ringer's lactate, bank blood or plasma expanders, or a combination. Vascular surgery is ordinarily contraindicated on hypotensive patients, but occasionally control of hemorrhage and revascularization of tissue is a prerequisite for control of shock. (2) A broad-spectrum antibiotic is given. (3) The adequacy of tetanus immunization is determined and tetanus toxoid is administered with or without tetanus immunoglobulin (human) as indicated. (4) Sympatholytic drugs and sympathetic blocks are contraindicated when there is arterial laceration or shock.

Infection, hemorrhage and reocclusion are the most frequent complications postoperatively and following discharge from the hospital.

Chronic Occlusive Arterial Disease

Chronic occlusive arterial disease has previously been regarded as a degenerative vascular disease that chiefly affects elderly males and men and women who have diabetes mellitus. More elderly people with chronic occlusive arterial disorders are seen now than in the past because the average life span is increasing. This condition is now being diagnosed with increasing frequency in younger, nondiabetic patients.

The clinician is increasingly apt to assess the circulatory reserve of the body's organs and extremities before making any conclusions regarding the choice of definitive medical or surgical treatment. Earlier and more accurate diagnosis has been made possible by various mechanical, electronic and laboratory facilities that were previously used only on an experimental basis. Nevertheless, confusion continues to exist regarding the complexities of possible diagnoses and therapeutic methods available in chronic occlusive disease.

Diagnosis

Arteriosclerosis obliterans is the most common peripheral chronic occlusive arterial disease. Symptoms are usually manifested in the lower extremities. Vasospastic conditions and vasculitis must be considered in the differential diagnosis. Any of these disorders may be complicated by infection, thrombosis or embolism. It is not uncommon for a patient to have multiple arterial occlusions, either partial or complete. They may occur in the symptomatic area as well as in the opposite lower extremity, the carotid, renal, coronary, subclavian and mesenteric arteries. These possibilities have a significant bearing on the diagnosis, prognosis and future course of treatment. It is important to note whether there is a family history of vascular disease: coronary disease or cerebral arterial disease, hypertension, diabetes, gangrene of an extremity or a hypercoagulable state. Other important aspects in the patient's history are age, sex, occupation, race, diet, smoking habits, hobbies and the presence of cardiac disease, hypertension, diabetes mellitus or anemia. Prior injury to any area of the body may also be pertinent. Neurological and intestinal complaints must be included, even though they may seem bizarre. Inquiry should be made about a history of ulceration or frostbite of the extremities. A reduction in exercise tolerance must be described, including the character, location, period of onset and duration, and aggravating conditions relating to the pain. Loss of sexual function in the male is an important indication of aortoiliac occlusive disease (Leriche's syndrome).

Pathology

The histopathological changes in atherosclerosis are primarily intimal, with extension into the inner media but avoidance of the outer media and adventitia. This process may begin by a platelet and fibrin thrombus repairing an intimal break or by liproproteins from the blood infiltrating the intimal lining. Both thrombus and lipoproteins may accumulate and form fibrosis and plaques, which in turn narrow the vessel lumen. When this process continues and is accompanied by subplaque hemorrhage and a superimposed mural thrombus, the vessel ultimately becomes occluded. Ulcerated atheroma occurring within a nonobstructed artery may be the origin of peripheral emboli that obstruct distal smaller caliber arteries. Such emboli contribute to limb ischemia by reducing the perfusion of the distal arterial network.[13]

Although the histopathological picture of chronic occlusive arterial disease may vary, the gross changes may be classified as follows:

1. *Segmental,* involving short distances of the aortoiliac, femoral popliteal, tibioperoneal, carotid, vertebral, subclavian, celiac, mesenteric and renal arteries. Treatment for these lesions is chiefly surgical. The etiology is primarily arteriosclerosis, but may occasionally be a previous injury, a localized arteritis of unknown origin or mechanical entrapment.

2. *Diffuse,* involving arteries throughout most or all of their length. Treatment may be surgical or medical depending on adequate distal arterial patency. The etiology is also chiefly arteriosclerosis, with an occasional case caused by a more extensive arteritis.

3. *Small vessel* disease associated with metabolic, allergic and hemato-

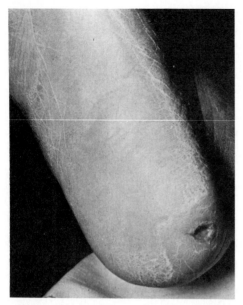

Figure 17–19 Ulceration of the heel in a diabetic patient. Although the ulceration is small and relatively painless, osteomyelitis is present and the patient required hospitalization for extensive débridement. Small vessel arterial disease alone or distal emboli from ulcerated atheroma, or both, in these patients frequently leads to the loss of the digits or parts of the foot, even when pedal pulses are present.

logical disorders. The diseases include diabetes mellitus (Figs. 17–19 and 17–20), collagen diseases, polycythemia vera, dysproteinemia, distal emboli from ulcerated atheroma, and other

conditions. Treatment for these disorders is chiefly medical.

The Lower Extremities

Arteriosclerosis obliterans is the commonest disease of the lower extremities. The symptoms of arteriosclerosis obliterans are entirely the result of ischemia of tissues. The symptoms are increased in relation to the proximity of the occluded artery, the extent of obstruction in the potential collaterals and the time involved in the development of the occlusion. The appearance of symptoms may be gradual and unnoticed or may be misinterpreted owing to the slow progression of occlusion. Symptoms may also be sudden in onset when a thrombus obliterates a relatively short segment of the artery. Sudden occlusion may not be interpreted as an acute process if excellent collateral channels are present. The disability period may be so short that the patient at first believes the symptoms will ultimately disappear. Symptoms may, however, stabilize to those noted in the slow process of arterial obliteration. A third pattern is observed when the occluded segment involves such a short area of the artery that symptoms are mild or absent. The previously mentioned abrupt episodes may occur in

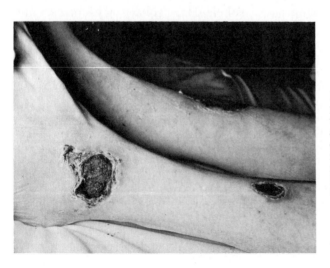

Figure 17–20 Ulcerations of the lower extremities in a diabetic patient, complicated by proximal arterial occlusions and small vessel arterial disease. Four attempts at débridement and skin grafting failed to heal the ulcers. Healing required proximal arterial surgery, bilateral lumbar sympathectomies and a fifth attempt at skin grafting.

sequence, with partial subsidence after each episode. However, the extremity becomes more symptomatic each time this occurs. Gradations of severity may be listed briefly as those patients who have (1) asymptomatic arteriosclerosis, (2) intermittent claudication, (3) nocturnal ischemic pain and (4) ischemic ulcers or gangrene (tissue loss).

Location of the Occlusion

Location of the occlusion will frequently determine the site and extent of the signs and symptoms. The sites may be in the aortoiliac, femoral popliteal or tibioperoneal arteries. When both high and low occlusions are present, high occlusion decreases the arterial flow to a certain degree and low occlusion further diminishes the blood flow. In isolated occlusions the prognosis is worse with the more distal occlusions. In aortoiliac artery occlusion the early course of the disease consists of an incomplete occlusion of one of the common iliac arteries (Fig. 17–21). This area later becomes completely occluded by thrombosis or dissection of blood beneath the atherosclerotic plaque. The process ultimately involves the other iliac artery and propagates upward toward the renal arteries. Occasionally only the terminal portion of the aorta is involved. The most common entity noted today is not the syndrome of bilateral aortic occlusion, first described by Leriche[52] in 1923, but a unilateral common iliac artery occlusion with early enroachment on the opposite common iliac vessel. This type of occlusion process is most commonly noted in men in the fifth and sixth decades of life. When both common iliac arteries or the abdominal aorta is occluded, impotence is common and the

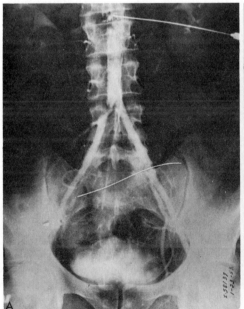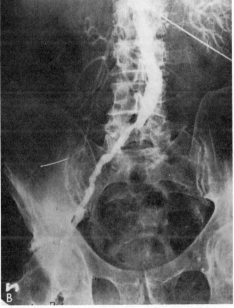

Figure 17–21 Arteriosclerosis obliterans. *A.* Localized occlusion of the right common iliac artery was treated with endarterectomy. *B.* Diffuse disease in this patient extended from the aorta down the left iliac artery, which was completely occluded, and it was also extensive in the right iliofemoral system. Surgery was not performed because of the diffuse nature of the disease. However, if symptoms and signs of lower limb ischemia are disabling, either a femoral-femoral or an axillofemoral bypass procedure is indicated when there is a distal patent run-off artery.

Leriche syndrome is present. Impotence may also occur with bilateral occlusion of both hypogastric arteries alone.

The most common site of occlusion is in the superficial femoral artery, beginning in Hunter's canal just proximal to the origin of the superior genicular artery. Occlusion extends proximally by thrombosis until the process reaches the area of the profunda femoris artery, which is the major collateral to the superior genicular artery and the distal vessels. Primary occlusion of the popliteal artery is seen more often in women and young men and is more frequently noted in the upper half of the vessel below its beginning at the exit of Hunter's canal. Popliteal occlusion may stop just proximal to the origin of the anterior tibial artery, or it may extend further to the tibioperoneal bifurcation. More extensive involvement may result in a diffuse, segmental disease involving the anterior tibial, posterior tibial and peroneal arteries. Multiple segmental occlusions occur far more commonly when the primary occlusion occurs below the inguinal ligament. This distribution is probably due to the slow flow rate present with distal occlusions compared with the high flow rate present through collaterals that are available with an aortoiliac occlusion.

About one third of superficial femoral artery occlusions will be bilateral within five years. However, the severity of occlusion in one extremity does not necessarily mirror that in the other.

Symptoms

Pain is the most significant early symptom that brings the patient to a physician. This symptom may be of four types: intermittent claudication, night cramps, superficial foot pain and ischemic or deep neuritic pain. The last two types are often grouped together as "rest pain." Only two of these types of pain, intermittent claudication and is-

chemic neuritis, are reproducible pains of arterial insufficiency. The types of pain caused by arterial insufficiency were discussed in detail in the introductory section of this chapter.

Occasionally venous congestion may be interpreted as claudication when the leg has the discomfort of heaviness or a "bursting" sensation. No relief occurs when the patient stops walking unless the extremity is elevated. In contrast, in arterial occlusion the claudication disappears within minutes after stopping, or even sooner, and elevation increases the pain. The past history and a physical examination should confirm the presence of deep venous obliterative disease.

Similarly, other conditions that may be identified as "pseudoclaudication" are osteoarthritis of the hip or knee and low neurospinal pain. Each can be readily excluded when the symptoms noted while taking a careful history and the signs found on physical examination do not match the severity and distribution of a complaint related to the arterial circulation.

Gout must be excluded since its presence is not uncommon in atherosclerotic patients.

Other rest pains that may be noted are pretrophic pain, pain of ulceration and gangrene and pain of disuse atrophy. All pain syndromes that occur in the extremity should be studied as to their physiological relationships and not grouped primarily according to their anatomical location or environment.

Signs

Physical findings in patients with arteriosclerosis obliterans are generally indistinguishable from the signs of occlusive arterial disease due to other conditions such as arteritis, arterial embolism and nongangrenous arterial thrombosis. When both extremities are involved it is uncommon for the changes to be symmetrical.

Color changes may be diagnostic of

decreased arterial circulation when pallor is noted in the distal portion of the limb. However, this is common in acute arterial occlusion but not in chronic occlusive arterial disease unless very advanced disease is present. The color of the feet appears normal in mild cases of arteriosclerosis obliterans. When advanced disease is present the foot may be red, especially when the extremity is dependent. This denotes a relaxed peripheral arteriolar bed where the vessel wall is receiving too little arterial blood to maintain its tone. Prognosis is poor if redness prevails when the extremity is horizontal. Testing for postural color changes is an excellent and simple means of obtaining valuable information concerning the degree of arterial occlusive disease. By elevating the legs to a 45 degree angle and rapidly flexing and extending the feet at the ankles, an impaired cutaneous circulation will present pallor on the plantar surface of the foot. Pallor on elevation, rubor on dependency and the presence of a normal color on a horizontal level demonstrates a mild-to-moderate arterial insufficiency. The two feet are compared with each other. The legs are elevated for two minutes and then suddenly placed in a dependent position. Failure of the color to return in 15 seconds denotes a moderate degree of arterial insufficiency. If the color changes are delayed for 30 seconds, arterial insufficiency is usually of a marked degree. A delay of 60 seconds indicates an advanced state of arterial occlusive disease. The time required for venous filling of the foot will provide similar information. Normally the superficial veins of the feet empty rapidly on elevation and refill within 10 to 12 seconds when the legs are placed in a dependent position. Significant prolongation of this time denotes occlusive arterial disease. This is a good means of measuring not only the status of arterial occlusive disease in the major vessels but also the small arteries when pedal pulses may be present. The tone of small cutaneous vessels may be evalu-

ated by pressing firmly on the skin of the toes for several seconds and removing the finger suddenly. Normally the pallor produced is momentary and the normal color returns in one to two seconds. When the color return is delayed for four to five seconds, circulatory impairment is present either from spasm or occlusive disease.

Skin temperature difference is suggestive of arterial insufficiency when one foot or the toes are lowered and compared with the other foot.

Muscle weakness denotes an extreme degree of arterial insufficiency. The presence of a foot drop should be detected by comparison of the dorsiflexion of both feet. When foot drop is present the patient should be informed of its presence so that trauma to the toes of the involved foot may be prevented. Similar observation should be made regarding stiffness of joints due to muscle weakness or prolonged disuse of the limb.

Trophic changes occur due to poor tissue nutrition. Hair distribution may be decreased or absent on the feet and toes. In more advanced cases the skin may appear shiny, and nail growth is retarded. The presence of edema in the foot and leg is usually a sign of advanced occlusive disease. It generally is noted in association with severe pain and gangrenous lesions. As previously stated, the patient with advanced disease usually finds it necessary to sit up for successive nights with his feet in a dependent position in an attempt to relieve the pain of ischemic neuritis.

Impaired arterial pulsation is the most significant finding on physical examination in occlusive arterial disease. A decreased or absent pulse will establish the presence of arterial disease and the location of the occlusion. Palpation of peripheral pulses is usually the first method of screening patients with symptoms suggestive of intermittent claudication when ruling out occlusive vascular disease. However, the presence of a pulse does not exclude the existence of arterial occlusion. Significant obstruction of an artery may be present in patients with palpable resting pedal pulses that disappear as claudication appears with exercise. In these patients collaterals are not sufficient to supply the flow necessary for the exercise performed. Failure to locate a pedal pulse by palpation identifies the *presence* of arterial disease. The absence of a popliteal pulse suggests that the occlusion may be relieved by surgery, since it identifies the *location* of obstruction in the femoral or iliac artery. The popliteal pulse is easily accessible behind the knee when the patient is supine and is located either in the midline or slightly lateral. The prone method of examination may also be used, with the knee flexed at 60 degrees and relaxed and the foot resting on the examiner's shoulder. The clinician who routinely palpates for a popliteal pulse will occasionally find a popliteal aneurysm. Popliteal aneurysms are of significance because of the risk of rupture and because they are the sources of emboli that cause distal arterial occlusion. Another cause for popliteal artery occlusion is a gastrocnemius entrapment when the popliteal artery is located laterally, traversing the lateral head of the gastrocnemius muscle.

There should be little concern when the dorsalis pedis pulse is absent. However, the congenital absence of a posterior tibial artery is very uncommon. When neither of these pulses is palpable a routine check should be made for a possible peroneal artery pulse, which — when present — lies just anterior to the lateral malleolus.

Auscultation can be a valuable procedure in checking the abdominal aorta and the iliac and proximal femoral arteries. In many cases of arterial disease of the extremity no bruits are heard because the occlusion is complete. However, when unilateral symptoms are present, the nonsymptomatic extremity will occasionally present a systolic murmur, which is an indication of early stenosis. In aortoiliac obstruction, auscultation over the femoral area may reveal the degree of stenosis.

Ancillary Diagnostic Studies

The diagnosis of chronic arterial occlusive disease is almost always possible by history and physical examination alone. Claudication with exercise and ischemic rest pain with recumbency are readily separated from nonvascular pain syndromes, and with the presence of pulse deficits, bruits or trophic ischemic changes there is usually little room for doubt. Therefore, ancillary studies are mainly used to (1) investigate the etiology of occlusive disease, (2) evaluate other major organ systems to determine the nature and severity of intercurrent disease that may affect operative risk and (3) determine the location, extent and functional severity of the occlusive disease itself. The usual practice is to obtain these studies on an inpatient basis, performing arteriography last, immediately prior to the intended operation.

The recognition by health insurance programs of the value of preadmission studies in either avoiding unnecessary hospitalization or reducing its duration may increase the use of these studies. For this reason, a discussion of the studies commonly included in the preoperative evaluation of candidates for arterial reconstructive surgery is presented in this chapter even though many will continue to be obtained after admission.

Detailed guidelines for the work-up of various vascular disorders requiring surgery have been prepared by a committee of the Society for Vascular Surgery[18] for Professional Standards Review Organization (PSRO) review purposes. They include indications for admission, anticipated length of hospitalization for preoperative evaluation, operation and postoperative care; expected services performed; routine and special diagnostic procedures; and special therapeutic and nursing requirements. A complete blood count, urinalysis, blood urea nitrogen, creatinine, multiphasic screening or biochemical profile, glucose tolerance test, EKG and chest x-ray are almost routinely advised. Patients with a history of myocardial infarction, congestive heart failure or angina and those with an abnormal EKG probably should have a stress EKG and possibly even coronary angiography. Similarly, screening tests for carotid artery occlusive disease, such as oculoplethysmography, the Doppler study of supraorbital hemodynamics, and common carotid artery velocity wave form analysis, are recommended in arteriosclerotic patients. The likelihood of such patients suffering a fatal myocardial infarction or cerebral vascular accident within five years of peripheral arterial reconstruction ranges from 20 to 50 per cent, the degree of risk correlating with the extent and severity of the peripheral arterial occlusive disease.

Obviously, if the underlying problem is atherosclerosis, serum cholesterol and triglyceride tests and lipoprotein electrophoresis should be ordered, and if thrombotic or embolic events have marked its course a coagulation profile should be obtained. Any intercurrent disease should be investigated on its own merits, but renal and pulmonary function should be routinely evaluated.

Invasive Diagnosis

With the development of noninvasive diagnostic techniques that can determine the location and functional severity of the occlusive lesions, *arteriography* is now normally reserved for patients with indications for surgery in order to provide the surgeon with a "road map" before embarking on the reconstructive procedure. Occasionally, arteriography will show that arterial reconstruction is not feasible because of the condition of the arterial tree distal to the major occlusion, but its main value is in establishing the most appropriate reconstructive procedure by visualizing the arteries proximal and distal to the obstruction. In this regard it should be remembered that the vast majority of patients whose symptoms

are severe enough to warrant surgery have a combination of occlusive lesions in series or in parallel. The most common lesion, superficial femoral artery occlusion, will not by itself produce very disabling symptoms if there has been sufficient time and stimulus for full collateral development.

Although arteriography techniques have improved, arteriograms must be interpreted with caution, for they usually supply anatomical information in only a single plane and little or no functional information. Haimovici[31] showed that anterior-posterior views of the iliac arteries were misleading in 40 per cent of cases, and in the face of superficial femoral occlusion, the patency of the popliteal artery and its branches was misjudged in 25 per cent of cases.

Overnight hospitalization is suggested if a translumbar aortogram or selective arteriography using a long catheter is performed. Translumbar aortography should not be performed in hypertensive patients or in those who have any tendency toward bleeding. The use of aspirin or sulfinpyrazone (Anturane) and even of low-dose heparin has been recommended to prevent clotting at the site where the long catheter is lodged during the procedure.

Noninvasive Diagnosis

Noninvasive diagnostic methods (1) allow the presence or absence of significant peripheral arterial occlusive disease (PAOD) to be established without arteriography, (2) provide functional information that aids in the selection and interpretation of arteriography, (3) place the indications for operation on a more objective basis, (4) aid in selecting the most appropriate procedure when multiple occlusive lesions are present and (5) allow the technical adequacy to be easily monitored.

DOPPLER EXAMINATION. The Doppler ultrasonic velocity detector gives information about the velocity and, by inference, about the flow of blood in accessible peripheral arteries. The Doppler signal may be processed with an audio frequency analyzer, recorded as a velocity wave form on a simple strip chart after passage through a zero crossing circuit or other frequency-to-voltage converter, or simply used to drive a speaker to produce audible sounds. All three methods share the same basic characteristics and, for most clinical work, the simpler audible signal suffices, although velocity wave form analyses have particular value in certain situations, which will be described later.

The velocity profile of an extremity artery normally has a sharp systolic peak followed by a variable degree of end-systolic reversal and a brief period of forward flow in early diastole. Because of the absence of significant end-diastolic arterial flow in the resting extremity, the velocity tracing rests on the zero baseline (Fig. 17–22). The normal arterial sound is triphasic in the lower extremity but biphasic in the upper extremity, where the end-systolic reversal is reduced or even absent. However, the first sound is always high-pitched. In contrast, below a *complete* obstruction there is only a single, broad, low-velocity wave whose equiv-

alent sound is therefore low-pitched and monophasic. Beyond a hemodynamically significant stenosis, the systolic downslope will be widened and irregular and often will cover up the second and third velocity components. In addition, since flow immediately distal to a significant stenosis may be continuous and turbulent, the Doppler sound at this point is like an amplified bruit and the velocity tracing, although still pulsatile, will be elevated above the zero baseline and contain minor irregularities representing turbulence. Thus, by simply surveying the major arteries in an extremity with a Doppler probe, one can determine from the characteristics of the arterial sounds whether flow is obstructed, post-stenotic or postobstructive.

SEGMENTAL LIMB SYSTOLIC PRESSURES.   The determination of segmental limb systolic pressures (SLP) is the single most valuable noninvasive diagnostic study for PAOD. Using multiple sphygmomanometer cuffs (e.g. on upper and lower thigh, calf and ankle) and employing a Doppler probe rather than the stethoscope to signal the return of flow during cuff deflation, the systolic pressure can be measured at multiple levels throughout the periph-

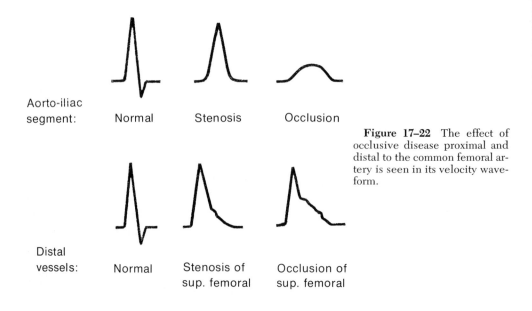

Aorto-iliac
segment: Normal   Stenosis   Occlusion

Figure 17–22 The effect of occlusive disease proximal and distal to the common femoral artery is seen in its velocity waveform.

Distal
vessels: Normal   Stenosis of   Occlusion of
                                  sup. femoral   sup. femoral

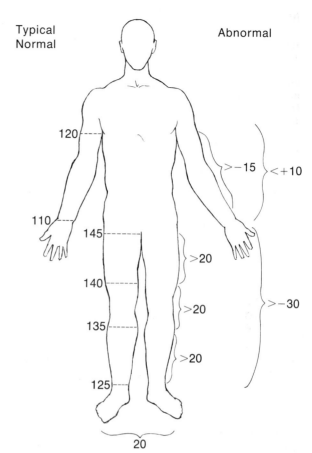

Typical Normal

Abnormal

120

>−15

<+10

110

145

>20

140

>20

>−30

135

>20

125

20

Figure 17–23 Segmental systolic pressures (mm Hg).

eral arterial tree and the presence of significant gradients between segments can be used to localize hemodynamically significant occlusive lesions. What constitutes a significant segmental pressure gradient has been established by a number of studies.[84] Typical normal SLP values are shown in Figure 17–23 along with the upper limits of normal for pressure gradients between different locations. As a general rule, a pressure gradient greater than 20 mm Hg between adjacent cuffs or between cuffs at the same level in the lower extremities indicates an occlusive lesion. A pressure drop greater than 15 mm Hg in the upper extremity or a 30 mm Hg drop in the lower extremity can also be considered abnormal. Because of the relatively greater girth of the upper thigh and the fact that

transmission of the standing arterial pressure wave down the aorta results in some systolic augmentation, the upper thigh systolic pressue should be at least 10 mm Hg higher than the brachial pressure if there is no aortoiliac occlusive disease. However, it must be kept in mind that dissipation of the pressure wave by an intervening aortic aneurysm may produce a similar effect.

If the proximal extent of a superficial femoral artery occlusion is high enough, the upper thigh cuff, which straddles the femoral bifurcation, may give a low value, suggesting proximal iliac occlusive disease. This is particularly true if a single large thigh cuff is used in an attempt to avoid the artifact produced by excessive thigh girth. Difficulty in determining the correct upper thigh pressure represents a serious weakness in this method, because iliac artery stenosis is hemodynamically more important than complete occlusion of the superficial femoral artery and should be the focus of reconstructive efforts if these two lesions coexist. In most cases an inflatable inguinal compressor will occlude the common femoral artery well above its bifurcation and eliminate this problem. At other times, direct pressure measurements may be necessary. These can be made at the clinic or bedside using the simple apparatus shown in Figure 17–24. A brachial-femoral mean pressure

gradient greater than 10 mm Hg at rest is considered significant. Such a pressure gradient can be accentuated by exercise, postischemic reactive hyperemia or vasodilator drugs. A drop in femoral artery pressure of greater than 20 per cent when hyperemia is provoked by one of these methods is considered abnormal. Femoral artery velocity wave form analysis, as described later, provides an alternative means of identifying occlusive lesions proximal or distal to the femoral artery.

An additional source of error in segmental limb pressure measurement is

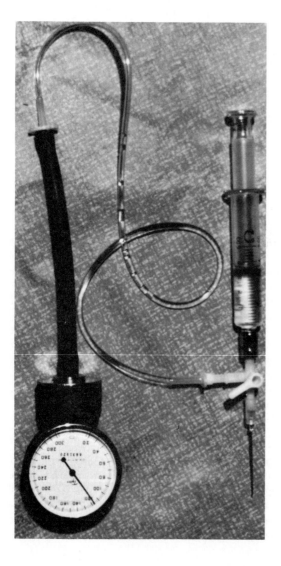

Figure 17–24 The basic equipment necessary for measuring intra-arterial mean pressure, as assembled, consists of a sphygmomanometer head, plastic extension tubing, a three-way stopcock, a 20 G needle and a 5 ml glass syringe filled with heparinized saline. (From: Rutherford, R. B.: A simplified method of obtaining mean intra-arterial pressure in the clinic or operating room. *In*: Rutherford, R. B. (ed.): Vascular Surgery. Philadelphia, W. B. Saunders Co., 1977, p. 134.)

the falsely high value produced by heavy calcification of peripheral arteries, as seen in diabetic and uremic patients. Even as much as 300 mm Hg pressure applied via the sphygmomanometer cuff may not occlude these rigid vessels. The knowledge that the patient had diabetes or renal insufficiency, the demonstration of heavy calcification in the peripheral vessels on x-ray and the abnormal pattern of rising segmental limb pressures as one proceeds peripherally should alert the examiner to this pitfall. In such cases, segmental pulse volume contours recorded plethysmographically provide a better impression of the arterial circulation at each level.

ANKLE PRESSURE RESPONSE TO PROVOKED HYPEREMIA. If there are obvious systolic pressure gradients at rest, further provocative tests are unnecessary. However, in patients with mild to moderate claudication, particularly if it is due to iliac artery stenosis, there may not be an obvious pressure gradient at rest but only during reactive hyperemia. The clinical cause of this phenomenon is the loss of pedal pulses following exercise. In most vascular diagnostic laboratories this is standardized by having the patient walk on a 12° inclined treadmill for five minutes at 2 mph, following which ankle pressures are serially monitored and compared with the pre-exercise level. A drop in ankle pressure greater than 20 per cent confirms the diagnosis of claudication, and the degree and duration of the drop correlate with the severity of the occlusive disease. This test is particularly useful in monitoring patients following arterial reconstruction both to test the adequacy of the procedure and to assure continued functional patency. Thus, if a femoral popliteal bypass restores ankle pressure to normal and if pressure does not drop significantly with treadmill exercise, the vessel is widely patent and there is good "run off." If such a patient subsequently develops a pressure gradient with exercise, arteriography is indicated, and if

anastomotic narrowing is revealed, a relatively simple procedure may save the graft before it progresses to complete occlusion and requires complete arterial reconstruction.

Because the systemic systolic pressure of patients varies, absolute values for segmental limb pressure do not allow adequate comparisons between patients or between serial measurements in the same patient. This is particularly true of hypertensive patients receiving drug therapy. Therefore, it is recommended that the recorded segmental limb pressures always be related to the highest brachial pressure, which is considered to represent systemic systolic pressure. The normal ankle-to-arm index has been found to be 1.14 ± 0.7.[77] Whenever this ratio is less than one, an occlusive lesion in that lower extremity should be suspected.

PLETHYSMOGRAPHY. For many years, the measurement of blood flow in the calf by venous occlusion plethysmography was the main noninvasive diagnostic test of arterial occlusive disease. Although this method is accurate, decreased flow usually does not occur at rest until the patient has progressed to the point of ischemic rest pain or actual tissue loss. Furthermore, even though this method can be made more sensitive by measuring blood flow before and during a period of reactive hyperemia, it does not correlate any better with the severity of the occlusive disease than the simpler measurement of ankle pressure response to provoked hyperemia. For that reason plethysmography, using either the strain gauge, impedance or volume displacement techniques, is now used mainly to record segmental pulse volume curves. These measurements are most valuable in studying digital circulation, assessing segmental circulation in diabetics and uremics, and detecting venous occlusive disease (see previous discussion).

VELOCITY WAVE FORM ANALYSIS. Although Gosling and associates[29] have established that comparison of the arterial velocity wave form at two adjacent locations in an extremity is a sensitive method of detecting occlusive lesions in the intervening segment, the technical requirements for simultaneous monitoring of two velocity wave forms has limited the application of this technique. However, Fronek[24] showed that the femoral artery velocity wave form alone could be helpful in distinguishing aortoiliac from femoral-popliteal occlusive disease. Subsequently, Nicolaides[61] identified those dimensions whose measurement allows this differentiation to be made with a high degree of accuracy. Figure 17–22 shows a normal femoral artery velocity wave form with its sharp systolic peak, end-systolic reversal and brief early diastolic flow. Even partial occlusion of the proximal iliac artery will cause broadening and irregularities on the downslope of the systolic peak, obliterating the end-systolic reversal. In contrast, distal occlusion (e.g., of the superficial femoral artery) reduces the systolic peak and accentuates the end-systolic reversal.

In summary, in the vast majority of cases, measurement of segmental limb pressures will localize a significant arterial occlusive lesion, and if it does not, the additional study of the ankle response to treadmill exercise, segmental pulse volume contours or the arterial velocity wave form should be diagnostic.

Treatment

The indications for medical and surgical teatment vary, depending on the area of the body in which arterial occlusive disease is present. Indications also depend on the patient's general medical status, the extent of arterial disease elsewhere and the patient's symptoms.

The patient must be evaluated regarding cerebral, renal and cardiac status before any major elective vascular reconstructive procedure is recommended. The extent of disease in these three systems has considerable bearing on the risk of surgery and on the patient's life expectancy.

The proper selection of patients for operative treatment is a cornerstone of clinical ability for the vascular surgeon, ranking in importance with technical skill. The surgeon must weigh carefully both the degree of disability and the natural or nonoperatively treated course of the underlying vascular disorder against the risk and projected benefits of the operation under consideration.

The degree of disability often constitutes only a relative indication when considered against the background of the patient's work and other normal activities. Elective vascular reconstruction may be recommended for relatively minor symptoms related to the carotid arteries, whereas claudication after walking 100 yards may not interfere with the rather sedentary lives of many retired people, so surgery would not be necessary. But to one who has worked long and hard in anticipation of a retirement filled with golf, fishing or hunting, the same degree of claudication constitutes a serious restriction. Claudication usually interferes significantly with the lives of most working people and is an accepted indication for surgery in this group. Similarly, abdominal angina may be sufficient indication for iliac or mesenteric artery reconstruction. Ischemic rest pain with dependent rubor, in contrast, is an utterly disabling pain that often cannot be controlled even with strong analgesics or narcotics and therefore is a universally accepted indication for surgery at any age.

NATURAL HISTORY. The natural history or nonoperatively treated course of the underlying condition adds a further dimension, as exemplified by these same examples. Peabody's Framingham study[70] reported that patients with intermittent claudication had approximately a 5 per cent risk of major amputation for gangrene within five years of the onset of this symptom, if treated expectantly, whereas within the same period 23 per cent developed symptoms of coronary insufficiency, 13 per cent suffered cerebrovascular accidents and 20 per cent died.

At least one-third of patients operated on for *advanced* arteriosclerosis obliterans involving the lower extremity will die of heart disease or stroke within five years. The degree of associated arteriosclerotic coronary disease must be considered, for a patent femoral-popliteal bypass can hardly be considered a success if relief of claudication unmasks the existence of angina pectoris. On the other hand, once arteriosclerosis obliterans has progressed to cause ischemic rest pain with dependent rubor, the eventual need for major amputation is high if arterial reconstruction is not undertaken.

One of the goals of reconstructive surgery is to prevent gangrene. Established gangrene was formerly considered only to be an indication for amputation. However, minor (e.g., digital) gangrene due to occlusive disease of major proximal arteries usually requires major proximal amputation to achieve primary healing. Therefore, we favor arterial reconstruction in these instances to prevent further tissue loss and to allow a limited débridement or spontaneous amputation to heal. Thus, the surgical attitude becomes more aggressive with increasing severity of peripheral arteriosclerotic occlusive disease.

RISK OF OPERATIVE PROCEDURE. The risk of the operative procedure, in terms of morbidity and mortality, must be weighed on the other side of the scale. Even though patients with arteriosclerosis are generally at a higher than average risk for their age, they tolerate operations limited to the extremities, neck or superficial layers of the trunk fairly well. Vascular procedures confined to these areas carry a relatively small risk. This risk is not greater than the risk attending the major amputation that might be required if arterial reconstruction is not undertaken. However, these patients would be exposed to risk which is three times higher if the arterial reconstruction is performed through the thoracic or abdominal cavity, as in the case of aortoiliac reconstruction.

In patients with two hemodynamically significant lesions, the proximal lesion is more important, even though the distal lesion may have a greater degree of occlusion. This knowledge had resulted in a greater percentage of aortoiliac bypass operations compared with femoropopliteal bypass procedures in patients with lesions in both areas. Fortunately, this apparent dilemma of having to shift towards the higher-risk operation has been avoided somewhat by the option now provided by the so-called "extra-anatomic" bypass procedures, e.g., the femoral-femoral or axillary-femoral bypass. Because of these and other alternatives, such as femoral profundoplasty, it is rare today for the vascular surgeon to be forced to turn down the patient with advanced arteriosclerosis because of the risk of reconstructive arterial surgery itself.

In predicting the risk and success of a vascular operation, the common practice of quoting large reported series may be misleading for several reasons. First, the surgeon may be more or less experienced than those reporting these results, depending on the degree to which the procedures were performed by experienced vascular surgeons or house staff-in-training. Second, the particular patient to whom this yardstick is being applied is not likely to fit exactly the average risk of a particular series. His or her risk for the same operation depends on the coexistence of other significant systemic disorders such as hypertension, diabetes or chronic obstructive pulmonary disease as well as on the degree of arteriosclerotic involvement of the coronary and cerebral arteries. The estimation of operative risk clearly must be individualized.

Third it is not uncommon for large series to extend back over a decade or longer and therefore they do not reflect accurately the more recent technical advances or the subtle but cumulative benefits of experience. It was during the sixties that vascular surgeons were obliged to inform patients of a 5 per cent and 15 per cent risk of loss of life and limb, respectively, for arterial reconstructive procedures on the lower extremity. Today, these risks have been greatly reduced. Aortic aneurysmectomy and carotid endarterectomy have experienced similar major reductions in morbidity and mortality during the same period. Increasingly frequent detection of small, asymptomatic abdominal aortic aneurysms has caused an apparent reduction in the risk of aneurysm rupture and even encouraged a more conservative attitude on the part of many physicians. Nevertheless, concomitant advances in anesthesia and preoperative, intraoperative and postoperative management have reduced the risk of elective aneurysmectomy by a factor of at least one third. Better preservation of renal function, avoidance of cross-clamping shock and the endoaneurysmal approach are important advances. Similarly, refinements in the methods of providing protection for the cerebral circulation during carotid endarterectomy and better case selection have reduced the rate of mortality and major morbidity (i.e., neurological deficit) from 8 to 10 per cent to less than 2 per cent each.

The oft-quoted 15 per cent five-year failure rate for arterial prosthesis partly reflects the incidence of anastomotic aneurysms and occlusion by sloughing pseudointima, complications more commonly associated with the era of silk sutures and tightly woven Dacron grafts. The rate of failure in the procedure to "harvest" a satisfactory saphenous vein graft for femoral-popliteal by-pass has been reduced

from 20 per cent to almost 5 per cent. Similarly, the frequency of late occlusion of these vein grafts because of atheromatous degeneration, intimal fibrosis, paravalvular stenosis or other conditions should decrease now that the causes of damage to the vein during its preparation for surgery have been recognized and can be avoided.

Clearly then, it is not possible to predict the future from the past with perfect accuracy. On the other hand, if the limitations of the data from such reported series are recognized, the information can still provide a better frame of reference than recent personal memory or anecdotal information. For this reason, the combined results of several major series of some of the more common vascular procedures are presented in Tables 17–6 to 17–9. While these averages do not truly represent current expectations for these procedures, they do present minimum standards against which one's own results may be compared and future results projected. In this regard, currently reported mortality rates for elective aortoiliac bypass grafting, whether for occlusive or aneurysmal disease, are in the range of 2 to 3 per cent. The amputation rate following reconstructive procedures for lower extremity ischemia should be less than 5 per cent, but the more distal the reconstructive procedure and the higher the ratio of desperate limb salvage cases to those with claudication only, the higher the amputation rate.

The indications for sympathectomy vary, but this procedure may be the only available means of increasing blood supply to the skin. It has been a useful means to relieve rest pain in some patients who have poor "run-off" from the popliteal artery, with only one or two branches of the popliteal artery patent. Sympathectomy is commonly performed as an adjunct to aortoiliac reconstruction and can usually be counted on to produce a warm foot immediately after operation. The possibility that sympathectomy can produce a "steal" syndrome is still debated. It appears that a unilateral sympathectomy can worsen the flow to one extremity by increasing the cutaneous blood flow on the sympathectomized side.

PREOPERATIVE IN-HOSPITAL EVALUATION. The preoperative in-hospital evaluation of patients for vascular surgery, including angiography, is dealt with following the discussion of case selection in order to emphasize the sequence and priorities observed in clinical practice, where patients normally are admitted after their probable candidacy for operative treatment has been

TABLE 17–6 Combined Results of Arterial Reconstruction for Chronic Occlusive Disease of the Lower Extremity[18]

PROCEDURE	REPORTS	CASES	EARLY MORTALITY (%)	PATENCY (%)	AMPUTATION (%)	LATE PATENCY (%)
Femoropopliteal Reconstruction						
Autogenous vein graft	7	1,100	2.3	91.0	5.0	72.1
Endarterectomy	4	443	1.4	84.6	10.5	68.7
Dacron prosthesis	2	1,401	1.3	86.8	5.7	71.2
Aortoiliac Reconstruction	8	4,050	4.7	94.3	3.3	86.3

TABLE 17–7 Operative Mortality for Abdominal Aortic Aneurysms— Combined Results[18]

CASE SELECTION	REPORTS	CASES	HOSPITAL MORTALITY (%)
Early Experience } same institutions	6	2,213	10.0
Recent Experience		1,051	4.7
Elective } same institutions	4	872	4.4
Emergency		308	43.2
All Institutions	21	4,214	9.2

TABLE 17–8 Combined Results of Amputations for Gangrene Secondary to Arterial Insufficiency[18]

LEVEL	REPORTS	CASES	OPERATIVE MORTALITY (%)	FAILURE TO HEAL (%)	REHABILITATION RATE (%)
Below Knee	14	2,280	8.0	19.3	71.0
Above Knee	8	1,039	29.2	11.2	43.7

TABLE 17–9 Results of Operative Treatment of Renovascular Hypertension[18]

REPORTS	CASES	COMPLETE CURE (%)	CURED OR IMPROVED (%)	OPERATIVE MORTALITY (%)
14	1,680	44.8	72.7	6.3

determined. This tentative decision is upheld in most cases, although occasionally the unexpected discovery of associated disease or a discouraging angiogram will reverse this judgment. More than a pertinent history and a physical examination relative to the vascular problem is required prior to operation. Assessment of the patient's operative risk is routinely made including cardiopulmonary and renal function. Guidelines for various vascular surgical disorders that could serve for PSRO review have been prepared by a committe of the Society for Vascular Surgery[25] and were discussed in the section on ancillary diagnostic studies. (See page 862.)

Special diagnostic procedures may be indicated, but the value of selectively employing objective, noninvasive methods of preoperative and postoperative monitoring is worthy of emphasis. These studies help to avoid misdiagnosis, gauge the extent and severity of the vascular disease prior to angiography, allowing that procedure to be employed more selectively, and provide a readily available means of assessing objectively the success of the operation itself.

Arteriographic studies on selected patients provide invaluable information regarding the location and extent of the disease, and occasionally this anatomical information is supplemented by qualitative impressions regarding the rate of blood flow. However, since it is often possible to diagnose the nature and location of the vascular lesion with reasonable certainty by physical examination alone, supplemented by some of the newer noninvasive diagnostic methods, the vascular surgeon usually obtains the arteriogram to study the condition of the vessels proximal and distal to the lesion. For example, when confronted with superficial femoral artery occlusion, the vascular surgeon wants to know whether there is occult iliac artery stenosis proximally, whether the profunda femoris is widely patent to provide maximal collateral

flow, and the condition of the popliteal and infrapopliteal arteries into which he or she may wish to graft. On the other hand if an abdominal aortic aneurysm is large enough to be felt easily, or if its calcific outline on a cross-table lateral film or on ultrasound studies indicates that it is at least 6 to 7 cm in diameter, there is no reason for aortography unless significant proximal (e.g., renal artery) or distal (e.g., iliofemoral) occlusive disease is suspected. In fact, since most abdominal aortic aneurysms are lined with intraluminal clot, their internal diameters often appear misleadingly normal on aortograms. In general, the more experienced the vascular surgeon, the less frequently he or she will request aortography for aortoiliac disease. This is particularly true now that measurements of segmental limb pressures are readily obtainable.

The vascular surgeon must confirm the existence, nature and extent of the vascular lesion and balance the disability it causes (or is likely to cause under nonoperative management) against the feasibility, risk and anticipated success of various operations. Only then can the patient or the referring physician be advised regarding the need for surgical intervention. The manner in which this evaluation is carried out and judgment is applied is the foundation for a successful practice in vascular surgery.

NONOPERATIVE (MEDICAL) MANAGEMENT. Nonoperative (medical) management is indicated in questionable cases and in those for which surgery would not be beneficial. The patient is educated about the long-term care for his extremities, using the following guidelines:

Instructions to Patients with Arterial Insufficiency

You have a condition that is going to require you to live carefully to prevent serious complications and to enable you to be comfortable. The name of the disease is arteriosclerosis obliterans. It means simply that the blood vessels carrying blood to your tissues are choked by an aging process also known as "hardening of the arteries." This is similar to the plumbing in a house that has become clogged with lime deposits over the years. The water will not flow as freely as it did when the pipes were new. Patience is required.

Unlike the pipes in your home, the vessels cannot be totally replaced. You must live with what you have. It is possible to live comfortably, provided that you are careful and follow certain simple rules. Details are of the utmost importance and must be followed. What would be a minor injury to someone else may well mean the loss of a leg for you.

1. Care of Other Diseases

If you have any other diseases be sure that they are under control. Diseases such as heart disease, diabetes or skin diseases are most important. Be sure to see your physician about these periodically.

2. Exercise

Walk at least two miles a day. The more you walk the more you will be able to walk. This does not mean two miles at a stretch but rather, walking interrupted by periods of rest prior to extremity fatigue or pain. Do not walk until the pain occurs and then stop for rest. You must exercise like an athlete, with rest before you develop extremity discomfort. Walking keeps the muscles in condition. A period of inactivity allows the muscles to waste away and they will not return to their former condition. If you follow this routine you should in a few weeks be capable of walking further distances before finding it necessary to stop for rest.

3. Guard Against Injury

When the circulation is good, small scratches heal promptly; when the circulation is not good a small scratch may become a large ulcer that will not heal in spite of good treatment. If you note anything wrong, see your doctor immediately; do not wait until it looks serious.

You may have noticed that the sensation in your legs and feet is not as good as it was previously. This may allow you to injure yourself without knowing it has occurred. One of the more common offenders is heat.

Burns caused by heating pads, lamps and hot water bottles are serious; none of these should be used at any time. In addition, pressure areas from shoes and socks may not be noted owing to this loss of sensation. A brief, thorough inspection after your daily foot bath is indicated.

4. Keep Yourself Warm

In cold weather keep yourself warm. Cold causes further constriction (spasm) of the blood vessls. This means that you must not only keep your feet and ankles warm but all of your body. Long underwear is excellent. One thing that is often forgotten is the head; your head exposes many vessels to cold, which may cause vessel constriction elsewhere in the body. Warm, dry, clean, well fitting socks are most important and should be considered as medicine.

5. Infection and Self-Treatment

There are only five things that should touch your feet and legs in the way of medicines. These are mild soap, water, 70 per cent alcohol, powder and PLAIN lanolin. You should NOT use anything else unless your doctor specifically orders it. "Put nothing on your feet that you wouldn't put in your eyes," excluding soap, alcohol and powder.

Infection occurs easily in legs and feet and must be guarded against at all times. A daily foot bath is imperative. The skin of your face is in good condition and you wash it every day. The skin of your feet and legs is not in good condition and you must wash your extremities every day — preferably twice daily. WHEN YOU WASH YOUR FACE, WASH YOUR FEET. Inspect them thoroughly after washing. If you see anything suspicious, such as itching between the toes, cracks between the toes, corns or calluses, see your doctor. DO NOT TRY TO TREAT IT YOURSELF.

6. Care of the Feet

a. *Shoes* should extend a half inch beyond the toes and be wide enough to allow all the toes to move. There should be no seams or other projections inside. They should be examined inside with your hand for small stones, nails and creases before putting them on each time. A torn lining should be removed or repaired. If possible two pairs of shoes should be used, to be worn on alternate days; allow them to dry and be aired before putting them on again.

b. *Socks* should be of ample size but should not bunch or wrinkle, thereby causing points of pressure. They should provide some cushioning of the sole and top of the foot against the shoe.

c. As mentioned before, a daily inspection of the feet should be made and anything suspicious such as itching or cracks between the toes should be reported to your doctor.

d. Again, a daily foot bath is a necessity. A thorough washing should be done using warm, but not hot, water and a mild soap, paying particular attention to the areas between the toes and around the nails. The feet should be thoroughly dried. A light oiling with lanolin at night and a dusting with a mild antifungal powder in the morning are important.

e. A word about corns and calluses, which are due to poorly fitting shoes: They should never be removed by you at home; it is absolutely necessary that they be taken care of by a trained person. Once they are removed, their recurrence should be prevented by properly fitted shoes. Therefore, if you have a corn or a callus have it examined by your doctor; do not cut it or treat it yourself.

f. *Toenails* must be properly cut and trimmed. Do not cut them yourself, especially if you have poor eyesight. To do so you must sit at an awkward angle. Your doctor or foot specialist is trained to see that they are properly managed. A small cut by the pressure of a toenail is just as important to you as a cut by any other means. If you find it necessary to trim your own toenails and you have good eyesight and no loss of sensation in your toes, the nails should always be trimmed straight across using a toenail clipper, never a razor blade or scissors.

7. GENERAL INSTRUCTIONS

All of these things you must do yourself. If you have any questions after reading this, be sure to ask your physician to clear up anything you do not understand. He or she will ask you questions to be certain that you do understand these instructions. They are important.

There are times when your physician will vary these instructions, give other medications or recommend other procedures. Follow his or her instructions to the letter. Remember that the attention you pay to details in the care of your feet may save them.

Arteritis

Inflammatory diseases of the arteries, which are referred to as arteritis, are difficult to classify. As a group, they occur more frequently than is generally realized and are often associated with underlying conditions such as the collagen diseases, thromboangiitis obliterans and allergies to proteins, toxins, antigens and some medications. Any area of the vascular system may be involved, but the inflammation usually involves small and medium-sized vessels. Diagnosis should be considered when medium-sized arteries are painful upon palpation. However, muscle biopsy including a small artery is frequently necessary for diagnosis except when arteritis is localized to major arteries.

Thromboangiitis Obliterans

Thromboangiitis obliterans, also known as Buerger's disease, is the most controversial disorder in the group.[32, 45] This disease has recently become much less common, probably because of a better understanding of arteriosclerosis obliterans. Numerous factors have been considered as the etiology of the disease.

Thromboangiitis obliterans occurs in patients with hypercoagulability and local arteritis due to a mechanical entrapment of the popliteal artery and vein in the adductor canal or the gastrocnemius muscle or of the subclavian artery and vein in the thoracic outlet area. It may also be caused by generalized vasculitis, resulting in peripheral gangrene. The exact cause is unknown and its identification as a specific disease is questioned by many clinicians.

However, when the signs and symptoms of chronic arterial occlusion occur and thromboangiitis obliterans is considered, tobacco smoking is found to be closely related by history and sensitivity tests to the development of the disease. There is no doubt that smoking has an aggravating influence on its progress. Another unusual feature is its predilection for white males. It occurs primarily betwen the ages of 20 and 40 years and is manifested by intense inflammation of the arteries and veins primarily and of the nerves secondarily. Thrombosis of the small and medium-sized arteries and veins progresses ultimately to larger vessels. Any or all of the arteries in the body may be involved, but the condition is predominately localized to the lower extremities.

DIAGNOSIS. Thromboangiitis obliterans is considered in a patient who has objective evidence of arterial occlusion in peripheral arteries, is a young male and an habitual smoker. Frequently there is a history of evidence of superficial thrombophlebitis, and the arterial occlusive process is progressive in each of the lower extremities and may also involve the upper extremities. Vasospasm often accompanies the condition, and Raynaud's phenomenon, with blanching, cyanosis or mottling of the skin of the part as well as excessive sweating, may be noted. The major difficulty in differential diagnosis is to determine whether chronic arterial occlusive disease is thromboangiitis obliterans or arteriosclerosis obliterans, especially in patients in their fifth decade.

Arteriograms are an essential diagnostic procedure to rule out arteriosclerotic segmental occlusion and to provide confirmatory evidence of thromboangiitis obliterans. The arterial pattern is that of multiple segmental occlusions in the smaller arteries of the extremities and of a tapered smooth vessel proximal to an occlusion without irregular arteriosclerotic plaques. A hypercoagulation panel is ordered on all patients, especially those who have now or have had superficial thrombophlebitis and those with a family history of arterial occlusion in a young male relative.

TREATMENT. Since the etiology of this condition is undetermined, treatment is directed toward symptomatic relief rather than specific therapy. It should be recognized that patients with thromboangiitis obliterans go through remissions and exacerbations.

ACUTE STAGE. Abstinence from *tobacco* is most important, and the clinician must try to persuade the patient to stop smoking. Sedatives and tranquilizing agents are of little benefit. Whiskey, 1 ounce four or five times a day, may be beneficial, but is never administered when tranquilizers have been prescribed.

Pain is relieved in a manner similar to that used for arteriosclerosis obliterans patients.

Edema usually indicates an advanced degree of ischemia, and its presence increases the amount of pain. Therefore, movement of the foot is encouraged and an oral diuretic is administered daily.

Treatment of infection is similar to the method described in the section on arteriosclerosis obliterans.

Anticoagulants, namely heparin, are prescribed subcutaneously in doses ranging from 10,000 to 20,000 units twice daily. Coagulation times are determined periodically to keep below 20 minutes just prior to the subsequent injection. Hypercoagulation studies should be done on all patients prior to the use of heparin, antiplatelet medication or any other drugs, especially Butazolidin, which may be prescribed for its anti-inflammatory characteristics.

Additional medical therapy should include routines similar to those described for arteriosclerosis obliterans, such as progressive ambulation, foot care and elevation of the head of the bed.

Surgery is not performed in the acute stage. However, if there is hyperesthesia and burning pain over the involved foot and if medical sympathetic denervation does not produce prolonged relief, sympathectomy is indicated. Amputation is avoided in the acute stage unless obvious irreversible ischemic changes are present. Prognosis is determined by the temperature of the foot and the trophic changes; if the foot is cool while appearing inflamed, the prognosis is poor. Diagnostic biopsy of a peripheral artery is contraindicated. In the past this disease responded poorly to all forms of treatment; present methods of care of the extremities have reduced the amputation rate.

CHRONIC STAGE. Thromboangiitis obliterans is primarily due to arterial occlusion, but it is frequently associated with and aggravated by vasospasm, which reduces collateral circulation to the part. Vascular flow improves and symptoms are usually relieved when the vasospastic component is released by a lumbar sympathectomy. The effects of sympathectomy may be more striking than in arteriosclerosis obliterans. Sympathectomy is done when the acute stage subsides and the foot improves; blanching on elevation diminishes and previously absent pulses may return.

Reconstructive procedures are rarely performed; however, arteriography should be routinely undertaken for proper evaluation of the disorder.

Collagen Diseases

Three collagen diseases may be considered when symptoms of peripheral chronic arterial occlusions occur and arteriosclerosis obliterans and thromboangiitis obliterans have been excluded. These diseases are periarteritis nodosa, disseminated lupus erythematosus and scleroderma.

Diagnosis of periarteritis nodosa is difficult and often requires an arterial biopsy. Raynaud's phenomenon may accompany the symptoms.

Disseminated lupus erythematosus may also be difficult to diagnose unless the characteristic "butterfly" skin eruption of erythema across the bridge of the nose and malar region is present. Biopsy of the involved area may be required to confirm the clinical diagnosis. A few patients may have symptoms and signs of Raynaud's phenomenon. Unlike periarteritis nodosa and thromboangiitis obliterans, alteration of peripheral pulses is uncommon and gangrenous changes are rare.

Scleroderma is not usually difficult to diagnose, especially when it is characterized in a diffuse induration of the skin and associated with vasomotor disturbances and visceral involvement. Raynaud's phenomenon frequently precedes the skin induration and trophic changes of the toes and fingers. Ulceration and even gangrene may occur at the tips of the digit. Peripheral pulses may be difficult to palpate because of vasospasm and the leathery and nonpliable character of the skin overlying the vessels. Therefore, the Doppler flow detector should be used to assess the occlusive arterial process. Occasionally calcinosis occurs as painful focal lesions over the joints of the extremities.

Other Forms of Arteritis

Other forms of arteritis are temporal arteritis, erythema nodosum, erythema induration of nodular vasculitis, steroid vasculitis and nonspecific arteritis.

Temporal arteritis and steroid vasculitis are especially important to a surgeon. Temporal arteritis, also called granulomatous or giant cell arteritis, may be diagnosed by the pain and tenderness that occur over the temporal arteries and is accompanied by diffuse headaches, fever, malaise and weakness. There may be redness and induration over the temporal artery as well as disappearance of the pulsations. The condition should not be taken lightly, for intracranial involvement may cause blindness. Biopsy of the temporal artery is frequently requested to confirm the diagnosis; dramatic relief of pain usually occurs. Steroid vasculitis may develop in patients who have been on cortisone or prednisone for several years. Leg ulcers may develop as a complication of the vasculitis.

Another group of arteritides includes those due to anatomic factors or to repetitious direct trauma, such as crutch arteritis, adductor canal arteritis or thrombosis, and to thoracic outlet syndromes resulting in arteritis and thrombosis.

Treatment for generalized arteritis is basically symptomatic and is directed toward removal of sensitizing factors. Steroid therapy should be avoided until all other therapy fails, or until the symptoms are persistent, or unless the process involves other than the superficial temporal artery, or if an acute episode develops. In acute episodes cortisone, 200 to 300 mg daily, or prednisone, 40 to 50 mg daily, is prescribed until symptomatic relief occurs; then the dosage is reduced until maintenance is established. The maintenance dose should be the smallest possible to achieve comfort and rehabilitation. Ultimate withdrawal of medication should be sought. Temporal and cranial arteritis should be treated with steroid therapy early, lest blindness ensue. Leg ulcers caused by steroid arteritis are treated by subcutaneous heparin, 10,000 to 15,000 units twice daily. In a few patients with periarteritis nodosa, sympathectomy may be necessary for relief of hyperesthesia and superficial pain as well as of any vasospasm in the ischemic part. Sympathectomy is not performed for any patients with scleroderma in spite of the belief that it may benefit the patient. Most surgeons who have performed a fairly representative number of sympathectomies on these patients agree that their results have not been beneficial.

Treatment of localized arteritis consists of removal of the anatomical cause of trauma and definitive therapy toward the specific artery involved.

Aneurysms

Abdominal Aortic Aneurysm

One of the most impressive achievements of medical progress in recent years has been the effective surgical treatment of abdominal aortic aneurysms. With the availability of aortic homografts and later synthetic cloth prostheses, the general consensus among the medical profession is that few individuals with abdominal aortic aneurysms should fail to have surgery for this potentially lethal lesion.[4, 75] Although the surgical mortality is reported to have been reduced to an acceptable level for both symptomatic and asymptomatic aneurysms, there is some doubt that this level of mortality has been achieved on a nationwide basis. Candidates for surgery are invariably advanced in years and always have systemic atherosclerosis. These individuals represent some of the poorest risks for a surgeon, especially when the surgery entails such an extensive operative assault as removal and replacement of an abdominal aortic aneurysm. The problem is compounded when the expanding and ruptured aortic aneurysm demands immediate surgery and does not permit selection. Every surgeon therefore must consider the general status of the patient in assessing operative risk and be qualified to understand the many problems of diagnosis and treatment that must be solved before operation is undertaken in the individual instance.

Clinical manifestations of abdominal aortic aneuryms are often difficult to separate from other symptoms that frequently appear in the sixth, seventh and eighth decades of life. The mean age of the occurrence of abdominal aortic aneurysms is 65 to 75 years of age.

Most of the lesions are asymptomatic when first diagnosed; however, some patients demonstrate a rapidly expanding or ruptured aortic aneurysm. Between these two extremes is a group of individuals who complain of vague abdominal symptoms. These are usually gastrointestinal in nature and are related to duodenal displacement by the aneurysm or to a change in bowel habits occurring from occlusion of the inferior mesenteric artery included in the aneurysmal dilatation. Back pain is common and is difficult to distinguish from symptoms of hypertrophic arthritis that may accompany the lesion.

An abdominal aortic aneurysm may be detected by palpation of a pulsatile mass anywhere in the abdomen but usually located to the left of the midline of the epigastrium and several centimeters below the umbilicus where the normal aorta bifurcates. Occasionally a significant pulsation can be transmitted through an abdominal mass, or the aorta may be easily palpated owing to marked curvature of the spinal column. A false impression of the presence of an aneurysm may occur in the hypertensive female patient in whom the aorta "buckles" from elongation and seems widened because of its tortuosity. Many aneurysms are first detected by radiologists when they review abdominal films obtained for other reasons. Calcification in the wall of the aneurysm is observed in the AP abdominal x-ray and may be more frequently found on a slightly over-exposed lateral film. Aortography is not ordered except when (1) a diagnosis of tortuous aorta is considered; (2) additional surgery for correction of a renal hypertension is contemplated and (3) severe distal chronic occlusive arterial disease is present and adequate patency beyond the occlusive area(s) may be a problem during and immediately following abdominal aorta surgery. Aortography is not routinely performed because the majority of abdominal aortic aneurysms are localized below the renal arteries, and even very large aneurysms may have an axial blood flow that appears normal on aortography. Ultrasound or CT scan is recommended not only to diagnose an abdominal aortic aneurysm but also to follow the size of the lesion. However, this equipment is not widely available.

Palpation of the pulsatile mass may elicit mild tenderness. When rapid expansion or rupture has already begun, tenderness is always present and severe rigidity of the abdominal musculature may develop, preventing detection of the underlying pulsatile abdominal mass.

Symptoms of rapid expansion or rupture may range from severe abdominal pain and immediate death to almost any symptom listed for acute abdominal conditions. A history of a past myocardial infarction is common, and symptoms of chronic occlusive disease of the lower extremities may be present in at least half of the patients. Unlike peripheral arterial aneurysms, abdominal aortic aneurysms are rarely the source of arterial emboli to the lower extremities.

Aneurysms may be *classified* as: (1) asymptomatic, when they are dormant and may enlarge to tremendous proportions without any significant complaints, (2) expanding, when they are potentially lethal or (3) ruptured, when death is inevitable without surgical correction.

The expanding aneurysm produces symptoms ranging from mild back, flank, hip and abdominal pain to severe pain related to the enlarging mass. No hemodynamic changes occur. Upon rupture, blood escapes from the aortic wall and may go (1) through the anterior wall into the peritoneal cavity, (2) into the retroperitoneal space or the mesentery and (3) into a hollow viscus such as the intestine or inferior vena cava.

Time of rupture prior to hospital admission is significant. Half of the patients presenting with a ruptured abdominal aneurysm survive for 24 hours, and a third have had symptoms of rupture for over 96 hours. Symptoms of expansion precede or accompany the rupture in about 60 per cent of patients, and these — together with symptoms of "double rupture" — have been described as characteristic of aneurysms. Diagnosis of a ruptured abdominal aortic aneurysm may be made by three findings: (1) presence of a palpable, pulsatile, midabdominal mass, (2) pain in the abdomen and back with radiation to the groin, genitalia, hip or thigh and (3) hemodynamic signs of continuous blood loss. With these findings, only a hematocrit, urinalysis and blood cross-matching should be obtained, for delay of surgical treatment by consultation on special studies may be fatal to the patient.

Selection of patients for operation is not always so clear-cut; an aneurysm should be considered as a malignant lesion and surgery should not be delayed. However, many patients with abdominal aortic aneurysms may have severe pulmonary disease as well as generalized atherosclerosis involving coronary, cerebral, mesenteric or renal arteries. Any of these conditions may lead to death or morbidity before the aneurysm ruptures, and elective removal of the aneurysm only assures the patient that he will not have a ruptured aneurysm.

Several questions should be answered before patients are electively selected for operation:

Is an abdominal aortic aneurysm significantly lethal to warrant surgery in all but a few patients? Even though the number of patients studied has been small and some reports are retrospective, there has been a fairly universal acceptance that an aneurysm will enlarge and rupture in a majority of patients within three years. All patients have a progression of their atherosclerosis, especially those who have symptomatic aneurysms, and a third have an even chance of dying from atherosclerotic disease or a ruptured aneurysm. The risk for surgery increases significantly in patients over 70 years of age and also depends upon the experience and capability of the surgeon performing the procedure.

Does aneurysmectomy restore to the patient the life expectancy he would have had without risking a potentially lethal lesion? Excluding surgery for ruptured aneurysms, which are obviously survival procedures, most experienced surgeons agree that life expectancy is as much as doubled for a five-year period.

What size abdominal aortic aneurysm is hazardous? The incidence of rupture increases in relation to its size. In lesions that are less than 7 cm in size the incidence of rupture is 4 per cent; the incidence of rupture rises to 82 per cent if the aneurysm is larger than 7 cm in diameter. The smallest measurable size for an aneurysm is 4.5 cm. Operative mortality rates for elective aneurysm surgery range from 5 to 18 per cent, while 34 to 85 per cent of those that are ruptured have a fatal outcome.

What are the criteria for operation? These can be listed as: (1) symptoms of pain or tenderness, suggesting impending rupture, (2) evidence of expansion, (3) associated iliac artery occlusive disease, (4) an aneurysm that is greater than 7 cm in size, (5) the occurrence of peripheral emboli, (6) patients who are less than 70 years of age and (7) aneurysms that have ruptured. Contrary to general belief, only a small percentage of patients expire immediately from exsanguination when an abdominal aorta ruptures. Obviously the ultimate outcome of the lesion varies with the location and rapidity of the hemorrhage. In a majority of patients a ruptured abdominal aorta leaks into the retroperitoneal or mesentary attachment areas for hours or even days. The average period between the onset of symptoms of rupture and death has been reported as ten hours. This is more than adequate time to hospitalize the patient and implement emergency surgery. In view of this common pattern, the high risk patient with an asymptomatic aneurysm may be examined only every two to three months. At each visit the size of the pulsatile mass is determined by measuring its distance from the umbilicus. A two-way scout film of the abdomen may be taken and the calcification in the wall noted. Ultrasound, as previously mentioned, is a valuable means of denoting any change in the size of the lesion. The patient is informed that he should contact his surgeon and make himself immediately available at the hospital if he experiences severe abdominal pain. This approach has been very successful for the few patients in this category in our clinic.

Improvement in monitoring, surgical technique and supportive therapy should result in a high incidence of survivors. Patients with symptomatic aneurysms should be operated upon; patients with asymptomatic aneurysms should have excision and replacement of the lesion according to the aforementioned guidelines. Otherwise, if they are included in a high risk group, they should be examined at regular intervals and should be counseled on the importance of abdominal symptoms.

Late complications following discharge include: (1) constipation frequently due to ischemic changes of the left colon, (2) occlusive distal arterial disease, (3) the development of a false or true aneurysm at the proximal suture line, (4) postsympathetic pain in the thighs on the tenth postoperative day if a lumbar sympathectomy was performed as an additional procedure and (5) aortoduodenal fistula, causing episodes of GI bleeding and bacteremia.

Anuria following abdominal aorta surgery should be evaluated for iatrogenic ureteral artery obstruction because of the close relationship of these excretory ducts to the aneurysm. Ureteral compression is so frequent preoperatively that a routine intravenous pyelogram is advised prior to surgery whenever possible.

Iliac Artery Aneurysm

Isolated aneurysms of the iliac arteries are rare; therefore intelligent and successful management depends upon a knowledge of their natural history.[55]

Aneurysms of the iliac arteries are an arteriosclerotic disease occurring most often in elderly males. They are generally extensions of an aneurysm of the lower abdominal aorta. Occasionally mycotic types occur; rarely they appear during or after pregnancy, and a few cases have been reported in children from a congenital weakness in the arterial wall. Their onset is insidious and their occult location in the pelvis may obscure the diagnosis. Rectal and vaginal examinations are often more informative than abdominal palpation. Most patients are asymptomatic when the aneurysm is diagnosed, for it may be found during examination for an unrelated condition. When symptoms are present the complaints usually are of abdominal and back pain. As with aneurysms elsewhere, iliac artery aneurysms continue to enlarge and elongate, and the enlargement continues until it impinges upon surrounding viscera or until it ruptures into the bowel or retroperitoneal area. When an asymptomatic aneurysm is diagnosed, operation may be elective unless there are specific contraindications. When aneurysms rupture, surgical intervention is mandatory.

Lower Extremity Aneurysm

Aneurysms of the lower extremities are much less common than abdominal aortic aneurysms. They are most frequently due to arteriosclerosis, especially in patients over 50 years of age. Additional causes are trauma, mycotic arteritis and necrotizing arteritis. Popliteal aneurysms occur more frequently than femoral aneurysms and are often bilateral (Fig. 17–25). Multiple aneurysms are frequently noted in the abdominal aorta, iliac and femoral arteries when the cause is arteriosclerosis or Marfan's syndrome and especially when a popliteal aneurysm is present. Occasionally multiple aneurysms of the superficial femoral artery may be observed, which are described as "rosary bead" aneurysms. It is interesting

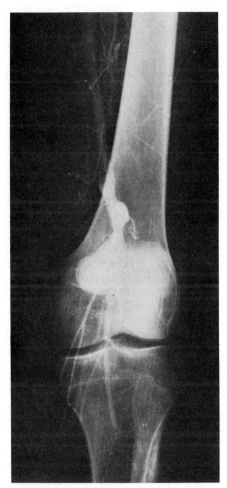

Figure 17-25 Popliteal artery aneurysm, as revealed by arteriography. These aneurysms frequently cause ischemic lesions of the digits because of embolization of fragments of thrombus. Treatment recommended is exclusion bypass with an autologous saphenous vein bypass graft.

that both the femoral and popliteal aneurysms occur at sites where muscles do not cover the vessel completely and where frequent flexion of the thigh and leg may weaken a diseased vessel. It has been postulated that the terminal portion of the superficial femoral artery is intermittently compressed by the tendinous hiatus of the adductor magnus muscle as it emerges from Hunter's canal to become the popliteal artery. This compression contributes to

the development of a poststenotic dilatation, which later develops into a popliteal aneurysm. A similar compression may be caused by the arcuate ligament behind the knee.

Diagnosis of femoral and popliteal aneurysms is usually made by palpation of a pulsatile swelling along the course of the artery. A normal pulsation may be transmitted through a mass of lymph nodes, tumor or abscess and should be considered in the differential diagnosis. If a pulsatile mass is thought to be an abscess it should not be incised until aneurysm has been excluded from the diagnosis.

When an aneurysm lies beneath a muscle mass such as the adductor magnus on the medial aspect of the thigh, the lesion(s) have been misdiagnosed as muscle ruptures. Elastic compression to the site may cause thrombosis of the aneurysm or distal emboli.

Pressure of an aneurysm on neighboring nerves may result in a characteristic radiation of pain. The first symptom of a popliteal aneurysm may be pain in the heel from pressure on the popliteal nerve. Both femoral and popliteal aneurysms may retard or obstruct adjacent venous return. Auscultation over the aneurysm may reveal a short systolic bruit; however, the majority of aneurysms do not have murmurs unless arterial stenosis with turbulence is present. If the murmur is a continuous to and fro machinelike bruit, an arteriovenous fistula must be present. Arteriography should be performed routinely for all peripheral arterial aneurysms to confirm the diagnosis and to establish the exact site and extent, the possible presence of more than one aneurysm, and the patency of the arterial system distal to the abnormally enlarged vessel.

Complications of lower extremity aneurysms are not uncommon and may result in loss of the limb or loss of life.

Femoral and popliteal aneurysms are usually asymptomatic until complications occur. Rupture of either is not common, but a distal embolism or a sudden thrombotic occlusion that may cause irreversible gangrene of the extremity is always a possibility. Therefore, elective treatment by excision and graft of a femoral aneurysm and an exclusion bypass procedure for a popliteal aneurysm is strongly recommended once the diagnosis is established. Multiple aneurysms in the vessels pose a problem in priorities and management; an abdominal aortic aneurysm should be approached surgically prior to the correction of lower extremity aneurysms.

The femoral artery aneurysm is more apt to be diagnosed early, since it is easily observed by the patient as a pulsatile mass in the groin. Popliteal aneurysms frequently go undiagnosed unless a complication occurs, since the popliteal artery is behind the knee and is not routinely palpated during the average physical examination. Its presence should be considered when a patient develops an ischemic toe or an ischemic spot on a toe with good pedal pulses and when no origin for emboli can be determined by history or physical examination.

Any patient who develops an acute thrombosis of a popliteal or femoral artery aneurysm has a poor prognosis for limb salvage unless distal thrombotic material is immediately removed at surgery and unless viability of the limb is maintained by a patent distal arterial bed proven by arteriography. Results depend upon the time of recognition, the time surgical intervention is undertaken, and the condition of the distal arterial vasculature. If good viability of the extremity is present and continues to be maintained, the operation may be scheduled as an elective procedure while the patient is maintained on subcutaneous heparin.

Visceral Arterial Aneurysm

Visceral arterial aneurysms are diagnosed much more frequently now than in the past because of increased awareness of these lesions, the widespread use of aortography and improved vascular surgical techniques.[82]

Any visceral vessel may develop an aneurysm. Although the three most common sites are the splenic, renal and hepatic arteries, aneurysms of the superior mesenteric, inferior mesenteric, pancreatic, pancreaticoduodenal, gastroduodenal, right gastroepiploic, celiac and cystic arteries have been reported.

Etiologically, visceral aneurysms have been listed as arteriosclerotic, congenital, mycotic, traumatic, dissecting and false aneurysm secondary to focal arteritis and to periarteritis nodosa. Multiple congenital visceral aneurysms are known to occur in the presence of polycystic disease of the kidneys, liver and other viscera.

Visceral aneurysms are usually asymptomatic until complications occur. Intra-abdominal rupture is a major complication that may be fatal if undiagnosed.

SPLENIC ARTERY. Aneurysm of the splenic artery is probably not as rare as was once thought. It is one of the most frequently occurring intra-abdominal aneurysms and is the only aneurysm that is found more often in women than in men. In the past, the overwhelming majority of cases were identified at operation or autopsy, and as a result, aneurysm of the splenic artery was associated with an extremely high mortality rate. In recent years opinions regarding the prognosis of splenic artery aneurysms have been encouraging. Although splenic artery aneurysm is not often seen, its importance should not be underestimated, for the alert physician may recognize it by its clinical pattern. Surgical intervention is indicated as an elective or life-saving measure.[68]

The precise cause of aneurysm of the splenic artery is unknown. The majority are atherosclerotic in origin, but a significant and interesting finding of localization of the arteriosclerosis to the splenic artery alone has been reported. The second most common cause is a congenital defect. A peculiar relationship may exist between the third trimester of pregnancy and the development of rupture of a pre-existing aneurysm of the splenic artery. Any pregnant or recently postpartum woman who develops upper abdominal pain, especially in the left upper quadrant, that is associated with signs of intraperitoneal bleeding, should be considered as a possible instance of splenic artery aneurysm. Surgical intervention is immediately indicated. There may also be some unexplained relationship to its occasional presence in patients with portal hypertension.

Several clinical features are sufficiently characteristic to suggest the presence of this lesion. The symptoms produced are of two types: those occurring before rupture and those occurring after rupture. The most common symptom before perforation is pain in the epigastrium or the left upper quadrant. Associated with this pain are a host of other symptoms, most of which are referable to the gastrointestinal tract. Most patients are asymptomatic, especially those in whom the aneurysm has been noted as an incidental finding during aortography, in a routine film of the abdomen or during surgery. Physical examination may reveal little besides tenderness in the upper abdomen. Other findings may be splenomegaly, a pulsatile tumor or a systolic murmur in the upper abdomen.

The most common clinical manifestation of splenic artery aneurysm is the typical calcification seen in roentgenograms of the abdomen. The calcified aneurysm appears as a round or oval shadow of increased density in the left upper quadrant or epigastrium. The periphery of this shadow is sharply delineated and the central portion presents a mottled appearance. If the patient is not asymptomatic, he should receive a translumbar aortogram to establish the diagnosis. Once the diagnosis is proved, surgical therapy is recommended.

The major complication is rupture, which commonly occurs in two stages — the so-called "double rupture," a common occurrence for all ruptured aneurysms. Following the first leak, the patient may improve clinically, and in this brief interlude the diagnosis and surgical treatment is lifesaving. Some time after the primary rupture, a secondary hemorrhage occurs into the greater peritoneal cavity, stomach or colon. Even with immediate surgery the mortality rate is exceedingly great.

RENAL ARTERY. Aneurysms of the renal artery must be managed surgically because of the complications they may cause within the kidney and their frequent association with hypertension. Unlike their splenic artery counterpart, renal artery aneurysms do not often rupture except during the third trimester of pregnancy or the early postpartum period. They are most commonly due to atherosclerosis, although some have a congenital origin. Multiple aneurysms may develop in the presence of fibromuscular hyperplasia. It is not uncommon for renal artery aneurysms to be found bilaterally. They rarely enlarge enough to be palpable, and although signet ring calcification does occur, it is unusual.

As with aneurysms elsewhere in the body, many patients with renal artery aneurysm are asymptomatic until complications develop. Since the aneurysms are usually saccular, a mural thrombus contained within the aneurysm may produce embolic infarctions in the kidney parenchyma. Another complication is the formation of a dissecting hematoma distal to the aneurysm. A majority of patients have hypertension as well as pain in the flank, lumbar region, lower back or upper abdomen and hematuria ranging from a few cells to a massive hemorrhage. Renal artery aneurysms caused by trauma may either rupture or form an arteriovenous fistula. The latter may be iatrogenic following mass ligation of both artery and vein during a nephrectomy.

Renal artery aneurysms are diagnosed much more frequently since translumbar aortograms have become routine for occlusive peripheral vascular disease and for any patients with hypertension. Radiographic studies should include excretory urography and nephrotomography. Once the diagnosis is made, immediate surgery is indicated. Previously, nephrectomy was the procedure of choice, but current techniques of vascular surgery can usually preserve renal function.

HEPATIC ARTERY. Hepatic artery aneurysms, like those of the splenic and renal arteries, have characteristic features that may lead to a definite diagnosis.

As in other aneurysms, the most common cause of hepatic artery aneurysm is arteriosclerosis. A variety of causes other than congenital have been implicated, including direct extension by an inflamed gallbladder, infected emboli, trauma from a previous biliary operation or an external penetrating injury.

The most frequent finding that leads to suspicion of the existence of a hepatic artery aneurysm is a triad of symptoms of jaundice, abdominal pain and gastrointestinal hemorrhage. Roentgenologically, there may be a calcification of the aneurysmal wall, a filling defect of the duodenum and narrowed duodenum cap. Occasionally a murmur may be present, and if the aneurysm enlarges sufficiently a pulsatile mass is found in the right upper quadrant. Any of these findings may suggest the need for aortography to establish the diagnosis.

The major complication is rupture into either the peritoneal cavity or the gastrointestinal tract. Several instances of rupture into the portal vein have been reported at operation or postmortem as a hepatic artery–portal vein fistula.

In view of the potential complications, surgery is advised. Collateral blood supply to the liver may be sufficient to allow resection of the artery without a graft replacement, although its use is recommended.

Mycotic Aneurysm

The term "mycotic" is used to identify those aneurysms that originate from inflammatory destruction of the arterial wall, especially the internal elastic lamina. The most common infection is of *intravascular origin.* These lesions may develop from: (1) infected emboli from endocarditis that lodge in the vessel lumen or in the vasa vasorum, (2) microorganisms deposited directly on the intima of the vessel or in the vasa vasorum, and (3) extension of infection from aortic or pulmonary valves to the proximal portion of the aorta or pulmonary artery. When the causative infection extends to the vessel from a contiguous or neighboring inflammatory process such as anastomotic or traumatic false aneurysms, the infection is classified as of *extravascular origin.* Very rarely, the lesion may result from a distant extravascular source of infection and is termed a "primary mycotic aneurysm." These lesions are not associated with any demonstrable intravascular inflammatory process or with any infection from surrounding tissue, but during the course of bacteremia an intimal defect caused by arteriosclerosis may permit the infection to obtain a foothold. Bacteremia may also cause secondary infection in congenital, traumatic and arteriosclerotic aneurysms and may result in aneurysmal rupture.

The course of the lesion depends on the virulence of the bacterial agent causing it. If it is highly virulent, the vessel wall is destroyed and rupture may occur before an aneurysm forms. This may happen less than two weeks after symptoms begin; however, symptoms are usually present for several weeks before the aneurysm ruptures, if it ruptures at all. Unfortunately, most of the aneurysms are located in visceral and cerebral arteries and in the aorta rather than peripherally. Circulatory impairment may be noted distally but gangrene is uncommon. Diagnosis is therefore determined by the presence of infection, chiefly bacterial endocarditis, and the rapid development of an inflamed painful pulsatile mass.

Treatment requires heavy doses of antibiotics, ligation of the artery if necessary to prevent exsanguination, or excision and restoration of vascular continuity if the infection is under control. It may be necessary to sacrifice the arterial supply to the involved part to save the patient's life. Extra-anatomical bypass grafts have been used successfully in these patients in order to avoid the area of infection. Owing to the widespread use of antibiotics, very few mycotic aneurysms may be encountered in afebrile patients in which the bacterial endocarditis has been at least temporarily arrested. Conversely, a mycotic aneurysm may be the focus for a fever of unknown origin. Excision of a mycotic aneurysm has been reported to have cured bacteremia.

Extracranial and Aortic Arch Occlusive Disease

Numerous descriptive terms are employed to identify the less common occlusive lesions of the great vessels arising from the aortic arch. The terms include nonspecific arteritis of Takayasu or pulseless disease, Martorell's syndrome, thrombotic obliteration of the aortic arch branches, and the aortic arch syndrome. Among the more common disorders are occlusion, stenosis or atherosclerotic ulceration of the extracranial and vertebral arteries. Each of these lesions may be present singularly or in combination with lesions of the aortic arch branches. The most common cause of partial or complete occlusion of the great vessels is arteriosclerosis. Less frequent causes are fibromuscular hyperplasia, arteritis, embolism and dissecting aneurysm.

Arteriosclerotic lesions usually occur at the origins and bifurcations of the brachiocephalic arteries. Usually these sites of atherosclerotic changes have progressed to a stenosis or occlusion in the first one or two centimeters of the great vessels, the first centimeter of the vertebral arteries and the first centimeter of the internal carotids at the common carotid bifurcations before they are detected. Many mild intermittent cerebral ischemic symptoms are the result of small emboli originating from friable thrombotic material within atherosclerotic ulcerations that have not advanced to the point of stenosis or occlusion of the vessel.

As with atherosclerotic lesions found elsewhere in the body, males are predominantly affected, and the usual age of occurrence is over 50 years. Younger males occasionally develop atherosclerotic lesions in a frequency similar to that which occurs in other sites of the arterial system. When symptoms occur in young women, however, the primary pathological change is commonly due to arteritis and usually occurs at the origins of the great trunks arising from the aortic arch.

Fibromuscular hyperplasia occurs infrequently and is usually present in the internal carotid artery. It has a corrugated or "string of beads" appearance on arteriography because of the irregular muscular hyperplasia and intervening pseudoaneurysms present in the vessel.

Dissecting aneurysm should be considered when clinical evidence of cerebral arterial insufficiency is present. An embolism lodged at the innominate or carotid bifurcation is an uncommon cause for cerebral ischemia, and when it occurs immediate surgery is required; otherwise irreversible brain damage ensues rapidly in many patients.

Any patient with symptoms and signs of cerebral insufficiency should be evaluated for lesions of the extracranial arteries as well as of the arteries originating from the aortic arch. Surgery for these lesions may be corrective as well as prophylactic, especially in patients with transient localized cerebral ischemia and in individuals who have an initial or recurrent stroke. Early diagnosis is essential, especially in a completed major stroke; some patients may be amenable to definitive surgical treatment if diagnosis and therapy are accomplished within a few hours after the symptoms occur.

Indications for surgery are:

(1) Transient focal cerebral ischemia in which patients have a correctable lesion of the carotid and vertebral arteries

(2) Aortic arch syndrome

Questionable indications for surgery are:

(1) An occasional patient with a completed stroke

(2) Extracranial embolic obstruction

(3) Asymptomatic stenosis of extracranial carotid artery, unless surgery is performed for another lesion

Contraindications for surgery are:

(1) A progressing or acute completed stroke

(2) Arteriographic evidence of both intracranial and extracranial stenosis or occlusion of the internal carotid and basilar arteries

(3) Complete occlusion of the internal carotid artery both intracranially and extracranially.

Transient Ischemic Attacks

Lesions that cause transient ischemic attacks occur in the area of the bifurcation of the common carotid artery and involve the internal carotid artery, the vertebral artery and occasionally the proximal segments of the branches of the aortic arch.

Approximately 50 per cent of the cases of cerebrovascular insufficiency result from extracranial lesions. A smaller number of these are due to a decrease in the blood flow resulting

from stenosis or occlusion of the internal carotid artery. However, the majority of transient cerebral ischemic attacks, or "little strokes," are due to small emboli arising from an atherosclerotic ulcer with or without the presence of internal carotid stenosis. Stenosis may occur from bleeding beneath an atherosclerotic plaque. A significantly high proportion of patients who have a stroke present a history of intermittent cerebral ischemic symptoms prior to the catastrophic neurological episode. Most commonly, the attack will affect either the ipsilateral hemisphere or the vision of the ipsilateral eye, or both. When the episode is limited to the vision field of one eye, the patient may experience a period of transient monocular blindness, identified as *amaurosis fugax*. The patient describes the process as an episode of partial or complete blindness in one eye lasting for a period of several minutes to an hour before vision is restored. Rarely the eye may become permanently blind.

DIAGNOSIS. The identification of transient ischemic attacks is usually not difficult when the symptoms are considered a prodromal evidence that a stroke may develop at a later date. A variety of symptoms may occur, such as brief episodes of lightheadedness and vertigo, blurring of vision or blindness, headaches, diplopia and short periods of paresthesia and paresis or incoordination of the extremities, especially on one side. These symptoms should not be ignored, for they may be the only clue that a lesion is present in the extracranial or aortic arch vessels.

A physical examination should first determine the blood pressure in both upper extremities and then evaluate the peripheral pulses. Next, bruits should be listened for in the vicinity of the carotid artery as well as over the subclavian artery. The area of stenosis may be located by a palpable decrease in or absence of carotid artery pulsations and by the presence of a bruit over the site. However, the finding of a bruit does not determine the severity of the stenosis, nor does the absence of this sound exclude the presence of a pathological change in the vessel wall. A bruit is not noted with an atherosclerotic ulcer unless stenosis is also present. Stenosis may progress to complete occlusion and the bruit disappears. Although the bruit frequently is systolic in phase, it may be continuous when the area of stenosis is extremely small. Bruits in the neck must be distinguished by requesting the patient to take several deep breaths and then to cease breathing. By so doing the examiner may more easily separate a carotid bruit from an aortic systolic murmur and a venous hum. Each has characteristic locations of intensity and sounds. An ECG is therefore routinely ordered to screen for past or present cardiac disease. A Doppler flowmeter may be used to screen those sounds heard by auscultation. Occasionally a thrill may be palpated over the bifurcation of the carotid artery. The firm mass of an atheroma also may be noted on palpation. The optic fundum should be examined carefully, especially in patients with amaurosis fugax, because the retinal arterial embolus may be seen and can be documented with a retinal camera. Before proceeding further, a standard complete neurological examination is essential to (1) establish whether the episode was a cerebral infarction or a transient attack, (2) determine if another lesion such as a brain tumor is present and (3) record a neurological baseline prior to surgery. An EEG will help to differentiate between a seizure disorder and transient ischemic attacks. Finally, brain scanning may be indicated to identify or evaluate the pressure of a "hot spot" or cerebral infarction.

Cerebral angiography is the most useful diagnostic procedure, since it determines the presence, location, number and severity of the lesions in the great vessels of the aortic arch, carotid and vertebrobasilar arterial systems. Angiography should be performed in patients with symptoms of transient ischemic attacks for whom surgery is contemplated. However, angiography is indicated for stroke patients only when the benefits from surgery are uncertain.

NONINVASIVE DIAGNOSTIC STUDIES. While complete arteriographic evaluation of the cerebral vessels remains the definitive and required diagnostic study prior to carotid artery surgery, the discomfort, expense and risk associated with this study preclude its use to screen or serially follow such patients. This combination of diagnostic need and therapeutic potential has spurred the search for discriminating noninvasive methods. Therefore, a discussion of the methodology and relative value of the following diagnostic approaches will be presented: evaluation of carotid bruits by auscultation and phonoangiography, ophthalmodynamometry and oculoplethysmography, frontal thermometry and Doppler study of supraorbital artery hemodynamics, carotid velocity wave form analysis and ultrasonic imaging.

Carotid Pulse and Bruits. Obviously, as mentioned before, it is important to feel the carotid pulse and to listen for bruits. Hearing a carotid bruit, particularly a high-pitched one that extends through systole and even into diastole, should indicate a significant carotid stenosis, for the turbulence it signals usually develops just before the point of critical stenosis. However, experience with atheromatous disease in humans does not conform precisely to this prediction. David[17] correlated arteriographic findings with the presence or absence of bruits and found that 12 per cent of 345 patients with an internal carotid artery stenosis of greater than 50 per cent diameter did not have bruits. Furthermore, 70 per cent of 121 patients with a stenosis of less than 50 per cent diameter did have bruits, whereas 28 per cent of 265 patients with no significant arteriographic narrowing also had bruits. In another study, 6 per cent of carotid bruits were due to stenosis of the external carotid artery. One reason for the absence of bruits in the face of high grade stenosis is that when there is good retrograde collateral flow, antegrade flow through the area of stenosis may drop off sharply, and the bruit may disappear before total occlusion occurs. Conversely, contralateral carotid artery occlusion may so stimulate flow through the ipsilateral side that a degree of occlusion that is normally not severe enough to cause turbulence and a bruit will do so.

Phonoangiography. An attempt has been made to improve the auscultation of bruits by placing a microphone at each of three levels over the course of the carotid artery in the neck, recording the sounds on an oscilloscope and making a permanent record of the display with a Polaroid camera. Kartchner and associates[48] have claimed an 86 per cent composite accuracy with 5 per cent false positive diagnoses and 9 per cent false negative diagnoses. Duncan and Lees[19] have added the sophistication of computer analysis of the audio frequency spectrum of the bruit, claiming that the frequency at which the bruit decreased in intensity provided a good index of the degree of carotid artery stenosis. In fact, by a double retrospective analysis of 50 out of 60 bruits, they were able to "predict" the diameter of the internal carotid narrowing to within 1 mm in 73 per cent of cases and to within 1.5 mm in 93 per cent of cases. In evaluating this approach, it must be remembered that the analysis was a retrospective one, involved expensive equipment and did not consider the almost 17 per cent of bruits that were not analyzable and, of course, that this technique would be of no value in the almost 30 per cent of patients with significant carotid artery stenosis who do not have bruits.

Ophthalmodynamometry. Since the ophthalmic artery is a direct branch of the internal carotid artery, the perfusion of the eye may serve as an index of internal carotid flow. This was exploited as early as 1917 by Brailliart (see Knox reference)[50] using ophthalmodyn-

amometry, a technique in which pressure is applied to the sclera while an ophthalmoscope is used to determine the pressure at which the retinal arteries first began to collapse (diastolic) and finally to occlude (systolic). In spite of a number of improvements in technique and interpretation, this method has not proved to be discriminating enough, as shown by Shapiro's study[80], in which there was a 77 per cent composite accuracy with 10 per cent false positive diagnoses and 13 per cent false negative diagnoses.

Oculoplethysmography. In oculoplethysmography a pulse volume contour of the eye is obtained by applying saline-filled glaucoma cups to the sclera and connecting these to a pressure transducer. As first introduced by Brockenbrough,[15] internal carotid artery occlusive disease was signaled by a unilateral reduction in the pulse contour. Simultaneous recordings of two ocular pulse contours and their differential, timed against external carotid flow signaled by an earlobe hemodensitometer, is a sophistication of the technique introduced by Kartchner and associates.[48] The detection of a unilateral pulse lag or delay, as reflected in the differential tracing, was found to be more sensitive than comparison of the magnitude of the pulse contours themselves. This technique is claimed to have a composite accuracy of 86 per cent with 4 per cent false negative diagnoses and 10 per cent false positive diagnoses, its main failing being in missing bilateral stenosis of approximately equal severity. It was uniformly accurate in detecting any unilateral stenosis sufficient to produce a drop in pressure or in flow.

Gee and colleagues[27] have developed a modification of the oculoplethysmography technique in which a vacuum of up to 300 mm Hg is applied to scleral cups and then progressively reduced until the pulse contour returns. The pressure at which this occurs can be correlated with intraocular pressure and in turn with ophthalmic pressure and, therefore, with internal carotid perfusion pressure. However, ocular pressure may not be reduced in the face of significant internal carotid artery occlusive disease if there is good collateralization from the contralateral side. Contralateral carotid compression (low in the neck to avoid the dangers associated with compression directly over the bifurcation) will allow this situation to be detected, because it will reduce contralateral ocular pressure, indicating that such pressure contributes significantly to its perfusion. Furthermore, ipsilateral common carotid arterial occlusion may also prove diagnostic if it does *not* cause a significantly reduced ipsilateral ocular pressure, indicating again that ocular perfusion is coming from the contralateral side. In addition, the ocular pressure following the latter maneuver is equivalent to retrograde or "stump" pressure and can serve to predict whether or not the internal carotid artery on that side can be ligated without neurological sequelae and whether or not carotid endarterectomy can be performed without need of a temporary shunt. In spite of its relative sensitivity, oculoplethysmography will not reliably detect degrees of stenosis that are not hemodynamically significant at rest. Thus, normal results do not rule out the presence of an ulcerated plaque that is not associated with a hemodynamically significant stenosis and, since most transient ischemic attacks and "petit strokes" are caused by embolism rather than by hypoperfusion, this represents a significant limitation.

Frontal Thermometry and Supraorbital Artery Hemodynamics. Austin and Sajid[3] in 1966 measured and compared the skin temperatures between the medial and lateral portions of the supraorbital ridge and found, in ten cases of *occlusion* of the internal carotid artery, that medial skin temperatures were lower on the occluded side compared with the ipsilateral lateral and contralateral medial temperatures. The explanation for this phenomenon lies in the fact that the medial portion of the supraorbital ridge is supplied by the supraorbital artery, a branch of the ophthalmic artery, which is in turn a branch of the internal carotid artery. The lateral supraorbital ridge is supplied by branches of the superficial temporal artery, which is the terminal extension of the external carotid artery.

However, in a large series of cases of both stenosis and occlusion of the internal carotid artery, Shapiro and associates[80] found that frontal thermometry was correct in identifying only 74 per cent of the cases, with 20 per cent false negative diagnoses and 6 per cent false positive diagnoses. It will not reliably detect stenosis or even some chronic occlusions of the internal carotid artery. Nevertheless, this approach was important because it led the way to a more discriminating test, namely, the study of *supraorbital artery hemodynamics* by directional Doppler velocity detector. The Doppler probe, placed over the supraorbital artery as it courses through the supraorbital notch, monitors the magnitude and direction of supraorbital arterial flow. Since this artery collateralizes with nearby branches of the superficial temporal artery, its flow will normally be upward and will increase in response to compression of the superficial temporal artery. In the face of occlusion or hemodynamically significant stenosis of the internal carotid artery, the probe will indicate that supraorbital flow is retrograde and diminishes with superficial temporal artery occlusion. The frontal artery, another branch of the ophthalmic artery that is located more medially near the bridge of the nose, displays similar hemodynamics but is not as readily influenced by superficial temporal artery compression. It is mainly used to confirm the direction of flow in that area.

Clinical evaluations of the sensitivity of this test unfortunately reflect mainly the severity of occlusive disease in the cases studied. That is, the test appears to be more accurate when total occlusions or high-grade stenoses dominate the series. Barnes and co-workers[8] increased the accuracy by using ipsilateral infraorbital and fascial and contralateral common carotid artery compression as additional maneuvers to clarify questionable cases. In their hands the test begins to become positive when 50 per cent stenosis is present, and with 75 per cent stenosis the test is 100 per cent accurate. However, it shares with oculoplethysmography the limitation that it will only detect hemodynamically significant occlusive disease.

Carotid Artery Velocity Wave Form Analysis. The *external* carotid artery, supplying high-resistance, low-flow vascular beds of muscle, skin and bone, has insignificant forward flow during late diastole. Its velocity tracing therefore rests on the zero baseline. In contrast, the internal carotid artery is a low-resistance, high-flow conduit whose velocity profile normally reflects the fact that significant flow persists throughout diastole. Because of the overlapping positions of these two arteries high in the neck, their diagnostic tracings are difficult to obtain. However, the velocity pattern of the more accessible common carotid artery accurately reflects the interrelationship between these two different outflow vessels. Normally it is dominated by the pattern of the internal carotid artery, through which over 80 per cent of the outflow normally passes. Thus, its velocity wave form also reflects considerable flow throughout diastole. However, with increasing degrees of internal carotid occlusive disease, the diastolic velocity steadily declines, and the pattern becomes more similar to that of the external carotid artery. Later there are reductions in the systolic velocity and in other dimensions.

Planiol and Purcelot[71] reported that the ratio of systolic velocity increase to peak systolic velocity (the difference being end-diastolic velocity) was diagnostic of internal carotid occlusive disease whenever it exceeded 0.75. Ruth-

erford and colleagues[76] found that, although this ratio alone was not a reliable index of carotid artery occlusive disease, when combined with other dimensions (end-diastolic velocity, peak systolic velocity, mean velocity, and others) in a weighted equation derived by discriminant analysis, it resulted in a "score" that predicted the degree of carotid occlusive disease with over 90 per cent accuracy. This test has the advantage of detecting lesser degrees of stenosis than the tests described previously, and it can be quickly and easily performed with relatively simple and inexpensive equipment. Its major disadvantages are the need to maximize the velocity tracings carefully, the possibility of overdiagnosis in the face of extensive arterial calcification at the site monitored, and the need to develop internal standards for normal and diseased carotid arteries for the Doppler probe and the recorder being used.

Ultrasonic Imaging. The diagnostic potential of ultrasonic imaging of the carotid arteries is being actively explored along several lines. One approach involves B-mode scanning but uses multiple transducers mounted on a rotating armature to provide a real-time image of adquate resolution. Unfortunately, because the B-mode technique depends upon differences in tissue reflectance, these instruments may not distinguish between flowing blood and intraluminal clot (false negative) or between luminal impingement and the sonic shadow of a calcific plaque (false positive).

Another ultrasonic imaging technique employs the Doppler principle. A 24-gate pulse Doppler probe is swept across or along the vessel, providing flow or no-flow information at 0.1-mm intervals. Using a sine-cosine potentiometer arm for orientation on a storage oscilloscope, the geometric dimensions of the lumen of a vessel can be "painted in" on the screen in either longitudinal or cross-sectional views. Barnes and associates[7] have clinically evaluated such a sono-arteriograph and found that it accurately diagnosed major occlusive lesions but tended to overdiagnose lesions associated with calcific plaques. These instruments also have the disadvantage of being expensive and requiring highly trained personnel for maintenance and performance.

In summary, we have two noninvasive tests (oculoplethysmography and the Doppler study of supraorbital artery hemodynamics) that will reliably diagnose hemodynamically significant occlusive lesions or identify a significant bruit (phonoangiography). In addition, two new ultrasonic approaches (velocity wave form analysis and sonoarteriography) may eventually prove reliable in detecting lesser lesions, even some ulcerated plaques.

However, none of these tests can be expected to eliminate completely the need for arteriography. In fact, it has been suggested that, since these tests cannot rule out the presence of small ulcerated plaques and since all symptomatic patients deserve arteriography even if the other tests are negative, there is no need for them at all. While there is some truth to this, these studies do appear to have clinical application in evaluating patients with asymptomatic carotid bruits and in screening patients with arteriosclerotic disease elsewhere, prior to angiographic study or major reconstructive arterial surgery. The new studies are also useful in evaluating patients with nonlateralizing cerebrovascular symptoms and as an aid in the decision regarding the need for cerebral angiography in patients whose clinical manifestations are either poorly documented or atypical or in whom the risk of cerebral angiography is usually high.

TREATMENT. Treatment of intermittent cerebral ischemic episodes must be individualized because the identification of the site and of the type of underlying pathology is often more important for the prevention of a future stroke than for the treatment of the existing one. The possibility of intracranial hemorrhage or tumor must always be kept in mind whenever the patient with stroke or intermittent ischemia is evaluated.

A useful approach is to divide the development of a stroke into three phases: Phase I includes the patient who recovers rapidly from transient ischemic attacks. Such a patient warrants thorough study to determine if surgery is indicated. Here the location, severity and accessibility of the vessel or vessels involved determines the procedure. If surgery is not advised, the hypercoagulability of the blood is inhibited with Coumadin or antiplatelet drugs. (See section on prophylactic anticoagulation.)

Phase II describes the patient who experiences an advancing stroke in which the localized neurological changes progress but the brain tissue remains viable temporarily. A rapid recovery demonstrates that the brain tissue is viable. Treatment requires immediate lowering of blood viscosity with low-molecular-weight dextran or heparin or with an antiplatelet drug such as aspirin, dipyridamole (Persantine) or sulfinpyrazone (Anturane). Many clinicians are reluctant to use heparin since it may cause hemorrhage into the infarcted brain. For the same reason some clinicians are against surgery to relieve the obstructed extracranial vessel. Others believe that either method of therapy is beneficial only if the procedure is undertaken early enough to precede cerebral infarction.

Phase III identifies the patient who has a progressive or acute completed stroke. In this individual a brain infarct has occurred and no method of treatment will restore blood flow to the damaged area.

Briefly, surgery is indicated principally for Phase I patients who are characterized by transient ischemic attacks. In Phase II patients, who have had a stroke with recovery, surgery is indicated if an infarction probably has not occurred. The procedure should usually be delayed for four to six weeks. Surgery is contraindicated in Phase III patients, in whom brain infarction is almost a certainty.

Aortic Arch Syndrome

Reduction in flow in the innominate, left carotid or left subclavian artery may be due to either of two mechanisms. The first mechanism is diminution or elimination of flow through these arteries as the result of pathological reduction in the vascular lumen. The second mechanism is termed the "vertebral-subclavian steal syndrome." Because the result of surgery in these patients is usually excellent, operation is indicated.

DIAGNOSIS. When pathological changes occur in the proximal portion of the innominate, left carotid and left subclavian arteries, blood supply may be decreased to the extracranial tissues, the intracranial tissues or the upper extremities, or a combination of these. Symptoms are similar to transient ischemic attacks. Syncope and convulsions may occur when the patient is placed in an upright position. Other findings are intermittent "claudication" of the forearm, decrease or absense of pulsations in the cervical carotid artery or in the upper extremity of the involved side, facial atrophy, optic atrophy and presenile cataracts.

The "steal" syndrome occurs in patients with stenosis or occlusion in the proximal left subclavian or innominate artery. In this syndrome, the patient is usually unaware of any problems in his upper limbs but has symptoms of cerebral vascular insufficiency, including lightheadedness or a feeling of "blacking out" after using the involved extremity above his head or when standing up quickly. The symptoms occur when pressure in the distal subclavian artery is less than that of the vertebral artery. In these patients, blood may flow in a reverse direction from the vertebral to the subclavian artery during exercise, which causes an increased demand for blood in the tissues and an increased flow through the vessel with the least resistance. The syndrome does not usually occur when significant occlusive lesions are present in all three of the great vessels of the aortic arch. Neurological changes are usually not present.

If a single arch vessel is occluded, it is usually the left subclavian. Occlusion of the innominate artery produces an additional possibility for "steal" from the cerebral circulation, since both the vertebral and the right common carotid arteries would have reversed flow to the right subclavian artery.

Besides diagnostic arteriography, supplementary findings include a discrepancy in the pulses and blood pressures between the two upper extremities and a bruit heard over the anterior chest, the supraclavicular fossa and the proximal course of the arch vessels involved. The bruit is heard with stenosis rather than occlusion.

A Doppler flowmeter may also be used to locate the area of stenosis proximal to the claudication. A "steal" syndrome may be confirmed by the use of two oscillometers. Recordings are made above the elbow of each limb while the carotid artery is compressed on the involved side. Plethysmography may be used as an alternate method.

TREATMENT. Treatment for the subclavian steal syndrome is surgical, anastomosing the distal subclavian-vertebral area to the carotid through a cervical incision. Bypass procedures are performed for occlusions of the carotid or innominate arteries. Results are good for patients with arteriosclerosis, but the long-term result for patients with arteritis is usually poor because of the generalized nature of the disease.

Vertebral Basilar Arterial Insufficiency

Vertebral artery disease can be divided into three categories: (1) patients with disease at the proximal orifice of the vessel who have no carotid artery disease, (2) patients with stenosis in both the vertebral and carotid arteries and (3) patients with a normal vertebral artery who have a proximal subclavian artery obstruction resulting in a "steal" syndrome.

Cerebral symptoms from vertebral artery occlusion are rare but do occur and may require surgery. However, when carotid artery occlusion or stenosis is present simultaneously, surgery for the carotid artery disease is usually performed.

Fibromuscular Hyperplasia

Fibromuscular hyperplasia is generally considered to be a disease of the renal arteries and is one of the causes of renovascular hypertension. However, it may also occur in the internal carotid artery as a separate condition or in both the renal and carotid arteries. It is characterized by a systolic bruit over the involved artery. When the internal carotid artery is affected, intermittent symptoms of cerebral dysfunction may occur, without progression to a stroke. It is confirmed upon angiography by the "string of beads" appearance of the internal carotid artery. There is stenosis of the lumen between each of the small dilated segments. Since the entire internal carotid vessel is often involved, definitive vascular surgery is difficult. It may be impossible to insert a bypass graft, but dilatation has been reported to be successful.[20]

Kinked Internal Carotid Artery

A kinked or buckled carotid artery occurs most frequently on the right side and is often incorrectly diagnosed as a carotid aneurysm because of the prominent pulse in the neck. The extracranial portion of the internal carotid artery may be obstructed owing to the high position of the aortic arch or elongation with resulting "volvulus," "buckling" or "kinking" of an artery that is fixed at either end. Some observers have re-

ported that the entity causes cerebral insufficiency.

Diagnosis is made by symptoms of cerebral insufficiency, a prominent pulsation in the neck, production or aggravation of symptoms by a change in position of head and neck and evidence of kinking confirmed by angiography. Generally the condition is considered benign. However, if an actual obstruction is demonstrated by arteriogram and no other cause for the symptomatology is noted, surgery is indicated.

Emergency Carotid Artery Surgery

Embolectomy is indicated only when immediate surgery can be performed. Otherwise, revascularization of an already infarcted brain may occur, resulting in a hemorrhagic infarct. The surgeon is rarely consulted early, so few operations are advised. There is also controversy regarding immediate surgery on a patient who has developed an acute neurological deficit that progresses or fails to recover. Most clinicians try to avoid surgery and manage the patient with a method similar to that for a completed stroke. At present there is no secure means of identifying which patient has an infarct and which has a simple ischemic area of the brain.

Emergency surgery is advised for patients with transient ischemic attacks whose arteriograms show a very small amount of flow through the stenotic area of the internal carotid artery. Emergency surgery is also indicated for patients whose bruit disappears after arteriography and those in whom arteriographic contrast medium shows extremely narrow or obstructed carotid artery lumen.

Asymptomatic Stenosis of Extracranial Carotid Artery

In the past, asymptomatic patients with a bruit over the bifurcation of the carotid artery or the first part of the subclavian artery were followed closely. However, a more aggressive approach has recently been employed, in which nonstenotic lesions associated with atherosclerotic ulcers and with transient ischemic attacks are removed. Surgery is also indicated for the asymptomatic patient with a stenotic carotid lesion. A more aggressive policy of prophylactic surgery is now recommended by many in order to lessen the likelihood of thrombosis and a resulting stroke. Patients who demonstrate early senile mental changes confirmed by relatives are classified as symptomatic. The totally asymptomatic lesion is still controversial and needs further study as to the benefits derived from prophylactic drugs versus definitive surgery. Since these studies will not solve the problem soon, individual approach is necessary for each patient before a policy is established.

CELIAC AXIS AND MESENTERIC VASCULAR DISEASE (ARTERIAL AND VENOUS)

Ischemic gastrointestinal disease may involve both the arterial and venous systems of the stomach and intestines. It may or may not be occlusive. Until recently, experience with mesenteric vascular disease was confined to the advanced state of massive midgut necrosis that necessitated extensive resection of small intestine and variable amounts of colon. This resulted in death or crippling gastrointestinal symptoms for most patients. Today, several ischemic bowel syndromes are considered, diagnosed and treated successfully.[10, 11]

Etiology and Pathogenesis

The clinical syndrome of chronic mesenteric arterial insufficiency is not common despite the high incidence of atherosclerosis in the vessels that supply the stomach and intestines. The acute occlusive process usually occurs in the orifice of the origin of the artery or in the proximal 1 to 2 cm of the artery and may be caused by an embolism, thrombosis or trauma. A nonocclusive type may also occur, producing infarction, but this is usually the result of extremely poor perfusion of the intestine secondary to shock.

Fibromuscular dysplasia may occur in the celiac, superior mesenteric and inferior mesenteric arterial systems, similar to that noted in renal and carotid artery stenosis. Aortic dissection may extend to or originate in the mesenteric vessels. Even though the celiac axis and the superior mesenteric arteries are the common sites for occlusion, the inferior mesenteric artery is most frequently reported to be occluded in aortic atherosclerosis or aneurysm. When the inferior mesenteric artery is not occluded, it may provide collateral circulation with the superior mesenteric artery and the branches of the hypogastric artery. Therefore, it may be the primary collateral vessel to the intestinal tract as well as to the extremities. This pattern of collateral arterial circulation should be recognized during aortography prior to abdominal aorta resection.

Other causes for mesenteric vascular occlusion are extrinsic compression of the celiac artery by the crus of the diaphragm or by the celiac ganglion. Occlusive lesions resulting from drugs such as methysergide maleate therapy and oral contraceptives are being reported with more frequency. Intestinal parasites have been reported as etiological agents, and patients with vasculitis from periarteritis nodosa and thromboangiitis obliterans may develop intestinal ischemia. All patients with mesenteric vascular occlusion due to arterial or venous thrombosis should have hypercoagulability studies similar to those advised for thromboembolism.

Necrosis of the intestine following sequential lumbar sympathectomy and ileofemoral bypass graft has been described when a marginal mesenteric arterial circulation was present. The phenomenon has been called the "aortoiliac steal" syndrome. Another postoperative mesenteric vascular syndrome that may result in bowel necrosis is the vasculitis that occasionally occurs following repair of a coarctation of the aorta.

Acute Mesenteric Ischemia

There are three distinct syndromes of acute mesenteric ischemia: acute mesenteric artery thrombosis, mesenteric ischemia without vascular occlusion and superior mesenteric artery embolus.

Acute Mesenteric Artery Thrombosis

This, like other acute atherosclerotic occlusive lesions of the peripheral vascular system, is commonly preceded by signs and symptoms of ischemic episodes. Many patients have a history of weight loss, postprandial pain, diarrhea and malabsorption with occult blood in the stool and the presence of an abdominal bruit prior to the episode when the abdominal pain becomes steady or colicky. This stage is followed by the classic signs of an intra-abdominal catastrophe, and symptoms of bowel necrosis develop, with abdominal distention, vomiting and bloody diarrhea. Fever, a marked leukocytosis and radiological evidence of dilated bowel loops are present in the late stages. The patient usually appears acutely ill. The abdominal pain is often so severe that narcotics do not bring significant relief.

There have been occasional reports of successful revascularization without bowel resection even on patients with generalized peritonitis for over 24 hours.

Patients who have survived massive small bowel resections for acute mesenteric vascular occlusion generally have malabsorption, steatorrhea and negative nitrogen balance. To improve the fat absorption in such patients, isocaloric substitution of medium-chain for long-chain dietary triglycerides has been found advantageous. Periodic hospitalization for hyperalimentation infusions has been advised. Home infusions have been used successfully in some patients.

Acute Embolic Occlusion

Acute embolic occlusion of mesenteric arteries should be suspected when there is a sudden onset of severe abdominal pain followed by a forceful evacuation of the bowel, with or without melena, plus a history of heart disease, dysrhythmias and evidence of peripheral embolization elsewhere. Acute mesenteric artery thrombosis is frequently fatal owing to the delay in diagnosis and treatment; the outcome of acute embolic occlusion to mesenteric arteries is potentially more favorable.

Other signs and symptoms of an embolic episode include vomiting, appearance of being severely ill out of proportion to physical findings, leukocytosis and an abdominal roentgenogram that shows absence of intestinal gas. Later signs simulate the symptoms of acute mesenteric artery thrombosis.

Since the embolus is usually lodged in the region of the midcolic artery, the first part of the jejunum appears normal at operation. In contrast, mesenteric thrombosis causes ischemia of the entire small intestine from the origin of the jejunum to the midtransverse colon. An embolus is relatively easy to remove from the midcolic artery; a thrombus is more difficult to extract when it lies at the origin of the superior mesenteric artery in the retroperitoneal area.

Acute Mesenteric Nonocclusive Ischemia

This is very difficult to differentiate from acute occlusive mesenteric vascular disease except by arteriography, absence of prodromal symptoms and the presence of a hemodynamic crisis resulting in a severe reduction in intestinal blood flow. The latter condition is caused by hypovolemic shock, prolonged use of vasopressor therapy, low cardiac output and congestive heart failure. Severe atherosclerotic stenosis of the mesenteric arterial vessel may or may not be present, but when present it contributes to the results. Therapy is directed toward improving the low cardiac output and not toward any surgical procedure. Mesenteric vascular dilatation by continuous epidural anesthesia should be initiated as well as local infiltration of an anesthetic at the base of the mesentery. Intra-arterial vasodilatation and anticoagulants are used to prevent blood sequestration.

Acute Inferior Mesenteric Artery Occlusion

This condition is much less common than superior mesenteric vascular ischemia. Occlusion of the inferior mesenteric artery may produce two syndromes of acute colorectal ischemia: spontaneous thrombosis and iatrogenic ischemia due to ligation of the artery during resection of the abdominal aorta for occlusive disease of an aneurysm.

Spontaneous thrombosis usually occurs in an elderly patient who has advanced generalized atherosclerotic disease. The patient complains of diarrhea and left lower quadrant pain of short duration. Leukocytosis is usually present. Proctoscopy reveals an edematous, pale or cyanotic friable rectal mucosa. Abdominal distention, shock, ileus and peritonitis occur as the ischemic process progresses. Immediate laparotomy is indicated.

Signs and symptoms of postoperative colorectal ischemia are identical to those of spontaneous thrombosis but are obscured during the postoperative period. Roentgenological findings are marked spasms and irritability with narrowing of the colon. A "thumb printing" appearance occurs from the thick-

ened and irregular mucosal folds and scalloping of the mucosal pattern. The mucosa may slough, and ulceration is noted. Treatment is identical to that advised for spontaneous thrombosis. However, some patients may develop a minor degree of ischemia resulting in edema and bleeding or sloughing of the mucous membrane only. Fibrosis and segmental strictures may form later, with constipation and a roentgenological picture of a pipestem or fibrotic left colon. The surgeon may prevent this condition by reconstituting the blood supply to the rectosigmoid colon following aortic resection.

Acute Mesenteric Venous Thrombosis

This is the cause of 15 to 25 per cent of all mesenteric vascular occlusions. It may occur simultaneously with venous thrombosis elsewhere in the body, such as portal vein thrombosis with cirrhosis of the liver, or with a hepatoma, intra-abdominal infection or injury to mesenteric veins. A hypercoagulable state may be present in any of these patients.

The signs and symptoms of this entity are similar to those of acute mesenteric venous occlusion, except that the progression of symptoms is slower. At operation, arterial occlusion presents a pale-appearing bowel, whereas venous occlusion presents an engorged, bluish, edematous bowel. Both sides of the circulation are occluded ultimately. Prognosis for venous thrombosis is generally better than for intestinal infarction resulting from arterial thrombosis. Treatment involves resection of the necrotic bowel followed by anticoagulation.

Chronic Intestinal Ischemia

Chronic visceral ischemia is known by many terms, including abdominal angina, splanchnic ischemia, intestinal angina, abdominal intermittent claudication and chronic occlusion syndrome of the mesenteric arteries. The classic symptoms are postprandial pain and weight loss. The diagnosis is often obscure, partly because the main intestinal arteries may become stenotic or almost completely occluded without the occurrence of any physiological change. The slow progression of atheromatous disease permits the progressive development of a profuse collateral circulation between the celiac and superior mesenteric arteries and the superior and inferior mesenteric arteries. At least two and frequently all three mesenteric artery systems usually must have severe occlusive disease in order to produce the abdominal angina syndrome. Stenosis of the celiac artery alone may produce severe symptoms in one individual, while another who has occlusion of both the celiac and superior artery may have no abdominal complaints.

Diagnosis is first suspected when the patient complains of postprandial pain accompanied by weight loss. Postprandial pain results from intermittent gastrointestinal ischemia and is frequently severely cramping in character. It may occur immediately after eating or be delayed for over thirty minutes. It may last for more than an hour, with radiation from the periumbilical region or the midepigastrium to the back. The severity of the pain often can be related to the size of the meal. The patient may restrict his food intake to lessen the pain. Weight loss may thus range from moderate to severe over a period of several months. Malabsorption may be a contributory factor to the weight loss. Flatulence, abdominal distention and a change in bowel habits may occur. Physical examination usually reveals an abdominal bruit and evidence of atherosclerosis in other areas of the body. The bruit is not diagnostic, since other abdominal atherosclerotic lesions may be present.

Diagnosis rests mainly on a clear arteriographic delineation of the major stenosis or occlusion in the mesenteric arteries. Lateral views are usually necessary to demonstrate the lesions in the proximal superior mesenteric and proximal celiac arteries. Collateral circulation patterns are a helpful finding for diagnosis, especially when the inferior mesenteric artery is tortuous and markedly dilated.

Almost all of the chronic visceral ischemic diseases exhibit external compression of the celiac axis by the crus of the diaphragm or by the celiac ganglion and atherosclerosis of the celiac axis and superior mesenteric arteries.

Treatment is primarily surgical and usually involves thromboendarterectomy, a prosthetic or autogenous vessel bypass, or reimplantation of the diseased vessel into the aorta. Surgical treatment may also require transection of the median arcuate ligament of the diaphragm or celiac ganglion as it courses over the celiac artery.

ARTERIOVENOUS FISTULAS

An arteriovenous fistula is a direct communication between an artery and a vein that permits the blood to bypass the capillary circulation. William Hunter first demonstrated the true nature of arteriovenous fistulas in 1757 when he observed an iatrogenic fistula that developed following a surgical puncture of the brachial artery and vein. Since this historic observation many clinicians and physiologists have studied these lesions, but not until 1968, when Holman published the results of his experimental studies, was there clarification of the physiological changes that may occur from abnormal arteriovenous communications.[40] He listed changes as follows:

Physiological Changes

a. *Immediate Effects*

(1) Both systolic and diastolic blood pressures are decreased.

(2) The pulse rate increases.

(3) The venous pressure increases distally as well as proximally to the fistula.

(4) The cardiac output increases in proportion to the size and location of the fistula.

(5) The heart and the proximal artery temporarily decrease in size owing to the diversion of blood from a high pressure system (arterial) to a low pressure system (venous), as seen in massive hemorrhage.

b. *Remote Effects*

(1) Part of the normal capillary bed is bypassed permanently because of the fistula.

(2) Total blood volume gradually increases in relation to the amount of flow through the fistula.

(3) Proximal vasculature, namely, the heart, artery and vein, dilate gradually because of increased volume of blood traversing the fistula into a low resistance system (venous).

(4) Extensive collateral circulation develops because the fistula has a low resistance to flow and the artery proximal to fistula constricts. The constricted artery contributes to an increased collateral circulation which in turn, because of the volume delivered, results in the artery dilating distal to the fistula.

(5) Heart musculature hypertrophies slightly owing to dilatation, overdistention and increased work load caused by an increased volume of flow.

(6) Pulse pressure widens when the lowered blood pressure recovers. The systolic pressure returns to its prefistula higher level and the diastolic pressure falls.

Physiological changes depend upon the size of the fistula, its location in the arterial tree and the patency of the vein proximal to the fistula. Variations therefore depend entirely upon the quantity of blood diverted through the fistula.

Closure of the Fistula

Closure of the fistula by compression or definitive repair produces the following changes:

a. *Immediate Effects*

(1) Both the systolic and diastolic blood pressures rise and then fall to readings above prefistula levels because the previously low peripheral resistance is eliminated, but the increased blood volume remains in the newly intact vascular system.

(2) Pulse rate and cardiac activity decrease.

(3) Venous pressure decreases proximal to the fistula.

(4) Cardiac output decreases markedly.

(5) Heart size increases for a short period owing to overdistention from the continued presence of an increased blood volume in the newly intact vascular system.

b. *Remote Effects*

(1) Blood pressure gradually returns to prefistula levels.

(2) Total blood volume gradually decreases to normal.

(3) Pulse rate gradually lowers to normal range.

(4) Dilatation in the vasculature proximal to the closed fistula, namely, the heart, artery and vein, gradually subsides but cardiac hypertrophy may be irreversible when the fistula is of a long duration.

Etiology

Arteriovenous fistulas may be congenital or acquired. The congenital type is the most frequently encountered.

Congenital arteriovenous fistulas may occur in any area of the body but are most often noted peripherally. Peripheral fistulas may be classified as: (1) hemangioma, (2) microfistulous arteriovenous aneurysm, (3) macrofistulous arteriovenous aneurysm, and (4) anomalous mature vascular channels. These classifications are based on the alterations that occur during the development of certain mesenchymal cells into mature blood vessels. Since both arteries and veins differentiate from a common capillary plexus, one vessel may function as the other in certain areas of the embryo and during specific stages of embryological life. In addition, it is always possible that any of the infinite number of communications that existed initially between arteries and veins may persist after birth, resulting in congenital arteriovenous fistulas.

Acquired arteriovenous fistulas most frequently result from penetrating wounds such as those from gunshot, stabbing, flying sharp objects or fragments of bone. A second cause is the spontaneous rupture of an arterial wall into the accompanying vein, as when a mycotic aneurysm ruptures into its neighboring vein. Iatrogenic arteriovenous fistulas may be produced inadvertently during surgery or diagnostic procedures involving major arteries or veins.

Sites of Arteriovenous Fistulas

Extremities

Congenital arteriovenous fistulas are most often noted in the extremities, mainly the legs. Any part of the limbs may be involved, including the bones. Usually the lesion has multiple channels that are diffuse or extensive. Even when multiple communications exist, the lesion may appear to be discrete or confined to a relatively small area.

Diagnostic features of congenital arteriovenous fistulas of the lower limbs include the presence of varicose veins. When varices are unilateral, are in an unusual location and present early in life for no apparent reason, one should suspect a congenital arteriovenous fistula. Further suspicion should be aroused when ulcerations develop on the distal part of the foot, a site where venous ulcers do not occur, and when elongation of the limb is noted. The communications may be so large that the varicosities pulsate. Increased warmth over the fistula may be expected. Pain localized to the site of the lesion usually indicates that thrombosis is occurring and may be considered a good prognostic sign. Bruits or thrills are usually not present, and the bradycardiac sign seldom can be demonstrated. The congenital fistula usually is not associated with cardiac effects except in infants. Some lesions become progressively larger at puberty or increase their arteriovenous components following minor trauma or exercise.

When surgery is being considered, arteriograms should be ordered routinely to determine the extent of the lesion. Frequently the presence of an arteriovenous fistula is demonstrated only by the early appearance of the venous phase of the arteriogram. Oxygen saturation samples may be taken from the vein proximal to the fistula and compared with a sample from a similar vein on the opposite limb. A Doppler flowmeter may be used to assist in the diagnosis and to delineate the limits of the lesion.

Treatment for congenital arteriovenous fistulas is often unsatisfactory. Surgery is discouraged unless the lesion can be demonstrated as discrete or localized, for the lesion is frequently found to be more extensive than contemplated, and complete excision is impossible. An approach that is too aggressive may result in the loss of a limb. Serious hemorrhage, extensive ulceration or infection may develop from extensive congenital arteriovenous fistula of an extremity. An amputation may be advisable in some patients with this type of lesion. One promising approach is the use of cryotherapy followed by a pressure dressing. This method of therapy initiates thrombosis within the vascular sinusoids and is not likely to cause permanent damage to tendons and nerves. The procedure is especially advised for hemangiomas of the hand (Fig. 17–26), and although a permanent cure does not result often, it may be used as a palliative procedure every few years. Sclerosing solutions and radiation therapy are useless.

Acquired arteriovenous fistulas are

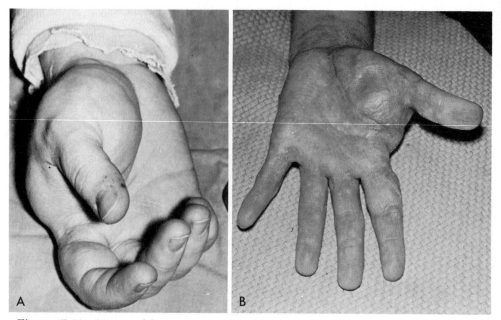

Figure 17–26 Congenital hemangioma of hand in 22 year old female. *A*. Note enlargement of thenar eminence and base of index finger. *B*. Results of intraoperative cryotherapy followed by pressure dressing. Multiple pregnancies necessitated palliative surgery every two to three years.

also most often noted in the extremities and are due almost invariably to trauma. The appearance of a fistula may be delayed for several days because of a hematoma at the site of communication between two vessels. The factors determining the volume flow through the fistula are the size of the opening, its location in the main arterial tree, the absence of fibrosis around the fistula and the duration of the fistula. These factors may be extensive enough to cause an increased blood volume, cardiac enlargement, cardiac failure and thrills localized to the fistula. Hemihypertrophy may be present if a fistula occurs at an early age before the epiphysis closes. Elevated venous pressure produces varicose veins that may pulsate, edema and skin pigmentation about the ankle and chronic induration similar to that seen in a postphlebitic syndrome. Distal ischemic changes, including gangrene, may occur when the fistula is large and collateral circulation is inadequate.

The skin is warmer in the area of the fistula than the skin of the opposite limb. However, the skin distally may be cooler than that of the companion extremity.

A machinelike murmur accentuated during systole is audible over the fistula, and a systolic thrill is palpable. Both are eliminated by pressure over the vein proximal to the fistula. Temporary closure of the fistula by compression causes the heart rate to slow and the diastolic pressure to increase — a positive Branham's sign. Other techniques used to locate the site of fistula are venous pressure (increased), oxygen saturation of the venous blood, thermography, flowmeter studies and arteriography.

Treatment involves some method of definitive repair. Excision of the fistula and reestablishment of the normal arterial and venous flow is preferred as early as possible. When minor vessels are involved, quadruple ligation and excision alone can be performed.

Aorto-inferior Vena Caval Fistulas

These may be spontaneous owing to rupture of an abdominal aortic aneurysm into the inferior vena cava or to trauma caused by a penetrating wound, including iatrogenic fistulas from lumbar disc operations.

Aorto-inferior vena caval fistulas require early diagnosis and repair. If they go unrecognized, the early fatality rate is high owing to their size and proximity to the heart. The physiological changes occur in an extreme degree, with possible additional findings such as massive swelling of the lower limbs and trunk and bleeding from the rectum and urinary tract.

If a patient undergoing surgical removal of an intervertebral disc has an unexplained drop in blood pressure or develops congestive heart failure postoperatively, he should be examined for the presence of an aorto-inferior vena caval or iliac arteriovenous fistula. An audible machinelike bruit in the lower abdomen is diagnostic. Emergency repair is advised in almost all patients.

Pulmonary Arteriovenous Fistulas

These may be congenital owing to persistence of embryological arteriovenous connections, or they may be acquired during pulmonary venous or arterial hypertension, specific types of obstructive lung disease, hepatic cirrhosis and certain infections such as *Schistosoma.*

Pulmonary arteriovenous fistulas may be separated into two groups — those with a pulmonary arterial blood supply, which are the most frequent, and those with a systemic blood supply.

The lesion with a pulmonary *arterial blood supply* causes a certain amount of the pulmonary circulation to bypass oxygenation in the lungs and flow directly into the left side of the heart and into the general circulation. This abnormal pulmonary blood flow pattern results in chronic arterial hypoxia, which produces symptoms of cyanosis, dyspnea, polycythemia and clubbing of the digits. The lesions may be single or multiple, and the majority occur superficially in the lower lobes of the lungs. Hereditary telangiectasis is a common finding. A continuous bruit with systolic accentuation at the time of deep inspiration is a diagnostic sign. The chest roentgenogram will usually show one or more well-circumscribed, noncalcified nodules with vessels connecting them to the hilum, and an angiogram confirms the diagnosis.

The pulmonary arteriovenous fistula with a *systemic blood supply* is very rare. The connecting vessel may be a bronchial, internal mammary or intercostal artery or the aorta. Collateral circulation may be so extensive that rib notching may develop. The signs and symptoms are those of a left-to-right shunt. The common complaint is dyspnea and easy fatigability. Diagnosis is confirmed by chest roentgenogram and angiograms.

The fistulas may be localized to the lung, or they may have associated abnormalities of hereditary telangiectasis of the skin, mucous membranes and other organs. The arterial supply is often multiple and may be bilateral. Surgery is advised if the fistulas are single, show localization when multiple or cause symptoms of progressive enlargement. However, sugery is not advised unless changes occur when the fistulas are multiple and diffuse, or single and asymptomatic.

Renal Arteriovenous Fistulas

These may occur with or without a functioning kidney distal to the fistula.

Fistulas associated with a functioning kidney may have a congenital acquired or idiopathic origin. Congenital lesions are angiomatous or cersoid in appearance and have multiple arteriovenous connections. Acquired fistulas result from hypernephroma, trauma, atherosclerosis or inflammation. The hypernephromatous lesions are due either to tumor invasion of the large vessels of the kidney or to the neoplasm becoming necrotic and forming arteriovenous communications within the tumor mass. Traumatic renal arteriovenous fistulas are caused by penetrating wounds and iatrogenic wounds following pyelolithotomy or percutaneous renal biopsy. Lesions from subacute bacterial endocarditis and other types of infection are rarely noted today.

Diagnosis is based on the existence of a continuous machinelike bruit localized to the renal area, diastolic hypertension, congestive heart failure and hematuria. Renal ischemia may occur from an infarct distal to the arteriovenous communication(s). An excretory urogram may be used as a screening procedure prior to the detailed renal arteriogram study that precedes surgery. Preservation of the kidney is desirable but is seldom accomplished owing to the extent of the lesion or the presence of renal infarcts.

Renal arteriovenous fistulas have been reported following nephrectomy and frequently have been blamed on mass ligation of both renal artery and vein during surgery. However, since not all of the patients reported had mass ligation of the vessels, it is thought that other factors contribute to renal arteriovenous fistulas. These factors include the formation of a hematoma or infection in the area of the pedicle or transfixion of the vessels without simple ligation.

Diagnosis is based on the presence of the aforementioned characteristic signs and symptoms noted for arteriovenous fistulas. Aortography is necessary to confirm the diagnosis and demonstrate the character of the lesion.

Portal Circulation Arteriovenous Fistulas

These are rare but should be considered whenever a patient is studied for portal hypertension. Congenital lesions frequently are associated with hereditary telangiectasis and are localized either within the liver parenchyma or in extrahepatic vessels. Gastrointestinal bleeding may occur because of rupture of the lesions in the submucosa. Acquired arteriovenous fistulas may result from spontaneous rupture of a visceral abdominal artery aneurysm into the portal circulation or may be iatrogenic following mass ligation of an artery and vein during splenectomy, gastrectomy or other intraabdominal surgery in which the vein accompanying the artery is part of the portal circulation. Penetrating or blunt trauma is also an etiological factor as with arteriovenous fistulas in other sites.

Clinical manifestations of portal hypertension occur, such as esophageal varices, ascites and splenomegaly. The diagnosis is suspected in the presence of the usual continuous bruit and confirmed by selective arteriography.

Surgery is indicated. Extrahepatic lesions require excision; revascularization of the vessels depends upon the site of the fistulas. Intrahepatic fistulas usually necessitate a hepatic lobectomy.

Arteriovenous Fistulas of the Neck and Face

These have become rare owing to the early aggressive surgical approach toward repair of traumatic injuries to vessels in this area of the body. Congenital arteriovenous fistulas are less common than acquired lesions. Vessels involved in acquired lesions are the common carotid artery and internal jugular vein and the thyroid, vertebral and subclavian arteries and veins. Penetrating wounds are the common cause, whether they result from violence or iatrogenically following surgery or a diagnostic procedure.

The usual history demonstrates evidence of a penetrating wound or surgery to the neck or face, followed by a hematoma that ultimately becomes pulsatile and presents an audible continuous bruit and palpable thrill. Neurological signs of cerebral ischemia may occur, and the patient complains of pain and a continuous disturbing sound in his head or neck. With a carotid artery and internal jugular vein communication it is common for the patient to develop a unilateral exophthalmus (Fig. 17–27). Occlusion of the carotid artery proximally abolishes the bruit and decreases the pulse, but the procedure may cause siphoning of the distal intracranial bed through the "thirsty" fistula, and syncope may occur. However, when the maneuver is performed carefully it helps to locate the precise site of the fistula. Arteriography is indicated to confirm the diagnosis and the character of the lesion.

Surgery is advised, since the morbid-

ity from these lesions is high. Excision with revascularization of the involved structures is indicated for carotid-jugular and subclavian lesions, while vertebral and isolated neck vessels with arteriovenous fistulas may be excised and ligated only.

Congenital arteriovenous fistulas of the head and neck are almost invariably multiple and often involve the underlying bone. The most frequent complaint is of a cosmetic nature, but hemorrhage or sudden enlargement with pain may occur. Surgery is frequently unsuccessful unless a radical resection is accomplished. Therefore the lesion is studied thoroughly prior to any surgical decision, and the patient is completely instructed as to the problems involved with and without operation.

Pelvic Arteriovenous Fistulas

Like other fistulas, these are divided into congenital and acquired types. Congenital fistulas have multiple arteriovenous connections with the branches of the internal iliac vessels and seldom cause hemodynamic changes in the systemic circulation. Symptomatology usually occurs just prior to menstruation or during pregnancy. When the uterus is involved, vaginal bleeding may occur at any time. Diagnosis is made by the presence of a pulsatile mass noted on pelvic examination and a continuous bruit over the lower abdomen. Arteriography should be performed to assist in establishing the site and size of the lesion before surgery is undertaken. If the patient is asymptomatic, surgery is not always suggested, since complete excision of the lesion may require extensive surgery.

Acquired arteriovenous fistulas result from penetrating trauma, including instances that occasionally develop following hysterectomy. They are thought to be caused by ligation of both artery and vein by transfixion without prior simple ligation. These fistulas usually

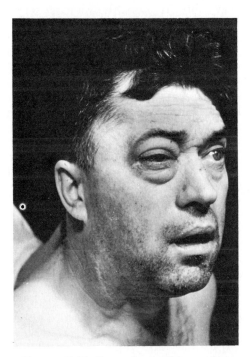

Figure 17–27 Internal carotid–internal jugular arteriovenous fistula causing unilateral exophthalmos. The fistula was created with the erroneous concept that it would improve cerebral ischemia. The fistula was later divided and the vessels repaired with a satisfactory result.

enlarge and produce hemodynamic changes. As with congenital arteriovenous lesions, the presence of a pelvic pulsatile mass and a continuous bruit is diagnostic. Arteriography is advised prior to surgery, which should be performed as soon as possible after diagnosis is made.

Diagnosis

The physical findings associated with arteriovenous fistulas, particularly the acquired variety, may make their diagnosis obvious. In other instances, particularly with congenital arteriovenous fistulas that are neither extensive nor long-standing, the clinical signs may be subtle or absent or consist of findings that may also be present in conditions other than arteriovenous fistula, such as hemangioma, unequal limb growth, varicose veins and others. It is in these same situations that arteriography is least reliable. The fistulas may not be apparent, and diagnosis may have to depend on subtle signs such as increased arborization of the arterial tree or rapid venous filling. Such findings not only fail to establish the diagnosis of fistula beyond doubt but also neither localize the fistula nor provide an estimate of its severity. On the other hand, application of three of the basic tests described in the section on noninvasive diagnosis of arterial occlusive disease can establish or rule out the diagnosis of arteriovenous fistulas reliably enough to eliminate the need for diagnostic arteriography. Clinical applications include determining the presence or absence of occult arteriovenous fistulas as the cause of asymmetrical limb growth, as a component of a more obvious vascular malformation (e.g., hemangioma) or as the cause of atypical or early onset of varicosities. Following trauma, these tests can differentiate between arteriovenous fistula and false aneurysm.

The reduced peripheral resistance associated with arteriovenous fistulas *decreases* mean pressure in the arterial tree proximal to the fistula but *increases* pulse pressure. Therefore, segmental limb *systolic* pressures proximal to the fistula will usually be *increased* compared with the contralateral (normal) extremity. Distal to the fistula, segmental limb pressures may be either normal or *decreased* if the fistula is "stealing" from distal arterial flow. Since an arteriovenous fistula will increase the volume changes normally produced by pulsatile arterial flow, segmental pulse contours obtained by strain gauge, impedance or volume displacement plethysmography will be uniformly greater proximal to the fistula. Distal to the fistula, the pulse volume tracings are often normal down to the digits, where they are usually decreased in magnitude. In addition, the proximal pulse contours have a sharper systolic peak without an anacrotic notch. However, the arterial velocity wave form is probably the most sensitive of these three screening tests. As mentioned previously, the second and third components of the wave form of an extremity artery normally include an end-systolic reversal and a brief period of early diastolic forward flow. End-diastolic flow is normally negligible, so that the velocity wave form rests on the zero baseline. The decreased peripheral resistance seen with arteriovenous fistulas eliminates reversed flow and increases forward flow, particularly during diastole. As a result, the end-diastolic velocity and the entire wave form are elevated above the zero baseline in direct proportion to the decrease in peripheral resistance. These findings are seen with the hyperemia associated with exercise, the relief of ischemia, vasodilator drugs, artificial warming of the extremity and with inflammation, as well as with arteriovenous fistulas and sympathectomy (which significantly increases arteriovenous shunt flow). However, in the absence of these other factors, the described findings are diagnostic of arteriovenous fistula.

Although not a noninvasive test, since it requires both arterial and venous puncture, the estimation of the degree of arteriovenous shunt flow by the labelled microsphere method may be extremely helpful in selected cases. In this technique, a suspension of ^{99m}Tc-labelled 135-micron human albumin microspheres, as used in radionuclide phlebography and lung scans, is injected into the main inflow artery to the extremity, while the lungs are monitored by a gamma camera or a rectilinear scintillation scanner. For one to estimate the degree of arteriovenous shunting in the extremity, it is only essential that the radioactivity incident to the arterial injection of microspheres be compared with that following a subsequent intravenous injection, 100 per cent of which will reach and be trapped by the lungs. In unanesthetized patients, this value is normally less than 3 per cent. This study not only establishes beyond reasonable doubt that there is anatomical arteriovenous shunting in an extremity but also provides an estimate of its degree as a basis for serial monitoring to determine the indications for, and results of, operative intervention.

LYMPHEDEMA

Lymphedema refers to the collection of lymph in the skin and subcutaneous tissues owing to an abnormality of the lymphatic system. It may be classified into primary and secondary types, both of which include several clinical symptoms. Primary lymphedema is thought to be caused by an inherent lymphatic disorder, while secondary lymphedema has an obstructive or akinetic cause. Early changes in the patient with classic lymphedema consist of dilatations of the lymphatics and widening of the tissue spaces owing to edema. Later the connective tissue proliferates and may show stages of inflammatory cell infiltration, pigmentation and scarring of the enlarged lymphatics.

The skin in lymphedema is normal or has a pale appearance. Edema does not occur in the skeletal muscle; it occurs only in the fascial planes and in the skin and subcutaneous tissue.

Normal lymphatics have the capacity to drain away free interstitial fluid. When protein-bound dye is injected into the subcutaneous tissue of an edematous leg, it passes very rapidly via the lymphatic channels toward the groin. Therefore, although fluid is rapidly entering the subcutaneous tissues, the lymphatics normally limit the amount of edema by returning the transudate to the circulation. The protein concentration of this normal edema fluid is low. The main characteristic of lymphedema fluid, however, is its very high protein content. This high protein content is responsible for the organization and fibrosis in the cutaneous and subcutaneous tissues, usually not seen in other cases of edema.

Etiology

In primary lymphedema lymphangiography demonstrates a developmental anatomical variation of the lymphatics. The lymphatic vessels are narrowed and few in number. Hyperplasia with dilated and tortuous lymphatic vessels is observed less frequently. Complete agenesis of the lymphatics and lymph glands is very rare. Females are more frequently affected than men (three to one), and no race is immune.

The predominant feature of secondary lymphedema is obstruction of the normal lymphatic flow, most commonly resulting from inflammation due to infection but often due to neoplastic disease and other causes.

Classification

a. Primary
   1. Congenital — at birth
   2. Lymphedema praecox — onset prior to 35 years

3. Lymphedema tarda — after 35 years
b. Secondary
   1. Obstructive
      (a) Lymphatic
         (1) Chronic infections — bacterial, parasitic, fungal
         (2) Malignant disease
         (3) Surgical resection of lymph glands
         (4) Injury
         (5) Irradiation — x-ray, radium
      (b) Venous
         (1) Normal or enlarged lymphatics
         (2) Hypoplastic or obstructed lymphatics
   2. Akinetic insufficiency
      (a) Causalgia
      (b) Paralysis

Primary Lymphedema

Congenital Lymphedema

Congenital lymphedema may be divided into two types: simple and hereditary. Simple lymphedema occurs at birth or shortly thereafter and involves only one member of a family. The hereditary type affects several members of a family and has become known as Milroy's disease,[57] although both the simple and hereditary types are often identified with this term.

The condition is mildly progressive until puberty, when it frequently becomes worse and may affect part or all of the upper or lower extremities, or both. Ulceration of the skin does not occur. There is an absence of pain, and recurrent attacks of infection seldom occur. Because the skin remains in good condition, the problem is cosmetic rather than functional. Kinmonth's[47] lymphography studies demonstrated hypoplasia of lymph channels in all three types of primary lymphedema, but complete aplasia and severe lymphangiectasia were much more frequent in the congenital group than in the other two types.

Patients with hypoplasia of the lymphatic channels show no other congenital changes in the lymphatic system. Congenital nonhereditary lymphedema is often combined with ovarian dysgenesis, in which case it is often bilateral and, unlike other forms of lymphedema, prone to regress spontaneously. The finding of other congenital anomalies is not unusual in patients with congenital lymphedema.

Lymphedema Praecox

The most common type of lymphedema, it characteristically occurs at puberty and has no familial history. It predominately affects females and is usually limited to the left lower extremity. The swelling begins spontaneously, usually with swelling of the foot or ankle, and spreads upward, increasing during prolonged standing, just prior to menstruation and during warm weather. It is frequently temporary at first. Elevation of the extremity produces temporary decrease of the edema but not disappearance. The amount and extent of the edema are determined by the degree of inherent lymphatic dysfunction present. In time the soft pitting edema progresses to pitting edema with fibrosis; ultimately, the extremity becomes unsightly and uncomfortable. Pain and ulceration do not occur and infection is infrequent.

Varicose veins rarely are noted in patients with lymphedema praecox.

Although the pathological basis of the disease is unknown, it is considered to be an inborn error, not only in the development of the lymphatics but in other organs of the body as well.

Lymphedema Tarda

Lymphedema tarda is the occurrence of primary lymphedema in patients over 35 years of age. This is probably no more than a delayed appearance of lymphedema praecox in patients who have a defective lymphatic system but are more resistant to precipitating factors such as venous entrapment by the common iliac artery. The influence of this factor in lymphedema tarda as well as in the other two types of primary lymphedema needs investigation to determine its incidence, its relationship to clinical findings and whether or not this group of patients needs to be reclassified as the secondary type. Another factor that needs investigation is the presence of microarteriovenous fistulas in the involved limb.

Edema in lymphedema tarda is usually less extensive and occasionally may be limited to the genitalia and thighs.

Differential Diagnosis

Edema due to renal or cardiac conditions or to hypoproteinemia must be excluded before primary lymphedema can be considered. However, any of these conditions may be a precipitating factor when abnormal lymphatics are present.

Premenstrual edema, pregnancy, and prolonged standing, especially in women, causes fluid to accumulate in the lower limbs. This type of edema disappears rapidly with elevation as well as with diuretics, and fibrosis does not occur. Malignant tumors of the abdomen, genitalia and kidney should be suspected in middle aged or older patients who have lymphedema.

Postphlebitic syndrome edema is differentiated by a history of deep vein thrombosis and pain, skin discoloration and ulceration.

Lipedema, when it occurs, is always present in women; it is bilateral and painful and the feet are not involved. Abnormal deposits of fat are present in the lower part of the body and in the lower limbs. Pitting is not present, the skin is soft and pliable, and edema disappears at rest.

Other conditions include pretibial edema from myxedema; arteriovenous fistula; Klippel-Trenaunay syndrome, in which there is elongation of bones,

hemangiomas of the skin and swelling of the leg; and edema due to certain drugs such as corticosteroids and progestin that subsides when the drugs are discontinued.

Diagnostic Studies

Lymphangiography, the intradermal injection of a blue dye or radiopaque contrast media into a lymph tract, demonstrates the lymphatic pathways. In primary lymphedema there may be hypoplasia, hyperplasia or agenesis. Secondary lymphedema is identified by the presence of multiple collateral channels, dermal backflow and changes in the regional lymph glands. When tumor involves lymph glands, it may completely replace the lymph nodes.

Phlebography of the lower extremities establishes a venous etiology for edema but is useless for patients who are thought to have primary lymphedema. On occasion the determination of the protein concentration of the edema fluid may help to establish a diagnosis. Controversy prevails as to the benefits of radioactive protein studies.

Complications

The chief complication of lymphedema is erysipelas. The slightest abrasion or laceration may introduce bacteria. Recurrent infections destroy additional lymphatics and the lymphedema progresses. Antibiotics should be prescribed and foot hygiene stressed.

Occasionally a lymph fistula may develop from a skin vesicle and drain for weeks, making ligation of the proximal lymph channels necessary.

Secondary Lymphedema

Secondary lymphedema is caused by obstruction of the lymphatic or venous systems or by an akinetic insufficiency of the extremity.

Lymphedema resulting from neoplastic invasion of lymph pathways is found in patients with malignant disease of the breast, uterine cervix, uterus, vulva, bladder, prostate gland, skin or bones. The clinical signs and symptoms of the primary malignant lesion may not precede the appearance of lymphedema. Therefore, a neoplasm must be ruled out if unexpected swelling of an extremity occurs, especially when the lymphedema develops after forty years of age. Other malignant conditions that may cause secondary lymphedema are Hodgkin's disease, lymphosarcoma and Kaposi's sarcoma. Many of these lesions may be complicated by simultaneous venous occlusion of the femoral or iliac veins.

Surgical removal of lymph nodes and lymph vessels for malignant disease of an extremity or following a radical mastectomy with a block dissection of the axillary lymph nodes may predispose to secondary lymphedema. Occasionally the upper extremity becomes edematous immediately after the operation and gradually progresses into a severely edematous limb termed *elephantiasis chirurgica*. However, in other patients there may be a delay of months or years before the extremity becomes edematous. Several explanations can be given for the discrepancy in the time before lymphedema occurs. Lymphedema that occurs immediately after surgery is probably caused by a complete excision of the lymphatic pathways. An axillary venous thrombosis can be a major contributory factor to the swelling. The later occurrence of swelling may be caused by lymphangitis and secondary obstruction of the remaining lymphatic channels due to a minor accident. A thoracic outlet syndrome prior to, shortly after or some time after surgery may be a contributory factor. Shoulder exercises and avoidance of prolonged periods of abduction help to lessen or eliminate edema from the extremity. Recurrence of tumor at a higher level or lymphangiosarcoma should be considered as an additional cause of late edema.

Radiation therapy is mentioned in the literature as provoking a fibrous reaction in the tissues within the area of treatment and producing further obliteration of lymphatic channels, thus aggravating or causing edema. We have not been able to prove conclusively that irradiation has been a primary contributor to edema. If it does participate significantly in the process, all other possibilities should be excluded before this mode of therapy is blamed.

Venous entrapment of the left common iliac vein by the right common iliac artery should be listed under secondary lymphedema even though it could be a contributory factor to lymphedema praecox or lymphedema tarda.

Obstructive lymphedema, which is more common than primary lymphedema, is caused by inflammation from infection more often than by malignant tumors or iatrogenic causes. Chronic or recurrent inflammation leads to occlusion of lymph channels by thrombosis, which in turn causes lymph stasis and results in fibrosis. With each successive infection the edema increases. The common offending organism is the streptococcus. However, fungus infection of the feet may contribute to recurrent attacks of infection, although edema from this cause is usually limited to the foot and ankle.

Parasitic invasion of lymphatic tracts is frequently seen in the Middle or Far East. The most common organism is filaria; the eggs and larvae provoke an inflammation in the lymph glands and vessels with ensuing fibrosis and obstruction of the normal flow of lymph. This type of lymphedema, referred to as *elephantiasis*, often involves the external genitalia and lower extremities with the development of a markedly deformed limb. In patients with elephantiasis, multiple projections identified as *lymphostatic verrucosis* may occur on the toes.

Patients with intolerable pain in an extremity, such as causalgia, or individuals with motor paralysis of a limb may develop secondary lymphedema because of immobility. These conditions cause an akinetic insufficiency within the lymph pathways owing to the accumulation of tissue fluid within the extremity. Without active movement of the limb, the lymph vessels have to transport a volume of fluid much higher than they are capable of handling. The lymph channels enlarge in a manner similar to that seen in lymphedema when the lymphatic pathways are obstructed. Consequently, the valves fail to close and valvular insufficiency of lymph circulation develops. In patients with prolonged lymphatic obstruction the vessels may disappear, either by lymphatic thrombosis or by perilymphatic fibrosis and contracture. The most serious complication of lymphedema is lymphangiosarcoma, which may develop in these obstructed lymphatics.

Any kind of burden on the lymphatics may upset the delicate balance between lymph formation and transport, whether it is due to venous stenosis from scars or arterial entrapment, thrombophlebitis causing a rise in capillary blood pressure, increased capillary permeability due to bacterial invasion, burns or other injuries, increased flow from microarteriovenous fistulas, occlusion of lymph channels by malignancies, block excision of lymph glands or lymphangitis.

Differential diagnosis of secondary lymphedema is made by lymphangiography, pelvic phlebography and determination of the protein concentration of the edema fluid after a detailed history and an evaluation of the clinical state of the patient is obtained. The possibility that the lymphedema is due to a malignant lesion must always be considered.

Treatment for Primary and Secondary Lymphedema

Lymphedema can usually be controlled medically by a combination of simple measures. Most patients do not have a major functional deformity and therefore surgery is usually unjustified. The cause of the lymphedema must first be established by the history, clinical assessment and specific examinations such as lymphograms, pelvic phlebograms and biopsy of the edematous tissue before therapy can begin.

Medical treatment must be instituted before fibrosis develops. Control of the edema is begun by using high daily doses of oral diuretics such as chlorothiazide and B-complex vitamins for a few days or a week or on a daily basis.

The lymphedematous extremity should be elevated whenever possible. The patient should use a portable pneumatic compression device for at least an hour each day until optimum results have been obtained. The edema can usually be reduced significantly; however, tissue hypertrophy will not be affected. Tailored elastic stockings or tights should be ordered when edema has been reduced to its least amount. A pure rubber bandage may be used over a cotton stocking until the elastic stocking is available. The same bandage may also be applied over the elastic stocking for those patients whose edema is more difficult to control.

Patients with postmastectomy lymphedema should support the limb in a sling during the day and exercise it as well as elevate it on pillows during the night. Bandages and a gauntlet elastic support should be applied during the day. The intermittent pneumatic compression machine should be used each day. Diuretics may be prescribed with the usual precautions taken to avoid hypokalemia and electrolyte disturbance. However, the use of diuretics has been somewhat disappointing.

Regular swimming exercises may be of benefit. The patient should avoid standing or sitting for long periods since limb movements propel the lymph. Encouragement of short intervals of elevation should be emphasized repeatedly.

Patients should be evaluated as to treatment response. Occasionally patients who have been under treatment for some time should stop using diuretics or elastic supports to determine if withdrawal of therapy is possible. For patients with advanced lymphedema in which fibrosis is present, treatment usually must be continued indefinitely.

Patients with an advanced type of lymphedema or an identifying cause such as venous entrapment should be considered for surgical therapy.

Traditional operations, such as the excision of all peripheral lymph-bearing subcutaneous tissue, have not met with prolonged success. These procedures are based on the theory that the lymph vessels below the muscle fascia are patent and subcutaneous fluid may be drained by these channels. These procedures are done in stages, one half of the leg at a time. Following surgery, the reduction of edema should be maintained by the same procedures mentioned in the nonsurgical management. More often than not the limb returns to its former size in a few years. Modifications of traditional surgical procedures have been performed, such as excising the skin with the subcutaneous tissue and muscle fascia and covering the defect with split thickness skin grafts.

Other operations include the implanting of nylon or silk threads in the subcutaneous tissue to provide new extralymphatic drainage channels, burying a shaved skin pedicle flap to enhance lymph drainage by transferring subcutaneous lymphatics into the deep compartment of the limb, implanting lymph vessels into lymph nodes by microsurgical technique, creating lymphaticovenous anastomosis and transposing omental tissue into the subcutaneous tissue. None of these procedures have been widely accepted.

When the common iliac vein·is entrapped by the right common iliac artery and there is elevation of the venous pressure inferior to the occlusion, a Silastic bridge is placed beneath the artery, after intimal adhesions within the

vein lumen are excised (Fig. 17–28). Trimble and associates have attained successful results in the majority of patients operated upon.[86]

Indications for surgery in primary and secondary lymphedema are: (1) failure to reduce the limb size in spite of adequate medical management, (2) functional impairment, (3) significant skin changes, (4) recurrent infections, (5) presence of a malignant lesion obstructing the lymphatics, (6) evidence of venous entrapment of the common iliac vein(s) or subclavian vein and resulting elevated venous pressure, (7) unsightly appearances, and (8) emotional problems related to the deformed limb.

Following excisional surgery, the limb must receive elastic support, and supplementary diuretics should be prescribed. If an aggressive postoperative program is not contemplated this type of surgery is ill-advised, for even with such a plan, excisional operation for lymphedema leaves much to be desired. However, patients who undergo the procedure have fewer incidences of infection than untreated patients.

Patients who have recurrent lym-

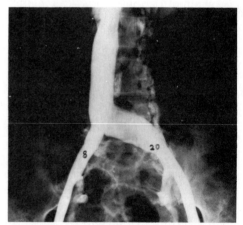

Figure 17–28 Venogram of inferior vena cava and iliac veins. Note defect of left common iliac vein from right common iliac artery and intimal adhesions. Pressure in left iliac vein was 20 mm Hg, while pressure in right iliac vein and inferior vena cava was 8 mm Hg.

phangitis, cellulitis or a minor open wound should receive vigorous antibiotic therapy routinely.

Lymph Collection in Wounds

Lymph collection in a wound, often identified as seroma, serum collection or lymphocele when chronic in nature, is a surgical complication that is of concern, especially if it occurs in the areas of the axilla, groin or adductor canal. The incidence is higher when transverse incisions have been performed or local venous occlusion is present. Treatment by repeated aspiration of the loculated amber-colored lymph fluid accompanied by a pressure dressing occasionally fails to eliminate the problem. In these patients the lymphocele requires excision and transfixion suture of the patent lymphatic vessel(s). The same may be necessary when a persistent lymph fistula is present; however, a pressure dressing often causes the lymphatic duct to clot, and lymph drainage ceases. Invariably lymphedema is present in these patients postoperatively and usually requires additional therapy.

MISCELLANEOUS PROBLEMS

Cold Injuries

Cold injuries produce peripheral vascular changes that cause characteristic symptoms and lesions.[37, 38, 69] The degree of injury from cold is the result of four environmental factors: temperature, moisture, wind and duration of exposure. Temperature and moisture determine the type of lesions that will develop, and the wind and duration of exposure determine how rapidly and how severely the lesion will appear. Cold injury may develop from prolonged exposure to relatively mild degrees of cold. The terms chilblain, trench foot, immersion foot, hypothermia and frostbite are not ways of classifying the degree of injury but of identifying the different modes of development.

Chilblain

The mildest form of cold injury is known as chilblain. It occurs after prolonged exposure of uncovered areas of the body in a climate that is moderately cold (60°F to freezing) and extremely humid. It is usually seen on the dorsal aspect of the hands of outdoor workers and on the anterior tibial surface of the lower extremities of young women. It is said to be common in the bare knees and cheeks of British schoolboys. Acute and chronic states are recognized. The chronic form, which is caused by repeated episodes of exposure, is termed pernio, Bazin's disease or erythrocyanosis. The local lesions are swollen and have a deep reddish purple discoloration. They form blisters that may ulcerate and produce pigmented scars after healing very slowly. The acute form has a bluish red color. It is swollen, hot and associated with itching and tenderness. Occasionally it may cause a burning pain. Treatment is symptomatic and includes advice that the patient dress warmly and prevent continued exposure. Anti-inflammatory and sympatholytic agents may be indicated to reduce pain and swelling.

Immersion or Trench Foot

Immersion or trench foot is seldom seen in civilian life. Its presence has been most frequently reported in sailors or soldiers who have wet feet for prolonged periods in temperatures ranging from 68°F to freezing. Dependency or immobility of the extremity and constriction by clothing or shoes are predisposing factors. Chilling and anoxia of the extremity accompanied by general body cooling and venous stasis results in nerve, muscle and blood vessel changes. As in patients with frostbite, it is not uncommon to observe that the patient has a previous history of personality instability, a labile peripheral vascular system and a marked tendency to perspire on the hands and feet. These individuals are characterized as sympathetic reactors and are often noted as problem cases in peripheral vascular clinics.

On first examination, the clinical manifestations include an ischemic, cold, swollen appearance of the feet and legs. Subjectively, there is a numb, tingling, itching and cramping pain and a mottled discoloration of the skin. Unlike frostbite, the tissues are resilient to palpation. The skin is soft and often very friable. This first stage is termed the prehyperemic phase. It may last for a few hours to several days and is followed by a hyperemic phase of several weeks. In this stage the pain may be severe; the feet are red, swollen and hot. Blisters appear, and ulcers and gangrene may occur. The third, or posthyperemic, phase is characterized by residual edema and deep pain. Superficial burning pain, hyperhidrosis and cold sensitivity are also present. This phase may continue for months or years.

Prevention requires education of the patient, chiefly those individuals who may experience a cold, wet environment. Rubber footwear should not be worn if possible, since it causes an extremely humid environment within the shoes. It is necessary to keep the feet dry at all times. Spare socks should be carried by people who are prone to wet feet or are in an environment where feet may easily become wet. Periodic elevation, massage and air drying are suggested, and constrictive clothing should be avoided.

Treatment is similar to that for frostbite except that thawing is not necessary.

Frostbite

PREDICTING OUTCOME. Because early physical findings in frostbitten limbs are notoriously deceptive, prognosis of ultimate tissue loss should be based on a system not solely dependent on the physician's examination.

The outcome of a given case of frostbite can be predicted with reasonable accuracy by knowing: the duration of exposure to the group temperature, the wind velocity and humidity, the type of protective clothing worn, and contact with metal or wetness that occurred, individual susceptibility such as a history of very moist hands and feet, and the blood supply to the area frozen. The patient's history and weather bureau data are essential means of evaluating methods of treatment and predicting tissue loss in most cases.[49]

FREEZING PROCESS. Freezing begins by the formation in the extracellular space of a small particle of ice that increases in size and number of crystals by drawing water from the cells into the extracellular space. It is supposed that the cell membrane is ruptured either by the mechanical compression of the ice crystals during freezing or by the rapid ingress of water into the cells during thawing. Many of the gross anatomical and cellular changes associated with freezing injury seem to occur largely during thawing, which makes the method of thawing important, since slow or gradual thawing may re-form larger crystals during the melting period, or red blood cell aggregation may initiate thrombosis of small distal vessels. Rapid rewarming, especially for deep frostbite, preserves the greatest amount of tissue and ultimately the most function.

Frostbite is the severest form of local cold injury. The injured area initially becomes white. Upon thawing, the sequence of response has three phases: (1) local skin erythema, (2) a wheal at the site of injury and (3) a flare in the marginal tissues.

CLASSIFICATION. Some clinicians prefer to classify frostbite into two types: *superficial*, which results in superficial dry freezing, and *deep freezing*, which is deep frostbite. However,

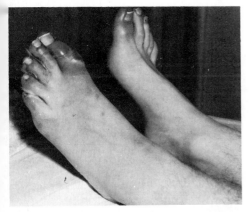

Figure 17–29 Frostbite: first and second degree at twenty-four hours. Following rewarming, second degree frostbite exhibits blister formation and first degree frostbite is erythematous. Sensation is preserved.

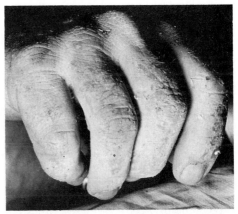

Figure 17–30 Frostbite: fourth degree, fourteen hours after rewarming. Absence of edema is an ominous sign, and it was correctly predicted that the fingers would be lost eventually because of total absence of sensation.

the commonly accepted classification of thermal tissue injury is preferred for cold injury as well as for burns (Figs. 17–29 through 17–32), and is as follows: first degree: erythema, swelling, burning and tingling without the formation of blisters; second degree: blister or bleb formation, edema, anesthesia and paresthesia that is marked by hyperemia on rewarming; third degree: full thickness injury with early edema, early necrosis and gangrene but without loss of a part; fourth degree: complete necrosis and loss of a part.

First and second degree frostbitten skin is cold and crisp. It may be moved freely over bony surfaces before it is thawed. Third and fourth degree frostbitten skin is not pliable over bony prominences and feels solid or wooden to palpation. However, all four types of cold injury may be similar on palpation after they are thawed. For this reason, Mills believes that these designations are academic clinically because the initial treatment, namely, rapid rewarming, is the same.[56]

PREDISPOSING FACTORS. Through the ages, beginning with Hippocrates' writings "on air, waters and places," certain types of people have been observed to have an increased suscepti-

bility to frostbite. As mentioned in the section on immersion or trench foot, the responses of these individuals (who are called sympathetic reactors) have verified the role of psychic and personality factors in frostbite. It is not uncommon

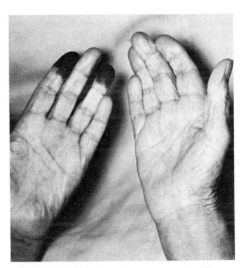

Figure 17–31 Frostbite: second degree, three weeks after injury. The blue skin eschar present subsequently peeled off, leaving normal tissue underneath. While it is true that the ischemia appears superficial in this patient, the point is made that surgical débridement of frostbite should not be aggressive unless wet gangrene appears.

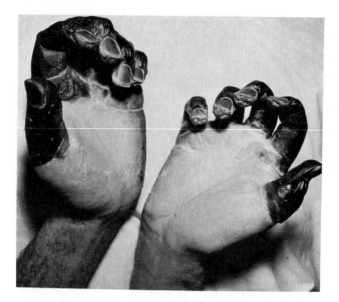

Figure 17–32 Frostbite: fourth degree, several weeks after injury. The desiccated necrotic digits eventually underwent autoamputation, which is the preferred method of treatment whenever possible. This method allows preservation of maximum length, since the deep tissues occasionally are viable for a greater distance than the epithelium. Skin grafting can be performed when necessary following autoamputation.

to observe that the patient who has developed frostbite after exposure to cold environment has had an increased incidence of neurasthenia, poor adjustment, poor motivation and excessive sweating. Since these people are inclined to place themselves in danger, it is essential that they be identified, educated about the hazards of a cold environment, and not be assigned to work in severe cold. They are readily recognized by their nonconforming habits and evidence of sweating on hands and feet. This does not imply that all patients with frostbite fit into this group; there are many cases in which exposure was quite unavoidable.

Another group exists that is not particularly susceptible but is apparently uninformed: the dedicated outdoor sports enthusiasts who participate in cross-country skiing, snowmobiling, ice fishing and hunting during cold weather. This group has increased in number with the growth in popularity of winter sports.

Racial susceptibility has not been clarified, but certain individuals, especially Eskimos and Arctic fishermen, apparently have developed a cold acclimatization at the cellular level. Studies on adaptation to cold by animals appear

quite convincing, but similar human response studies have been inconclusive.

ENVIRONMENTAL FACTORS. The depth of cold penetration into the tissues and the duration of exposure of the affected part to the cold environment are the final determinants of the severity of frostbite. This conclusion, as previously mentioned, is based on inquiries from weather stations in the area where the exposure occurred. Inquiries must be made regarding the ambient temperature and other environmental factors that increase heat loss by either conduction or convection. A temperature of 22°F or below apparently produces the highest incidence of frostbite (see Table 9–2).

The type of clothing worn is obviously important. Studies have shown that wool cloth beneath an outer garment of closely woven windproof fabric makes excellent use of the insulating properties of still air.

Proper headgear and footwear are extremely important. Gloves should be worn at all times, especially when hands must come in contact with metallic objects.

A sound educational program should be continually stressed for individuals who live in or are transient in cold regions. The failure to cover properly some specific area of the body often determines the pattern of injury.

EARLY TREATMENT. Superficial frostbite should be thawed immediately to reduce the total time of cold exposure and lessen the potential of a freezing injury.

Simple methods are often effective: to thaw the face, place a warm hand over the area until the face becomes painful; fingers are best treated by placing the hand in the opposite axilla; and feet can be warmed by placing them on the abdomen of a companion beneath the clothing. When hot objects are used, extreme caution should be taken to avoid burning of the insensitive cold part. Rubbing or otherwise applying snow or slush to the part is absolutely contraindicated.

When deep frostbite has occurred the core body temperature should first be raised. Constricting clothing or boots should be loosened to avoid circulatory loss. Rapid rewarming is not recommended until the patient reaches a medical facility. This avoids the possibility of a frozen part being thawed and then refrozen, which is likely to cause the loss of some of the part.

After arrival at the hospital, immediate measures are taken in the Emergency Department to raise the body temperature to normal. Vital signs are monitored and treatment for shock is initiated after inserting a central venous pressure catheter and drawing blood for routine analysis, including pH, blood gases and electrolyte determinations. An electrocardiogram should be taken and interpreted immediately. Bradycardia and dysrhythmias are life-threatening and should be continuously monitored and treated as indicated.

If the patient is suffering only from frostbite and has no cardiorespiratory problems, rapid thawing is begun by immersion of the part(s) in a whirlpool bath for two or more hours at 104° to 107.5°F (40 to 42°C) until the distal vascular bed shows flushing. The prognosis is favorable if there is prompt return of sensitivity in the skin and large pink blisters extending to the digit tips appear. Unfavorable prognostic signs are additional trauma to the cold-injured part(s), ruptured blebs, purple or reddish-blue blebs, cold and cyanotic digits distal to the blebs and complete absence of edema after severe injury. Thawing is painful. Rewarming may require the use of analgesics or intra-arterial or intravenous injection of 25 mg of tolazaline hydrochloride (Priscoline) or 0.6 mg of dihydro ergot alkaloids (Hydergine). These may be used at the physician's discretion.

Patients who show evidence of hypothermia of the legs or of the entire body should be hospitalized with bed rest until body temperature has returned to normal, edema subsides and the blebs dry. Cold injury that does not result in a lowering of the body temperature and frostbite that is localized only to the hands, ears or nose do not require more than a short hospital admission or treatment in the Emergency Department. In these patients the same procedures are instituted at home or on an outpatient basis as for patients admitted to the hospital.

The frozen areas are cleansed with antiseptic soap and water if the extremity was already thawed when first seen. Aseptic precautions are taken in the hospital, using sterile sheets, footboard, cotton between the toes and reverse isolation until the blebs are dry. Frostbitten fingers are covered with sterile dressings with cotton or sterile lamb's wool between the digits. Blebs should not be ruptured. Tetanus prophylaxis is administered either by a toxoid booster or human antitoxin. The injured parts are immersed in a whirlpool at body temperature with antiseptic soap for 20 minutes twice a day, and the patient is encouraged to move every joint of every part not only while in the whirlpool but also during the intervening waking hours.

If digital circulation appears to be impaired and digital motion is limited by the constricting black eschar, lateral escharotomy is undertaken during the second or third week. Débridement or amputation is not instituted until the skin begins to separate. This may require as long as four months. By this time the black eschar will have peeled off or the digits will have become shrunken and mummified and be considered for amputation. "Frozen in January, peel in March and amputate in July" is an often-quoted axiom. Antibiotics are administered if superimposed infection develops.

SUMMARY. Since most patients with superficial or deep frostbite have been warmed before medical treatment is sought, physicians working in the Emergency Department should accept the responsibility of educating the lay public and ambulance and rescue personnel. All individuals engaged in prehospital emergency care should be trained in the technique of rapid rewarming. If the geographical site of cold injury is far enough away from the hospital to delay treatment significantly, emergency health personnel should begin rapid thawing procedures. If refreezing may occur or adequate warming equipment is unavailable, thawing must not be done until the patient arrives at the hospital. Dry heat should never be used for thawing, for the already injured tissues may easily be burned.

Reimplantation of an Extremity

An Emergency Department that receives a large number of traumatized patients will occasionally have patients who are referred for reimplantation of a dismembered extremity. It is rare to have both the patient and the dismembered part meet the criteria for reimplantation. Before an Emergency Department physician alerts a specialty service, he or she must recognize that certain guidelines for the procedure of reimplantation must be reviewed before this treatment is initiated.

General Criteria

The optimum limb for reimplantation is one that has been dismembered cleanly in a young patient at a site between the midarm and the base of the fingers. An avulsed arm should not be reimplanted when the major nerves and vessels were avulsed several centimeters away from the limb. Furthermore, it is contraindicated to reimplant an extremity that has a severely comminuted fracture or is crushed distally, or where there is a double amputation. Rarely should a single finger or fingertip be reimplanted. At present, reimplantation of lower extremity amputation is confined to those circumstances that are ideal and to cases of bilateral limb amputation.[54]

When a severed part does not accompany the patient, transportation personnel are advised to obtain any tissue left at the scene of the accident. If the tissue is not used for reimplantation, the skin on the part may be available for grafting at the amputated site or elsewhere on the body.

The dismembered extremity must have the potential of viability; that is, the extremity must reach the hospital within twelve hours after injury, having been kept cold by being placed in a plastic bag and then in ice water.

Tissue destruction of the dismembered part and of the patient's amputated stump must not be extensive.

The candidate must be young.

The patient must have been in good physical and mental health prior to the accident.

The plan must be explained thoroughly to the patient and his relatives and they must agree to every aspect of the undertaking.

Team A (responsible for the patient) and Team B (responsible for the severed extremity) are designated, and necessary liaison between the two teams is established. The teams should include a general surgeon, a vascular surgeon, a neurosurgeon and an orthopedic surgeon, respectively.

After team assignments are made in the Emergency Department, both the patient and the severed extremity are transported to the operating room.

Only those hospitals designated as comprehensive trauma centers and experienced in the techniques should undertake a limb reimplantation. All other hospitals should arrange for transfer of the patient and of the refrigerated limb to a hospital with these qualifications.

Thoracic Outlet Compression Syndrome

Much of the confusion regarding the diagnosis and treatment of shoulder girdle compression syndromes has abated since 1962 when Falconer and Li and Claggett reported their experience with first rib resection for severe thoracic outlet compression syndrome. This syndrome grouped together all of the possible causes for neurovascular signs and symptoms of the upper extremities, including scalenus anticus, costoclavicular, cervical rib, hyperabduction, shoulder-hand, fractured clavicle, effort vein thrombosis and pneumatic hammer syndromes. The authors advised that the first rib be resected in patients who were unresponsive to physiotherapy, traction and collars and even to scalenotomies. Their studies and reports of other workers have shown that all shoulder girdle compression syndromes have one problem in common — compression of the brachial plexus and the subclavian artery and vein, usually between the clavicle and the first rib (Fig. 17–33). Therefore, the thoracic outlet compression syndrome should be considered in all neurological and vascular complaints of the upper extremities.[63]

Resection of the first rib for thoracic outlet compression syndrome was cautiously accepted at first because the two surgical approaches available at the time, namely, the supraclavicular and the parascapular, were complicated, traumatic and somewhat hazardous and provided limited exposure. However, since the introduction of the relatively simple transaxillary approach by Roos in 1966, first rib resection has been used almost to excess. We believe that only about one patient out of five with shoulder girdle complaints should be considered for surgery. The remainder either respond to physiotherapy or have symptoms so mild that surgery is not indicated.

Symptoms

Symptoms may be grouped into neurological and vascular complaints. The most common neurological symptom is aching pain in the side or back of the neck, extending across the shoulder and down the arm into the forearm and hand. The pain may radiate in all directions from the point of compression. Numbness and tingling are frequently experienced in the hand, usually located to a C_8–T_1 distribution, and fine coordination may be affected. Any sustained upper extremity activity aggravates the pain and causes paresthesias and weakness. These activities include combing hair, painting, throwing a baseball or football or any other use of the hands above shoulder level, reaching, using a typewriter, holding a newspaper, telephone or steering wheel, and backpacking. The pain is usually not noticed until after the arm is used. It may be particularly troublesome at night, often causing the patient to awaken.

Vascular complaints may be divided into arterial and venous symptoms. Arterial symptoms range from coolness, cold sensitivity and pallor of the hand on elevation to Raynaud's phenomenon or occlusion of the subclavian artery. Venous symptoms vary from edema, stiffness of the fingers and venous engorgement in certain elevated arm po-

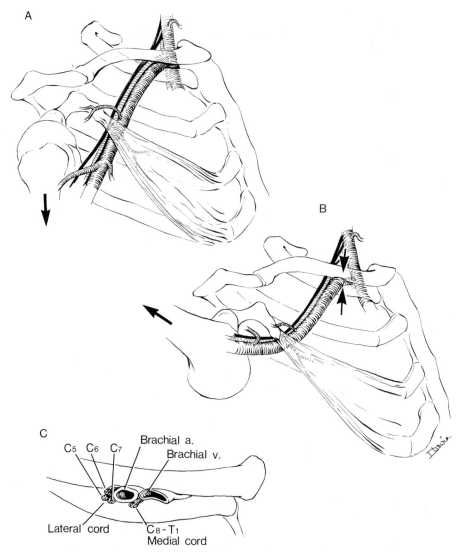

Figure 17–33 Pathological anatomy in thoracic outlet compression.

sitions of shoulder depression when carrying heavy objects to acute thrombophlebitis of the subclavian or axillary vein (Fig. 17–34).

The onset of symptoms may be either spontaneous or post-traumatic. Most patients with spontaneous symptoms are thin females in their twenties or thirties, while male patients usually have a muscular body build. The post-traumatic group may include anyone who has received an injury to the shoulder, clavicle or neck. Any severe jerking injury to the shoulder or neck, such as the so-called "whiplash" auto injury, may precipitate the outlet syndrome. The appearance of arm symptoms may be delayed for several days, weeks or even months after the injury, and the symptoms tend to respond poorly to physical therapy. Other examples of traumatic etiology of the syn-

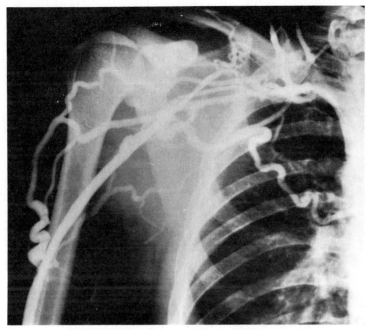

Figure 17-34 Subclavian vein thrombosis due to thoracic outlet entrapment. The patient also had hypercoagulability causing priapism. Treatment was given with heparin followed by first rib resection.

drome are brachial plexus palsy following arm abduction and long-term exposure to vibrating tools.

Patients may present mild, moderate or severe forms of the syndrome. The mild complaints include occasional numbness and tingling of the extremity, especially at night and most often in patients who sleep with their arms above shoulder level. They do not seek or need medical attention. The moderate group has pain in the neck, shoulder, arm and hand for which they seek diagnosis and care. The severe form has limitation of ordinary activities, pain and loss of sleep. Complications such as Raynaud's phenomenon, emboli, thrombophlebitis or muscle atrophy may also occur in the severe category.

Many of the symptoms described by patients are so similar that a diagnosis can often be considered from the history alone. However, confirmation must be made by physical examination.

Signs

Signs may be divided into vascular and neurological changes. The compression of the brachial plexus and subclavian vessels is demonstrated with the arm in a 90-degree, abduction–external rotation (AER) position, without shoulder elevation. With this maneuver the clavicle swings posteriorly and inferiorly from its fixed fulcrum at the sternoclavicular joint, creating a scissorlike entrapment of the plexus and subclavian vessels against the first rib and producing a decreased or absent radial pulse, a blood pressure fall of 15 mm Hg or greater, and a bruit of the subclavian artery either above or below the clavicle. With both arms elevated in the 90-degree AER position and the subclavian artery partially occluded, the fingers are flexed rapidly to demonstrate the "claudication test." Forearm pain and finger paresthesias occur within a few seconds in an extremity with an outlet syndrome, and the arm will soon collapse from fatigue and discomfort. An extremity without arterial compression may be exercised for over a minute with little or no distress. Positive findings with these maneuvers do not necessarily identify the patient as having a thoracic outlet compression syndrome. However, these tests assist in confirming the diagnosis in individuals whose pulse is obliterated at less than 90-degree abduction and who identify the level of abduction as the position at which their complaints are reproduced and in patients who have neurological complaints without vascular signs. It is possible to produce pulse obliteration or murmurs in the subclavian artery in various positions of the head and arm in many normal individuals, especially young women. This suggests that even in the normal adult the thoracic outlet is limited to little more than enough space to permit the passage of the subclavian vessels and the brachial plexus. A change in posture such as an abnormal descent of the shoulder girdle in adults, a fractured clavicle, hypertrophy of the scalene muscles, a large scalene tubercle on the first rib, a cervical rib or any other condition that may compromise the reserve space available predisposes to a thoracic outlet compression syndrome.

Neurological signs include reproduction of the symptoms by thumb pressure in the supraclavicular fossa over the subclavian artery and brachial plexus, tenderness to tapping in the same site, pinprick hyperesthesia in the hand (most often in the C_8–T_1 (ulnar) dermatome), weakness of the interosseous muscles of the hand innervated by the ulnar nerve, and weakness of the biceps and triceps muscles and the hand grip. Normal tendon reflexes are usually present, and nerve conduction times of the ulnar and median nerves are almost always normal. The ulnar nerve is more often involved than the radial and medial nerves because it is formed from the C_8–T_1 cervical roots, the lowest cord of the brachial plexus.

This portion of the cord lies directly on the first rib and therefore may receive the greatest compression in the bony "scissor blade" of the clavicle against the rib.

Differential Diagnosis

Differential diagnosis includes herniated cervical disc, cervical spondylosis, carpal tunnel syndrome, bursitis, capsulitis, tendinitis, shoulder or wrist arteritis, myositis, angina pectoris, multiple sclerosis and carcinoma involving the brachial plexus. Each entity may be confused with a thoracic outlet compression syndrome. Appropriate studies including x-rays must be used to differentiate these disorders.

Treatment

Treatment first considered is a means to enlarge the thoracic outlet by improving posture and exercises to strengthen shoulder suspensory muscles. The patient should be told about the anatomical reason for the complaints, that is, the scissors effect of the clavicle and first rib upon the neurovascular structures in the outlet area. To relieve this, the patient is instructed to elevate both shoulders and push them forward when passing through a doorway or when stopped for a traffic light when in an automobile. Soon the patient unconsciously reverses the abnormal descent of the shoulder girdle, and symptoms lessen or disappear. Additional measures for relief of symptoms are traction, heat, ultrasonic treatments and rest from all activities. These measures are beneficial to most patients in the mild to moderate categories.

When conservative measures fail, surgery may be considered but usually only after nonoperative means of treatment have been used for at least three months. Surgery requires the removal of the first rib. This allows the plexus and vessels to drop slightly, and the clavicle then has no hard surface against which to trap these structures. The preferred approach for rib removal is via the axillary route. If definitive vascular surgery is necessary, the clavicular approach may be incorporated as a separate incision.

Complications may be an occasional wound infection, a brachial plexus injury from refraction, or residual hyperesthesia when the upper thoracic sympathetic ganglia have not been removed. Other complications include residual neck pain because the entire posterior portion of the rib (and the cervical rib when present) was not included in the resection, and postsympathectomy neuralgia over the anterior superior portion of the chest and shoulder on approximately the tenth postoperative day. The latter may be relieved by sympatholytic drugs as reported elsewhere in this chapter.

Sympathetic Disorders

The diagnosis and treatment of disorders of the sympathetic nervous system has had a colorful and interesting history for more than a century. The first classic description of pain related to the sympathetic nervous system was made in 1864 by Mitchell, Morehouse and Keen, who reported burning pain in soldiers with gunshot wounds of peripheral nerves, an entity that Mitchell eight years later termed causalgia.[58] Sympathetic ablation as therapy for specific disorders was advocated by Jennisco in 1897 and by Jaboulay two years later.[43, 44] They advised periarterial sympathectomy as a method of treatment for epilepsy, glaucoma, migraine and ulceration of the feet. Following their reports, the leading advocate for the diagnosis and treatment of sympathetic disorders was René Leriche, who published many articles on the subject beginning in 1913. Sympathectomy achieved widespread popularity for peripheral vascular diseases about thirty years ago, but this popularity was lost when ganglionic blocks were introduced and reconstructive vascular surgery was developed a decade later.

Diagnosis

Diagnosis of sympathetic disorders is based on careful clinical evaluation of vascular and neurological changes due to congenital or familial conditions, vascular diseases, trauma, metabolic abnormalities, infections or combinations of these.

There are *four primary reasons* for treating conditions that are related to overactivity or underactivity of the sympathetic nervous system: (1) the presence of vasospasm, (2) the need for small collateral channels when there is obstruction of a major arterial vessel, (3) the relief of causalgic type pain and (4) the elimination of hyperhidrosis.

Clinicians frequently have widely divergent opinions about the value of therapy involving the sympathetic nervous system because some patients fail to achieve the expected results from treatment. Therapy involving the sympathetic nervous system has much to offer patients when the *limitations* are clearly understood and properly ordered. A sound knowledge of the variations in the anatomy of the sympathetic nervous system and of the pathophysiology of the patient's condition is essential before treatment can be advised. The results of treatment may be influenced by improper choice of drug, inappropriate technique used in blocking sympathetic ganglia, improperly performed sympathectomy and the failure to appraise clinical results by objective measurements.

Relief of pain is one of the most interesting and dramatic responses to medical or surgical sympathetic therapy, specifically in patients who have causalgia or causalgic type pain that is burning, hypersensitive, numb and superficial in nature. No relief of deep pain of somatic root origin should be expected.

The beneficial effects of sympathectomy are not always permanent in vasospastic and occlusive arterial disease. Another problem is that sympathectomy may produce unexpected bizarre pain syndromes postoperatively in patients with causalgia.

Sympathectomy for vasospastic conditions such as Raynaud's phenomenon consistently fails to have the same lasting effect in the upper extremities that it has in the lower extremities. Sympathectomy may produce dramatic improvement in the initial postoperative period when performed for Raynaud's phenomenon, which is secondary to other diseases. However, its effect is generally so short-lived that the procedure is considered of little value, especially when scleroderma is present. For the primary type of Raynaud's disease, sympathectomy is valuable for relief of pain but is not necessarily useful for the abnormal color changes that frequently recur postoperatively.

The dependent rubor in severe occlusive disease is due to paralytic vasodilatation or chronic hyperemia in the small peripheral vessels and therefore sympathectomy is not indicated. However, the procedure may be warranted for causalgic type pain in patients with chronic arterial occlusive disease. An intra-arterial sympatholytic drug such as Priscoline may identify the type of pain that may be relieved by surgery.

Since arteriosclerosis obliterans is a progressive disease, the development of a rich collateral bed does not change the possibility of further thrombosis of the vessel. Any patient with rapid progression of disease usually has the poorest effect from a sympathectomy.

The means by which sympathetic tone returns is obscure. It has been suggested that "intrinsic tone" or increased sensitivity to circulatory catecholamines develops. Reserpine has been found to reduce the catecholamine content of the tissues.

There also has been much published about *regeneration* of sympathetic nerve fibers postoperatively. There are several proposed theories as to why autonomic activity returns following sympathectomy. Regeneration has been classified as early (within one year) or late (after a year or more). Theories for early return of sympathetic activity are: (1) the sympathectomy was not adequate, (2) an anatomically complete sympathectomy cannot be performed, since the sympathetic trunks frequently have anatomical variations, and (3) the sympathetic pathways readjust when fibers cross over from the contralateral side. One theory for late regeneration is that the remaining intact fibers of the sympathetic nervous system respond to a stimulus produced by nearby degenerating fibers. Fine branches develop from these fibers and contact the adventitial cells of remaining axons to reach the degenerated structures. Theories to explain early or late regenerations are: (1) the disease for which the sympathectomy was performed may progress and the resulting reduction in blood flow may be considered (erroneously) to be caused by a regeneration of a sectioned sympathetic change, and (2) the vessels are hypersensitive to circulatory catecholamines, the amino-oxidase content of the arterial wall is lowered and the normal synthesis of acetylcholine in the arterial wall is eliminated.

"Regeneration" is most often noted, and is considered more significant, in patients under forty who underwent sympathectomy two or more years prior to the return of sympathetic tone. The earlier the return of symptoms, the more likely that an inadequate sympathectomy was performed; reoperation may be indicated for these patients.

Occasionally one hears of a patient who was relieved of *intermittent claudication* following a lumbar sympathectomy. However, there is overwhelming evidence that sympathectomy is not useful for uncomplicated intermittent claudication. Any improvement results indirectly from the relief of foot symptoms as well as from the manner in which the patient ambulates.

Sympathectomy should not be advised for patients who have no chance for revascularization of the extremity or for those whose bizarre pain patterns *might* be relieved by sympathectomy. The *"hope for improvement"* is not a logical reason for performing a sympathectomy, especially in a patient whose extremity is doomed to amputation. Sympathectomy also should not be performed when definitive vascular surgery is indicated.

Indications for Sympathetic Denervation

These can be divided into three groups of disorders: vascular, neurological or both. Selection of patients is therefore based on careful clinical evaluation of these systems.[65]

VASCULAR DISORDERS. These are evaluated first according to the presence and degree of peripheral arterial flow, by utilizing one or more of the diagnostic studies previously described in the section on chronic occlusive arterial disease. Collateral circulation may simply be determined by the degree of blanching on elevation, the extent of cutaneous congestion on dependency, and the time of venous filling in the toes and foot. Blanching of the toes and forefoot should not occur in less than 120 seconds; upon dependency, flushing time should be 20 seconds or less in the same area and venous filling should be 30 seconds or less. A constant red or purplish red color on a dependent foot denotes poor collateral circulation, and sympathectomy to improve vascular flow is contraindicated.

The presence or absence of vasospasm should be recorded. The simplest method is to block the posterior tibial nerve inferior to the medial malleolus. An increase in toe temperature and improvement in its cutaneous

circulation denotes a probably successful result following sympathectomy. Plethysmographic studies, as previously described, provide an additional means of evaluating an active vasoconstrictor mechanism.

Sympathetic blocks may be used to select patients for sympathectomy — the stellate ganglionic block for the upper extremity or the lumbar sympathetic block for the lower limb. Both procedures are unreliable if the block is technically incomplete. The validity of the test depends on the expertise of the clinician performing the block, the absence of anatomical variables in the sympathetic ganglia and the use of instruments and tests that identify specific physiologic changes in the extremity following the procedure. Horner's syndrome occurs after a successful block of the sympathetic impulses to the cervical chain. However, Horner's syndrome does not prove that the postganglionic sympathetic fibers supplying the involved upper limb were anesthetized. This needs to be verified by demonstrating the absence of sudomotor activity with a skin resistor or by evaluating the digital blood flow with a plethysmograph or by recording temperature changes with a thermocouple in a temperature-controlled room. Tests for the accuracy of the procedure are also required when a lumbar sympathetic block is performed. When digital temperature or blood flow decreases, a sympathectomy is not advised. Neither spinal nor epidural anesthesia should be utilized to evaluate pain problems related to the sympathetic nervous system, since somatic root and sympathetic type pain patterns cannot be differentiated.

Unless a definite positive response is obtained by one test, multiple tests for patient selection should be performed. The optimum test is the one that is the simplest and most frequently utilized by a clinician who thoroughly understands the patient's problem and the limitations of the diagnostic procedure.

CAUSALGIA. Causalgia or causalgic type pain may develop from injury, infection, venous or arterial disorders or peripheral nerve conditions. Although the pain has many interesting aspects, it is most often characterized as a superficial burning pain with hyperesthesia localized to the involved site or part. It may occur on any surface of the body but is most often localized to an extremity. Therefore, clinicians who treat vascular disease see it in patients with vascular disorders and in patients referred for consultation about pain of possible vascular etiology. Relief for these patients rests on an accurate diagnosis and adequate medical or surgical sympathetic denervation.

Various names are used to identify "causalgia." The common names are acute atrophy of bone, Sudeck's atrophy, traumatic angiospasm, reflex nervous dystrophy, post-traumatic osteoporosis, minor causalgia, neurovasospastic phenomenon and chronic traumatic edema. The pain may be totally related to the sympathetic nervous system or to a combination of somatic root pain and sympathetic pain. Similar types of pain are seen in vascular disorders such as Raynaud's phenomenon, thoracic outlet compression syndrome, postsympathetic neuralgia, pain of arterial or venous etiology associated with rest pain, and postphlebitic ulcers, frostbite, and so on. In some of these conditions the vascular signs may be of minor importance; the pain is the major complaint for which the patient is requesting relief. Proper therapy depends upon consideration of the vascular changes as well as of the character of the pain preoperatively and postoperatively.

The most outstanding *symptom* of causalgia or causalgic pain is *burning type of superficial pain.* The superficial aspect is emphasized to differentiate it from deep pain that has a somatic root origin, e.g., traumatic neuritis, abscess, ischemic neuritis, neuromas, and so forth. Other descriptions of causalgia are "throbbing" or "vise-like."

The pain may occur instantaneously, but most often it is delayed for days or weeks. On the extremity, the pain referral is distal and occupies chiefly the palm of the hand, the fingers, toes or the plantar surface of the foot.

Hyperesthesia is the second most conspicuous complaint and may be localized to a sensory nerve. Frequently there is an area of numbness closely related to the area of hyperesthesia.

Increased sweating of the involved hand or foot may be very marked in traumatic or vasospastic disorders. Often a past history of sweating can be obtained.

Vasomotor changes may vary from vasoconstriction to vasodilatation. The involved part may be warm and erythematous initially and may later manifest vasoconstriction, being pale, cool and wet. Patients with arteriosclerosis obliterans commonly show a shiny, scaling, dry foot.

Additional signs may include stiffness of joints, swelling and roentgenological evidence of spotty osteoporosis.

Diagnosis is based on a history of an overactive sympathetic nervous system, with superficial burning pain exceeding the expected amount and hyperesthesia localized to a sensory nerve.

Diagnosis may be readily established by injecting Priscoline, 25 mg, or Hydergine, 0.6 mg, intravenously or into the proximal artery. Prior to the injection the patient is told to classify his pain as 100 per cent, and after several minutes he will be requested to determine what percentage of the original pain remains. The pain is evaluated by stroking the area of complaint before and after the injection. If over 50 per cent relief is obtained for 30 minutes or more, one can conclude that at least part of the pain is related to the sympathetic nervous system. A similar method may be used to monitor the results following oral intake of sympatholytic drugs or a sympathetic block. Any residual pain may or may not be related to the somatic root.

HYPERHIDROSIS. This is a rare pathological condition of excessive perspiration limited to the palmar surfaces of the hands, the feet and the axilla. Patients are usually young, nervous individuals with serious psychological and social problems. The sweating may be extremely annoying, embarrassing and even incapacitating in certain occupations. When the patient is under a nervous strain, water may literally drip from his fingers and cause him to avoid handshaking, piano playing, typewriting or touching objects such as delicate materials. When the patient's feet are involved, his socks and shoes are so wet that they become foul-smelling, and the skin easily becomes macerated and subject to fungus infections.

Relief seldom is obtained by either medical treatment or psychotherapy; however, when these approaches have failed, surgical removal of the sympathetic nerve pathways is indicated and produces relief. When all four extremities are involved and more than two extremity sympathectomies are being considered, they should be staged at six month intervals to allow readjustment of thigh and arm sudomotor activity. No more than three extremities should be denervated.

PHANTOM LIMB PAIN. This pain often is described as causalgic in type. When pain is localized to the distal portion of the phantom limb and is described as burning and superficial in character, the same approach to diagnosis and treatment as described previously for causalgia is taken. Stump pain is not related to the sympathetic nervous system.

ADDITIONAL CONDITIONS. Additional conditions for which some method of sympathetic denervation may be considered are herpetic neuralgia, postparalytic pain and rheumatoid arthritis.

Treatment

Prompt diagnosis and treatment lessens the likelihood of fixed patterns of pain, which cause dysfunction and atrophy of the part.

The nature of the disease, the physiological basis for the pain and the possibility of therapeutic relief are explained to the patient in an attempt to obtain his cooperation. This patient-doctor understanding is best obtained by injecting one of the sympatholytic drugs in the manner previously described. Following a favorable response to an intra-arterial or intravenous sympatholytic drug, the physician prescribes an oral sympatholytic drug such as Hydergine, 0.5 to 1.5 mg four to six times a day, or Dibenzyline, 10 mg three times a day. Each medication is adjusted to patient response and usually is advised just prior to bedtime when the pain is often most severe.

A paravertebral sympathetic block is indicated when previously described diagnostic methods are short-lived, the pain does not lessen, the medications cause too many side effects or permanent relief from pain does not seem to be forthcoming. The block is routinely checked for adequacy by confirming the absence of sweating by gross evaluation or a skin resistance apparatus.

When pain relief occurs for four or more hours following any of these methods, the treatment is repeated as often as is feasible.

A sympathectomy is indicated when drug therapy or intermittent paravertebral sympathetic blocks fail to elicit progressive improvement in a few weeks, when the pain is so severe that other methods of therapy seem unwarranted, or when additional indications for sympathectomy are present. These include diffuse small vessel involvement, ischemic slow-healing superficial ulcers, the need for development of small collateral channels, or vasospasm. Occasionally a sympathectomy may be justified to relieve the pain in a patient with dependent rubor. However, the procedure is contraindicated unless the major portion of intolerable pain is demonstrably sympathetic in origin.

Postsympathectomy Pain Syndromes

Unexpected postoperative pain patterns may develop in patients who have a sympathectomy. These pain patterns may be separated into five types according to the time of occurrence and site of origin.[67]

Type 1 is the recurrence of the preoperative pain approximately six days after an apparently adequate sympathectomy and during the period when the temperature of the foot lessens. It seems to occur only in patients with severe ischemia who have disabling rest pain and dependent rubor. Sympathectomy is ordinarily contraindicated in such patients to improve circulation but may on occasion be done for pain. Possible explanations for the pain are: hypersensitivity of the vessels to circulatory catecholamines or to an unknown hormone or an intrinsic change in the smooth muscle. Injection of Priscoline, 25 mg, into the proximal femoral artery is effective treatment for this type of pain.

Type 2 is the reappearance of the preoperative pain within three months after supposedly adequate sympathectomy. Possible reasons for the recurrence are: a readjustment of the sympathetic pathways, a less than adequate sympathectomy or similar causes as listed under Type 1. A more extensive sympathectomy unilaterally or bilaterally is required for relief.

Type 3 is the reappearance of the preoperative pain one year or more after an adequate sympathectomy. This type probably is due to "regeneration" or to the readjustment of the sympathetic pathways. Treatment is the same as was advised preoperatively for the pain and may require a higher sympathetic block, a contralateral sympathectomy if the block relieved the pain, or a more extensive sympathectomy.

Type 4 is the most common syndrome and is identified as postsympathectomy neuralgia. The pain usually occurs about ten days postoperatively, proximal to the preoperative site of pain. It manifests itself as a causalgic type of pain and is localized chiefly to the lateral, anterior or medial areas of the thigh. It often includes the buttocks, with a deep pain in the sacroiliac area of the involved side. It is possibly due to irritation of the preganglionic fibers on the anterior spinal nerve during surgery. The pain is usually limited for a period of three months. Sympatholytic drugs may be used orally, intravenously or intra-arterially on the involved side to relieve the complaints.

Type 5 is the appearance of pain in the operative site months following surgery. The pain is localized to a sensory nerve that was traumatized during operation and is termed postsympathectomy causalgia. Relief is obtained by the methods previously described for medical sympathetic denervation.

If the clinician following the patient postoperatively does not understand these pain patterns, he or she may unjustly consider the sympathectomy as a failure or the sequelae too severe and frequent to advise sympathectomy for other patients. One very intriguing aspect of these pain syndromes is that their incidence is extremely high in patients undergoing sympathectomy for causalgic type pain.

Chronic Leg Ulcers

Chronic leg ulcers have concerned clinicians since early times because of their common occurrence and the difficulty of their cure. Chronic ulcers of the extremities are almost always a symptom or complication of another illness. Although most leg ulcers are secondary to the venous or arterial disease, some result from insufficient innervation of tissues, ulcerating neoplasms, blood disorders, endocrine disturbances or other local and systemic diseases. Careful analysis of these various etiologies may help to establish a rational system of treatment. Sometimes the diagnosis is obvious. More often, the history needs to be more detailed and the examination may necessitate specific laboratory procedures such as biopsy, culture, angiography and other means to uncover a systemic disease. The location of the ulcer, its appearance, the degree of pain and the number of lesions present are important aspects in distinguishing one type of ulcer from another (see Table 17–2). Some characteristic features of several types of chronic ulcers are listed here to assist the clinician in determining the correct diagnosis and the factors that influence healing of the ulcer.

Venous Ulcers

In 1868 John Gay[26] wrote that "ulceration is not a direct consequence of varicosity but of other conditions of the venous system of which varicosity is not infrequently a complication." Over one hundred years later some clinicians continue to believe that postphlebitic leg ulcers require that varices be injected, ligated or excised. However, many individuals with severe varices do not suffer from ulceration, and patients with chronic venous insufficiency and ulceration of the legs often do not have varicose veins. There is no noticeable difference between ulcers with or without varicose veins. There are a few venous leg ulcers that have a "venous lake" beneath the lesion and a few with an identifiable vein "feeding" the ulcer through a nearby perforator. There are also those that can be termed "varicose vein ulcer" due to trauma, infection or localized minute arteriovenous con-

nections. But attention must be directed to the essential problem of hydraulics, namely, the leg muscle pump. This leg pump is an efficient system in normal people but it has such little reserve that standing for long periods in one position will cause edema of the ankles. Venous return may be impaired by arterial insufficiency, arteriovenous fistula, defects in the relay pumping mechanism and venous obstruction due to structural defects, functional changes or both. Chronic venous insufficiency, therefore, may occur from thrombosis in the deep veins with or without recanalization; incompetency of the deep, perforating and superficial vein valves; failure of muscle contraction owing to knee or ankle joint changes from arthritis; prolonged dependency and immobility of the lower limb; or from a combination of these causes as well as from arterial insufficiency affecting the capillary flow.

Rarely does a postphlebitic ulcer appear earlier than two years following deep vein thrombophlebitis. The mean period is usually seven years. The appearance of a venous ulcer is preceded by edema, induration and reddened pigmentation of the skin in the medial malleolar region, accompanied by a sensation of distention and severe itching. This may progress to pain upon walking or bathing. Ultimately a superficial single ulcer develops over a thrombosed vein.

Complications occur when the ulcer is permitted to remain open and develop repeated infections. Further induration and scarring occurs, producing the chronically edematous leg and reducing the possibility of early healing. This chronic tissue inflammation often leads to calcific changes in the surrounding tissues and the foot is drawn into an equinus position. Hemorrhage seldom occurs in a large ulcer but is frequent in smaller lesions.

Chronic venous ulcers rarely become malignant unless they have failed to heal in fifteen or more years.

Patients with a history of repeated episodes of thrombophlebitis and patients with recurrent ulcers should be investigated for hypercoagulability. Treatment of chronic venous ulcers has been discussed previously in this chapter.

Arteriovenous Fistula Ulcers

Leg ulcers may occur from arteriovenous fistula. This vascular short circuit bypasses the capillary system and delivers a higher pressure to the veins. Venous hypertension causes ulcers as well as skin pigmentation, induration and varicosities. The diagnosis and treatment of these ulcers, whether the fistula is congenital or the result of trauma, has been discussed in the previous section on arteriovenous fistula.

Dependency and Immobility Ulcers

Ulcers of dependency and immobility occur in the aged arthritic, in people with chronic congestive heart failure and in patients with any other condition that results in limited ambulation.

Immobility and dependency of the limbs in patients with severe arthritis may cause edema complicated by ulcers, which are usually located in the lower third of the legs, often in the region of the malleoli.

Patients with chronic heart failure and respiratory difficulties may be obliged to remain seated both day and night with their legs dependent. This dependency and immobility results in venous hypertension of the limbs, which causes ulcers of the legs when combined with excessive leg edema, hypoproteinemia, distention and skin fissures. These ulcers tend to weep copiously and become infected.

Therapy includes elevation of the leg to lessen edema, cardiac medication, diuretics and application of Unna's paste boots even after the ulcers have healed.

Traumatic Ulcers

Traumatic ulcers of the legs are common and may be self-induced or neurotropic in origin.

Pain may be of diagnostic importance in an ulcer related to trauma. Ischemic ulcers are the most painful, especially hypertensive ischemic ulcers. Dependency decreases the pain of an ischemic ulcer. Venous ulcers and most of the other ulcers mentioned here are usually only mildly painful. Neurotropic ulcers are easily identifiable by their lack of pain. Wound care includes débridement, moist soaks and antibiotics. Unna's paste boots that are changed periodically may be of therapeutic value.

Arteriosclerotic Ulcers

Arteriosclerosis obliterans of the lower extremities may produce a spontaneous, isolated ischemic ulcer. However, the ulcer is usually initiated by trauma. The ulcers are localized most frequently in the digits, occasionally in the foot, and more rarely in the leg. They are almost always unilateral on the extremity, which is pulseless and cool. There is usually a prior history of intermittent claudication. Pain is often lessened by dependency, and the ulcer has a pale gray base.

So-called "senile ulcers" are ischemic lesions due to arteriosclerosis of the small vessels in the skin. There is neither obliteration of the pedal pulses nor a history of intermittent claudication. The most important factor in their appearance is some insignificant trauma. They occur most often in people in the eighth or ninth decade of life.

Treatment is the same as that described in the section on arterial diseases. A senile ulcer may not heal until a lumbar sympathectomy is performed.

Unna's paste boots are also recommended for senile ulcers.

Hypertensive Ulcers

Hypertensive ischemic ulcers occur as the result of obliterative lesions of the small arterioles. They begin with the appearance of a pigmented or purpuric spot of variable extent or a reddened spot that becomes cyanotic in a few days. An ischemic superficial necrosis then occurs, from which an ulcer with a grayish base is formed. Frequently the ulcer is bilateral and symmetrical and located on the anterior lateral or posterolateral aspect of the leg near the junction of the middle and lower thirds. The ulcer may be very painful and resistant to treatment. No visible circulatory changes are present and there is seldom any edema. Lumbar sympathectomy relieves the pain and promotes healing. Treatment of the hypertension is indicated.

Diabetic Ulcers

In diabetic individuals arteriosclerotic ulcers are not uncommon and ulcerated plaques *(necrobiosis lipoidica)* may occasionally be seen. Small vessel disease is often present in diabetics. These patients may develop one or more isolated areas of ischemia on the leg, presenting a chronic black eschar with little or no inflammation. Pedal pulses are usually present and there is no history of intermittent claudication.

The recommended treatment is a lumbar sympathectomy. Attempts to excise and graft the ischemic lesion invariably fail unless a healthy bed for grafting can be identified during surgery.

Corticosteroid Ulcers

Patients may present with necrotic, punched-out ulcerations on an extrem-ity after receiving corticosteroids for arthritis for 15 or more years. These lesions are seldom painful except in the base of the ulcer. Treatment requires débridement, application of wound-stimulating ointments, and heparin injected twice daily into the subcutaneous tissue of the abdominal wall. Most of these ulcers ultimately heal with this regimen. The lesion is caused by an obliterative arteritis. Unna's paste boots may be of therapeutic value.

Neurotropic Ulcers

These ulcers develop from repeated trauma to the extremities of patients with myelopathies and neuropathies such as syringomyelia, transverse myelitis, tumors or injuries of the spinal cord. Ulcers also occur from peripheral nerve disturbances such as neuritis, leprosy, injuries or tumors of nerves. The ulcers develop as plantar lesions on the toes, or over bony prominences on the leg, ankle or foot. They are usually single, indolent, deep and infected.

Routine wound care and antibiotics are advised.

Vasculitis Ulcers

There are a number of systemic diseases that are characterized by generalized vasculitis. Among these conditions are lupus erythematosus, necrotizing angiitis, periarteritis nodosa, rheumatoid arthritis and allergic vasculitis. Proliferative and degenerative inflammation of the capillaries and arterioles occasionally develops in one or more areas of the leg, resulting in necrosis and ulceration. Scleroderma ulcers are found on the toes, feet and bony prominences. Leg ulcers from vasculitis are frequently localized in the lower third of the leg but occasionally may present at a higher level. They may be single but are usually multiple; they are small in size with bluish-purple, indurated edges and are mildly painful (see Fig. 17–4). Treatment is directed toward the specific disease and usually requires corticosteroids. Subcutaneous heparin is administered in the abdominal wall.

Hematological Ulcers

The most common hematological ulcers derive from sickle cell disease. They may occur on the foot, ankle or leg and are caused by ischemia secondary to thrombosis of small arterioles. Treatment is usually successful when Unna's paste boots are applied periodically (Fig. 17–35).

Other hematological conditions that may cause leg ulcers are spherocytic anemia, thalassemia, polycythemia vera, leukemia and dysproteinemias such as macroglobulinemia and cryoglobulinemia.

Treatment is directed toward the underlying disease and the ulcer is handled in a mannner similar to that described for a postphlebitic ulcer. Antibiotics are usually indicated.

Frostbite Ulcers

Ulceration from frostbite occurs on the digits and feet. However, leg ulcers (chilblains) may occasionally develop, most frequently in young female children or adolescents. Diagnosis and treatment have been discussed in the frostbite section earlier in this chapter.

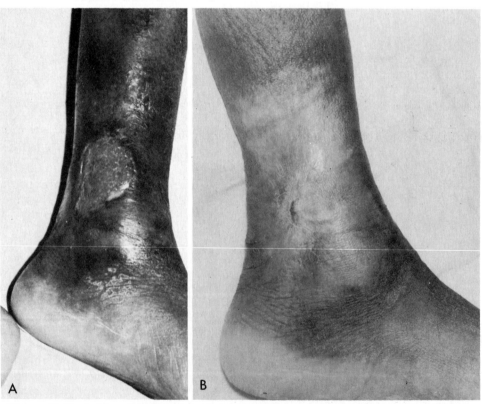

Figure 17–35 Sickle cell ulcer (A) healed following several applications of Unna's paste boot (B).

Miscellaneous Ulcers

A number of systemic or nonvascular diseases may cause leg ulcerations. Among these are reactions to drugs such as bromides, ergot and methotrexate; infections, including fungus, syphilis, tuberculosis and other bacterial organisms; metabolic conditions such as pyoderma gangrenosa (associated with chronic ulcerative colitis), Gaucher's disease, gout and porphyria cutanea tarda; tumors such as basal cell epithelioma, Kaposi's hemorrhagic sarcoma, squamous carcinoma, lymphoma, hemangiolymphangioma and malignant melanoma; and many other isolated conditions.

General Measures of Treatment

Excluding the treatment required for the underlying disease, most leg ulcers require a variety of approaches, each related to specific findings noted on examination of the lesion and the limb. The number of dyes, antiseptics, ointments and other materials used for local treatment is endless. Generally the simplest and least expensive form of therapy is the most successful. Antibiotics are seldom used in leg ulcers unless cellulitis, diabetes, ischemia or a blood dyscrasia is present. Antifungal drugs are frequently used, since most leg ulcers contain fungi that are synergistic with the bacterial organisms inhabiting the ulcer.

All predisposing factors must be investigated and eliminated when possible. Diabetes must be controlled, arterial circulation reestablished when considered to have a reasonable chance of being successful, anemia corrected, hypercoagulability averted, and so on.

The application of heat from any source to an ulcerated extremity is absolutely contraindicated. Moist soaks that utilize body heat are less hazardous and more logical.

Chronic or indolent ulcers should be cleansed frequently with saline soaks and exposed for a couple of hours daily to prevent maceration. Biopsy should be considered, for various neoplasms will cause chronic ulcers (see *Miscellaneous Ulcers*). When circulation is adequate and edema is present, the affected extremity should be elevated above body level until the edema subsides. If enzymatic ointments are used for chemical débridement, mechanical débridement must not be abandoned. Ointments that stimulate the growth of healthy granulations are advised for nonischemic limb ulcers. However, the ointment should produce no harm to surrounding tissues, or "daughter" ulcers may appear. A fungicide soak such as potassium permanganate (1:10,000) applied for 30 minutes three times a day for three days should routinely be used prior to the application of an Unna's paste boot.

Ischemic ulcers should be kept dry to discourage bacterial growth. Aqueous solutions of Mercurochrome or tannic acid are good drying agents. A logical policy is to keep moist ulcers moist and dry ulcers dry when gross infection is not evident and there is some doubt regarding the cause of the ulcer.

When the patient is ambulatory and there is adequate arterial circulation to the limb, elastic support stockings represent a practical approach. This treatment should be accompanied by leg elevation for short periods prior to the development of swelling. Unna's paste boots may be substituted for elastic stockings. Diuretics may help the patient to keep the limb free of swelling. Subcutaneous heparin is frequently prescribed for patients who have vascular ulcers that are refractory to other forms of palliative treatment. Anti-inflammatory agents or sympatholytic drugs are prescribed for pain. See the section on sympathetic nervous system disorders.

Surgical procedures are usually discouraged. However, skin grafts may be applied to large chronic venous ulcers, and lumbar sympathectomy may be utilized for small vessel disease and causalgic type pain. Arterial revascularization is utilized for proximal occlusions of large arteries, and Achilles tendon lengthening is recommended for equinus deformity that limits the use of the leg pump. Palliative measures should be utilized on an outpatient basis before surgery is considered.

The time required to heal chronic leg ulcers varies according to the size of the ulcer, the local condition of the tissues, the nature of the underlying disease and the general physical condition of the patient. Few ulcers are totally refractory to treatment.

THE CLOTTING PROCESS

Intravascular thrombosis is not only one of the most frequent causes of death but also a major contributor to the chronic disability of a significant percentage of the population.

There is a balanced relationship between factors that increase the activity of clotting and naturally occurring clotting inhibitors that retard intravascular clotting. For example, fibrinolytic activity may be spontaneously increased, reduced or even absent. It is difficult

but not impossible to measure hypercoagulability in clinical situations. Hypercoagulability may be periodic or cyclical or may occur in response to environmental stimuli.

In the wake of thrombosis, the consumption of clotting factors and release of inhibitors may render the patient normal or hypercoagulable when tested. Several clotting parameters must be checked simultaneously and serially. Areas of interest include studies to explain the reasons for anticoagulant failure; screening for potential "clotters"; methods to identify cases of intravascular clotting; studies of the hypercoagulability potential of certain drugs, e.g., oral contraceptives; and many others.

The coagulation of blood is the result of an enzymatic chain reaction in which activators, precursors, activated enzymes, inhibitors and additional components, such as calcium, participate.

Basic Steps in the Coagulation Process

The three phases of clotting are: Phase I, initiating events resulting in the formation of activated factor X; Phase II, conversion of prothrombin to

TABLE 17–10   Origin of Clotting Factors

Factors Present in Blood Before Clotting	Clotting Factor[1]	Factors Formed During Clotting
fibrinogen[2]	I	fibrin
prothrombin[2]	II	thrombin (active for short period, then neutralized by antithrombins)
calcium	IV	
proaccelerin[2] ?	V	
proconvertin[2]	VII	
antihemophilic globulin (AHG)	VIII	These clotting factors are "activated."
plasma thromboplastin component (PTC)[2]	IX	
Stuart-Prower factor[2]	X	
plasma thromboplastin antecedent (PTA)[2]	XI	
Hageman factor	XII	platelet factor 3[2] (released)
fibrin stabilizing factor[2] ?	XIII	blood thromboplastin, III
platelets		activated factor X + factor V + phospholipids + Ca++ complex

[1]The clotting factors have Roman numerals; platelet factors have Arabic numerals.
[2]Clotting factors that originate in liver.

TABLE 17–11   Fate of Clotting Factors

FACTORS CONSUMED DURING CLOTTING (*Relatively Little Present in Serum*)		FACTORS NOT CONSUMED DURING CLOTTING (*Serum Relatively Rich in These Factors*)	
antihemophilic globulin (antihemophilic factor, AHF)	VIII	proconvertin	VII
		plasma thromboplastin component	IX
proaccelerin	V	Stuart-Prower factor	X
prothrombin	II		
fibrinogen	I		

thrombin; and Phase III, conversion of fibrinogen to fibrin, followed by polymerization and stabilization.

Clotting Factors

To help classify the complex mechanisms of blood coagulation, von Kaulla[87] has separated the factors of the clotting system according to three major considerations: origin, fate and stability.

1. ORIGIN OF CLOTTING FACTORS (Table 17–10). The liver manufactures several clotting factors. The origin of most of the others is unknown. At present, investigators are attempting to determine the organ or organs that synthesize antihemophilic globulin. The best current information is that vascular endothelium makes factor VIII. Therefore, theoretically any organ transplanted into a hemophiliac patient may cure his disease.

2. FATE OF CLOTTING FACTORS (Table 17–11). The fate of clotting factors circulating in human blood is partly unknown. It has been established that the liver clears plasminogen activator and activated factor X. Some clearing occurs in the reticuloendothelial system and some of the clotting factors can enter the extravascular space.

3. STABILITY OF CLOTTING FACTORS (Table 17–12). Two aspects of the stability of the clotting factors that are important for therapy are (1) the "shelf" life and (2) the biological half-life. "*Shelf*" *life* is the term given to the duration of stability of clotting factors in shed blood and in isolated factors derived from shed blood. Shelf life can be modified by storage conditions. An example is factor VIII, antihemophilic globulin. This highly unstable factor can be stabilized for more than one year by proper treatment. *Biological half-life* of a clotting factor is determined on the basis of serial blood specimens drawn from a patient who has received a transfusion of blood or a blood fraction. Biological half-life is

TABLE 17–12   Stability of Clotting Factors[1]

FACTORS STABLE IN SHED BLOOD		FACTORS UNSTABLE IN SHED BLOOD (*Unless Certain Techniques of Conservation Are Used*)	
		Platelets (loss of viability) antihemophilic globulin	VIII
plasma thromboplastin component (PTC)	IX		
plasma thromboplastin antecedent (PTA)	XI		
Stuart-Prower factor	X	prothrombin	II
proconvertin	VII	proaccelerin	V
fibrinogen	I		
plasminogen (fibrinolytic enzyme system)		free plasminogen activator	

[1]Important for selection of blood or blood product: fresh blood or fresh frozen plasma vs. "bank blood" or blood products, platelet concentrates and factor VIII preparations.

the length of time until the immediate post-transfusion value has decreased 50 per cent. Biological half-lives vary for each factor from a few hours to several days.

Dynamic Relationships Between Clotting Factors and Clotting Inhibitors

Clotting factors, which may be grouped as to origin, fate and stability, have relationships to each other as well as to the naturally occurring clotting inhibitors. The relationships are dynamic, and the activity or concentration of one or more of them may change very rapidly under physiological or pathological stimuli.

These dramatic changes are noted chiefly in hospitalized patients and therefore will not be described here. However, there are many examples of changes in the clotting mechanism that develop slowly over a period of weeks or months. Patients with these conditions are often seen on an outpatient basis. It is therefore essential that they be identified early in the process of change. Examples include:

1. Liver disease, with a reduction of components of the prothrombin complex (factors II, VII, IX and X).

2. Kidney disease, in which there may be disturbances of platelet function or loss of factor IX, or both.

3. Collagen disease, in which there is an appearance of clotting inhibitors.

4. Cancer of the prostate, which may show an increase of fibrinolytic activity and thrombocytopenia.

5. Release of tissue thromboplastin in many malignancies.

Phase I. Initiating Events and Blood Activated Factor X Formation

INITIATING EVENTS. Two events initiate extravascular hemostasis and

pathological intravascular blood coagulation. Of *primary importance* is the contact of blood with rough wettable surfaces. This event plays a prominent role in the initiation of normal blood coagulation and hemostasis and also may induce pathological intravascular clotting. When the smooth nonwettable surface of the vascular endothelial lining is damaged, the collagen-containing basement membrane is exposed. This exposed membrane initiates the clotting mechanism by activating factor XII, triggering release of platelet factor 3 from the platelets. It may also activate erythrocyte erythroplastin, which is a partial thromboplastin. Normal endothelial surfaces are nonthrombotic, but when damaged or denuded they cause platelet adherence because of exposure of subendothelial connective tissue. The platelet sequence consists essentially of adhesion, release of constituents such as ADP, secondary aggregation and enhancement of fibrin stabilization. Antiplatelet drugs have significant prophylactic value against arterial thrombosis but not against venous thrombosis. Of *secondary importance* is the admixture of tissue (extrinsic) phospholipids found in almost all human tissues that play an auxiliary role in normal hemostasis and an important role in some instances of diffuse intravascular clotting. Tissue phospholipids will produce an erroneous result in studies of coagulation *in vitro* if the blood specimen is contaminated with tissue fluids. This is particularly true when a question of hypercoagulability is involved.

Blood samples withdrawn for coagulation studies should be done through an 18 gauge needle with a free flow of blood using a two-syringe technique. The citrate should be adjusted when the hematocrit is very high or low, i.e., especially over 60 or below 20. The blood should be transported to the laboratory chilled in ice for prompt (within two hours) analysis.

BLOOD ACTIVATED FACTOR X FOR-

MATION. This is the result of the first phase of coagulation. The reaction is initiated when Hageman factor XII is activated by contact with rough surfaces. This factor interacts with factor XI in a chain reaction that eventually results in the formation of blood (intrinsic) activated factor X (Xa). Other factors that participate in formation of Xa are plasma thromboplastin antecedent (XI), plasma thromboplastin component (IX) and antihemophilic globulin (VIII). For this chain reaction to follow its proper course, calcium ions are required and phospholipids are released from platelets as platelet factor 3.

All components of the normal "intrinsic" process of blood clotting are derived from blood, except the rough wettable surfaces that are primary initiating factors in coagulation. Activated factor Xa evolves during the process and converts prothrombin into thrombin.

The "extrinsic" pathway of blood coagulation occurs when extravascular or extrinsic material ("tissue phospholipid") is mixed with blood. The extrinsic clotting chain reaction that follows is shorter than the intrinsic pathway, because factors XII, XI, IX and VIII are bypassed. In addition, platelets are not required. Tissue phospholipid probably forms a complex with factor VII and Ca^{++} that activates factor X in converting prothrombin into thrombin. Factor V accelerates the action of Xa on prothrombin.

er hypercoagulability. The extrinsic clotting system contributes to thrombin formation in extravasated blood, and consequently it is important in hemostasis. Prothrombin was the first member of the so-called prothrombin complex to be discovered. All factors of the prothrombin complex that are related to prothrombin conversion into thrombin are synthesized by the liver. Clotting factors that are synthesized by the liver only drop to low levels in the presence of severe liver disease. In addition to the prothrombin complex, fibrinogen I and antithrombin III levels decrease in liver disease.

Vitamin K is required for biosynthesis in four of the five factors of the prothrombin complex: prothrombin II, proconvertin VII, Christmas factor IX and Stuart-Prower factor X. Each of these is reduced in prothrombin-reducing agents such as coumarin drugs (Coumadin and dicumarol, among others). Prothrombin II and proconvertin VII are also reduced in patients with liver disease. Proaccelerin (factor V) is not reduced by prothrombin-depressing agents but is reduced by severe liver disease. Hemorrhagic diathesis is produced by severe isolated or combined deficiency of the factors of the prothrombin complex. Bile must be present in order for vitamin K to be absorbed from the intestinal tract. Prolongation in prothrombin time is caused by absence or nonabsorption of vitamin K or by the congenital or acquired absence of any of the factors of the prothrombin complex.

Phase II. Thrombin Formation

Thrombin formation is the second basic step in the coagulation process. Thrombin is formed by conversion of prothrombin into thrombin by factor Xa. This requires about ten seconds. The combined kinetics of the first and second phase of clotting are measured in the thrombin generation test, which measures the amount of thrombin formed. It is a useful method to discov-

Phase III. Fibrin Formation

Fibrin formation is the third and final step in blood coagulation. It depends primarily on thrombin concentration. Thrombin is a proteolytic enzyme that hydrolyzes peptide bonds in the fibrinogen molecule, permitting them to form the fibrin monomer. Fibrin monomers combine to form fibrin polymers, from which the fibrin network is produced. In many pathological conditions, fibrin monomers can be found in the circulating blood.

Fibrin stabilizing factor is required in the formation of a firm and physiologically useful clot. Fibrin stabilizing factor is probably a transaminase, requiring calcium and thrombin for its activity. This factor is totally missing in rare congenital cases and is markedly reduced in some diseases. A weak clot is then formed that does not become well organized. Poor wound healing results and bleeding may occur within a few hours to days after any type of trauma. The usual clotting tests are normal in these patients, except for fibrin stabilizing factor XIII.

A normal clot consists of a fibrin network that incorporates proteins, erythrocytes, leucocytes and platelets. A grey clot consisting of platelets occurs in the artery, while a red clot involving erythrocytes in coagulum develops in the vein. *Clot retraction* occurs when a platelet substance known as thromboasthenin interacts with fibrin fibers, slowly drawing them together, a process termed syneresis. Clot retraction depends in part on the presence of normal platelets. Poor or absent clot retraction *in vitro* is an indication of a low platelet count or an abnormal platelet function. Clot is organized *in vivo* by the ingrowth of fibroblasts with a few days unless a pathological condition results in fibrinolysis. Normal hemostasis requires the passage of time for development or remodeling of a clot, for firmness and adherence to tissue and wound surfaces. *A good firm clot may not develop in the presence of a low fibrinogen level, deficiency of fibrin stabilizing factor, fibrinolysis, a reduced platelet count or poor platelet function.*

In summary, the three phases of clotting are: the initiating events and the formation of activated factor X (Xa) (Phase I): conversion of prothrombin to thrombin (Phase II); and conversion of fibrinogen to fibrin, followed by stabili-

zation of fibrin (Phase III). Calcium is required for each of these phases, and removal of calcium results in uncoagulability of the blood.

Endogenous Inhibition of Clotting

Studies indicate that some intravascular fibrin formation proceeds slowly on a continuous basis. This process is controlled by endogenous clotting inhibitors and by the fibrinolytic enzyme system. Clotting inhibitors are theoretically necessary to prevent the clotting process from spreading beyond the area where it is required. However, if endogenous clotting inhibitors increase, a more or less pronounced hemorrhagic diathesis may develop. When the activity of endogenous clotting inhibitors is reduced beyond a certain point, there is increasing evidence that a potential danger of intravascular clotting exists. The key factor in this phenomenon is antithrombin III.

Endogenous clotting inhibitors are known as antithrombins and antithromboplastins. The *antithrombins* are: antithrombin I — the fibrin clot which absorbs thrombin; antithrombin II — the thrombin inhibitor which immediately neutralizes thrombin; antithrombin III — a serum antithrombin which progressively neutralizes thrombin; (antithrombin IV is no longer recognized as a specific entity); antithrombin V — pathological macroglobulins which interfere with fibrin polymerization; and antithrombin VI — a pathological mixture of fibrinolytic breakdown products derived from fibrinogen or fibrin, which may interfere with fibrin polymerization. Markedly reduced antithrombin III levels have been found in families with hereditary thrombophilia. Another natural inhibitor is heparin, which is present in very small amounts in blood. This inhibitor needs a cofactor for its anticoagulant activity, which is probably antithrombin III. Blood normally contains antiheparin activity known as platelet factor 4 or antiheparin platelet factor, which is derived from the thrombocytes. Heparin inhibits thrombin and factor X and probably also interferes with the activation of factor IX by factor XI.[33]

Endogenous clotting inhibitors are generally called "circulating anticoagulants."

Predisposing Factors

The clinician's interest in the etiology of venous thrombosis should focus initially on the prevention of this disease. An account of "clotting very quickly" may occasionally be extracted from the patient's history. Examples include a history of trival trauma that has been accompanied by clots or an erythematous area on the skin suggestive of phlebitis. A past history of one or more bouts of minor or major thrombophlebitis may be elicited. An additional aspect is a family history of clotting tendency. These patients should be considered for special laboratory studies. The most common predisposing factor is the patient's presenting disease.

Associated diseases that commonly accompany venous thrombosis include pneumonia, typhoid fever, septicemia, chronic ulcerative colitis, carcinoma, lymphoma and localized and generalized cardiovascular disease. Other associated conditions are seen in a wide variety of obstetrical and surgical illnesses. A high incidence of venous thrombosis is noted in various forms of trauma, including venipuncture or prolonged intravenous cannulation, advancing age, prolonged debilitating illness and rapid changes in the hemodynamics of the body during shock or dehydration. The predisposing factors also include drug abuse and the use of contraceptive medications. Surgery was formerly followed by a high incidence of venous thrombosis. The incidence is now lower, probably as a result of improved preoperative intraoperative and postoperative hemodynamics; that is, by aggressive intravenous therapy with better monitoring.

Hypercoagulability

Identification of Individuals Who Have a Tendency to Intravascular Clotting

Patients with evidence of repeated thromboembolism have previously been studied by various individual coagulation tests. Most of these tests failed to detect "chronic clotters," and "clotters" were therefore usually best identified by their history alone. Recently, however, there has been renewed interest in these tests because of the thromboembolic events that have occurred in association with use of oral contraceptive drugs. *Clinicians should realize that it is naive to attempt to use a single test for the evaluation of hypercoagulability of the blood.* Widely different triggering events and resulting alterations occur in the clotting process that predispose to intravascular thrombosis. Entirely different coagulation procedures are required to reveal the danger of intravascular clotting in amaurosis fugax, which may be due solely to an increased spontaneous aggregation of platelets, as compared with the recurrent thrombophlebitis of a disseminated carcinoma, in which necrosing cells may cause massive penetration of phospholipid material into the circulation. Appropriate therapy may be determined after identifying the abnormal clotting parameters. In these two examples aspirin might prevent the platelet aggregation in amaurosis fugax, while thromboembolic complications of disseminated carcinoma would necessitate adequate levels of heparin. Endogenous clotting factors have received little attention until recently, when it was found that a normal level of antithrombin III activity is important to prevent thromboembolism. It is believed that many other endogenous factors are important in preventing thromboembolism.

Even if the laboratory detects the existence of hypercoagulability *in vitro*, it should not be stated that the patient will develop intravascular thrombosis. It does, however, warn the clinician of the patient's propensity to clot. The predisposing events or factors are the catalysts that convert a clotting tendency into an actual thromboembolism. A combination of tests identified as the *hypercoagulability panel* for outpatients (disseminated intravascular coagulation tests are omitted) is required to screen the various parameters of the coagulation system to produce meaningful results for the clinician. These tests include: (1) *thrombin generation test,* (2) *thromboelastography,* (3) *platelet aggregation* (may be increased in amaurosis fugax, transient ischemic attacks and recurrent vertigo), (4) *platelet count* (a high count reveals clotting tendency while a low count may indicate hypercoagulability, diffuse intravascular coagulation, or both), (5) *circulating soluble fibrin monomers,* sometimes called fibrin split products (their presence indicates a preliminary stage of clotting), (6) *fibrinogen* (if high, hypercoagulability is enhanced; if low, disseminated intravascular coagulation is suggested) and (7) *antithrombin III activity* (in which a low level indicates reduced protection against clotting. All oral contraceptives cause the level to be low, so other tests are required in that case. Antithrombin III activity is deficient in hereditary "clotters," high in infants and children, decreasing to normal by early twenties; if subnormal or normal in coumarin-treated patients, then subcutaneous heparin is the drug of choice. In liver disease it may be low or absent.)

Any patient receiving oral contraceptives or having any other predisposing condition should be treated cautiously. In iatrogenic hypercoagulability from "the Pill," it is necessary to stop the drug at least three weeks before elective surgery. Mass laboratory screening of patients for hypercoagulability is not practical and is not advised. Clinical screening is essential for all patients but specific conditions warrant further study by the laboratory.

Prophylactic Anticoagulation

The *indications* for the use of anticoagulants are twofold: as *prophylaxis* to prevent *in vivo* thrombosis and *therapeutically* to stop thrombotic progression. Heparin is the agent most often given initially when therapeutic anticoagulation is indicated, while coumarin drugs, dextran and antiplatelet drugs are reserved for prophylaxis. Heparin may also be indicated prophylactically for specific patients in low dosage. Defibrinogenating agents such as urokinase have been utilized therapeutically in both venous and arterial disease but are still investigational. Since anticoagulants are seldom ordered therapeutically for outpatients, only those agents used for prophylaxis will be discussed.

In recent years more attention has been directed towards the use of prophylactic anticoagulant agents in the postoperative patient, the trauma patient, the patient with serious disease, the patient with evidence of hypercoagulation and those individuals who have occlusive arteriosclerotic disease, especially of the carotid arteries. This has resulted in forthcoming efforts to lessen the incidence of *in vivo* thrombosis which may occur in outpatients as well.

LOW DOSE HEPARIN. The rationale behind "low dose heparin" is that, by preventing the cascade effect of the coagulation process, a much smaller amount of heparin can be effective prophylactically than would be required therapeutically. Heparin enhances the activity of antithrombin III, one unit of which, in turn, inhibits 32 units of factor Xa, preventing in turn the potential generation of 16,000 units of thrombin.

Thus, it has been suggested[88] that 1 microgram of heparin given prophylactically is worth 1330 micrograms of heparin applied therapeutically (after the coagulation cascade has begun). It has now been demonstrated beyond doubt, by large, well-controlled clinical trials using the radioactive fibrinogen detection of deep venous thrombosis as an end point,[46] that 5000 units of heparin administered subcutaneously every 12 hours does have a significant prophylactic effect. At this dose, clotting studies are usually entirely normal. Given every 8 hours, the same dose will begin to prolong the partial thromboplastin time and will also lead to a small but definite incidence of spontaneous bleeding.

Clinical trials have also shown that this regimen will decrease not only the number and size of postoperative pulmonary emboli but also the frequency of fatal pulmonary embolism. However, a significant percentage of treated patients will develop wound hematomas.

Heparin administered by this subcutaneous route results in extremely variable plasma heparin levels. It has been shown[62] that if the plasma heparin level exceeded 0.2 units per ml, there was a 47 per cent wound bleeding rate, whereas at lower levels it was only 11 per cent (compared with a control level of 12 per cent). Unfortunately, there are no good bedside tests to predict heparin levels. Finally, although these low doses of heparin have been shown to be effective in preventing deep venous thrombosis in patients undergoing routine surgical procedures, they will *not* effectively prevent it in those circumstances in which prophylaxis is most needed, where the stimulus for thrombosis is greatest. For example, low dose heparin will not satisfactorily protect patients undergoing major extremity surgery or the victims of extensive extremity trauma, and if the dose is increased to achieve protection, significant wound bleeding occurs.

DEXTRAN. To date, there have been 30 well-controlled studies in the literature on dextran prophylaxis against deep venous thrombosis.[12] Twenty-seven used dextran 40 and three used dextran 70. The effectiveness of each of these preparations appears to be essentially equal. It has now been established that when dextran is given after surgery it offers no protection, but when given during surgery it provides significant protection. Six of the studies were venographic and all six showed a decreased incidence of deep venous thrombosis. Fourteen of the studies used radioactive fibrinogen scans as the end point, and only six of these showed a significant decrease in deep venous thrombosis, suggesting that dextran probably protects against the propagation of small venous thrombi into large ones. Regarding its prophylactic effect against fatal pulmonary emboli, 36 out of 1801 control patients had fatal pulmonary emboli, whereas only 6 out of 1722 dextran 40–treated patients had fatal emboli. With dextran 70, 8 out of 408 control patients and 1 out of 400 treated patients had fatal pulmonary emboli.

The effect of dextran has been considered to be due to (1) hemodilution, (2) coating of the platelets and (3) negative charge to the endothelial wall. Bergentz[12] has concluded that it functions mainly through its interference with the action of factor VIII and that in essence, a dose of over 1.5 grams per kilogram (approximately 1 liter) produces a temporary von Willebrand's disease.

COUMARIN DRUGS. Although prophylaxis against deep venous thrombosis by vitamin K antagonists was first reported in 1941, it was not until 1951 that the first controlled trial was reported, and another eight years passed before Sevitt and Gallagher[79] reported their landmark study. In this study, 43 out of 150 control patients developed deep venous thrombosis, compared with only 4 out of 150 in the coumarin-treated group. Later studies showed comparative protection rates.[78]

Coumarin drugs sequentially depress factors VII, IX, X and XI, but their effect is dependent on the patient's nutrition and liver function and on the dose prescribed. Initially, the patient is given 15 to 20 mg orally on a daily basis until the prothrombin time is twice the control time that is the therapeutic range. Prophylactically this range is a few seconds less. The use of coumarin prophylactically has been most successful against arterial emboli in patients with cardiac disease, especially in those with rheumatic mitral stenosis and those with prosthetic heart valves. Prolonged use is indicated. Unless low dose heparin is used for the most serious venous thromboembolic conditons, it is almost routine to prescribe a coumarin drug prophylactically for three to six months.

A large number of drugs may augment the effect of a coumarin drug on prothrombin time. A few of the common drugs are antibiotics, salicylic acid, phenylbutazone (Butazolidin), tolbutamide and diazoxide. A decrease in the effect on prothrombin time may be noted in patients with diabetes and hyperlipemia, in patients taking adrenocortical steroids or oral contraceptives and in those who have a heavy ingestion of vitamin K.

ANTIPLATELET DRUGS. Until recently, the major role played by platelets in the clotting process has been ignored, in terms of prophylactic anticoagulation, in favor of drugs that either deplete clotting factors or enhance their natural inhibitors. Normal endothelial surfaces are nonthrombogenic, but when damaged or denuded they cause platelet adherence because of subendothelial connective tissue. The platelet sequence consists of adhesion, release of constituents such as ADP, secondary aggregation and enhancement of fibrin stabilization.

It is now generally accepted that antiplatelet drugs have significant prophylactic value against arterial thrombosis but not against venous thrombosis. Using a triple tracer technique (^{51}Cr-labeled platelets, ^{131}I-labeled fibrinogen and ^{125}I-labeled plasminogen), Harker[34] has shown that venous thrombosis is associated with equivalent utilization rates for all three substances but that in arterial thrombosis there is a disproportionately high rate of platelet consumption. The fact that endothelial surface abnormalities are more common in arterial diseases, particularly arteriosclerosis, may explain these observations. In addition, three lines of investigation suggest an important role for platelets in atherogenesis: (1) in homocystine-treated hypercholesterolemic baboons the atheromatous lesions observed can be prevented by antiplatelet drugs,[35] (2) in arterial injury preparations, no secondary plaques were formed in animals receiving antiplatelet drugs,[59] and (3) pigs with von Willebrand's disease did not develop the same atheromatous lesions that age- and sex-matched controls did when placed on an atherogenic diet.[14]

Antiplatelet drugs also appear to reduce the frequency of thromboembolic complications in other settings. For example, they appear to decrease the frequency of amaurosis fugax[21, 36] and, to a lesser extent, other types of transient ischemic attacks. However, they have not been shown to prevent the later developement of a major stroke. Nor have they been found effective in preventing arterial embolization to the extremities (the "blue toe" syndrome).[51] On the basis of this information, it is felt that antiplatelet drugs can be expected to be effective only in controlling embolic events produced by small ulcerated plaques, i.e., those not associated with a significant degree of stenosis. Such drugs will not be effective against large ulcerated plaques or stenosis sufficient enough to cause turbulence. Nevertheless, these drugs are of value when administered after endarterectomy or arterial reconstructive procedures until re-endothelialization has occurred.

Antiplatelet drugs have different

actions.[41] The nonsteroidal, anti-inflammatory drugs, such as aspirin and sulfinpyrazone, inhibit platelet release and reduce the secondary phase of platelet aggregation but have no effect on the primary platelet adhesion, whereas pyrimidine compounds, such as dipyridamole, mainly inhibit primary platelet aggregation.

There is some disagreement regarding the relative efficacy of the three most popular antiplatelet drugs now in use. Sulfinpyrazone (200 mg q.i.d.) and aspirin (300 mg q.i.d.) seem to be the most effective *single* agents, followed by dipyridamole (100 mg q.i.d.). The first two drugs may produce undesirable gastrointestinal side effects, while the third often causes excessive vasodilation at the recommended dose. The combination of aspirin (300 mg) with a reduced dose of dipyridamole (25 mg) taken q.i.d. may prove to be better tolerated and less expensive than and as effective as sulfinpyrazone.

COMPLICATIONS. The most common complication in prophylactic anticoagulation is hemorrhage, particularly from heparin. The most frequent occurrences are in postmenopausal women, in patients with severe hypertension and following injury or a surgical procedure. Hemorrhage is also the most common complication of coumarin drugs. With these drugs hematuria is the most frequent occurrence, especially in patients with cystitis. A very uncommon yet serious complication is an acute abdomen ("coumarin belly") from petechial or ecchymotic bleeding into the peritoneum or bowel wall. These patients require repeated examination to evaluate the indication for surgery. Hemorrhagic complications resulting from the use of either heparin or coumarin drugs is due to overdosage. Antiplatelet drug may also cause bleeding. The usual site is gastrointestinal.

Sensitive reaction is the second most common complication. The impurities in heparin may cause bronchiole constriction, lacrimation and urticaria. Long-term use may result in alopecia

and osteoporosis. The latter may be a serious complication. It is most often noted in patients who have congenital hypercoagulopathy and are receiving heavy doses of heparin over a prolonged period. The side effects of coumarin drugs include urticaria, dermatitis, alopecia, diarrhea and fever. Antiplatelet drug hypersensitivity varies with the type of drug prescribed. Aspirin frequently causes gastritis. Dipyridamole, which is also a coronary artery dilator, may produce headaches, dermatitis, dizziness and gastrointestinal upset. Sulfinpyrazone, which inhibits renal tubular reabsorption of uric acid, may initiate gastrointestinal disturbances, fever and dermatitis.[81]

Caution should be taken about withdrawal of prophylactic heparin or of coumarin drugs. Discontinuance should not be abrupt but should take place over a period of several days owing to the possibility of a "rebound" clotting phenomenon.

REFERENCES

1. Abbott, W. M., Mione, P. J., and Austen, W. G.: Effect of venous interruption on arterial circulation. Surg. Forum, 25:246–247, 1974.
2. Anderson, C. B.: Mycotic aneurysms. In Rutherford, R. B. (ed.): Vascular Surgery. Philadelphia, W. B. Saunders Co., pp. 709–721, 1977.
3. Austin, J. H., and Sajid, M. H.: Direct thermometry in ophthalmic-internal carotid blood flow. Arch. Neurol., 15:376–392, 1966.
4. Baker, A. G., Jr., and Roberts, B.: Long-term survival following abdominal aortic aneurysmectomy. JAMA, 212:445–450, 1970.
5. Barker, W. F.: Surgical treatment of peripheral vascular disease. New York, McGraw-Hill Book Co., 1962.
6. Barnes, R W.: Venous strain-gauge plethysmography. In Rutherford, R. B. (ed.): Vascular Surgery. Philadelphia, W. B. Saunders Co., 1977, pp. 191–200.
7. Barnes, R. W., Bone, G. E., Reinertson, J., et al.: Noninvasive ultrasonic carotid angiography: Prospective validation by contrast arteriography. Surgery, 80:328–335, 1976.
8. Barnes, R. W., Russel, H. E., Bone, G. E., et

al.: Doppler cerebrovascular examination: improved results with refinements in technique. Stroke, 8:468–471, 1977.

9. Bauer, G. A.: A roentgenological and clinical study of the sequels of thrombosis. Acta Chir. Scand. (Suppl.), 74, p. 1, 1942.

10. Bergan, J. J., and Yao, J. S.T.: Acute intestinal ischemia. *In* Rutherford, R. B. (ed.): Vascular Surgery. Philadelphia, W. B. Saunders Co., 1977, pp. 825–842.

11. Bergan, J. J., and Yao, J. S. T.: Chronic intestinal ischemia. *In* Rutherford, R. B. (ed.): Vascular Surgery. Philadelphia, W. B. Saunders Co., 1977, pp. 843–851.

12. Bergentz, S. E.: Dextran prophylaxis in venous thrombosis. *In* Bergan, J. J., and Yao, J. S. T. (eds.): Venous Problems. Chicago, Year Book Publishers, 1978.

13. Bernhard, V. M.: The management of chronic occlusive arterial disease affecting the lower extremities. *In* Rutherford, R. B. (ed.): Vascular Surgery, Philadelphia, W. B. Saunders Co., 1977, pp. 487–496.

14. Bowie, E. J. W., Fuster, V., Owen, C. A., Jr., et al.: Proceedings: resistance to the development of spontaneous atherosclerosis in pigs with von Willebrand's disease. Thromb. Diath. Haemorrh., 34:599, 1975.

15. Brockenbrough, E. C.: Screening for the prevention of stroke: use of a Doppler flowmeter. Information and Education Research Support Unit of Washington-Alaska Regional Medical Program, 1969. (Monograph)

16. Cranley, J. J., Canos, A. J., and Sull, W. J.: The diagnosis of deep venous thrombosis. Arch. Surg., 111:34–36, 1976.

17. David, T. E., Humphries, A. W., Young, J. R., et al.: A correlation of neck bruits and arteriosclerotic carotid arteries. Arch. Surg., 107:729–731, 1973.

18. DeWeese, J. A., Blaisdell, F. W., and Foster, J. H.: Optimal resources for vascular surgery. Arch. Surg., 105:948–961, 1972.

19. Duncan, G. W., Gruber, J. O., Dewey, C. F., Jr., et al.: Evaluation of carotid stenosis by phonangiography. N. Engl. J. Med., 293:1124–1128, 1975.

20. Ehrenfeld, W. K.: Fibromuscular dysplasia of the carotid artery. *In* Rutherford, R. B., (ed.): Vascular Surgery. Philadelphia, W. B. Saunders Co., 1977, pp. 1123–1129.

21. Evans, G.: Effect of drugs that suppress platelet surface interaction on incidence of amaurosis fugax and transient cerebral ischemia. Surg. Forum, 23:239–241, 1972.

22. Farmer, D. A., and Smithwick, R. H.: Thromboembolic disease. Angiology, 1:291–301, 1950.

23. Folse, R., and Alexander, R. H.: Directional flow detection for localizing venous valvular incompetency. Surgery, 67:114–121, 1970.

24. Fronek, A., Johansen, K. H., Dilley, R. B., et al.: Noninvasive physiologic tests in the diagnosis and characterization of peripheral arterial occlusive disease. Am. J. Surg., 126:205–214, 1973.

25. Garrett, W. E., Wylie, E. J., and DeWeese, J. A.: Proposed vascular surgical guidelines for screening. Bull. Am. Col. Surg., p. 6, June 1974.

26. Gay, J.: On varicose diseases of the lower extremities. The Lettsomian Lectures of 1867. London, Churchill, 1868.

27. Gee, W., Smith, C. A., Hinson, C. E., et al.: Ocular pneumoplethysmography in carotid artery disease. Med. Instrum., 8:244–248, 1974.

28. Gius, J. A.: Arteriovenous anastomoses and varicose veins. Arch. Surg., 81:299–310, 1960.

29. Gosling, R. G., King, D. H., Newman, D. L., and Woodcock, J. P.: Transcutaneous measurement of arterial blood-velocity by ultrasound. J. Ultrasonics. USI Conf. Papers 16–23, 1969.

30. Haeger, K.: Problems of acute deep venous thrombosis. I. The interpretation of signs and symptoms. Angiology, 20:219–223, 1969.

31. Haimovici, H., and Steinman, C.: Aortoiliac angiographic patterns associated with femoropopliteal occlusive disease: significance in reconstructive arterial surgery. Surgery, 65:232–240, 1969.

32. Haimovici, H.: Thromboangiitis obliterans: a nosologic reappraisal. J. Cardiovasc. Surg., 4:83–86, 1963.

33. Hamstra, R.: Personal communication.

34. Harker, L. A.: Inhibitors of platelet function in the prevention of arterial thrombosis. *In* Jensen, K. G., and Killman, S. (eds.): Antiplatelet Drugs and Thrombosis. Copenhagen, Munksgaard, 1976, pp. 105–124.

35. Harker, L. A., Ross, R., Slichter, S. J., and Scott, R. C.: Homocystine-induced arteriosclerosis. J. Clin. Invest., 58:731–741, 1976.

36. Harrison, M. J. G., Marshall, J., Meadows, J. C., et al.: Effect of aspirin in amaurosis fugax. Lancet, 2:743–744, 1971.

37. Hedblom, E. E.: Disturbances due to cold. Conn, H. F. (ed.): Current Therapy. Philadelphia, W. B. Saunders Co., 1971, pp. 766–771.

38. Hermann, G., Schechter, D. C., Owens, J. C., Starzl, T. E.: The problem of frostbite in civilian medical practice. Surg. Clin. North Am., 43:519–536, 1963.

39. Hobbs, J. T.: The treatment of varicose veins by sclerosing therapy. *In* Rutherford, R. B. (ed.): Vascular Surgery. Philadelphia, W. B. Saunders Co., 1977, pp. 1153–1168.

40. Holman, E.: Abnormal arteriovenous communications: peripheral and intracardiac acquired and congenital, 2nd ed. Springfield, Ill., Charles C Thomas, 1968.

41. Holmsen, H.: Classification and possible mechanisms of action of some drugs that

inhibit platelet aggregation. *In* Jensen, K. G., and Killman, S. (eds.): Antiplatelet Drugs and Thrombosis. Copenhagen, Munksgaard, 1976, pp. 50–80.

42. Hull, R., Van Aken, W. G., Hirsh, J., et al.: Impedance plethysmography using the occlusive cuff technique in the diagnosis of venous thrombosis. Circulation, 53:696–700, 1976.

43. Jaboulay, M.: Le traitement de quelques trouble trophiques du pied et de la jambe par la denudation de l'artere femorale et la distension des nerfs vasculaires. Lyon. Médical, 91:467, 1899.

44. Jennesco, T.: Rescetia totala di bilaterala a simpaticului cervical in cazuri: de epilepsi si gusa exoftalmica. Romania Med., 4:479, 1896. Translated in Zentralblatt für Chirurgie, 24:33, 1897.

45. Juergens, J. L.: Thromboangiitis obliterans. *In* Rutherford, R. B. (ed.): Vascular Surgery. Philadelphia, W. B. Saunders Co., 1977, 593–596.

46. Kakkar, V. V., Field, E. S., Nicolaides, A. N., et al.: Low doses of heparin in prevention of deep-vein thrombosis. Lancet, 2:669–671, 1971.

47. Kinmonth, J. B., Taylor, G. W., Tracy, G. D., and Marsh, J. D.: Primary lymphoedema: clinical and lymphangiographic studies of a series of 107 patients in which the lower limbs were affected. Br. J. Surg., 45 (189): 1–9, 1957.

48. Kartchner, M. M., McRae, L. P., and Morrison, F. D.: Noninvasive detection and evaluation of carotid occlusive disease. Arch. Surg., 106:528–535, 1973.

49. Knize, D. M., Weatherley-White, R. C., Paton, B. C., et al.: Prognostic factors in the management of frostbite, J. Trauma, 9:749–759, 1969.

50. Knox, D. L.: Ocular aspects of cervical vascular disease. Surv. Ophthalmol., 13:245–262, 1969.

51. Kwaan, J. H., Molen, R. V., Stemmer, E. A., et al.: Peripheral embolism resulting from unsuspected atheromatous aortic plaques. Surgery, 78:583–588, 1975.

52. Leriche, R.: Des obliterations arterielles hautes (obliteration de la terminaison de l'aorte) comme cause des insuffisances circulatoires des membres inferieurs. Bull. Soc. Chir., 49:1404, 1923.

53. Luke, J. C.: The pathology and treatment of the postphlebitic leg and its complications. Can. Med Assoc, J., 61:270–275, 1949.

54. Malt, R. A., and Smith, R. J.: Limb replantation: selection of patients and technical considerations. *In* Rutherford, R. B., (ed.): Vascular Surgery. Philadelphia, W. B.)Saunders Co., 1977, pp. 471–476.

55. Markowitz, A. M., and Norman, J. C.: Aneurysms of the iliac artery. Ann. Surg., 154:777–787, 1961.

56. Mills, W. J., Jr.: Out in the cold. Emergency Medicine, 8(1):134–147, Jan. 1976.

57. Milroy, W. F.: Chronic hereditary edema: Milroy's disease. JAMA, 91:1172–1175, 1928.

58. Mitchell, S. W., Morehouse, G. R., and Keen, W. W.: Gunshot Wounds and Other Injuries of Nerves. Philadelphia, J. B. Lippincott Co., 1864.

59. Moore, S., Friedman, R. H., Singal, D. P., et al.: Inhibition of injury-induced thromboatherosclerotic lesions by antiplatelet serum in rabbits. Thromb. Haemostas., 35:70–81, 1976.

60. Mullick, S. C., Wheeler, H. B., and Songster, G. F.: Diagnosis of deep venous thrombosis by measurement of electrical impedance. Am. J. Surg., 119:417–422, 1970.

61. Nicolaides, A. N., Angelides, N., Fernades, J., et al.: The value of Doppler blood velocity tracings in the detection of aortoiliac and femoropopliteal disease in patients with intermittent claudication. Proceedings of International Cardiovascular Congress on Noninvasive Diagnosis. Scottsdale, Arizona, March 1977.

62. Nicolaides, A. N.: The current status of small-dose subcutaneous heparin in the prevention of venous thromboembolism. *In* Bergan, J. J., and Yao, J. S. T. (eds.): Venous Problems. Chicago, Year Book Medical Publishers, 1978.

63. Owens, J. C.: Thoracic outlet compression syndromes. *In* Haimovici, H., (ed.): Vascular Surgery: Principles and Techniques. New York, McGraw-Hill, pp. 733–760, 1976.

64. Owens, J.: The management of arterial trauma. Surg. Clin. North Am., 43:371–385, 1963.

65. Owens, J. C.: Indications for lumbar sympathectomy. *In* Dale, W. A. (ed.): Management of Arterial Occlusive Disease. Chicago, Year Book Medical Publishers, 1971.

66. Owens, J. C., and Anderson, L. L.: Indications for surgical treatment of the postphlebitic syndrome. Surgery, 41:81–93, 1957.

67. Owens, J. C.: Complications of sympathectomy. *In* Beebe, H. G., (ed.): Complications of Vascular Surgery. Philadelphia, J. B. Lippincott Co., 1973, pp. 201–241.

68. Owens, J. C., and Coffey, R. J.: Collective review: aneurysm of splenic artery, including a report of six additional cases. International Abstracts of Surgery, 97:313–335, 1953.

69. Owens, J. C.: Treatment of cold injuries. Postgrad. Med., 48:160–165, 1970.

70. Peabody, C. N., Kannel, W. B., and McNamara, P. M.: Intermittent claudication: surgical significance. Arch. Surg., 109:693–697, 1974.

71. Planiol, T., and Purcelot, L.: Doppler effect

study of the carotid circulation. *In* de Vlieger, M., White, D. N., and McCready, V. W., (eds.): Proceedings of the Second World Congress on Ultrasonics in Medicine, Rotterdam, June 4–8, 1973. New York, American Elsevier Publishing Co., 1975.

72. Porter, J. M.: Raynaud's syndrome and associated vasospastic conditions of the extremities. *In* Rutherford, R. B. (ed.): Vascular Surgery. Philadelphia, W. B. Saunders Co., 1977, pp. 597–604.

73. Raines J.: Vascular laboratory evaluations using the pulse volume recorder. *In* Rutherford, R. B. (ed.): Vascular Surgery. Philadelphia, W. B. Saunders Co., 1977, pp. 57–71.

74. Roos, D. B.: Transaxillary approach for first rib resection to relieve thoracic outlet syndrome. Ann. Surg., *163*:354–458, 1966.

75. Rutherford, R. B.: Infrarenal aortic aneurysms. *In* Rutherford, R. B., (ed.): Vascular Surgery. Philadelphia, W. B. Saunders Co., 1977, pp. 639–654.

76. Rutherford, R. B., Hiatt, W. R., and Kreutzer, E. W.: The use of velocity waveform analysis in the diagnosis of carotid artery occlusive disease. Surgery, 82:695–702, 1977.

77. Rutherford, R. B.: Personal communication.

78. Salzman, E. W.: Prevention of venous thromboembolism by oral anticoagulants and drugs affecting platelet function. *In* Bergan, J. J., and Yao, J. S. T., (eds.): Venous Problems. Chicago, Year Book Medical Publishers, 1978.

79. Sevitt, S., and Gallagher, N. C.: Prevention of venous thrombosis and pulmonary embolism in injured patients. Lancet, 2:981–989, 1959.

80. Shapiro, H. M., Laurence, N. G., Mishkin, M., et al.: Direct thermometry, ophthalmodynamometry, auscultation and palpation in extracranial cerebrovascular disease: an evaluation of rapid diagnostic methods. Stroke, *1*:205–218, 1970.

81. Silver, D.: Anticoagulant therapy. *In* Rutherford, R. B. (ed.): Vascular Surgery. Philadelphia, W. B. Saunders Co., 1977, pp. 301–308.

82. Stanley, J. C.: Splanchnic artery aneurysms. *In* Rutherford, R. B., (ed.): Vascular Surgery. Philadelphia, W. B. Saunders Co., 1977, pp. 673–685.

83. Sumner, D. S.: Evaluation of the venous circulation using the ultrasonic Doppler velocity detector. *In* Rutherford, R. B. (ed.): Vascular Surgery. Philadelphia, W. B. Saunders Co., 1977, pp. 179–189.

84. Sumner, D. S.: Noninvasive measurement of segmental arterial pressure. *In* Rutherford, R. B., (ed.): Vascular Surgery. Philadelphia, W. B. Saunders Co., 1977, 115–131.

85. Thal, E. R., and Perry, M. O.: Peripheral and abdominal vascular injuries. *In* Rutherford, R. B., (ed.): Philadelphia, W. B. Saunders Co., 1977, pp. 433–450.

86. Trimble, C., Bernstein, E. F., Pomerantz, M., et al.: A prosthetic bridging device to relieve iliac venous compression. Surg. Forum, 23:249–251, 1972.

87. Von Kaulla, K. N., and von Kaulla, E.: Elementary coagulation facts. Denver, University of Colorado School of Medicine, 1971.

88. Wessler, S.: Hypercoagulability and its contribution to venous thromboembolic disease. *In* Bergan, J. J., and Yao, J. S. T., (eds.): Venous Problems. Chicago, Year Book Medical Publishers, 1978.

89. Wheeler, H. B., O'Donnell, J. A., Anderson, F. A., et al.: Bedside screening for venous thrombosis using occlusive impedance phlebography. Angiology, 26:199–209, 1975.

90. Wright, C. B., and Swan, K. G.: Hemodynamics of venous occlusion in the canine hindlimb. Surgery, 73:141–146, 1973.

18 The Abdomen and Gastrointestinal Tract

ALEX M. STONE, M.D.,
GEORGE J. HILL, II, M.D.,
and LESLIE WISE, M.D.

INTRODUCTION

The general surgeon is charged with responsibility for surgical diseases of the abdominal viscera, including the gastrointestinal tract, mesentery, peritoneum and abdominal wall. Symptoms and signs mimicking gastrointestinal disease arise in major vascular structures, the chest, urogenital organs, musculature, spinal cord and peripheral nerves and the lymphatic systems. An appropriately wide differential diagnosis must be kept in mind when dealing with an abdominal complaint.

The treatment of most surgical diseases of the abdomen is beyond the scope of outpatient surgery and generally requires in-hospital care. Outpatient care is generally restricted to preadmission diagnosis and postoperative follow-up. There are a few conditions, however, that may be cared for on an outpatient or short hospital stay regimen.

It is of primary importance for the physician who initially sees the outpatient having abdominal complaints to make a decision on the urgency of the problem at hand. Certain pathological entities require immediate surgery, but some may not require surgery at all. Although this statement would seem apparent to the most casual observer, such decisions are not always so obvious.

A careful history should be taken and a thorough physical examination completed before elective surgery is performed. However, an urgent need for surgery or the presence of several simultaneous emergencies may restrict the surgeon's goal of completeness. No matter how busy one is, however, one should always review the pertinent details of the history and personally confirm the important aspects of the physical examination. There is little justification for planning to spend several hours in the operating room without performing a careful review of the case prior to surgery. An unwary surgeon will not be prepared to encounter an unexpected carcinoma, a fallopian tube abscess or a ureteral calculus. A subsequent review of the history will often reveal the details that were overlooked when the patient was hustled off to surgery. Appropriate laboratory and radiological tests must also be considered and used as guides in confirming the clinical diagnosis and the necessity for surgery.

It should be recognized that surgery is at times a diagnostic as well as a therapeutic procedure.[2, 11, 39] Occasionally, laparotomy is less dangerous to the patient than a long delay due to a series of diagnostic tests that have little chance of arriving at a definitive diagnosis. It should be realized that, especially in the acutely ill patient, any diagnostic tests ordered should not unduly delay the initiation of appropriate therapy.

A sick patient with abdominal complaints should be carefully supervised during the initial period in the hospital. Regardless of the duration of illness, close professional observation is indicated until definitive treatment is instituted and the patient has shown definite improvement. The elderly patient with chronic small bowel obstruction due to carcinoma of the cecum may vomit and aspirate while undergoing a simple x-ray of the abdomen in the Outpatient Department. The patient with toxic megacolon may go into shock while waiting in line to have a venipuncture at the outpatient laboratory. The surgeon in the Outpatient Department must be aware of these possibilities. A nasogastric tube may be unpleasant for a sick, distended patient to swallow. But if the surgeon inserts the tube before the patient leaves for the x-ray department, he may be rewarded by having the gastrointestinal contents drained into a basin instead of into the patient's bronchial tree.

EVALUATION OF ABDOMINAL EMERGENCIES

Symptoms

Symptoms of illness may be observations that are narrated in the history or extracted by questioning the patient. Although some symptoms are so specific that the diagnosis is clear or the necessity for surgery is obvious, most are relatively nonspecific. Symptoms must therefore be judged in the context of the entire history and physical examination to arrive at an appropriate decision.[8]

A careful record should be made of *pain*. Inquiry should be made into the acute, chronic or relapsing nature of pain and the duration of episodes if it is recurrent. Acute pain is perhaps more likely to be an urgent surgical problem than chronic pain, but a patient with a myocardial infarction should not be operated upon with the mistaken opinion that he has acute cholecystitis. "Mild" pain must be viewed in the light of the individual who describes it. If he is concerned about cancer he may minimize the symptoms; if he is obese he may have a localized infection well protected by fat; and if he is stoic he may inadvertently mask the seriousness of his condition. Radiation of pain is frequently a helpful sign,[24] since subdiaphragmatic inflammation may radiate to the shoulder, pancreatic lesions radiate to the back and ureteral colic may radiate to the testicle. A past history of related abdominal pain may be important, even though the patient is unaware of its significance. The patient with gallstone ileus may have suffered from indigestion and biliary colic for years, but may not reveal it except on direct questioning.

The patient may be aware of a *mass*, and if so the physician can usually confirm this on examination. However, even in the absence of palpable mass, this history may provide an important clue. The mass is usually frustratingly evanescent in patients with intermittent intussusception due to cecal tumors, and patients with hernias also may give a history of an intermittent mass that appears only after vigorous exercise or a long period of time spent in the erect position. A mass in the mesentery, greater omentum or in the intestines may be apparent to the patient but not palpable when he later visits the physician, the mass having shifted on its mobile mesentery. The history of a definite intra-abdominal mass should be taken seriously when narrated by a stable, intelligent patient or parent of a child. A series of visits should be arranged for sequential examinations, until it is clear that the mass did not reappear or a diagnosis has finally been made.

Weight loss is not, by itself, a condition that warrants surgery, but it may be an ominous indication of serious illness. Cancer is perhaps the most common serious illness associated with weight loss, but the surgeon and patient may be gratified to discover that chronic peptic ulcer, chronic appendiceal abscess or some such benign disease is the cause of loss of appetite and weight. The loss in weight may be more apparent to the patient than to the doctor, as when a heavy patient begins to find it easy to maintain an "ideal" weight, without calorie counting. Yet any history of loss of weight should be taken seriously, especially when associated with specific abdominal symptoms and signs.

Diarrhea and *constipation* are rarely obvious indications of surgical disease, although a change in bowel habits often seems clear in retrospect when a diagnosis of cancer of the colon has been made. In practice, constipation and diarrhea are usually problems for the internist or pediatrician, and the surgeon is not consulted until surgical disease is finally apparent or suspected. Diarrhea with surgical implications may be the florid bloody mucus of fulminant ulcerative colitis or the explosive hyperperistalsis due to chronic incomplete small bowel obstruction. It may be seen in gastrojejunocolic fistula and associated with the gastric hypersecretion produced by stimulation from the islet cell tumors of the pancreas described by Zollinger and Ellison.[53] It may be the result of protein, water, electrolyte or mucus loss from Ménétrier's disease of the stomach[44] or villous adenoma of the rectum. It may be due to massive gastrointestinal bleeding, "diarrhea" being the complaint of the patient just prior to fainting from blood loss. Constipation may be so subtle that only the patient is aware of a change. It may be complete but of such recent onset that the physician is lulled into complacency until the cecum ruptures. Cecal distention is a dangerous complication of colonic obstruction, which occurs in patients with *competent* ileocecal valves. Constipation is a common complaint of aging patients and may have no pathological significance. The most common surgical diseases causing constipation are diverticulitis and carcinoma of the rectosigmoid.

Complaints of intestinal *"gas"* are nonspecific, but may be troublesome enough to warrant gastrointestinal x-rays, especially if it is persistent or associated with other symptoms. The patient may describe belching, flatulence, borborygmi, cramps or "indigestion." In the majority of these patients the symptoms are due to relatively benign pathological conditions or to anxiety and aerophagia. However, carcinoma of the gastrointestinal tract may also cause chronic distention and hyperperistalsis. Pancreatic enzyme secretion may be blocked by obstruction from chronic inflammation of the pancreas, thus interfering with digestion in the small bowel. The consequences include steatorrhea, diarrhea, excessive intestinal gas and alterations in bacterial flora of the gut. Indigestion, or "heartburn," is thoroughly nonspecific but is often the presenting symptom in "surgical" conditions such as peptic ulcer, hiatus hernia, chronic cholecystitis, hepatoma and other cancers of upper abdominal viscera.

Tenderness may be mentioned by the patient and should be carefully considered by the surgeon. Abdominal pain is too common a problem to bring each case to a surgeon's attention. But a history of well-localized tenderness is a significant consideration for surgeons, and the point of maximum tenderness may give an important clue to the organ in which the condition is located.[4] Especially significant is tenderness at the right costal margin (cholecystitis), right lower quadrant (appendicitis) and left lower quadrant (diverticulitis). Epigastric tenderness is usually associated with benign peptic ulcer. Flank tenderness is sometimes a serious indication of penetrating intra-abdominal disease (appendicitis, carcinoma, diverticulitis), but it usually is a sign of conditions involving the genitourinary or musculoskeletal system. Bilateral lower abdominal tenderness is common in acute pelvic inflammatory disease, which usually can be confirmed by the presence of normal peristalsis and characteristic findings of tenderness or a tubal mass on pelvic examination.

Abnormal stools may be significant to surgeons, especially if associated with weight loss and change in frequency of bowel movements. Small pencil-thin hard stools are often described by patients with lesions of the descending and sigmoid colon. Narrow stools streaked with blood or mucus are the hallmark of carcinoma of the rectum, but all too often they are ascribed initially to hemorrhoids. Watery bowel movements may be present in patients with ulcerative colitis, Crohn's disease and in patients with villous adenomas of the colorectum. The presence of blood and mucus is more ominous and a thorough diagnostic evaluation, including sigmoidoscopy, barium enema and occasionally colonoscopy, is indicated to establish the diagnosis. Foul smelling bowel movements may be due to blood ("tarry" stools), pancreatic insufficiency or the change in intestinal flora associated with a "blind loop" syndrome. The history of passage of worms may lead to suspicion of ascariasis in a child with biliary or small bowel obstruction and may thereby suggest a trial of medical therapy instead of laparotomy.

Increased girth is a common problem in our affluent society and may be a sign of cirrhosis as well as obesity. But several surgical conditions often begin with such a history, including ascites from metastatic cancer and distention from chronic distal small bowel obstruction.

Fatigue is the most nonspecific of complaints. *Fever,* like fatigue, is relatively nonspecific, but if documented and apparently not factitious, it may be due to a condition that occasionally can only be uncovered at laparotomy.[2, 11, 39] Diseases range from lymphoma and tuberculosis to retroperitoneal abscess. In many cases, surgery may not only be diagnostic but also therapeutic.

Vomiting should always be viewed by a surgeon as a potentially serious symptom. Even if the cause is a non-surgical lesion (acute alcoholism, gastroenteritis), persistent vomiting may cause lower esophageal ulceration and, occasionally, even rupture (Mallory-Weiss syndrome). Prolonged vomiting may lead to serious electrolyte disturbances that must be corrected appropriately. Hypokalemic hypochloremic *alkalosis* occurs from peptic ulcers that obstruct the pylorus or first portion of the duodenum. Metabolic *acidosis* may result from chronic loss of small bowel contents from vomiting.

When vomiting is constant, the likelihood of a surgical lesion is increased, but nonsurgical lesions should still be considered, including myocardial infarction, uremia and drug toxicity. If vomiting is present without nausea, increased intracranial pressure from primary or metastatic brain tumor should be suspected. The appearance and odor of vomitus is of great importance. The presence of massive bloody vomitus should be an obvious indication for prompt surgical consultation. Fecal odor or appearance is usually associated with intestinal obstruction.

Signs

Signs of disease are revealed on physical examination. The surgeon's skills must include the ability to perform a complete examination of all areas of the body. If major surgery is contemplated, or if a minor problem is raised which has a complex differential diagnosis, the surgeon should not be content with an examination of the abdomen but should perform a complete, though possibly limited, examination of the rest of the patient.

The examination of the abdomen should ordinarily be systematic, thorough and unhurried, although the approach may be altered in the presence of localized tenderness or obvious urgency. It should always include pelvic and rectal examination. The rectosigmoid should be studied by sigmoidoscopy when indicated, especially during evaluation of gastrointestinal bleeding, diarrhea and anal or rectal pain. A stool specimen should be tested for occult blood.

Inspection of the abdomen will reveal abnormalities in abdominal contour or the presence of localized masses and hyperperistalsis. *Auscultation* is most effective if performed in the quiet period before the intestines are displaced by palpation. The quality, quantity and pitch of peristalsis should be noted. Patients suspected of having tumors or vascular lesions should be examed for a bruit. *Percussion* is useful to outline solid masses, such as the liver edge or tumors. Tympany may be suggestive of free intra-abdominal air obliterating the liver

**TABLE 18–1   Regional Anatomy of the Abdomen from a
Practical Point of View**

Region	Landmarks	Contents and Organs from which Symptoms are Referred
Right upper quadrant (right subcostal; RUQ)	Superior to umbilicus and right to midline	Liver Gallbladder Bile ducts Duodenum (1st and 2nd parts) Lesser sac Pylorus Right kidney Right adrenal gland Right colon and hepatic flexure Head of pancreas
Epigastrium (subxiphoid)	Upper third of area between midclavicular lines	Stomach; duodenum (3rd and 4th parts) Distal esophagus Celiac artery Pancreas, body Transverse colon
Left upper quadrant (left subcostal; LUQ)	Superior to umbilicus and left of midline	Spleen Splenic flexure and upper left colon Left adrenal gland Left kidney Tail of pancreas
Periumbilical (midabdomen)	Middle third of area between midclavicular lines	Pancreas, body Transverse colon Duodenum (3rd and 4th parts) Superior mesenteric artery Greater omentum Abdominal aorta Small bowel (Appendicitis symptoms appear here)
Right lower quadrant (right iliac; RLQ)	Inferior to umbilicus and right of midline	Appendix Cecum Right ureter Right Fallopian tube and ovary Right iliac lymph nodes Right iliac artery
Suprapubic	Lower third of area between midclavicular lines	Bladder Uterus Appendix (occasionally) Right or left ovary and Fallopian tube Transverse colon, omentum and small bowel (occasionally)
Left lower quadrant (left iliac; LLQ)	Inferior to umbilicus and left of midline	Sigmoid colon and rectosigmoid junction Left ureter Left Fallopian tube and ovary Left iliac lymph nodes Left iliac artery

TABLE 18–1   Regional Anatomy of the Abdomen from a
Practical Point of View (*Continued*)

Region	Landmarks	Contents and Organs from which Symptoms are Referred
Other regions of the abdomen are:		
Groins	Approximately 4 cm superior and inferior to Poupart's (inguinal) ligament	Inguinal and femoral hernias Lymph nodes Femoral nerve (entrapment) Common femoral artery and vein Iliopsoas muscle
Flanks	Superior to iliac crest and lateral to anterior axillary line	Kidneys Ureters Adrenals Iliopsoas muscle Retroperitoneal appendix Retroperitoneal sigmoid colon Tail of pancreas (left)

edge or distended viscera filled with fluid and gas. Percussion is also useful as a gentle form of palpation to localize areas of tenderness, especially in apprehensive patients. *Palpation* may be done with one hand or two, using either the fingertips or palms, depending on the organ being evaluated and the preference of the examiner. The "succussion splash" of a chronically distended stomach is best elicited with two hands, whereas one hand lying on the other is frequently the best method of ballottement of deep masses. Experienced surgeons frequently "walk" gently around the abdomen with their fingertips in the examination of patients with localized tenderness.

A useful maneuver to distinguish anxiety and hypochondriasis from true abdominal tenderness is to use the stethoscope for palpation of the abdomen. The surgeon should appear to listen through the stethoscope and the patient will then attempt to remain quiet and relaxed as pressure is applied. If the patient truly has abdominal tenderness it will be apparent, but the hypochondriac will often let the surgeon press deeply into his abdomen with the stethoscope.

Palpation of the abdomen usually begins in the right upper quadrant. Keeping in mind the structures normally present in each area and the potential pathological conditions in each organ (Table 18–1), the surgeon next systematically examines the epigastrium, the left upper quadrant, the midabdomen and the lower abdomen from right to left. The groin is examined for hernias, lymph nodes, and the quality of vascular pulsations. The examination concludes with a rectal and pelvic examination.

The usual pattern of palpation is modified when the patient is known to have a tender or painful area in the abdomen. In this situation, the most tender area is usually examined last, to avoid disturbing the patient prematurely.

The patient with acute cholecystitis may be unable to inspire deeply when the surgeon is pressing at the right costal margin, a phenomenon known as "Murphy's sign." Costovertebral angle tenderness frequently indicates the presence of pyelonephritis. Involuntary contraction ("spasm") of the abdominal musculature may be present over areas of inflammation, whereas guarding (voluntary contraction of muscle) may be either the response to a factitious complaint or a protective mechanism to avoid pain during examination.

Although it is true that pain may be referred to a distant region, the location of the symptom or sign is the single most useful guide to identification of a diseased organ.

Unfortunately, general agreement has not been reached regarding the terms that are used to describe the surface area and regions of the abdomen. The classic definitions of the anatomists have been modified greatly in practice in the United States, and precise definitions of the regions of the abdomen are now rarely given by surgeons in practice. Variations in body habitus produce considerable variation in the surface features of anatomy, and the underlying organs are also relatively inconstant.

Pain may be *referred* out of the abdomen from many diseases of abdominal organs. Common examples are:

Right shoulder — Liver, diaphragm
Left shoulder — Spleen, diaphragm
Back   — Pancreas, kidneys
Groin   — Ureter, tubes and ovaries,
                 appendix
Legs   — intervertebral disk, nerve root,
                 lumbar abscess, obturator
                 hernia

Laboratory Procedures

A complete blood count will probably be automatically performed on all patients with abdominal complaints. Of prime interest is the white blood cell count which, though nonspecific, is usually indicative of an inflammatory process when significantly elevated. A hematocrit or hemoglobin or both should be done; the presence of anemia is suggestive of chronic bleeding or other debilitating disease. Hemoconcentration is consistent with numerous inflammatory conditions of the abdomen in which there is a decrease in circulating plasma volume with loss of fluid to third space areas.

Urinalysis should be routinely per-formed on all patients with acute abdominal complaints. The greatest number of patients with extraperitoneal causes of abdominal pain ultimately turn out to have symptoms referable to the urinary tract. Diabetes mellitus may be apparent after routine urinalysis. Acetonuria may be present, caused by the ketoacidosis of diabetes mellitus, but it is more likely due to starvation or prolonged vomiting from other causes. White blood cells and bacteria present on microscopic examination reflect urinary tract infections. Red cells are frequently associated with calculi, but may also be present with urinary tract infection or neoplasms of the genitourinary tract. The specific gravity of the urine is generally a good indication of the state of hydration of the patient prior to visiting the office or emergency room.

An elevated serum amylase level is most frequently associated with acute pancreatitis. The absolute level of serum amylase is not necessarily proportional to the severity of the disease.[37] Hyperamylasemia may also be associated with a variety of other intraabdominal processes, including perforated viscera, cholecystitis and choledocholithiasis. It also may be elevated with several nonabdominal conditions such as parotiditis or orchitis.

A sickle cell preparation should be done in all black patients with abdominal pain. Although sickling can be a primary cause of abdominal pain it should be remembered that the presence of sickle cell trait or sickle cell anemia does not necessarily mean that another intra-abdominal problem is not present.

Emergency Radiological Evaluation

Radiological procedures are helpful and occasionally diagnostic in patients having acute abdominal complaints. Since these patients are frequently quite ill, attention should be directed to easily obtained radiographical findings before proceeding to more esoteric invasive techniques.

Attention should be first directed to the chest x-ray. Chest conditions that can be confused with acute abdominal problems can frequently be visualized on the chest x-ray (Fig. 18–1). Pneumonia, atelectasis and pleural effusions are easily visualized. The most significant abdominal finding is the presence of "free air" under the diaphragm (Fig. 18–2). Chest x-rays in patients with acute abdominal problems should be routinely taken with the patient in a standing position. In a patient with a perforation of the gastrointestinal tract the air rises and can be seen outlining the leaf of the diaphragm. This is most easily seen on the right, where the liver keeps the air-filled viscera out of the way. It is incumbent on the physician caring for the patient to be certain that the chest x-ray was taken with the patient in a standing position. Frequently, patients with severe abdominal catastrophies are quite ill and have difficulty standing for the x-ray procedure. A useful hint as to whether the patient was standing is the presence of an air-fluid level in the stomach which can frequently be visualized on the chest x-ray. Many radiology departments mark their films with a free floating lead weight that will sink to the bottom when the patient is standing. It should be emphasized that the absence of free air does not exclude a perforation of the gastrointestinal tract. The most common cause of free air is a perforated duodenal ulcer. In cases in

Figure 18–1 Pulmonary embolus causing "acute abdomen." Forty-six year old man with past history of active duodenal ulcer one year previously and fracture of patella three months previously. Acute onset of severe abdominal pain, rigidity and mild dyspnea. No peristalsis. Upright chest x-ray normal (A). After some debate among attending physicians, patient was not operated upon. Symptoms persisted, rales developed, and right basilar infiltrate appeared in 48 hours (B). Pulmonary angiogram (C) at 1.75 seconds demonstrated major occlusion in right main pulmonary artery and distal occlusions in branches of left pulmonary artery. Inferior vena cava plication was performed. Abdominal symptoms and signs slowly subsided.

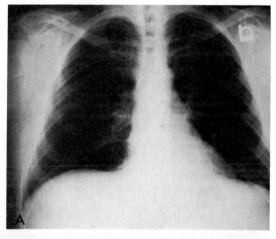

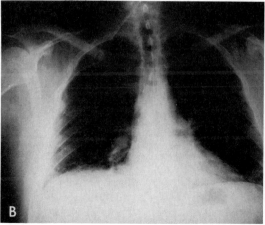

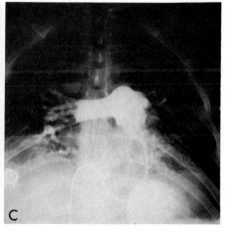

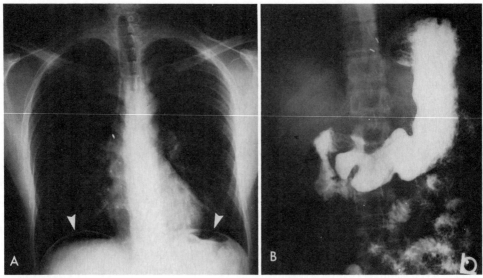

Figure 18–2 Perforated duodenal ulcer with free air. Thirty-two year old transient laborer. Ulcer symptoms for many years. Acute onset of abdominal pain, rigid abdomen, no peristalsis. Upright chest film (A) taken three hours after onset of pain shows free air under left and right diaphragm (arrows). Small gas bubble in stomach is inferior and medial to subdiaphragmatic collection. Patient underwent immediate operation (pyloroplasty and vagotomy) and had an uneventful course. GI series seven weeks later (B) shows normal gastric emptying and typical cloverleaf post-pyloroplasty deformity of antrum and pylorus.

which the patient is unable to be upright for the performance of the chest x-ray, a cross-table lateral decubitus examination can be ordered. Needless to say, the same care must be taken to be sure that the study was performed properly. If the history and clinical findings are suggestive of perforated duodenal ulcer, but no free air can be demonstrated and the diagnosis is in doubt, then the stomach may be inflated with air via a nasogastric tube, which will frequently produce visible free air on the chest plate. If this is still not diagnostic, a water-soluble radiopaque solution can also be placed in the stomach and occasionally will demonstrate the leak (Fig. 18–3).

Most patients with abdominal complaints will have films taken of the abdomen both in the recumbent and in the erect positions. These must be scanned generally and then carefully studied in order not to miss the diagnosis. In the right upper quadrant, a radiopaque gallstone may be visible on the flat film (Fig. 18–4). Approximately 20 per cent of all gallstones are visible on flat plates. In contrast, approximately 80 per cent of all stones in the urinary tract are visible on flat plates. Occasionally, the entire gallbladder may be calcified, the so called "porcelain gallbladder." The latter condition carries with it a higher risk of carcinoma of the gallbladder.[35] Air may be present in the biliary tree outlining the biliary ducts (Fig. 18–5). This is diagnostic of a communication between the biliary tree and the gastrointestinal tract. It will be seen normally in any patient who has had a choledochoduodenostomy or a cholecystojejunostomy constructed. All patients having air spontaneously in the biliary tree should be checked for the development of intestinal obstruction from blockage of the distal ileum by a gallstone. Occasionally this may also be visible on abdominal x-ray.

Rarely, a fecalith of the appendix can be visualized in the right lower quad-

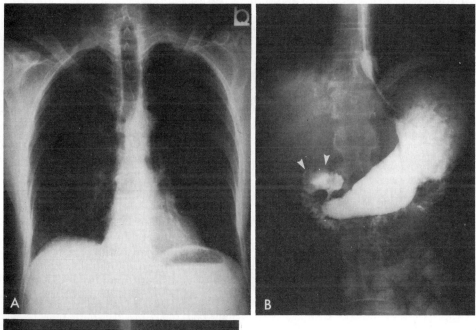

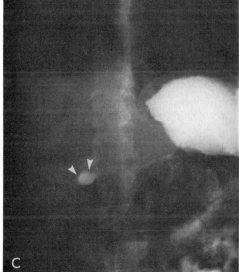

Figure 18–3 Perforated duodenal ulcer — no free air. Fifty-two year old businessman with well-documented past history of peptic ulcer disease and previous myocardial infarctions. Developed acute episgastric pain, hypotension, arrhythmia. Upright chest film showed no free air on two occasions (A). EKGs showed changes consistent with new infarction. After 12 hours, blood pressure was declining and pain was worse. Upper GI series with Gastrografin showed apparent leak (arrow) from duodenum (B), confirmed on film taken 30 minutes later (C) (arrow). He underwent immediate laparotomy, plication of perforation into lesser sac, and had an uneventful postoperative course.

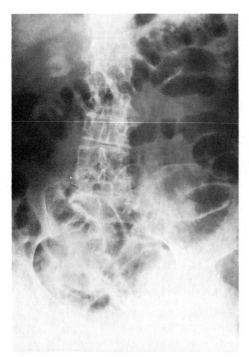

Figure 18–4 Radiopaque gallstone in patient with acute cholecystitis.

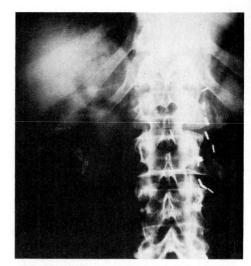

Figure 18–5 Gallstone ileus. Note air outlining the biliary ducts.

rant. In these patients the appendix proximal to the fecalith can occasionally be visualized, filled with intraluminal air. A radiopaque ureteral calculus can occasionally be seen on a flat plate (Fig. 18–6A) and is an important sign of a nonoperative condition producing abdominal pain. If the history is suggestive of ureteral colic, a confirmative intravenous pyelogram should also be performed. This may reveal hydronephrosis secondary to partial obstruction of the distal ureter by a calculus (Fig. 18–6B).

The clinical diagnosis of mechanical small bowel obstruction should be confirmed on plain and upright films of the abdomen. The presence of multiple dilated loops of small bowel with multiple fluid levels and no gas in the colon is diagnostic (Figs. 18–7A and B), and usually no other studies are necessary prior to initiation of therapy.

The clinical diagnosis of large bowel obstruction can also be confirmed on the flat and upright films. Frequently there is dilated small bowel along with the widely dilated colon when the pressure in the colon rises to levels such that small bowel peristalsis is unable to force more fluid or gas into the colon. The most frequent cause of large bowel obstruction, in our society, is a sigmoid carcinoma. This can be confirmed on barium enema examination. Sigmoid volvulus is another cause of large bowel obstruction (Fig. 18–8). Barium enema performed in these patients shows a characteristic inverted funnel sign as the barium column flows through the rectum to the twist in the sigmoid. This can often be reduced nonoperatively, with surgery postponed until it can be performed electively.[51] Cecal volvulus is a somewhat rarer cause of large intestinal obstruction, but with a characteristic plain and upright abdominal film (Fig. 18–9). Generally, the colon is massively dilated and, because of the torsion, the cecum is located in the left upper quadrant of the abdomen. Cecal volvulus is a surgical emergency.[25]

Text continued on page 960

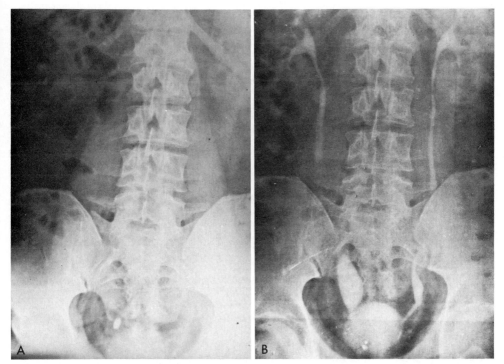

Figure 18–6 Radiopaque ureteral calculus. *A,* Calculus can be seen in right lower quadrant. *B.* An intravenous pyelogram in the same patient shows right hydroureter.

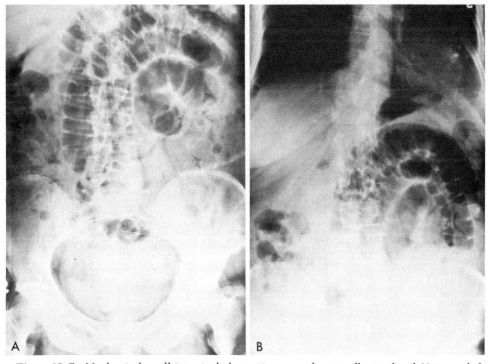

Figure 18–7 Mechanical small intestinal obstruction secondary to adhesive band. Note stepladder pattern of dilated small bowel with multiple fluid levels. *A.* Flat abdominal film. *B.* Upright abdominal film, showing multiple fluid levels.

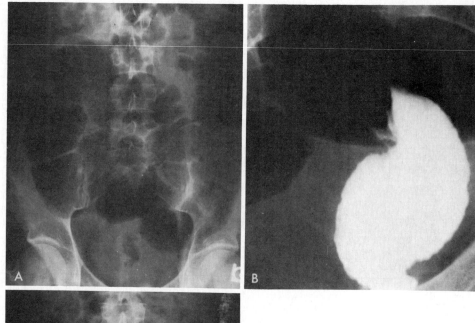

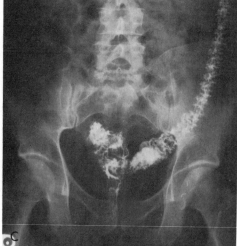

Figure 18–8 Sigmoid volvulus. Twenty-eight year old man, slightly retarded and chronically constipated. No previous history of volvulus. Constipation and distention when admitted to Emergency Room. Abdominal x-ray shows massive colonic distention and small amount of air in rectum, presumably from a self-administered enema (A). Barium enema showed characteristic inverted funnel as contrast medium was introduced (B). Volvulus was immediately reduced by the barium enema, which then revealed a redundant loop of sigmoid colon (C). Sigmoid resection was performed electively and postoperative course was benign.

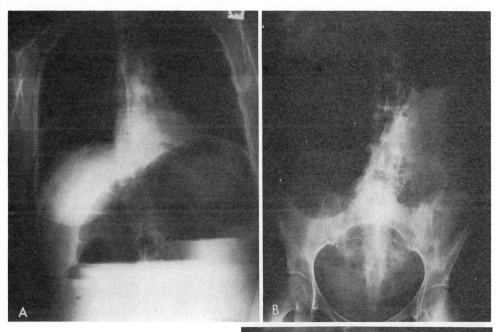

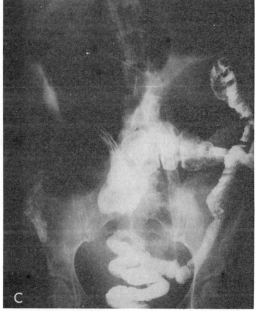

Figure 18–9 Cecal volvulus. Fifty-nine year old woman, a recluse who could not relate a history, was brought to Emergency Room with an acute abdomen. X-rays of chest (A) and abdomen (B) showed massive dilatation of colon. Diagnosis was immediately clarified by barium enema (C), which showed typical tapered narrowing of barium column at hepatic flexure due to cecal volvulus. Laparotomy was immediately performed and the gangrenous, perforated right colon was resected. She eventually recovered after a stormy postoperative course.

IMMEDIATE MANAGEMENT OF ACUTE ABDOMINAL EMERGENCIES

Upper Gastrointestinal Bleeding

Upper gastrointestinal bleeding is usually defined as bleeding proximal to the ligament of Treitz. This may be manifested by melena (the passage of tarry stools) or hematemesis (vomiting of blood). Upper gastrointestinal bleeding generally requires hospitalization, with rapid diagnostic work-up and appropriate therapy.

The etiologies of upper gastrointestinal tract bleeding from a series of 1500 cases are reviewed in Table 18–2.[33] Peptic ulceration is by far the most common cause, and of these, duodenal ulcer is approximately three times as common as gastric ulcer. Massive bleeding is the first symptom in approximately 15 per cent of patients with peptic ulcer. The bleeding is caused by erosion of the ulcer process into a local artery, most commonly a branch of the gastroduodenal artery. Most bleeding ulcers are surrounded by local inflammatory changes that tend to hinder spontaneous hemostasis. The vast majority of bleeding ulcers stop bleeding spontaneously, especially in younger patients whose arteries are more elastic than those of older patients.

Esophagogastric varices occur in patients with cirrhosis or extrahepatic obstruction of the portal vein. Although in some private hospitals these lesions account for less than 10 per cent of upper gastrointestinal bleeding, the percentage is much greater in hospitals with large indigent populations in which the incidence of alcoholism is greater than in the population at large. Bleeding varices are the most important cause of massive hematemesis in the child, the etiology of which is extrahepatic portal vein obstruction. It should be remembered that, although varices are the most common cause of massive upper gastrointestinal bleeding in cirrhotics, there is also a much higher incidence of duodenal ulcer, gastritis, and Mallory-Weiss bleeding in these patients. The demonstration of cirrhosis is not necessarily diagnostic of bleeding varices.

Gastritis is associated with acute ulcerations and erosions of the stomach which may produce hemorrhage. Alcohol, aspirin, steroids and other drugs have been implicated as etiological factors. The role of stress, as in war casualties, intensive care patients or sepsis has also been extensively investigated. Generally, the majority of patients bleeding from alcoholic gastritis will stop spontaneously in the absence of other etiological factors, while true "stress" bleeding is a difficult therapeutic problem.

TABLE 18–2   Etiology of Upper Gastrointestinal Bleeding (1500 Cases)*

DIAGNOSIS	%
Duodenal ulcer	27
Gastric ulcer	13
Esophagogastric varices	20
Erosive gastritis	13
Erosive esophagitis	8
Mallory-Weiss syndrome	5
Stomal (anastomotic) ulcer	3
Gastric cancer	1
Miscellaneous	3
Undetermined	7

*From Palmer, E. D.: Upper Gastrointestinal Hemorrhage. Springfield, Charles C Thomas, 1970.

Hiatal hernia with reflux esophagitis may be associated with occult bleeding, but is only rarely a cause of hematemesis or massive bleeding.

Tumors of the stomach may rarely be associated with massive upper gastrointestinal bleeding. Usually there is a history of occult bleeding and anemia. The majority of these patients can be controlled with conservative therapy and operated upon electively. Mallory-Weiss syndrome is bleeding from a small esophagogastric mucosal tear caused by violent retching and vomiting. Alcoholics, pregnant women and nonalcoholics vomiting from binge drinking are the usual patients with this condition.

The ease and accuracy of diagnosis of upper gastrointestinal bleeding has markedly advanced in the last few years, owing to the advent of selective angiography and fiberoptic gastroduodenoscopy. A careful history should be taken, concentrating on previous incidence of abdominal pain or ulcer disease. A history of consuming alcholic beverages is also pertinent. The history should also include questions about drugs the patient might be taking. Physical examination should be directed toward determining the vital signs and looking for various stigmata of diseases associated with upper gastrointestinal bleeding, such as cirrhosis.

RAPID TREATMENT AND SPECIAL DIAGNOSTIC PROCEDURES. The vast majority of patients with upper gastrointestinal hemorrhage require admission to the hospital. In all patients, one or more large bore intravenous lines should be started. Blood should be typed and cross matched. Initial therapy should begin restoring vital signs to normal with infusion of electrolyte solutions until blood is ready. Anemia may be assessed by determination of the hematocrit and hemoglobin, but it should be remembered that with rapid bleeding the extent of hemorrhage may not be reflected in the hematocrit level, since it takes several hours for this to equilibrate.

A nasogastric tube should be used in all patients with upper gastrointestinal bleeding. The stomach should be irrigated with cold normal saline. This generally will determine whether there is fresh bleeding proximal to the pylorus. With slow bleeding between the pylorus and the ligament of Treitz there may be no reflux of blood into the stomach. After the patient is successfully resuscitated from hypovolemia, fiberoptic endoscopy, selective angiography or both should be performed for diagnosis, depending on the rapidity of hemorrhage. If the rate of hemorrhage is rapid, selective angiography is likely to be of more value, since under these conditions it is very difficult to see the source of bleeding with endoscopy. On the other hand, with relatively slow bleeding (less than 100 ml per hour), angiography will probably not demonstrate pooling of blood, whereas gastroduodenoscopy will probably indicate the source of bleeding.[52] Both emergency endoscopy and selective angiography are now available at most larger hospitals and this has led to an increased diagnostic accuracy.

Lower Gastrointestinal Bleeding

Bleeding distal to the ligament of Treitz may be accompanied by guaiac positive stools, melanotic stools, or even by the passage of frank blood from the rectum (hematochezia). Although a large number of clinical conditions may result in lower gastrointestinal tract bleeding, the vast majority of them fall into relatively few categories.

SMALL BOWEL BLEEDING. Meckel's diverticulitis, regional enteritis and intussusception represent the most common causes of small bowel bleeding, followed by various benign or malignant neoplasms, polyps or hemangiomas. It is generally extremely difficult to make the diagnosis on an outpatient basis; indeed the diagnosis may occasionally be difficult even at

TABLE 18–3   Gastrointestinal and Intraperitoneal Causes of Abdominal Pain*

I. INFLAMMATION

   A. Peritoneum
     1. Chemical and nonbacterial peritonitis – perforated peptic ulcer, gallbladder, ruptured ovarian cyst, mittelschmerz
     2. Bacterial peritonitis
       a. Primary peritonitis – pneumococcal, streptococcal, tuberculous
       b. Perforated hollow viscus – stomach, intestine, biliary tract

   B. Hollow intestinal organs
     1. Appendicitis
     2. Cholecystitis
     3. Peptic ulceration
     4. Gastroenteritis
     5. Regional enteritis
     6. Meckel's diverticulitis
     7. Colitis – ulcerative, bacterial, amebic
     8. Diverticulitis

   C. Solid viscera
     1. Pancreatitis
     2. Hepatitis
     3. Hepatic abscess
     4. Splenic abscess

   D. Mesentery
     1. Lymphadenitis

   E. Pelvic organs
     1. Pelvic inflammatory disease
     2. Tubo-ovarian abscess
     3. Endometritis

*From Schwartz, S. I., and Storer, E. H.: Manifestations of gastrointestinal disease. *In* Schwartz, et al. (Eds.): Principles of Surgery, 2nd Ed. New York, McGraw-Hill, 1974.

laparotomy. Occasionally, the diagnosis of a Meckel's diverticulum with ectopic gastric mucosa can be made by technetium scanning.[23]

COLONIC BLEEDING. The most common colonic causes of bleeding in order of decreasing incidence include carcinoma, diverticulosis, inflammatory bowel disease and polyps. Although carcinoma represents the most common cause, the bleeding associated with this lesion is rarely massive and it usually stops spontaneously.

Diverticulosis is the most common cause of *massive* rectal bleeding. This is related to erosion of vessels in the neck of a diverticulum. Occasionally, bleeding from diverticulosis is so massive that emergency surgical intervention is required. If the bleeding can be demonstrated on selective angiography, segmental resection can be performed; otherwise, total colectomy with ileoproctostomy should be done.[26]

Inflammatory bowel disease is also a relatively common cause of rectal bleeding. This is usually mild; rarely, however, massive hemorrhage may occur that may necessitate emergency resection. There is some controversy as to whether these patients should have a total proctocolectomy or a subtotal colectomy with ileostomy and mucous fistula performed.

RECTAL BLEEDING. This is manifested by blood coating the stool or on the toilet tissue after a bowel move-

TABLE 18–3 Gastrointestinal and Intraperitoneal Causes of Abdominal Pain *(Continued)*

II. MECHANICAL [OBSTRUCTION, ACUTE DISTENSION]
    A. Hollow intestinal organs
        1. Intestinal obstruction—adhesions, hernia, tumor, volvulus, intussusception
        2. Biliary obstruction—calculi, tumor, choledochal cyst, hematobilia

    B. Solid viscera
        1. Acute spenomegaly
        2. Acute hepatomegaly—cardiac failure, Budd-Chiari syndrome

    C. Mesentery
        1. Omental torsion

    D. Pelvic
        1. Ovarian cyst
        2. Torsion or degeneration of fibroid
        3. Ectopic pregnancy

III. VASCULAR
    A. Intraperitoneal bleeding
        1. Ruptured liver
        2. Ruptured spleen
        3. Ruptured mesentery
        4. Ruptured ectopic pregnancy
        5. Ruptured aortic, splenic or hepatic aneurysm

    B. Ischemia
        1. Mesenteric thrombosis
        2. Hepatic infarction—toxemia, purpura
        3. Splenic infarction
        4. Omental ischemia

IV. MISCELLANEOUS
    A. Endometriosis

ment. The most common causes include benign anorectal disease such as hemorrhoids, anal fissures and proctitis and is discussed at greater length in Chapter 21. It should be emphasized that the presence of anorectal disease does not mean that the patient does not have more serious colonic pathological conditions and all patients with rectal bleeding should have a work-up consisting of sigmoidoscopy and barium enema if bleeding is persistent.

The Acute Abdomen

The causes of acute abdomen are summarized in Table 18–3. Most of these conditions require hospitalization and as such are beyond the scope of this book. The primary problem confronting the emergency room physician or office practitioner is to separate the surgical from the nonsurgical conditions that also may cause severe abdominal pain (Table 18–4).[42] Many of these conditions also require hospitalization. Patients with severe abdominal pain should be considered surgical emergencies until proven otherwise. It is incumbent on the physician to consider surgery unless the pain can be definitely ascribed as secondary to a nonsurgical cause. It should be kept in mind that it is occasionally necessary to operate on patients with acute abdominal pain before making a diagnosis, since the risk of missing a serious remediable pathological condition

TABLE 18–4   Extraperitoneal Causes of Abdominal Pain*

CARDIOPULMONARY
  Pneumonia
  Empyema
  Myocardial ischemia
  Active rheumatic heart disease
	VASCULAR
	  Dissection, rupture or expansion
	    of aortic aneurysm
	  Periarteritis

BLOOD
  Leukemia
  Sickle cell crisis
	METABOLIC
	  Uremia
	  Diabetic acidosis
	  Porphyria
	  Addisonian crisis

NEUROGENIC
  Spinal cord tumors
  Osteomyelitis of spine
  Tabes dorsalis
  Herpes zoster
  Abdominal epilepsy
	TOXINS
	  Bacterial (tetanus)
	  Insect bites
	  Venoms
	  Drugs
	  Lead poisoning

GENITOURINARY
  Nephritis
  Pyelitis
  Perinephric abscesses
  Ureteral obstruction
    (calculi, tumors)
  Prostatitis
  Seminal vesiculitis
  Epididymitis
	ABDOMINAL WALL
	  Intramuscular hematoma
	
	PSYCHOGENIC

*From Schwartz, S. I., and Storer, E. H.: Manifestations of gastrointestinal disease. *In* Schwartz et al. (Eds.): Principles of Surgery, 2nd Ed. New York, McGraw-Hill, 1974.

may be greater than the risk of an "unnecessary" surgery.

A note is required here about ruptured abdominal aneurysms: Any patient in the older age group who presents with abdominal pain or back pain and is hypotensive should be considered as having a possible case of ruptured abdominal aneurysm. With careful palpation the aneurysm can frequently be felt. This may be masked by a large retroperitoneal hematoma. A rim of calcium surrounding the aneurysm may be seen on a lateral film of the abdomen or abdominal flat plate. In any patient in whom the clinical diagnosis of ruptured aneurysm is confirmed, plans for emergency surgery should be made without delay. One of the major contributing factors to death from this condition is the inordinate delay in diagnosis and initiation of therapy. If the diagnosis is made in the emergency room, several large bore intravenous infusions should be started and the patient should be cross matched for large volumes of blood (ten units or more). Operation should be undertaken without delay.

Intestinal Obstruction

Mechanical intestinal obstruction is one of the most common surgical emergencies. Although a large number of pathophysiological entities may cause intestinal obstruction (Table 18–5),[42] surgically they can be divided into two main types: small intestinal obstruction and large intestinal obstruction.

SMALL BOWEL OBSTRUCTION. This usually involves colicky abdominal pain, vomiting, abdominal distention and failure to pass feces and flatus. Initially, crampy abdominal pain is felt by the patient. This is generally accompanied by vomiting of gastric contents. If the obstruction is not relieved the pain continues and abdominal distention becomes apparent. Vomiting then becomes more continuous. The character of the vomitus may become feculent. The diagnosis generally can be confirmed on plain and upright films of the abdomen.

Although a large number of clinical conditions can produce small bowel obstruction, the vast majority fall into two categories. In patients who have had previous abdominal surgery the most common cause is mechanical obstruction from adhesive band constriction. In patients who have not had

TABLE 18–5   Mechanisms of Intestinal Obstructions*

A. MECHANICAL OBSTRUCTION OF THE LUMEN
   Obturation of the lumen
       Meconium
       Intussusception
       Gallstones
       Impactions – fecal, barium, bezoar, worms
   Lesions of the bowel
       Congenital
           Atresia and stenosis
           Imperforate anus
           Duplications
           Meckel's diverticulum
       Traumatic
       Inflammatory
           Regional enteritis
           Diverticulitis
           Chronic ulcerative colitis
       Neoplastic
       Miscellaneous
           K+-induced stricture
           Radiation stricture
           Endometriosis
   Lesions extrinsic to bowel
       Adhesive band constriction or angulation by adhesion
       Hernia and wound dehiscence
       Extrinsic masses
           Annular pancreas
           Anomalous vessels
           Abscesses and hematomas
           Neoplasms
   Volvulus

B. INADEQUATE PROPULSIVE MOTILITY
   Neuromuscular defects
       Megacolon
       Paralytic ileus
           Abdominal causes
               Intestinal distension
               Peritonitis
               Retroperitoneal lesions
           Systemic causes
               Electrolyte imbalance
               Toxemias
       Spastic ileus

C. VASCULAR OCCLUSION
   Arterial
   Venous

*From Schwartz, S. I., and Storer, E. H.: Manifestations of gastrointestinal disease. *In* Schwartz et al. (Eds.): Principles of Surgery, 2nd Ed. New York, McGraw-Hill, 1974.

prior abdominal surgery, incarcerated hernia is the most common cause.

Physiologically, intestinal obstruction results in the accumulation of large quantities of fluid within the lumen of the bowel. Fluid is also lost by vomiting. This rapidly depletes the extracellular fluid space, which may lead to hemoconcentration, hypovolemia, renal insufficiency and death. Occlusion of the blood supply to a segment of bowel in addition to obstruction is known as strangulated obstruction. This is the most serious complication of intestinal obstruction and failure to relieve the obstruction will result in necrosis of the segment of small bowel.

The treatment of small bowel obstruction consists of resuscitation of the patient with fluid and electrolyte therapy, decompression and surgical intervention. Once the diagnosis of small bowel obstruction is confirmed, plans should be made to operate on these patients following resuscitation.[42] A nasogastric tube should be placed in the stomach for decompression of the stomach and blood specimens should be sent for determination of the complete blood count, blood urea nitrogen (BUN) and electrolytes. Intravenous therapy should be started. In severely dehydrated patients a Foley catheter should be placed in the bladder. Fluid resuscitation should be rapidly commenced and should continue until there is adequate urine output, the central venous pressure approaches normal and vital signs are maintained. The initial hematocrit reading may be high because of dehydration and this should return towards normal. The BUN should also fall. Infusion of potassium is usually necessary but should not be started until a good urinary output is assured. When the patient has adequate fluid balance, the operation should be undertaken. The time for resuscitation should be measured in hours and not in days. Some surgeons will treat patients who have adhesive band obstruction with-

out the features of strangulation with gastric decompression for 6 to 12 hours. If the pain disappears and there are no signs of peritonitis, decompression is continued for a further 48 hours or so, and in some patients surgery will not be necessary. Strangulated obstruction, however, always requires surgical therapy immediately following resuscitation.

Some surgeons advocate the use of long intestinal tubes (Miller-Abbott or Cantor tubes) for the treatment of non-strangulating adhesion obstruction. This method of therapy has gradually lost favor in recent years with the lowered mortality rate of laparotomy. Most surgeons now recommend early operation for acute small intestinal obstruction. The principal indications for primary intubation therapy are obstruction in the immediate postoperative period, the treatment of obstruction in a patient who had multiple previous laparotomies for obstruction or small bowel obstruction associated with generalized carcinomatosis.

LARGE BOWEL OBSTRUCTION. The signs in patients with large bowel obstruction are usually less dramatic than in those with small bowel obstruction. Patients usually present with constipation and progressive abdominal distention. Pain may be present but it is generally not a striking feature. The majority of cases of large bowel obstruction are caused by carcinoma, followed by diverticulitis and then volvulus. The clinical diagnosis can generally be confirmed by a flat plate of the abdomen. The diagnosis may be further elucidated with a barium or Hypaque enema. Surgical therapy will depend on the etiology of the obstruction. Generally, in cases of colon obstruction, the fluid and electrolyte derangements are not as great as with small bowel obstruction. The major emergency is related to the fact that, with progressive distention, rupture of the cecum may occur. Therefore, in cases of colonic obstruction the primary emergency is to decompress the distended cecum and to divert the intestinal contents via a colostomy. Obstruction secondary to sigmoid volvulus can generally be decompressed by means of a sigmoidoscope and rectal tube with later operative repair.[51]

Abdominal Trauma

Significant abdominal trauma, in general, warrants a period of close observation in a holding area, such as the "overnight ward." For abdominal gun-

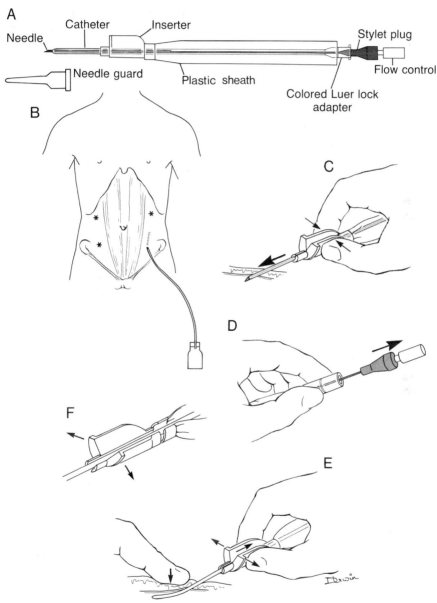

Figure 18–10 Therapeutic paracentesis. Sterile radiopaque Teflon catheter is inserted percutaneously into one of the four abdominal quadrants, following percussion of abdomen to identify and avoid gas-filled viscera. We prefer a catheter and needle unit in which needle is *inside* the catheter. The needle can safely be withdrawn after insertion into the abdomen. Suitable catheters are: Deseret E-Z Cath, 16 ga., 12 inches, Cat. No. 2254; and Deseret Angiocath, 16 ga., 5¼ inches, Cat. No. 2854.

shot wounds, exploratory laparotomy is the safest approach.[34] Abdominal stab wounds are routinely explored at some institutions and selectively explored at other institutions, depending on the clinical course of the patient, the results of peritoneal lavage, or both.[34, 41] Blunt trauma produces the greatest problems in management, for it is often difficult to assess the likelihood of intra-abdominal damage. It is necessary to remember that the amount of force, the duration of the period of injury and the nature of the trauma may give clues to the likelihood of intra-abdominal lesions. A deep abdominal abrasion from a seat belt after an auto crash at high speed is a sign of sufficient trauma to rupture viscera in the abdomen.[50] Paracentesis (Fig. 18–10) may indicate a need for prompt surgery, but a "negative" tap in such a patient does not rule out the possibility of significant injury.[34] Blast injury commonly causes ruptured viscera. The problem is to assess the severity of the blast and the proximity of the patient to it. Fractured ribs may be a sign of trauma severe enough to rupture spleen, liver or other organs — especially in children, whose ribs are less liable to fracture than the brittle ribs of adults.

SURGICAL DISEASES OF SPECIFIC ORGANS

Abdominal Wall

Tumors of the abdominal wall may be treated on an inpatient or an outpatient basis, depending on the size and type of the lesion. All melanomas, in general, warrant hospitalization. Congenital defects and hernias almost always require hospitalization for definitive repair. Useful preparation in the outpatient clinic includes instruction for reduction in weight, evaluation of cough and a search for prostatic obstruction or constipation, if any of these predisposing causes for hernia are present.

Inguinal hernia[28, 31] may be "indirect" (a congenital weakness of the internal inguinal ring) or "direct" (an acquired weakness of the floor of the inguinal canal). Distinction can frequently be made on the basis of the age of the patient and the location of the hernia. Direct hernias are uncommon in young men and usually do not descend into the scrotum. It is, however, of little practical importance to distinguish between these two types of hernias preoperatively. The distinction can be made at the time of surgery on the basis of location in reference to the deep inferior epigastric vessels. Indirect hernias arise lateral to the epigastric vessels and direct hernias occur medial to the vessels. Hesselbach's triangle, the classic site of direct hernias, is bounded by the epigastric vessels, Poupart's ligament and the lateral border of the rectus abdominis muscle. The repair of an inguinal hernia must, in either case, include closure of the defect and establishment of a secure floor of the inguinal canal. Recurrent inguinal hernias nearly always begin as a defect adjacent to the pubic tubercule (in the "direct" area). Inguinal hernias may be operated upon under general, spinal or local anesthesia.

Femoral hernia may present in the groin, simulating an inguinal hernia, but it usually produces a relatively lower (inferior) bulge. The neck of the bulge is below the inguinal ligament. Femoral hernia is more common in women than men and is rarely seen in young people. Femoral hernias frequently become incarcerated, even when small. A small, hard groin mass, which appears to be a lymph node, should immediately raise the question of an incarcerated femoral hernia, especially if it is tender and irreducible. Incarceration of one wall of the bowel (Richter's hernia) is not uncommon. A Richter's type of hernia requires immediate hospitalization and surgical repair.

Umbilical hernia is relatively uncommon in adults, although it is a significant cosmetic and psychological problem in children (see Chapter 23). In adults the hernia is usually paraumbilical and incarceration and strangulation are much more likely than in children. Surgical repair is recommended in adults, since the likelihood of complications is greatly increased. Frequently, however, only omentum or preperitoneal fat will be found in the hernia.

Other types of abdominal wall hernias are relatively uncommon. Paraspinal (lumbar) hernias occur in the triangle of Petit.[31, 32] Spigelian hernias occur along the lateral border of the rectus muscle. Obturator canal hernias may present with discomfort in the buttocks.

Ventral hernias are common complications of partial or complete postoperative wound disruption, in which case they are termed incisional hernias. They also occur occasionally in the linea alba on a congenital basis. All of these hernias should be recognizable to the outpatient surgeon, but should be treated only on an inpatient basis.

Intercostal nerve entrapment may occasionally produce pain and a small tender mass that simulates a spigelian hernia at the lateral margin of the rectus sheath. A test for this diagnosis is local infiltration with anesthetic, which can be performed in the Outpatient Clinic. If the symptoms recede temporarily and then return, exploration of the area should be carried out. The nerve should be freed up from the entrapment, or resected if a neuroma has developed.

Peritoneum

If the surgeon is consulted because of a diagnosis of peritonitis, he will undoubtedly hospitalize the patient and initiate therapy, which usually leads to surgery with appropriate drainage, resection or repair. Occasionally, a patient may be extremely ill and the diagnosis unclear. The emergency work-up of the acute abdomen has been reviewed earlier in the chapter.

Intraperitoneal fluid accumulation may be a chronic, recurring problem, and therapeutic paracentesis may provide useful palliation. Recurrent ascites may be a complication of hepatic vein thrombosis, cirrhosis, metastatic cancer or miliary tuberculosis. These forms of ascites can usually be distinguished easily from chylous ascites and pseudomyxoma peritonei, each of which may be more suitably treated by exploratory laparotomy to attempt correction of the primary problem.

Liver

The patient with surgical disease of the liver will usually have either a right upper quadrant mass, jaundice, pain, fever or various combinations of these problems.

A right upper quadrant mass may be due to hepatomegaly, an enlarged gallbladder, a tumor of or adjacent to the liver or a host of less common conditions. Occasionally, the liver may be made more easily palpable as the result of pulmonary emphysema and flattening of the diaphragm, but this will rarely produce symptoms of right upper quadrant discomfort. The liver may be enlarged as the result of metastatic disease, cardiac congestive failure, hepatic vein thrombosis or cirrhosis. Diffuse disease such as hepatitis or cholangitis may cause liver enlargement, pain, tenderness, jaundice and fever. Liver abscess may also present with a right upper quadrant mass.

If the liver is grossly nodular and the patient is cachectic, a careful search for the primary tumor should be made before liver biopsy is undertaken. If the patient is otherwise well, it may be most expeditious simply to biopsy the liver percutaneously or with the aid of the laparoscope. A significant degree of jaundice or abnormal clotting parameters are contraindications to need-

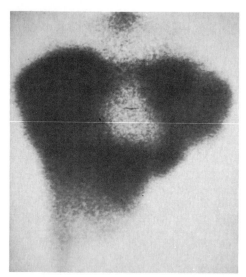

Figure 18–11 Liver scan. 14 cm hepatoma in medial segment of the left lobe, seen preoperatively with ^{99}Tc scan.

le biopsy. The patient *must* be closely observed for several hours afterward. If the patient has a solitary tumor, hospitalization for an open liver biopsy and appropriate therapy is recom-

mended. Occasionally an enlarged or displaced liver lobe may be discovered and may lead to concern. Riedel's lobe is a classic trap for the unwary.

A liver scan is often very helpful in defining the size and location of lesions (Fig. 18–11). Selective arteriography is also helpful in identifying the number and size of hepatic lesions. Transfemoral, celiac and mesenteric arteriograms (Fig. 18–12) may be performed on an outpatient basis if the patient is observed for signs of intestinal ischemia or bleeding for a few hours after the study.

In the series of major liver tumors reported by Malt and colleagues[27] 26 out of 63 were found to be benign and excision was curative. The most common benign tumors are hamartomas and hemangiomas. The use of oral contraceptives is associated with benign liver cell adenomas.[1] Malignant tumors include metastatic tumors and solitary or multicentric hepatomas.

Jaundice raises questions of hepatitis, cirrhosis, hepatomas, cholangitis,

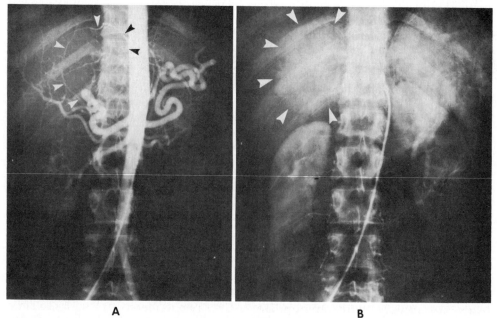

A   B

Figure 18–12 Hepatic arteriography. Celiac artery injection of case in Fig. 18–11, shows displacement (arrows) of arterial branches in early phase *(A)* and venous tumor "blush" (arrows) in late phase *(B)*.

common duct stones, carcinoma of the pancreas, metastatic carcinoma and toxic drug reactions. It is rarely suitable to study and treat the patient with jaundice of unknown etiology on an outpatient basis, so the work-up of this condition involves prompt hospitalization.

If the patient has previously undergone biliary tract surgery, the presence of common duct stones or stricture is a likely possibility, and the operations required may be formidable procedures. The rate of mortality in reoperation is approximately ten times higher than that in first operations on the biliary tract.[16]

Right upper quadrant pain is more commonly due to disease of the gallbladder than to liver disease, but all of the lesions that produce hepatomegaly can also cause pain. Hematobilia is one such condition. Although it usually occurs as a complication of injury to the liver, it may occur from a benign or malignant tumor. The presentation may be in the form of intermittent gastrointestinal bleeding of unknown origin, and the presence of pain due to distention of the biliary tree may be the only clue to the site of bleeding. Selective arteriography will usually reveal a lesion if it is performed when bleeding is active or if a mass is present within the liver. Post-traumatic hematobilia usually requires hepatic resection, although healing has been reported without surgery.[19] Hematobilia also occurs as a rare, usually end-stage complication of carcinoma of the gallbladder, bile ducts or pancreas.

Fever of unknown origin may be the result of diffuse or localized infection of the liver or its surrounding tissues. Many of these patients will also have pain, tenderness, a mass, jaundice or all of these. Any patient with a fever of unknown origin should have a careful liver function evaluation and should be considered for a liver scan and possible arteriography. If there is any reason to suspect liver abscess, spot films or tomograms of the liver may show the telltale gas bubbles or air fluid levels that localize the abscess. Sonography is frequently helpful in making the diagnosis.

Liver abscess may occur as a result of cholangitis, amoebae, or echinococcus cysts, by metastatic spread from elsewhere in the body (especially the portal system or pelvis), or on an idiopathic basis. Elevation of alkaline phosphatase and a solitary defect on liver scan may provide the essential clues to diagnosis. Amoebic abscess is rare in the United States, except in those who have lived or travelled in Mexico or the tropics. The treatment is usually medical, Flagyl being the preferred drug at the present time, since it is equally effective as and less toxic than emetine. Echinococcus cysts are encountered in specific geographical regions where the cycle of the dog tapeworm has been established. These lesions are not uncommon in Alaskan Eskimos and Indians. The patients should ordinarily be hospitalized for drainage.

The evaluation of the patient with possible liver disease should be done with the differential diagnosis in mind, so that appropriate questions, examinations and tests are requested and performed. The patient should be questioned regarding his exposure to hepatic toxins, alcohol, injections and jaundiced persons. He should be asked if he is known to have had gallstones or has had fatty food intolerance, dark urine or clay-colored stools. A careful record should be made of the size of the liver on physical examination, indicating its edge in relationship to the costal margin and umbilicus. Its size should be estimated in centimeters (not finger-breadths) from the costal margin at specific points (for example, xiphoid line, midclavicular line, anterior axillary line). The presence or absence of tenderness, irregularity, firmness and mobility should be recorded. The patient should be observed for palmar erythema, asterixis and spider angiomata of the skin. Masses or tenderness in other areas of the body may be a definite clue to the origin of liver disease, especially if a rectal cancer or superclavicular nodes are palpated. Intravenous cholangiograms can be performed on an outpatient basis, but they usually contribute little in patients with a serum bilirubin over 4 mg per 100 ml. An oral cholecystogram does not usually visualize the biliary tract if the serum bilirubin is greater than 3 mg per 100 ml. Intravenous cholangiography also has definite hazards, including anaphylaxis.

Diaphragm

Hiatus hernia is the most common surgical disease of the diaphragm. Sliding hiatus hernia is observed in up to 10 per cent of gastrointestinal series in which it is looked for. Paraesophageal hiatus hernia is much less common but is more likely to produce symptoms or incarceration than a sliding hernia. Sliding hernia should be treated medically until it is obvious that symptoms ("heartburn," regurgitation, dysphagia) or complications (aspiration pneumonia, esophagitis) will not subside without surgery. Esophagitis may progress to stricture, which may require surgery. Dilatation by bougie may provide long-term success in cases in which the stricture is mild. The decision to recommend surgical repair for reflux esophagitis should be based not only on symptoms and intractability, but also on documentation of acid reflux in esophageal studies that can be performed on an outpatient basis. Hiatus hernia may be relatively asymptomatic and discovered only incidentally in the course of a gastrointestinal work-up for gallstones or sigmoid diverticulitis (Saint's triad).

Rupture of the central tendon of the diaphragm may occur as the result of trauma, and can be followed by incar-

ceration of stomach or colon within the chest.[12] Symptoms of intrathoracic borborygmi and "heartburn" during defecation may be bizarre consequences of this lesion which should be corrected by surgery. Diaphragmatic rupture is more common on the left side than on the right. Intrathoracic displacement of the liver through a ruptured right diaphragm may cause acute embarrassment of hepatic or pulmonary function if unrecognized. Rupture of the right diaphragm may be erroneously diagnosed as a hemothorax, in which case an attempt may inadvertently be made to insert a chest tube into the intrathoracic liver.[46]

Subphrenic abscess is usually the consequence of previous surgery or trauma and may become apparent only after the patient has been discharged from the hospital. The diagnosis should be suspected in the patient with low grade intermittent fever, recurrent pleural effusion and leukocytosis. Other signs may include subcostal or costovertebral ache and tenderness, a paralyzed or sluggish motion of the diaphragm, displacement of the liver or spleen, a defect on the liver-spleen scan or a subphrenic accumulation of air. Displacement of the stomach may be apparent on plain abdominal x-ray or a gastrointestinal series. When the diagnosis is strongly suspected, the patient should be admitted for final preoperative studies and surgical drainage (Fig. 18–13).

Fenestration of the diaphragm is the result of a congenital weakness that causes a bulge in the center of one of the hemidiaphragms. It is usually of no functional significance.

Tumors of the diaphragm are rare. Sarcomas may occur in this organ. More common, however, are metastatic tumors or local invasion from cancer in adjacent organs. The prognosis is very poor. The diagnosis of a neoplasm involving the diaphragm can frequently be suspected from inspection of the chest film.

Biliary Tract

Gallstones represent the major surgical problem in the biliary tract, and may produce complications of acute cholecystitis, carcinoma, obstructive jaundice, gallstone ileus, biliary cirrhosis and pancreatitis. Acute cholecystitis has a particularly high rate of mortality in the aged population, dia-

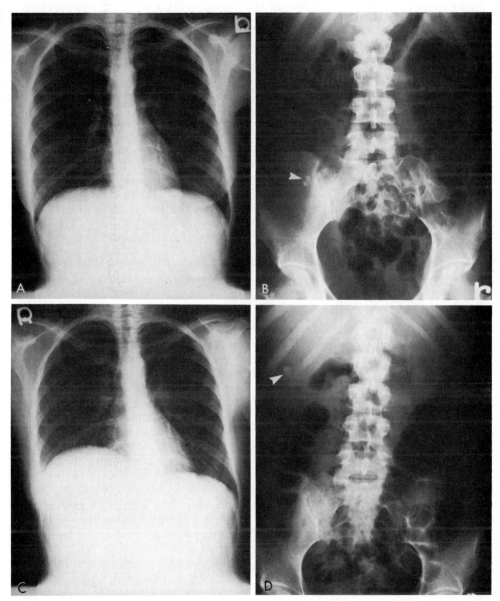

Figure 18–13 Subphrenic abscess caused by an unrecognized fecalith of the appendix. *A.* Normal chest x-ray when admitted with acute appendicitis in January 1971. *B.* Abdominal x-ray showing fecalith (arrow) in appendiceal abscess, January 1971. Fecalith was not seen at this time and was not removed. *C.* Elevated right diaphragm, June 1971. *D.* Abdominal x-ray, June 1971. Laminated fecalith is now visible in RUQ (arrow).

Illustration continued on the following page

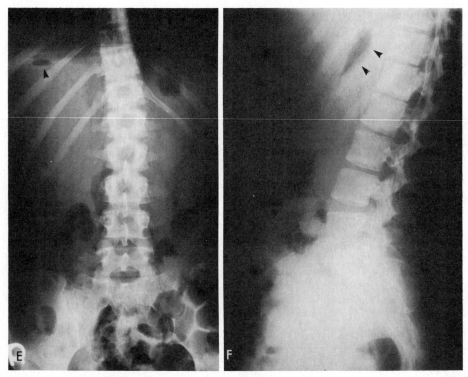

Figure 18–13 *(Continued)*. *E.* Upright film shows subphrenic air-fluid level (arrow). *F.* Lateral film shows location of subphrenic abscess (arrow). Patient recovered promptly following rib resection, drainage and removal of fecalith.

betics and patients with leukemia. It occurs with increased frequency in families with congenital spherocytic anemias. It has been suggested that truncal vagotomy and drainage is followed by an increased incidence of gallstones, possibly as the result of poor emptying of the gallbladder.

Gallstones should be suspected in patients who have intolerance to fried or fatty foods or who describe "bloating" or dyspepsia after ingestion of cabbage, cucumbers, cauliflower or onions. Many patients will have a long history of mild complaints, while others will have only one or two severe episodes of pain before seeking medical attention. The disease may first present as an episode of acute cholecystitis with fever and right upper quadrant pain. Most of these patients will improve following conservative therapy with intravenous fluids, naso-

gastric suction, antibiotics and sedatives. Morphine should not be administered since it produces spasm of the sphincter of Oddi.

The presence of gallstones is a sufficient indication for cholecystectomy in patients who are otherwise well, since the complications of gallstones are usually more hazardous than the risk of surgery. Common duct exploration should be added to the operation if there are clear signs of common duct stones, stricture, obstruction or if jaundice is present. If there is a significant past history consistent with obstruction, operative cholangiography should always be performed, and if the duct system is not completely normal, exploration is carried out. The risk of the operation is increased very little by common duct exploration, although if stones are present in the duct, the overall morbidity and mortality are increased somewhat. Multiple small stones are more hazardous than a single large calculus, since small stones are more likely to escape detection and become lodged in the common duct.

The overall rate of mortality for cholecystectomy is approximately 1 to 2 per cent, but should be less than 0.5 per cent in elective operations in otherwise healthy individuals. The mortality in 1090 consecutive cholecystectomies reported by Seltzer was 1.6 per cent.[45] The mortality for all operations on the biliary tract in 2358 patients reported by Glenn and McSherry was 1.7 per cent.[16] Glenn, McSherry and Dineen also reported an overall nonfatal complication rate of 6.9 per cent in 3217 patients with biliary tract operations for nonmalignant disease.[17]

The diagnosis of gallstone disease is made in most cases by oral cholecystography. The stones may be so small that they can be seen only when dye has coated them and they layer out on an upright film. Very few false positives are seen — that is, cases in which gallstones are believed to be visualized on x-ray but are not found at the time of surgery. On the other hand, failure to visualize the gallbladder does not prove that the organ is diseased. It may concentrate the dye if the test tablets are administered for two or three more days. Temporary failure to function occurs during episodes of acute illness, such as with an active peptic ulcer or pancreatitis. The reverse situation may also be true, and a "normal" oral cholecystogram may be present in a patient who actually has small gallstones. If the patient has a good history for recurrent biliary colic, exploration and even cholecystectomy may be indicated, since very small stones may not even be palpable intraoperatively and will be revealed only when the gallbladder is opened. In cases of acute cholecystitis or jaundice, the oral cholecystogram is of little or no help, since the gallbladder will not be visualized. Occasionally, an intravenous cholangiogram or sono-

gram is helpful in such patients. We routinely obtain an alkaline phosphatase in patients suspected of having gallstone disease, since mild or transient obstruction of the common duct will cause elevation in alkaline phosphatase. Serum bilirubin should also be obtained, since subclinical jaundice may occur and this would be an indication for further study of the common duct.

Other diseases of the biliary tract frequently present a dilemma for the surgeon, especially if they are completely asymptomatic or if the patient is a poor operative risk. Occasionally, an oral cholecystogram demonstrates a small, immobile radiolucent defect in the fundus. This frequently represents a polyp or, rarely, an adenoma. It should be possible to rule out the presence of a gallstone by repositioning the patient and obtaining another x-ray. These patients usually should be operated on simply to rule out the presence of carcinoma, since virtually the only cases of cancer of the gallbladder that are cured occur in patients in whom a small, localized, asymptomatic cancer is present and is removed completely with a cholecystectomy. The annual rate of mortality for cancer of the gallbladder is actually almost as high as that for benign disease of the gallbladder, in spite of the rarity of this tumor. Calcification in the wall of the gallbladder (porcelain gallbladder) is another uncommon condition (Fig. 18–14) that probably warrants an operation in otherwise healthy patients, because of an increased risk of carcinoma.[35]

The elderly patient with asymptomatic or nearly asymptomatic cholelithiasis presents a philosophical problem for the surgeon. In properly selected elderly patients, the rate of mortality for elective cholecystectomy is only slightly higher than that for the population at large.[22]

Trauma to the gallbladder or common duct may rupture the biliary tract, leading to acute bile peritonitis. This

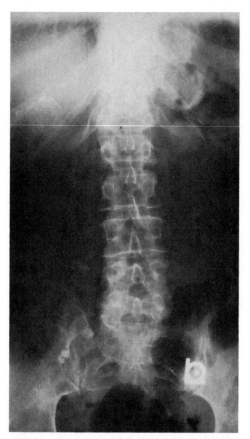

Figure 18–14 Calcification in gallbladder wall. Seventy-four year old woman with recurrent myocardial infarctions and chronic obstructive pulmonary disease. Abdominal x-ray obtained when calcification was accidentally observed during chest fluoroscopy. No symptoms related to gallbladder. Operation was not advised.

condition is increasingly common as the result of seat belt injuries in high speed automobile accidents. Stab wounds and gunshot wounds may lacerate the biliary tract, and any patient who has bile-stained retroperitoneal tissues or free bile observed at laparotomy must have the source of the bile determined or disaster will usually result in the postoperative period.

Stricture of the common bile duct or hepatic ducts may occur from trauma, carcinoma or on a congenital basis. Most of these cases, however, are the result of prior surgical damage to the biliary tree. Reconstructive surgery for correction or palliation is usually a complex matter.

The exact cause of the postcholecystectomy syndrome is unknown, but the symptoms may be the same as those for which cholecystectomy was performed initially. A proper work-up of such patients should include cardiac, neurological, pancreatic, gastric, colonic, renal and psychiatric studies. Occasionally, such patients are found to have new or retained stones in the common duct. Some have had incomplete cholecystectomies or a long residual cystic duct stump in which stones may form. This complication sometimes may be diagnosed by an intravenous cholangiogram.

Stomach and Duodenum

Peptic ulcer disease is the cause of most of the surgical problems related to the stomach and duodenum. Duodenal ulcers, benign gastric ulcers, gastritis, esophagitis and a multitude of complications provide a steady series of challenges for the outpatient surgeon. In addition, cancer, trauma and congenital abnormalities may also be seen in these organs.

The etiology of peptic ulcer is still not completely understood. The parietal and chief cells of the fundus of the stomach secrete hydrogen and pepsin, respectively, in response to stimulation both by the hormone gastrin and by the vagus nerves. Gastrin is released from the gastric antrum when the antrum is distended by food or liquid or is bathed in an alkaline medium. The vagal response is triggered by the sensation of hunger and hypoglycemia. It may therefore be initiated by endogenous or exogenous insulin. Gastric mucus probably plays a role in protecting the gastric mucosa from the digestive effects of acid and pepsin in the stomach, and the alkaline secretions of bile, pancreatic juice and Brunner's glands normally protect the duodenum from acid digestion.

Men have higher gastric acid production than women, and peptic ulcer disease is more frequent in men than in women. In general, patients with duodenal ulcers have higher gastric acid outputs than do normal controls. Patients with benign gastric ulcers generally have lower acid outputs than normal controls and patients with carcinoma of the stomach. Gastric acid production decreases in the last few decades of life, but complications from previously active peptic ulcers may occur after acidity has decreased to low levels. The most common complications of peptic ulcers are bleeding, pain, obstruction and perforation, and these are the most common indications for operation. Gastric ulcers on the greater curvature have a higher incidence of malignancy than those on the lesser curvature and are therefore subject to greater scrutiny and earlier operation than ulcers on the lesser curvature.

Duodenal ulcers most commonly occur in the first and second portions of the duodenum. Anterior ulcers are more likely to be complicated by perforation, whereas posterior ulcers tend to penetrate into the pancreas and may erode into branches of the gastroduodenal artery, causing bleeding. Typically, the symptoms of duodenal ulcer are intermittent epigastric pain and tenderness, especially aggravated by anxiety and hunger, and relieved with rest, food and antacids. Frequently, a predisposing stimulus can be found, such as a family problem or other psychological conflicts. The symptoms are often aggravated by alcohol and smoking. Occasionally, drug ingestion may be the inciting cause. Aspirin, indomethacin and phenylbutazone are the most common offenders at the present time.

Benign gastric ulcers frequently have a history similar to that of duodenal ulcers, but in many instances there is no clear history of pain related to hunger and anxiety and relieved by food and antacids. Giant benign gastric ulcers sometimes occur in the presence of only moderate amounts of gastric acidity. Occasionally, patients with duodenal ulcers will develop gastric outlet obstruction and simultaneous ulcerations in the stomach.

Investigation of the patient with presumed peptic ulcer disease involves obtaining a careful history and physical examination, followed by the necessary laboratory tests to document and confirm the diagnosis. In most cases the history will be characteristic. Physical examination frequently reveals only epigastric tenderness in the patient with an acute peptic ulcer. If there is gastric outlet obstruction a succussion splash may be present and vomiting will have occurred intermittently. The stool and vomitus should be examined for gross and occult blood.

Useful laboratory tests include an upper gastrointestinal x-ray series, in which the esophagus, cardia, stomach and duodenum should be evaluated. Fluoroscopy will often be more useful than the plain films in revealing spasm and irritability of the duodenum. The fiberoptic gastroscope can be used in the Outpatient Department; a record of the appearance of the ulcer may be obtained on color film and biopsy may be performed.

The medical management of peptic ulcer disease includes the use of antacids, anticholinergics and sedatives; bland diet with frequent feedings; elimination of tobacco and alcohol; and correction of underlying psychological stress, if it can be identified. Recently carbenoxolone was shown to be of value in the acceleration of healing of gastric ulcers, and Cimetidine, an H_2-blocker, is a valuable agent in the treatment of duodenal ulcers.

The operation performed for duodenal ulcer is selected by the surgeon on the basis of his experience and the findings present at surgery. Truncal vagotomy and simple drainage is the easiest and least hazardous operation, but the recurrence rate following this operation is somewhat higher than that following vagotomy and antrectomy. Antrectomy as performed in most institutions is simply a distal 50 per cent gastrectomy. More recently, highly selective (parietal cell) vagotomy without drainage has been suggested as the operation of choice. This operation results in an approximately 8 per cent recurrence rate, but the rates of mortality and morbidity of the procedure and its late side effects are minimal. The operation of choice for a chronic gastric ulcer is a partial gastrectomy.

The evaluation of a patient who has acute upper abdominal pain can be complex, and occasionally it is impossible to determine preoperatively whether or not the patient has a perforated ulcer. The diagnosis of the acute abdomen has been discussed earlier. Acute upper gastrointestinal bleeding is likewise not necessarily due to a peptic ulcer, even in patients with a long history of a peptic ulcer.

The virulent ulcer diathesis caused by Zollinger-Ellison tumors may be suspected on the basis of repeated episodes of ulceration and high acid outputs. These patients should be treated by total gastrectomy.

Gastritis may occur as a mild irritative lesion of the gastric mucosa, or it may be ulcerative, with bleeding or even perforation. Common presentations in the Outpatient Department include pain (similar to that of acute duodenal ulcer) or bleeding, which may be mild to massive. Among the most common inciting causes are ingestion of alcohol or other drugs, severe stress, major burns and increased intracerebral pressure. Gastritis may appear as a consequence of acute, excessive ingestion of alcohol or in chronic intemperate use of alcohol, the mechanism postulated being diminished conjugation of endogenous histamine by the intoxicated or cirrhotic liver, leading to locally increased concentrations of this gastric secretagogue. The four other common toxic compounds which at present are significant causes of gastri-

tis are corticosteroids, aspirin, phenylbutazone (Butazolidin) and indomethacin (Indocin). Acute hemorrhagic gastric ulcerations due to burns (Curling's ulcer) or cranial pathology (Cushing's ulcer) are not commonly seen in outpatients. The treatment for acute hemorrhagic gastritis is not completely satisfactory. Hospitalization is required, and iced saline lavage is usually tried initially. Selective catheterization with Pitressin infusion into the bleeding vessel may stop the hemorrhage. If conservative measures fail, operation is indicated.

Adenocarcinoma of the stomach is declining in frequency in the United States, but it is still a major concern in every patient who has a gastric ulcer that does not heal promptly and completely by medical therapy. Patients with pernicious anemia have histamine-fast achlorhydria and an increased incidence of carcinoma of the stomach. Other malignancies of the stomach include lymphocytic lymphosarcoma, reticulum cell sarcoma, leiomyosarcoma and carcinoid tumors. The most common benign tumor of the stomach is leiomyoma, which may be grossly and microscopically identical to leiomyosarcoma, except that the malignant variant is usually larger and metastasizes. All malignancies of the stomach tend to present in the same way, with bleeding, dyspepsia, weight loss, perforation, obstruction or by signs of metastases in distant locations.

Giant hypertrophic "gastritis" (Ménétrier's disease) may simulate a tumor in its presentation. This condition is one in which large folds of gastric mucosa develop, secreting excess mucus. The upper gastrointestinal series may look similar to a diffuse lymphosarcoma of the stomach, but the diagnosis can usually be made by gastroscopy and biopsy. The patient may be depleted by loss of water, protein and electrolytes from the hypertrophic mucosa.[44]

Bezoars may cause epigastric discomfort or even obstruction and perforation. Foreign bodies may be ingested accidentally or deliberately by children and may occasionally need to be removed surgically. Psychotic patients will often swallow large masses of objects, which may be removed by gastrotomy. Fruit pulp bezoars causing gastric outlet obstruction may be seen in raw citrus fruit eaters who have undergone a gastrojejunostomy or pyloroplasty.

Duodenal diverticulum is a relatively common condition, but rarely produces complications that require operation.

Duodenal trauma is a common sequela of severe blunt trauma, especially from automobile accidents. The possibility of a retroperitoneal rupture must be considered in all such patients, even when peristalsis remains present. The presence of blood in the stomach or air in the retroperitoneal tissues should lead to strong suspicion of this lesion. The temptation is to assume that the blood was due to facial trauma and was swallowed by the patient and that the little air bubbles present on x-ray really are not extraluminal. However, when the question has seriously been raised, it is best to perform an exploratory laparotomy and inspect the entire retroperitoneal duodenum. Gastric trauma is easier to diagnose, since the stomach is usually injured only by violent force or penetrating injury, in which case exploratory operation is obviously indicated. The injury to the stomach is usually visible, since the stomach is anteriorly located and has no retroperitoneal component like the duodenum.

Preparation for elective surgery of the stomach and duodenum may often be performed on an outpatient basis. It should be remembered, however, that large fungating gastric cancers may be infected with clostridium and other anaerobes. The elderly patient with a chronic obstructing ulcer and a distended stomach should not be expected to "open up," and thereby avoid the need for surgery. This kind of patient should be hospitalized and intubated for the few days required for preoperative preparation. Intubation serves to decompress the stomach, reducing the danger of aspiration and allowing the stomach to regain some of its normal tone. Preparation is also directed at restoration of a normal metabolic state, correcting the hypochloremic, hypokalemic alkalosis which is usually present.

Syndromes following surgery of the stomach and duodenum may be challenging for the outpatient surgeon. Occasionally the problem may be solved by a gastrointestinal series, which may demonstrate partial stomal obstruction or a marginal ulcer. It should be remembered, however, that stomal (marginal) ulcer may be difficult to visualize on a gastrointestinal series and may only be recognized by gastroscopy. Bile reflux gastritis is a recognized complication of gastrectomy, gastroenterostomy or pyloroplasty, and, if significant enough, corrective surgery may be required. The three main syndromes that may follow gastric surgery are marginal ulceration, diarrhea and the dumping syndrome.

Evaluation of postvagotomy marginal ulcerations should include a Hollander test, which is the insulin stimulatory test for vagal function. In the presence of an intact vagal nerve, administration of insulin will stimulate release of gastric acid. The test requires that adequate hypoglycemia be obtained and that the patient be able to form gastric acid, since an *increase* in acid is measured in the test. The Hollander test is the best test for an intact cephalic phase of digestion and can be performed in the Outpatient Department if trained personnel are available to watch for symptoms of hypoglycemia, so that glucose can be given promptly to reverse the symptoms. Hollander's test is performed as follows:[21]

A light diet is given the previous day. The patient is fasted overnight. A nasogastric tube is introduced and its location in a dependent part of the body of the stomach is confirmed by fluoroscopy. Regular insulin (15 units) is administered intravenously after aspiration of the stomach for basal sample and collection of basal blood sugar specimen. The stomach is aspirated every 15 minutes and blood sugar specimens are obtained every 30 minutes for two hours. Specimens are analyzed for total acid (pH less than 7.0). A *positive* test is a well-defined rise in acid secretion. The blood sugar must fall to 50 mg per cent or less in order to constitute an adequate stimulus for the cephalic phase of secretion.

Many patients have an increased frequency of bowel movements after gastric surgery, particularly if the operation has included truncal vagotomy. The diarrhea may vary from mild and transient to prolonged, severe and even disabling. Diarrhea develops in approximately 25 per cent of patients following truncal vagotomy with any form of drainage (i.e., antrectomy, gastroenterostomy or pyloroplasty), but in only about 6 per cent of those who had partial gastrectomy without vagotomy. It should be noted that in most cases the diarrhea is mild and episodic; in only about 4 per cent of patients is the diarrhea severe and troublesome after truncal vagotomy. Severe diarrhea after partial gastrectomy without vagotomy is extremely rare. The incidence of diarrhea following selective vagotomy and drainage is about 12.5 per cent. Again, it is usually mild, but in about 2 per cent it is severe. Following highly selective vagotomy without drainage the incidence of diarrhea is no higher than that in the general population.

The dumping syndrome is an annoying complication of gastric surgery. Its relation to meals permits classification into early and late varieties. The symptomatology of the early postprandial dumping syndrome has two components: (1) vasomotor symptoms — flushing, sweating, palpitation, tachycardia, weakness, fainting; and (2) gastrointestinal symptoms — epigastric fullness, nausea, borborygmi, intestinal cramps, diarrhea.

The clinical features of the *late* postprandial dumping syndrome are similar to, but not identical with, the vasomotor symptoms of the early postprandial dumping syndrome.

A major factor responsible for dumping seems to be the loss of pyloric control of gastric emptying. Its incidence after highly selective vagotomy without drainage, therefore, is essentially the same as in normal controls.

Spleen

Splenectomy is performed for a number of reasons and is virtually the

TABLE 18–6 Postprandial Dumping Syndrome

FEATURES	EARLY	LATE
Incidence	8% – 20%	1% – 6%
Relation to meals	Immediately afterward	1½ to 3 hours after meals
Duration of attack	30–40 minutes	30–40 minutes
Relief by	Lying down	More food, glucose
Aggravated by	More food	Exercise
Precipitating factor	Bulk of food, especially liquids	Carbohydrates
Chief symptoms	Sweating, tachycardia, epigastric fullness; occasionally colic, diarrhea	Tremor, faintness, epigastric emptiness, nausea

only operation performed on the spleen. Few patients are subjected to long-term evaluation by surgeons prior to splenectomy, for elective splenectomy is usually recommended only after evaluation by a hematologist. The surgeon's major responsibility is to assess the risks and determine when the patient is in optimum condition for the operation.

Hypersplenism may be produced by any disease that causes enlargement of the spleen, including lymphosarcoma and storage diseases. If hypersplenism becomes a major continuing problem, splenectomy may be indicated even if the spleen is not enlarged on physical examination. Hypersplenism is recognized by an increased rate of hemolysis of red cells, leukopenia and thrombocytopenia. Patients with idiopathic thrombocytopenic purpura are greatly improved or cured by splenectomy in up to 50 per cent of cases. Splenectomy cures the anemia and symptoms of hereditary spherocytosis, although the underlying abnormality in the red cell membrane is unchanged. Hypersplenism in rheumatoid arthritis (Felty's syndrome) is a well-established indication for operation.

Pain or discomfort is usually not the major indication for splenectomy, but it may be the deciding factor in patients with gigantic splenomegaly, as in lymphoma.

Splenectomy for diagnostic purposes has recently been utilized for the staging of lymphomas and Hodgkin's disease. The efficacy of the procedure in clarifying the stage cannot be questioned seriously, but the safety and ultimate benefit to the patient must still be regarded as under investigation.[10]

Trauma is the indication for most emergency splenectomies. The spleen is easily injured, and even a small laceration of the capsule or tear at the splenic pedicle will usually be treated better by splenectomy than by sutures or pressure in the faint hope that bleeding will stop. Patients who have blood loss from abdominal injuries should have the spleen examined carefully regardless of the nature and location of the injury, since force is so easily transmitted to this delicate organ. One of the most common indications for splenectomy is, sadly, a small iatrogenic laceration in the splenic capsule or short gastric vessels during the performance of hiatus herniorrhaphy or vagotomy.

Other indications for splenectomy or procedures on the spleen include its resection during radical surgery on the stomach, left kidney and adrenal, and colon. It is usually removed in the course of a distal or total pancreatectomy and as a part of the splenorenal shunt for portal hypertension. Splenectomy has also been recommended in some centers prior to renal transplantation.

Diagnostic dilemmas include the left upper quadrant discomfort of patients with rapidly enlarging spleens in malaria and infectious mononucleosis, and the possibility of delayed rupture of the spleen following trauma. While it is true that accidental rupture of the spleen during trivial trauma has been reported in these conditions, the incidence in fact is very low. For this reason, left upper quadrant discomfort in such patients is not an indication for immediate splenectomy. The diagnosis of "delayed post-traumatic rupture" of the spleen may often require considerable judgment. Bleeding may occur from a spleen 10 to 14 days after injury, but in most cases there has been premonitory evidence of injury through a fall in hematocrit and evidence of hemoperitoneum or fractured ribs.

The late sequelae of splenectomy are relatively minor in most cases, but recent work suggests increased susceptibility to infections, especially in children.[13, 18] Failure to clear the aging blood cells can be recognized in the peripheral smear of otherwise normal patients who have undergone splenectomy. Transient elevations in platelet count may produce alarm when the count exceeds one million platelets per ml, and such patients should usually be anticoagulated for a few weeks, initially with heparin, followed by Coumadin.

Pancreas.

Pancreatic disease most commonly presents with pain — epigastric, periumbilical or back pain in most cases. Pancreatitis (acute or chronic), traumatic injury to the pancreas, adenocarcinoma of the pancreas, abscess and pseudocyst are the most common pancreatic problems seen by the surgeon in adults. Other conditions, less commonly seen, are ectopic pancreas, islet cell adenoma and pancreatic exocrine insufficiency following pancreatectomy.

Acute edematous pancreatitis may mimic almost any other disease of the upper abdomen, but classically it presents with midabdominal pain and tenderness, fever, elevation in the serum amylase and ileus. Predisposing causes include alcohol ingestion, gallstones, mumps, penetrating peptic ulcer or a large meal. The disease is also seen with increased frequency in patients with chronic renal disease, in cases of homotransplantation and in patients on high doses of corticosteroids. In these conditions, the diagnosis may be more difficult because the serum amylase may also be elevated by decreased renal clearance. In patients with acute pancreatitis, the initial treatment should begin in the emergency room with insertion of a nasogastric tube and institution of intravenous fluids. The loss of plasma into the abdomen may be exceedingly rapid, and untreated patients may show signs of hypotension or dehydration within only a few hours. The overall rate of mortality from acute edematous pancreatitis is approximately 5 per cent.

Acute hemorrhagic pancreatitis is a more serious manifestation of acute pancreatitis. It may be rapidly fatal, or it may have a protracted course leading to necrosis of portions of the pancreas and delayed recovery or death from retroperitoneal abscess and hemorrhage.[37] The mortality rates reported range from 50 to 100 per cent. The antecedent causes and treatment are the same as for acute edematous pancreatitis. Occasionally, laparotomy may be performed to rule out other causes of the acute abdomen; however, the patients subjected to surgery appear to have an increased rate of mortality.[37]

Chronic relapsing pancreatitis may develop after one or more episodes of acute pancreatitis. These patients have recurrent episodes of abdominal pain similar to acute pancreatitis, but without signs of life-threatening illness. Many of these patients are alcoholics and chronic users of tranquilizing and narcotic drugs. Amylase elevation may occur with episodes of pain. Stippled pancreatic calcification becomes apparent through deposits of calcium soaps on the surface of the pancreas and stones in the pancreatic ducts. It is the responsibility of the outpatient surgeon to recognize this disease and identify the patients, usually with x-rays of the abdomen that are examined carefully for pancreatic calcification. All patients with biliary tract stones and pancreatitis should have their gallbladders removed, because gallstones are a predisposing factor for recurrent pancreatitis. Preoperative work-up should include a GI series and small bowel follow-through with cross-table lateral films to search for pseudocyst. The patients should also have an oral cholecystogram (and possibly an IV cholangiogram) to exclude biliary tract calculi and postinflammatory obstruction of the sphincter of Oddi and ampulla of Vater.

Adenocarcinoma of the pancreas is an increasingly common and highly fatal malignancy. Less than 10 per cent of patients with carcinoma of the head of the pancreas survive for five years. Carcinomas of the ampulla of Vater, which present with jaundice and occult bleeding, have a 35 per cent five year survival rate following pancreatoduodenectomy (Whipple operation). Adenocarcinomas of the head, body and tail of the pancreas have a dismal prognosis in spite of partial or total pancreatectomy. The mortality for the radical operation is high, and metastases may become apparent soon after surgery. Nevertheless, the patient suspected of carcinoma of the pancreas should be admitted for thorough evaluation. Appropriate studies include evaluation of the C-loop of the duodenum (first, second and third portions) on GI series, liver function tests, and CAT (computerized axial tomography) scan of the abdomen. Conflicting opinions regarding radical versus conservative operations for carcinoma of the head of the pancreas have been expressed.[9, 48]

Hormone-producing tumors of the pancreas include islet cell adenomas (insulin or glucagon), Zollinger-Ellison tumors (gastrin) and carcinoids (serotonin). The diagnosis of these neoplasms is usually made because of their peripheral symptoms, which may be present long before surgery. The presence of Whipple's triad (hypoglycemia, symptoms of hypoglycemia when the blood sugar is low and correction of the symptoms by raising the blood sugar) should lead to a search for an islet cell tumor. The study should include selective arteriography, which has been increasingly useful in identifying these tumors. In the presence of recurring episodes of hypoglycemia with syncope or psychosis, exploration of the pancreas may be indicated, even in the absence of a positive tumor blush on arteriography.

Zollinger-Ellison tumor should be suspected in every patient with a virulent peptic ulcer diathesis or recurrent peptic ulcers with high gastric acid production. It is the responsibility of the outpatient surgeon to think of the problem and request a fasting serum gastrin assay when seeing a patient

with a severe or recurrent peptic ulcer. Glucagon-secreting adenomas are unusual but should be suspected in patients with diabetes mellitus that is unresponsive to therapy. Carcinoid tumors of the pancreas may present all of the manifestations of other carcinoids. All of the functioning pancreatic adenomas may be relatively slow growing, and repeated resection of metastases may be indicated to control symptoms on a palliative basis.

The postoperative management of the partially pancreatectomized patient presents relatively little difficulty in insulin regulation, but some patients become diabetic. Those who do so can be managed as mild diabetics, with regular or NPH insulin or both, administered after observation of urine sugars. They are usually well regulated by the time they leave the hospital, but should be rechecked at clinic visits. If total pancreatectomy has been done, the resultant diabetes is more brittle. The exocrine management of the patient with a total pancreatectomy is sometimes a greater problem and requires considerable patience. Several preparations of pancreatic extract are available. The control of steatorrhea is an easily recognizable guide to dosage.

Esophagus

The terminal intra-abdominal portion of the esophagus is of concern in the differential diagnosis of abdominal complaints, for it may be the seat of a variety of conditions presenting as pain, dysphagia, bleeding or shock. These and other aspects of esophageal problems are also discussed in Chapter 16.

The most common problems of the distal esophagus are caused by reflux esophagitis. Regurgitation of acid may cause ulceration and fibrosis. The initial symptoms may be substernal discomfort and "water brash" regurgitation, although the patient may present with weakness from anemia and occult GI bleeding may be found. Later, persistent "burning" discomfort may be noted, followed by dysphagia. Occasionally a startling presentation occurs when a patient has swallowed a large piece of meat that fails to pass the cardioesophageal junction. The diagnosis should then be confirmed by a Hypaque swallow. The obstruction may be relieved with the ingestion of a teaspoon of papain paste (prepared from proteinase from Carica papaya) or a household meat tenderizer mixed in water, taken every four to six hours. Proteolytic treatment should only be used if the obstructing bolus is known to be meat alone, without bone. Impacted meat containing bone fragments should be removed carefully through the esophagoscope. Esophagoscopy should later be performed in all cases to rule out carcinoma. Medical therapy for reflux esophagitis may preclude surgery if it is instituted before irreversible stricture has occurred. The treatment consists of elevation of the head of the bed on six-inch blocks of wood, a bland diet and antacids. Esophageal dilatation may restore a narrow esophagus to a satisfactory lumen and may be attempted before scheduling a surgical procedure. Bougies are also useful in postoperative treatment, if a too-snug hiatus herniorrhaphy has been performed. The Hurst (mercury-filled) bougies are generally the safest and most useful for outpatient treatment.

Other problems of the lower esophagus which may present with symptoms similar to hiatus hernia include the following, which can usually be distinguished on a barium swallow: achalasia (failure of the cardioesophageal junction to open properly during swallowing); carcinoma; scleroderma (a leathery, ineffective esophagus, associated with other aspects of this collagen disease); and chronic stricture from lye ingestion. The indications for surgery and the results of operations in these conditions have been reviewed in Chapter 16.

Bleeding from the esophagus may range from massive to minimal, even when due to esophageal varices. All patients suspected of bleeding from esophageal varices should be admitted to the hospital for diagnosis and therapy. If the patient is exsanguinating in the E.R., an attempt should be made to arrest bleeding with a Sengstaken-Blakemore tube.

Rupture of the esophagus may be either insidious or obvious. The most common cause is endoscopic instrumentation or dilation, and for this reason it should be a particular concern of the outpatient surgeon. In these cases it is frequently a localized perforation that initially causes only discomfort and a low grade fever. The diagnosis should be confirmed by contrast radiography with a water-soluble contrast medium, for example, gastrografin. Free perforation is usually a devastating event and should lead to immediate hospitalization. Esophageal perforation may be caused by strenuous vomiting, blunt or penetrating trauma to the chest or upper abdomen or carcinoma (which may be either adenocarcinoma of the stomach or squamous carcinoma of the distal esophagus). Free perforation into the chest or mediastinum requires immediate drainage.

Small Intestine

Diseases of the small intestine are frequently difficult to recognize. Some conditions require immediate surgery in cases in which obstruction, volvulus, perforation or peritonitis is apparent. Mesenteric vascular disease is apt to be insidious in many cases, except in the classic situation of rheumatic heart disease, arterial fibrillation, sudden onset of abdominal pain and melena — the result of an embolus to the superior mesenteric artery.

Small bowel obstruction can usually be suspected in cases of abdominal distention, hyperperistalsis, crampy abdominal pain and failure to pass flatus and feces. The work-up and therapy of intestinal obstruction is discussed earlier in the chapter.

Bleeding from the small bowel may be a troublesome diagnostic problem, especially if it is slow and intermittent. If immediate placement of a nasogastric tube rules out gastric bleeding, a selective angiogram may be helpful. All too frequently, however, gastrointestinal bleeding from the small bowel ceases prior to angiography, and the bleeding site may then be difficult or impossible to locate, even at laparotomy. In the work-up of patients with chronic anemia of unknown etiology, with or without demonstration of occult blood in the stools, small bowel bleeding should be considered. Causes may include benign or malignant tumors (especially adenocarcinoma) or vascular malformations such as hemangioma and arteriovenous malformation. In these cases, fluorescein may localize the bleeding site. The patient should be given a soft string to swallow, tied to a small washer, which is allowed to advance through the bowel until the washer is in the colon. When bleeding occurs again, 5 ml of fluorescein solution is injected intravenously. The string is then withdrawn and examined under ultraviolet light (the Woods' lamp of the dermatologist) for fluorescence. If rapid GI bleeding is occurring from an unknown source, hospitalization is obviously indicated, and a selective mesenteric arteriogram should be performed as soon as possible.

The most common chronic disease of the small bowel is regional enteritis. In general, regional enteritis (Crohn's disease) is a disease of slow onset and progression, in which granulomatous changes begin in the musculature, serosa and mesentery of the ileum. As the disease progresses, the mucosa becomes involved, with ulcerations and strictures (Fig. 18–15). Crohn's disease may involve any part of the gastrointestinal tract. The disease may first present as an inflammatory lesion of the colon (granulomatous colitis). "Skip" areas are common, so conservative surgery is indicated when operations must be performed. Approximately one -third of patients who are operated upon will require no further treatment; approximately one-third will continue to have intermittent symptoms; and one-third will eventually develop another complication that requires surgery. The diagnosis is made by barium follow-through examination of the small bowel in patients who have crampy episodes of pain, low grade fever, weight loss and intermittent diarrhea. If surgery is utilized for Crohn's disease it should be reserved for complications resistant to medical management, including obstruction, perforation, bleeding and intractable pain associated with a palpable mass.

Other chronic diseases of the small bowel may be diagnosed by laparotomy; these include Whipple's disease, sprue and lymphosarcoma. The increased effectiveness and safety of transoral small bowel biopsy with a tube has rendered many of these operations unnecessary. Enzyme determinations have clarified the nature of many illnesses, especially chronic milk "allergy" in adults, associated with mucosal lactase deficiency.

Pneumatosis cystoides intestinalis is a condition in which air is present in the wall of the bowel, most commonly the jejunum. In adults it is frequently asymptomatic and is discovered incidentally during abdominal radiography performed for a variety of reasons. It may be associated with peptic ulcer, carcinoma of the stomach and rupture of pulmonary blebs. In children, however, it is usually caused by severe enterocolitis, which requires emergency surgery.[47]

Congenital abnormalities of the small intestine are not commonly encountered in adults. Ectopic gastric mucosa in a Meckel's diverticulum may cause bleeding or perforation. The diagnosis can occasionally be made by technetium pertechnetate scanning.[23] Malrotation may present for the first time in adults, although the diagnosis can usually be suspected by the presence of other anomalies.

Recent developments in pharmacol-

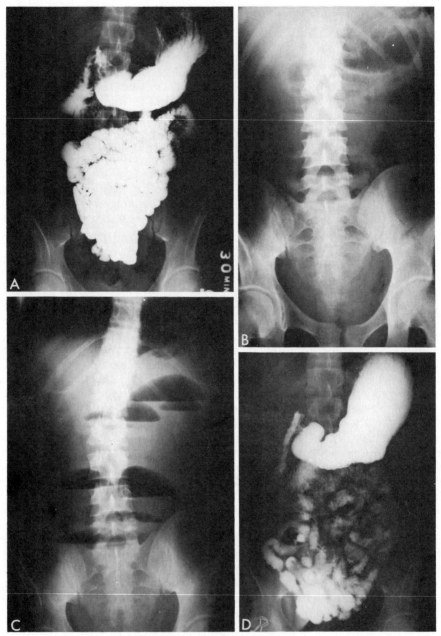

Figure 18–15 Regional ileitis. Twenty-one year old man with recurrent abdominal pain, diarrhea, and gastrointestinal x-rays characteristic of extensive regional ileitis. The typical features seen are *(A)* entrapment of the small bowel in a mass of inflammatory tissue with shortened mesentery and abnormal mucosal pattern. Small bowel transit is rapid, but entry into colon is greatly delayed. In the next five months he had several episodes of partial small bowel obstruction and finally appeared with distention and vomiting. Flat film showed only enlarged gas-filled loops of intestine *(B),* but upright film showed the air fluid "stepladder" that is characteristic of complete small bowel obstruction *(C).* He underwent lysis of adhesions, resection of the distal ileum and construction of an end ileostomy. He has subsequently gained weight and had only mild symptoms, which have not required hospitalization. Vitamin B-12 absorption is normal, indicating adequate function of residual ileum. Small bowel x-ray nine months postoperatively *(D)* shows increased mobility in small bowel, improved mucosal pattern and normal transit time.

ogy have produced new chronic and acute diseases that must be remembered in patients with abdominal pain. These include ulceration and obstruction from enteric-coated tablets containing potassium salts and mesenteric vasculitis from oral contraceptives. Corticosteroid therapy has been associated with idiopathic mesenteric vasculitis (arterial and venous), causing acute or chronic gastrointestinal bleeding or small bowel infarction. The majority of these patients can be identified by other signs of collagen-vascular or autoimmune disease, but occasionally idiopathic thrombophlebitis of the mesenteric vessels is the first serious indication of the presence of such diseases.

During the past decade, many small bowel bypass operations have been performed to treat morbid, exogenous obesity and hypercholesterolemia. In patients with congenital hypercholesterolemia, an average 40 per cent decrease in serum cholesterol is produced.[5] Jejunoileostomy has produced remarkable reduction in weight in patients with intractable obesity.[43] Complications of this procedure, however, may include electrolyte depletion, gallstones, urinary calculi and severe liver dysfunction, including cirrhosis.[49] Patients proposed for operations to control obesity should be evaluated independently by a surgeon, an internist and a psychiatrist, and close long-term postoperative follow-up is mandatory.

Mesentery

The mesentery is rarely identified preoperatively as the primary location of disease. Some mesenteric diseases, however, should be considered as possible causes of obscure abdominal pain, fever, gastrointestinal bleeding and abdominal masses. The mesenteric diseases most commonly encountered are lesions of the vessels and lymph nodes.

In each case, surgery is ordinarily required to confirm the diagnosis or to initiate definitive therapy.

Mesenteric arterial vascular obstruction may be acute (embolus, or thrombosis due to low arterial flow). Gangrene and death will ensue unless immediate surgery is performed and repair is possible. Chronic intestinal ischemia due to arteriosclerosis may cause the rare syndrome of intestinal angina (pain and nausea after meals). This diagnosis should be confirmed by selective arteriography and the disease may be alleviated by arterial reconstruction. Mesenteric venous obstruction may be insidious, and it usually progresses to infarction before it is recognized. In patients with a history of idiopathic thrombophlebitis and hypercoagulability, the illness may be aborted by medical therapy. Treatment should be initiated in the hospital, controlled with studies of coagulation parameters. It is the responsibility of the outpatient surgeon to suspect this condition. Segmental mesenteric infarction has been reported in females taking oral contraceptives.[40]

Mesenteric lymph nodes may be involved with a wide variety of infections and neoplasms and are occasionally the key to the diagnosis of an obscure illness. In fever of unknown origin, for example, laparotomy should be considered when all else has failed to provide a diagnosis.[2, 11, 39] Biopsy in such cases may reveal lymphosarcoma, tuberculosis or occult carcinoma. Arrangements should be made preoperatively to obtain cultures of the nodes for bacteria, fungi, acid-fast organisms and viruses, if a virus laboratory is available. Frozen section should also be obtained so that additional tissue can be removed if the pathologist suggests it.

Mesenteric adenitis is relatively uncommon in adults, and when laparotomy for appendicitis in adults reveals only this condition, a thorough exploration should be performed in addition to diagnostic biopsy of the nodes.

Appendix

This structure has been a source of great misery for humans, and its elective removal is frequently performed in the course of uncomplicated laparotomy for a wide variety of conditions. The major disease of the appendix which provokes concern is acute appendicitis, but pinworm infestation, malignant carcinoid tumors, adenocarcinoma and mucocele with pseudomyxoma peritonei are also problems that can originate or persist in the appendix. A fecalith in the appendix is a sign of potential trouble (Fig. 18–13) and some surgeons regard it as an indication for appendectomy, particularly in the younger age group.

Acute appendicitis should be suspected in every instance of right lower quadrant abdominal pain. Severe right lower abdominal pain, however, may also be due to bowel infarction, ruptured ovarian cyst, ectopic pregnancy and so on. The typical symptoms of appendicitis usually appear over a period of somewhat less than 24 hours, involving a sequence of midabdominal pain shifting to the right lower abdomen, nausea or anorexia, constipation (or occasionally diarrhea), low grade fever and mild leukocytosis. Such a patient usually can be admitted for a few hours' observation before a decision is made to operate. The delay is sometimes an important means of differentiating nonsurgical diseases from appendicitis, including simple constipation, "mittelschmerz" (pain from rupture of the ovarian follicle) and gastroenteritis. If appendicitis is strongly suspected, appendectomy should be advised.

Carcinoid tumors of the appendix are usually found incidentally at laparotomy. These are the most common and also the most curable type of carcinoids. Simple appendectomy is ordinarily sufficient, unless the lesion is larger than 2 cm, in which case right colon resection is indicated.[29] Pseudomyxoma peritonei is usually caused by rela-

tively slow-growing tumors of the appendix or ovary. The primary tumor should be removed if it is still in place when the patient presents with pseudomyxoma.[6] An unruptured mucocele of the appendix is unlikely to be diagnosed preoperatively, and should be removed with caution if encountered unexpectedly. Adenocarcinoma of the base of the appendix should be treated as a carcinoma of the cecum. A difficult preoperative diagnosis may be posed by the turned-in appendiceal stump, which may have the smooth, convex surface of a small benign tumor of the cecum.

Colon

The major concern of the surgeon with respect to the colon is cancer. Surgeons are called upon to evaluate and treat many emergencies of the colon, such as bleeding, obstruction, perforation, volvulus and impaction. Regardless of the certainty of diagnosis of a nonmalignant condition, the wise surgeon always keeps in mind the possibility that a cancer is also present. This thinking is based on the knowledge that, next to skin cancer, carcinoma of the colon and rectum is the most common cancer of humans, and only half of its victims are salvaged even with aggressive surgery, radiation therapy and chemotherapy. Rectal examinations should be performed as part of all complete physical examinations and should be a part of all abdominal examinations. A stool specimen should be obtained and examined personally by the surgeon for occult blood during every rectal examination. A sigmoidoscopy, followed by barium enema, should be performed for rather liberal indications, knowing the high incidence of colorectal cancer in our population.

Carcinoma of the colon occurs most commonly in the rectum and distal sigmoid colon. Constipation is a common symptom of carcinoma of the sigmoid. This tumor may leave streaks of blood and mucus on the bowel movements.

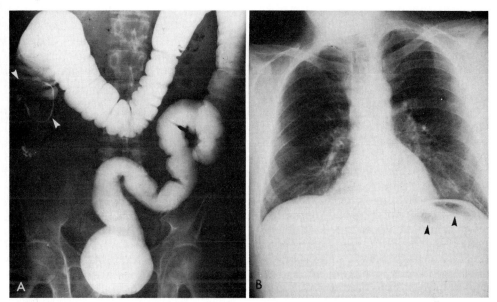

Figure 18–16 Carcinoma of the cecum with perforation and death. Fifty-one year old male psychiatric outpatient with mild bloating and indigestion for several months. GI series normal. Barium enema *(A)* was read as "normal." Patient developed acute collapse 25 days later and was admitted to Emergency Room. Chest x-ray *(B)*, taken during resuscitation, was read as "normal." Patient subsequently complained of abdominal pain and review of x-rays showed cecal lesion (arrows, *A*) and double left subdiaphragmatic air shadow (arrows, *B*) characteristic of gastric bubble and free air. At laparotomy, gangrenous perforated carcinoma of cecum and generalized peritonitis were found. Patient died of septicemia postoperatively.

Carcinoma of the cecum may be relatively silent for a long time (Fig. 18–16). It may grow to a large size before perforating or causing obstruction, and it will frequently produce severe anemia from occult bleeding without obvious change in the color, consistency or frequency of bowel movements. Carcinoma should be strongly suspected in flat or napkin-ring lesions of the colon. It is present, unsuspected preoperatively, in 3 per cent of resections for diverticulitis.[4] Carcinoma is a significant risk in patients with ulcerative colitis for more than ten years. The early diagnosis of colonic carcinoma is important, for curability decreases as the disease spreads through the layers of the colon. With lesions confined to the mucosa, 85 per cent of patients may be cured. However, only 50 per cent are cured when all layers of the colon are invaded, and only 15 per cent when lymph nodes or adjacent organs are involved. The carcinoembryonic antigen (CEA) described in association with colon cancer may provide a useful serological test for early cancer. It is being utilized on an experimental basis to follow the progress of the disease.

Colonic polyps are a troublesome problem, since sessile polyps may be malignant and even pedunculated adenomatous polyps are not free of this possibility. In general, polypectomy can be recommended for polyps over 1 cm in size; most pedunculated polyps can be removed via a colonoscope. A definite demonstration of the polyp on two successive barium enemas or visualization with the colonoscope is mandatory, however, since a ball of feces may mimic a polyp.

Villous adenomas are sessile polypoid tumors that occur most frequently in the distal sigmoid and rectum. Although frequently benign on surface biopsy, they must be excised completely for diagnostic evaluation. Areas of malignancy are frequently found when they are examined completely under the microscope. If malignant, they should be treated as an adenocarcinoma in that particular location. Villous adenomas frequently present with massive loss of fluid, mucus, protein and potassium.

Multiple familial polyposis is a premalignant disease. Patients with a family history of this condition should be scheduled for colectomy in their twenties or as soon thereafter as possible. Patients with polyposis or ulcerative colitis who have ileorectal anastomoses must have the entire residual rectum visualized through a sigmoidoscope at intervals of three to six months. Resection of the rectum is ideal for protection from cancer, but many patients will not consent to it.

Ulcerative colitis is a disease that requires considerable judgment in management. Although the dangers of complications are readily apparent (for example, carcinoma, toxic megacolon), the patients are not usually willing to accept total proctocolectomy when the disease is first diagnosed. The surgeon may help in providing consultation, sigmoidoscopy (and cautious rectal biopsy to establish the diagnosis) and management of the perianal problems which may arise. A recommendation of surgery should be made when the surgeon firmly believes that it is advisable (rather than too early, or after the patient is moribund). Elective total proctocolectomy with ileostomy is recommended for patients with a history of ulcerative colitis for ten or more years, because carcinoma becomes a significant risk after this length of time. Toxic megacolon occurs in less than 4 per cent of patients with ulcerative colitis, but it can unfortunately be masked by steroid therapy until perforation and peritonitis have developed. Emergency surgical therapy is generally indicated for its treatment.

Patients with stomas may be referred to the local community's "Ostomy As-

sociation," which will provide routine postoperative counseling. Ileostomy dysfunction (cramps and diarrhea) commonly results from stricture at the level of fascia or skin. It is an indication for hospitalization if digital examination confirms the existence of a stricture. Herniation of the small intestine may occur adjacent to the terminal ileum and is a cause of "ileostomy dysfunction" or acute bowel obstruction in some patients.

Granulomatous colitis (Crohn's disease) is an inflammatory disease of the muscularis and mesentery of the colon, with secondary erosion of the mucosa. This condition is contrasted to ulcerative colitis in which ulceration begins in the mucosa, forming pseudopolyps and penetrating outward into the muscularis. In about 10 per cent of cases it may be difficult to distinguish granulomatous from ulcerative colitis.

Volvulus of the colon is an uncommon but dramatic problem which occurs most commonly in psychotic or elderly patients. The x-ray findings and therapy are discussed earlier in the chapter. Nonoperative reduction may be sufficient therapy unless a second episode occurs. Even in properly selected patients, the emergency resection for sigmoid volvulus has a high rate of mortality. Severe coexisting disease has been reported in 90 per cent of these patients.

Trauma to the colon is a major surgical problem, and if strongly suspected it is sufficient indication for laparotomy. Rupture of the sigmoid colon may occur during sigmoidoscopy. The relative benignancy of the condition in the first few minutes or hours should not lull the surgeon into complacency. The safest procedure is a proximal colostomy and closure of the defect, or exteriorization of the lacerated segment of the colon. Free intraperitoneal air may occasionally be discovered in a patient who feels well. The condition may be caused by escape of air from the wall of the intestinal tract in patients with pneumatosis intestinalis.

Diverticulosis is a common cause of colonic bleeding. In some cases, a small artery at the base of diverticulum may produce significant hemorrhage. Diverticulosis, especially in elderly patients, may also be complicated by diverticulitis or obstruction. The disease may present for the first time with one of these major complications. If the patient has had more than one episode of definite diverticulitis, and is a reasonably good operative risk, elective resection of the involved area is recommended.[26]

Preparation for colon surgery is best done in the hospital, where both a mechanical preparation and antibiotic reduction in fecal bacteria can best be accomplished. The advantages and disadvantages of the various types of bowel preparations are beyond the scope of this chapter and the reader is referred elsewhere.[7, 30] It is recommended that a final plain x-ray of the abdomen be obtained prior to surgery if preparation is done as an outpatient, to exclude signs of residual feces.

Colostomy care is a subject for outpatient consideration, for few patients are perfectly adjusted to a colostomy by the time they leave the hospital after surgery. A left-sided colostomy can usually be managed eventually with only a cloth compress covering the matured stoma. Careful guidance and encouragement of the patient is necessary to achieve this goal. Whether or not to irrigate is a question of preference for the patient. Avoidance of the irrigations will eliminate the serious hazard of colonic perforation by the irrigating catheter. However, it is easier to obtain regularity of colostomy function with irrigation. A colostomy of the transverse or right colon may be a chore to manage because of the fluid nature of the feces and the need to wear an appliance at all times.

The ideal size of a matured colostomy stoma is determined by the adequacy of its function. The surgeon should not be dismayed if the stoma admits only his little finger, if it has functioned well for a long time. On the other hand, most well-functioning colostomies in adult patients will accept two joints of the index finger if a little patience is used in performing the examination. The postoperative evaluation of a colostomy patient should include digital examination of his colostomy. Colostomy stricture may occur at the skin or fascia level. A skin stricture may be resected under local anesthesia in the clinic; however, bleeding may be unexpectedly brisk, and assistance should be available. A stricture at the fascial level requires hospitalization and general or spinal anesthesia with relaxation for repair.

POSTOPERATIVE WOUND CARE AND COMPLICATIONS

Routine

The majority of abdominal incisions heal primarily without difficulty. Skin sutures are placed in wounds to provide strength until the natural healing processes will keep the wound together during normal activity. In the case of abdominal wounds this generally requires approximately one week, at which time the skin sutures are removed. It should be emphasized, however, that the skin incision has not reached its maximum tensile strength at this time but can be separated if excess tension is applied perpendicularly to the axis of the wound. The wound can be disrupted in this manner for two weeks or more after the initial wounding. A clean, uninfected wound that separates because of undue trauma in the postoperative period should not be a cause of undue concern. The wound should be inspected to be certain that is does not communicate with a dehiscence of the musculofascial layers or with an abscess. A culture of the healing surfaces should be taken. If the surfaces are clean, contain no obviously infected material and there is no musculofascial defect, the wound can be closed by applying tapes perpendicularly across the wound, holding the skin edges in a redundant position. It is not necessary to resuture the epidermis. These wounds will heal at a faster than normal rate, and the tapes may generally be removed after one to two weeks.

Because of a high incidence of wound infection, many surgeons do not close traumatic wounds or heavily contaminated wounds during the initial operative procedure. This is especially true with wounds received during military conflicts. The wounds are kept open using packing and are closed secondarily several days later if no infection occurs and the patient is doing well and is afebrile. Usually these wounds are closed before the patient leaves the hospital. Decision for closure can be made when granulation tissue begins to develop on the fat edges and there is no excessive drainage from the wound. The skin is apposed using strips of tape placed transversely across the wound. Alternatively, skin sutures may be placed by the operating surgeon at the initial procedure and left untied. If this is the case, these sutures can be tied at the appropriate time. Generally, the sutures should be removed during the seventh to tenth postoperative days.

Wound Infection

Wound infection may become apparent any time from immediately following surgery to long afterwards. Most commonly, however, wound infection becomes apparent between the fourth and tenth postoperative days. Usually it is preceded by increased wound pain, temperature, wound swelling and/or systemic manifestations of sepsis. As the liquefied area nears the surface, there is a gradually appreciated area of "fluctuance," which is a soft, liquid-filled cavity palpable under the incision. In patients who are on antibiotic prophylaxis, the symptoms of wound infection may be less apparent and may

occur later in the postoperative course than previously recognized in the preantibiotic era.

When a wound infection becomes apparent, it should be drained as soon as possible. In the case of minor wound infections this can be done in the office or in the emergency room. The skin overlying the fluctuant area is suitably anesthetized and a small incision is made. The pus is expressed and a culture and sensitivity test is taken. The wound can then be irrigated with either hydrogen peroxide or saline. It is packed with either plain gauze or gauze impregnated with iodoform. This keeps the skin edges from reclosing and ensures free drainage. Depending on the size of the wound infection and the amount of drainage, the dressings need to be changed frequently for several days and less frequently thereafter. In the case of a minor wound infection, the defect will gradually granulate in until it is completely closed.

Occasionally, a wound infection is of such major extent that the wound must be opened in its entirety from end to end. In these patients the wound must be packed open with a gauze pack. This may require rehospitalization and, rarely, general anesthesia. In most cases, the defect will heal over the course of several weeks by secondary intention.

Sometimes a wound infection is only the first sign of an anastomotic leak from the alimentary tract. This usually becomes clear following incision and drainage, when the character of the drainage changes from purulent to biliary, gastric, pancreatic, or feculent appearing material. It is somewhat more unusual for a fistula to be found in patients discharged after a routine postoperative course, since patients developing major fistulae are usually quite sick in the immediate postoperative period and are still in the hospital when the fistula becomes apparent. Usually fistulae from the GI tract will spontaneously close, depending on the site of fistulization, the presence or absence of distal obstruction, the proximity of the origin of the fistula to the skin and the presence of active disease at the site of origin of the fistula. The passing of gas via a wound infection is usually an indication that a fistula is present. The treatment of fistulae from the gastrointestinal tract is outside the scope of this chapter and can range from local therapy with spontaneous closure to intravenous hyperalimentation followed by extensive secondary operative procedures.

Wound Dehiscence and Evisceration

Wound dehiscence implies separation of all or part of the musculofascial abdominal wound closure. The majority of cases can be ascribed to two etiologies. The most common is wound infection. Because of necrotizing infection, there is a loss of tensile strength in the musculofascial layers with subsequent separation of the layers and extrusion of whatever suture material is in place. The second most common cause is a technical error in the closure of the wound. This is due to improper placement of the sutures or tying the sutures too loose or too tight. Other predisposing factors include increased intra-abdominal tension (for example, associated with pregnancy, constipation, chronic cough, urinary obstruction) and malnutrition.

Treatment depends on the size of the dehiscence and whether or not there has been extrusion of the intra-abdominal contents (evisceration). When evisceration is present the wound should be covered with a sterile dressing and the patient should be immediately admitted to the hospital for secondary closure of the abdominal wall. Even when there is a small dehiscence without evisceration, the patient should be hospitalized. If the dehiscence follows infection, any bowel or omentum present underneath the incision is usually adherent to the parietal peritoneum and prevents evisceration. These wounds can be packed with sterile packing and managed in a way similar to an uncomplicated wound infection. Any loose wires or sharp material in the wound must be removed to prevent perforation of intra-abdominal contents. Care must be used in applying packing to prevent injury to the underlying viscera.

After spontaneous closure of a dehiscence, a ventral hernia will be present. This can be demonstrated in the patient by simple examination of the abdominal wall. Frequently there is obvious protrusion of the intra-abdominal contents in a hernia sac palpable directly under the skin layer. With time, the size of the hernia gradually increases. These hernias can usually be easily reduced — that is, the intra-abdominal contents can be pushed back into the abdomen by simple pressure. When a ventral hernia occurs, plans should be made for elective repair when the patient fully recovers from the primary operative procedure and there is no remaining infection.

Suture Sinus

Following wound infection or dehiscence patients may continue to drain small amounts of purulent material from the wound for prolonged periods. The drainage often originates in infected suture material, which serves as a foreign body nidus for continuing infection. This is particularly prolonged when braided nonabsorbable suture material is used and the infection becomes firmly established within the interstices of the suture material. A suture sinus can be an extremely annoying postoperative problem for the patient and the surgeon. It frequently will drain indefinitely until the infected suture material is removed. The incidence of this complication has decreased significantly in recent years because of the increased popularity of single layer closure of abdominal wounds, using monofilament stainless steel wire that will not serve as a nidus for infection.

Suture material may be extracted from wounds long after they are closed without reoperation. The simplest method of doing this is using ordinary metal crochet hooks which have been autoclaved. These are introduced through the suture sinus (Fig. 18–17A) until they are looped around the suture. The suture is then pulled up onto the abdominal wall through the skin. At this point it is grasped with a clamp (Fig. 18–17B) and then cut and removed (Fig. 18–17C). Anesthesia is usually not needed, but the procedure is somewhat uncomfortable for the patient. Following removal of the infected suture the wound will generally close spontaneously.

A more recent development for removing buried infected sutures is the Glatzer hook (Fig. 18–18A).[36] This instrument has a blunt hook on the end, similar to a crochet hook. The suture is hooked first (Fig. 18–18B) and immobilized (Fig. 18–18C). By next turning the knob on the top of the instrument, the suture is cut in its position without having to pull it to the skin surface (Fig. 18–18D). The apparatus with the suture attached is then removed with less pain for the patient.

SHORT HOSPITAL STAY ABDOMINAL PROCEDURES

Inguinal Hernia Repair

The most common major elective surgical procedure performed in the

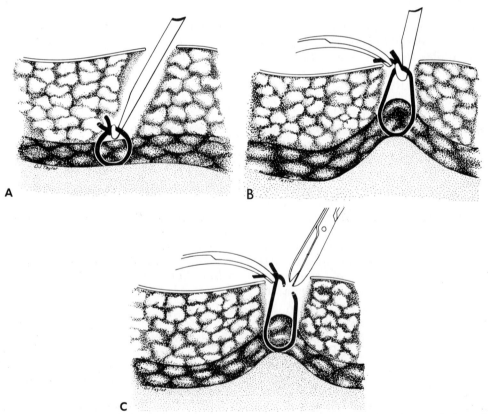

Figure 18–17 Retrieval of buried suture from suture sinus via crochet hook technique. *A* Buried suture hooked with crochet hook. *B* Suture pulled to skin level and clamped. *C*. Suture cut and removed.

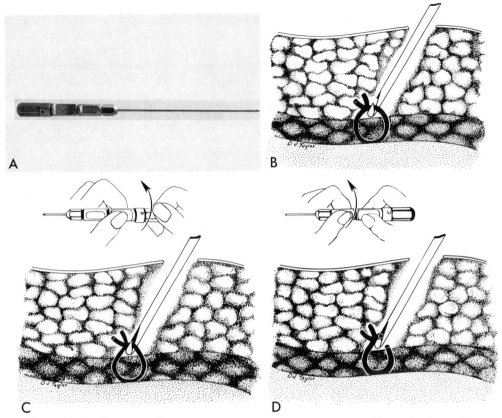

Figure 18–18 Retrieval of buried suture from suture sinus using a Glatzer hook. *A.* Glatzer Hook. *B.* Buried suture hooked with the Glatzer instrument. *C.* Suture immobilized on hook. *D.* Suture cut in place and removed.

United States today is inguinal hernia repair. Most surgeons admit their patients for inguinal herniorrhaphy one day prior to surgery for performance of preoperative testing, perform the operation under anesthesia and discharge their patients five to eight days following surgery. This results in an inordinate use of hospital beds for the routine repair of uncomplicated inguinal hernias. For many years, the repair of infant hernias has been done on a semi-outpatient basis. Until recently the need for longer in-hospital therapy for adult inguinal hernias had not been questioned.

There have been reports recently from several groups emphasizing that adult inguinal hernias can be repaired and the patients discharged after a short hospital stay.[3, 14, 15] Inguinal herniorrhaphy by an anterior transversalis fascia repair using local anesthesia is advocated by these groups. The largest number of patients operated upon with this technique are reported from the Shouldice Hospital in Toronto, Canada. It would appear to us that standard Poupart's or Cooper's ligament repairs could also be done under local anesthesia utilizing short hospital stay.

OPERATIVE PROCEDURE (Fig. 18–19). The patient is given suitable preoperative sedation. Local infiltration anesthesia is induced by infiltrating along the incision line. An anterior groin incision is made parallel to the inguinal ligament. The cord is explored and a high ligation and excision of an indirect hernial sac (if present) is performed, as with all groin hernia repairs. Additional local anesthetic agent is injected underneath the transversalis fascia layer. The first step in the repair of the inguinal floor consists of division of the transversalis fascia parallel to the inguinal ligament from the pubic tubercle to the internal ring (Figs. 18–19*A* and *B*). This should be continued deeper until the yellow preperitoneal fat pouts out. The preperitoneal fat is then pushed cephalad and medially, exposing the combined fibers of the transversalis fascia and the transversus abdominis underneath the medial flap. This is visible as a white line. If there is a large direct hernial sac it generally is inverted when dissecting away the preperitoneal fat. A continuous suture is used to appose this combined transversalis fascia to the previously divided

lateral lip of transversalis fascia (Fig. 18–19*C*). The suture is begun at the pubic tubercle medially and continues laterally to recreate a snug internal inguinal ring. Laterally, these sutures must be placed with care in order to avoid entering the femoral or epigastric vessels. If present, the excess medial leaf of transversalis fascia containing the direct hernia sac is excised. The previously placed suture is then doubled back on itself medially, this time suturing the free leaf of transversalis fascia medially to the shelving edge of the inguinal ligament laterally (Fig. 18–19*D*). The suture is tied to itself at the most medial portion of the

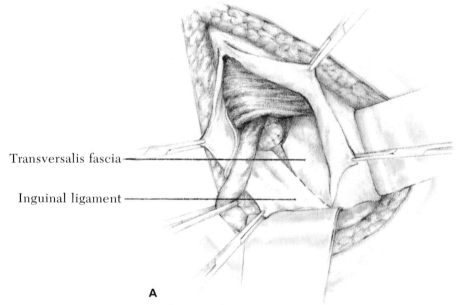

Transversalis fascia

Inguinal ligament

A

Figure 18–19 Anterior transversalis inguinal hernia repair. A. Anterior aspect of posterior wall of right inguinal canal, showing site and direction of division of transversalis fascia commencing laterally at internal ring. B. Anterior aspect of posterior wall of right inguinal canal, showing division of transversalis fascia completed from internal ring to pubic bone, with medial flap mobilized. C. Anterior aspect of posterior wall of right inguinal canal, showing first suture line approaching internal ring after commencing at pubic bone. D. Anterior aspect of posterior wall of right inguinal canal, showing second suture line returning to pubic bone after reversing at the internal ring, overlapping medial flap anterior to lateral flap. E. Schematic representation of anterior transversalis inguinal hernia repair.[3]

    Step (1) The lateral cut edge of the transversalis fascia (a$_1$) is sutured to the undersurface of the medial edge (a$_2$) and to the transversus abdominis muscle (b).

    Step (2) The medial cut edge of the transversalis fascia (a$_2$) is sutured to the lateral margin of the transversalis ("iliopubic tract") and to the shelf of the inguinal ligament (e).

    Step (3) Internal oblique (c) and conjoined muscle are sutured to the undersurface of the external oblique (d).

    Step (4) The cord is replaced under the external oblique.

    (Reprinted with permission from Glassow, F.: The Shoudice Repair of Inguinal Hernia. *In* R. L. Varco and J. P. Delaney (Eds.): Controversy in Surgery. Philadelphia, W. B. Saunders Co., 1976.)

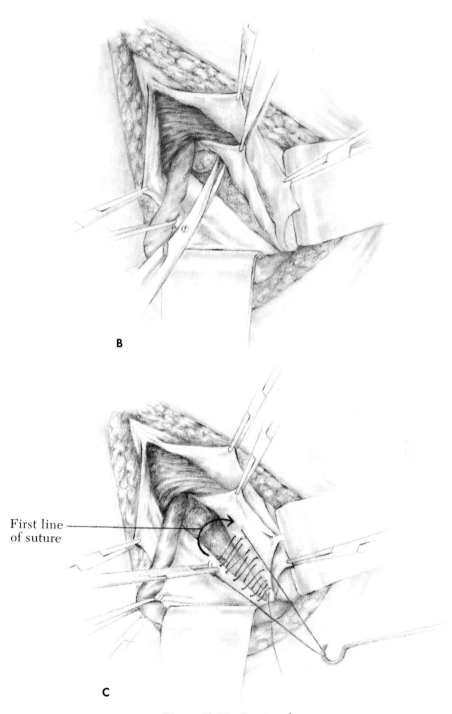

B

First line of suture

C

Figure 18–19 *Continued.*

Illustration continued on the following page

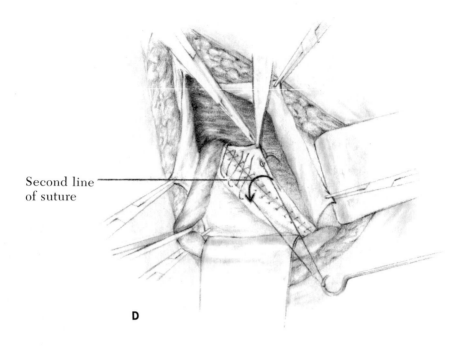

Second line
of suture

D

PRE-OPERATIVE

**excess direct sac
to be excised**

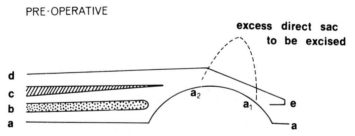

d

c

b

a

a_2

a_1

e

a

POST-OPERATIVE

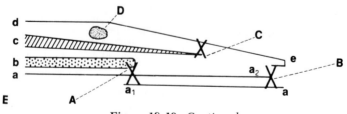

d

c

b

a

D

C

B

A

a_1

a_2

e

a

E

Figure 18–19 *Continued.*

wound. A third layer of continuous monofilament suture is then used to approximate the internal oblique muscle and conjoined tendon to the inguinal ligament (Fig. 18–19E). Relaxing incisions are not necessary. The cord is placed back underneath the external oblique fascia and the superficial groin layers are closed as in other hernia repairs. This operation can be done under local anesthesia in all but the most obese or nervous patients without undue difficulty.

Patients are allowed to be up and about as soon as the intraoperative sedation has been metabolized. There are essentially no limits to activity postoperatively except that which would cause an inordinate amount of pain at the incision. If bilateral hernias are present, the second side is generally repaired on the third day following the initial surgery, or at a later date. The patients are discharged from the hospital on the second or third day following surgery. From our own experience they could probably be discharged even sooner.

In our hospital, with the anterior transversalis fascia repair, a recurrence rate of 1.2 per cent was found for primary inguinal hernia repairs.[3] This is much lower than the recurrence rates reported from most other institutions performing hernia repairs by the standard Bassini or McVay techniques.[4]

Since there are no controlled alternate patient studies as yet available comparing anterior transversalis fascia repair to other techniques, it cannot be said definitively which is superior. The data reported by Berliner and colleagues[3] and by Glassow[14, 15] suggest that anterior transversalis repair is an excellent technique. There is no question that these hernia repairs, performed under local anesthesia, result in a short hospital stay.

Laparoscopy

In recent years laparoscopy (peritoneoscopy) has become popular as a diagnostic and therapeutic tool for gynecologists. The procedure was extensively tried in the past by general surgeons; however, it fell into disrepute because of technical problems such as poor light source and limited visual field. The gradually decreasing rates of morbidity and mortality associated with diagnostic laparotomy have also been discouraging the advocates of laparoscopy. In recent years, however, technical improvements such as fiberoptic lighting have increased the capability of the procedure. Laparoscopy has recently been extensively utilized by general surgeons in Europe and Japan and also in the United States. The surfaces of organs can be visualized but no palpation can be done. It is often difficult to visualize organs that are not in fixed positions; therefore, it is easy to visualize the liver or the gynecological structures, but it may be difficult to visualize lesions situated on the outer surface of the small bowel.

TECHNIQUE. At present, most laparoscopic procedures are performed on patients in the hospital operating room, usually under general anesthesia. However, they could also be performed with local anesthesia and sedation. This procedure can be done on an outpatient or short-stay hospital admission. The performance of the procedure is fairly standardized (Fig. 18–20A–D). The abdomen is prepared and draped by standard techniques. A pneumoperitoneum is then established using carbon dioxide from a controlled source. A Verres needle is inserted into the abdomen and carbon dioxide is introduced via an insufflator. Generally between the 2.5 and 3.5 liters of carbon dioxide are required to have enough space to perform the procedure. The adequacy of insufflation can be estimated clinically by the degree of tympany on percussion of the abdomen. A 1 centimeter infraumbilical incision is made through the skin. A trocar is then introduced into the abdominal cavity. This is relatively safe because of the space present between the viscera and the abdominal wall caused by the previously produced pneumoperitoneum. The trocar is removed and the laparoscope is in-

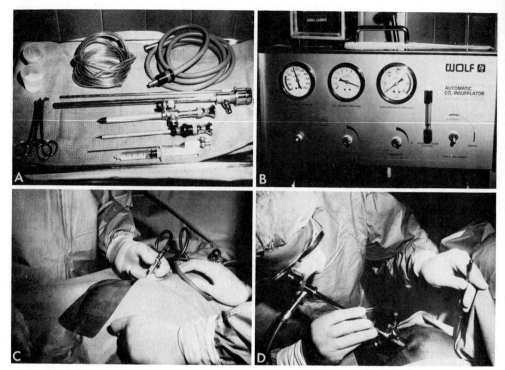

Figure 18–20   Laparoscopy. *A.* Instruments. *B.* Insufflator. *C.* Insufflation. *D.* Examination.

serted through the cannula. The fiberoptic light source is then attached. An additional smaller cannula with a probe is inserted through a stab wound at another point in the abdomen, depending on the expected pathological findings. This probe is used for manipulation of bowel loops, measurement of visualized structures and for biopsy.

RESULTS OF LAPAROSCOPY. As far as the general surgeon is concerned, laparoscopy is most adaptable for intra-abdominal diagnosis and for the evaluation of the liver for metastases. An isolated liver nodule, which is often missed by a closed liver biopsy, can be visualized and accurately biopsied under laparoscopic control. Laparotomy may also be useful in the evaluation of selected blunt and penetrating abdominal trauma cases. Since the indications for laparotomy in many of these patients are clear, laparoscopy may be superfluous in some; however, in patients with equivocal indications for abdominal exploration, laparoscopy could be useful.

Another role for laparoscopy is in the differentiation of pelvic inflammatory disease from acute appendicitis. It is also of value as a diagnostic modality in extremely poor risk patients in whom the mortality from laparotomy is great and no tissue diagnosis is available. Diagnostic accuracy reported in several series is as high as 90 per cent.[20, 38]

Average bedrest required following laparoscopy is three to four hours. The patient may be discharged from the hospital the same day or the following day if findings do not necessitate further therapeutic procedures. In properly selected cases, laparoscopy can often resolve a diagnostic problem, determine the extent of the disease and permit initiation of appropriate therapy.

CONCLUSION

There is probably no other field in which both the art and science of surgery are so important than that of diseases of the abdomen and gastrointestinal tract. Many rules and suggestions may be studied as guides to therapy. Nevertheless, the young surgeon must always be ready to ask for advice from colleagues when the problem is unusual. In lonely clinics or remote regions, the conclusion may be especially difficult. But inevitably, the moment of decision will come. The surgeon must decide whether to operate; if there is hesitation the patient may slip into an irreversible condition and an unnecessary death.

REFERENCES

1. Baek, S., Sloane, C. E., and Futterman, S. C.: Benign liver cell adenoma associated with the use of oral contraceptives. Ann. Surg., *183*:239–242, 1976.
2. Ben-Shoshan, M., Gius, J. A., and Smith, I. M.: Exploratory laparotomy for fever of unknown origin. Surg. Gynecol. Obstet., *132*:994–996, 1971.
3. Berliner, S., Burson, L., Katz, P., and Wise, L.: An anterior transversalis fascia repair for adult inguinal hernias. Am. J. Surg., *135*:633–636, 1978.
4. Botsford, T. W., and Wilson, R. E.: The Acute Abdomen. Philadelphia, W. B. Saunders Co., 1969.
5. Buchwald, H., Moore, R. B., and Varco, R. L.: Ten years clinical experience with partial ileal bypass in management of the hyperlipidemias. Ann Surg., *180*:384–392, 1974.
6. Byron, R. L., Yonemoto, R. H., King, R. M., Lamb, E. J., Amromin, G. D., Solomon, R. D., and Gildenhorn, V. B.: The management of pseudo-myxoma peritonei secondary to ruptured mucocele of the appendix. Surg. Gynecol. Obstet., *122*:509–512, 1966.
7. Cohn, I.: Intestinal Antispepsis. Springfield, Charles C Thomas, 1968.
8. Cope, Z.: The Early Diagnosis of the Acute Abdomen. 13th Ed. London, Oxford University Press, 1968.
9. Crile, G., Jr.: Advantages of bypass operations over radical pancreatoduodenectomy in the treatment of pancreatic carcinoma. Surg. Gynecol. Obstet., *130*:1049–1053, 1970.
10. Devlin, H. B., Evans, D. S., and Birkhead, J. S.: Elective splenectomy for primary hematologic and splenic disease. Surg. Gynecol. Obstet., *131*:273–276, 1970.
11. Dexor, D., and Knauft, R. D.: Exploratory laparotomy for abdominal pain of un-

12. Ebert, P. A., Gaertner, R. A., and Zuidema, G. D.: Traumatic diaphragmatic hernia. Surg. Gynecol. Obstet., *125*:59–65, 1967.
13. Ein, S. H., Shandling, B., Simpson, J. S., Stephens, C. A., Bandi, S. K., Biggar, W. D., and Freedman, M. H.: The morbidity and mortality of splenectomy in childhood. Ann. Surg., *185*:307–310, 1977.
14. Glassow, F.: The surgical repair of inguinal and femoral hernias. Can. Med. Assoc. J., *108*:308–313, 1973.
15. Glassow, F.: The Shouldice Repair of Inguinal Hernia. In Varco, R. L., and Delaney, J. P. (Eds.): Controversy in Surgery. Philadelphia, W. B. Saunders Co., 1976.
16. Glenn, F., and McSherry, C. K.: Secondary abdominal operations for symptoms following biliary tract surgery. Surg. Gynecol. Obstet., *121*:979–988, 1965.
17. Glenn, F., McSherry, C. K., and Dineen, P.: Morbidity of surgical treatment for nonmalignant biliary tract disease. Surg. Gynecol. Obstet., *126*:15–26, 1968.
18. Haller, J. A., Jr., and Jones, E. L.: Effect of splenectomy on immunity and resistance to major infections in early childhood: Clinical and experimental study. Ann. Surg., *163*:902–908, 1966.
19. Hendren, W. H., Warshaw, A. L., Fleischli, D. J., and Bartlett, M. K.: Traumatic hemobilia: Non-operative management with healing documented by serial angiography. Ann. Surg., *174*:991–993, 1971.
20. Herbsman, H., Gardner, B., and Alfonso, A.: The value of laparoscopy in general surgery. J. Reprod. Med., *18*:235–240, 1977.
21. Hollander, F.: The insulin test for the presence of intact nerve fibers after vagal operations for peptic ulcer. Gastroenterology, 7:607–614, 1946.
22. Ibach, J. R., Jr., Hume, H. A., and Erb, W. H.: Cholecystectomy in the aged. Surg. Gynecol. Obstet., *126*:523–528, 1968.
23. Jewett, T. C., Duszynski, D. O., and Allen, J. E.: The visualization of Meckel's diverticulum with ^{99}Tc-pertechnetate. Surgery, 68:567–570, 1970.
24. Jones, C. M.: Digestive Tract Pain, Diagnosis and Treatment. New York, MacMillan Co., 1928.
25. Large, A. M.: Partial intermittent volvulus of the cecum. Ann. Surg., *167*:609–611, 1968.
26. Localio, S. A., and Stahl, W. M.: Diverticular disease of the alimentary tract. Curr. Probl. Surg., 1–78, December 1967.
27. Malt, R. A., Hershberg, R. A., and Miller, W. L.: Experience with benign tumors of the liver. Surg. Gynecol. Obstet., *130*:285–291, 1970.
28. McVay, C. B.: Hernia: The Pathologic Anat-

omy of the More Common Hernias and their Anatomic Repair. Springfield, Charles C Thomas, 1954.

29. Morgan, I. G., Marks, C., and Hearn, D.: Carcinoid tumors of the gastrointestinal tract. Ann. Surg., *180*:720–727, 1974.

30. Nichols, R. L., and Condon, R. E.: Preoperative preparation of the colon. Surg. Gynecol. Obstet., *132*:323–337, 1971.

31. Nyhus, L. M., and Harkins, H. M.: Hernia. Philadelphia, J. B. Lippincott Co., 1964.

32. Orcutt, T. W.: Hernia of the superior lumbar triangle. Ann. Surg., *173*:294–297, 1971.

33. Palmer, E. D.: Upper Gastrointestinal Hemorrhage. Springfield, Charles C Thomas, 1970.

34. Perry, J. F., Jr.: Blunt and penetrating abdominal injuries. Curr. Probl. Surg., May 1970.

35. Polk, H. C.: Carcinoma and the calcified gallbladder. Gastroenterology, *50*:582–585, 1966.

36. Ragins, H., and Glatzer, S. G.: A nonoperative approach to subcutaneous removal of stubborn sutures from wound granulomas. Am. J. Surg., *133*:393–395, 1977.

37. Ranson, J. H. C., Rifkind, K. M., Roses, D. F., Fink, S. D., Eng, K., and Spencer, F. C.: Prognostic signs and the role of operative management in acute pancreatitis. Surg. Gynecol. Obstet., *139*:69–81, 1974.

38. Robinson, H. B., and Smith, G. W.: Applications for laparoscopy in general surgery. Surg. Gynecol. Obstet., *143*:829–834, 1976.

39. Rothman, D. L., Schwartz, S. I., and Adams, J. T.: Diagnostic laparotomy for fever or abdominal pain of unknown origin. Am. J. Surg., *133*:273–275, 1977.

40. Ruoff, M., and Ranson, J. H. C.: Persistent hypercoagulability after venous mesenteric infarction and oral contraceptive. N.Y. State J. Med., *73*:791–793, 1973.

41. Ryzoff, R. I., Shaftan, G. W., and Herbsman, H.: Selective conservatism in penetrating abdominal trauma. Surgery, *59*:650–653, 1966.

42. Schwartz, S. I., and Storer, E. H.: Manifestations of gastrointestinal disease. *In*

Schwartz, et al. (Eds.): Principles of Surgery. New York, McGraw-Hill, 1974.

43. Scott, M. W., Jr., Law, D. M., IV, Sandstead, H. M., Lanier, V. C., Jr., and Younger, R. K.: Jejuno-ileal shunt in surgical treatment of morbid obesity. Ann. Surg., *171*:770–782, 1970.

44. Scott, M. W., Jr., Shull, H. J., Law, D. H., IV, Burko, H., and Page, D. L.: Surgical management of Menetrier's disease with protein-losing gastropathy. Ann. Surg., *181*:765–777, 1975.

45. Seltzer, M. H., and Rosato, F. E.: Mortality following cholecystectomy. Surg. Gynecol. Obstet., *130*:64–66, 1970.

46. Stone, A. M., Pearson, W., Lansdown, F., and Tice, D. A.: Spontaneous rupture of the diaphragm. Ann. Thor. Surg., *9*:479–482, 1970.

47. Stone, H. H., Webb, H. W., Larson, R. A., Wright, H. K., and Cleveland, J. C.: Pneumatosis intestinalis of infancy. Surg. Gynecol. Obstet., *130*:806–812, 1970.

48. Warren, K. W., Choe, D. S., Plaza, J., and Relihan, M.: Results of radical resection for periampullary cancer. Ann. Surg., *181*:534–540, 1975.

49. Wise, L.: The iatrogenic short bowel syndrome: The surgical treatment of morbid exogenous obesity. *In* Ballinger, W. F., and Drapanas, T. (Eds.): Practice of Surgery. St. Louis, C. V. Mosby Co., 1975.

50. Witte, C. L.: Mesentery and bowel injury from automobile seat belts. Ann. Surg., *167*:486–492, 1968.

51. Wuepper, K. D., Otterman, M. G., and Stahlgren, L. H.: Appraisal of operative and nonoperative treatment of sigmoid volvulus. Surg. Gynecol. Obstet., *122*:84–88, 1966.

52. Yajko, R. D., Norton, L. W., and Eiseman, B.: Current management of upper gastrointestinal bleeding. Ann. Surg., *181*:474–480, 1975.

53. Zollinger, R. M., and Ellison, E. R.: Primary peptic ulceration of the jejunum associated with islet cell tumors of the pancreas. Ann. Surg., *142*:709–723, 1955.

19 Urology

RICHARD A. BLATH, M.D.,
and WILLIAM R. FAIR, M.D.

Introduction

Urology is the surgical specialty concerned with the male genitourinary system and the female urinary tract. This broad field involves patients of all ages with many different problems and symptoms. Some urgent problems that are seen by the Emergency Room staff include minor and major trauma, urinary retention, blood in the urine, acute scrotal diseases and renal colic. The symptoms may be severe or mild and the diagnosis may be immediately apparent or thoroughly obscure. The major features of differential diagnosis, outpatient evaluation and immediate treatment for each of these problems will be considered in this chapter.

Ambulatory urology involves the patient with nonurgent problems, such as genital lesions, infertility, impotence and problems of urinary control. In addition, outpatient evaluation of high blood pressure and renal lesions is accomplished. A series of diagnostic steps must be followed to arrive at the correct diagnosis and treatment.

With the recent growth of short stay surgery, elective outpatient operations are increasing. Both diagnosis and treatment of a variety of acute and

---

TABLE 19–1   Genitourinary Investigative Procedures

EXCRETORY UROGRAM (INTRAVENOUS PYELOGRAM—IVP)
   Renal concentration, excretion of intravenously administered contrast medium. Anatomical but not a functional study.
   Rapid Sequence (Hypertensive): Includes early films (30 sec, 1 min), revealing time and concentration discrepancy between kidneys which may suggest reduced renal artery flow.
   Infusion: Large dose of contrast medium allowing visualization of kidneys despite elevated BUN and poor preparation. One ml per pound contrast medium with 1 ml per pound normal saline, rapidly infused.
CYSTOGRAM
   Antegrade: Bladder visualization associated with routine or infusion IVP.
   Retrograde: Through urethral catheter or accompanying retrograde urethrogram.
   Voiding: May accompany retrograde study; may reveal reflux, diverticulum or valve.
   Double Exposure: Occasionally helpful in demonstration and staging bladder tumors; does not replace cystoscopy/biopsy.
URETHROGRAM
   Voiding: Accompanies cystogram; helpful in demonstrating valves, diverticula, fistulae.
   Retrograde: Isolated procedure; assists investigation of urethral trauma, stricture, congenital defects.
   Cine: Accompanies cine cystograms; dynamic study of voiding; assists investigation of stricture, valves, fistulae, diverticula.
URETEROPYELOGRAM
   Retrograde: Accompanies cystoscopy; delineates ureter and renal pelvis.
RENAL CYSTOGRAM
   Accompanies IVP and fluoroscopy; aspiration of cyst fluid and insertion of contrast medium; assists differentiation between renal cyst and tumor; accompanied by cytology of aspirate.
NEPHROTOMOGRAM
   Accompanies IVP; elucidates mass lesions (cyst vs. tumor).
ARTERIOGRAM
   Translumbar: Percutaneous injection of constant medium into lumbar aorta.
   Seldinger: Percutaneous transfemoral arterial catheterization and advancement.
   Midstream Aortic: Outlines aorta and major branches.
   Selective Renal: Selective fluoroscopic catheterization of renal arteries; occasionally used for infusing chemotherapeutic agents.
   Selective Adrenal: Selective fluoroscopic catheterization of adrenal arteries.
   Selective Hypogastric: Selective fluoroscopic catheterization of hypogastric arteries; occasionally helpful in staging bladder tumor; occasionally used to infuse chemotherapeutic agents.
   Epinephrine: Preceding contrast injections; normal vessels constrict and do not feel well; neoplastic vessels do not constrict but remain unchanged.

chronic problems can be dealt with on an ambulatory basis. Anesthesia of the genital organs and techniques for local and regional procedures will be discussed. Urology is unique in its reliance upon endoscopy and specialized radiographic techniques. These methods are listed and briefly discussed in Table 19–1.

ANESTHESIA

Penile Block (Fig. 19–1)

Most minor surgical procedures performed on the penis require only an infiltration of a local anesthetic. These operations include circumcision, dorsal preputial slit, meatotomy, cutaneous biopsy and reduction of paraphimosis. Innervation of the foreskin is by the dorsal cutaneous nerves, which traverse the penile shaft at the one o'clock and eleven o'clock positions. Appropriate infiltration at these areas in the base of the penis will usually afford total distal anesthesia. A circumferential subcutaneous infiltration is also advisable to ensure adequate local anesthesia. After routine cleansing and draping of the penis, an appropriate agent is used. Lidocaine, 1 per cent solution, is recommended and will provide excellent anesthesia for a one to two hour period. Infiltrations with

---

TABLE 19–1   Genitourinary Investigative Procedures (*Continued*)

INFERIOR VENA CAVAGRAM
   Percutaneous transfemoral venous catheterization; outlines displacement, effacement, obstruction, compromise of inferior vena cava by lymph nodes, tumor thrombus.
RENAL VENOGRAM
   Selective: Extension of interior vena cavagram.
   Differential Collections: Including renin levels (renal hypertension), epinephrine levels (pheochromocytoma).
VASOGRAM
   After surgical exposure of vas deferens, needle or catheter cannulation, contrast injection; to demonstrate displacement, obstruction, inflammation, neoplasia of vas deferens or seminal vesicle.
LYMPHANGIOGRAM
   Pedal: Contrast migration from pedal lymphatics to iliac, lumbar, periaortic, renal hilar nodes; useful for evaluation of staging of testis tumor, gynecological tumor, etc.
UROFLOWMETRY WITH/WITHOUT CATHETER
   Time/volume evaluation of urine flow; normal flow exceeds 20 cc per minute; may assist evaluation of surgical results.
CYSTOMETROGRAM (BETHANECOL TEST)
   Dynamic study of bladder pressure plotted against time and volume; significant subjective component; assists evaluation of neurogenic bladder.
ELECTROMYOGRAPHY (RECTAL SPHINCTER, PERIANAL)
   Helpful in determining muscle activity (innervation) in neurological lesion affecting lower urinary tract function.
URETHRAL PRESSURE PROFILE (U.P.P.)
   Method of measuring pressure changes throughout the entire urethral length; beneficial in voiding disorders, incontinence, sphincter abnormalities.
ISOTOPE STUDIES
   Renogram: ^{131}I-labeled Hippuran: differential concentration/decay curve; helpful in evaluating differential renal function, blood flow, obstruction.
   Renal Scan: ^{131}I Hippuran or graphic demonstration of differential "hot" and "cold" renal lesions (infarct, tumor, cyst).
TESTIS SCAN
   Use of ^{99}Tc pertechnetate to measure flow through testis; in diagnosis of torsion and epididymitis.
ULTRASOUND
   Use of high frequency sound waves to delineate renal and pelvic mass lesions (cystic vs. solid).
COMPUTERIZED TOMOGRAPHY (CAT SCAN)
   X-ray system that uses different tissue attenuation coefficients to display body organs. Useful in diagnosing mass lesions and perhaps in tumor staging.

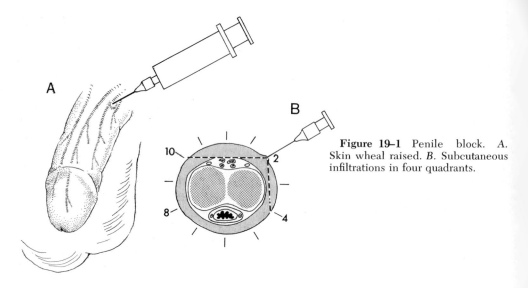

Figure 19–1 Penile block. *A.* Skin wheal raised. *B.* Subcutaneous infiltrations in four quadrants.

solutions containing epinephrine are contraindicated in the penis because of the risk of injection directly into the corporal bodies. After producing the skin wheal subcutaneously, the needle is advanced through the skin and is aspirated to ensure that the corporal bodies have not been entered. Penile nerve blocks are performed using 3 to 5 ml of anesthetic solution. After a short delay, a touch test will confirm total cutaneous anesthesia, although additional infiltration at the frenulum will occasionally be necessary.

Spermatic Cord and Testicular Anesthesia (Fig. 19–2)

Inflammatory and traumatic lesions of the testis and epididymis may be extremely painful. In order to both relieve the patient's discomfort and allow for adequate physical examination by the physician, a spermatic cord block is often essential.

The testis is innervated by the superior spermatic nerve, arising at the level of T10. The hypogastric nerve plexus gives rise to the middle and spermatic nerves, which supply both the testis and the epididymis. These nerves run through the external inguinal ring in the spermatic cord. To relieve pain in the testes and epididymis, these nerves can be anesthetized by a spermatic cord block.

With the patient lying in a supine position, a sterile area is prepared. The spermatic cord is located in the superior and anterior portion of the scrotum and is grasped with one hand. A skin wheal is raised in the overlying scrotal skin and the needle is slowly advanced into the spermatic cord. After aspiration ensures that no blood vessels have been entered, 5 to 10 ml of an appropriate local anesthetic is injected. Within moments, the patient should experience complete relief of pain and the clinician may proceed with careful examination of the testis. The relief of autonomic vasospasm by this local anesthetic may aid in the resolution of inflammation and is occasionally of great benefit in the treatment of acute epididymitis.

EMERGENCY UROLOGY

Trauma to the Genitourinary System

Emergency Room care of an individual who has sustained injury to the ab-

A

Location of block   B

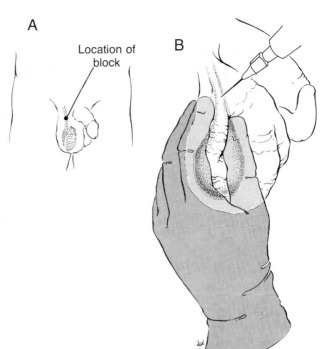

Figure 19–2 Spermatic cord block. *A.* Area of insertion of needle for spermatic cord infiltration. *B.* Spermatic cord is grasped above the testis with thumb and forefinger and infiltrated through a skin wheal with 5–10 cc of appropriate local anesthetic.

domen, flank, back or genital regions necessitates prompt urological investigation. The most common symptom of injury to the genitourinary tract is hematuria. Since this may indicate either a mild contusion or major catastrophic injury, complete evaluation is required.

Most patients with urological trauma also have other injuries. Urological evaluation must be undertaken concurrently with the investigation of other organ systems and in conjunction with resuscitative efforts. A rapid yet thorough technique has been devised to adequately assess all potentially serious urological injuries in a minimum amount of time.

After initial resuscitation with intravenous fluids, a rapid overall evaluation should be made to assess the patient's general condition. If no urethral injury is suspected, an attempt should be made to pass a Foley catheter into the bladder and the urine should be examined. If a catheter cannot be easily passed, an immediate retrograde urethrogram will show the presence

and site of urethral trauma. If a pelvic fracture, or other injuries that may suggest a urethral injury, is present, a retrograde urethrogram must be performed *before* attempting to pass a catheter. In the presence of hematuria, a rapid physical examination is made. The flanks are specifically examined for an enlarging renal mass, ecchymosis or back tenderness. The suprapubic area is inspected for tenderness and the genital region is also examined for the presence of any hematoma formation.

After an initial abdominal x-ray is performed to detect free subdiaphragmatic air, fractures or soft tissue injury, a rapid radiographic investigation follows. The bladder is filled with a 100 ml solution of dilute contrast material and intravenous contrast simultaneously is infused in a bolus dose of 1 ml per pound of body weight. A subsequent roentgenogram will demonstrate vascular flow to both kidneys, the size and position of the kidneys and also reveal bladder integrity. The bladder is then emptied of contrast and a five minute roentgenogram taken in the supine and oblique positions will assess renal or ureteral injury and also demonstrate vesical extravasation. Subsequent arteriograms or retrograde studies may be done if indicated. In many trauma centers it is routine practice to inject 50 to 75 ml of contrast media at the time the initial IV is started. A single abdominal film five to ten minutes after injection will, as a minimum, reveal the presence of two kidneys, and major urinary extravasation can be readily identified.

Renal Trauma

The most common cause of blunt renal trauma is automobile accidents. Isolated renal injuries are infrequent and are usually associated with trauma to the spleen, liver and mesentery. The extent of renal injury is determined with the use of intravenous urography. This study is also valuable to determine function in the contralateral kidney. Minor injury consists of renal contusions and superficial capsular tears with perirenal hematoma. The collecting system is intact, and there is no urinary extravasation or parenchymal fragmentation. These patients are treated conservatively with broad-spectrum antibiotics, bed rest and sedation until the hematuria clears.

Moderate renal injury exists in the presence of urinary extravasation from trauma to the collecting system or fracture with laceration of the renal parenchyma.[9] Controversy exists over whether these cases should undergo conservative therapy or an aggressive surgical approach. If the patient's condition is unstable, hypotension is prolonged and an enlarging flank mass occurs, then exploration is mandatory. In the presence of stable vital signs and no evidence of deterioration, an initial conservative approach may be undertaken.

Injury to the renal pedicle can result in a tear of the renal artery or vein.

This is a major renal injury and the patients are often in shock. When urography reveals a nonfunctioning kidney, emergency renal arteriography is indicated to search for a ruptured vessel or an intimal tear. Immediate surgery is required to prevent hemorrhage or renal loss.

All penetrating injuries that involve the kidney require exploration. Low velocity wounds, such as knife wounds, may need only superficial débridement and drainage. High velocity missile wounds often devitalize large amounts of renal parenchyma and require extensive débridement, heminephrectomy or nephrectomy.

Long-term complications from renal trauma include hypertension from segmental renal artery stenosis, arteriovenous fistula formation and renal atrophy.

Trauma to the Renal Pelvis and Ureter

The renal pelvis may be injured in association with injury to the kidney resulting in a leak of urine into the perirenal tissue. If the peritoneum is torn, urine will leak into the peritoneal cavity and peritoneal irritation will result. If the tear is small, spontaneous healing may result. Perirenal urinary extravasation is not a definitive indication for immediate exploration. On the other hand, a steadily increasing flank mass needs to be explored and the urinoma drained.

Damage to the ureter is often iatrogenic in surgical or gynecological procedures, although external trauma produces one-half of all ureteral injuries. These are best diagnosed by a retrograde ureterogram, and surgery is necessary for débridement and reconstruction.

Bladder contusion produces hematuria, and with a complete transmural tear no urine will be obtained upon catheterization. A cystogram is diagnostic and indicates both the degree and site of injury.

Trauma to the Bladder

A ruptured bladder associated with a fracture of the pelvis usually occurs extraperitoneally. A small extraperitoneal extravasation can be adequately treated by an indwelling urethral catheter. In the absence of a fractured pelvis, bladder injury is often intraperitoneal and may result from a sudden deceleration. This usually occurs in the presence of an overdistended bladder and has been related to automobile seat belts. Intraperitoneal bladder rupture should always be treated with exploration, for bowel may herniate through the ruptured bladder opening. Immediate suturing and drainage by a suprapubic catheter is recommended.

Trauma to the Urethra

Blood at the external urinary meatus, inability to void or a tense, distended, discolored penis or perineum indicates injury to the urethra. Prompt retrograde urethrography will demonstrate the site and extent of injury. No urethral instrumentation or catheterization should be done, for there is danger of converting an incomplete tear into a complete rupture. Urethral injuries may be divided into proximally and distally located areas of trauma.

Injury to the proximal urethra occurs at the level of the puboprostatic ligament and results in a tear of the prostatic and membranous urethra. This most commonly occurs with pelvic fractures as the urethra is sheared by bone chips. Rectal examination reveals boggy hemorrhage in the prostatic fossa and elevation of the prostate. The patient is unable to void. A cystogram shows a "tear drop" configuration of the bladder from the pelvic hematoma. A catheter cannot be passed into the bladder, and any attempt to do so will worsen the injury. Treatment involves surgical intervention with the placement of a suprapubic cystostomy tube. Controversy exists on whether to rea-

lign the injury and accomplish primary repair, attempt to establish urethral continuity with sounds and urethral catheters or perform simple diversion with a urethroplasty planned in the future. Complications of prostate injuries are significant — incontinence in 25 per cent and stricture formation in 40 per cent of cases.

A straddle injury results in trauma to the anterior urethra. Urinary extravasation will occur if the injury is distal to the urogenital diaphragm or triangular ligament. While rupture of Buck's fascia will result in extravasation within the boundaries of the penis, a tear of Colles' fascia will result in urinary extravasation throughout the scrotum and onto the abdominal wall. The patient should not attempt to void because urinary extravasation will increase. Treatment consists of initial ice packs and pressure. Surgery is necessary to evacuate the hematoma and urinoma and adequately debride and drain the area. Proximal suprapubic urinary diversion is often necessary. Primary identification of the injury site and urethral reanastomosis is indicated. Prophylactic antibiotics are frequently beneficial.

FAILURE OF URINATION

When faced with a patient who presents with an inability to produce urine, the physician must determine:
  (1) whether the patient is producing urine or is actually anuric,
  (2) whether his condition represents an acute or chronic retention, and
  (3) how best to make a diagnosis and relieve the problem.

Acute Retention

Although acute urinary retention may appear abruptly, as in a patient with a vesical calculus or bladder tumor obstructing the bladder neck, most patients have a preceding history of voiding difficulty. This includes decreasing size and force of the urinary stream, hesitancy, dribbling and nocturia. In these patients a physiological balance has been created between an increased urethral pressure and an increased vesical effort allowing them to maintain a satisfactory voiding pattern. Any situation that interferes with optimal bladder contraction will upset this balance, and the bladder will not be able to overcome an increased outlet resistance. The result of this unbalanced state is acute urinary retention.

Typical precipitating events include alcoholic overindulgence, a lengthy motor trip, a state of increased fluid intake or other similar circumstances. These patients have extreme supravesical discomfort and pain, and physical examination reveals an enlarged, distended bladder. In patients who have longstanding benign prostatic hypertrophy, a firm, smooth, symmetrically enlarged prostate can be palpated on rectal examination. While an enlarged prostate is the most common cause of acute urinary retention, this condition can also exist in patients with bladder calculi, vesical neoplasms and urethral strictures.

The patient with acute urinary retention is extremely uncomfortable, and the goal of treatment should be immediate relief of the obstruction. This is most easily accomplished by passage of a urethral catheter and complete decompression of the bladder (Fig. 19–3). Following decompression, the catheter may be removed and prompt restoration of the predistention voiding pattern will occasionally occur. However, all patients with acute urinary retention do have uropathology; therefore, a complete urological evaluation including intravenous urography and cystoscopy should be performed. Occasionally urethral obstruction will be so marked as to resist easy passage of a urethral catheter. In these circumstances, the passage of a Coudé catheter may prove successful

if the obstruction is an enlarged prostate or a median bar. Another alternative is to use a sterile, flexible wire catheter guide placed inside the urethral catheter. This guide gives the catheter a semirigid curve and increased rigidity, approximating a Van Buren sound. With the addition of perineal or rectal pressure as an added guide, successful passage into the bladder may be accomplished. When a urethral stricture is present, successful catheterization with a flexible No. 16 or No. 18 French catheter will be unsuccessful. When this occurs, the physician should try a smaller diameter catheter or attempt to pass urethral filiforms. These filiforms, in size No. 3 or No. 4 French, will often circumvent the stricture and allow the physician to dilate the urethra with consecutively larger followers.

Suprapubic Cystostomy

If the patient's bladder can be readily palpated above the pubic symphysis, but the urethra cannot be catheterized because of strictures or other disease, consideration must be given to placement of a suprapubic catheter. Many of these are commercially available, including the Cystocath and Bonano suprapubic tubes. The procedure can be done in the office or in the Emergency Room, using only local anesthesia. It is imperative that this procedure only be attempted when the bladder is easily palpable. It is contraindicated in patients who have had prior lower abdominal surgery, because of the possibility of bowel adhering to the anterior vesical surface.

Local anesthetic is infiltrated into the skin in the midline, approximately two finger breadths above the pubic symphysis. The available apparatus consists of a No. 13 or No. 16 French polyethylene cannula around a trocar needle. This trocar is passed through the area of anesthesia in a direct caudal fashion at a 45 degree angle behind the pubic symphysis until urine returns.

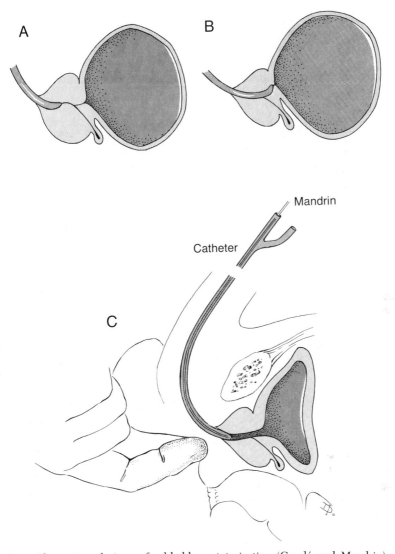

Figure 19-3 Alternate techniques for bladder cateterization (Coudé and Mandrin). *A.* and *B.* Coudé-tipped catheter more easily maneuvered through posterior urethra in the presence of enlarged middle lobe of prostate *(A)* or median bar at vesical neck *(B)*. *C.* Mandrin guide technique. Lubricated mandrin is inserted inside catheter and bent into desired shape. Catheter is then inserted, as a urethral sound (see Fig. 19-11), with perineal digital pressure aiding advancement through posterior urethra.

The catheter is then threaded over the needle until urine is seen in its lumen, at which time the needle is removed. The catheter can then be secured with a suture. A local antibiotic ointment of Neomycin or Betadine is placed over the skin and a sterile dressing is applied. As an alternative to urethral catheterization, a single suprapubic aspiration using a No. 18 or No. 20 French spinal needle can be used for the treatment of acute retention. The method used when a urethral sound can be passed is shown in Figure 19-4.

Acute urinary retention occurs in females. When a woman comes to the Emergency Room and is unable to urinate, it often indicates a conversion reaction in a depressed or hysterical

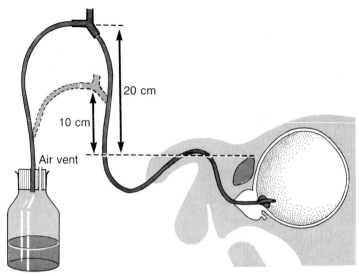

Figure 19-4 Gradual vesical decompression. Drainage tubing attached to catheter through Y-adapter open to the air. Adapter initially placed 20 cm for 24 hours, lowered 10 cm for 24 hours, then placed to gravity drainage.

patient. Other causes include urethral stenosis, urinary tract infection, vesical calculus or malignancy.

Anuria

If the patient is not producing any urine, does not have a distended bladder and has no urine in the bladder at the time of urethral catheterization, then supravesical renal failure must be investigated. Prerenal causes of anuria or oliguria include marked dehydration, shock, congestive heart failure, hemorrhage and thyrotoxicosis. These may be excluded by assessing the patient's general condition. In the absence of heavy metal poisoning, drug toxicity, hypotension or long-standing kidney disease, primary renal failure may also be excluded. Under these circumstances, a critical condition exists if obstruction of a solitary kidney or bilateral simultaneous urinary tract obstruction has occurred. These patients are true emergencies and urinary decompression must be achieved rapidly to prevent the damage of pressure atrophy and hydronephrosis. The etiological factors of such a condition include

retroperitoneal disease (retroperitoneal fibrosis or malignancies), trauma or calculus disease involving a single collecting system.

Emergency investigation is carried out with excretory urography and retrograde pyelography if needed. In most instances these studies will define the site and etiological factors of the obstruction. If the patient is not a candidate for emergency definitive surgery, percutaneous renal decompression and drainage may be carried out under local anesthesia. Ultrasonography has been extremely beneficial in aiding in the location of a distended renal pelvis and assisting in the placement of a percutaneous nephrostomy tube.

Percutaneous Nephrostomy[13]

With the patient prone on an examining table, B-mode ultrasonography is used to locate the distended renal pelvis. The site of needle entry is usually 2 to 3 cm below the 12th rib and 4 to 6 cm lateral to the spinous processes. This area is identified with ultrasound and marked, and the area is then cleansed and anesthetized with Xylocaine. If ultrasound is not available, the procedure can easily be accomplished after injecting radiopaque contrast material intravenously and observing the renal pelvis under fluoroscopy. Using the images obtained as a guide, a No. 18 to No. 20 gauge French spinal needle is slowly advanced toward the renal pelvis. When the kidney and collecting system have been entered, the needle moves with respiration and urine can be readily aspirated. Contrast solution may be introduced through the needle to confirm its position fluoroscopically and assist in lateral maneuvers. After localizing the renal pelvis, a thin guidewire is introduced through this needle and allowed to pass into the renal pelvis. With the guidewire in place, the spinal needle is removed. A fascia cutting needle is placed over the guidewire and inserted through the fascia of the flank. This needle is then removed and a No. 12 French polyethylene arterial catheter is inserted over the guidewire and advanced into the renal pelvis, at least 2 cm beyond the guidewire tip. This catheter can be previously shaped into a corkscrew or "J" so that additional length may be placed into the renal pelvis to prevent accidental withdrawal. The guidewire is finally removed and the catheter is attached to drainage and sutured to the skin. Antegrade pyelography may then be accomplished through this catheter for additional diagnostic information. This procedure is relatively safe and can be accomplished with either an intrarenal or extrarenal pelvis.

Chronic Urinary Retention

Though chronic urinary retention is generally seen in older patients with a long history of prostatism, it may occur in patients of any age who have long-standing urethral stricture or neurogenic bladder dysfunction. These patients have urinary frequency, dribbling, nocturia and occasional incontinence. Examination often reveals a large, distended urinary bladder that can be percussed above the level of the umbilicus. The patients are not uncomfortable. With a chronic increase in intravesicular pressure there may also be hydroureter and hydronephrosis. Renal failure and uremia can occur, causing an elevation in serum creatinine and blood urea nitrogen. Urinary tract infections complicate the picture. Chronic outlet obstruction is most often due to an enlarged prostate or urethral stricture. However, a neurogenic bladder of the flaccid or paralytic type is also a frequent cause.

Vesical decompression in these patients is accomplished in the same manner as in patients with acute obstruction. Complications can occur after acute decompression of chronic retention and these must be watched for carefully. After the removal of the large amount of clear urine, vesical hemorrhage may occur. This is called hemorrhage *ex vacuo* and is caused by the acute engorgement and decompression of venous channels within the bladder wall. With diuresis, the bleeding will spontaneously clear.

Postobstructive diuresis may also occur. This syndrome involves an obligatory salt and water loss from the kidneys in response to tubular dysfunction after sudden renal decompression. In these patients, salt and water are lost in amounts far greater than would occur under normal circumstances. Intermittent clamping and releasing of the catheter was initially thought to control this problem. However, it is now felt that the catheter should be allowed to drain freely and any electrolyte or fluid losses should be replaced, intravenously if necessary. The postobstructive diuresis may be of massive proportions, ranging up to 2 liters of fluid an hour. When this occurs the patient becomes extremely dehydrated, and emergency measures must be undertaken. Vital signs, urinary output, weight and central venous pressure should be monitored frequently. The etiological factor of this phenomenon was once thought to be an osmotic diuresis from high serum urea or creatinine levels; however, it has recently been proven to result from tubular dysfunction. The renal tubules are unable to reabsorb adequate amounts of water and electrolytes, primarily sodium. An obligatory diuresis results, lasting up to 72 hours and always self-terminating. If the patient can be supported through the time of severe diuresis, the syndrome is reversible. Urinary volume and electrolytes should be observed, and should be replaced with an intravenous solution comparable in composition. After the initial 24 hour diuretic period, intravenous fluids can be slowly curtailed to prevent overhydration.

Intermittent Catheterization

In patients with acute urinary retention who are unable to withstand surgery, or in patients with chronic urinary retention who have a long-standing vesical dysfunction, continued catheterization may be indicated. Constant urethral catheterization with a Foley-type catheter for an extended period of time is acceptable, but multiple complications can develop. These include purulent urethritis, erosion of the glans penis in the male or urethral stretching and dilatation in the female, calculus formation around the catheter and the development of urinary tract infections. While a suprapubic catheter avoids the urethral complications, a foreign body is still present within the bladder, resulting in an increased incidence of infection and stone formation. An excellent alternative, providing long-term bladder decompression, is the use of intermittent catheterization.[6] This is especially advantageous in patients with a neurogenic bladder or those who are not candidates for surgical relief of outlet obstruction. With the use of intermittent catheterization, the incidence and severity of urinary tract infections is decreased and overdistention of the bladder is prevented. The patient is catheter-free and can ambulate without the use of a drainage bag. In addition, the procedure can be performed by the patient in the privacy of a bathroom or public commode.

Prior to institution of intermittent catheterization, urinary tract infections should be treated with appropriate antibiotics. To prevent overdistention of the bladder during the night, the patient should be restricted to 2500 cc of fluid between 6 A.M. and 6 P.M. and should have no fluids from 6 P.M. until the next morning. A catheterization schedule should be initiated every four hours. As the residual urine decreases in volume, the time schedule can be lengthened to every six hours or longer. If the residual urine is consistently over 500 cc on a four hour schedule, consideration should be given to catheterizing the patient every three hours.

Instruction in intermittent catheterization can be given to the patient by either a physician, a trained nurse or a urologic assistant. The male patient is initially taught to catheterize himself in the supine position, and, with experience, can accomplish the procedure either sitting or standing by the commode. The female is instructed to catheterize herself in the sitting position. In women, initial instruction is done using a mirror placed at the feet so that the patient may become accustomed to the anatomy and the location of the urethra. Catheterization in the male patient is performed with a No. 16 or No. 18 French reusable catheter. In the female, because of a short urethra, a No. 16 or No. 18 metal urethral sound or catheter is most beneficial. Under either condition, a clean, but not necessarily sterile, technique is used. The catheter or sound is washed in a soap solution and kept accessible at all times. It may be maintained in a container of acetic acid, vinegar or soap solution, or may be left dry in a polyethylene bag. At the time of catheterization, the patient removes the catheter or sound and washes his hands and the catheter in warm, soapy solution for three to five minutes. The urethral meatus is also cleansed with a soap solution and the catheter is well lubricated with sterile surgical lubricant. The catheter is then gently inserted by the patient until urine is obtained. There should never be an attempt by the patient to force the catheter into place. When urine ceases to flow, the catheter is simply removed and placed back within its container. The local instillation of a small amount of neomycin-polymyxin solution prior to removing the catheter will virtually eliminate the risk of a catheter induced infection. The patient should be instructed to see his physician if catheterization cannot be accomplished or if bleeding, pain or discomfort occur.

Intermittent catheterization has proven to be extremely safe, simple and convenient for the patient with a chronic bladder dysfunction. Naturally, it is not applicable in the presence of urethral strictures or marked bladder outlet obstruction when the patient will have difficulty entering the bladder. The incidence of urinary tract infections has been greatly reduced and many patients may be off antibiotics for years with a successful intermittent catheterization program.

HEMATURIA

The sudden presence of blood in the urine is alarming to the patient, and rapid diagnosis is essential to treat the disease and relieve the patient's anxiety. In a patient with gross hematuria, many items must be considered. These include the age and sex of the patient, the presence of predisposing factors, associated urological and nonurological symptoms, as well as whether blood is in the entire urinary stream or just in a portion of the stream. The etiology of blood in the urine involves careful examination of the entire urinary tract from the renal cortex to the meatus.

The causes of hematuria may be categorized as infection, calculus disease, trauma, neoplasm, glomerulopathy, blood dyscrasia and vascular insults. Under all circumstances a systematic, rational approach must be used to make the correct diagnosis and initiate treatment. While it is a well-documented fact that certain diseases involve patients in different population groups (as in young women developing acute hemorrhagic cystitis), it must be kept in mind that any patient who presents with an emergency condition of bleeding may have any condition in the above categories.

The initial step in patient evaluation is to obtain a thorough personal history. The presence of any known blood dyscrasias, a history of preceding blunt or sharp trauma and the location of abdominal, flank or back pains are all-important questions that must be answered. Ingestion of drugs, such as Coumadin or phenacetin, may cause hematuria. Any recent or long-standing urological complaints must be uncovered. Infection is often accompanied by urinary frequency, urgency and dysuria. Renal glomerulopathies may be associated with a recent upper respiratory infection, weight gain and peripheral swelling. Physical examination is equally important and may direct the physician to the source of the urinary bleeding. Easy bruisability and enlarged joints are frequently seen in hemophiliacs. The presence of back or costovertebral angle discomfort should arouse suspicions of renal etiology and it indicates renal lithiasis or neoplasm. Abdominal examination may reveal a palpable abdominal mass indicating a renal malignancy in adults or a Wilms' tumor in children. Tenderness in the bladder area may indicate cystitis or vesical neoplasms. A careful genital examination can reveal meatal stenosis, a urethral discharge, frequently seen in urethritis, or evidence of blunt genital trauma. The prostate examination can show firmness of adenocarcinoma of the prostate or the tender bogginess of prostatitis.

After the initial patient evaluation is complete, a three glass urine specimen is obtained. The patient is instructed to void the first 10 cc into the first glass. He is then instructed to continue voiding and a midstream clean-catch specimen is obtained in a second bottle. The termination portion of the stream is then placed in a third glass. All specimens are then examined for the presence of microscopical or macroscopical blood, white blood cells and bacteria. The presence of blood in the initial or terminal specimens and its absence in the midstream indicates that the origin of the disease is distal to the bladder neck. This implies a urethral or prostatic origin as in urethritis, prostatitis, benign prostatic hypertrophy (BPH) or adenocarcinoma of the prostate. If all three specimens show equal amounts of blood, then the patient has "total hematuria." This indicates bleeding proximal to the bladder neck involving the bladder, ureters, kidneys or vascular system.

Other initial laboratory examinations that are beneficial include serum prothrombin time, partial thromboplastin time, bleeding and clotting times, complete blood count, sickle cell preparation, renal function studies and tuberculin skin test. A urine culture should always be obtained and the urine examined for albumin, red cell casts and oval fat bodies.

When gross hematuria is accompanied by dysuria, suprapubic pain and/or frequency and urgency, a tentative diagnosis of urinary tract infection may be made. This can be further substantiated by the presence of white blood cells or bacteria in the urinary sediment. In these patients initial treatment with antibiotics can be instituted, and the hematuria should disappear within a 48 hour period. In all other patients with gross hematuria,

including patients with obvious genital or urinary trauma, urological and radiographic investigation should be initiated immediately. It is an axiom of urology that middle-aged patients with the sudden onset of total and painless hematuria have a bladder malignancy until proven otherwise.

Radiographic investigation should begin with the intravenous urogram searching for renal masses, ureteral or vesical calculi or filling defects in the renal pelvis, ureter or bladder, relating to blood clots or neoplasia. Delayed function and an enlarged silhouette are often seen in renal vein thrombosis. Renal tuberculosis, papillary necrosis, nephrolithiasis and other rare upper tract diseases can only be diagnosed with proper urographical technique. (Evaluation of trauma patients is discussed under a separate heading.) If the excretory urogram is not fruitful, urethroscopy and cystoscopy should be performed. Inflammation, calculus disease and malignancies of the urethra, prostate and bladder can be seen under direct vision. If these areas do not indicate the presence of bleeding, the right and left ureteral orifices should be observed, noting the presence of blood emanating from either or both. If hematuria is noted from a single ureteral orifice, a retrograde ureterogram and pyelogram should be obtained.

With proper radiographic and bacteriological techniques, most cases of hematuria can be diagnosed, including genitourinary malignancies, trauma, infections and urinary lithiasis. Bilateral hematuria seen from both ureteral orifices often implies glomerulopathy or blood dyscrasia. Further evaluation of the latter includes coagulation studies and hemoglobin electrophoresis. Blood count and bone marrow studies can reveal acute leukemia and thrombocytopenia as a cause of hematuria. Acute or chronic glomerulonephritis can be evaluated by obtaining 24 hour urine collections for creatinine and protein, serum titers for antistreptolysin and rheumatoid factors, lupus preparations and antinuclear antibody titers.

Occasionally all of the above examinations are negative and the patient continues to have hematuria. When this occurs, the clinician is left with a difficult puzzle to solve and the answer may only be obtained by invasive techniques, such as renal arteriography, to search for small renal cortical adenomas or arteriovenous fistulae. A renal biopsy will aid in the diagnosis of glomerulonephritis. While both of these techniques carry a slight risk to the patient, the clinician must decide whether this risk is worth the possible information gained. It is often necessary to make an accurate diagnosis of hematuria to relieve the patient's anxiety or assess the conditions for insurance purposes.

Total gross painless hematuria can be seen after stress or exercise, especially in young, athletic individuals. This is frequently encountered after extreme athletic exertion, such as playing basketball, football or in wrestling. It usually disappears within a 24 hour period. However, a routine investigation should always be performed to exclude any infections or malignancies.

HEMATOSPERMIA

The occurrence of blood in the semen or ejaculate can be a frightening and distressing symptom.[12] In most instances, hematospermia is an isolated sign and the patient is otherwise asymptomatic. If blood in the semen is associated with other urological complaints such as dysuria, hesitancy or hematuria, then urological investigations including excretory urography and diagnostic endoscopy should be performed. The urine should be examined microscopically and routine bacteriological and tuberculosis cultures should be obtained. In symptomatic patients, causes for hemospermia include malignancies of the seminal ves-

icles or prostate, prostatitis, trauma, hyperplasia of the seminal vesicles, cysts of the utricle, blood dyscrasias and masturbation. In a patient who is symptom-free and has had a recent change in his sexual activity, a single episode of hemospermia needs no further evaluation.

In the few patients in whom hemospermia persists despite a normal urological evaluation, a five to seven day course of diethylstilbestrol, 1 mg t.i.d., is often effective.

RENAL CALCULUS DISEASE

Clinical Presentation

Renal calculus disease occurs most frequently in white males during the second, third and fourth decades of life and usually presents with intermittent, acute, severe, colicky pain along the course of the urinary tract.[11, 13] Renal colic, when associated with microscopical hematuria, should lead the physician to the diagnosis of renal or ureteral lithiasis. Prompt medical attention is often needed to relieve the patient's suffering and also to prevent complications of hydronephrosis, pyelonephritis, sepsis and renal dysfunction. The pain originates in the flank and is associated with a dull ache or pressure in the area of the costovertebral angle. As the calculus progresses down the urinary tract and into the bladder, the pain will appropriately shift from the flank into the groin, radiating into the ipsilateral testis, or labium majus, and then to the medial aspect of the thigh. Nausea and vomiting are frequently present. The patient is extremely restless, constantly changing positions in an attempt to relieve the discomfort. The pain is episodic in nature, waxing and waning as ureteral peristalsis attempts to propel urine past a calculus blocking the lumen. As the stone enters the bladder, the pain may be suddenly relieved, only to be replaced again by urinary tenesmus and dysuria as the calculus is passed through the urethra and out the meatus.

On examination, the patient will exhibit tenderness in the costovertebral angle. Abdominal and peritoneal signs of guarding and rebound tenderness are occasionally present. At times the patient is diaphoretic and has a tachycardia. When fever or chills are present, an associated pyelonephritis must be considered.

Routine laboratory values will usually be normal, although a mild leukocytosis may be present. Urinalysis reveals microscopical hematuria in more than 80 per cent of cases, and crystals will occasionally be noted in the sediment. Identification of these crystals may correlate with the stone composition. The presence of large numbers of leukocytes in the urine may signify an associated urinary tract infection. When a calculus totally obstructs the ureter, the urine sediment can be normal, showing no red blood cells, white blood cells or crystals. As time permits, additional laboratory data should be obtained, including serum levels of calcium, phosphorus, uric acid, electrolytes, blood urea nitrogen and creatinine. Subsequent urinary studies should include a 24 hour urine collection for calcium oxalate, uric acid, urinary pH measurements and qualitative assays for cystine or other amino acids. A urine culture should always be obtained, especially when pyuria is present or when the patient appears toxic.

Roentgenographical evaluation is crucial to the diagnosis and therapy of patients with renal calculus disease. An initial scout film is helpful to determine the size and position of radiopaque calculi; however, 10 per cent of all stones are radiolucent and will be invisible on this x-ray. Any patient who is suspected of having renal calculus disease should have an emergency intravenous urogram to confirm the size and position of the stone as well as the degree of obstruction in the ipsilateral side and the condition of the contralateral collecting system. Frequently, delayed films will be necessary in order to adequately evaluate the renal system and document the position of the offending calculus. Renal calculi will most commonly obstruct at the levels of the ureteropelvic junction, the iliac crest with crossing vessels and the ureterovesical junction. Although these sites represent the narrowest portions of the ureteral lumen, it is the actual passage and peristalsis of the stone down the ureter which creates the extreme pain and discomfort. If the exact position of the calculus cannot be ascertained by routine intravenous urography, retrograde pyelograms may be necessary.

After the initial examination and radiographic evaluations are complete, patient management and therapy are initiated. Hospital admission is indicated when:

(1) the patient is septic with fever, chills or both,

(2) nausea and vomiting are so severe that intravenous hydration must be administered,

(3) pain is so severe that parenteral analgesics are required,

(4) when the obstruction occurs in a solitary kidney or

(5) if the stone is of large size.

The calculi within the ureter can be measured on the x-ray film. A stone measuring less than 6 mm in diameter will pass spontaneously in 90 per cent of patients, while a calculus greater than 6 mm will pass spontaneously in only 10 per cent of patients. Patients with small calculi may be followed clinically as outpatients with subsequent x-rays and excretory urograms to monitor the progress of the calculus. When a large stone is seen and there is dilatation of the ureter or renal pelvis above it, consideration must be given to admission and eventual surgery.

For outpatient treatment, adequate oral analgesia should be supplied and the patient should be instructed to consume fluids and be active in the hope that the calculus will pass. The urine should be strained through a gauze at all times in the hope of retrieving a passed stone and sending it for chemical analysis. Acute management of renal colic often requires administration of narcotics (morphine, Demerol, Dilaudid), which are nearly always useful. Antispasmodics and anticholinergic drugs are of limited value.

Pathogenesis

Evaluation of all patients who have passed renal calculi is vital and may be done on an ambulatory basis. Though 60 per cent of all renal calculi are idiopathic in origin, many instances of stone disease are associated with an increase in urinary crystalloid content. Hypercalciuric states are the most common predisposing phenomenon. A urinary calcium excretion of more than 375 mg per 24 hours (males) or 300 mg per 24 hrs (females) on a regular diet is strongly suggestive of idiopathic hypercalciuria. Hypercalciuria is also associated with hyperparathyroidism, renal tubular acidosis and vitamin D intoxication. Hyperoxaluric conditions prevail in patients who have had an increased ingestion of oxalate, primary hyperoxaluria, in patients with gastrointestinal diseases such as regional enteritis or in patients who have had an intestinal bypass procedure for extreme obesity.

Increased production of uric acid is seen in patients with gout, myeloproliferative disorders and in those maintained on antimetabolic drugs. Those patients with chronic diarrhea and individuals with an ileostomy may have hyperuricosuria and form radiolucent uric acid calculi. Struvite stones (magnesium ammonium phosphate) are associated with urea splitting microorganisms and are commonly seen in conjunction with Proteus infections. These patients often have a large staghorn calculus; portions of this stone may fragment and pass down the collecting system, causing renal colic.

Treatment

After the initial therapy, consideration must be given to preventing further episodes of renal stone formation. Regardless of the type of stone, dilution of urine by increasing water intake, particularly at night, is an important component of any long-term treatment regimen. Surgical procedures may be required to relieve urinary stasis, and antibiotics may be necessary to treat infections. An alteration in urine pH has been used in an attempt to increase the solubility of urine crystals. Urinary acidification is thought to be beneficial in treating struvite and calcium phosphate calculi.

Urinary alkalinization with sodium bicarbonate, to elevate the pH to 7.0 or greater, has proved beneficial in the treatment of patients with uric acid stones. In addition, these patients should be placed on allopurinol, 300 per day, to decrease uric acid output. In the syndrome of idiopathic hypercalciuria, hydrochlorothiazide, 50 mg b.i.d., has been found to decrease calcium clearance and increase the urinary excretion of magnesium, a potential inhibitor of stone formation. Oral phosphates may also lower urinary calcium levels and may be administered in the form of cellulose phosphate or orthophosphate. Cystine calculi can be managed by hydration with 4000 ml of fluid a day, urinary alkalinization and the administration of penicillamine when necessary. When renal tubular acidosis has been diagnosed, the urine should be alkalinized with sodium bicarbonate or

Shohl's solution (magnesium citrate–calcium carbonate).

Occasionally ureteral obstruction by other materials, such as a blood clot or sloughed renal papilla, may cause renal colic. In these cases, hospitalization is usually warranted to evaluate the underlying condition. Both blood clots and sloughed renal papilla should pass spontaneously. However, retrograde ureterograms may be necessary to make the diagnosis, as both of these substances are radiolucent.

ACUTE INTRASCROTAL DISORDERS

In the absence of genital injury with its well advertised signs — ecchymoses, hematoma or puncture wounds — the acute onset of testicular pain in any male is urological emergency and requires rapid and accurate diagnosis. Differential diagnosis of an acute unilateral process includes torsion of the spermatic cord, torsion of a testicular appendage, acute epididymitis or orchitis, strangulated inguinal hernia, scrotal abscess and hemorrhage into a neoplasm. All of these disorders can present with sudden and severe testicular pain and prompt evaluation is mandatory. Because torsion of the spermatic cord may result in testicular ischemia and necrosis, this diagnosis must always be suspected. Acute epididymitis may occur at any age, although it usually involves males who are past the first decade of life.

Torsion of the Spermatic Cord (Fig. 19–5)

This disorder may occur in any age group but it primarily affects children and young adolescents. Two types of torsion may occur: intravaginal and extravaginal. Extravaginal torsion occurs when the entire tunica vagin-

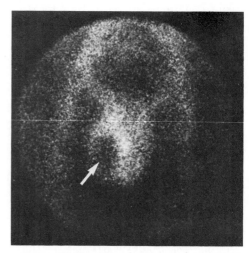

Figure 19–5 Torsion of spermatic cord. ^{99}Tc scan in patient with torsion of right testis, showing decreased blood supply (arrow) on side with pain.

alis with its contained testis and spermatic cord structures twists within the scrotum. This primarily occurs in newborns owing to a greater mobility of the cord. Any neonate with a scrotal mass may need emergency exploration in order to preserve testicular viability. Intravaginal torsion is more common and occurs in a testis that lacks the normal epididymal attachment of the tunica vaginalis ("bell-clapper testes"). In these patients, the testis is allowed to swing freely within the tunica vaginalis and becomes twisted.

Although trauma and exertion may contribute to the development of spermatic cord torsion, the twisting can occur spontaneously while the patient is at rest or during sleep. Other factors reported to contribute to testicular torsion are cryptorchidism, Marfan's syndrome and Henoch-Schönlein purpura. Sudden onset of unilateral testicular pain is often associated with abdominal pain, nausea and vomiting. The testis on the involved side is usually retracted and higher than the contralateral testis. There is a marked absence of any other signs and symptoms. The patient usually denies any voiding symptoms including dysuria, urgency and frequency, and blood counts and urinalyses are unremarkable.

Upon examination the testis appears diffusely enlarged and tender. The spermatic cord is also enlarged and painful to palpation. The normal cleavage plane between the testis and epididymis cannot be felt and the overlying scrotal skin appears normal. Occasionally a reactive hydrocele may form, making examination more difficult.

As the spermatic cord twists a full two or three revolutions, vascular obstruction to the testis occurs. Venous circulation is interrupted, causing edema in the cord. This in turn will result in increased pressure within the cord and eventually stop arterial flow. The need for prompt detorsion is obvious. If accomplished early, manual external derotation is often successful.[5] Because the right testis rotates clockwise and the left testis twists counterclockwise, reversing these maneuvers will often accomplish detorsion. Multiple revolutions must be made to completely detorse a twisted testis but when this is accomplished the pain is dramatically relieved. Even if this procedure is successful, surgical intervention is needed because recurrent torsion is likely.

Since testicular ischemia will result in damage after a period of 24 to 36 hours, rapid diagnosis is important. Radionucleotide imaging of the scrotum or a testicular scan has been of great benefit in differentiating testicular torsion from other intrascrotal disorders.[4] After the injection of radioactive material (technetium pertechnetate), the genital area is scanned. In cases of testicular torsion there will be a decreased blood supply on the side of the pain (Fig. 19–5), while in episodes of acute epididymitis, orchitis or abscess formation, the blood supply will be equal or increased (Fig. 19–6).

Ultrasound of testes using the Doppler apparatus can also be of benefit when comparing the audible pulses of one testis to the other. Blood flow will be decreased in the presence of spermatic cord torsion.

The diagnosis of testicular torsion requires prompt surgical exploration with detorsion of the involved testis. When testicular necrosis has occurred, orchiectomy is indicated. In matters of questionable viability, the testis should be left in situ, for recovery may occur. Intrascrotal fixation of both tests should always be performed, since the developmental anomaly predisposing to torsion may exist bilaterally. The necessity for prompt intervention is demonstrated by statistics indicating an 85 per cent salvage rate in patients explored within 24 hours of onset of symptoms. This falls to only 25 per cent if the surgery is delayed for more than 72 hours.

Acute Epididymitis (Fig. 19–6)

An epididymitis is the most common intrascrotal inflammation seen in

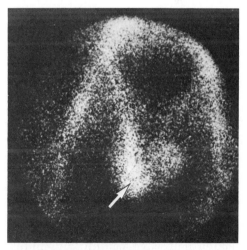

Figure 19–6 Epididymitis. ^{99}Tc scan in patient with epididymitis of right testis, showing increased blood supply (arrow) on side with pain.

the adult. Though this disorder seldom occurs prior to the third decade, it may occur in children or adolescents. Acute epididymitis in young men may be related to vesical outlet obstruction, ectopic ureters or urinary tract infections. Epididymal inflammation is often associated with dysuria, urgency, and frequency, and in those cases a bacterial infection may be the cause. In many young adults there is no urinary symptomatology and the disease may originate from reflux of sterile urine along the vas deferens during straining or heavy exercise. Chronic infections of the epididymis by syphilis or tuberculosis are rare.

Acute epididymitis presents with sharp, though not precipitous, unilateral testicular pain and tenderness. When the patient is initially examined, this pain will be localized to the epididymis at the posterior and inferior aspect of the testis (globus minor). Swelling and induration of the epididymis will occur as the disease progresses. Further enlargement and induration of the epididymis obliterates the normal epididymal testicular sulcus. Under these circumstances, the epididymis and testes may appear as a single mass. However, the testis in itself is not painful. If the progression of the disease proceeds unchecked, epididymo-orchitis may result, with a painful and enlarged testicular mass within a reddened and edematous scrotal sac. Pain and tenderness may be intense, frequently extending along the entire spermatic cord. In some cases adequate clinical evaluation is impossible, and a spermatic cord block is required for examination. Manual elevation of the testes frequently produces symptomatic relief (Prehn's sign).

The patient with a urinary tract infection may have voiding difficulties. Fever, chills and leukocytosis are common. Urine sediment will reveal numerous white cells and bacteria.

Urine cultures should be obtained on all patients. In young adults the differential diagnosis between acute epididymitis and spermatic cord torsion may be difficult. A radionucleotide study of the scrotum or a testes scan will be beneficial in distinguishing these patients. Blood flow to the involved side will be increased in the presence of inflammation. Occasionally this differentiation is difficult to make, and prompt exploration may be required to rule out testicular torsion.

The treatment of acute epididymitis begins with oral or parenteral antibiotics, according to the condition of the patient. If urine cultures are negative, antibiotic therapy may be discontinued. Complete bedrest is recommended during the acute stage of the disease. Scrotal elevation will usually provide significant relief in conjunction with local applications of heat or cold. Effective elevation is provided by placing a pillow between the legs and under the scrotum or by construcing a bridge of broad strips of adhesive tape passed between the upper anterior thighs. When the patient is ambulatory, a scrotal support should be worn at all times. Analgesia and antiinflammatory measures may be required. Frequently administered aspirin and oxyphenbutazone (Tandearil) can be beneficial. After the acute inflammation has subsided the patient is allowed to ambulate slowly. Though the pain and local symptoms will usually subside after three to five days, complete resolution of the enlargement and induration takes weeks or months. Repeated episodes of epididymitis, often in conjunction with sepsis, raises the possibility of a resistant or recurrent urinary tract infection and a predisposing cause should be suspected.

If treatment is delayed or inadequate, a testicular abscess may result, noted as fluctuance of the testes on examination. Tuberculosis must always be considered under these circumstances. Drainage of a testicular abscess is not adequate and orchiectomy must be accomplished. Recurrent episodes of epididymitis can be prevented by performing a bilateral vasectomy or epididymectomy.

Torsion of a Testicular Appendage

Patients with a torsion of either the appendix testes or appendix epididymis show symptoms similar to individuals with torsion of the testes or with acute epididymitis. Severe unilateral testicular pain is present and tenderness is localized over the upper pole of the involved testis. This pain is usually sudden in onset and radiates up into the lower abdomen. Hemiscrotal edema and a reactive hydrocele may form and become extensive. There is a marked absence of associated urological symptoms. The patients lack the fever and chills frequently seen with acute epididymitis and have a normal urine sediment and blood cell count.

The incidence of at least one unilateral epididymal or testicular appendage has been reported as 75 per cent. The appendix testes, a remnant of the embryological Müllerian duct structures, account for over 95 per cent of the appendiceal torsions. Both the appendix testes and appendix epididymis reside near the junction of the globus major of the epididymis and the superior pole of the testis anteriorly.

Examination of patients with acute torsion of a testicular appendage will reveal a tenderness immediately over the globus major, accompanied by a hard, pea-sized mass representing the torsed appendage. Transillumination occasionally reveals a bluish dot in the region of the upper pole of the testis, the "blue-dot sign." If a definite diagnosis can be made, these patients are treated conservatively with bedrest and ice packs. The involved appendage will infarct and later calcify, forming a free floating intrascro-

tal mass. If a definitive diagnosis cannot be made, nuclear scanning of the scrotum will be beneficial. In the absence of a firm diagnosis, emergency exploration to rule out a potential testicular torsion is indicated.

Abscess of the Scrotal Skin

A subcutaneous collection of purulent material may form in an epidermoid cyst or hair follicle within the scrotal skin. This lesion commonly occurs in young men past adolescence. In contrast to a periurethral abscess, there is a marked absence of any voiding or urinary symptoms. A slowly enlarging, tender, fluctuant mass will develop on the inferior portion of the scrotum. Intrascrotal contents including testes, epididymis and spermatic cord will be uninvolved. These patients are in extreme discomfort and have difficulty ambulating. The most common etiological organism in the abscess is a *Staphylococcus* and proper treatment involves incision and drainage with irrigation of debris. After bacteriological cultures, the incised area is packed with gauze and the patient is instructed in local wound care, including warm baths and frequent dressing changes. An appropriate antibiotic is given.

Periurethral Abscess

A periurethral collection of pus represents extravasation of infected urine in the perineum and requires a prompt diagnosis and definitive treatment. Periurethral abscesses are seen in older men and usually are preceded by recurrent urinary tract infections and urethral strictures. As the bladder empties against an increased urethral resistance, infected urine is forced through a small rent in the urethral wall, resulting in perineal contamination. Bacteria proliferate in a closed space and result in a midline perineal mass. These patients often have fever and chills and marked voiding symptoms, distinguishing them from patients with a subcutaneous scrotal abscess. A retrograde urethrogram will demonstrate the degree and site of the stricture and the urinary extravasation. The mass is in the perineal midline and no true fluctuance is present. Urinalysis will reveal leukocytes and, frequently, bacteria.

In the presence of urinary extravasation, simple incision and drainage is not adequate and will result in a urethrocutaneous fistula. In addition to parenteral antibiotics, thorough vesical decompression must be accomplished to allow the urethra to heal. A urethral catheter is inappropriate because the stricture makes passage difficult and the presence of a foreign body will perpetuate the infection and prevent proper healing. These patients should be treated with suprapubic urinary diversion and drainage of the abscess. After the infection has subsided and urethral integrity has been re-established, the stricture may be treated by dilation, internal urethrotomy or urethroplasty. A recurring periurethral abscess or persistent urethrocutaneous fistula is highly suggestive of genital tuberculosis or an occult carcinoma of the urethra.

PHIMOSIS AND PARAPHIMOSIS

A narrow opening in the prepuce that prevents it from being drawn back over the glans is called phimosis. Paraphimosis exists when the prepuce is retracted sufficiently proximal to the glans penis to allow for development of circumferential edema. Reduction then becomes progressively difficult and painful. Paraphimosis may occur in an unconscious or debilitated patient in whom the prepuce was retracted to allow for cleansing or catheterization, and also in infants whose mothers have been instructed to retract the foreskin for cleansing. If left untreated, venous return from the glans penis will be impeded, causing increased edema and swelling of the glans. As this edema progresses, the constrictive band of foreskin becomes tighter and results in ischemia.

Treatment of paraphimosis consists of several maneuvers performed sequentially until reduction occurs (Fig. 19–7). The first technique involves placing the thumbs on the glans, producing countertraction against the second and third fingers of both hands placed on either side and behind the preputial contraction ring. Counterpressure is then applied until reduction occurs. The applica-

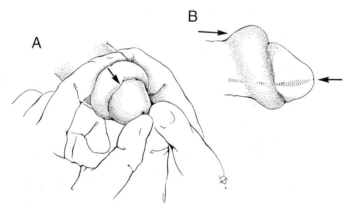

Figure 19–7 Reduction of paraphimosis. *A.* Manual reduction, demonstrating counter-pressure between thumbs and fingers *(B).*

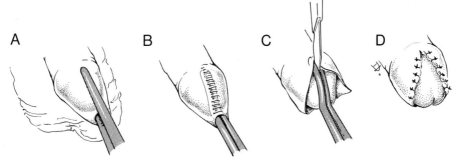

Figure 19–8 Preputial dorsal slit. *A.* Application of hemostat in vertical midline to depth of ½ to 1 cm distal to corona. *B.* Insertion of grooved director. *C.* Incision of clamped tissue. *D.* Application of absorbable suture. A running hemostatic suture is usually preferable to the interrupted stitches shown here.

tion of liquid soap or mineral oil about the corona will ease this maneuver. Circumferential or quandrantal injection of hyaluronidase around the constricting band may facilitate reduction. Occasionally, constant manual pressure on the glans will induce decompression of the edema fluid, making reduction easier. Success has also been obtained with the application of Babcock clamps to the retraction ring, exerting gentle and continuous traction. If all of these maneuvers fail, a dorsal slit is usually successful. Figure 19–8 shows a dorsal slit being performed for phimosis. For paraphimosis, a 2 or 3 cm midline dorsal vertical incision is carried from a point proximal to the constricting ring across this band and onto the distal aspect of the edematous foreskin. The raw edges can be secured with sutures to prevent hemorrhage. If paraphimosis recurs, circumcision should be performed.

PRIAPISM

This is a relatively rare condition of persistent painful erection, often totally unrelated to sexual activity.[7] The onset may be initiated by sexual stimulation, although priapism affects only the corpora cavernosa and spares the corpora spongiosum and glans penis. If treatment is delayed or unsuccessful, impotence is the common sequela.

The pathophysiology of priapism has not been clarified and its natural history has never been fully documented. Fifty per cent of such cases are idiopathic in origin. Several causative factors related to priapism are sickle cell disease or trait, anticoagulation with warfarin or Coumadin, trauma, cancer of the bladder or prostate involving the penis, syphilis, polycythemia and leukemia.

A general therapeutic policy in the treatment of priapism is an immediate search for and treatment of any etiological factor. In idiopathic priapism, initial medical therapy includes sedation, analgesia, ice packs and enemas. If these initial steps are unsuccessful the patient may undergo epidural anesthesia, the administration of proteolytic enzymes and infusion of low molecular weight dextran. When the response to these measures is poor and there is no contraindication to an operation, aspiration of the corpora is done with heparin under spinal anesthesia. If this aspiration fails to cause detumescence, a surgical shunt of the cavernosus-saphenous vein or cavernosum-corpus spongiosum type should be performed immediately. In spite of the use of the best medical and surgical therapy, one-half of the cases result in long-term impotence.

AMBULATORY UROLOGY

Venereal Diseases

Gonococcal Urethritis

Gonorrhea is the most commonly reported communicable disease in the U.S.A. The number of reported cases of gonorrhea in the United States has tripled in the decade from 1966 to 1976 and it is recognized that many cases of the disease go unreported, so that the true incidence is probably several times higher. It has been estimated that up to 80 per cent of gonorrhea infected women are asymptomatic and the greatest problem in controlling the spread of gonorrhea is the existence of a vast reservoir of asymptomatic and hence unidentified infections in the female population. Ten to twenty per cent of infected females may have some complaints of vaginal discharge, dysuria, lower abdominal pains or other non-specific complaints. In fact, there are no signs or symptoms specifically diagnostic of gonorrhea in women.

In men, gonococcal urethritis typically occurs three to five days after exposure. Male patients with gonorrhea are symptomatic in the vast majority of cases and present with a clinical picture that is easily recognizable on gross examination. The patient usually complains of a yellowish urethral discharge that is often profuse, accompanied by dysuria and increased frequency of urination. He may occasionally experience symptoms of epididymitis and prostatitis and, more rarely, systemic symptoms including arthritis (most commonly involving the wrist, ankle and knee), ophthalmia, endocarditis, hepatitis and meningitis.

DIAGNOSIS. Women:

(1) Specimens should be obtained from the endocervical and anal canals and inoculated separately onto modified Thayer-Martin medium (MTM). In a screening situation only culture specimens from the endocervical canal may be required.

(2) All women treated for gonorrhea should have repeat culture done as a test for cure.

(3) Oropharyngeal specimens should be obtained from all patients suspected of having disseminated gonococcal infections or pharyngeal gonococcal infections and should be inoculated on an MTM medium. Once pharyngeal gonococcal infection has been demonstrated, at least two pharyngeal specimens should be obtained after treatment in order to document cure.

Gram stain or fluorescent antibody stain smears are *not recommended* for the diagnosis of gonorrhea in women. Although Gram stain smears from the endocervical canal may be quite specific when examined by well trained personnel, they are not sensitive enough to rule out gonorrhea. Neither Gram stain nor fluorescent antibody stain smears are recommended as a test of cure in women.

Men:

(1) The microscopic demonstration of typical gram-negative intracellular diplococci on a smear of a urethral exudate constitutes sufficient basis for the diagnosis of gonorrhea. Prepare the slide by *rolling* the swab on the slide. *Do not* rub the swab on the slide, because microscopic morphology will be distorted. If gram-negative diplococci cannot be identified on direct smear of the discharge, a culture specimen should be obtained from the anterior urethra and inoculated on MTM medium.

(2) In homosexual men, additional culture specimens should be obtained from the anal canal and the oropharynx and inoculated on MTM medium.

(3) Tests to determine the ade-

quacy of treatment and ensure cure are recommended for all men treated for gonorrhea, and all sites that were found to be infected before therapy should be re-treated. This is accomplished by inoculating a culture specimen from these sites on MTM medium.

(4) As in women, once pharyngeal gonococcal infection has been demonstrated, at least two pharyngeal specimens should be obtained after treatment in order to document cure.

(5) Fluorescent antibody staining of smears of the urethral discharge is not recommended in men and a negative gram stain of the discharge should not be accepted as evidence of cure.

Any patient with the presumptive diagnosis of gonococcal urethritis should receive immediate antibiotic therapy without waiting for diagnostic confirmation. The advice of some authorities is to treat prophylactically any female exposed to gonorrhea regardless of the absence of symptoms and a negative culture.

All patients treated for gonorrhea should undergo serological testing for syphilis at the time of treatment and a follow-up test each month for four months to detect syphilis that might have been partially masked by therapy for the gonorrhea. Treatment schedules recommended by the U.S. Department of Health, Education and Welfare Center for Disease Control are outlined in Table 19–2.

Syphilis

With some 80,000 cases reported annually and an estimated 540,000 unreported, syphilis ranks fourth in frequency among communicable diseases in the United States. The resurgence of this disease and its medical and social implications present a serious problem that demands astute medical attention, investigation and therapy.

CLINICAL COURSE. During development the disease progresses from primary and secondary syphilis, marked by mucocutaneous lesions, to tertiary noninfectious stages during which the infection is latent but produces granulomatous complications that may involve any organ or system.

The primary stage of syphilis becomes apparent after an incubation period that may range from 10 to 90 days. The primary lesion (chancre) appears at the site of the inoculation, usually within three weeks after the infection. The site of the primary lesion may be extragenital (for example, in the rectum, perineal area, oral mucosa or breast), so it may often be overlooked. The typical chancre of primary syphilis is solitary, indurated and painless, with a smooth base. Atypical lesions are common, and therefore all genital lesions and suspicious extragenital lesions should be examined for *Treponema pallidum*. Regional adenopathy is common. A positive darkfield microscopic examination establishes the diagnosis, but a negative result requires repeat examination on three consecutive days. Since only 25 per cent of patients have positive serological studies during the first week of the appearance of the chancre, such studies may be positive or negative at the time of the darkfield examination. This figure increases by 25 per cent with each successive week so that by the fourth week, virtually all patients will have a positive serological reaction. Failure to demonstrate *T. pallidum* on darkfield examination does not totally exclude the diagnosis of syphilis, since not enough organisms may be present for an adequate examination. Repeated examination or aspiration of an enlarged regional lymph node is necessary to demonstrate the organism in some patients. At the time of the patient's initial visit, a reagin test for syphilis (VDRL or RPR) should

TABLE 19–2 Recommended Treatment Schedule For Gonorrhea

Since the efficacy of penicillin therapy for gonorrhea was first demonstrated in 1943, there has been an increasing problem of resistance of the organism to penicillin. Until recently this resistance was relative, not absolute, and required increasing dosages of penicillin to effect a cure. However, in 1976, a new strain of gonorrhea was introduced into the U.S. which is totally resistant to penicillin. This organism is called Penicillinase Producing Neisseria Gonorrhoeae (PPNG), which produces a beta-lactamase or penicillinase that destroys penicillin. The presence of PPNG makes a "test of cure" culture mandatory for all patients treated for gonorrhea. If the patient has not responded to therapy with penicillin, ampicillin or tetracycline, spectinomycin therapy should be given as outlined below.

UNCOMPLICATED GONORRHEA IN MEN AND WOMEN
The treatment of choice is aqueous procaine penicillin G, 4,800,000 units IM, divided into at least two doses and injected at different sites at one visit, together with 1 gm probenecid by mouth just before the injection.

Prophylactic or epidemiological treatment for gonorrhea (male or female) is accomplished with the same treatment schedules as for the uncomplicated gonorrhea.

ALTERNATIVE REGIMENS
(1) Patients in whom oral therapy is preferred: Ampicillin, 3.5 gm by mouth, plus 1 gm probenecid by mouth at the same time. There is evidence that this regimen may be slightly less effective than the IM penicillin.

(2) Patients who are allergic to the penicillins or probenecid: Tetracycline hydrochloride, 1.5 gm initially, by mouth, followed by 0.5 gm, by mouth, 4 times per day for 4 days. (Total dosage: 9.5 gm). Other tetracyclines are not more effective than tetracycline hydrochloride. All tetracyclines are ineffective as single dose therapy.

TREATMENT AND COMPLICATIONS
Test of cure cultures are mandatory at approximately five to seven days after therapy, as discussed above. In the male, a Gram stain is adequate if positive; otherwise a culture specimen should be obtained from the anterior urethra. In the female, a culture specimen should be obtained from both the endocervical and anal canals.

A positive culture after adequate treatment with the regimens outlined above using procaine penicillin G, ampicillin or tetracycline therapy is an indication that the organism is a penicillinase-producing *Neisseria gonorrhoeae.* Patients should be re-treated with spectinomycin hydrochloride, 2 gm IM, in one injection. Test of cure cultures should again be performed 7 to 14 days after treatment.

NOT RECOMMENDED
Although long acting forms of penicillin (such as benzathine penicillin G) are effective in the therapy of syphilis, they have *no* place in the treatment of gonorrhea. In addition, oral penicillin preparations such as penicillin V are not recommended for treatment of gonococcal infections.

SEROLOGICAL TESTS FOR SYPHILIS
All patients treated for gonorrhea should have a serological test for syphilis at the time of treatment. Seronegative patients without clinical signs of syphilis who are receiving the recommended parenteral penicillin schedule need not have follow-up serological tests for syphilis. Patients treated with ampicillin, spectinomycin or tetracycline should have a follow-up serological test after three months to detect any inadequately treated syphilis.

Patients with gonorrhea who also have syphilis should be given additional treatment appropriate to the stage of syphilis.

(U.S. Public Health Service, Center for Disease Control, 1976.)

be obtained. Patients with typical lesions and a reactive reagin test should be treated for primary syphilis even if the darkfield examination is negative. Treponemal serological tests are *not* recommended in the presence of a nonreactive test, regardless of the nature of the lesion. If the initial reagin test is nonreactive, repeat tests should be performed one week, one month and three months later. Nonreactive reagin tests over three months exclude syphilis as the cause of the lesion.

Secondary syphilis generally appears within six months, typically six to eight weeks after exposure, at which time the chancre is usually healing. The patients may have highly variable skin lesions, usually bilaterally symmetrical, macular, papular or papulosquamous in appearance. Mucous membrane lesions, lymphadenopathy, fever, alopecia or local organ involvement are not uncommon. The demonstration of *T. pallidum* in material from lesions and lymph nodes in such patients provides proof of syphilitic infection. A reagin test should be obtained in all patients suspected of having syphilis. Patients are considered to have syphilis if they have a reactive serological test and a physical examination consistent with the disease, even if the direct tests for spirochetes are negative. Patients with atypical findings or VDRL titers of less than 1:16 should have repeat reagin tests and a treponemal test to confirm syphilitic infection. Virtually all patients with secondary syphilis have reactive reagin tests. Therefore, the diagnosis of secondary syphilis is extremely unlikely if a reagin test for syphilis is nonreactive.

Patients with early syphilis should be seen at three month intervals for at least one year following diagnosis. At each visit a quantitative reagin test for syphilis should be obtained. The reagin titer declines in most patients during the course of the one year follow-up, until little or no reaction is detected.

A cerebrospinal fluid examination should be done on those patients who receive therapy other than the recommended penicillin regimen. Treatment schedules recommended by the U.S. Department of Health, Education and Welfare Center for Disease Control are outlined in Table 19–3.

Lymphogranuloma Venereum (Lymphopathia Venereum: Tropical Bubo)

This disease is caused by *Chlamydia trachomatis*. Following an incubation period of 3 to 30 days, a typical initial sign is a small, local, papular vesicle that heals spontaneously and is often overlooked. The patient usually shows unilateral, painful, inguinal adenopathy with nodes palpable both above and below the inguinal ligaments. Systemic symptoms that often appear during the initial stage of infection include arthralgia, abdominal pain, fever, chills and headache. Suppuration and fistula formation from the regional lymph nodes frequently occur. Diagnosis relies upon the sexual history, the appearance and the evolution of the lesions and serological studies. Syphilis is excluded by a negative darkfield examination. A positive complement fixation test against *C. trachomatis* is diagnostic. Severe scarring in the urethra or rectum may occur in the late stages of this disease. Tetracycline, 0.5 gm 4 times a day orally, is the treatment of choice.

Chancroid (Soft Chancre)

Chancroid is caused by *Hemophilus ducreyi* and is highly contagious if wounds or abrasions are present. Although lesions are usually genital, oral inoculation is common and extragenital lesions occur. Clinically, the lesions appear following an incubation period of one to five days and present as multiple soft tender papules which soon thereafter become pustular in appearance. The pustules then rupture, leaving a dirty, painful ulcer with a grayish base and undermined indurated edges, the so-called "soft chancre." Both the lesions and the associated adenopathy, often more pronounced on one side, are quite painful. The diagnosis relies on the history, gross appearance of the lesion by direct stain, smear or cultures. Some chancroid patients have low titer, false positive serological tests for syphilis. A significant incidence of treatment failure has shown the need for protracted treatment pro-

TABLE 19-3 Recommended Treatment Schedule For Syphilis

EARLY SYPHILIS (Primary, secondary, latent syphilis of less than one year's duration)
Rx: Benzathine Penicillin G, 2,400,000 units total by intramuscular injection at a single session.
Because effective therapy is given at a single visit, benzathine penicillin G is the drug of choice.
Or: Aqueous Penicillin G, 4,800,000 units total; 600,000 units by intramuscular injection daily for 8 days.
Or: Procaine Penicillin G in oil with 2% monostearate (PAM), 4,800,000 units by intramuscular injection; 2,400,000 units at the first visit and 1,200,000 units at each of two subsequent visits three days apart. (PAM is no longer available for use in the United States.)

Patients Allergic to Penicillin:
Rx: Tetracycline hydrochloride, 500 mg 4 times a day, by mouth, for 15 days. Food and some dairy products interfere with the absorption of tetracycline. *All forms of tetracycline should be given one hour before or two hours after meals.*
Or: Erythromycin (stearate, ethylsuccinate or base), 500 mg 4 times a day, by mouth, for 15 days.

SYPHILIS OF MORE THAN ONE YEAR'S DURATION (Latent syphilis of undetermined origin of more than one year's duration, cardiovascular, late benign, neurosyphilis)
Rx: Benzathine penicillin, 7,200,000 units total; 2,000,000 units by intramuscular injection, once weekly for three successive weeks.
Or: Aqueous procaine penicillin G, 9,000,000 units total; 600,000 units by intramuscular injection, daily for 15 days.
Although therapy is recommended for established cardiovascular syphilis, there is little evidence that antibiotics reverse the pathology associated with this disease.
Cerebrospinal fluid examination is mandatory in patients with suspected symptomatic neurosyphilis. This examination is also desirable in other patients with syphilis of greater than one year's duration, to exclude asymptomatic neurosyphilis.

Patients Allergic to Penicillin:
Rx: Tetracycline hydrochloride, 500 mg, 4 times a day, by mouth, for 30 days.
Or: Erythromycin (stearate, ethylsuccinate or base), 500 mg, 4 times a day, by mouth, for 30 days.

SYPHILIS IN PREGNANCY
Syphilis in pregnancy should be managed in the same manner as in the nonpregnant patient. Urgency of treatment is the keynote of therapy. Erythromycin estolate and tetracycline are not recommended for syphilitic infections in pregnant women because of potential adverse effects on mother and fetus.

FOLLOW-UP AND RE-TREATMENT
All patients with early syphilis and congenital syphilis should have a repeat quantitative nontreponemal test 3, 6, and 12 months after treatment. Patients with syphilis of more than one year's duration should have a repeat serological test 24 months after treatment. Careful follow-up is particularly important in patients treated with antibiotics other than penicillin. An examination of the cerebrospinal fluid should be planned as part of the last follow-up visit after treatment with alternative antibiotics.
All patients with neurosyphilis must be carefully followed with serological testing for at least three years. Follow-up of these patients should include clinical re-evaluation at six month intervals and repeat cerebrospinal fluid examinations, particularly in patients treated with alternative antibiotics.
The possibility of reinfection should always be considered when re-treating patients with early syphilis. A spinal fluid examination should be performed before re-treatment unless reinfection and a diagnosis of early syphilis can be established.
Re-treatment should be considered when
(1) Clinical signs or symptoms of syphilis persist or recur.
(2) There is a sustained fourfold increase in the titer of a nontreponemal test.
(3) An initial high titer nontreponemal test fails to decrease fourfold within a year.
Patients should be re-treated with the schedules recommended for syphilis of more than one year's duration.

EPIDEMIOLOGICAL TREATMENT
Patients who have been exposed to infectious syphilis within the preceding three months and other patients who, on epidemiological grounds, are at high risk for syphilis should be treated as for early syphilis. Every effort should be made to establish the diagnosis in these cases.

(U.S. Public Health Service, Center for Disease Control, 1976.)

grams. Treatment consists of intravenous cephalothin, 3 gm daily for 5 to 15 days.

Herpes Genitalis

Herpes genitalis is an infection due to Type 2 herpes simplex virus. The incidence of infections with this virus has increased precipitously over the past twenty years. Before 1965, this disease was not often seen or considered in the differential diagnosis of venereal diseases. At present it is, in some areas, more common than gonorrhea. There is an extremely high prevalence of the disease among females. Epidemiological studies indicate that from 10 to 30 per cent of the total female population may have been infected at some time with Type 2 herpes simplex virus.

The incubation period ranges from three to six days. Typically, the patient presents with 2 to 3 mm vulvar or penile vesicular lesions that burst within one to four days. Spontaneous healing usually occurs within one to three weeks. During the primary stage, nonsuppurative inguinal lymphadenopathy is often present. The diagnosis can be made by careful clinical observation. In females in whom the lesions may be limited to the cervix, the simplest method is to prepare a standard Pap smear for the exudate of the herpetic lesions. Multinucleated giant cells with nuclear inclusion bodies are characteristic of herpes virus infection. The therapy of this disease is limited to improved hygiene and specific treatment of superinfection. It is important to advise patients to abstain from intercourse or to use condoms during the active and convalescent stages of infection.

There is a strong association between herpes genitalis infection and cervical carcinoma. More than 90 per cent of women with invasive carcinoma of the cervix are found to have Type 2 herpes simplex virus. Thus, patients with herpes cervicitis are clearly at risk; annual Pap smears throughout the life of the patient are recommended for all women with genital herpetic infection.

There is no specific therapy for herpes genitalis. Recently some authors have advocated the application of ether to the vesicles as a specific therapy to destroy the herpes virus.

Condyloma Acuminata

Condyloma acuminata is characterized by verrucal warts of viral etiology occurring on the mucous membranes and skin of the genitalia, including the penis, scrotum, perineum and anus. Lesions most commonly occur under the prepuce in the male, and involvement of the frenulum and urethral meatus is not uncommon. Sexual transmission occurs, and an incubation period of several weeks to months may be present. Diagnosis relies exclusively on clinical appearance. Treatment may include surgical excision, electrocautery or, most effectively, local application of 10 to 25 per cent podophyllin suspension in tincture of benzoin. Application of podophyllin should be accompanied by instructions for local soap and water cleansing after four hours to prevent chemical burn. In the presence of meatal lesions, panendoscopy is essential to rule out intraurethral involvement, in which case endoscopic electrofulguration is indicated.

Molluscum Contagiosum

This is a viral disease that may occur anywhere on the body. Genital occurrence may rely on venereal contact, however. Following an incubation period of three to six weeks, waxy, firm, smooth umbilicated elevations of various sizes develop. Diagnosis relies on clinical appearance and histopathological changes, while therapy may include electrodesiccation, curettement, surgical excision or application of liquid nitrogen.

Other Infections[14]

Nongonococcal Urethritis

Nonspecific or nongonococcal urethritis (NGU) is the most prevalent sexually transmitted disease in some parts of the world. The symptoms are similar to those of gonorrhea, although the urethral discharge seen with NGU is typically clear, watery and scant. Most patients also have some mild urethritis with minimal dysuria, frequency and, rarely, hematuria.

The etiology of NGU is not known with certainty, although *Chlamydia* and T-mycoplasma *(Ureaplasma urealyticum)* probably account for the majority of cases.

The diagnosis of NGU is most often made as a result of excluding gonorrhea as the cause of the patient's symptoms. In addition to the Gram stain and culture for gonococcus, routine aerobic cultures of the urethra (or of the first 5 ml of a voided urine specimen) should be done to rule out a bacterial urethritis. The same specimen should be examined microscopically to exclude a *Trichomonas* infection.

In the absence of a positive bacterial culture, treatment effective against *Chlamydia* and *Ureaplasma* should be instituted. Most patients respond well to minocycline (Minocrin), 100 mg b.i.d., or doxycycline (Vibramycin), 100 mg b.i.d. for five days. Occasionally, additional therapy at one-half the above dosage is required for an additional 14 to 21 days to completely clear all symptoms.

Prostatitis

Chronic abacterial prostatitis is a clinical entity seldom associated with bacteriological invasion and the pathology typically associated with acute inflammation disorders. It usually involves patients in the fourth to sixth decades, and may also occur following interruption of an active sexual pattern. Acute local or systemic symptoms are seldom severe. Symptoms of vague perineal discomfort, mild symptoms of prostatism or vesical irritability and reduced sexual potency are frequently experienced. Urinalysis may be negative, but examination of the prostatic fluid will often show increased numbers of fat-laden macrophages, the "oval fat bodies" thought to be an indication of chronic inflammation.

The rectal examination will occasionally reveal a moderately enlarged prostate with a "boggy" consistency, but often it will be indistinguishable from a normal gland found in the asymptomatic male. The number of white blood cells per high power field, often used to make the diagnosis of prostatitis, is of little value. Many specimens from normal males will show >15 WBC/HPF; furthermore, the number of white cells in the prostatic fluid specimens will vary markedly from sample to sample in the same individual.

The treatment of chronic abacterial prostatis, or "prostatosis," as it is often referred to, is as varied as the agents reported to induce it. Reestablishment of normal sexual activity, hot sitz baths, antibiotics, anticholinergics, antispasmodics, antihistamines, analgesics and tranquilizers have all been reported as effective. Many urologists, in the belief that "congestion" is the primary problem, treat prostatosis with a series of prostatic massages. Why this is more effective than a normal ejaculation is not clear. In the author's opinion, many patients receive psychological gratification from prostatic massage which may help relieve their symptoms, but the actual physiological benefits are minimal and the routine use of prostatic massage, except for obtaining prostatic secretion for examination and culture, should be discouraged.

Chronic bacterial prostatitis is a much less common condition that is due to an infection with a bacterial pathogen, usually *Escherichia coli*, *Proteus*, *Klebsiella* or *Staphylococcus*. Patients with this condition are generally asymptomatic until the bacteria within the prostate seed the bladder and a urinary tract infection ensues. With infection the patient often complains of malaise, anorexia, fatigue, fever, chills, arthralgia, nausea, frequency, dysuria, nocturia and hematuria. The bacterial pathogen can be cultured from the urine. In between episodes of urinary tract infection, the diagnosis of bacterial prostatitis can be made by culturing urine specimens obtained before and after prostatic massage. If the bacterial colony count in the post-massage specimen exceeds the number in the initial specimen by tenfold or greater, the diagnosis is established. When asymptomatic, the prostatic examination is unremarkable and cannot be relied upon in making the diagnosis.

The treatment of chronic bacterial prostatitis is complicated by the fact that most available antimicrobial agents do not penetrate into the prostatic fluid; hence, they will not eradicate the infection. If the infecting organism is sensitive to trimethoprim-sulfamethoxazole (TMP-SMX) (Bactrim, Septra), this combination given as two tablets twice daily for six to twelve weeks will totally cure about one-third of cases. Other agents will be effective in a smaller percentage of cases. Many individuals with chronic bacterial prostatitis can only be kept symptom-free by prolonged low dose maintenance chemotherapy. Nitrofurantoin (50 to 100 mg daily) or TMP-SMX (1 tablet nightly) is extremely effective in this regard.

Cystitis

Cystitis is a common entity among females and is due to a bacterial infec-tion in the bladder. Gram-negative bacteria (*E. coli*, *Proteus*, *Klebsiella*, *Pseudomonas*) account for the majority of bladder infections, although about 5 per cent are due to gram-positive organisms, chiefly *Staphylococcus*. The symptoms of cystitis may be summarized as those of an "irritated bladder," with frequency, urgency, dysuria, nocturia, suprapubic discomfort and a sensation of incomplete bladder emptying present in the typical case. In addition, painful hematuria is a frequent complaint, particularly in the so-called "honeymoon cystitis" seen in young, sexually active females.

The presence of a bladder infection can often be suspected from an examination of the spun urine sediment. Typically, many WBC's and motile rod-shaped bacteria are observed. The diagnosis can only be made if a urine culture reveals more than 10^5 organisms per ml. The presence of irritable bladder symptoms in the absence of a positive urine culture demands a thorough urological investigation to rule out such entities as interstitial cystitis, neurogenic bladder or even an infiltrating bladder tumor. It is a wise rule to investigate every patient with hematuria, gross or microscopic. However, in younger patients, when the clinical impression is overwhelmingly in favor of an infectious etiology, it is often reasonable to treat the bacteriuria and then re-evaluate the urinalysis after treatment is completed. The presence of hematuria in the absence of an infection is an indication of the first magnitude for an evaluation of the entire genitourinary tract.

The treatment of cystitis is dictated by the results of the urine culture and sensitivity. In women experiencing their first or second infection, virtually any of the commonly used antimicrobials will be effective (sulfisoxazole, nitrofurantoin, nalidixic acid, penicillin, ampicillin and so on). In patients with multiple recurrences of infection it is often necessary to withhold therapy until the appropriate antimicrobial can be chosen on sensitivity testing.

Pyelonephritis

This is a disorder requiring prompt and adequate management. The clinical syndrome of acute pyelonephritis includes fever, chills, flank pain, malaise, anorexia, diaphoresis, nausea and vomiting. Symptoms of lower tract irritability may or may not be present. Severe systemic symptoms may require that the patient be hospitalized. Treatment with appropriate antibiotics in addition to general supportive measures is essential and should be continued for 10 to 14 days. If the patient is severely ill, the initiation of empirical therapy with parenteral gentamycin plus ampicillin is advised. This combination will be effective against virtually all of the common urinary tract pathogens. When the results of sensitivity testing are available, therapy can be switched to the appropriate oral agent.

An intravenous pyelogram is necessary to exclude the possibility of an acute obstruction of the kidneys or ureters. In the presence of an obstructed kidney, immediate drainage (percutaneous nephrostomy, ureteral catheterization), is mandatory.

Chronic pyelonephritis frequently does not produce localizing symptoms. Severe renal damage may already be present before the diagnosis is apparent. The only symptoms may be "failure to thrive," chronic lethargy and malaise. The diagnosis is made by the finding of cortical scarring and blunted calyces on intravenous urography. Once the diagnosis has been established, a complete evaluation of renal function is mandatory. Every attempt should be made to determine the rate of deterioration of renal function and a search should be made to find and eliminate contributing factors.

Central to preventing further loss of renal function is achieving sterile urine. Periodic urine cultures are required and any infection must be promptly treated. In some patients long-term maintenance therapy with nitrofurantoin or a sulfa drug may be required. Any anatomical factor (stone, obstruction) contributing to the persistence of the infection should be eliminated.

The Prevention of Recurrent Bacteriuria in Women

It now appears clear that the first incident in the chain of events necessary for the establishment of a urinary tract infection in females is that the organism must establish itself and colonize the vaginal vestibule. This probably explains the well known association of recurrent cystitis with sexual intercourse. The bacteria are massaged from the vaginal site into the bladder and grow readily in the urine. The other important recent finding that has helped our understanding of the prevention of recurrent infection has been the observation that more than 90 per cent of infections in females are *reinfections* with a totally new organism, not relapses from an incompletely treated infection or from a chronic focus of infection somewhere in the GU tract. An understanding of these two facts is helpful in explaining an approach to the prevention of recurrent bacteriuria.

The age-old advice of having the patient empty the bladder immediately after intercourse to eliminate any bacteria that may have entered the bladder is still sound and is effective in many women. When prolonged maintenance chemotherapy is indicated, its rational use would demand that (1) it will not cause the development of resistant bacteria in the bowel flora (the ultimate reservoir of all urinary tract pathogens), or (2) it would eliminate gram-negative bacteria from the vagina and prevent their colonization. The long-term administration of sulfa drugs for the prevention of recurrent lower tract infection is to be avoided. Within seven to ten days after the initiation of therapy with most sulfas, the majority of fecal organisms are resistant to the drug. Nitrofurantoin, 50 to 100 mg nightly, is extremely effective in preventing reinfections in most women. Trimethoprim-sulfamethoxazole may be useful in those patients not controlled by maintenance nitrofurantoin. One-half tablet nightly should be prescribed. By virtue of the fact that trimethoprim will concentrate in the vaginal secretions, this agent will virtually eliminate gram-negative bacteria from the vagina and markedly reduce the incidence of recurrent infections. Some women prefer to take a single tablet of an appropriate antibiotic (nitrofurantoin, TMP-SMX, ampicillin and so on) immediately following sexual intercourse rather than a daily dosage.

Pediatric Infections

Urinary tract infections in children beyond the neonatal period occur almost entirely in little girls. A number of surveys have confirmed that at any given time about 1 per cent of school age female children will have significant bacteriuria. The diagnosis and management of urinary tract infections in children is similar to that outlined for adults. Because of the greater incidence of abnormalities noted on radiography in children with infection, as opposed to adults, more complete evaluation is warranted. In little girls, the presence of fever and flank or abdominal pain with a urinary tract infection, or at least three documented episodes of cystitis, is an indication for the performance of an intravenous pyelogram. If the IVP is normal, no further investigation is needed. If upper tract disease is present, a voiding cystourethrogram and a cystoscopy, to assess the presence of vesicoureteral reflux or other abnormalities, are indicated. The evaluation and treatment of reflux is beyond the scope of this chapter and will not be discussed further.

A more common problem in the management of recurrent urinary tract infections is the absence of any demonstrable anatomical abnormality. Here the physician must be guided by the clinical situation encountered. Certainly, long-term suppressive antimicrobial therapy is not warranted in the child with a single infection. However, after the third or fourth episode of bacteriuria, serious consideration must be given to twelve months or more of suppressive medication. The authors prefer nitrofurantoin, 20 to 25 mg nightly. The sulfa drugs encourage the rapid development of resistance in the fecal flora and are less than optimal for long-term use.

Enuresis

Nocturnal bedwetting becomes a significant problem when it continues beyond the age of three years.[18] Most of these children have never achieved initial control and are described as primary enuretics. One-fourth of children have a dry period of several months or years and then revert to bedwetting. This is characterized as secondary enuresis. Important points that may indicate the etiology of the problem should be noted while obtaining the child's history. The presence of a familial tendency towards bedwetting is frequently seen with parents or siblings having enuresis after the first decade of life. In children with a strong family history of enuresis, continued bedwetting probably represents a familial neurological lag in maturation. These children often will not respond to treatment until they mature significantly.

Most enuretics have difficulty with control only when sleeping; however, the presence of daytime wetting, incontinence, urgency and frequency is significant. These individuals may have an uninhibited neurogenic bladder with frequent involuntary contractions. The presence of pain with voiding and dysuria is suggestive of urinary tract infections.

In all cases, a thorough physical examination, urinalysis and urine culture should be obtained. True meatal stenosis in boys can cause enuresis. The physical examination should include observation of the urinary stream, abdominal and genital examination and evaluation of neurological integrity. The latter can be inspected by examining the spinal area, checking peripheral refluxes, evaluating perineal sensation and performing a careful rectal examination to evaluate anal sphincter tone. The most common cause of primary enuresis is delayed maturation of bladder innervation. The child maintains an infantile type of neurogenic bladder with uninhibited spontaneous contractions. Other causes include sleep disorders and psychological problems. From an organic standpoint, urinary tract infections, congenital urinary anomalies and bladder outlet obstructions can all produce bedwetting. In secondary enuresis environmental factors must be considered. These children are often suffering from nervousness and anxiety related to instability in the home, new environmental stress, pressures at school or other emotional trauma.

In the presence of primary enuresis, a detailed extensive evaluation with cystometrograms and radiographs is not indicated. When other symptomatology is present, such as daytime incontinence, frequency and urgency, an underlying anatomical etiology is suspected and full clinical evaluation is warranted.

While no single therapeutic plan has proven universally successful in treating enuresis, a variety of approaches are available. A private physician-child talk is often helpful. The child will realize that the physician is concerned with his problem and in turn will be better able to relate his anxieties and feelings. Physicians should attempt to instill confidence in the patient that the enuresis can be cured in time and that the child must take part in his own therapy.

Initial steps at controlling enuresis include water deprivation four hours before bedtime, having the child double-void prior to sleeping, and waking the child in the middle of the night to void. The system of positive reinforcement may be established in the family, rewarding the child for having a dry bed in the morning. In this way the child is actively involved in his own therapy and is rewarded for a positive achievement.

Drug therapy has been remarkably successful in treating cases of primary enuresis. Functional bladder capacity increases and uninhibited bladder contractions occur less frequently. Imipramine is a drug of choice for enuresis, given in a dosage of 25 mg for children aged four to eight years, and 50 mg for older children. If nocturnal enuresis is the only problem, the drug should be given at dinner time. If the child also has daytime incontinence, an additional 25 mg of imipramine may be given in the morning. Oxybutynin (Ditropan) is also an anticholinergic drug that has been of great benefit in treating enuretic patients.

If all other measures fail, the parents may initiate a trial of negative conditioning therapy. An alarm system is connected to a special sheet upon which the child sleeps. At the time of bedwetting, an electronically triggered buzzer harshly awakens the child. Repeated awakenings act as negative reinforcement, and enuresis will decrease in 75 to 80 per cent of cases.

Cryptorchidism

The undescended testis is the most common anomaly of the male reproductive system and usually presents in the pediatric age group.[10] In true cryptorchidism the testis is arrested in its normal path of descent and lies in an intraabdominal or inguinal position. This must be distinguished from an ectopic testis, which has properly descended through the external inguinal ring but has failed to enter the scrotum, and a retractile testis, which is within the scrotum but readily retracts to the inguinal region during manipulation or cold. The retractile testis requires no therapy and will become lodged in the scrotum as the child passes through puberty. An ectopic testis does not require therapy except for comfort or cosmetic purposes.

The failure of normal testicular descent may be related to inadequate gonadotropin stimulation, mechanical obstructions at the inguinal canal, absence of a well-developed gubernaculum or primary testicular dysgenesis. Cryptorchidism is associated with other congenital abnormalities including the prune-belly syndrome, hypospadias and chromosomal anomalies.

Undescended testes have a higher incidence of malignancy than normal testes developing in the scrotum. In addition, bilateral cryptorchidism results in sterility. For these reasons it is important to diagnose and institute appropriate therapy for cryptorchidism when the child is young.

Since testicular retraction occurs with manipulation, physical examination should be performed in a warm room and with good patient rapport. Simple observation may reveal two testicles within the scrotal sac. A true cryptorchid testis may be palpated within the inguinal canal and attempts at manipulating the testis into the scrotum are unsuccesfful. Upper urinary tract abnormalities may be associated with bilateral cryptorchidism and these patients should have radiographic evaluation.

Five per cent of all male neonates have unilateral cryptorchidism. By the age of one year most of these testes have descended, resulting in a 1 per cent incidence of true cryptorchidism at the age of two years. These patients should be treated aggressively to avoid the resultant oligospermia seen in patients with long-term undescended testes. A trial of human chorionic gonadotropin (HCG) may be given in young children. A dosage of 1000 units every other day for ten treatments is suggested, with the best results being seen in bilateral cryptorchidism. If this measure is unsuccessful, orchiopexy should be performed. Continued follow-up and examination are necessary throughout the patient's life, for the undescended testis has an increased incidence of malignancy despite a successful surgical procedure. Therapy should be performed before the age of five years to prevent abnormal spermatogenesis. When seen after puberty, consideration should be given to performing an orchiectomy and placing a testicular prosthesis in the scrotum. In bilateral cryptorchidism, parents should be counseled that sterility is likely.

NEUROGENIC VESICAL DYSFUNCTION

Individuals with a neurogenic bladder are as diverse as the child with an uninhibited bladder and an elderly patient with bladder contractions following a stroke. Abnormalities of neuromuscular innervation to the bladder may be associated with spinal cord injury or tumors, multiple sclerosis, syringomyelia, the peripheral neuropathy of heavy metal poisoning or diabetes, polio, tabes dorsalis and myelomeningocele. Many of these conditions are obvious to the clinician and have definite central and peripheral neurological findings. It is unusual for neurogenic bladder dysfunction to be an isolated clinical finding. Rather it is a symptom in a picture of greater neurological disease.

Ambulatory patients with neurogenic bladders will usually complain of difficulty voiding and chronic urinary retention, or the loss of urine and incontinence. In either situation, an accurate voiding history must be obtained, including the presence of neurological disease and drug therapy. The patient's voiding habits must be fully understood and emphasis placed on the occurrence of enuresis, daytime incontinence and the presence of urgency, frequency or dribbling. Physical examination should involve a careful neurological evaluation including examination of the back, motor and sensory function and the integrity of spinal reflex arcs. Routine radiographic evaluation should detect the presence of spina bifida or sacral dysgenesis.

Neurogenic Bladder

Any interference with the normal conduction of nerve impulses over neurons concerned with urination will produce a neurogenic bladder. Bladders so affected may be of many types. For complete evaluation of any neurovesical dysfunction, a cystometrogram should be performed, often in conjunction with a urethral pressure profile, electromyelography and measurements of sphincter pressures. For routine outpatient evaluation, a simplified method of evaluating patients with suspected neurogenic abnormalities has been devised (Table 19–4).

Patients with a normal innervation of the bladder and perineum should be able to void completely with a residual less than 50 cc. Perineal sensation should be intact, and the bulbocavernosus reflex arc should be present. The latter test involves pressure on the glans penis or clitoris resulting in rectal sphincter muscle contraction. A normally innervated bladder should have a total capacity of 350 to 500 cc and should be able to distinguish pressure and temperature. Upon sudden stimulation with ice water, a spontaneous involuntary contraction should not occur. The performance of these simple tests can adquately distinguish different classes of neurogenic bladders.

Individuals with a large bladder capacity who retain a large amount of residual urine are said to have a flaccid or paralytic bladder. If perineal sensation is absent, this may be further subclassified as a sensory paralytic bladder, often seen in patients with diabetes mellitus. The absence of a bulbocavernosus reflex indicates interruption of the spinal reflex arc, frequently resulting from injury to the autonomic nervous system from pelvic surgery. Patients with a paralytic type of neurogenic bladder demonstrate chronic retention and have difficulty in emptying. Overflow incontinence, recurrent urinary tract infections and bladder calculi are frequently seen. These patients may be treated with intermittent catheterization, abdominal pressure (Credé) maneuvers, double voiding and the administration of Urecholine (bethanechol) in doses up to 200 mg a day.

Uninhibited bladder contractions are seen in patients with central nervous system lesions or spinal cord lesions above the level of T10. In these circumstances spontaneous bladder contractions occur, causing urinary incontinence. The bladder is characteristically small with a decreased volume. Intro-

TABLE 19–4 Neurogenic Bladder Evaluation

Type of Bladder	Bladder Capacity	Residual Urine	Urge to Void	Uninhibited Contractions	Perineal Sensation	Bulbocavernosus Reflex	Ice Water Test
Normal	350–500 cc	0–50 cc	100–250 cc	Absent	Present	Present	Negative
Uninhibited	50–100 cc	0 cc	20–50 cc	Present	Present	Present	Positive
Reflex	50–150 cc	50–100 cc	Absent	Present	Absent	Hyperactive	Positive
Motor paralytic	500–1700 cc	>300 cc	200–400 cc	Absent	Present	Variable	Negative
Sensory paralytic	500–1700 cc	>300 cc	Absent	Absent	Absent	Variable	Negative
Autonomic	500–1700 cc	>300 cc	Absent	Absent	Absent	Absent	Negative

duction of ice water into the bladder results in an uninhibited spontaneous contraction and involuntary voiding (positive ice water test). These patients may be greatly helped by anticholinergic drugs which decrease spasticity and allow for a greater bladder volume, such as atropine, Pro-Banthine, and oxybutynin (Ditropan).

Incontinence

Urinary incontinence is the involuntary leaking of urine. A careful history must be obtained to note if the urine leakage is intermittent or constant.

Constant day- and nighttime leakage of urine in adults or children is unusual and indicates underlying pathology. Total incontinence can occur in the the presence of an ectopic ureteral orifice in the female. In these cases, an intravenous pyelogram will show a duplicated collecting system, and an ectopic orifice may be seen in the urethra or vagina during endoscopy. Total urinary incontinence in the male may occur in the presence of injury to the sphincter mechanism following prostate surgery, or in the female after gynecological surgery that has caused a urinary fistula.

Intermittent incontinence may represent overflow of chronic urinary retention caused by obstruction or neurogenic dysfunction. The bladder is constantly full and cannot completely empty. Overdistention results in a dripping type of incontinence and is easily diagnosed by passage of a catheter and measurement of the residual urine volume. Urgency incontinence is associated with an uninhibited neurogenic bladder or lower urinary tract infections.

Incontinence with coughing, straining, or lifting is termed stress incontinence. This is most commonly seen in females and results from weakening of the anterior vaginal musculature, loss of the angle between the urethra and bladder and a shortened urethra. Loss of urine occurs with exertion or any increase in intra-abdominal pressure. Cystoscopic, radiographic and neurological evaluations of the bladder are unremarkable and cultures are negative. Definitive diagnosis is confirmed by performing a Marshall test. With the patient in the lithotomy or standing position, the bladder is filled to capacity. Upon removal of the catheter, urine can be actively retained, but leakage occurs with coughing. In addition, the placement of the examiner's fingers on either side of the urethra with upward pressure (to elevate and lengthen the urethra) will stop the incontinence. Treatment consists of a urethral suspension by the suprapubic or vaginal approach.

EVALUATION OF RENAL MASSES

Whenever a renal mass is noted on an intravenous urogram, additional studies must be performed to rule out malignancies. Though renal cancers frequently present with flank pain, hematuria or a palpable mass, 20 per cent of tumors are noted on studies done for other purposes, such as hypertension or urinary tract infections. A peripheral or central mass of the renal parenchyma may represent a simple renal cyst, multilocular cyst, carbuncle, neoplasm or pseudotumor.

After performing intravenous urography, nephrotomograms should be done to determine the precise size and location of the mass; a simple cyst will often show a "beak" or "claw" sign. Simple renal cysts are common and are frequently seen in urograms in older patients. When the nephrotomogram is suggestive of a renal cyst, needle puncture of the mass may be done immediately. Under most circumstances, renal ultrasonography is performed to determine whether the mass is sonolucent.[2] In the presence of a cystic mass, a presumptive diagnosis of renal cyst may be made, and percutaneous cyst aspiration should be performed. The fluid of a simple cyst is straw-colored and clear. Specimens should be sent for cytology and culture. There is no evidence that assays for LDH, protein or fat staining can reliably predict renal malignancies.

In the absence of a sonolucent mass or a clear, yellow cyst aspirate, selective renal arteriograms should be performed. This may be accomplished by cholinergic or adrenergic stimulation to better delineate the vasculature of the mass. Simple cysts, multilocular cysts, renal carbuncles and pseudotumors all have distinguishing arteriographical characteristics. Arteriovenous fistulae can be easily demonstrated and hemangiomas located. Hypervascularity or neovascularity represents angiomyolipoma or renal cell carcinoma. A papillary renal cell carcinoma may masquerade as an avascular renal mass and appear cystic on arteriography. These tumors show a solid or indeterminate pattern on ultrasonography and needle puncture yields bloody fluid. An inferior vena cavagram will demonstrate involvement of the renal vein with tumor.

Surgical exploration is indicated for any mass showing hypervascularity or neovascularity on arteriography and for any mass yielding bloody fluid on aspiration. A radical nephrectomy is performed for renal carcinomas. Peripheral renal cysts do not require operative intervention, however, although centrally located cysts may cause hydronephrosis or renal vascular hypertension by compression of the ureter and renal artery respectively. Under these circumstances, exploration and unroofing of the cyst is indicated.

INFERTILITY IN THE MALE

Seven per cent of all adult males have an abnormal semen analysis and are infertile. Investigation may be performed simultaneously with gynecological evaluation of the female or it can be reserved until after female examination documents a normal anatomical and physiological function.[1]

In obtaining an accurate sexual history, the presence of mumps orchitis, venereal disease, prostatitis or epididymitis should be documented. Radiation and surgery involving the scrotum, inguinal areas, prostate, bladder or retroperitoneal space may also cause infertility. A history of the patient's sexual activity and ability should preferably be obtained from the female partner. Drug intake can also affect the sperm count. Nitrofurantoin decreases sperm motility and viability. Antihypertensive and psychotherapeutic drugs may result in loss of sympathetic and parasympathetic tone, resulting in retrograde ejaculation. Such medications include guanethidine, hydralazine, chlorpromazine and L-dopa.

On physical examination the location and size of the testes are important. A past history of cryptorchidism or the presence of an undescended testis is related to ipsilateral decreased spermatogenesis. Small testicles, less than 2 cm in length, may be associated with Klinefelter's syndrome. Hypospadias not only makes erection and penetration difficult, but it also prevents direct deposit of the sperm at the cervical os.

The presence of a varicocele of any size is responsible for abnormal sperm maturation in 40 per cent of all infertility cases. A search for a varicocele is important. Patients should be standing for three to five minutes prior to the examination and should perform a Valsalva maneuver during palpation. The size of the varicocele is not important, for even small dilated veins may result in infertility.

Laboratory tests include serum or urine LH, FSH and serum testosterone. Hormonal abnormalities indicate malfunction of the pituitary-testicular axis. Patients suspected of having Klinefelter's syndrome should have buccal smears and karyotype if indicated. On occasion, endocrinopathies such as diabetes mellitus or thyroid disease cause infertility.

The most important laboratory examination in evaluating the infertile male is the semen analysis. It should be collected after three days of abstinence and deposited in a wide-mouth glass container. For accuracy, a semenogram should be performed within one-half hour after collection. Normal sperm volume is 2 to 5 cc and normal count is greater than 20 million per cc. The motility should be greater than 80 per cent immediately and greater than 50 per cent after one hour. A Blom stain for viability and a count of abnormal forms should be performed. All sperm should be active, and greater than 80 per cent should be normally formed. Fructose analysis will confirm the presence of seminovesical fluid in the ejaculate. Liquefaction should occur promptly. A postcoital catheterized urine specimen should be examined. The presence of active spermatozoa indicates possible retrograde ejaculation.

In the presence of azoospermia, further investigation may consist of performing a seminovasogram and testes biopsy.

Treatment is highly individualized, depending on abnormalities found. In patients with a normal seminogram, couples are reinstructed as to proper timing and positions for intercourse. When the semen volume is high and the first portion of a split ejaculum has been found to be the better fraction, many patients have achieved pregnancy by the use of a coital technique in which the husband withdraws his penis from the vagina after release of the first portion of the ejaculum. This technique is used during the fertile portion of the menstrual cycle and only when the husband has a high volume of semen.

In patients with a clearly demonstrable varicocele, high ligation of the ipsilateral spermatic vein may improve the semen analysis in 85 per cent of individuals. Sperm count, motility and viability may increase within three to four months after surgery and a pregnancy rate as high as 60 per cent has been reported. Good results will occur when the patient has mild oligospermia and when testicular biopsy demonstrates sloughing and disorganization within the seminiferous tubules. In the presence of obstruction of the vas deferens or the epididymis, surgical reanastomosis and bypass of the obstruction can be successful.

Drug treatment for the oligospermic patient who has no physical findings is of uncertain benefit. A trial of low dose testosterone is given to males with demonstrated low serum androgen levels. Another treatment involves administration of high dose testosterone for three to four weeks until the sperm count is depressed. Testosterone is then discontinued at the time of ovulation, in the hope that rebound spermatogenesis will produce normal levels of motile sperm. Clomiphene citrate has been used empirically in a cyclic regimen of 25 mg per day for 25 days in a small series. Other drugs include intramuscular HCG, arginine and steroids.

When retrograde ejaculation is suspected following retroperitoneal or prostate surgery, the use of ephedrine may be of benefit. This adrenergic drug acts to close the internal sphincter during ejaculation and prevent backflow of semen into the bladder.

In those couples who have been attempting pregnancy for at least two years and when both partners have normal tests, the presence of antispermatozoa antibodies should be considered. When the female has antisperm antibodies, the husband uses a condom for six months and antibody levels decline. Small oral doses of prednisolone have also been beneficial. Thirty per cent of men who have had reversal of a vasectomy have sperm agglutinating antibodies in their serum. These men may develop normal sperm counts but pregnancy will not result. Oral steroids can be used in treating these patients.

The overall success rate in treating infertility is 45 per cent. Certain patients cannot be aided and no drugs or surgery are indicated. This group includes men with Klinefelter's syndrome, a history of bilateral mumps orchitis, radiation or bilateral cryptorchidism. In the "Sertoli cell only" syndrome, or germinal cell aplasia, spermatogonia are absent from seminiferous tubules. These patients can be counseled on adoption facilities.

IMPOTENCE

The inability to obtain and maintain an erection is a not uncommon complaint of middle-aged males. The etiology may be organic or functional. Diabetes, vascular insufficiency, heavy metal poisoning, or neurological diseases such as multiple sclerosis or myasthenia gravis may produce impotence. Surgical procedures such as cystectomy, radical prostatectomy or sympathectomy may also contribute to organic causes. In true organic impotence, the patient is totally unable to obtain erection or penetration. Vascular or neurogenic disease is present and the patient is impotent in spite of any stimulation.

The ability to achieve an erection upon arising in the morning with a full bladder indicates that the patient does not have organic impotence. Tactile or visual stimuli will also produce erections in patients with a functional disorder. Many psychological factors produce an emotional state of anxiety and hinder a male's ability to perform sexually. These include alcoholism, difficulties with employment, marital instability or other problems that create a nervous or anxious mental condition.

While the treatment of psychological impotence may involve extensive psychotherapy or sexual therapy, organic impotence will not respond to these methods. Occasionally, the administration of testosterone results in increased sexual performance. In cases of anatomical abnormalities producing impotence, a penile prosthesis may be surgically inserted.

INVESTIGATION OF RENAL HYPERTENSION

In view of the extensive literature dealing with the indications and use of rapid sequence pyelography, radioisotope renograms, aortography, split renal function studies and the differential renal vein renin ratios, the physician dealing with the hypertensive patient must exercise care and judgment in deciding when and how to pursue a diagnosis of renovascular hypertension in the individual patient.

The first question the physician must ask himself is: If a renal artery stenosis is found to be the cause of the hypertension in a given individual, is the patient in satisfactory physical condition for surgery to be carried out and will he agree to a surgical approach? Obviously, in older patients with hypertension as a manifestation of generalized arteriosclerotic disease, and with high blood pressure easily controlled by medication, the physician may elect to continue medical therapy for as long as the patient tolerates it. Also, in young women on oral contraceptive medication, the wise physician will suspend investigation until he has examined the woman several months after the birth control pills have been discontinued. The association between oral contraceptives and high renin hypertension is well documented and this should be the first diagnosis considered when dealing with the young female hypertensive patient.

If, after careful consideration of the question, the physician is of the opinion that surgery would be warranted if a correctable lesion is diagnosed, the first test ordered should be the rapid sequence (hypertensive) IVP. The "rapid sequence" urogram can be of considerable value as a screening test to select those individuals to be investigated in more detail for a possible renovascular etiology of their hypertension. The most common abnormality seen in patients with proven renovascular hypertension, and the most reliable feature in distinguishing essential hypertension from unilateral renovascular disease, is a delay in the calyceal appearance time on the side of the involved kidney. For this reason, failure to obtain early films one to four minutes after injection of the contrast agent means that the most valuable information to be obtained from the urogram is lost. The other major abnormalities in the urogram of patients with proven RVH — disparity in renal size and later hyperconcentration of contrast on the affected side — occur with much less frequency. The routine use of the *conventional urogram* (in which the first film is obtained 5 minutes or more following the injection of the contrast agent) in evaluating patients for the etiology of their hypertension is inadequate, a waste of time and money and is ethically indefensible in the light of current knowledge. Ancillary urographical features such as ureteral notching caused by collateral circulation to the kidney via ureteral vessels, a decreased volume of the collecting system and thin, "spidery" calyces or hyperconcentration of the contrast on the involved side (as a consequence of excessive water reabsorption), while occasionally helpful in a given patient are, in general, unreliable diagnostic aids.

If available, a renogram capable of quantitating differential renal function should also be performed as part of the initial evaluation.

One should proceed to a renal arteriogram in both frontal and oblique projections in patients with an abnormal IVP, renogram or both; in all young patients (less than 25 years of age); or in patients in whom it is not possible to control the blood pressure on a medical regimen that is acceptable to the patient without seriously impairing the quality of his life. If the arteriogram demonstrates a renal artery lesion, this lesion must be assessed for its functional significance before a rational decision with respect to surgery can be reached. The relative ease of sampling renal venous blood makes the use of the renal vein renin ratios very appealing as the next investigative step. If the peripheral and renal vein renin determinations do not afford convincing evidence of significant renal ischemia in a patient with radiographic evidence of unilateral renal artery stenosis, split renal function studies (Table 19–5) should be performed to more accurately and reliably diagnose possible renovascular hypertension. Although they are rather complicated and time consuming, split function studies are invaluable for confirming the diagnosis

TABLE 19–5 Individual Kidney Function Tests for Evaluation of Hypertension*

Preparation

For one week prior to the test, a normal sodium diet is taken, and all diuretic medications are discontinued if possible. On the morning of the test, breakfast is omitted. Beginning two hours before cystoscopy, the patient is hydrated with 240 ml of water by mouth or 120 ml of 5 per cent dextrose and water intravenously at half-hour intervals, continuing throughout the test. General anesthesia is usually necessary in children. Saddle block or adequate urethral anesthesia will usually suffice in adults.

Catheterization

The ureters are catheterized through a No. 24

Brown-Buerger cystoscope. The possibility of postcatheterization edema should be considered, and for this reason only the kidney suspected of being abnormal should be catheterized in some patients. This complication is more common in males than females. The other kidney in these patients can be drained through a bladder catheter.

Collection of Specimens

Urine collection is started 15 minutes after insertion of the catheters. The normal kidney should excrete 1 ml per minute or more. Collection periods are timed to the nearest 15 seconds, and should allow for collection of at least 20–30 ml of urine from the better kidney in each period.

*Adapted from Protocol of the Cooperative Renal Hypertension Study Group.

Table continued on the following page.

TABLE 19–5 Individual Kidney Function Tests for
Evaluation of Hypertension *(Continued)*

Urine is collected directly into 50 ml graduated cylinders, for at least three collection periods. The bladder is emptied and measured at the end of each collection period. Blood specimens include appropriate pre-infusion and mid-collection period specimens as well as a final specimen at the end of the test. A record is made of blood pressure every 15 minutes, and each urine specimen should have its color and volume recorded before it is centrifuged for chemical analysis.

RAPOPORT TEST (Tubular Rejection Fraction Ratio)

This is the shortest and simplest of the split function tests. Urine is measured for sodium and creatinine. Glomerular filtration rate (GFR) is calculated for each kidney, utilizing a blood specimen obtained at the midpoint of each urine collection, and the formula:

$$GFR = C_{cr} = \frac{U_{cr} \times \dot{V}}{P_{cr}}$$

C_{cr} Creatinine clearance (ml/min)

U_{cr} Urinary creatinine concentration (mg/ml)

$\dot{V}$ Urinary flow (ml/min)

P_{cr} Plasma creatinine concentration (mg/ml)

The tubular-rejection-fraction of sodium (TRFNa) of the left kidney is divided by that of the right. The result is Tubular Rejection Fraction Ratio (TRFR):

$$TRFR = \frac{L\ U_{Na}}{L\ U_{Cr}} \times \frac{R\ U_{Cr}}{L\ U_{Na}}$$

A positive test consists of a TRFR of less than 0.7 or greater than 1.5. A low TRFR (0.6 or less) indicates involvement of the right renal artery.

HOWARD TEST

Urine from each kidney is measured for volume, sodium and creatinine. For volume and sodium the formula used is:

$$\frac{normal - diseased}{normal} \times 100$$

For creatinine calculations, the formula used is:

$$\frac{diseased - normal}{diseased} \times 100$$

A positive test consists of (1) reduction of 40 per cent or more in urine volume, coupled with 15 per cent or more reduction in sodium concentration; or (2) reduction of 40 per cent or more in urine volume, with creatinine concentration at least 50 per cent higher from the affected kidney than from the nonaffected kidney.

STAMEY TEST (Urea-PAH)

Salicylates, penicillin, chlorothiazide and sulfonamides must not be administered for 48 hours prior to this test, and procaine must not be used during the procedure. These substances interfere with determination of para-amino hippurate (PAH). Ten ml of blood is needed for determination of PAH in the blood specimens.

A single priming dose of PAH is given intravenously. The desired plasma concentration of PAH is 2.5 mg/100 ml. The volume of 20 per cent PAH injected is determined by multiplying the patient's weight by 0.04. For example, a 70 kg man would receive 2.8 ml of 20 per cent PAH solution.

Urea is given in an 8 per cent solution at the rate of 10 ml per minute. The solution used is a "urea-PAH-ADH solution." It is prepared by withdrawing 160 ml of saline from a 1000 ml bottle of normal saline; 60 ml are discarded and 50 ml are injected into each of two 40 gm bottles of crystalline urea U.S.P. The saline-urea mixture from the small bottles is reinjected into the liter bottle of saline. PAH must then be added to this bottle to maintain a plasma level of approximately 2.5 mg per cent during the test. The amount of 20 per cent PAH added depends on the patient's renal function. If the serum creatinine is 2.0 mg per cent or less, 5.3 ml of PAH solution is added; if the serum creatinine is greater than 2.0 mg per cent, 2.6 ml of PAH is added.

Collection periods are begun 45 minutes after the urea-PAH-ADH infusion has been started. Each collection lasts at least 10 minutes, and a urine flow of at least 2 ml per minute is necessary. At least 30 ml of urine must be obtained from each ureter during each collection period. A blood specimen for PAH should be obtained in the midpoint of each urine collection period, or at least at the midpoint of the second collection period.

Because the patient has received an osmotic diuresis in this test, the bladder should be catheterized for at least six hours after the test, and he should receive 2000 ml of 5 per cent dextrose in water at a rate of 300 ml per hour.

A positive test consists of at least a 3:1 difference in urine flow rates and a 100 per cent or greater difference in PAH concentrations. Flow rate is *decreased* on the affected side and PAH concentration is *increased* on the affected side. A 2:1 difference (decrease) in urine flow rate on the affected side and an increase of less than 100 per cent in PAH concentration on the affected side are compatible with any of the following:

1. Essential hypertension with disparity in nephrosclerosis
2. Segmental renal hypertension (branch lesion) in one kidney
3. Bilateral renal arterial stenosis with disparity in ischemia.

and planning the surgical approach in those cases in which the renal vein renin determination is inconclusive.

FEMALE UROLOGY

Irritable Bladder Syndrome

This syndrome is the most common condition of the urethra or bladder in females. It is also termed urethral syndrome or urethrotrigonitis. It is characterized by intermittent episodes of burning, dysuria, suprapubic pain, urgency, frequency and occasional incontinence and dysuria. The patients may have a pelvic or rectal discomfort often associated wtih great anxiety for symptomatic relief.

Physical findings, urinalysis and cultures are negative. Excretory urography is completely normal. Endoscopy may reveal an inflammatory pseudomembrane or vascular injection involving the urinary trigone compatible with trigonitis. The vesical neck and urethra may exhibit pseudopolypoid changes, edema and erythema, indicative of chronic urethritis. The physician must exclude other diseases, including interstitial cystitis and urinary tuberculosis.

Specific treatment involves the use of sedatives and antispasmodics in combination to break the cycle of nervousness and irritability that causes spastic bladder contractions. Urethral dilatations are usually not helpful and may cause bladder infections by introducing pathogenic urethral bacteria, unless an antimicrobial agent is instilled into the bladder at the time of dilatation. Repair of cystoceles that cause no residual urine and are asymptomatic does not adequately treat the problem. In addition, removal of asymptomatic caruncles or indiscriminate fulguration of urethral polyps in the bladder neck is useless. Other procedures have never been shown to be of significant benefit, including internal urethrotomy and urethrolysis, external meatotomy and resection or incision of the bladder neck. When true strictures or bladder neck contractions do occur, some of these procedures are justified; however, these conditions are rare.

Urethral Caruncle

This lesion represents a chronic granuloma frequently seen in women with multiple voiding symptoms. A patient with the irritable bladder syndrome is likely to have a caruncle removed in the hope of relieving her symptoms, but the caruncle is usually not responsible for urinary complaints. The urinalysis and cultures are always negative and cystoscopy is normal. Caruncles frequently respond to local administration of estrogen creams and operation is rarely indicated. Most caruncles are best left untreated and the patient simply reassured. When bleeding or discomfort is great, surgical intervention may be necessary. The lesion can be cauterized with the coagulating electrode or can be surgically removed. The latter maneuver requires amputating the lesion from the urethral mucosa and approximating the edges with 4-0 chromic sutures.

Urethral Diverticulum

Women with a urethral diverticulum complain classically of post-void dribbling. Other symptoms include recurrent cystitis, dyspareunia, urgency and nocturia. The physical finding is a fluctuant mass in the anterior vaginal wall. Digital compression of this mass results in a discharge of pus or urine from the urethral meatus. Definitive diagnosis can be obtained by performing retrograde urethrography using the double balloon catheter. Cystoscopy reveals the exact location and size of the diverticulum. Treatment involves surgical excision using a transvaginal approach.

OUTPATIENT OPERATIVE PROCEDURES

Circumcision (Fig. 23–11)

Circumcision is the most common operative procedure performed on males in the United States. In newborns and infants, the Gomco clamp or Plastibell is typically used in performing circumcision. If the procedure has not been done at birth, elective circumcision is usually deferred until the child is older than one year of age in order to avoid potential anesthetic problems.

The technique of circumcision in children is illustrated in Figure 23–11. Children usually undergo general anesthesia, while adults can have a local penile block (Fig. 19–1). After the appropriate preparation and draping, a vertical midline incision is made on the prepuce, care being taken to avoid injury to the urethra and glans penis. The dorsal slit is carried proximally on the foreskin to an area approximately 1 cm from the corona sulcus. A similar incision is made on the ventral surface along the midline raphe and extending to the frenulum. Troublesome bleeding at the frenular attachment may be controlled by a horizontal mattress suture. With the prepuce divided into two hemispheres, excision of the redundant foreskin can be easily and accurately performed. Undue tension should be avoided during excision of the foreskin to prevent removal of excess prepuce. The glans should be gently retracted to one side so the corona is entirely within view. Using a smooth single cut of the scissors blade, the redundant foreskin is amputated. In this manner, a hemi-circumcision is done in a single maneuver rather than a series of small maneuvers that can result in scalloping. After completing the circumcision, bleeding vessels are identified and secured with electrocoagulation or chromic ties. The edges of the foreskin are then reapproximated using absorbable sutures. Interrupted sutures are placed circumferentially, with each stitch bisecting the remaining distance. Using this technique, more than a dozen sutures are seldom required. The incision is then protected with an antibiotic ointment and Vaseline gauze. The patient should be observed for several hours to be sure that there is no delayed hemorrhage. The dressing can be removed on the following day and warm baths instituted. Intercourse should be avoided until the suture line is well healed.

Meatotomy (Figure 19–9)

Urethral meatal stenosis is usually an acquired problem. In children and infants who have been circumcised, narrowing of the meatus is seen as a result of recurrent episodes of meatitis. Frequently the meatus will be reduced to a pinpoint opening, causing a slow, weak stream and prolonged voiding. Meatotomy is painful in children and should be performed under general anesthesia. After adequate preparation, the meatus is calibrated with Bougie-à-boules. A small straight clamp is then placed within the meatus on the ventral aspect of the glans and allowed to remain in place for a minute. An avascular area is created and the meatotomy is performed. Subsequent calibration should allow for passage of a No. 14 or No. 16 French bougie. Sutures are rarely needed. The parents must be instructed to spread the meatus open daily so that the raw edges will not approximate.

Meatal stenosis in the adult is generally the result of a fibrous narrowing due to inflammation of chronic irritation. It is commonly seen following episodes of indwelling catheterization. Meatotomy can be performed under a local anesthesia in the adult male. A local anesthetic is introduced into the lateral and ventral aspects of the meatus and down the midline to the frenulum. A straight hemostat is ap-

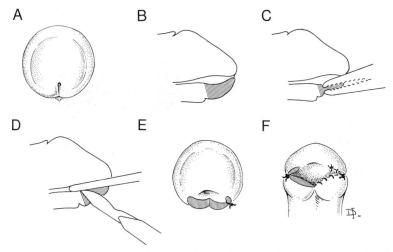

Figure 19-9 Urethral meatotomy in the male. *A.* Urethral meatal stenosis. *B.* Depth of meatotomy (shaded area). *C.* Application of hemostat. *D.* Incision of clamped tissue over grooved director or metal sound. *E, F.* Suture of neomeatus laterally to each corona to impede coaptation.

plied for several minutes and the tissue is crushed. After performing the meatotomy, bleeding is minimal and may be controlled with application of a silver nitrate stick or a suture ligature of 3-0 chromic.

Urethral meatotomy in the female is of questionable benefit. True urethral stenosis in women is rare and usually can be treated with urethral dilations. Meatotomy is not indicated for the treatment of recurrent urinary tract infections, cystitis or urethritis.

Vasectomy (Figure 19–10)

A vasectomy is performed for elective sterilization and for the prevention of retrograde epididymitis. Vasectomy has been commonly employed at the time of a prostatectomy to decrease the incidence of postoperative epididymitis.

More commonly, vasectomy is being chosen as an elective sterilization procedure by young couples who wish to limit the size of their families. The operative procedure is virtually foolproof and avoids expense, inconvenience, hospitalization and discomfort associated with other methods of contraception. The operation should always

be preceded by lengthy counseling between the couple and the physician. During this time the couple is informed that vasectomy is essentially a totally irreversible and permanent procedure. (Though reanastomosis is possible, the patient should be informed that vasectomy reversal is a difficult procedure and is not always successful.) All risks and complications should be thoroughly explained. Emphasis is placed on the fact that sterility is not immediate and that contraceptive measures should be continued until ten to twelve ejaculations have occurred to allow for emission of any viable sperm distal to the point of vas interruption. A semen specimen is analyzed six to eight weeks after vasectomy to ensure azoospermia. Finally, it should be emphasized that spontaneous recanalization occurs rarely despite the use of a proper surgical technique. The patient must be willing to accept this at his own risk. Permission for elective vasectomy as a sterilization procedure should include witnessed signatures of both husband and wife.

The surgical procedure (Fig. 19–10) should be preceded by shaving the scrotum and base of the penis. After routine sterile preparation, the vas def-

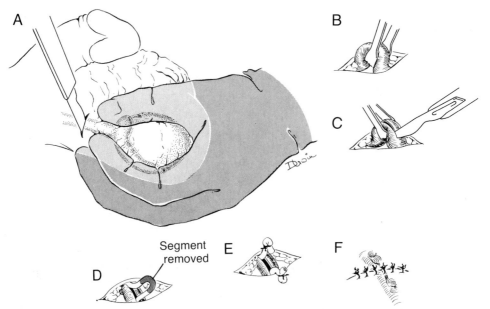

Figure 19–10 Vasectomy technique. *A.* Incision over vas deferens after anesthetic infiltration of skin and spermatic cord. *B.* Vas deferens, in its fibrous sheath, grasped with Allis clamp and delivered through incision. *C.* Longitudinal incision in fibrous sheath, exposing vas deferens. *D.* Vas deferens delivered with fine-toothed forceps. Segment excised (shaded area). *E.* Vasal remnants suture ligated. *F.* Scrotal skin closed with interrupted absorbable sutures.

erens is isolated on either side through the scrotal skin. The scrotal skin is infiltrated with Xylocaine. A 1 cm transverse incision is made over the anesthetized area and the vas deferens is isolated with a hemostat. An Allis clamp is introduced through the incision and the vas is grasped and delivered into the wound. The fibrous investment of the vas is incised longitudinally, and the vas is then grasped with a fine-tooth forceps. After withdrawing a 2 to 3 cm portion of the vas, each end is clamped with a hemostat and a section is removed. The cut edges are then turned upon themselves and ligated with nonabsorbable suture material such as silk or Mersilene. An alternative method is to introduce a needle-tip electrode through the lumen of the vas and coagulate the distal centimeter of tissue. Care must be taken to assure local hemostasis to prevent development of a hematoma. The vasal remnants are then returned to the normal intrascrotal position, and

the scrotal incision is closed with 3-0 chromic suture. At the time of discharge, the patient is instructed to wear a scrotal support and to use ice packs on the wound for the initial 24 hours. Warm baths may then be taken to alleviate the pain, discomfort and swelling. Antibiotics are given optionally. Vigorous activity should be avoided for two to three days to discourage any capillary bleeding.

Hydrocelectomy

Small or moderately large hydroceles are rarely symptomatic and seldom require excision or decompression. When the patient complains of discomfort or heaviness, surgical resection is indicated. The procedure is usually brief and benign, with minimal morbidity and a rapid convalescence.

In children, hydroceles are commonly associated with communicating hernias via a patent processus vaginalis. Operation for children with a hydrocele may be performed on a short-stay surgery basis. After the induction of anesthesia, the groin is prepared and an inguinal incision is made. After opening the external oblique muscle, care is taken not to injure the ilioinguinal or iliohypogastric nerves. The patent processus vaginalis is isolated and the structures of the spermatic cord and vas deferens are also carefully isolated and preserved. The hernia sac is dissected free and high ligation is performed on the internal inguinal ring. The hydrocele is drained and will not recur.

To ensure proper diagnosis in the adult, the hydrocele must be smooth, firm and translucent to light. A scrotal approach is used and the procedure is commonly done under spinal anesthetic. The scrotal skin is opened horizontally and the hydrocele sac is isolated. Upon perforating the sac, clear, straw-colored fluid is removed. The redundant tunica vaginalis is then either excised or wrapped around the spermatic cord. In either case, the transected edges of the sac are closed with 3-0 chromic sutures to prevent recurrence of the hydrocele. A small drain is routinely left in place and is removed 24 hours after the procedure. In those patients who are unable to undergo a complete hydrocelectomy, percutaneous aspiration of hydrocele fluid can be performed to relieve discomfort. The hydrocele fluid will reaccumulate in three to six months and repeated aspirations are necessary.

MANAGEMENT OF URETHRAL STRICTURE

Straddle injuries usually produce strictures of the bulbous urethra, while those accompanying deceleration injuries and pelvic fracture most commonly involve the area of the membranous urethra. Strictures associated with gonococcal urethritis usually involve the bulbous and proximal pendulous urethra. Strictures due to urethritis from indwelling catheters typically involve the distal pendulous urethra at the level of the fossa navicularis and the urethral meatus. Strictures associated with periurethral abscess due to pressure necrosis from chronic indwelliing catheters usually involve the proximal bulbous urethra and distal pendulous urethra at the penoscrotal junction.

Evaluation and treatment of urethral stricture will depend upon the site and severity of the lesion. This may bear little relationship to the symptoms experienced or the sequelae produced. Symptoms may range from urinary tract infection and outflow obstruction to vesicoureteral reflux and deterioration of the upper urinary tract. Urethral meatal strictures may be managed by dilatation and internal urethrotomy. An alternate technique is careful insertion of a No. 11 scalpel blade through the meatus and stricture. Meatotomy is frequently necessary before the scalpel blade can be introduced. Ultimately, dilatation is carried out to the diameter of a No. 24 French with bougie or metal sound. This technique should be performed only by experienced personnel using adequate local anesthesia. More proximal urethral strictures require thorough investigation prior to intervention, including bougie-à-boule calibration in the less severe strictures. Calibration yields information regarding the site, density, pliability and extent of the fibrous obstructions. More severe strictures and those not amenable to such calibration are best delineated preoperatively by urethrography. Vesical outlet obstruction due to prostatic disease and stricture at the vesical neck are best investigated cystographically and endoscopically.

Nonoperative management of urethral strictures includes the use of urethral sounding, filiforms and followers and internal urethrotomy.

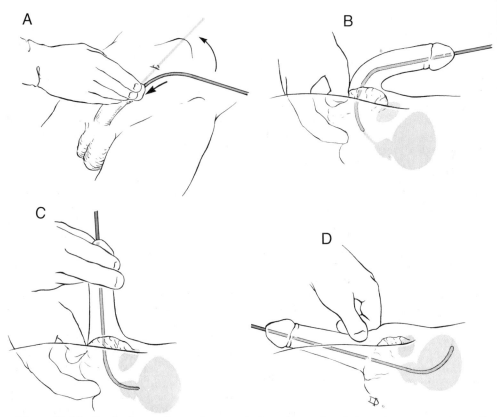

Figure 19–11 Urethral sounding technique. *A.* Sound introduced through meatus with handle over left iliac crest to facilitate passage. *B.* Sound maneuvered to midline vertical position, and advanced to the level of the urethral bulb. *C.* Sound maneuvered gently to horizontal position to facilitate advancement through external sphincter and vesical neck. Digital perineal pressure may assist. *D.* Sound advances through vesical neck.

Urethral Sounding (Fig. 19–11)

This procedure should be preceded by filling the urethra with a water-soluble lubricant such as K-Y Jelly or Lubrasporin, or a topical anesthetic such as Xylocaine jelly. In apprehensive male patients, a topical anesthetic is usually not so useful as intravenous sedation with Valium. In females, urethral sounding is relatively quick and painless, especially if preceded by application for a few seconds of Xylocaine jelly on a sterile cotton swab.

Filiforms and Followers

With dense and tortuous strictures it may be necessary to employ filiforms and followers to carry out therapeutic dilation or incision. Urethral filiforms are merely flexible guides of small caliber and varying tips (olive or pigtail, for instance) that may be introduced into the urethra until an obstruction is met or until the urethral lumen at the level of obstruction is encountered and traversed. If obstruction is met, the filiform is left in place and another inserted. This process is repeated until the obstruction is traversed, at which point the final filiform is maintained in position while the others are removed (Fig. 19–12). Each filiform has a proximal fitting to which can be attached appropriate followers of varying dimensions for dilation, including the Phillips woven silk catheters and the LeFort metal sounds (Fig. 19–13). Beginning

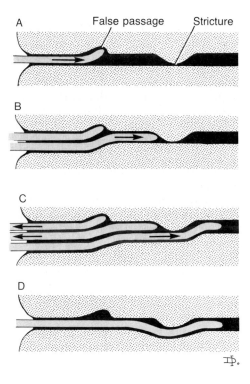

Figure 19-12 Insertion of urethral filiform guide. Insertion of multiple filiform guides will obliterate false passages *(A, B)*, while further diameters allow passage through strictured urethral segments *(C)*. The vesical filiform is then stabilized while the remaining filiforms are removed.

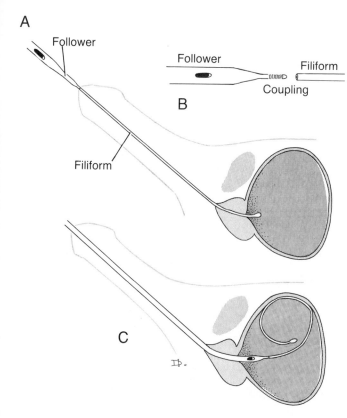

Figure 19-13 Insertion of filiforms and follower. *A.* Filiform guide advanced into bladder. *B.* Follower (draining catheter or dilating sound) attached to filiform. *C.* Follower advanced into bladder.

with an appropriate small caliber follower, the area of the stricture is sequentially dilated with the replaceable followers until an adequate caliber has been attained or until the operator's experience indicates that further dilation would be hazardous. A similar technique is employed for relief of urinary retention associated with urethral strictures that preclude easy catheterization. It is to be emphasized that such a maneuver should be performed under the strictest aseptic technique, with attention to the patient's comfort and anxiety and with maximum observation for potential infection and sepsis. Antibiotics are essential following the procedure, and the patient should be instructed to notify the physician immediately upon experiencing any prodromal symptoms of septicemia. In employing the LeFort follower, gentle digital perineal pressure will assist in diverting the instrument anteriorly away from the rectum and through the vesical neck. At no time should exertion be used with any dilating instrument.

Internal Urethrotomy

Longer or more proximal areas of fibrous strictures and those that respond poorly to repeated dilations are often more responsive to internal urethrotomy. This technique utilizes the Otis urethrotome (Fig. 19–14), which combines a variable caliber and a nontraumatic, movable cutting blade restricted to a single plane. After routine preparation of the patient in the lithotomy position, the instrument is introduced in its smallest caliber, and the knife is withdrawn from its shielded position along its track. Depending upon the severity of the stricture, inci-

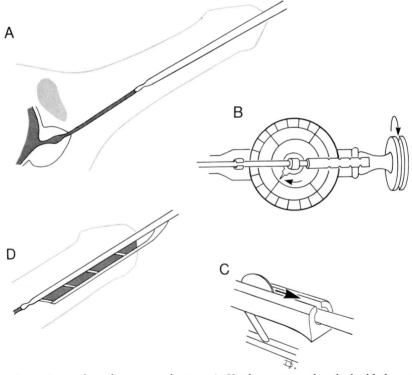

Figure 19–14 Internal urethrotomy technique. *A.* Urethrotome in closed, shielded position advanced through area of stricture. *B.* Dilator gauge advanced to desired setting, resulting in urethral dilatation (*C*). *D.* Withdrawal of the unshielded urethrotome, resulting in incision of the strictured area.

sions may be repeated at the three, nine and twelve o'clock positions. The incision is deepened as necessary until urethroscopy reveals that the stricture is completely cut and that normal red panurethral tissue can be visualized beneath the scar. A No. 24 French retention catheter of inert material should be left in place for three to six weeks to prevent the coaption of the incisions, and routine attention to catheter hygiene should be observed.

OUTPATIENT UROLOGICAL PROCEDURES

Cystoscopy

Outpatient urological practice utilizes cystoscopy extensively for diagnosis and, to a lesser extent, for therapy. Cystoscopy should be performed only under the supervision of an experienced urologist with full understanding of the hazards of the procedure. When properly performed, outpatient cystoscopy can be helpful in providing immediate answers to diagnostic questions. It eliminates the cost and time of hospitalization in patients with certain types of recurrent bladder disease that are amenable to either biopsy or fulguration. The indications for cystoscopy may include voiding dysfunctions such as vesical irritability, reduced size of the urinary stream, infection, nocturia, incomplete emptying, hematuria and suprapubic pain. There is essentially no contraindication to cystoscopy in adult patients who require a urological evaluation, but extreme care should be taken in patients on anticoagulation medication. Individuals with acute, ongoing urinary tract infections should not have a cystoscopy without appropriate antibiotic coverage because of the hazard of producing bacteremia.

Cystoscopy requires right angle and Foroblique lenses and obturators. These are available in multiple sizes for both children and adults —

#12, 14, 16, 17, 20 and 22 French. The instruments are stored in a liquid germicide such as Cytal and are rinsed in sterile water immediately before use.

The patient undergoing cystoscopy should be in the lithotomy position. After preparing the genitalia, the urethra can be locally anesthetized with regional administration of Xylocaine lubricant. Intravenous diazepam (Valium), 5 to 10 mg, will produce significant relaxation and amnesia. In the male, the instrument is always passed with the Foroblique lens in place and advanced under direct vision so that the entire urethra is visualized as the urethroscope is passed. The process of passing the cystoscope blindly with the obturator in place is hazardous and is to be condemned. The Foroblique panendoscope lens is useful for evaluating the posterior bladder wall, the prostatic urethra and the remaining portions of the urethra. The entire bladder is always inspected with the right angle cystoscope lens. The areas of the trigone, bladder neck, urethral orifices, lateral walls and dome are closely inspected. Biopsy may be performed cautiously with the cold biopsy alligator forceps or a transurethral cautery loop. Since proper treatment of most lesions involves the complete removal of the lesion, it is usually wise to admit a patient to the hospital to perform any deep biopsy or complete resection. Deep biopsies are often associated with moderate amounts of bleeding, and a urethral catheter may be needed until the bleeding ceases.

Vesicolithalopaxy

Bladder calculi can be easily visualized on cystoscopy and can usually be removed on a short-stay or outpatient basis. Calcium oxalate and calcium phosphate stones form in the presence of outlet obstruction and are usually associated with prostatic hypertrophy or urethral strictures. The presence of a foreign body in the bladder, such as an indwelling urethral catheter, often promotes infection and is associated with struvite (magnesium ammonium phosphate) calculi. These stones are extremely soft and can be easily crushed and evacuated. Uric acid stones are seen in patients with hyperuricosuria and in individuals from the Middle East and Far Eastern countries.

The lithotrite, or stone crusher, is a urological instrument that has been used for ages. Present instruments include the Bigelow and Lowsley lithotrites. After preparing the genital area and administering anesthesia, the instrument is introduced into the bladder. The stone may be directly visualized and engaged within the jaws of the lithotrite. The jaws are then closed and the stone is crushed into the bladder and the stone fragments are irrigated. It is vital that all stone fragments be evacuated to prevent leaving a nidus for further stone formation. Infection should be treated with adequate antibiotics.

Recently, a great interest has arisen in an electronic, ultrasonic lithotrite. This is composed of a "black box" that emits an ultrasonic wave through a probe. Under direct cystoscopic vision, this probe is passed through the urethra until it comes in contact with the bladder calculus. Ultrasonic waves then act to fragment and disintegrate the calculus. All particles are evacuated with an obturator or sheath. Injury to the urethra and the bladder mucosa is minimal.

Needle Biopsy of the Prostate (Fig. 19–15)

The importance of a digital rectal exam cannot be overemphasized, particularly in men over the age of 40. Prostatic cancer ranks as the most common malignant visceral tumor in men and is responsible for over 20,000 deaths a year.

Any patient demonstrating nodularity, induration or asymmetry of the prostate gland requires investigation by prostate biopsy whether the patient is symptomatic or asymptomatic. Four methods of biopsy are available. Open perineal biopsy is reserved for clinical confirmation of malignant disease prior to a total prostatectomy in patients potentially amenable to surgical cure. Transurethral resection is restricted to patients in whom urethral obstruction requires relief. Either of the aforementioned methods may be used if needle biopsy is unsuccessful and suspicion remains high. The remaining techniques are transrectal and transperineal needle biopsy.

Needle biopsy of the prostate can be performed in the outpatient department, with a local infiltration anesthesia, by any physician who is acquainted with the technique and familiar with the local anatomy. The accuracy of needle biopsy is reported to range from 70 to 95 per cent. Biopsy is performed using the Franklin modification of the Vim-Silverman biopsy needle or the Travenol disposal biopsy needle.

The technique (Fig. 19–15) involves placing the patient in the extreme lithotomy position, with the perineum essentially parallel to the floor. A lubricated finger is placed in the rectum to isolate the prostate and palpate the desired area of biopsy. In the transperineal technique, a skin wheal is raised in the midline two finger-breadths anterior to the rectum at the approximate site of needle insertion. This infiltration is continued as the needle is advanced toward the prostate gland. With the rectal finger guiding the biopsy needle to the suspicious area, several cores of tissue are removed for pathological inspection. With the transrectal technique, the biopsy needle is introduced into the rectum and is guided by the index finger until it reaches the lesion. No local anesthesia is required using this technique and adequate tissue is removed for biopsy.

Because occult malignancy may be present in all areas of the prostate, it is

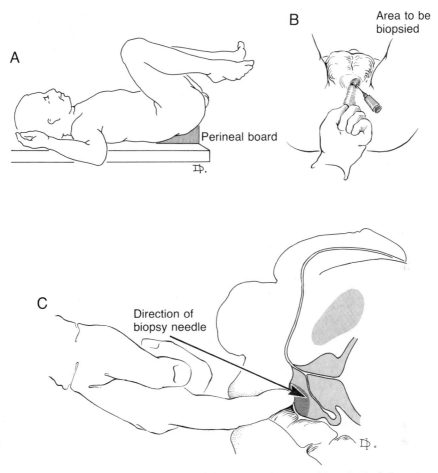

Figure 19–15 Prostate biopsy. *A.* Extreme lithotomy with perineal board (shaded area). *B.* After perineal skin wheal is raised, rectal finger guides infiltrating needle to the suspicious prostatic area. Prostatic capsule is infiltrated at this area. *C.* Lateral view, demonstrating direction of biopsy needle.

wise to remove tissue from the opposite prostatic lobe even though it feels normal. Hematuria occurs frequently and is usually mild and self limited. When significant gross hematuria occurs, the patient should be admitted to the hospital. Continued bleeding may indicate intravascular fibrinolysis or a disseminated coagulopathy. These syndromes most commonly occur in association with malignant glands and may be so severe as to require intravenous fluids or transfusions. Efflux of urine from the needle indicates that the bladder was inadvertently punctured. In such cases, antibiotics should

be given for two to three days, although urethral catheterization is rarely needed in patients with borderline outlet obstruction. Urinary retention may occur following needle biopsy because of prostatic tissue edema. Seeding of the needle tract with tumor cells is an extremely rare occurrence.

Biopsy of Lesions of the Scrotum or Penis

Any raised or ulcerated lesions of the glans, prepuce or skin of the penis or scrotum present a difficult clinical diagnosis. Serological tests for syphilis and darkfield microscopic examination should be performed routinely. Obvious lesions such as condylomata acuminata are treated appropriately. Cases in which an exact clinical diagnosis cannot be made require biopsy. Large fungating lesions of the glans penis or prepuce should be biopsied in the operating room after the patient has been hospitalized. If the biopsy is positive, definitive surgery is indicated.

Painless or superficial lesions may represent Bowen's disease, Paget's disease, erythroplasia of Queyrat, myeloma, Buschke-Lowenstein tumor or carcinoma. These lesions are differentiated by pathological examination. Biopsy involves local anesthetic infiltration, followed by a wedge excision of the lesion. Genital skin is reapproximated with an absorbable suture material.

Percutaneous Renal Biopsy (Fig. 19–16)

This procedure is a reasonably safe and efficient means to obtain renal tissue for pathological evaluation in patients of all ages. Since general anesthesia is seldom necessary when sedation is adequate, percutaneous biopsy may be performed in the outpatient department. The most common indications for renal biopsy are hematuria, proteinuria, hypertension, uremia and nephrotic syndrome. Renal biopsy is also performed to aid in the diagnosis of lupus erythematosus and other collagen vascular diseases. Renal pathological findings provide a guide to a prudent and rational therapeutic approach and may indicate eventual prognosis.

An oral or intravenous waterload of approximately 3 per cent of body weight should be given during the two hours prior to biopsy. A similar oral or intravenous volume should be given postoperatively. This will produce sufficient diuresis to allow monitoring of the urine and also will reduce clot formation that may cause renal colic. Excretory urography, hemoglobin, hematocrit and coagulation studies are routinely obtained preoperatively.

The biopsy is performed with the guide of fluoroscopy or ultrasonography. Whenever possible, the right kidney is selected because of its lower position. The patient is placed prone and a sandbag is placed under the abdomen in order to elevate and fix the kidney in position. Many techniques have been used to localize the kidney, including the application of lead markers and sterile needles to the skin. The

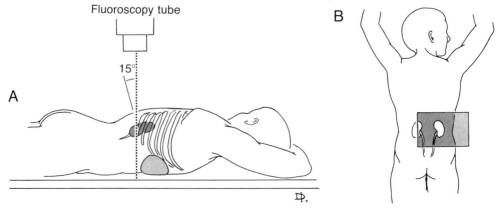

Figure 19–16 Percutaneous renal biopsy. *A.* Patient in prone position with sandbag under lower rib cage on side of biopsy (preferably right) to stabilize kidney. Fluoroscopy tube indicated. Arrow indicates 15° cranial angulation of biopsy needle. *B.* X-ray grid in place to localize kidney for biopsy.

procedure routinely involves intravenous administration of contrast medium for visualization of the kidney and collecting system. If renal perfusion is poor and a nephrogram is not seen, the biopsy may be performed using B-mode ultrasound.

The procedure includes adequate prebiopsy sedation, routine skin preparation and the use of the Franklin modification of the Vim-Silverman needle or Travenol disposable biopsy needle. Using fluoroscopic control, the needle is advanced and should ideally be inserted in the peripheral aspect of the lower pole of the kidney. The patient is requested to stop breathing while the needle is advanced past the renal fascia and capsule and into renal parenchyma. If the needle has engaged renal tissue, subsequent breathing will result in a to-and-fro movement of the needle hub. One or two biopsy specimens are obtained and can be immediately inspected under a hand lens to ensure the presence of glomeruli. Ten to twelve glomeruli are sufficient for diagnosis. The specimen is immediately handed to a pathology technician in the fresh state. Routine tissue processing involves preservation of the specimen for histology, electron microscopy and immunopathology staining.

Postbiopsy care involves temporary bedrest and observation of serial urine specimens for blood. A hematocrit and hemoglobin should be determined four to six hours after biopsy. Immediate complications are renal colic, perirenal hematoma and vesicle clot retention. Leakage of urine through the collecting system usually heals immediately. Rare complications include entrance into the pleural space, spleen, liver, bowel and major blood vessels. Microscopic hematuria is common and generally self limited. Gross hematuria may be immediate or delayed and will usually subside with bedrest, although blood transfusions are occasionally necessary. Any patient with postbiopsy pain after 24 hours should undergo intravenous urography to assess renal function, vascular integrity and obstructive uropathy. Arteriovenous fistula formation may produce significant hypertension, particularly in children. If this does not subside spontaneously with the passage of time, further investigation and possible surgery may be indicated.

Contraindications to percutaneous renal biopsy are the presence of a solitary kidney, a hemorrhagic diathesis or a cutaneous lesion near the biopsy site. In addition, if inadequate biopsy specimens are obtained after three repeated attempts because of atrophic or hypoplastic kidneys or excessive abdominal girth, the procedure should be terminated. In these instances, an open surgical biopsy is performed.

VASOGRAM AND TESTIS BIOPSY

Infertility problems in the male should be initially evaluated with an adequate history and physical examination, followed by multiple semen analyses. In patients with azoospermia, a vasogram or testis biopsy may be indicated. Trauma to the genital tract, gonorrhea, tuberculosis or epididymitis may result in fibrosis or scar tissue within the vas deferens, seminal vesicles or epididymis. In these individuals, a bilateral vasogram and seminal vesiculogram are necessary to demonstrate patency. The determination of seminal fructose is often helpful. Fructose is produced by the seminal vesicles; an absence of fructose in the ejaculate indicates congenital absence of the seminal vesicles (and also the vasa deferentia) or a complete block of the vasa, usually at the level of the ejaculatory duct.

The vasogram is done in the cytoscopy suite on a short-stay basis. Regional or spinal anesthesia is preferred and radiographic facilities are required. After adequate anesthesia and preparation of the genitalia, the vas deferens is isolated using the same technique as in a vasectomy (Fig. 19–13). With the vas deferens held taut by a tape, 3 to 5 cc of radiographic contrast material are carefully injected into the lumen of the vas with a No. 25 gauge needle. This injection is done both proximally and distally and subsequent x-rays should demonstrate proximal backflow of contrast to the epididymis. Distal flow of contrast will outline the vas deferens and seminal vesicles. Contrast should be present in the bladder and indicates that the ampulla and ejaculatory ducts are patent. After closure of the initial scrotal incision, the contralateral vas deferens is isolated. The procedure is repeated using radiographic contrast material and the No. 25 gauge needle. To demonstrate patency of the ampulla and ejaculatory ducts on the contralateral side, methylene blue is mixed with the contrast material prior to injection. After the radiographs are complete, a small catheter is inserted in the bladder and the retrieval of blue dye indicates patency of the system. Those patients who show anatomical strictures, fibrosis or scars can be surgically treated with a vaso-epididymostomy.

A testis biopsy is indicated in patients with no obvious historical, physical or congenital problems to explain aspermia or marked oligospermia. A biopsy may also be confirmatory evidence of sterility in patients with pelvic radiation, bilateral mumps orchiditis and Klinefelter's syndrome. Biopsy is often done in conjunction with a vasogram. After adequate anesthesia and scrotal preparation, a small incision is made in the scrotal skin and the tunica vaginalis is opened. Any fluid present should be allowed to drain freely from within the tunica vaginalis. The testis is grasped firmly and a 1 mm incision is made in the tunica albuginea. With pressure, seminiferous tubules are extruded. Great care is taken to preserve tubular integrity and the tissue is never grasped with forceps or clamps.

A sharp iris or dissecting scissors is used to slice off the protruding tubules. The specimen should be placed in Bouin's solution for good tissue preservation. A testicular incision is then closed with 4-0 chromic gut suture. The scrotal incision is closed. No drains are needed. After microscopic examination of the testicular biopsy, individual patients can be counseled appropriately.

FEMALE UROLOGY

Many minor conditions of the bladder and urethra are seen in women. Nevertheless, it is usually wise for the physician to take a comprehensive history of the patient including all systems, with particular attention given to psychological and sexual problems relating to urinary symptoms. Dysuria and burning with urination are extremely common. Urinary urgency and frequency may be associated with organic or functional disorders. Intermittency of stream, decreased force and difficulty in the initiation of voiding may suggest significant uropathology. While all of these symptoms are commonly seen in functional disorders, care must be taken to exlude infection or other true pathology. Incontinence of urine has several causes and is discussed elsewhere in this chapter.

A general physical examination is routine and includes particular attention to neurological evaluation. The urine specimen should be examined microscopically and appropriate cultures obtained. Even if the symptoms and physical findings indicate a simple vesical or urethral problem, a thorough investigation should always be considered. Some situations require excretory urography, postvoiding films and residual urine measurements. Occasionally voiding cystourethrograms and cystoscopy are needed. In other cases measurements of urine flow, urethral pressures and cystometrograms are needed.

TABLE 19–6 Gram-Negative Sepsis

EVALUATION	MANAGEMENT

1. Vital signs
  Acute temperature elevation
  Hypotension
  Tachycardia, bradycardia
  Restlessness
  Disorientation
  Air hunger
  Rigors
  Diaphoresis, dry skin
2. Central venous pressure (<6 cm H_2O; often <2 cm H_2O)
3. Urine output (oliguria, reflecting lowered splanchnic perfusion)
4. Pulse pressure lowered (reflecting lowered cardiac output)
5. Chest x-ray (pneumonia, atelectasis, pulmonary edema, embolism)
6. Electrocardiogram (dysrhythmia, ischemia-infaction, pericardial tamponade, pulmonary hypertension)
7. Urinalysis (infection, crystalluria, hematuria, clot, casts, tissue)
8. Blood and urine cultures
9. Laboratory data:
  Hemogram — anemia, hemolysis
  Electrolytes — hyponatremia, hypercalcemia, acidosis, hypocalcemia
  Blood sugar
  BUN, creatinine
  Serial platelet count
	1. Early recongition; prompt aggressive intervention
	2. Rapid fluid replenishment
	  Blood, colloid, saline, Ringer's solution
	  Monitor CVP, which reflects volume status and cardiac efficiency
	  Monitor BP, urine output, chest auscultation
	3. Antibiotics
	  Penicillin (20–60 × 10^6 u/d IV) or cephalothin (1.0 gm IV q 4–6 h)
	  Kanamycin (500 mg IM q 12 h) — Proteus
	  Sodium colistimethate (15 mg IM q 12 h) — Pseudomonas
	  Gentamycin
	  Carbenicillin
	  (Observe indicators of drug intolerances and renal impairment)
	4. Steroids — hydrocortisone (100–500 mg IV stat; 100 mg IV q h)
	  Methylprednisolone (250 mg IV q 4–6 h)
	  (add prophylactic oral antacid therapy)
	5. Oxygen (nasal, mask)
	6. Antifebrile measures (hypothermia blanket)
	7. Sodium bicarbonate IV
	8. Digitalis for cardiac dysrhythmias with rising CVP, pulmonary congestion, hypotension
	9. Isoproterenol (2.5–5 mg/250–500 cc normal saline; titrate infusion for effect)
	  Pulse rate <120
	10. Furosemide (40–80 mg IM or IV; observe response, repeat, increase prn)
	11. Chlorpromazine or phenoxybenzamine to assist micro-circulation
	12. Heparin (in presence of evidence of diffuse intravascular coagulation)

Fibrinogen level Fibrin split products ⎱ useful for the recognition of diffuse intravascular coagulation	

Acute bacteriological infections of the urinary tract are common in all women and should be treated with appropriate antibiotics as discussed earlier. Recurrent episodes of infection require total investigation and perhaps suppressive antibiotic therapy.

SEPTICEMIA

Sepsis and shock may result from gram-negative bacillary infection arising in any organ of the genitourinary system. These infections demand early recognition and immediate, vigorous, thorough and expectant therapy. Such management can be adequately performed only in the hospital. Gram-negative sepsis requires intensive, round-the-clock work by qualified personnel until the crisis has passed. The details of evaluation and management in gram-negative septic shock are summarized in Table 19–6.

ACUTE INTRASCROTAL INFECTION
(Epididymitis and Orchitis)

Acute inflammatory conditions of intrascrotal organs are discussed in conjunction with other acute intrascrotal disorders.

EXTERNAL GENITAL LESIONS

The skin of the external genitalia is subject to many inflammatory, infectious and neoplastic processes. Suspicious lesions on the glans may represent venereal disease or penile malignancies. In the absence of a positive serological test, a biopsy should be obtained under regional or general anesthesia. Infections of the glans penis or abscesses of the scrotal skin must be treated aggressively with appropriate antibiotics. Acute balanitis involves inflammation, edema and occasional ulceration of the prepuce and glans penis. The etiological agents involve a saprophytic infection with *Vibrio*, a nonsyphilitic spirochete, and *Streptococcus*. Treatment consists of frequent exposure to air, local cleansing and penicillin. A spreading necrotic infection of the scrotum and perineal tissue is termed Fournier's gangrene. This rare and potentially fatal infection is often seen in diabetics or individuals with urinary tract infection. Treatment involves hospitalization, parenteral antibiotics and aggressive débridement.

Condylomata acuminata, or venereal warts, are caused by a transmissible virus and arise in the coronal sulcus and glans. They can occasionally spread to the meatus and involve the entire urethral mucosa. Initial treatment involves topical application of podophyllin. If lesions recur, electrocautery or surgery may be required. Because of the venereal characteristics of the disease, all sexual contacts should be inspected and treated.

The scrotum and genital areas are frequently involved with infestations of fungus and parasites. Pediculosis pubis involves colonization of the pubic area with the crab louse and is treated with Kwell shampoo (gamma benzoate hexachloride). Scabies appears as intensely pruritic papules caused by the mite Sarcoptes. Therapy consists of 25 per cent benzyl benzoate emulsion or Kwell.

Fungal infections generally result in the formation of inflamed scaly patches. Tinea cruris ("jock itch") is caused by a dermophyte and involves the scrotum and surfaces of the thigh and perineum. The condition is aggravated by perspiration and physical activity. Treatment consists of topical agents, such as Tinactin, Micatin or Lotramin cream. Tinea versicolor is a superficial lesion characterized by brown pigmented patches and is effectively treated with selenium (Selsun) applications. *Candida albicans* (monilia) is responsible for most cases of intertrigo, an inflammatory, oozing condition frequently seen in children and termed "diaper dermatitis." Treatment consists of frequent diaper changes, cleansing and nystatin cream.

Dermatitis involving the genital skin can be caused by a reaction to topical drugs or to contact with oils, detergents, fabrics and powders. Treatment is directed toward elimination of the offending agent. Other dermatological conditions, such as psoriasis, lichen planus and seborrheic dermatitis, can also involve the scrotal or penile skin.

Raised or ulcerated lesions may represent syphilis, melanoma, Paget's disease, erythroplasia of Queyrat or carcinoma. All questionable areas should be biopsied.

PEDIATRIC UROLOGY

The most common pediatric problems seen in ambulatory or outpatient clinics involve urinary tract infections, meatal stenosis, undescended testes and bedwetting. Pediatric urinary tract infections, including cystitis and pyelonpehritis, are discussed elsewhere in this chapter. Uncircumcised boys may develop a marked inflammation beneath a phimotic foreskin. This is characterized by edema, erythema and a purulent discharge. The child often complains of pain on urination and may have urinary frequency and urgency resulting from irritation to the meatus. Balanitis is treated with local antibiotic ointments, oral antibiotics and frequent warm baths. The most common offending organism is *Staphylococcus*. If recurring episodes develop, circumcision should be performed.

Meatal stenosis is common in young boys who have been circumcised. The meatus is pinpoint in character and will not admit a No. 10 French pediatric feeding tube. The child voids with a small, weak stream and takes a long time to empty his bladder. If this diagnosis cannot be made by clinical means, a voiding urethrogram will demonstrate the stenosis with proximal urethral dilatation. A meatotomy can be done on an outpatient basis with excellent results.

REFERENCES

1. Amelar, R. D., and Dubin, L.: Basic and practical aspects of the etiology and management of male infertility. Urol. Dig., May 1975, p. 19.
2. Doust. V. L., Doust, B. D., and Redman, H. C.: Evaluation of ultrasonic B-mode scanning in the diagnosis of renal masses. Am. J. Roentgenol., *117*:112, 1973.
3. Fowler, E., Meares, E. M., Jr., and Goldin, A. R. L.: Percutaneous nephrostomy: techniques, indications and results. Urology, 6:428, 1975.
4. Hahn. L. C., Nadel, N. S., Gitter, M. H., et al: Testicular scanning: new modality for preoperative diagnosis of testicular torsion. J. Urol., *113*:60, 1975.
5. King, L. M., Sekaran, S. K., Saur, D., et al: Untwisting in delayed treatment of torsion of the testis. J. Urol., *112*:217, 1974.
6. Lapides, J., Diokno, A. C., Gould, F. R., et al: Further observation on self-catheterization. J. Urol., *116*:169, 1976.
7. Laroque, M. A., and Cosgrove, M. D.: Priapism; a review of 46 cases. J. Urol., *112*:771, 1974.
8. Perlmutter, A.: Enuresis. In Kelalis, P. P., and King, L. R. (Eds.): Clinical Pediatric Urology. Philadelphia, W. B. Saunders Co., 1976, p. 166.
9. Peterson, N. E., and Staples, D.: Blunt renal injury of intermediate degree. Urology, 9:11, 1977.
10. Pinch, L., Aceto, T., Jr., and Meyer-Bahlbung, H. F. L.: Cryptorchidism: a pediatric review. Urol. Clin. North Am., *1*:573, 1974.
11. Thomas, W. C., Jr.: Clinical concepts of renal calculus disease. J. Urol., *113*:423, 1975.
12. Trolley, D. A., and Castro, J. E.: Hemospermia. Urology, 6:331, 1975.
13. Williams, H. E. L.: Nephrolithiasis. N. Engl. J. Med., *290*:33, 1974.
14. Stamey, T. A.: Urinary Infections. Baltimore, Williams and Wilkins Co., 1972.

Female Genitourinary Tract and Obstetrics 20

JAMES R. JONES, M.D.,
and EKKEHARD KEMMANN, M.D.

INTRODUCTION

Most of the work of the gynecologist-obstetrician is done in an office or outpatient setting. The evaluation of problems such as genital bleeding, infection and pain and the control of reproductive function make up the greatest part of the daily work of the gynecologist. The obstetrician usually would choose delivery in a controlled, fully equipped environment, but ideal situations are not always possible and furthermore, a small but determined group of patients prefers deliveries outside of the hospital. The use of outpatient and overnight facilities deserves and obtains more attention these days. The pressure of medical economics will further increase this trend. This chapter tries to delineate the scope of outpatient obstetrics and gynecology. For further discussion the reader is referred to texts listed at the end of the chapter.[18, 24]

Gynecology

GYNECOLOGICAL BLEEDING

Unexpected or extensive genital bleeding is alarming and usually prompts the patient to seek medical advice on an emergency basis. Although bleeding is frequently due to endocrine factors (nonovulation), presumption of this overlooks the potentially more dangerous neoplastic and pregnancy disorders. A thorough history and physical examination, including a pelvic examination, is necessary. The approach to gynecological bleeding is modified to some extent by the age of the patient.

Bleeding in Children

Prepubescent females may bleed because of vaginal irritation (secondary to infection or a foreign body), elevated estrogen levels (due to functional ovarian tumors, precocious puberty, the ingestion of mother's contraceptive pills, or other reasons) or neoplasm. When encountering uterine bleeding in a child it is important to determine whether there are any other signs of sex hormone activity (e.g., breast or pubic hair development). If any are found, the child should be referred for complete endocrinological evaluation.

Gynecological Examination of Children

Although usually accomplishable in the office, examination may be done with the patient under general anesthesia or under meperidine-diazepam analgesia. The abdomen is palpated for pelvic masses and the external genitalia are inspected. The vagina can be examined completely by using a nasal speculum and a cotton-tipped applicator. The presence of intravaginal foreign bodies should be excluded. The cervix should be visualized, and cultures for *Neisseria gonorrhoeae* should be taken on Transgrow medium or on Thayer-Martin plates. A wet mount (with added KOH) should be examined for moniliasis. A rectal examination is carried out to rule out pelvic masses.

Pubescent Bleeding

Menstrual cyclicity is usually not established in the female until one or two years after menarche. Prior to its establishment, adolescents may have excessive and erratic uterine bleeding, occasionally associated with a secondary anemia. If the pelvic examination is normal, the possibility of local endometrial pathology is remote. When dealing with acyclic bleeding the use of dilatation and curettage (D & C) is not advisable.

Treatment of juvenile bleeders is hormonal and is best accomplished by administration of estrogen-progestin combination birth control pills, such as Ortho-Novum 1/50, Norinyl 1 + 50, and Demulen. Initially, such a combination pill is given q.i.d. or more often for five days to stop endometrial shedding.[30] An orderly menstrual bleeding will follow and regular cyclic treatment may then be instituted. It is our opinion that cyclic therapy should not be continued for more than three to six months.

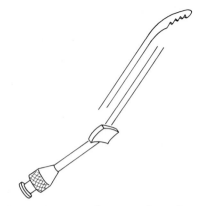

Figure 20–1 Novak curette for endometrial biopsy.

tion created by an attached 10 ml syringe and applied during a short scraping movement with the curette. The tissue is placed in formalin and inspected to assure that a sufficient quantity was obtained for histological examination.

Bleeding in the Reproductive Years

In this group of patients it is most important to exclude a gestational event (abortion, ectopic pregnancy, trophoblastic disease, and so on) or a neoplasm as the cause of bleeding. Bleeding disorders in the reproductive years are usually due to nonovulation and require further specific evaluation. An endometrial biopsy may be helpful in defining local pathology.

Endometrial Biopsy

This diagnostic procedure can be done in the office without anesthesia. After pelvic examination the anterior lip of the cervix is grasped and the cervico-uterine axis is straightened. The biopsy curette (Novak curette; Fig. 20–1) is introduced into the cavity and tissue is sampled from the uterine walls (a four-quadrant sampling). The tissue sample is obtained with the aid of a small amount of suc-

Perimenopausal Bleeding

In a woman over 35 years of age with hypermenorrhea or intermenstrual bleeding the possibility of endometrial cancer is significant. Thus, for diagnostic purposes the procedure of choice is a fractional dilatation and curettage (D & C). A D & C will usually stop the bleeding temporarily and allow for a specific tissue diagnosis.

Fractional D & C

A dilatation and curettage is done under aseptic conditions. Because of cervical dilatation, anesthesia is required and can be local (paracervical block) or general. The major complication of D & C is uterine perforation, which usually can be handled expectantly. Patients can be discharged within a few hours after a D & C.

The patient is placed in lithotomy position, then prepared and draped.

A perineal shaving is not needed. Pelvic examination is made and the uterine position is noted. The cervix is visualized, with its anterior lip grasped with a tenaculum. The endocervix is curetted with an endocervical curette to obtain the first specimen. The cervico-uterine axis is straightened and the cervix is dilated using a set of Hegar dilators, usually up to size 18 (Fig. 20–2). The uterus is sounded and its depth is recorded (normal being 6 to 8 cm), and a uterine curette is manipulated in a clockwise scraping movement, thus removing the endometrial tissue as the second specimen. The tissue is caught in a wet sponge that has been placed in the posterior vaginal fornix.

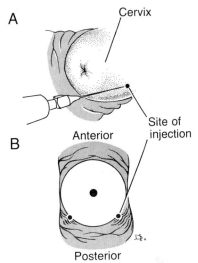

Figure 20–3 Uterosacral block. *A.* Sites of injection in the uterosacral ligaments are 4:00 and 8:00 with the patient in the lithotomy position. *B.* Gentle traction on the cervix permits identification of the uterosacral ligaments. 5 to 10 ml of 1% lidocaine are injected with a 22 gauge, 3½ inch spinal needle. Each uterosacral ligament is injected to a depth of 0.5 cm.

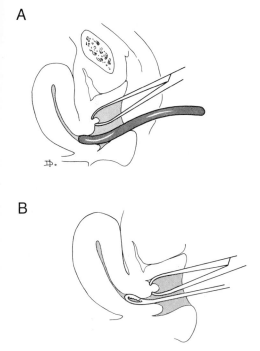

Figure 20–2 Dilatation and curettage of the uterus. *A.* Progressively larger Hegar dilators are used to overcome resistance at internal os. Forcep type dilators should not be used. *B.* The largest sharp curette which can be passed through the endocervix is passed to the fundus. Strips of endometrium are removed from the uterine cavity in a clockwise fashion. The illustration shows the curette in the endocervix, which should be curetted as a separate specimen prior to introduction of the curette to the fundus.

The cavity is re-explored for polyps, which may be missed with the curetting. After removal of the instruments a final pelvic examination is carried out. Bleeding that occurs from the procedure is minor and self-limited.

PARACERVICAL BLOCK. Paracervical block is satisfactory anesthesia for most procedures requiring dilatation of the cervix. Minor dilatation of the cervix, such as that required for endometrial biopsy, is tolerated well by most patients without anesthesia.

A speculum is placed into the vagina and the cervix is grasped with a tenaculum. Gentle traction on the cervix will usually identify the uterosacral ligaments, which are at the 4 o'clock and 8 o'clock positions. A 10 ml syringe with a 22 gauge, 3½ inch spinal needle is used. Five to 10 ml of 1 per cent lidocaine is injected into each uterosacral ligament after the needle has been inserted ½ cm into the ligament. A submucosal swelling should be visible at the injection site. The needle is introduced about 2 cm from the external os (Fig.

20–3). Aspiration on the syringe is important before injecting the solution in order to avoid a sudden intravenous injection in this highly vascular area.

Postmenopausal Bleeding

Any genital bleeding in the postmenopausal woman is abnormal and deserves evaluation. On occasion atrophic vaginitis may be the only problem, and it is amenable to local application of estrogen cream. Cervical neoplasia must be ruled out by visual and cytologic examination. Frequently the bleeding is uterine. A fractional D & C is the diagnostic procedure of choice.

GENITAL INFECTIONS

Vulvovaginitis

Vulvovaginitis, manifested by discharge, irritation and itching, is a common gynecological complaint that is amenable to outpatient evaluation and treatment.

Most vulvovaginitis is the result of a specific vaginal infection with *Candida albicans, Trichomonas vaginalis* or *Hemophilus vaginalis.* The specific clinical criteria for these vaginitides, as compared with physiological vaginal discharge, are shown in Table 20–1.

The specific diagnosis is frequently confirmed by wet mounts that are immediately examined. Cultures are usually not necessary but can be carried out with specific media.

Candida infection can often be recognized as white plaques adherent to the vaginal walls and the cervix. Candida can be identified microscopically by the presence of spores and mycelia, which are recognizable after KOH is added to the wet mount (Fig. 20–4). Contributing factors for candidiasis are antibiotic, estrogen and immunosuppressant therapy, diabetes mellitus and debilitating diseases. Treatment consists of local or systemic administration of nystatin and elimination of contributing factors.

Trichomoniasis is easily identified in a saline wet mount as an active, ciliated, tear-shaped protozoan (Fig. 20–5). Treatment is with metronidazole and should also be given to the patient's sexual partner to prevent recurrent infection.

Hemophilus vaginitis is diagnosed by the identification of "clue" cells — exfoliated vaginal cells stippled with minute cocci (Fig. 20–6). Triple sulpha cream is appropriate treatment.

A number of other entities may cause vulvovaginitis:

FOREIGN BODY. Diagnosis is usually evident on examination. This problem is not uncommon in children.

HERPES GENITALIS. This often-recurrent virus infection may cause herpetic lesions that become secondarily infected by bacteria. Treatment consists of antibiotic ointment. The herpetic infection itself, which is characterized by vesicle formation and pain, is extremely difficult to treat. Silver nitrate applications may

TABLE 20–1 Clinical Characteristics of Vaginal Discharge

CAUSE	COLOR	CONSISTENCY	ODOR	VAGINAL pH	REMARK
Physiological	clear	thin to mucoid	none	3.5	increased at ovulation
Candida	white	curd-like	musty	4.5	itching predominant
Trichomonas	yellow-green	frothy	fetid	5.0	often urinary symptoms
Hemophilus	milky	viscid	acrid	5.5	"clue cells"

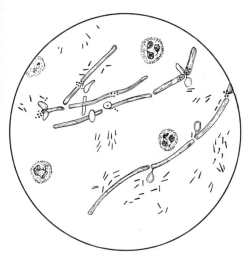

Figure 20–4 Candida albicans spores and mycelia as seen on a wet smear. Leukocytes and Döderlein's bacilli are also present. (From: Kistner, R. W.: Gynecology: Principles and Practice, 2nd ed. Chicago, Year Book Medical Publishers, 1971, p. 84.)

ameliorate specific vesicular areas. Fortunately, antibodies are formed and the disorder tends to be self-limited. When active herpes genitalis infection is diagnosed during late pregnancy a vaginal delivery should be avoided, because contact with the herpetic infection is life-threatening to the newborn.[20]

CONDYLOMATA ACUMINATA. These are multiple warts that may develop over extensive portions of the vagina, cervix, vulva and perineum. Associated vaginal infections should also be treated. Smaller warts can be eradicated by multiple applications of 20 per cent podophyllin in tincture of benzoin. The medication should be washed off after six hours. Larger lesions may have to be removed surgically under anesthesia. Lesions are desiccated with electrocoagulation and excised with a sharp knife. Recently, the use of cryosurgery (see following section) has become popular. Lesions are frozen for a few seconds, depending on their size and the instrument used, and no further treatment is necessary. The approach is safe and simple.

ATROPHIC VAGINITIS. Inadequate estrogen production may lead to chronic vaginal infection and dyspareunia. Cytology reveals a lack of cornified vaginal epithelium. Treatment consists of local estrogen supplementation.

Chronic Cervicitis

An alkaline discharge of the cervix may disrupt the normal vaginal flora.

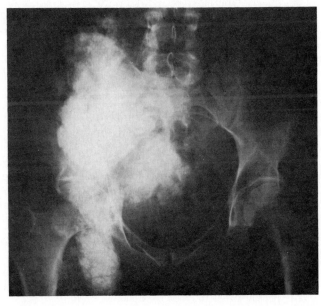

Figure 20–5 Wet smear preparation showing trichomonads, leukocytes and exfoliated vaginal cells. (From: Kistner, R. W.: Gynecology: Principles and Practice, 2nd ed. Chicago, Year Book Medical Publishers, 1971, p. 81.)

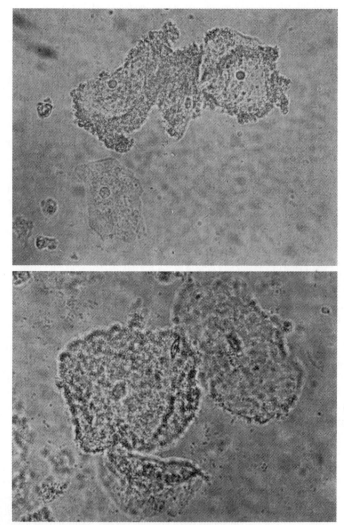

Figure 20–6   Wet mount showing "clue cells," epithelial cells stippled with *Hemophilus vaginalis* organisms. (From: Gardner, H. L., and Dukes, C. D.: *Hemophilus vaginalis* vaginitis: A newly defined specific infection previously classified "non-specific." Am. J. Obstet. Gynecol., 69:970, 1955.)

In chronic cervicitis the cervix is usually everted and a columnar cell surface extends around the external os. If cytologic and colposcopic examinations confirm the benign character of the condition, local destruction by heat or freezing aids in the healing of such a cervical erosion.[19]

strips are cauterized over the everted surface (Fig. 20–7). No anesthesia is necessary. The postoperative healing process may be facilitated by the use of a vaginal antibiotic cream. Care should be taken not to perform excessive cauterization, which may result in cervical stenosis.

Cervical Cauterization

The cervix is visualized, and with a nasal cautery tip six to eight radial

Cryosurgery

Cryosurgical treatment may be used for chronic cervicitis and cervi-

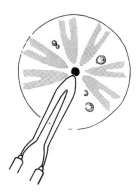

Figure 20–7 Cervical cauterization. Nasal cautery tip is introduced into the endocervical canal. Six or eight radial strips are cauterized over the eroded surface. "Actual" cautery is used, with a glowing red cautery tip.

cal eversions. Usually no anesthetic is required. The probe of the freezing unit is inserted into the os and should include most of the ectocervix, including the abnormal areas. After the tip is applied the cooling agent is allowed to flow through the probe. The effective freezing temperature is achieved within 5 to 30 seconds and varies with different instruments. The length of application depends on the instrument used and the local anatomy but is usually about two minutes. The patient should be aware that over the next three weeks an increased watery discharge is to be expected. The discharge is rich in potassium, and on occasion slight, generalized muscle weakness may be noted. Follow-up examination should ascertain adequate healing. Cervical stenosis is extremely rare.[21]

Gonorrhea

As a sexually communicable disease, gonorrhea is usually found during the reproductive years, but gonorrheic vulvovaginitis may also occur in children and postmenopausal adults. A large proportion of infected patients, male or female, may have minor or no clinical problems and are "carriers." Early clinical manifesta-

tions in the female include vaginal discharge, abnormal uterine bleeding and signs of lower urinary tract infection. In 17 per cent of these individuals the disease may advance into the upper genital tract, resulting in pelvic inflammatory disease (PID).

The most effective method of diagnosis is a culture utilizing Thayer-Martin media. Culture sites should include the cervix, but other contact areas (such as the anus and pharynx) may yield positive cultures. Thayer-Martin cultures need immediate incubation at 35 to 36° C in a 6 to 10 per cent CO_2 atmosphere. To overcome this problem the "Transgrow" system has been developed. Repeat cultures are necessary to confirm eradication of the *Neisseria gonorrhoeae*. Screening for syphilis should be carried out on all patients with gonorrhea.

The treatment of gonorrhea is outlined in Table 20–2. Sequelae of gonorrheal infection may necessitate surgical intervention.

TABLE 20–2   Treatment of Gonorrhea[1]

RECOMMENDED TREATMENT

Parenteral
 4,800,000 units of aqueous procaine penicillin G in two intramuscular injections administered at one visit, together with 1 gm of probenecid administered orally 30 minutes before the injection.

or

Oral
 3.5 gm of ampicillin and 1 gm of probenecid administered simultaneously.

ALTERNATIVE TREATMENT
 (For patients in whom penicillin, ampicillin or probenecid is contraindicated.)

Parenteral
 Spectinomycin dihydrochloride pentahydrate in one intramuscular injection, 2 grams for males and 4 grams for females.

or

Oral
 1.5 gm of tetracycline hydrochloride in an initial dose, followed by 0.5 gm four times a day until a total dose of 9.5 gm has been administered.

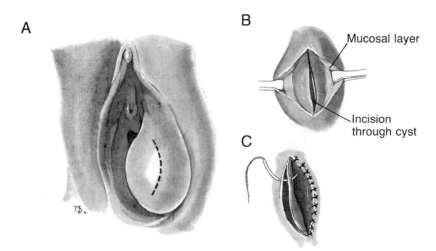

Figure 20–8   Marsupialization of Bartholin's cyst. *A*. Longitudinal incision is made along muco-cutaneous junction of vulva and vagina, overlying the cyst. *B*. Incision is carried down through cyst wall and contents are drained. *C*. Cyst lining is everted and sutured to skin, with interrupted 3-0 chromic catgut sutures.

Bartholin's Abscess

Infection of the Bartholin's duct may lead to obstruction and abscess formation. A nontender Bartholin cyst may be found as the result of chronic infection. Not all Bartholin's abscesses are due to gonorrhea.

Although simple incision and drainage of the Bartholin's abscess will give immediate relief, this procedure is not recommended because of the high recurrence rate and subsequent cyst formation associated with it. The most effective treatment is marsupialization of the Bartholin's gland. This is also preferable to excision of the Bartholin's gland.

MARSUPIALIZATION. After cleansing, local anesthesia (1 per cent lidocaine) is applied to the intended line of incision at the mucocutaneous junction of the affected labium minora. A stab incision is extended into a wide incision, as shown in Figure 20–8. After drainage of the contents of the cyst or abscess, the cavity is irrigated with saline. The lining of the cyst is everted and sutured to the skin with interrupted 000-chromic

catgut. No drains are necessary, but sitz baths are advised.

Pelvic Abscess

Abscess formation may occur behind the uterus or within tubes and ovaries. Persistence of a pelvic abscess in spite of hospitalization and vigorous antibiotic therapy is an ominous sign that it may require surgical excision. This is an unfortunate circumstance, since the most effective approach is removal of all affected organs (uterus, tubes and ovaries) when the abscess is secondary to gonorrhea. When infected tissue is left behind, the recurrence rate is high.

NEOPLASM

The diagnosis of neoplasm depends on the histological examination of a tissue specimen. Biopsy material from the vulva, vagina, cervix and endometrium can be obtained in the Outpatient Clinic. The treatment of gynecological malignancy is best given in centers specializing in gynecological oncology.

Vulva

Postmenopausal women who complain of vulvar irritation and itching should be tested with toluidine blue staining of the vulva. After cleansing with 1 per cent acetic acid, a solution of 1 per cent toluidine blue stain is sponged over the vulva and perineum. The toluidine blue stain is removed with another acetic acid rinse. Areas that retain the stain contain excessive nuclear material, should be considered potentially malignant, and therefore should be biopsied.

Vulvar Biopsy

Toluidine-stained areas, nonhealing ulcerations and any suspicious vulvar or perineal lesions should be biopsied to rule out cancer. After the vulva is cleansed, the skin next to the biopsy area is locally anesthetized. A dermatological punch biopsy instrument (Fig. 20–9) is used to remove tissue, preferably from the margin of the lesion. The instrument is rotated on the skin and, when lifted, the biopsy tissue can be removed. Pressure, or an astringent solution, will usually suffice to stop any bleeding.

Excisional Biopsy

Small or subcutaneous lesions may be removed by excisional biopsy. Although such lesions may be asymptomatic, their removal is indicated to rule out neoplasia. Common lesions are sebaceous cysts and hydroadenomas. After cleansing and local anesthetic infiltration of the area, an elliptical incision is made around the lesion. The lesion is grasped with an Allis clamp and freed by blunt and sharp dissection. Bleeding points as well as the basal vascular pedicle of

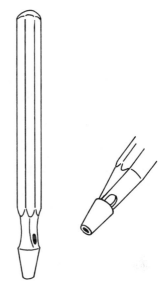

Figure 20–9 Punch biopsy instruments for vulvar biopsy.

the growth are tied (000-chromic). After removal of the lesion the skin is closed with 000 nylon.

Vagina

The discovery that maternal exposure to diethylstilbestrol (DES) may be associated with vaginal cancer and adenosis in the female offspring makes it mandatory to examine thoroughly all children with vaginal bleeding or persistent discharge. "DES daughters" may exhibit characteristic lesions such as transverse vaginal and cervical ridges, cervical collar, vaginal hood and cockscomb on the cervix. Staining with Lugol's solution (Schiller test) may reveal abnormal areas. The exocervix and the vagina have glycogen-containing squamous epithelium, and when this epithelium is replaced by columnar or abnormal epithelium (adenosis) the iodine stain is not retained after washing with saline. Nonstaining areas should be examined by colposcopy and biopsied.[11]

Cervix

Pap Smear

The cornerstone in the routine evaluation of the normal-appearing cervix is the cytological evaluation of cells from the squamocolumnar junction — the "Pap" test. A yearly cervical smear should be obtained for all women who are sexually active and all women over the age of 20. The equipment consists of clean glass slides, a nonabsorbent cotton-tip applicator or a cervical spatula, and a container of equal parts of 95 per cent alcohol and ether. The unlubricated speculum exposes the cervix, and the applicator is used to scrape cells from the endocervix and the squamocolumnar junction. The cells are transferred to the slide by rolling the applicator on the glass or scraping the glass with the spatula. A fine film of cells is thus obtained. Thick or bloody films should be avoided. The slide is immediately placed in the container with the alcohol-ether fixative. If the estrogen status of a patient is to be evaluated cytologically, a second slide containing cells from the lateral vaginal walls is prepared in the same fashion. After fixation of about two hours the slides may be removed, dried and sent to a cytology laboratory.

Cervical Biopsy

If a suspicious cervical lesion is found, a cervical punch biopsy should be taken (Fig. 20–10). A variety of biopsy instruments are available. Except in pregnancy, biopsy sites of the cervix rarely need any attention. However, if continuous bleeding is encountered, electrocautery or a 000-chromic suture is adequate for hemostasis.

Colposcopy

If a woman has atypical or suspicious cervical cells on cytological ex-

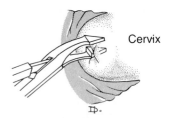

Figure 20–10 Cervical punch biopsy (Schubert forceps). Biopsy must include squamocolumnar junction. With this instrument, it is possible to include tissue within the endocervical canal in the biopsy.

amination, inspection of the cervix with a colposcope is helpful if the examiner is experienced with using one.[16] The status of the cervix is assessed under magnification. After the vascular pattern has been enhanced through the application of acetic acid, the optimal biopsy site can be chosen from the most suspicious area. Suspicious tissue is removed with a Kervokian biopsy forceps, and endocervical curettage specimens are obtained. Colposcopy may give the experienced observer sufficient information to obviate more extensive diagnostic procedures such as a cone biopsy. Colposcopy is an outpatient procedure and requires no anesthesia.

Cone Biopsy

Cone biopsy of the cervix is used most often with patients whose cells are abnormal and who have no gross or colposcopically visible lesion of the cervix. The cone biopsy removes the entire squamocolumnar junction, allowing the pathologist to examine a wide selection of tissue. Cold knife cone biopsy should be performed rather than the older methods of cone biopsy using a cautery instrument. At all times except during pregnancy, this procedure is combined with dilatation and curettage of the uterus to establish the source of the abnormal cells and the extent of the disease.

While it is possible to accomplish this procedure under local anesthesia or paracervical block, it is preferable to use regional or general anesthesia. Shaving the perineum is unnecessary and only causes the patient undue discomfort after the procedure. The patient is placed in the dorsal lithotomy position, and the perineum and vagina are prepared with an appropriate skin antiseptic. Care should be taken during the preparation to avoid the cervix and upper vagina so that superficial cells will not be dislodged. Pelvic examination should be done to confirm the preoperative findings. A weighted speculum is placed in the vagina to depress the posterior vaginal wall, and narrow retractors are utilized to visualize the remainder of the vagina and cervix. With a tenaculum on the anterior lip of the cervix, the cervix and vagina are stained with Lugol's solution or Gram's iodine. The cervical canal and the uterine cavity should be probed gently with a uterine sound to determine the direction of the cervical canal before biopsy. Before an incision is made in the cervix, hemostasis should be accomplished by placing a single 0-chromic suture in each lateral portion of the cervix to occlude the major blood supply to the area. These sutures are left quite long so that they can be used for traction during the procedure. A conelike incision is made in the cervix with a scalpel blade, the margins of the cone including all non-staining areas. A shallow incision is carried far enough to include the squamocolumnar junction but not the internal os, which has previously been identified using the uterine sound. After the initial incision is made, the upper limits of the cone biopsy can be removed from the cervix with curved scissors (Fig. 20–11). Any bleeding points on the cervix should be controlled with figure-of-8 0-chromic sutures. If a large portion of the cervix is removed with the cone, the Sturmdorf mattress suture will help reconstitute the epithelium and at the same time control bleeding (Fig. 20–12).

Antibiotics, packing and douches are unnecessary following a cone biopsy. The patient should be advised to abstain from intercourse for one month, and she should be seen by the physician two weeks and six weeks after the procedure so that the cervical canal can be sounded to prevent stenosis or adhesions.

A small percentage of patients who have a cone biopsy will develop excessive postoperative bleeding. Usually this occurs about ten days after the procedure when the eschar is expelled. In these cases the bleeding areas must be resutured or cauterized.

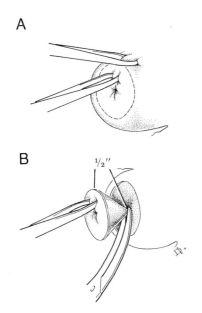

A

B

½"

Figure 20–11 Cervical cone biopsy #2: Removal of specimen. *A.* The cervix is grasped with a tenaculum. Circular scalpel incision should include squamocolumnar junction, but not the internal os. *B.* Removal of specimen is completed with curved Mayo scissors.

Endometrium

Cancer of the endometrium is found most commonly in perimenopausal and postmenopausal women

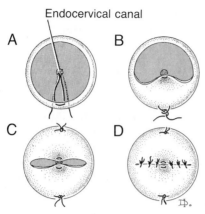

Endocervical canal

Figure 20–12   Cervical cone biopsy #3: Closure with Sturmdorf mattress suture. *A.* An 0-chromic suture on a heavy, curved, noncutting needle is passed from the posterior aspect of the *portio vaginalis* to the apex of the cone in the endocervical canal. The suture is then brought back to the superficial margin of the biopsy. It is returned to the apex of the cone and again brought out to the *portio vaginalis*. *B.* The suture is tied, inverting the mucosa over the biopsy site. *C.* Similar suture is placed anteriorly. *D.* Additional sutures may be used as necessary for hemostasis and to close the mucosal defect.

and usually signals its presence with abnormal uterine bleeding. The diagnostic procedures, i.e., endometrial biopsy and D and C, have been described in previous sections. In addition, it may be advisable to perform periodic endometrial biopsies in nonbleeding patients who are known to be at risk for endometrial cancer (for example, patients receiving long-term estrogen medication, nonovulatory patients, those with a past history of endometrial hyperplasia, and others). Various types of endometrial aspirators have been developed. However, their use should be limited to "screening" since their accuracy is not at the level of the D and C or the endometrial biopsy.

Patients in whom a diagnosis of adenomatous endometrial hyperplasia has been made should be followed (and perhaps treated) carefully. Although not a neoplasia, adenomatous hyperplasia is a precancerous lesion.[10]

Ovary

Ovarian cancer has the poorest prognosis of all gynecological malignancies. Many attempts have been made to identify "markers" (carcinoembryonic antigen, human chorionic gonadotropin, and others) for ovarian cancer, but these are still inconclusive. The pelvic examination remains the single most effective method of detection.

Ovarian enlargement (cystic or solid) in a postmenopausal woman or a prepubescent child demands immediate and aggressive investigation. Solid ovarian enlargement in a woman of any age requires a definitive diagnosis. Unilateral cystic ovarian enlargement in the reproductive-age woman can be due to either "functional" or neoplastic cysts. Functional cysts rarely exceed 6 cm, and their size definitely changes from menstrual cycle to menstrual cycle. Neoplastic cysts stay the same or increase in size and, of course, require laparotomy.

PELVIC PAIN

Pelvic pain is a common complaint in women. The character and timing of the pain generally dictate its designation. Premenstrual pelvic "heaviness" is usually referred to as "pelvic congestion"; crampy pain directly associated with the period is called dysmenorrhea; vaginal discomfort or abdominal pain during sexual intercourse is termed dyspareunia; and vaginal "heaviness" is usually found with pelvic relaxation syndromes. Since pelvic relaxation will be covered in the next section, this discussion will be concerned with pelvic congestion, dysmenorrhea and dyspareunia.

Pelvic Congestion

The symptoms of pelvic congestion are usually perceived as lower abdominal "heaviness" preceding (by as much as two weeks) the menstrual period. In general, this syndrome is found in young women and women approaching the menopause (perimenopause). Some degree of pelvic discomfort prior to the period is entirely normal and reflects the normal changes of circulating estrogens and progesterones. The pelvic congestion syndrome refers not to this expected discomfort but rather to an incapacitating degree of premenstrual lower abdominal pain.

The etiology of pelvic congestion is unknown. Clearly it is related to changes in circulating hormones, but why these affect some patients profoundly and others not at all is obscure. It has been anecdotally observed that pelvic congestion is often associated with a lack of childbearing or sexual intercourse. In the perimenopausal woman a case may be made for venous congestion and the formation of pelvic varicosities as possible causes.

Whatever the etiology of pelvic congestion may be, the diagnosis is usually made by excluding other factors such as chronic pelvic infection, ovarian cysts, endometriosis and leiomyomata uteri. In patients for whom the discomfort is significant and prevents normal day-to-day living, laparoscopy may be carried out to establish the diagnosis. Treatment for pelvic congestion is symptomatic and often frustrating. Unfortunately, once confirmed, there is little that can be done for pelvic congestion. Diuretics have been used but with little success. Replacement therapy (cycling with an oral contraceptive) has been employed extensively but is not universally effective. In addition, oral contraceptives probably should be used only infrequently, and with very specific indication, in women more than 35 years old. Pelvic congestion is frequently seen in the obese patient, and some very satisfying results have been obtained with significant

weight reduction. Exercise (jogging, tennis, walking, and so on) is frequently an excellent adjunctive therapy. Rarely, if ever, is surgery indicated unless a specific lesion is found.

Dysmenorrhea

Abdominal discomfort associated with the menstrual period is normal, but dysmenorrhea can be incapacitating and requires specific therapy. Dysmenorrhea is divided into primary and secondary types.

PRIMARY DYSMENORRHEA. Primary dysmenorrhea is that syndrome of lower abdominal menstrual pain that is not associated with a discernible pelvic cause. This is the typical dysmenorrhea experienced by many women in their early reproductive years. It is generally ascribed to a uterocervical dysfunction, i.e., the lack of synchrony between fundal contractions and cervical passage of the menstrual fluid. The diagnosis of primary dysmenorrhea is usually made by exclusion. Generally the patient will complain of crampy abdominal pain that is coincident with the first day of bleeding. It may continue for the second day but rarely beyond that. In the etiology of dysmenorrhea the release of excessive amounts of prostaglandins has been suggested.[10]

The treatment of primary dysmenorrhea can be symptomatic or specific. Frequently, relief can be obtained with analgesics (codeine, acetophenetidin and aspirin, and others); however, this palliative therapy is not effective over an extended period of time, since dysmenorrhea is frequently progressive. Cyclic therapy (using oral contraceptives in the usual manner) is more specific and most often will eliminate dysmenorrhea. It is conceded that long-term cyclic therapy in the young patient is not desirable. For this reason, our usual approach is to prescribe oral contraceptives for only three or four months and then to discontinue the treatment. Once the patient realizes that the discomfort can be attenuated she is generally more capable of handling the dysmenorrhea by her own devices. The oral contraceptive has indeed proved to be an excellent therapeutic modality for these patients, but its use must be limited on the basis of need.

SECONDARY DYSMENORRHEA. Secondary dysmenorrhea is menstrual or premenstrual pain that is associated with a pelvic lesion (ovarian cyst, adhesions, or other conditions). Obviously, in this instance removal of the pelvic lesion is the key to success.

One of the most common causes of secondary dysmenorrhea is endometriosis. Endometriosis is defined as the growth of endometrium-like tissue outside of the uterine cavity, e.g., on the ovaries, the posterior broad ligaments, the cul-de-sac and uterosacral ligaments or potentially in any other area of the abdominal cavity or even outside it. These endometriotic lesions are hormone-dependent (estrogen and progestin), and therefore their size may vary with the circulating steroid levels. Just prior to the fall in estrogen and progestin levels that causes menstruation, the lesions are maximally stimulated and therefore may cause considerable discomfort. With menstruation and the marked decrease in hormone levels, the endometrial implants decrease in size and the pain may be lessened. This continuous cycle of stimulation and quiescence coupled with the "burning out" of older lesions may lead to cicatrization and adhesion formation, causing continuous pain not related to menstruation. Other sequelae of endometriosis may be infertility and dyspareunia. Occasionally, an endometrial lesion in an ovary (called endometrioma or "chocolate cyst") can grow to considerable size, and the patient presents with the findings and symptoms of an ovarian cyst.

Although it is recommended that the diagnosis of endometriosis be confirmed by biopsy, the pelvic examination can be suggestive. In the patient with progressive dysmenorrhea and no previous history of infection, the finding of thickening in the adnexa or of an irregularity of the uterosacral ligaments is highly suggestive of endometriosis. When suspected, the patient should have laparoscopy and appropriate biopsies for confirmation of the diagnosis.

The treatment of endometriosis depends upon the extent of the disorder and the patient's reproductive plans. For a young patient with the reproductive years ahead of her, the most appropriate therapy is probably hormonal. To this purpose danazol (Danocrine), a mildly androgenic suppressor of gonadotropins, is most efficient. Danazol (400 to 800 mg per day for six to nine months) leads to a state of temporary ovarian suppression referred to as "pseudomenopause" and usually provides good relief but not a permanent cure. Other medical therapies, such as high doses of oral contraceptives, are less desirable because of the numerous side effects. In the young patient with extensive endometriosis, conservative resection under observation of the reproductive functions may become necessary. A total abdominal hysterectomy (usually with bilateral salpingo-oophorectomy) would be indicated for disabling or extensive endometriosis, especially if maintenance of reproductive capability is no longer important to the patient.

Dyspareunia

Pain with sexual intercourse is clinically divided into "insertional" and "bumping" types. Insertional dyspareunia is usually described as vaginal pain (or burning or irritation) upon insertion of the penis. Its cause may be vaginismus, vaginal infections, cervical or vaginal tumors or atrophic vaginitis. Therapy depends upon the specific findings. Bumping dyspareunia, that is, abdominal pain associated with the penis (or a finger or a vibrator) making contact with the cervix, is due to intra-abdominal pathology — ovarian cysts, endometriosis, leiomyomata uteri, pelvic inflammatory disease, and so on. Treatment is directed at the underlying pathology.

PELVIC RELAXATION

The general term "pelvic relaxation" refers to prolapse of the uterus, cystocele, rectocele and enterocele. All these entities need not be present concomitantly, but the specific diagnosis is important in the choice of corrective procedures and the ultimate outcome.

The major supportive structures for the uterus, upper vagina and bladder are various condensations of the endopelvic fascia. The uterus and upper vagina are supported by the base of the broad ligaments (the cardinal or Mackenrodt's ligaments), which attach to the lateral portion of the lower fundus and the upper cervix and vagina and insert at the lateral pelvic wall. The condensation of the endopelvic fascia beneath the vaginal mucosa, which spreads from the symphysis pubis, bladder and cervix (perivesical fascia), is the primary supporting fascia for the bladder and urethra. Although there is a thickening of the fascia beneath the vaginal mucosa overlapping the rectum (rectovaginal fascia), the major support of the rectum is the levator ani muscle. The pouch of Douglas (the cul-de-sac) in the normal patient is rather shortened and is prevented from bulging into the vagina by the uterosacral ligaments.

A cystourethrocele results from a herniation of the bladder and the urethra through a defect in the perivesical fascia. A rectocele is usually accompanied by a disruption in the levator ani muscle and the rectovaginal fascia. Prolapse of the uterus is most frequently secondary to weakening and attenuation of the cardinal ligaments. An enterocele, that is, herniation of peritoneum and small bowel through the pouch of Douglas into the vagina, generally results from disruption of the cardinal ligaments and attenuation of the uterosacral ligaments. The basic cause of the endopelvic defects is the trauma associated with childbirth. Rarely, one will see a nulliparous patient whose pelvic relaxation has a congenital or familial basis. Pre-existing pelvic relaxation is commonly accentuated during the postmenopausal years.

The symptoms of pelvic relaxation are quite variable. Most commonly a multiparous patient will have some aspects of pelvic relaxation but will be completely asymptomatic. In this instance, no surgical therapy should be recommended.

Cystocele, prolapse and rectocele may cause the patient to present because of "protrusion," and occasionally uterine prolapse is associated with back pain. Pelvic relaxation rarely causes abdominal pain. Difficulty with sexual intercourse (loss of sensation, poor penetrance) is a rather common complaint. Probably the most disconcerting and, in some instances, incapacitating symptom is that of urinary stress incontinence, which frequently accompanies a cystourethrocele. The patient specifically complains of an involuntary loss of urine caused by an increase in intra-abdominal pressure from laughing, sneezing, exertion, bending over or other movements. Characteristically, there is no loss of urine when sleeping or when simply sitting or standing. Chronic prolapse of the uterus can result in a very severe and extensive drying and ulceration of the cervix. In severely incapacitated patients, especially those who are bedridden, one will occasionally see entrapment of the uterus (and perhaps of the entire vaginal tube) outside the introitus with resultant edema, excoriation and severe pain.

The diagnosis of pelvic relaxation is usually quite obvious. However, the evaluation of a cystourethrocele and its relationship to urinary stress incontinence requires a detailed cystometric examination.

Cystometric Examination

The basic pathology of urinary stress incontinence is not cystourethrocele but rather a flattening, or "loss," of the posterior urethrovesical angle. Therefore, urinary stress incontinence is occasionally found with little in the way of pelvic relaxation. Conversely, a large cystourethrocele may be found without accompanying stress incontinence. Other causes of urinary incontinence, such as cystitis, a neurogenic bladder or a vesicovaginal fistula, must be ruled out. Evaluation of the patient's urinary stress incontinence can be accomplished by having her void and immediately inserting a Foley catheter. The volume of residual urine is measured and a specimen is obtained for culture and urinalysis. If more than 50 ml of residual urine are found, the diagnosis of a neurogenic bladder must be ruled out before performing surgery. A 1000-ml bottle of normal saline solution is attached to the catheter. As the solution fills the patient's bladder, she acknowledges the first sensation of bladder fullness (150 to 200 ml) and the point at which she feels her bladder can hold no more (500 to 700 ml). If the patient's first urge to void is at 50 ml or less, she should be suspected of having trigonitis or a small, spastic bladder. If the bladder capacity is over 700 ml, a flaccid, neurogenic bladder may be the problem, and more sophisticated urological investigation should be undertaken before any pelvic surgery is performed.

After the bladder capacity has been reached, saline is drained from the catheter until 250 ml of solution remain within the bladder, and the catheter is removed. In the lithotomy position, if the patient loses urine when she coughs, the examiner inserts two fingers into the vagina, elevating the urethrovesical angle beneath the symphysis pubis. Care should be taken not to occlude the urethra. If urine is not expelled when the patient coughs again, one of the surgical procedures to elevate the posterior urethrovesical angle will probably be successful in correcting the incontinence. The test should be repeated in an upright position if incontinence cannot be demonstrated when the patient is lying down. If loss of urine when coughing cannot be demonstrated with 250 ml of saline in the bladder, the diagnosis of stress incontinence due to poor anatomical support should be questioned. In these circumstances, attempts at surgical correction will not improve the patient's symptoms and, in fact, may aggravate her problem.

A further refinement in identifying the type of stress incontinence and measuring the posterior urethrovesical angle is the bead-chain cystogram.

Evaluation of Uterine Prolapse

The clinical extent of the prolapse is categorized as follows (Fig. 20–13): first degree prolapse is one in which the cervix comes to, or approaches, the introitus; in second degree prolapse, the cervix protrudes through the introitus; and in third degree (complete) prolapse, the entire uterus (cervix and fundus) is external to the vaginal introitus. Although usually a straightforward diagnosis, uterine prolapse can be confused with cervical hypertrophy. This can be resolved by locating the uterosacral ligaments. The uterosacral ligaments insert posteriorly at the upper portion of the cervix, and hypertrophy of the cervix occurs below the insertion of the ligaments. Thus with uterine prolapse alone, the ligaments will be close to the introitus, whereas with cervical hypertrophy the uterosa-

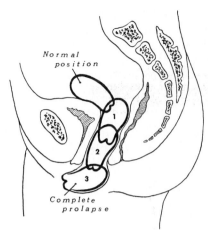

Figure 20–13 Diagrammatic representation of the degrees of uterine prolapse. (From: Parsons, L., and Sommers, S. C.: Gynecology, 2nd ed. Philadelphia, W. B. Saunders Co., 1978, p. 1442.)

cral ligaments will be high in the vagina.

An enterocele is usually quite difficult to diagnose in the office. It is most often associated with uterine prolapse and rectocele. The diagnosis is most commonly made at the time of surgery when the posterior wall is opened and the protruding peritoneal sac is exposed. It is absolutely critical to repair the enterocele, since its continued presence can result in vaginal prolapse. The treatment of pelvic relaxation is usually surgical, with the underlying principle being repair of the endopelvic fascial defects.

In cystourethrocele the perivesical fascia is exposed and the defect is closed (anterior colporrhaphy); the same is done with the periurethral fascia (Kelly plication). When urinary stress incontinence is associated, it is important to reconstruct the posterior urethrovesical angle. On occasion (generally after failure of the vaginal approach), an abdominal procedure is utilized in which the angle is restored by various "sling" or stabilizing operations (Marshall-Marchetti procedure, Ball procedure, and others).

The usual surgical correction of prolapse is a vaginal hysterectomy with shortening and reattachment of the cardinal ligaments to the lateral cuff. In the young patient who desires to have more children (in whom uterine prolapse occurs only infrequently), or in the very elderly patient with third-degree prolapse in whom there is little in the way of cardinal ligaments to reconstruct, a Manchester-Fothergill procedure may be carried out.

The key to repair of a rectocele (posterior colporrhaphy) is repair of the levator ani muscle and closure of the fascia. As discussed previously, it is essential that an enterocele be located, the peritoneal sac ligated and excised, and the uterosacral ligaments closed. There is little agreement about or success with the repair of vaginal prolapse.

On occasion, in the very elderly and debilitated patient, various vaginal pessaries may be used to correct pelvic relaxation (Fig. 20–14). Whenever possible, however, the best approach is surgical. In young patients or in pa-

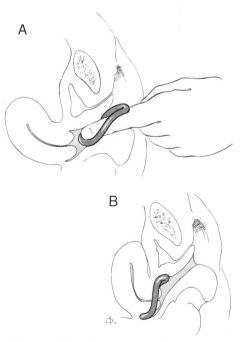

Figure 20–14 Pessaries: Smith-Hodge type. A. Pessary is inserted behind cervix. B. Pessary in place.

tients with small amounts of pelvic relaxation, various perineal muscle exercises can be helpful. These exercises
consist in the patient's voluntarily contracting the pubococcygeus muscle
with its visceral extensions. This is accomplished by instructing the patient
to contract her vaginal muscles as
though she were stopping a bowel
movement or the flow of urine. Once
she has learned it, the patient continues
this exercise for 10 to 20 minutes
several times a day.

Finally, it must be remembered that
additional factors such as obesity,
chronic lung disease, heavy smoking
and other conditions can contribute
significantly to a poor surgical outcome.

FAMILY PLANNING

Contraception

Present contraceptives vary widely
in use-effectiveness (Table 20–3). Selection of the "best" method depends
on the patient's age, her medical, obstetrical and sexual histories and her personal attitudes.

The diaphragm and the intrauterine
device (IUD) require specific fitting
procedures.

TABLE 20–3   Use-Failure Rates of
Contraceptive Methods*
(Pregnancies per 100 Woman-Years)[22]

METHOD	USE-FAILURE RATE
Oral contraceptives	2–5
Intrauterine device	3–6
Progestin injection	5–10
Diaphragm	15–20
Condom	15–20
Foam	30
Calendar rhythm	35
Withdrawal	20–25
No method	80

*From: Page, E. W., Villee, C. A., and Villee,
D. B.: Human Reproduction, 2nd ed. Philadelphia,
W. B. Saunders Co., 1976, p. 89.

Diaphragm

Diaphragms are manufactured in a
number of sizes, and as a rule the largest size that is comfortably accomodat-
ed by the vagina is the one that should
be prescribed. In our experience most
patients tolerate a 75 or 80 mm diaphragm well. The diaphragm is always
used with contraceptive jelly and is left
in place for about eight hours after intercourse.

FITTING OF DIAPHRAGM. Either a
fitting set of flexible rings or a set of
diaphragms of progressive size (65 to 85
mm) should be used for fitting. The
well-lubricated diaphragm is squeezed
together and introduced into the vagina
with the convex side directed inferiorly. It is moved along the vagina until
the posterior portion of the ring is positioned behind the cervix, in the posteri-
or vaginal fornix. The anterior portion
of the ring should slide snugly behind
the lower border of the symphysis. The
patient should examine herself, feel the
cervix and confirm that the cervix is
covered; there should be no discomfort
at all when the diaphragm is in place.
The patient is taught to insert and remove the diaphragm herself and is instructed about proper maintenance and
storage.

Intrauterine Device

Many types of IUDs are available,
but the physician is best advised to
become completely familiar with one
or two of them. The major complication
is perforation, which usually occurs at
the time of insertion and is related to
the physician's lack of experience.

Side effects of IUDs are excessive
bleeding, pain and a possible increase
in the incidence of pelvic infection.
Retention rates are lower and side effects higher in nulliparas and patients with abnormal uteri (congenital
malformation, fibroids); therefore,
these patients are not considered prime
candidates for these devices. The FDA

requires that any patient in whom an IUD is inserted must read and understand a specific patient brochure provided with each device.

INSERTION TECHNIQUE. A pelvic examination is done to rule out the presence of pelvic infection or anatomical abnormalities. The most appropriate time for insertion is at the end of a menstrual period. The cervix is cleansed and the uterocervical axis is straightened by grasping the anterior cervix with a tenaculum. The uterus is sounded and the depth of the cavity is noted. The plastic inserter is introduced and the device is released into the fundus. Two types of inserters are currently used. More recent developments favor an inserter that is progressed to the fundus, the depth of which is known from the sounding. When the inserter is pulled back the device is released (release technique, Fig. 20–15). Older types of IUD (e.g., the Lippes Loop) have an inserter that is moved only into the lower uterine cavity. Then the device is pushed forward with the plunger and finally released (push-in technique, Fig. 20–16). After removal of the inserter the presence of the device in the cavity is indicated by a thread protruding from the cervix. It should be cut to a length of 2 to 3 cm from the cervical os.

REMOVAL OF IUD. This is usually accomplished simply by bringing the cervix and the uterus into a straight axis using traction on a cervical tenaculum and then grasping the thread with a Kelly clamp and exerting gentle but steady traction on the device. If a patient is found to be pregnant while wearing an IUD, the device should be removed.

"LOST IUD." If the thread of the IUD is not visible, either the IUD has been expelled or it is in a misplaced intrauterine or intra-abdominal position. Exploration of the endocervical canal with a cotton-tipped applicator may reveal the string. Exploration of the uterine cavity with a Randall stone forceps or an alligator forceps may be successful in delivering a malpositioned intrauterine IUD. If this examination does not reveal that the IUD is in the uterus, additional localization methods should be used. A plain film of the abdomen will reveal whether an IUD is present in the pelvis. A hysterosalpingogram will outline the intrauterine or extrauterine device. If located *in utero,* an IUD may be removed by D and C, with hysteroscopy or under fluoroscopy with an alligator forceps. If the IUD is found to be intra-abdominal, removal via laparoscopy is quite often successful.

PELVIC INFECTION SECONDARY TO IUD. Although relatively minor pelvic infections (endometritis, vaginitis) are fairly common in patients with an IUD, pelvic abscess occurs infrequently. These are sometimes unilateral, affecting only one adnexal area. They are treated with antibiotics and rarely with surgical excision. Because of the relatively localized nature of an IUD abscess as compared with gonorrhea, less extensive surgery can usually be carried out.

Oral Contraceptives

Birth control pills have proven to be highly effective, efficient and convenient. They also exemplify the problems that arise when a relatively safe drug is given to a large population.

Oral contraceptives available in the U.S. are usually of the "combination" type, containing an estrogen (either mestranol or ethinyl estradiol) and a progestin. Side effects are usually minor and consist of facial pigmentation, nausea, depression and edema. Glucose tolerance may be decreased and triglyceride and phospholipid levels may be elevated. An increase in renin and renin substrate may lead to reversible hypertension in some women. Patients taking oral contraceptives are more likely to suffer from gallbladder disease. Hepatoma development has been associated with oral

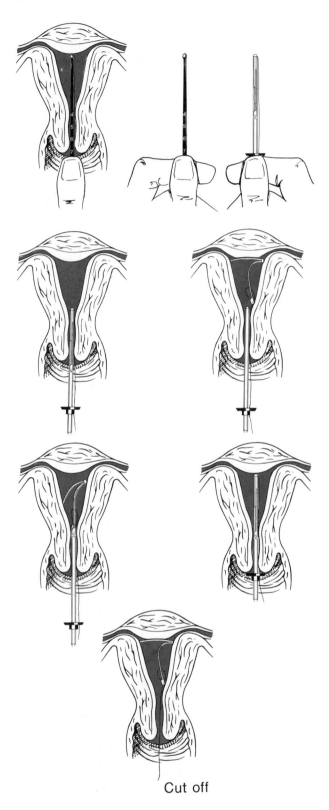

Cut off

Figure 20–15 Release technique for IUD insertion. With this method, the inserting tube is placed to the fundus, and the tube withdrawn, releasing the IUD.

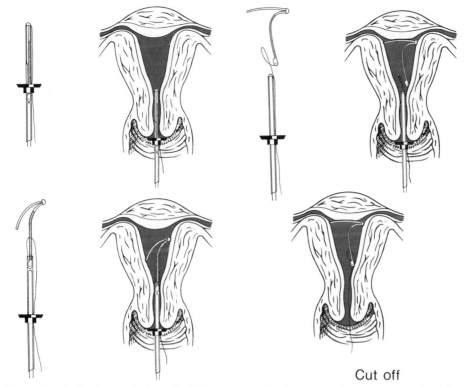

Cut off

Figure 20–16 Push-in technique for IUD insertion. The inserting tube is inserted only to the end of the endocervical canal and the IUD is then pushed into the uterine cavity.

contraceptive use. A number of collaborative studies indicate that the rate of thromboembolic disease is increased about sevenfold in oral contraceptive users. Problems may arise from superficial or deep vein thrombosis, pulmonary embolism, thrombolic or hemorrhagic stroke and myocardial infarction. Smoking has been identified as an additive factor in the development of thromboembolic disease. Another risk factor is age, and it appears that after the age of 35 the Pill is a poor choice of contraceptive. There is no reason to believe that oral contraceptives are a risk factor in the development of genital or breast cancer.

It appears that the thromboembolic phenomena are primarily related to the estrogen component of the contraceptives. Thus, most agents currently used are "low" in estrogens, e.g., they may contain 30 to 50 μg of ethinyl estradiol. When prescribing oral contraceptives, it is quite rational to start with the lowest estrogen dose available.[29] Contraindications to the use of oral contraceptives are given in Table 20–4.

When oral contraceptives are first started it is often recommended that an adjunct contraceptive method be used for the first ten days. Manufacturers provide 21 or 28 day packages, the latter containing seven hormonally inert tablets to keep the patient in the habit of taking one pill a day. Preferably, the pill should be taken in the evening, and if one is missed, then two pills should be taken the next day. If more than five pills are missed the contraceptive effect is essentially lost. Examinations at regular intervals include breast, liver and genital examinations, blood pressure recording and cervical smears.

TABLE 20–4 Contraindications for Oral Contraceptives

ABSOLUTE

History of thromboembolic disease
Known or suspected breast cancer or estrogen-
    dependent cancer
Undiagnosed genital bleeding
Congenital hyperlipidemia
Pregnancy and breast feeding
Liver impairment

RELATIVE

Heavy smoking
Age over 35
Hypertension
Epilepsy, migraine headaches
Gallbladder disease
Emotional problems
Leiomyomata uteri
Renal dysfunction
Varicosities

An alternative type of oral contraceptive is the "progestin only" pill. Although they are highly effective and avoid the side effects caused by estrogens, "progestin only" pills are not widely used because of the high incidence of breakthrough bleeding.

Sterilization

Sterilization should only be advised if the patient has completed her reproductive goals and understands that sterilization procedures are permanent and, for all practical purposes, irreversible. Classic laparotomy methods that required hospitalization have increasingly been replaced with methods that can be performed in an advanced outpatient setting, where the patient is discharged either the same day or after an overnight stay. However, because of potential unexpected findings and serious acute complications, full hospital facilities should be within reach. Current female sterilization procedures consist of tubal occlusion techniques performed via laparoscopy or mini-laparotomy.

Laparoscopy

A number of methods are used. The tubes can be closed mechanically by the application of various devices (Silastic band, Hulka clip) or can be destroyed by electrocoagulation.[23]

LAPAROSCOPIC PROCEDURE (Fig. 20–17). At laparoscopy the surgeon can observe the pelvic organs and has surgical access specifically to the uterus, fallopian tubes and ovaries. Indications for laparoscopy are suspected ectopic pregnancy, suspected endometriosis, unexplained chronic pelvic pain and unexplained infertility. In addition, laparoscopy serves as a method for tubal sterilization. Contraindications to laparoscopy are cardiopulmonary deficiency, intestinal obstruction, extensive intraperitoneal adhesions, intra-abdominal hernias, generalized peritoneal infection and obesity (more than 200 lb overweight). A major complication is hemorrhage from lacerated vessels of the abdominal wall, mesentery, pelvis or retroperitoneum. Iliac or aortic punctures or lacerations may occur owing to improper penetration by the gas needle or the trocar. Other complications are preperitoneal emphysema, puncture of intraabdominal organs and gas embolism. The procedure is performed under strict aseptic conditions with the supervision of an experienced laparoscopist. General anesthesia is preferable because patients are placed in deep Trendelenburg position. Laparoscopy can be done in ambulatory centers but the potential complications require rapid access to full hospital facilities.

The specific equipment for laparoscopy includes a gas insufflation needle (Verres), a telescope with a sheath and a trocar, a gas insufflation machine connected to a carbon dioxide source and a fibro-optic attachment.

The patient is placed in semilithotomy position and anesthesia is induced. The vagina and abdomen are prepared for surgery and the bladder is emptied. After pelvic examination a

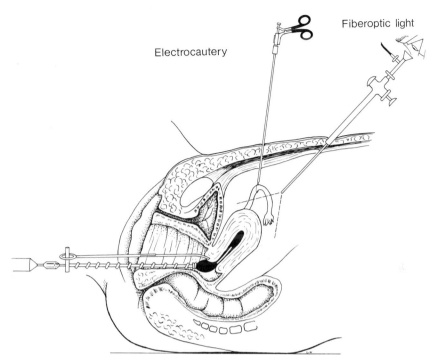

Electrocautery

Fiberoptic light

Figure 20–17   Laparoscopy technique. Note the laparoscope has been inserted immediately infraumbilically with a second probe just above the symphysis. The suprapubic probe can be used for cauterization or other manipulations of the tubes.

tenaculum with a Cohen cannula is placed on the cervix for uterine manipulation. The patient is placed in the Trendelenburg position. Through an infraumbilical stab incision the Verres needle is introduced into the peritoneal cavity; its thrust is straight towards the fascia and then angled toward the center of the pelvis. An aspirate is obtained using an attached syringe and is checked for blood or intestinal contents. Carbon dioxide is insufflated at a rate of not more than one liter per minute with control of the intra-abdominal pressure (which should not exceed 30 mm Hg). After insufflation of about three liters of gas, the abdomen should be globally distended and typanitic and liver dullness should have disappeared. The needle is then replaced by the trocar, which is pushed for 2 cm beneath the skin and then thrust downward into the abdominal cavity directed toward the center of the pelvis.

Through the sheath the telescope is introduced and observation may begin. Ancillary instruments can be introduced either alongside a specially constructed laparoscope (single-puncture technique) or through a second puncture. The two-puncture technique requires a second small tocar with sheath, which may be inserted in the midline of the lower abdomen. In this manner, calibrated probes, grasping forceps, scissors, biopsy forceps and various other instruments can be introduced. After termination of the procedure, the abdomen is partially deflated and the skin is closed with a subcutaneous absorbable suture.

Postoperative discomfort is usually minimal. Sometimes shoulder pain is noted. The patient can be discharged the same day or after an overnight stay.

Each tubal occlusion technique has specific instruments that are introduced into the abdomen, usually through the two-puncture technique. Clear identification of the fallopian tube is essential and can only be accomplished by visualization of the fimbriated end. Occlusion techniques are applied to the isthmic portion of the tube. Complications arise owing to improper application of the clips or band. In using electrocoagulation techniques, thermal injury to bowel and abdominal wall are potential problems. Failure of sterilization may be due to an overlooked pregnancy at the time of the procedure, to incomplete occlusion or recanalization of the tubes or to occlusion of structures other than the fallopian tubes (i.e., round ligaments).

Mini-Laparotomy

Mini-laparotomy does not require any specialized equipment; standard surgical techniques are used. The procedure can be done under local infiltration anesthesia or general anesthesia. Contraindications are obesity, pelvic infection or adhesions, uterine enlargement or fixed retroversion and pregnancy. Complications include uterine perforation and bladder or bowel injury. The inability to visualize the fallopian tubes or to stop accidental tubal bleeding may necessitate enlargement of the incision.

The basic principle of the procedure is that, with a sound or a uterine elevator, the uterus is brought against the abdominal wall so that the fallopian tubes can be reached and occluded through a small abdominal incision.[12]

MINI-LAPAROTOMY PROCEDURE (Fig. 20–18). Patient is placed in semilithotomy position, prepared and draped. The bladder is emptied. Pelvic examination is done and a Vitoon uterine elevator is introduced into the anteriorized uterus. By means of a 3 cm transverse suprapubic incision through skin, subcutaneous tissue and fascia, the rectus muscles are reached. These are retracted laterally. The peritoneum

is identified and incised transversely. Army-Navy retractors are used to provide lateral traction. By gentle manipulation of the uterine elevator the uterus is brought upward and forward so that the tubes appear in the incision separately. A modified Pomeroy tubal ligation is carried out. The midsection of each tube is picked up with a Babcock clamp and a kink is formed. At a distance of 2.5 cm from the kink, the lateral and medial portions of the tubes are crushed with a Kocher clamp and ligated with a figure-of-8 0-plain catgut suture. The loop portion of the tube is excised. The peritoneum, fascia and skin are closed in layers. Instead of the Pomeroy procedure, other methods of tubal occlusion such as electrocoagulation or application of a Silastic band are often used.

In the sterilization procedures discussed here, the intrinsic failure rate is approximately two pregnancies or less in 1000 patients.

INFERTILITY

It is estimated that 10 to 15 per cent of couples who desire children will ultimately consult a physician because of infertility or subfertility. About half of these couples will demonstrate an abnormal female factor and about one-third will show a significant abnormality in the male. Frequently more than one factor, involving both partners, will be found. In about 10 per cent of infertile couples, no abnormalities will be found even after the most extensive of investigations.

There is no "standard" infertility work-up. What is described here gives an overview of many infertility factors, their significance and possible treatments.

Infertility in the Female

The major causes of infertility in the female are nonovulation, tubal obstruc-

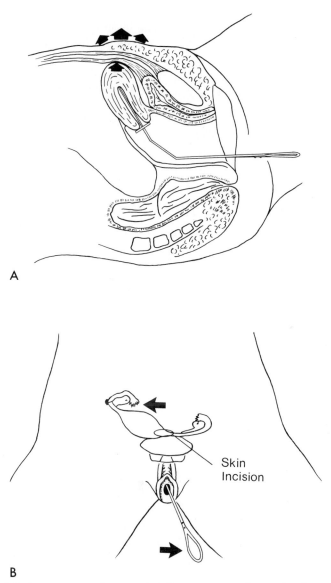

A

B

Figure 20–18 Minilaparotomy technique. *A.* A Vitoon uterine elevator has been inserted into the uterus and the fundus is pressed against the anterior abdominal wall. *B.* A small suprapubic transverse incision is made over the point where the fundus bulges the anterior abdominal wall and then the uterus is moved laterally to gain access to the tubes on each side. (From: Contemporary Obstetrics and Gynecology, *11*:114, 1978.)

tion and failure of proper implantation of the fertilized egg.

Determination of Ovulation

There is only one absolute test of ovulation and that is pregnancy. The following tests are tests of implied ovulation; essentially they depend not on the release of the oocyte but rather upon the associated estrogen and progesterone production.

MENSTRUAL HISTORY. When a patient becomes nonovulatory she usually notices a disruption of the menstrual pattern and the development of either irregular menses or amenorrhea.

Amenorrhea is divided into primary and secondary types. Primary amenorrhea is defined as the lack of spontaneous menses after the completion of the seventeenth year. Secondary amenorrhea is amenorrhea occurring at some point after spontaneous periods have been established.

PREMENSTRUAL SYMPTOMS. Generally the cyclic (ovulatory) patient experiences a fullness of the breasts, "bloating" and some emotional irritability for about ten days prior to the expected period. These premenstrual symptoms (molimina) are excellent hallmarks of endocrinological normalcy.

BASAL BODY TEMPERATURE. There is an increase of 0.5 to 0.7 degree F in the basal body temperature (BBT) from the follicular to the luteal phase. This shift in temperature can be noted best from basal conditions. In about one third of cycles, a fall (about 0.3 degree F) in temperature may occur prior to the rise.

ENDOMETRIAL BIOPSY. Generally, the finding of a secretory endometrium is indicative of ovulation. However, obtaining an endometrial biopsy carries with it the risk of interrupting a pregnancy. It is our opinion that there are sufficient other tests to preclude the use of endometrial biopsy in most infertility patients.

VAGINAL CYTOLOGY. The se-

quence of changes in vaginal exfoliative cell morphology from the follicular phase to the luteal phase can be followed by noting the alterations in cornification, cellular folding, nuclear characteristics and the presence or absence of leukocytes. This approach, however, is one of hindsight and cannot be predictive. In addition, a number of vaginal infections (trichomonal, nonspecific vaginitis) can interfere with the interpretations of vaginal cytology.

SPINNBARKEIT. At the time of ovulation the cervical mucus thread may be stretched to 10 cm or more. After ovulation there is thickening and increase in density of cervical mucus.

FERN TEST (Fig. 20–19). When this test is done using secretions obtained from the cervix during the proliferative phase, a ferning reaction will take place when the mucus dries on a slide. The fern-like pattern disappears in the presence of progesterone. Hence, it is the disappearance of ferning that indicates that ovulation has occurred.

PREGNANEDIOL AND PROGESTERONE. Progesterone is partially excreted in the urine as pregnanediol. In the follicular phase the output of pregnanediol rarely exceeds 1 mg per 24 hours. This test is expensive and time-consuming and affords no immediate answers. A more specific test is the weekly determination of plasma progesterone. Levels above 4 ng per ml are found in the luteal phase.

There are many causes for failure of ovulation. The specific diagnosis is usually made by extensive testing, and a discussion of these tests is not within the scope of this chapter.

Induction of Ovulation

Within the past few years a number of highly effective methods of inducing ovulation have evolved.

CLOMIPHENE CITRATE (CLOMID). This is an oral medication that acts as an antiestrogen to "push" the patient's pituitary to produce FSH and LH, thereby prompting ovulation. Ob-

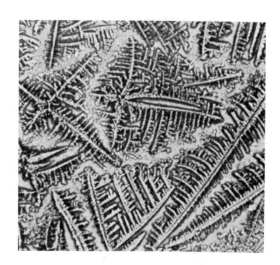

Figure 20–19 Fern test. The crystallization of cervical mucus into a fern-like pattern. This is the result of unopposed estrogen exposure. (From: Jeffcoate, T. N.: Principles of Gynecology, 4th ed. New York, Appleton-Century-Crofts, 1975, p. 94.)

viously, clomiphene requires a potentially normal pituitary.[30]

REPLACEMENT WITH FSH AND LH (PERGONAL). The use of human FSH and LH to induce ovulation has been one of the most important advances in infertility treatment in the past 20 years. It is usually limited to those patients who have a loss of pituitary function, but it is also used extensively in patients in whom clomiphene has failed. Pergonal is given by injection for 10 to 14 consecutive days, after which ovulation is induced with human chorionic gonadotropin (hCG). Although it is a very potent and successful method of treatment, the use of Pergonal should be limited to a very few clinics that have the ability to monitor the patient's daily estrogen response (plasma or urinary estrogen determinations).

WEDGE RESECTION OF THE OVARIES. This method, which consists in surgically removing about one-half to two-thirds of each ovary, is limited to patients with large polycystic ovaries. Wedge resection should only be carried out in patients who are interested in immediate pregnancy and in whom other methods of inducing ovulation have failed. The possibility of postoperative adhesion formation severely restricts the usefulness of this procedure.

Evaluation of Fallopian Tubes

Obstruction of the fallopian tubes may result from pelvic infections, congenital abnormalities, previous pelvic surgery or endometriosis. Depending upon the location and the extent of the damage to the tube or tubes, tuboplasty may be of help.

After a number of years of experience with tuboplasties it is clear that, although reconstruction can be carried out, successful pregnancy rates do not parallel the "surgical cure" rates.

The most essential point in the repair of tubal obstruction is the precise diagnosis of the obstruction. For many years the Rubin test (an office procedure in which carbon dioxide is injected into the uterus through the cervix) was used in diagnosing tubal obstruction. Today it is felt that the Rubin test is frequently misleading, and other studies must be carried out.

Hysterosalpingography (HSG)

HSG consists of the injection of radiopaque material into the cervix to outline the uterine cavity and the fallopian tubes. Thus, both intrauterine and tubal problems can be defined (Fig. 20–20).

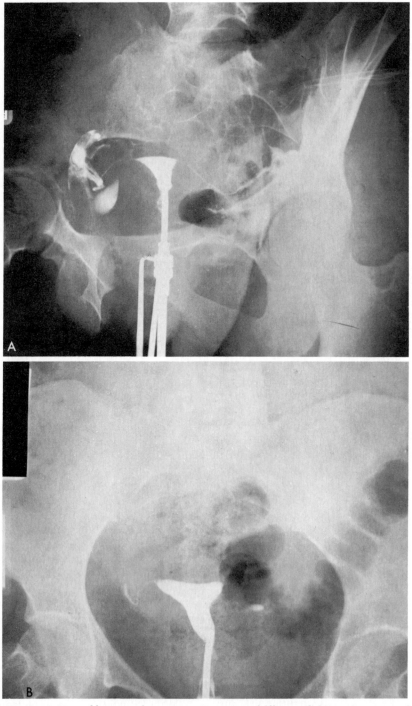

Figure 20–20   *A*. Normal hysterosalpingogram. Note normal filling and shape of uterus. Radiopaque material is found to be filling both tubes and spilling freely into the peritoneal cavity. *B*. Hysterosalpingogram in patient with bilateral tubal ligation. Note normal configuration of uterus and filling of tubes to their mid-portion where the flow of dye abruptly terminates.

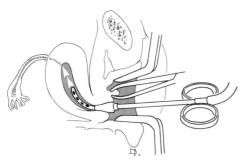

Figure 20–21 Technique for instillation of CO_2 or contrast material into uterus and fallopian tubes. Traction is placed on cervix with tenaculum. Olive-tipped cannula is inserted into cervix to achieve air-tight apposition of cervix to the olive portion. CO_2 or contrast material is introduced, depending on the test desired, as described in the text.

PROCEDURE FOR HSG. A laxative or enema on the evening prior to the procedure is advisable. A scout film of the abdomen and pelvis is taken prior to beginning the procedure. The patient is placed in a comfortable lithotomy position on the x-ray table, and a speculum is introduced into the vagina. The anterior lip of the cervix is grasped with a tenaculum and the cervix is cleansed. A sterile olive-tipped cannula is filled with contrast medium, and air bubbles are eliminated from the cannula and syringe. The cannula is inserted in the cervix and secured either by hand or by attaching the cannula to a special clamp on the tenaculum (Fig. 20–21).

The contrast medium used should be water-soluble. The water-soluble material is rapidly absorbed and is not associated with the rare but perplexing complication of oil granuloma. Oil-soluble material may cause fatal embolism.

After proper placement of the cannula, 1 to 2 ml of medium are slowly injected into the uterus, and the first film is exposed. It is preferable that films be taken during fluoroscopic observation of the progress of the procedure. A second film is taken after filling of the tubes is noted. If these films fail to visualize both fallopian tubes well, the patient is turned to either oblique position and, after further injection of 1 to 3 ml, a picture is made to visualize adequately the fallopian tube that may have been obscured by the position of the uterus. Defects in the uterine cavity must be differentiated from air bubbles by persistence of the defect on all films. Spilling of the material into the peritoneal cavity is evidence of tubal patency. One must still be suspicious of peritubal pathology if the passage of the contrast material into the peritoneal cavity is delayed or if the material becomes restricted to one area. When using water-soluble medium, a 10-minute delayed film will be satisfactory for determining peritoneal spilling of the contrast material.

Complications of this procedure are uterine perforation, exacerbation of pelvic inflammation and intravascular injection of contrast material if excessive force is used during the injection. The ideal time for performing hysterosalpingography is the preovulatory period.

Laparoscopy

Using this technique for visualization of the pelvic viscera (as outlined previously), methylene blue is injected into the cervix via a Cohen cannula during the laparoscopy, and the passage of the dye through the tubes is observed. In addition, tubo-ovarian relationships can be assessed and pelvic adhesions, not seen on HSG, can be visualized.

In general, in any patient in whom a tubal factor is suspected as the cause of infertility, both HSG and laparoscopy should be carried out. Laparoscopy is also suggested in infertile women in whom the previous investigation has not revealed the cause of infertility.

Tuboplasty is usually not carried out if there is another cause of infertility in addition to the tubal obstruction. The overall success rate of tuboplasty varies from 5 per cent to 40 per cent, depending upon the type of tuboplasty, the cause and extent of tubal damage and the skill of the surgeon.

Uterine Evaluation

The uterine cavity may be so distorted from previous infections, congenital abnormalities or fibroids that the egg cannot implant successfully. These abnormalities are usually detected with HSG, but on occasion hysteroscopy may be helpful to define the problem.

HYSTEROSCOPY PROCEDURE. Hysteroscopy enables the observer to inspect the uterine cavity and to perform minor operative procedures. Hysteroscopy can be done in an outpatient setting and requires only a paracervical block and occasional supplemental analgesia. Its major complication is cervical or uterine perforation. Hysteroscopy should only be done by an experienced examiner. Indications for hysteroscopic operations are limited to intrauterine abnormalities such as synechiae, septum formation and leiomyomata. In addition, IUDs that have resisted ordinary attempts can be removed under hysteroscopic control. Pelvic infection, hemorrhage, cervical stenosis and pregnancy are contraindications to the use of hysteroscopy.[28] The uterine cavity must be distended for observation, and a variety of media can be used for this purpose. The easiest method is the use of 50 ml of 32 per cent dextran 70 in a syringe connected to the stopcock of the sheath of the hysteroscope. The telescope-mounted sheath is introduced into the uterine cavity after cervical dilatation. Sufficient dextran is injected to distend the cavity, and the cavity is illuminated via a fibro-optic system.

The most common uterine surgery carried out for infertility is the myomectomy. Myomectomy should be performed only for those patients in whom one is reasonably certain that fibroids are the cause of infertility.

There are a number of miscellaneous and more difficult to define factors that should be mentioned.

Postcoital Test

CERVIX. The adequacy of the cervix and its mucus is usually investigated by means of a postcoital test (PCT). This is carried out by asking the couple to have intercourse around the time of ovulation. Within eight hours a small sample of the cervical mucus is examined under the microscope. Although there are no definite standards, at least ten motile sperm per high-power field should be seen. An adequate PCT indicates adequate coital technique, appropriate cervical mucus and probably no significant cervical infection.

IMMUNE FACTORS. It seems clear that a very small but definite number of infertility problems are caused by an immune factor, either in the female or the male.[25] This factor may cause the sperm to agglutinate or to be immobilized. This entire area requires much further research before we can firmly state its relative importance.

Infertility in the Male

Any investigation of an infertile couple must include a history and physical examination of the male partner as well as a sperm analysis. In the history, certain factors that may depress the sperm analysis reversibly, such as stress (usually related to work or emotional difficulties), excessive smoking or alcoholism and recent infections (both viral and bacterial) should be excluded. In addition, a complete history of genital infections, sexual adequacy and groin trauma is of obvious importance. Certain childhood viral infections (especially mumps) can result in compromise of testicular function.

The most important test is of course the sperm analysis. Sperm is best collected by masturbation after two to three days of abstinence and should be analyzed within two hours. A normal sperm sample shows:

Volume: 2–5 ml

Concentration: more than 20 million sperm per ml

Motility: more than 60 per cent with normal movement

Morphology: more than 60 per cent normal-appearing sperm

If any of these factors is abnormal, fertility may be reduced. A single sperm analysis is not adequate, and repeat testing should be done after four weeks. Results from a sperm analysis may be abnormal for many reasons.

ENDOCRINE-METABOLIC PROBLEMS. These include such problems as hypopituitarism, adrenogenital syndrome, hypothyroidism, diabetes mellitus and the Klinefelter syndrome.

VARICOCELE. For reasons that are by no means clear, varicocele can result in a depressed sperm count with some abnormally shaped sperm ("tapered" forms). Varicocelectomy, when carried out in the selected patient, can be very successful (up to 50 per cent pregnancy rates).[7] In our experience, fertility is unaffected by varicocelectomy in patients with markedly low sperm counts.

TESTICULAR FAILURE. In a fairly large group of infertile males the only diagnosis that can be made is of testicular failure. The cause is not clear, and thus therapy is nonspecific and rarely helps.

CRYPTORCHISM. Intra-abdominal testes that persist till after puberty are usually sterile. In a child with cryptorchism it is essential that this condition be diagnosed and treated promptly. Even when childhood treatment of cryptorchism is successful, about one-quarter of such males will have infertility problems later.

EXPOSURE TO DES. There is some evidence that some of the male offspring of women treated with diethylstilbestrol (DES) during pregnancy may have infertility problems.[11] The precise effect of DES on males has not been delineated, although it appears to compromise the function both of the testes and of the testicular ducts.

Unfortunately, it is quite true that infertility in the male is frequently untreatable. When faced with this rather bleak prospect the couple must come to the ultimate decision — whether to abandon hope and "settle" into a future of childlessness or to attempt some alternative method. In the recent past, the obvious alternative was adoption. Today, with the liberalization of abortion laws, adoption is more difficult. A reasonable option is artificial insemination using donor sperm (AID). When carried out properly, AID is quite successful. It is a relatively simple procedure, requiring very little time and money when compared with adoption. The major difficulty with AID is the decision to do it. Careful and sensitive counseling of the infertile couple is critical.

RAPE

Rape is carnal knowledge, through compulsion, of a nonconsenting female.[26] Individual state laws may specify whether "carnal knowledge" means penile penetration or complete coitus. Statutory rape refers to acts of carnal knowledge to which the female is unable to consent (i.e., minors). By definition, any sexual violence by a husband against his wife is not considered to be rape but an aspect of wife abuse.

Rape is probably the most frequently committed violent crime; however, relatively few assailants are brought to trial. Convictions are unlikely if the medical examination is conducted in a superficial or careless manner. The examiner not only manages the medical problems of the victim but establishes an authoritative record of the history and physical findings that will be used in the judicial process. The physician is not asked to decide whether rape occurred and should refrain from making this nonmedical decision. It is prudent to have a third party present during the examination.

The violent character of rape may lead to both nongenital and genital injuries. Major physical injuries, which may consist of head trauma, fractures, intra-abdominal lacerations and stab wounds, require emergency medical care. A major genital trauma is a laceration of the vaginal vault with possible prolapse of intestines.

A detailed history is obtained using the victim's own words. It includes a description of the assault and of the perpetrator, and the time, place and circumstances of occurrence. The sexual contact should be described, including possible oral or anal penetration. The history is incomplete without data on the victim's menstrual pattern, previous sexual activity and contraceptive practices.

The physical examination should describe the mental state of the patient and the possible influence of alcohol and drugs. The absence or presence of nongenital trauma (bruises, abrasions, hematoma) is recorded. Clothes are inspected for blood and semen stains. Genital examination describes the presence or absence of injury to the external and lower genital organs. The hymen is inspected to determine whether it is present, intact, with or without evidence of tears, or absent. Wet-mount specimens of the vaginal pool (and rectal pool if necessary) are examined under the microscope for the presence or absence of active or dead sperm. Two further specimens are also collected from the vaginal pool for permanent cytology and for acid phosphatase testing. The history and physical examination may suggest other areas of collection. Dried blood and semen are collected and processed for identification (blood grouping) or frozen until this examination is possible. Clothes with suspicious stains of semen or blood should be collected for the same purpose. The mons pubis may be combed for the detection of hair from the rapist. The examining physician is responsible for the proper transfer of

TABLE 20–5   Postcoital Pregnancy Prevention (To be given within 72 hours of exposure)

Diethylstilbestrol 25–50 mg b.i.d. for 5 days
Ethinyl estradiol 1–5 mg q.i.d. for 5 days
Premarin 2.5–10 mg t.i.d. for 5 days
Premarin 40 mg I.V. single dose

collected specimens to the pathologist and should obtain signed receipts.

Prevention of infection is paramount and consists primarily of prophylaxis against gonorrhea and syphilis. VDRL testing and cultures for *Neisseria gonorrhoeae* from the cervix and other areas of contact should be obtained. Prophylactic treatment follows the guidelines described previously. The VDRL test should be repeated in four weeks. A follow-up examination is necessary to exclude the presence of *Trichomonas vaginalis* and to ascertain the patient's recovery.

Postcoital Pregnancy Prevention

Protection against pregnancy is crucial if the assault occurred during the unprotected midcycle of a woman in her reproductive years. A variety of estrogen treatments have been used successfully. Although accompanied by unpleasant side effects such as nausea and bleeding, these regimens are quite reliable if used within 72 hours. Various preventive regimens are listed in Table 20–5.

Victims will manage the emotional trauma of rape in a variety of ways. In addition to an understanding and sympathetic attitude, the physician may provide a mild sedative or tranquilizer initially, and more extensive emotional evaluation and treatment should be offered. Rape crisis centers (RCC) and organizations such as Women Organized Against Rape (WOAR) may offer substantive practical and emotional support.

Obstetrics

PREGNANCY TESTS

Because of their recent proliferation, it is reasonable to discuss the various types of pregnancy tests in terms of what it is they measure and the advantages and disadvantages of each. The older (and less reliable) pregnancy tests using a classic bioassay (mouse, rabbit or frog tests, for example) are rarely used. Current pregnancy tests are either immunological or membrane-binding methods. All pregnancy tests measure human chorionic gonadotropin (hCG), which is a glycoprotein produced by the syncytiotrophoblastic tissue and is secreted in large quantities throughout pregnancy. In fact, hCG is detectable about three to four days prior to the missed period, shortly after endometrial implantation.

Both luteinizing hormone (LH) and hCG are glycoproteins constructed of an alpha- and beta-subunit. Since the subunits are similar in LH and hCG, most pregnancy tests cannot distinguish between the two. The beta-subunits, however, are specific for LH and hCG, and this provides a method of differentiating between them.

IMMUNOLOGICAL TESTS (GRAVINDEX, PREGNOSTICON). These are the most commonly used pregnancy tests and are capable of detecting hCG at a concentration of approximately 1000 IU per liter of urine. They are rapidly performed and usually become positive from about the fortieth day after the last menstrual period.

The immunological tests detect the entire hCG molecule (both alpha and beta chains) and therefore also are capable of detecting LH. The tests are set to become positive at the 1000 IU per liter level so as to avoid confusion with LH. LH is excreted in large quantities in the urine of postmenopausal (or castrate) patients, and thus when pregnancy tests are carried out on these patients they may indicate a pregnancy erroneously.

RADIOIMMUNOASSAY hCG. As a pregnancy test, this assay offers no advantages over the nonradiation immunological methods. It is cumbersome, expensive and requires two to four days to carry out. It also does not distinguish between hCG and LH.

BETA-SUBUNIT hCG. This radioimmunoassay is specific for hCG and does not cross-react with LH. The most common usage of beta-subunit hCG is in the follow-up of patients with trophoblastic disease (hydatidiform mole, choriocarcinoma, and so on) when the levels drop below those detectable by the standard immunological pregnancy tests. Results are obtained in two to four days.

RADIORECEPTOR hCG (RR-hCG). Corpus luteal membrane has receptors for both LH and hCG. In this test the amount of hCG (or LH) present in a sample can be correlated to the displacement of hCG tracer from the membrane. This is a remarkably sensitive test and can detect as little as 2 mIU per ml of hCG in plasma. Results can be obtained in less than three hours. It must be remembered, however, that this assay can also detect LH. By using the RR-hCG assay it has been shown that hCG begins to rise in maternal blood three to four days prior to the missed period. This could provide a very early test for pregnancy.

ABORTION

Spontaneous Abortion

Abortion is defined as termination of a pregnancy prior to "viability" of the fetus. Survival of a fetus of less than 500 gm or 20 weeks' gestation is exceedingly rare, and therefore it is widely agreed that abortion encompasses pregnancy termination prior to the twentieth week. By far the largest number of abortions today are voluntary. These are discussed in the second half of this section.

Although there are many varieties of spontaneous abortions, clinically we are concerned with four types: threatened, incomplete, missed and septic abortions.

THREATENED ABORTION. This is defined as bleeding (spotting, staining, frank bleeding) in early pregnancy. When the bleeding is confined to spotting or staining and is unaccompanied by uterine contractions (pain), about half of such pregnancies will remain intact. When bleeding is heavy or accompanied by pain, the prognosis is poor. In general the treatment for threatened abortion is to "wait and see." There is no firm evidence that progestins or other hormonal therapies are effective in averting a pregnancy loss; there is much evidence that progestins frequently cause "missed" abortion. It does seem reasonable to limit the patient's physical activity and to proscribe intercourse, douching and other potentially harmful activities.

INCOMPLETE ABORTION. If the patient has passed placental or fetal tissue or if her internal cervical os is found to be open, this is by definition an incomplete abortion. If it occurs in very early pregnancy (one of less than eight weeks' duration) it is highly probable that the patient will empty the uterus completely, decrease in bleeding and complete the abortion. If bleeding persists and completion is not obvious, or if the pregnancy is of longer than eight weeks' duration, the patient should be admitted to the hospital and given oxytocin (10 IU per liter of intravenous fluids), and a curettage should be carried out. The curettage can be accomplished best using suction curettage, as described later in the chapter.

In all abortions in Rh negative pa-

tients, Rh_0 (D antigen) immune globulin (RhoGAM) should be administered. For pregnancies that terminate before 12 weeks, a mini-dose of immune globulin (MICRhoGAM) is available.

MISSED ABORTION. As noted previously, this is found fairly frequently in patients designated as having a "threatened" abortion who receive hormonal therapy. It may also occur without a history of medication. In the typical missed abortion, the uterine size progresses for some time, bleeding occurs, and no further uterine growth is noted. In fact, shrinkage of the uterus is frequently found. The most appropriate therapy is to do nothing and wait until the patient begins the abortion herself. These patients should be followed up with tests of serum fibrinogen levels, since a small number, usually after retaining a missed abortion more than one month, may develop a fibrinogen depletion syndrome. The most common clinical approach is to watch the patient for two weeks and, if abortion has not occurred, admit her to the hospital, start an oxytocin infusion, and complete the abortion with a D and C.

SEPTIC ABORTION. Fortunately, with the wide availability of legal elective abortions, septic (criminal) abortions have decreased in frequency. The diagnosis is made clinically by the findings of bleeding, usually an open internal os, lower abdominal pain, fever and exquisite tenderness of the uterus and frequently of the adnexa. This is a dangerous condition requiring immediate attention. The usual approach is hospitalization, the obtaining of uterine blood and urine cultures and the starting of intravenous antibiotics and oxytocin. When it is felt that the infection has stabilized, a curettage is carried out. Matched blood should always be available for the treatment of hypovolemia. The major problem in septic abortions is the danger of septic shock with renal shut-down. When the uterine culture samples are obtained,

Gram stain slides should be investigated immediately, looking for the presence of clostridia. Clostridial infections demand much more aggressive surgical therapy — hysterectomy and bilateral salpingo-oophorectomy. Essentially all affected and necrotic tissue must be removed to prevent hemolysis, renal failure and shock.

OTHER TYPES OF ABORTION. "Habitual" abortion is the term generally applied to a patient who has had three or more consecutive abortions. In these circumstances it is highly appropriate that chromosomal karyotyping be carried out on both husband and wife (and the abortus if possible). In addition, other contributing factors such as chronic infection (pyelonephritis, severe cervicitis, uterine abnormalities and others) and debilitating disorders must be ruled out. Reproductive endocrinopathies are rarely the cause. In the vast majority of patients, no etiology will be found for the repetitive abortions. In fact, even after three abortions, the patient's chance of aborting again with the next pregnancy is only slightly greater than that of the normal population.

One type of repetitive abortion, usually occurring between the twelfth and twenty-fourth weeks of pregnancy, is that associated with incompetency of the internal cervical os. In this condition, which frequently is related to previous cervical trauma (D and C, obstetrical laceration, or other trauma), the internal os begins to dilate early in the pregnancy, and there is rupture of the membranes, uterine contractions and delivery. Diagnosis of an incompetent cervical os is usually made from the history and by having followed the patient through one or two of these abortions. A hysterosalpingogram can be done between pregnancies and will often (but not always) demonstrate a patulous internal os. The most appropriate therapy for incompetency is a cervical cerclage (Shirodkar or McDonald procedure) carried out after the eighth week of the next pregnancy.

The suture should not be placed if rupture of the membranes has occurred. If cerclage is successful, the patient will go to term with the suture intact. The cerclage suture is usually removed in early labor and the patient delivers vaginally. On occasion, the suture is electively left intact or is difficult to remove, and in these circumstances a cesarean section is performed.

Trophoblastic Disease

Placental tissue may evolve into a hydatidiform mole or its malignant counterpart, choriocarcinoma. The entire spectrum of trophoblastic tumor formation frequently presents as an abortion, with the characteristic grape-like tissue expelled. This entity is highly dangerous and is best handled at a center experienced in treating trophoblastic disorders. After definitive surgery or chemotherapy, or both, has been carried out, the levels of hCG in these patients are determined at frequent intervals for two years. The usual method of following the hCG levels is by means of the urinary immunological pregnancy tests until the level of excretion of hCG falls below 1000 IU per liter and the test becomes negative. Thereafter, the radioimmunoassay for beta-subunit hCG is utilized until hCG is no longer detectable.[14] During this recovery period, patients should be advised not to become pregnant.

Induced Abortion

First Trimester Abortion

MENSTRUAL REGULATION. Menstrual regulation differs from the classic curettage techniques in that the procedure is done in the office within two weeks after the missed period and cervical dilatation is unnecessary.[4] The development of highly sensitive pregnancy tests based on the radioreceptor assay for hCG allows the detection of pregnancy as early as two to three days before the missed period.

Procedure. The patient is placed in lithotomy position and prepared. A paracervical block may be used. With a tenaculum placed on the anterior cervical lip, the cervicouterine axis is straightened. A 5 or 6 mm flexible cannula is introduced and the uterine contents are aspirated via a suction pump (less than 75 mm Hg pressure) or a 50 cc syringe.

SUCTION CURETTAGE. This is the usual technique for first trimester abortion.[2] It is also the method of choice for evacuation of the uterus in patients with an incomplete abortion. Either paracervical block or general anesthesia is indicated. The procedure is applicable in an ambulatory setting, although it is done most commonly on an in-patient basis.

Procedure. The patient is placed in lithotomy position, prepared and draped, and a pelvic examination is performed to determine the size and position of the uterus. The cervix is grasped anteriorly with a tenaculum and the cervicouterine axis is straightened. The cervix is dilated with Hegar dilators. The uterus is explored with an ovarian forceps and larger pieces of tissue are removed mechanically. Suction cannulas vary in size; usually 8 to 10 mm cannulas are adequate. Suction can be controlled by the manual release of an opening in the suction tubing. Pressure at the tip increases when this opening is occluded by the fingertip and should not exceed 50 mm Hg. While introducing the curette, suction should not be applied. In the uterine cavity the suction tip is withdrawn gently toward the cervix, clockwise, in a scraping fashion, while the suction is operating. This method is efficient and provokes less bleeding than does a sharp curettage. The patient can be discharged within hours.

The major complication of curetting techniques is uterine perforation. Unless this results in hemorrhage or lac-

eration of intestinal structures 24 hour observation is usually sufficient. Other complications include infection, incomplete evacuation and occasionally the later development of uterine synechiae.

Second Trimester Abortion

AMNIOCENTESIS (SALINE). Abortion in the second trimester is usually accomplished using the amniocentesis technique. Legal guidelines define whether or not this procedure can be done in an outpatient setting. Since clinical estimates of gestational age are subject to error, it is recommended that sonographic fetal size determination be obtained. About 150 to 200 ml of amniotic fluid are withdrawn and replaced with an equal volume of 20 per cent NaCl solution.[15] After a latency period of about 24 to 30 hours, labor and delivery can be expected. Once labor starts, oxytocin administration may begin at a rate of 20 to 50 mU per minute.

Technique. After the patient voids, a pelvic examination is done to determine the size of the uterus. The uterus must be at least 14 gestational weeks in size before amniocentesis is attempted. The skin is prepared with an antiseptic solution and the skin and subcutaneous tissue are infiltrated with a local anesthetic agent about one inch above the symphysis pubis in the midline. An 18 gauge, 3½ inch spinal needle is inserted through the skin into the uterus. There is a characteristic change in resistance when the needle enters the amniotic cavity. The assistant attaches a syringe to the needle, and the amniotic fluid is withdrawn. There are no unusual precautions that the patient must observe following this procedure. In about 10 per cent of cases, fluid is not obtained in the first attempt. In these situations, the patient returns in one week and the procedure is repeated.

A serious complication consists in the accidental maternal injection of the salt solution. During injection the position of the needle should be repeatedly checked by aspiration of amniotic fluid. Early warning signs of maternal injection include abdominal or pelvic pain, a feeling of heat, tingling of fingers, headache and intense thirst. Later signs include severe headache, convulsions, lethargy and hypernatremia. Intravasation leads to hyperosmotic crisis with hemolysis, disseminated intravascular coagulopathy and cerebral dehydration. Other major complications include heart failure, peritonitis and septic shock. Minor problems are fever reaction and retained products of conception.

The use of hypertonic saline is contraindicated in patients with cardiac disorders, hypertension, hemoglobinopathies and convulsive disorders. Because of the potentially serious side effects, only experienced physicians should attempt intra-amniotic pregnancy termination.

PROSTAGLANDIN. Prostaglandin $F_{2\alpha}$ has been approved by the FDA for use in second trimester pregnancy termination. Prostaglandins are administered into the amniotic sac after 16 weeks of gestation following the technique just described but without removal of large amounts of amniotic fluid. The dose is 40 mg prostaglandin $F_{2\alpha}$, which is injected after an initial test dose of 5 mg.

Side effects are nausea and vomiting. Intravascular accidental injection causes hot flushes, hypertension, fever and occasionally bronchospasm. Complications frequently include the retention of the placenta, which requires removal in the operating room. Other complications are infection, cervical fistula and fever reaction.

If the uterus is not too large (16 weeks of gestation or less), some physicians have reported that suction curettage can be used safely and effectively.[8] In order to diminish the risk of uterine perforation, an ovarian or sponge stick forceps is used prior to suction to reduce the intrauterine mass.

ECTOPIC PREGNANCY

An ectopic pregnancy is a gynecological emergency. Most ectopically implanted pregnancies occur in the middle portions of the fallopian tube, but they may also occur in other parts of the tube, in the ovary and in the abdomen. Since almost all common ectopic pregnancies are tubal, we will confine our remarks to these.

The incidence of tubal pregnancy is increased (1:80 normal pregnancies) in urban areas that have a high incidence of gonorrhea and low (1:400) in rural regions of the country. Some of the causes of tubal pregnancy are previous pelvic inflammatory disease, congenital abnormalities of the tubes, endometriosis and transperitoneal migration of the ovum. Once implanted in the tube, a fertilized ovum may proceed to a tubal abortion or to a tubal rupture. In either event, intra-abdominal bleeding occurs and surgical intervention is mandatory.

The clinical features of a tubal pregnancy are amenorrhea followed by unusual vaginal bleeding and abdominal pain. The amenorrhea is caused by peristence of the corpus luteum secondary to the tubal pregnancy's production of hCG. A basic diagnostic point is that careful history-taking will quite commonly discover an abnormality in the usual menstrual cycle. Abdominal pain is the most consistent finding. It is usually referred to one or both lower quadrants and is initially due to distention of the tube with the pregnancy and blood.

As the tubal pregnancy progresses the pain is secondary to free blood in the abdomen and the classic acute abdomen develops. It is not uncommon that the patient also complains of referred shoulder pain, fainting, urinary frequency, dysuria and rectal tenesmus. Sudden collapse and shock may occur.

The findings on general physical examination vary from those of a normal female with no symptoms to severe hypovolemic shock. These patients are almost always afebrile. There may be signs of an early pregnancy (Montgomery follicles in the areolae of the breasts, cyanotic cervix, positive pregnancy test). At pelvic examination pain is elicited on movement of the cervix and tenderness is noted in one or both adnexa. The pain is usually so severe that guarding is extensive, and it is quite difficult to palpate a mass. The hematocrit may be normal in the early ectopic pregnancy. The usual immunological pregnancy tests are positive in about 70 per cent of patients. Pelvic sonography is occasionally helpful, primarily by indicating the absence of an intrauterine pregnancy in a patient who has signs of pregnancy and abdominal pain. Probably the most important diagnostic tool is the laparoscope. Obviously, laparoscopy should not be carried out in the patient with hypovolemic collapse and, by the same token, a patient with a suspected tubal pregnancy should not be sent home to "see what happens." Laparoscopy has the advantage of allowing one to view the entire pelvic contents and to make appropriate decisions.

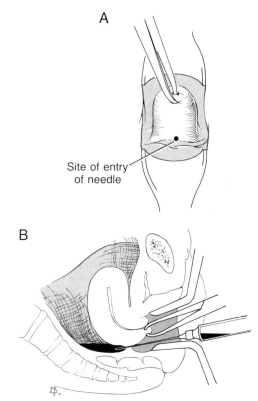

Figure 20–22 Culdocentesis. *A.* Traction on posterior lip of cervix exposes posterior cul-de-sac. *B.* Syringe containing 1 ml of saline or local anesthetic is attached to 18 gauge 3½ inch needle. Needle is introduced into posterior cul-de-sac. Fluid is injected to clear tissue from the needle, followed by aspiration of cul-de-sac contents. Needle is introduced parallel to the sacrum, to avoid entry into uterus or rectum.

Culdocentesis

Culdocentesis is a method for determining the presence of free blood in the abdomen. Anesthesia and analgesia are unnecessary for the procedure. A bimanual pelvic examination is performed prior to it.

A speculum is inserted into the vagina, and the posterior lip of the cervix is grasped with a tenaculum. The cervix is elevated, allowing adequate visualization of the cul-de-sac. A 3½ inch 18 gauge needle is attached to a syringe containing 1 ml of saline or local anesthetic solution. The needle is then advanced through the vaginal mucosa into the cul-de-sac with a single deliberate motion (Fig. 20–22). At this point, the patient will experience a sudden but brief pain when the needle traverses the peritoneum. The patient should then be positioned so that any abdominal fluid will pool in the cul-de-sac of Douglas. The solution within the syringe is injected so as to clear the needle, and the needle is then withdrawn slowly while aspirating the contents of the cul-de-sac with the syringe. In normal patients, a small amount of yellowish peritoneal fluid can be obtained. A hematocrit should be performed on any bloody fluid. If it is less than 10 per cent, needle trauma of the uterus or of adjacent structures or a ruptured ovarian cyst must be suspected. If the hematocrit is greater than 10 per cent, the source of intraabdominal bleeding must be determined by surgical exploration. No special precautions are necessary following culdocentesis. One contraindication to the procedure is a mass that is fixed in the cul-de-sac.

Diagnostic curettage is occasionally helpful if there is a question of abortion of an intrauterine pregnancy. If the curettage specimens show decidual tissue only, ectopic pregnancy is likely. Specific morphological changes in the endometrium, known as the Arias-Stella reaction, have been associated with both intrauterine and extrauterine pregnancy. This reaction has been called an anaplasia of pregnancy because of its characteristic hyperchromatic nuclear clumping, marked cellular atypism, mitotic activity and polyploidy. It may be present in 10 to 25 per cent of pregnant women. Since the findings from curettage are equivocal in so many patients and since a normal intrauterine pregnancy may be interrupted, curettage is definitely not advised as a routine diagnostic procedure.

The management of the patient with an ectopic pregnancy centers on blood replacement and surgery. In the severely hypovolemic patient surgery must begin as soon as whole blood is being replaced. The response to surgery and ligation of the bleeding area is quite dramatic. The surgery may consist of salpingectomy (with or without cornual resection) or salpingostomy, in which an attempt is made to conserve the affected tube.

The differential diagnosis of a tubal pregnancy usually includes salpingitis, incomplete or threatened abortion, appendicitis, bleeding corpus luteal cyst and diverticulitis.

OUTPATIENT OBSTETRICS

Fetal Evaluation

In the majority of patients the development and well-being of the fetus can be assessed using rather simple clinical observations: progressive and appropriate enlargement of the uterus, periodic auscultation of fetal heart tones and determination of fetal position, lie, presentation, and so on. The uterine enlargement should be consonant with the period of amenorrhea. The patient's noting of the first-felt fetal movements (16 to 18 weeks in the multipara, 18 to 20 weeks in the primigravida) is also helpful in the designation of the length of gestation.

Recently, ultrasonography has been used to determine the fetal biparietal diameter, which can be correlated (± 2 weeks) with fetal age. Ultrasonography has been helpful in the diagnosis of early pregnancy, ectopic pregnancy, hydatid mole, fetal abnormalities, fetal death and placental localization.[17]

Fetal-placental well-being can also be estimated by the use of serial determinations of urinary estriol (E_3). E_3 is a secretory product of the maternal and fetal adrenal and liver and of the placenta. In instances of "high risk" pregnancy, frequent assays showing a stable or increasing output of E_3 reassure that the fetal-placental unit is intact and maturing appropriately.[3] Other tests of fetal well-being are serial determinations of human placental lactogen, plasma estriol or urinary or plasma estetrol.

Amniocentesis

The removal of a sample of amniotic fluid via amniocentesis has been shown to be helpful in fetal evaluation.[27] Amniocentesis technique was described in the section on abortion; however, for this purpose a smaller needle gauge (22) should be chosen. The size of puncture is dictated by the placental site and the position of the fetus and ideally should be aimed at the small parts of the fetus so as to avoid placental injury. Many physicians prefer to localize the placenta and fetal parts with sonography prior to amniocentesis in order to minimize potential harm to the fetus.

Complications such as placental bleeding, fetomaternal transfusion (and therefore the possibility of isoimmunization), cord injury and fetal puncture may arise. Other problems are the potential induction of labor and the possibility of infection. The risk in amniocentesis is generally thought to be minimal (less than 1 per cent). The following are indications for diagnostic amniocentesis:

GENETIC EVALUATION. Between 14 to 18 weeks of gestation, amniotic fluid may be removed for determination of a large number of genetic disorders, chromosomal studies and sex determination.

ISOIMMUNIZATION. If a risk of fetal-maternal blood group incompatibility has been determined and if screening titers suggest a fetal endangerment, amniocentesis techniques are useful to assess the situation. The concentration of unconjugated bilirubin titers in conjunction with fetal age will usually direct the further approach, be it expectation, intrafetal transfusion or delivery.

DETERMINATION OF FETAL MATURATION. The lecithin-sphyngomyelin (L:S) ratio has evolved as the most valuable test for fetal maturity. A ratio of more than 2 indicates that the lung has reached a certain degree of maturity and that therefore the possibility of the delivered fetus developing respiratory distress syndrome is minimal.[5] Other less commonly used tests of maturity measure creatinine concentration and percentage of fat-stained cells. Injection of radiopaque dye into the amniotic cavity has been used in amniography to outline fetal and placental contour.

Fetal Monitoring

Alpha-fetoprotein determination from the amniotic fluid has become a valuable tool in the detection of neural tube defects and other congenital-genetic disorders of the fetus.

During labor, fetal monitoring systems determine the rate of fetal cardiac activity and its alterations in relation to uterine activity. The normal fetal heart rate can be measured by external devices transabdominally or, after rupture of the membranes, by internal equipment attached to the fetal presenting part.[13] In addition, in the latter situation the fetus is accessible for pH determinations, which may complement the results from the heart rate pattern. The interpretation of heart rate–uterine relationships should be carried out by experienced obstetricians.

OXYTOCIN CHALLENGE TEST. Recently, these same principles have been applied for the assessment of the fetus before the patient goes into labor.[6] Recordings of fetal heart rate and uterine activity are started and the patient is given highly diluted oxytocin intravenously in an attempt to initiate uterine contractions. Once defined contractions are established, observations of the response of the fetal heart rate changes are made. Fetal well-being is usually assured temporarily in the absence of any ominous fetal heart rate response.

Extramural Delivery

Out-of-hospital ("extramural") deliveries are inevitable. They may result from geographical isolation, very rapid labor or a host of transportation-related problems. The following section deals with the management of these obstetrical emergencies.

The physician attending such a patient should have available the following equipment:

Clean towels and receiving blanket
Sterile gloves (several pairs)
Rubber half-sheet
Stethoscope
Sphygmomanometer
Cord clamps or umbilical tape
Soft rubber bulb suction apparatus

Labor

When the patient is in labor a vaginal examination is performed with a sterile glove. The dilatation and effacement of the cervix and the position of the presenting part are determined. If the presentation of the fetus is anything other than vertex, every effort should be made to transport the patient to an obstetrical unit. This is usually quite possible, since other presentations (breech, brow, face, shoulder and so on) generally result in a slower, less progressive labor. In order to minimize the possibility of amnionitis, as few vaginal examinations as possible are carried out after the initial examination. This is particularly important after rupture of the membranes has occurred. If the cervix has not become fully dilated in 12 hours after the onset of labor in a primigravida (8 hours in a multipara), pelvic contraction or an abnormality of uterine contractions should be suspected. The same is true if there is no progress in cervical dilatation or descent of the presenting part in a two-hour period. In either case, one should prepare to transfer the patient to a hospital.

Throughout the first stage of labor the fetal heart rate is determined every 30 minutes. Any persistent change of fetal heart rate to more than 160 per minute or less than 120 per minute indicates possible fetal distress. The patient should be turned on her left side to allow adequate venous return through the inferior vena cava. Oxygen, if available, should be administered. If this does not improve fetal heart tones, preparation should be made to transfer the patient to an obstetrical unit. If the fetal heart rate does improve secondary to these maneuvers, it is also strongly suggested the patient be removed to an obstetrical area, since these alterations in fetal heart rate may presage even more profound and less reversible alterations later in the labor and during delivery.

If at any time during labor the blood pressure reaches levels of 140/100 mm Hg and the deep tendon reflexes are hyperactive, one should suspect pre-eclampsia and attempt to remove the patient to a hospital if at all possible.

The second stage of labor (the time from full dilatation to delivery) should last no longer than two hours in the primigravida and one hour in a multiparous patient. A second stage of labor lasting longer than these limits suggests pelvic contraction or abnormal presentation of the fetus (brow, face, shoulder or compound presentation).

Delivery

When delivery is imminent, as evidenced by perineal crowning of the presenting part, the delivery area should be prepared. A rubber half-sheet is applied to the bed or table, and the perineum is washed with soap and water. The infant is delivered with the patient on her back with knees flexed and the physician standing at the foot of the bed or table. During this time the patient is encouraged to "bear down" with each contraction, bringing into play the increased forces of abdominal contractions. These pushing efforts of the patient can be made more effective by allowing the patient to grasp her flexed knees and bring her head forward during the contractions.

As the head distends the perineum, counterpressure should be applied to prevent an explosive exit of the head that may result in extensive vaginal lacerations. If the head is carefully controlled at this point, usually only a small perineal laceration near the midline will result. When the head is delivered, the mouth and nares of the infant are gently aspirated with a soft rubber bulb suction. With the next contraction gentle downward traction will bring the anterior shoulder under the symphysis pubis. By then directing the head toward the symphysis, the posterior shoulder will deliver over the perineum, and the remainder of the birth is inevitable.

The umbilical cord is clamped or tied and cut about 1 inch from the abdomen. A rapid evaluation of the baby will indicate whether there is a need for resuscitation. A baby who is breathing spontaneously and has a vigorous cry, good tone, a plethoric or pink appearance and a pulse rate higher than 100 per minute requires no further resuscitation. If the baby does not breathe spontaneously and has poor tone, a mottled blue and pale color and a pulse rate less than 100, resuscitative efforts should be instituted at once. Mouth-to-mouth resuscitation will suffice if intubation equipment is not at hand. In most depressed infants who have no congenital abnormalities, maintenance of ventilation and body warmth will result in rapid improvement in a few moments. After the infant's condition is stable, body temperature should be maintained by wrapping the child in a blanket.

Third Stage of Labor: Delivery of the Placenta

Gentle traction on the umbilical cord will suffice to deliver the placenta after it has descended into the lower uterine segment. Descent of the placenta into the lower uterine segment can be diagnosed by enlargement of the fundus, usually a gush of blood vaginally, and a 4 or 5 cm lengthening of the umbilical cord. If the placenta has not been delivered within 30 minutes, a hand wearing a sterile glove should be inserted into the uterus. This is best accomplished with the patient under general anesthesia and therefore in a hospital. If the cervix is tightly closed or if the placenta within the uterus seems adherent, further, more vigorous efforts to remove the placenta should await the patient's transfer to an obstetrical unit. Hemorrhage at this stage can be catastrophic. Gentle massage of the uterine fundus will improve uterine tone.

The perineum and cervix are inspected for lacerations. Any significant lacerations should be repaired in the hospital.

Immediate Postpartum Period

Care during the immediate puerperium includes frequent observations to detect hemorrhage from uterine atony, prolonged urinary retention, hypertension or postpartum eclampsia. Urinary retention manifested by a distended bladder and inability to void, and usually due to urethral edema or reflex perineal pain, requires catheterization. Hypertension is a sign of potential postpartum eclampsia. Patients with uterine atony with hemorrhage, urinary retention or postpartum hypertension deserve hospitalization.

Early ambulation of postpartum patients should be encouraged in order to avoid venous stasis, which may lead to thrombophlebitis or pulmonary embolism.

Elective Nonhospital Delivery

It is estimated that for the past five years registered nonhospital deliveries have increased at a rate of 0.1 per cent per year. The facilities in which these births occur range from well-equipped, physician-attended "birthing centers" that are closely associated with a hospital to remote, minimally equipped, lay midwife–directed home deliveries. Although a number of studies from the United States have appeared, the small number of patients and the large number of variables make it difficult to generalize on the safety and efficacy of elective nonhospital deliveries. The European literature, in general, is somewhat negative in terms of "domiciliary" obstetric experiences.

It is quite astonishing that, without adequate data, the medical community has been capable of making highly emotional statements on both sides of the issue. What is clear, however, is the fact that, if nonhospital deliveries are to be established, the requirements and facilities must be more extensive than those outlined previously for "simple," involuntary extramural deliveries.

Selection of Patients

This is of course a critical issue. It would be obstetrical folly to accept all patients into a nonhospital delivery system. One can anticipate that from 5 to 15 per cent of the home delivery population will be screened out during the initial or early antepartum care. The following are general considerations that, to the authors, would constitute ineligibility for nonhospital delivery. This list is by no means complete, but simply a guide.

1. Maternal age: A patient of age 16 or less or 35 or older is a high-risk patient.
2. Parity: Para 5 or more.
3. History of previous obstetrical problems:
   Hemorrhage
   Complicated labor
   Operative delivery (forceps, cesarean section)
   Rh sensitization
   Severe pre-eclampsia or eclampsia
   Premature delivery or rupture of membranes
   Low or excessive birth weight infants
   Unexplained fetal deaths
   Multiple congenital abnormalities
   Extensive cervical or vaginal laceration(s)
4. History of major medical or surgical disorders:
   Diabetes mellitus
   Hypertension
   Heart disease
   Kidney disease
   Clotting problems

Colostomy or ileostomy
Myomectomy
Repair for pelvic relaxation
Drug addiction

In the course of the present pregnancy, even after compulsory screening, another 10 per cent of the maternal population will ultimately require hospitalization. Some indications for interrupting the nonhospital care are bleeding, hydramnios, malpresentation (including breech), multiple pregnancy, dysfunctional labor, meconium staining, alterations in fetal heart rate, amnionitis, intercurrent disease and other problems.

Antepartal care should be the same whether in-hospital or out-of-hospital delivery is anticipated. A physician should talk with and examine the patient during the antepartal course and should be readily available at any time. It is imperative that typed and cross-matched blood also be readily accessible.

In addition to the previously listed items required for an extramural delivery, the following should also be available in a structured nonhospital delivery system:

Intravenous needles, tubing and solution
Oxygen
Low outlet forceps
Urethral catheter
Infant laryngoscope
Infant endotracheal tube
Magnesium sulfate (50 per cent solution in 10 ml vials)
Calcium gluconate (10 per cent solution in 10 ml vials)
Lidocaine (1 per cent)
Antibiotic ophthalmic ointment (1 gm tube)
RhoGAM
Meperidine
Urine "dipsticks" for testing acetone, glucose and protein levels
Oxytocin (10 units per 1 ml vial)
Methylergonovine (0.2 mg per 1 ml vial)

Portable scale
Alcohol sponges
Syringes (2 ml, 10 ml)
Needles (22 gauge)
Mayo-type scissors
Needle holder
4 Kelly clamps
Chromic 000 sutures on noncutting
  needles

Structured nonhospital deliveries may differ from the involuntary extramural deliveries in a number of ways.

1. Intravenous fluids can be administered.

2. Forcep deliveries, when indicated, can be carried out to a limited extent.

3. The treatment of mild preeclampsia can be initiated and maintained with magnesium sulfate. In this regard, calcium gluconate (or its equivalent) must be available in the event of magnesium overdose. If hypertension (a blood pressure of 140/90 or greater, or a 30 mm Hg rise in systolic pressure, or a 10 mm Hg rise in diastolic pressure) with active deep tendon reflexes or proteinuria greater than "trace," is noted, magnesium sulfate therapy should be started (10 ml of 50 per cent solution given as a deep intramuscular injection into each buttock; total dose 10 gm). Thereafter, 5 gm of magnesium sulfate are given every four hours throughout labor and delivery and for 24 hours after delivery as long as reflexes are active. Hypertension developing postpartum is also an indication for magnesium sulfate therapy.

4. Lacerations can be repaired. This is usually carried out with interrupted 000-chromic sutures after local infiltration with 1 per cent lidocaine. Two-layer closures are quite satisfactory, with the first sutures approximating the submucosal and subcutaneous tissues. If it appears that the external anal sphincter or the rectal mucosa has been lacerated (third- and fourth-degree lacerations, respectively), the laceration must be repaired meticu-

lously in a three-layer closure with interrupted 000-chromic sutures. The closure begins with approximation of the rectal submucosa in two layers. One should avoid placing sutures through the rectal mucosa. The ends of the external anal sphincter are identified, and several sutures are placed in the surrounding capsule to approximate the torn ends of the muscle. Sutures within the muscle itself are unnecessary. The remainder of the perineum and vagina are closed in two layers. Antibiotics and laxatives are unnecessary following an episiotomy repair or the repair of a third- or fourth-degree laceration. Enemas or rectal tubes should not be used. Cervical lacerations, because of the difficulty in exposing them and identifying their extent, are best repaired in an obstetrical surgical suite.

5. More rigorous resuscitation of the newborn can be attempted using the laryngoscope and endotracheal tube.

6. Obstetrical analgesia can be administered (usually meperidine, 100 mg IM)

7. Oxytocin (10 units) or methylergonovine (0.2 mg) can be given intramuscularly after the delivery of the placenta to prevent uterine atony. Methylergonovine should not be given to a patient with hypertension.

8. Urinary retention can be relieved by urethral catheterization.

Obstetrics, regardless of current popular beliefs and fads, remains an emergency type of service. Although it is infrequent, severe and catastrophic hemorrhage can occur — and in an extraordinarily short period of time. The lack of an immediately responsive blood blank is a major drawback to nonhospital-planned deliveries. Maternal death due to exsanguination because of a lack of immediately available blood can and will hapen; it is inevitable.

Perhaps the best solution is a change in hospital obstetrics. The depersonalization, the excessive instrumentation, the indiscriminate use of drugs and the alienation of the family from the birth process can all be altered within the hospital itself by the use of family rooms and birthing rooms and by encouraging family participation. This would seem the most rational approach.

REFERENCES

1. American College of Obstetricians and Gynecologists: Gonorrhea—Diagnosis and Therapy in the Female. Technical Bulletin No. 28, 1974.
2. Andolsek, L.: The Ljubljana Abortion Study 1971–1973. Bethesda, Md., National Institutes of Health Center for Population Research, 1974.
3. Beling, C.: Estrogens. *In* Fuchs, F., and Klopper, A. (eds.): Endocrinology of Pregnancy, 2nd ed. New York, Harper & Row, 1977.
4. Brenner, W. E., Edelman, D. A., and Kessel, E.: Menstrual regulation in the United States: a preliminary report. Fertil. Steril., 26:289–295, 1975.
5. Ekelund, L., Arvidson, G., and Astedt, B.: Amniotic fluid lecithin and its fatty acid composition in respiratory distress syndrome. J. Obstet. Gyaecol. Brit. Commonw., 80:912–917, 1973.
6. Freeman, R. K.: The use of the oxytocin challenge test for antepartum clinical evaluation of uteroplacental respiratory function. Am. J. Obstet. Gynecol., 121:481–489, 1975.
7. Greenberg, S. G.: Varicocele and male infertility. Fertil. Steril., 28:699–706, 1977.
8. Grimes, D. A., Schultz, K. F., Cates, W., Jr., et al.: Midtrimester abortion by dilatation and evacuation. N. Engl. J. Med., 296:1141–1145, 1977.
9. Gusberg, S. B., and Kaplin, A. L.: Precursors of corpus cancer. Am. J. Obstet. Gynecol., 87:662–678, 1963.
10. Halbert, D. R., Demers, L. M., and Jones, D. E. D.: Dysmenorrhea and prostaglandins. Obstet. Gynecol. Surv., 31:77–81, 1976.
11. Herbst, A. L. (ed.): Intrauterine Exposure to Diethylstilbestrol in the Human. Proceedings of Symposium on DES. Chicago, American College of Obstetricians and Gynecologists, 1978.
12. Hibbard, L. T.: The minilap approach to sterilization. Contemp. Obstet. Gynecol., 11:113–117, 1978.
13. Hon, E. H.: Fetal heart rate monitoring. *In* Gluck, L.(ed.): Modern Perinatal Medicine. Chicago, Year Book Medical Publishers, 1974.
14. Jones, W. B., Lewis, J. L., Jr., and Lehr, M.: Monitor of chemotherapy in gestational trophoblastic neoplasm by radioimmunoassay of the beta-subunit of human chorionic gonadotropin. Am. J. Obstet. Gynecol., 121:699–673, 1975.
15. Kerenyi, T. D., Mandelman, N., and Sherman, D. G.: Five thousand consecutive saline abortions. Am J. Obstet. Gynecol., 116:593–600, 1973.
16. Kolstad, P., and Stafl, A.: Atlas of Colposcopy. Baltimore, University Park Press, 1972.
17. Kratochwil, A.: The state of ultrasound diagnosis in perinatal medicine. J. Perinat. Med., 3:75–88, 1975.
18. Mattingly, R. F.: Te Linde's Operative Gynecology, 5th ed. Philadelphia, J. B. Lippincott Company, 1977.
19. Miller, J. F., and Elstein, M.: A comparison of electrocautery and cryocautery for the treatment of cervical erosions and chronic cervicitis. J. Obstet. Gynaecol. Brit. Commonw., 80:658–663, 1973.
20. Nahmias, A. J., Alford, C. A., and Korones, S. B.: Infection of the newborn with herpes virus hominis. Adv. Pediatr., 17:185–226, 1970.
21. Ostergard, D. R., Townsend, D. E., and Hirose, F. M.: The long-term effects of cryosurgery of the uterine cervix. J. Cryosurg., 2:17–22, 1969.
22. Page, E. W., Villee, C. A., and Villee, D. B.: Human Reproduction. Philadelphia, W. B. Saunders Co., 1976, p. 89.
23. Phillips, J. M., and Keith, L. (eds.): Gynecological Laparoscopy: Principles and Techniques. New York, Stratton Intercontinental Medical Book Corp., 1974.
24. Pritchard, J. A., and MacDonald, P. C.: Williams Obstetrics, 15th ed. New York, Appleton-Century-Crofts, 1976.
25. Ruemke, P., van Amstel, N., Meser, E. M., et al.: Prognosis of fertility of men with spermagglutinins in the serum. Fertil. Steril., 25:393–398, 1974.
26. Schiff, A.: Rape. Med. Aspects Hum. Sexuality, 6:76–84, May 1972.
27. Schwarz, R. H.: Amniocentesis. Clin. Obstet. Gynecol., 18:1–22, 1975.
28. Siegler, A. M., and Kemmann, E.: Hysteroscopy. Obstet. Gynecol. Surv., 30:567–588, 1975.
29. Speroff, L.: Which birth control pill should be prescribed? Fertil. Steril., 27:997–1008, 1976.
30. Speroff, L., Glass, R. H., and Kase, N. G.: Clinical Gynecologic Endocrinology and Infertility. Baltimore, Williams & Wilkins Co., 1975.

Anus and Rectum 21

J. E. L. SALES, M.A., M. Chir., F.R.C.S.

1108

INTRODUCTION

Anorectal conditions requiring treatment are a common outpatient problem. This chapter describes the diagnostic evaluations and surgical procedures which may be carried out in outpatients. The chief complication of most of these surgical procedures is reactionary hemorrhage. It is, therefore, important to warn the patient that bleeding may occur and to provide facilities, especially at night, for its emergency treatment.

ANATOMY

This section describes the anatomy of the anorectal region. It is not intended to be a comprehensive account, but those aspects of the anatomy which are of practical importance in examination and surgery of the region are described in detail.

The Rectum

The rectum starts in front of the third piece of the sacrum at the rectosigmoid junction. It follows the curvature of the sacrum and coccyx inferiorly and anteriorly until at 1½ inches anterior to the coccyx it makes a right-angled bend posteriorly to become the anal canal (Fig. 21–1). It is approximately 5 inches (12.5 cm) long. In addition to its anteroposterior curvature, it has three lateral curves, one right and two left, which produce shelves within the rectum — the valves of Houston (Fig. 21–2).

The upper third of the rectum is covered with peritoneum anteriorly and laterally, the middle third anteriorly only. The lower third, which is dilated to form the ampulla of the rectum, lies below the level of the rectovesical pouch and is therefore devoid of peritoneum (Fig. 21–2). The distance from the anal verge to the rectovesical pouch is 3 inches (7½ cm).

The rectum is lined with columnar epithelium, which is pink in color. In the normal bowel, the submucosal vessels can be seen clearly through the mucosa.

The Anal Canal

The anal canal in the adult is approximately 1½ inches long, and it extends

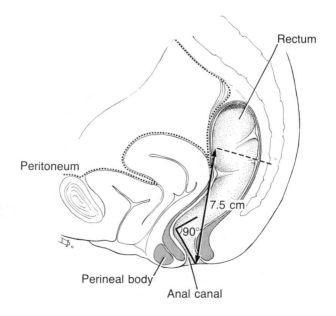

Figure 21–1 Sagittal section of the female pelvis showing the relationship of the peritoneum and pelvic structures to the rectum.

Rectum

Peritoneum

7.5 cm

90°

Perineal body

Anal canal

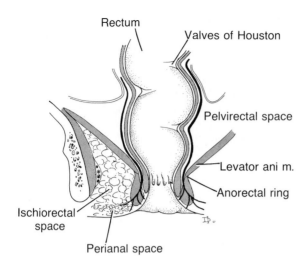

Figure 21–2 Coronal section of the pelvis showing the rectal curves and the tissue spaces surrounding the rectum and anal canal.

from the anal verge to its junction with the rectum at the level of the anorectal ring (Fig. 21–3). The lining of the canal may be divided into two parts: an upper or proximal mucosal, and lower or distal cutaneous, and these are separated by the dentate line some ¾ inch from the anal verge.

The mucosa of the upper anal canal is folded into approximately ten longitudinal folds — the anal columns. These become less distinct with increasing age of the patient. The distal ends of these columns fuse to form the anal valves, and behind each is a small pocket, the anal sinus or crypt (Fig. 21–3). The mucosa is principally simple columnar epithelium in type and appears plum-colored owing to the un-derlying internal hemorrhoidal venous plexus.

Below the dentate line, the canal is lined by stratified squamous epithelium, which contains no hair follicles or sebaceous glands. It merges with normal skin at the anal verge.

Anal Glands

These small branching glands, usually four to eight in number, open into the anal crypts and extend for a variable distance into the anal muscu-lature (Fig. 21–3). They are lined with stratified columnar epithelium and do not secrete. However, it has been suggested that infection occurring in these

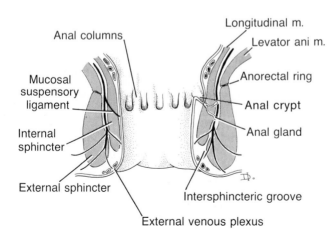

Figure 21–3 The anatomy of the anal canal and anorectal ring. The dentate line is the row of anal crypts which separates the stratified squamous epithelium of the anal canal from the columnar epithelium of the rectum.

glands is the underlying cause in the majority of cases of anal fistula.[34] Nesselrod[31] believes that anal crypt gland infection is also a principal cause of hemorrhoids and fissure. This view, however, is not generally accepted.

The Anal Sphincters

The Internal Sphincter

This is a thick cylinder of smooth muscle surrounding the anal canal. It is a localized thickened portion of the circular muscle of the rectum, extending just distal to the dentate line. It has a well-marked and palpable rounded lower edge.

The External Sphincter

This is composed of striated muscle, surrounding the internal sphincter and extending distally to it. It blends with the puborectalis superiorly, inferiorly it is inserted into the perianal body and posteriorly with the anococcygeal raphe. There is no suggestion histologically that it is divided into three separate parts as traditionally described.[14] Its lower border can be felt on digital examination just inferior and lateral to that of the internal sphincter. There is a palpable interval between the two

sphincters in the wall of the anal canal, the so-called intersphincteric or intermuscular groove.

The Longitudinal Muscle

This is a continuation of the longitudinal muscle of the rectum. It passes downward between the internal and external sphincters. At its lower end it splits up into many fibers which pass through the lower borders of the internal and external sphincters. Some fibers passing through the internal sphincter bind the anal mucosa firmly to the sphincter just below the dentate line, the mucosal suspensory ligament[33] (Fig. 21–3). Although the presence of a definite ligament is disputed, the mucosa is firmly bound at this point and this forms the boundary between the internal and external hemorrhoids — the interhemorrhoidal groove (see Fig. 21–8). The fibers passing through the external sphincter are inserted into the skin of the anus and perianal region, and this constitutes the corrugator cutis ani.

The Levator Ani Muscles

This group of muscles which form the pelvic diaphragm also constitute part of the anal sphincter mechanism (Figs. 21–2 and 21–4). The two major

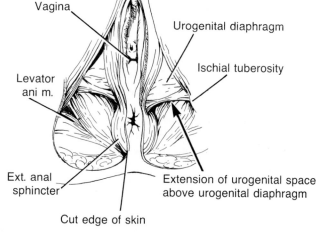

Figure 21–4 The female perineum.

Vagina

Urogenital diaphragm

Ischial tuberosity

Levator ani m.

Ext. anal sphincter

Extension of urogenital space above urogenital diaphragm

Cut edge of skin

parts of the muscle are:
(1) Iliococcygeus
(2) Pubococcygeus

These arise from the pelvic wall fascia and pubis and are inserted into the lower pieces of the sacrum, fusing with the muscle of the opposite side to form the anococcygeal raphe. The innermost fibers of the pubococcygeus are usually separately described as the puborectalis. They arise from the posterior aspect of the pubis and form a sling around the anorectal junction, producing the anorectal angle. At the anorectal junction, these fibers combine with those of the internal and external sphincters to form the anorectal ring (Fig. 21–3). This ring of muscle, which is stronger laterally and posteriorly than it is anteriorly, constitutes the principal part of the anal sphincter mechanism.

Although the internal and external sphincters are important in the preservation of continence, they can, if necessary, be divided with no loss of normal control. If, however, the anorectal ring is completely divided, incontinence results. It is therefore vitally important to identify this ring of muscle before performing any surgery.

Tissue Spaces

There are several tissue spaces related to the anal canal which are important, as they are frequent sites of infection.

The Ischiorectal Fossa

This is a wedge-shaped space filling the lateral part of the anal triangle and extending forward above the urogenital triangle (Fig. 21–4). Its lateral wall is formed by the fascia over the lower part of obturator externus, the falciform margin of the sacrotuberous ligament and the ischial tuberosities. Me-

dially, the two fossae are separated by the perineal body, the anal canal and the anococcygeal body. The roof is formed by the levator ani muscles. The fossa is filled with coarsely lobulated fat into which the anal canal can expand during defecation. It is important to remember that infections of this space may also involve the extension of the fossa above the urogenital diaphragm. The inferior rectal artery and vein and inferior rectal nerve (S3,4) arise from the neurovascular bundle in the pudendal canal, cross the floor of the fossa to supply the external sphincter, the posterior part of levator ani and the perianal skin.

The Perianal Space

This is the subcutaneous space which extends from the lower part of the anal canal to the buttocks (Fig. 21–2). The fat in the space is finely lobulated in contrast to that of the ischiorectal space, since the lobules are separated by fibrous septa. Whether there is a definite layer of fascia separating these two spaces is disputed. Infection or hematomas in this space give rise to considerable tension and hence are exquisitely painful.

The Submucous Space

This lies under the mucosa of the upper two-thirds of the anal canal. It contains the internal hemorrhoidal plexus and is the site of sclerosant injections in the treatment of hemorrhoids (see Fig. 21–8).

The Pelvirectal Space

This is a potential space containing connective tissue lying between the peritoneal floor of the pelvis and the upper surface of the levator ani muscles (Fig. 21–2). On rare occasions, it is the site of infection.

Blood Supply to Rectum and Anal Canal

Arterial Supply

The principal arterial blood supply to the rectum and anal canal is the superior rectal artery, which is the terminal branch of the inferior mesenteric artery. At the rectosigmoid junction it divides into right and left branches, which run forward around the rectum and branch into it. The branches of the superior rectal artery then pierce the muscle layer and run into the submucosa. The right branch divides into two parts while the left remains single, and these branches continue as far as the anal columns. This arrangement accounts for the position in which the primary hemorrhoids occur in the anal canal (see Fig. 21–8 *B*). The middle rectal arteries are variable in size. They arise from the internal iliac and pass to the rectum in the lateral ligaments. The inferior rectal artery arises from the internal pudendal artery in the pudendal canal, crosses the ischiorectal fossa and supplies the anal canal below the dentate line and the perianal skin. It anastomoses with the superior rectal artery.

Venous Drainage

This follows the arterial supply. The submucosal hemorrhoidal plexus of the anal canal above the dentate line and the plexus in the rectal wall drain into the superior rectal veins. These veins unite at the level of the rectosigmoid junction to form a single superior rectal vein which drains into the inferior mesenteric vein. The middle rectal veins chiefly drain the muscular wall of the rectal ampulla and end in the internal iliac veins. The inferior rectal vein drains the anal canal below the dentate line to the pudendal vein. The venous plexus which lies between the lower border of the external sphincter and the perianal skin is called the external hemorrhoidal plexus (see Fig. 21–8 *A*). The rectal veins do not contain valves and the hemorrhoidal veins therefore easily become distended in the presence of proximal obstruction. Hemorrhoidal varices thus occur in patients with portal hypertension, which raises the pressure in the superior rectal vein, and in pregnancy, in which the gravid uterus raises pressure generally throughout the hemorrhoidal venous system.

Lymphatic Drainage

Lymphatic drainage also follows the arterial supply and therefore flows principally upward. The lymphatic plexuses of the rectal wall and upper anal canal drain into the pararectal nodes which lie behind the rectum, and then to the superior rectal and inferior mesenteric nodes. The lymphatics following the middle rectal vessels drain into the internal iliac nodes. The upper part of the anal canal also drains into the internal iliac nodes by lymphatics which pierce the levator ani. The anal canal below the dentate line drains via the cutaneous lymphatics to the inguinal nodes.

Nerve Supply

Rectum and Anal Canal

The rectum and upper anal canal is supplied by the rectal plexus, which is derived from the pelvic plexus. It contains sympathetic and parasympathetic fibers. The parasympathetic nerves, derived from the pelvic splanchnic nerves (S2–4) contain both afferent and efferent fibers. The afferent nerves are sensory from the rectum, while the efferent are motor. The anal canal below the dentate line is innervated by the inferior rectal nerve (S2, 3 and 4).

Anal Sphincters

The levator ani muscles are innervated on their pelvic aspect by branches from S4 and on the perianal aspect by the inferior rectal nerve.

The internal sphincter has sympathetic and parasympathetic innervation. The sympathetic system is motor and the parasympathetic system is inhibitory. The voluntary external sphincter is supplied by the perineal branch of the inferior rectal nerve (S4).

HISTORY

The patient frequently finds difficulty in describing his symptoms accurately. Therefore, although a well-taken history is essential, it usually is of less significance than a careful clinical examination. It is advisable and quicker then, to take the history in the form of a series of leading questions put to the patient. Most clinics have a form pre-printed for this purpose. The main symptoms about which the patient must be asked are:

(1) *Nature of complaint* and its duration.

(2) *Bleeding.* When it occurs, amount, whether bright or dark red and whether or not it is mixed with the stool.

(3) *Pain.* Its nature, location (i.e., whether it occurs in anus, rectum or abdomen) and its relationship to defecation.

(4) *Prolapse.* Whether it occurs with defecation or at other times. Whether it will reduce spontaneously or must be replaced.

(5) *Swelling.* Mode of onset, duration and degree of pain, if any. Any discharge of blood or pus.

(6) *Pruritus.* Is it constant or does it occur only after defecation? Is it worse at night? Does it involve the vulva, groins or toes?

(7) *Incontinence.* Its degree and nature.

(8) *Bowel habit.* Any recent change in habit. Constipation or diarrhea. If diarrhea, its frequency and presence of any associated blood or mucus.

(9) *Micturition.* Any recent evidence of cystitis or pneumaturia.

(10) *General health.* Any recent deterioration, loss of appetite or weight.

(11) *Past history.* Illnesses, allergies or previous operations.

(12) *Family history.* Any history of bowel diseases.

(13) *Therapy.* Any drugs being taken. Any anal suppositories or creams being used.

EXAMINATION

A general physical examination must be carried out. It is important to remember that anorectal symptoms can be a manifestation of systemic disease. The principal points that should be noted in the examination are:

(1) General condition, any weight loss or evidence of anemia.

(2) Cardiopulmonary status, including an evaluation of the patient for anesthesia and consideration of the relative risks of the various types of anesthesia that could be used.

(3) Abdomen — presence of any distention, fluid, tenderness or masses.

(4) Lymphadenopathy, cervical and inguinal.

When the general examination has been completed, the rectal examination should be carried out.

Position for Rectal Examination

The three positions for rectal examination are shown in Figure 21–5 *A*, *B* and *C*: (1) Left lateral or Sims' position; (2) Knee-shoulder; and (3) Prone on proctoscopic table.

The position one uses for the examination depends, of course, on personal preference. I feel that the left lateral is the best, both for the comfort of the patient and for the performance of the examination.

A   Left lateral or Sims' position

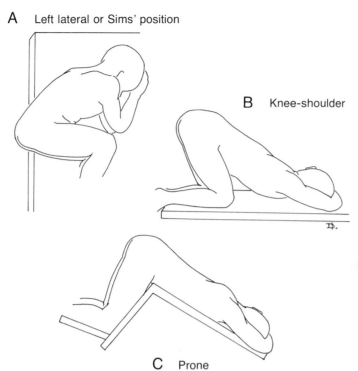

B   Knee-shoulder

C   Prone

Figure 21–5 Rectal examination. *A.* Left lateral (Sims') position. *B.* Knee-shoulder position. *C.* Prone position.

Inspection

It is most important to examine the perianal region carefully, as many of the common anal conditions can be diagnosed on inspection alone. Rubber gloves should be worn on both hands at all times. The chief points to notice are:

(1) The condition of the perianal skin. Notice whether there are any skin changes, their extent and characteristics and whether there are any other skin lesions on the body. Are there scars from previous operations?

(2) Note whether there is any discharge. If so, what is its nature and origin? A careful look for a fistulous opening must be made if the discharge is purulent. If there is a fecal leak and soiling of clothes, note whether this is due to poor hygiene or incontinence.

(3) The presence of swellings, e.g., perianal hematoma, external hemorrhoids, skin and sentinel tags, condylomata acuminata and so on.

(4) The tone of the sphincters, which may be gauged by lateral separation of the buttocks. If lax, the patient should be asked to strain down to see whether there is any prolapse. If there is spasm, note whether there is a fissure present.

Rectal Examination

A well-lubricated finger cot must be used over the glove. The perianal region should first be gently and carefully palpated for evidence of tenderness and induration.

The finger should then be gently inserted into the anal canal. It is very important to tell the patient exactly what you are going to do in order to retain his confidence and keep him relaxed. Relaxation is facilitated by asking him to breathe slowly and deeply through the mouth. He should be warned that it may be uncomfortable. If an acute anal fissure is present with spasm of the sphincter, the examination should be postponed. When the finger is in the anal canal, the tone of the sphincters and any narrowing of the canal must be noted. The perianal structures should then be palpated between finger and thumb for any evidence of inflammation, and also to determine the direction of a fistulous tract if present. The finger should then be advanced into the rectum. The depth to which the finger can be inserted depends on its length and the size of the patient, but usually it is some 8 to 10 cm.

The lumen of the rectum should first be examined for fecal contents and for any evidence of stricture. Hard feces may sometimes feel like a tumor but usually can be indented. The rectal wall is next carefully palpated. It is good practice to start with an assessment of the prostate in the male and cervix in the female in order to get one's bearings in the rectum. The finger is then swept round the bowel wall to detect any irregularity, e.g., the cobblestone mucosa of Crohn's disease, polyps, soft villous adenoma. The indurated edge of a carcinoma has a characteristic feel. Its site, extent and mobility should be assessed. Pedunculated polyps may be difficult to feel if they have a long stalk. It is very important to feel posteriorly just above the anorectal ring, as lesions in this site may easily be missed on endoscopy.

The extrarectal structures should be palpated, starting with the rectouterine or rectovesical pouch. This should be a bimanual examination. In the female, the size and position of the uterus and the presence of any adnexal swellings should be determined. Are there any swellings in the sigmoid colon or secondary carcinoma deposits in the pouch? Laterally and posteriorly the walls of the pelvis, sacrum and coccyx should then be palpated.

Finally, on withdrawal of the finger, the color and consistency of the fecus, and the presence of any blood, mucus or pus, should be noted. The feces should also be tested chemically for the presence of occult blood with guaiac, benzidine or Hematest.

PROCTOSCOPY

The patient is put in the left lateral or Sims' position. The upper or right buttock is retracted with the left hand. The proctoscope is held in the right hand with the handle in a horizontal position pointing toward the patient's back in the line of the natal cleft. The obturator is held in position by the right thumb. The proctoscope, which must be well lubricated, is gently inserted in the direction of the umbilicus. Once fully inserted, the handle is grasped by the left hand and the obturator is removed with the right. Cotton wool pledgets held in long nontoothed forceps can be used to clean the anal canal of excess mucus or feces.

When the proctoscope is fully inserted, it lies above the anorectal ring (Fig. 21–6 A). On removing the obturator,

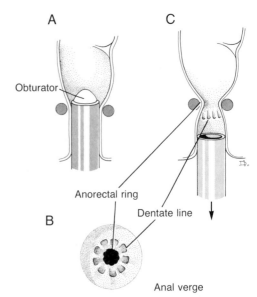

Figure 21–6 Technique of proctoscopy. A–C. Views of anal canal seen on withdrawal of the proctoscope.

the lumen of the rectum is examined. A note is made of the color and consistency of the feces, and whether or not any blood or mucus is present in or around the stool. The mucosa is next examined for any inflammatory changes, as shown by changes in color, ease of bleeding, ulceration or edema. Occasionally, low-lying tumors can be seen and a biopsy can be undertaken. The proctoscope is then slowly withdrawn. As it passes from the rectum into the anal canal, the anorectal ring closes above it (Fig. 21–6 *B* and *C*). The upper canal is surrounded by the submucous hemorrhoidal plexus, which gives it a plum color. If hemorrhoids are present, they will be visible in the lumen as bulges of varying sizes. It is advisable to ask the patient to strain down gently at this point to ascertain the degree of prolapse of any hemorrhoids or to detect any potential prolapse. The anal valves are usually clearly visible and a note should be made of any hypertrophied papillae or fibrous polyps arising in this area. Below the valves, a fissure, if present, may be seen in the midline posteriorly. The internal opening of a fistulous tract usually occurs at the level of the anal valves, and this may be confirmed by pressing on the tract either by finger or proctoscope, at which time a bead of pus will appear at the opening.

SIGMOIDOSCOPY

A sigmoidoscopy must be carried out in all cases.

Bowel Preparation

Sigmoidoscopy is best carried out, if possible, without any previous bowel preparation by laxatives and enemas. These produce fluid stools which irritate the rectal mucosa with resulting congestion and excess mucus production. This leads to obvious problems with the procedure and often to difficulties in diagnosis. Ideally, the patient should be asked to have a bowel movement a few hours prior to the examination. If the bowel is so loaded that examination is impossible, the patient should be sent away to defecate with the help of a suppository or return at a suitable time after a bowel action with or without the aid of laxatives.

Technique

The patient may be placed for this examination in one of the following positions (Fig. 21–5): (1) Left lateral or Sims' position; (2) Knee-shoulder; (3) Prone on the sigmoidoscopy couch.

The left lateral is probably the most convenient and comfortable position for the patient. In order to prevent complications caused by blind passage of the instrument, a digital examination must always be carried out prior to instrumentation. The digital examination must be done to exclude a stricture or any gross pathology in the anal canal and lower rectum. A well-lubricated sigmoidoscope should then be gently introduced in the direction of the umbilicus (Fig. 21–7, position 1). The progress of the sigmoidoscope will be stopped by the anterior wall of the rectum just above the anorectal ring. The obturator should then be withdrawn, and the light and bellows attached. Further progress of the sigmoidoscope must be performed under direct vision. Using the minimum of inflation with the bellows, the sigmoidoscope should be gently advanced up the rectum following the sacral curve past the valves of Houston (Fig. 21–7, position 2). Any small amounts of feces obstructing the passage or impeding a view of the mucosa should be cleared with pledgets of cotton wool held in long alligator forceps. Liquid stool may be removed by a suction tube. It is important not to overinflate the rectum, as this produces an intense desire

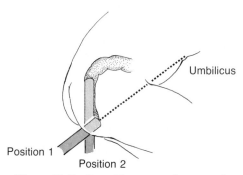

Figure 21–7 Sigmoidoscopy, showing the axis of the instrument required following insertion into the rectum.

to defecate, which may unsettle the patient and make him uncooperative. The rectosigmoid junction is reached when the sigmoidoscope has been inserted to about 15 cm. Here the bowel bends at an acute angle into the left iliac fossa. It is usually possible to pass it into the sigmoid colon by gentle inflation and manipulation of the sigmoidoscope. In some cases, however, there may be acute angulation of the bowel at this point due to a short mesosigmoid. The rectum may also be narrow due to spasm or rigid due to inflammatory changes produced by, for example, diverticulitis or extracolonic pelvic pathologic process. It is then difficult, and often very distressing to the patient, to try and negotiate the bend. Force should not be used, and in these cases the procedure should be abandoned at this level. A barium enema may be used to display the sigmoid colon.

During the procedure, usually when withdrawing, great care should be taken to examine all parts of the rectum and the visible sigmoid colon, and the following points must be noted:

(1) Distance to which the instrument was inserted.

(2) The nature of the feces in the rectum and whether or not there is any blood, pus or excess mucus present in or on the stool.

(3) The state of the mucosa and the nature and extent of any inflammatory changes., i.e. color, friability, edema,

ulceration and extent of bleeding when rubbed with a cotton pledget.

(4) The presence of any intraluminal polyps, villous adenomas or carcinomas, their size and their level measured from the anal verge.

(5) Mobility of gut wall when inflated and whether there is any evidence of rigidity in the wall.

If, for reasons such as nervousness of the patient or excessive pain and discomfort, sigmoidoscopy is unsatisfactory, the procedure should be carried out under general anesthetic.

RECTAL BIOPSY

A biopsy must be performed for all suspicious lesions of the rectum before making a tissue diagnosis. Biopsy may also be used as a follow-up procedure in chronic ulcerative colitis when the development of histological precancerous changes in the rectum reflects the general condition of the colonic mucosa.[30]

Punch Biopsy

This may be used for mucosal lesions, small sessile polyps and carcinomas.

TECHNIQUE. The forceps are introduced through the sigmoidoscope under direct vision. The lesion is grasped and the handles closed to cut the biopsy. This usually is easy in friable lesions, but is sometimes difficult when normal mucosa is included in the biopsy sample. In these cases, the forceps should be rotated so that the sample is twisted off the surrounding mucosa. Great care should be taken when making biopsies above the peritoneal reflection, as perforation is a risk.

A disadvantage of this technique is that it often provides the pathologist with a damaged piece of tissue which is difficult to assess.

Suction Biopsy

This method is preferable for inflammatory lesions when the mucosa is friable. It provides a relatively undamaged piece of mucosa for histological examination.

TECHNIQUE. The Truelove-Salt or Dick instrument should be used. A sigmoidoscope is passed and the site of biopsy is selected. The biopsy instrument is then passed, suction applied and the tissue taken. The piece of tissue obtained should always be orientated by the examiner before fixation so that the pathologist can take a truly transverse section. This can best be done by pressing it on to a ground glass slide or piece of blotting paper with the epithelium uppermost to prevent curling.

COMPLICATIONS. The site of the biopsy must be carefully inspected after removal of the tissue. If there is excessive bleeding, then a pledget of cotton wool soaked in 1:1000 solution of epinephrine should be applied to the site and held in position for a few minutes until the bleeding stops. The patient should not be sent home for at least an hour or until further examination after this time shows that the bleeding has completely stopped. Rarely, blood transfusion may be required for persistent bleeding.

Incisional Biopsy

This method is used to confirm the diagnosis of Hirschsprung's disease. A strip of mucosa, submucosa and muscle is excised from the rectal wall and anal canal below the peritoneal reflection.

TECHNIQUE. The bowel should be prepared with enemas before the operation, a procedure which should be carried out under a general anesthetic with the patient in the lithotomy position. A bivalve speculum is placed in the anal canal and a chromic catgut stitch is then inserted into the left posterior wall 1 inch above the anorectal ring. Another catgut stitch is inserted vertically below in the anal canal just above the dentate line. Traction is then applied to both sutures to raise a ridge of rectal wall. A strip of mucosa, submucosa and muscle approximately 5 mm wide is excised. The defect is closed with a running chromic catgut stitch. The patient may go home after recovering from the anesthetic.

COMPLICATIONS. Bleeding may occur. This should be stopped either by direct pressure through a proctoscope or underrunning the bleeding point with a catgut stitch.

Anal and Perianal Biopsy

Any lesion in this area should be subjected to biopsy by taking a small wedge of tissue with a scalpel after previously infiltrating the area with a local anesthetic. A hemostatic catgut stitch may be inserted afterwards if necessary.

INVESTIGATIONS

Further tests may be required to establish the diagnosis. The principal ones are:

1. RADIOLOGY. A barium enema should be carried out if a lesion is suspected higher in the colon or to find the extent of a mucosal lesion or polyposis present in the rectum. The barium enema with air contrast is the most accurate technique for assessing the colon. If facilities are available, an "instant" barium enema[40] may be performed without preparation for immediate information regarding the extent of the mucosal lesions seen on sigmoidoscopy. A barium meal and follow-through should be carried out for small bowel lesions. Sigmoidoscopy should *always* be performed before barium enema to rule out the presence of a lesion in the rectosigmoid colon. If a constricting rectal or sigmoid lesion is

present, barium must be instilled with great caution to prevent impaction which may require an emergency colostomy for decompression. Likewise, proctosigmoidoscopy and barium enema should precede barium meal and small bowel examination to prevent inadvertent impaction of barium above a lesion of colon or rectum.

Barium enema should not usually be performed on the same day as a biopsy of the rectum, in order to prevent the occurrence of perforations.

2. EXAMINATION OF STOOLS. Stools should be examined for cysts, ova, protozoa and occult blood.

HEMORRHOIDS ("PILES")

Hemorrhoids are varicosities of the venous plexus lying in the wall of the anal canal. They may be classified according to their site of origin (Fig. 21–8):

1. INTERNAL. These are varicosities of the internal hemorrhoidal plexus in the submucous space of the upper anal canal above the mucosal suspensory ligament. They are covered with columnar epithelium.

2. EXTERNAL. These arise in the external hemorrhoidal plexus of the lower third of the anal canal and anal verge. They are therefore covered by skin.

Internal Hemorrhoids

Internal hemorrhoids are one of the commonest conditions requiring surgical treatment. It is difficult to estimate their true incidence, as they are often asymptomatic and patients are frequently reluctant to consult the doctor about them. They may occur at any age, but the incidence increases over the age of 50 years. Men are more commonly affected than women, although temporary prominence of hemorrhoids is a common complaint of pregnant women. Primary hemorrhoids arise in the left lateral, right anterior and right posterior positions (Fig. 21–8 B) which corresponds to the anatomical position of the terminal branches of the superior hemorrhoidal artery. Secondary and daughter piles, however, occur between them.

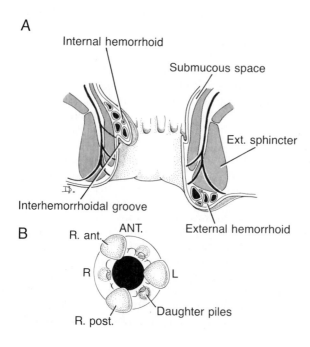

Figure 21–8 Hemorrhoids — anatomical location. *A*. Anatomical relationship of internal and external hemorrhoids. *B*. Arrangement of primary internal and accessory hemorrhoids as seen from below.

Classification

They are classified according to their size:

First degree: bleed but do not prolapse.

Second degree: prolapse on defecation but return spontaneously.

Third degree: prolapse on defecation or spontaneously and have to be replaced manually.

Clinical Features

Hemorrhoids commonly present with bleeding and prolapse.

BLEEDING. This occurs during and after defecation. It is bright red and is not mixed with the stool. It usually is only a small amount, but occasionally can be profuse, particularly from a prolapsed bleeding hemorrhoid. Bleeding may occur without defecation and stain the underclothes. It is important to remember that chronic blood loss from hemorrhoids is a common cause of hypochromic anemia.

PROLAPSE. This usually occurs when straining at stool. Third degree hemorrhoids may prolapse on walking or coughing. Prolapse is painless unless thrombosis occurs.

DISCHARGE A mucous discharge is common in patients with prolapsed piles. There may also be a fecal leak.

Examination

A general examination should be carried out to exclude anemia and primary cause for the hemorrhoids, e.g., abdominal tumors, pregnancy or portal hypertension. Inspection of the perianal tissue will reveal the extent of any external hemorrhoids, skin tags, third degree hemorrhoids and pruritic skin changes.

A rectal examination will exclude a rectal carcinoma, as hemorrhoids are not palpable unless thrombosed.

Proctoscopy determines the size and degree of prolapse. The proctoscope should be inserted above the anorectal ring, then slowly withdrawn. The patient should be asked to strain down and the degree of prolapse noted.

Sigmoidoscopy must be carried out in all cases to exclude any lesion in the rectum and lower sigmoid.

If there has been any recent alteration in bowel habit, a barium enema must be carried out to exclude a colonic lesion before the hemorrhoids are treated.

Complications

THROMBOSIS (STRANGULATED HEMORRHOIDS). This may occur in second degree or third degree hemorrhoids. They prolapse and are gripped by the anal sphincters, producing thrombosis in the hemorrhoids and edema of the perianal tissues. It is a very painful condition which may be aggravated by simultaneous thrombosis of external hemorrhoids.

Rectal examination reveals the prolapsed internal hemorrhoids with marked edema of the perianal tissues. Proctoscopy and sigmoidoscopy should not be attempted until the condition has resolved.

The majority will resolve spontaneously. If untreated, a few will sclerose and slough ("autohemorrhoidectomy"). Occasionally, abscess formation may occur as a result of secondary infection.

Treatment

There are four effective, safe methods for the outpatient treatment of uncomplicated hemorrhoids:

(1) injection of sclerosants;

(2) ligation (Blaisdell-Barron technique);

(3) cryosurgery; and

(4) manual dilatation of anus (Lord's procedure).

Before treatment is started, any constipation should be corrected by diet and bulk laxatives, so as to establish a regular bowel habit.

Injection Therapy

The aim of injections is to produce a submucosal fibrosis around the vessels of the internal hemorrhoidal plexus, which obliterates them and thereby causes the hemorrhoid to shrink. The most effective solutions commonly used are 5 per cent phenol in almond or arachis oil, 5 per cent aqueous solution of quinine urea hydrochloride, or 50 per cent glucose in water. Quinine urea should be avoided in pregnant women because of reputed danger of inducing miscarriage.

Indications

This technique is suitable for all first degree and the smaller second degree hemorrhoids. In these cases it will give either a complete cure or a prolonged relief from symptoms. It may be used also as a temporary palliative measure in third degree hemorrhoids.

Contraindications

(1) When there are associated pathological conditions in the anal canal or rectum, e.g., anal fissure or fistula.

(2) If there are strangulated hemorrhoids present.

(3) When the submucosal tissue plane is completely fibrosed following several injections. Further injections are liable to produce mucosal ulceration.

Preoperative Preparation

The rectum should be empty before injections are given, although this is not absolutely necessary.

Technique

The procedure is described with the patient supine, in the lithotomy position, although the prone or Buie position may also be used.

The sclerosant must be injected into the submucous space over the pedicle of the hemorrhoid, which lies immediately above the level of the anorectal ring. The technique is illustrated in Fig. 21–9 A. The proctoscope is inserted into the rectum and then withdrawn until its tip lies just below the anorectal ring. Then at 3, 7 and 11 o'clock, the sclerosant is injected slowly into the submucosal space, approximately 5 ml of phenol in almond oil. The injection should continue until the distended mucosa blanches and the small capillary vessels become visible over it. If a 5 per cent aqueous solution of quinine urea hydrochloride is used, 1 ml is

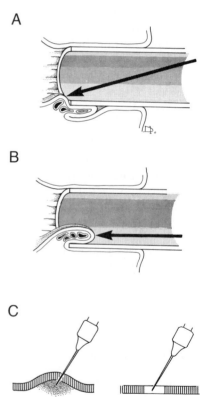

Figure 21–9 Techniques of injecting hemorrhoids. *A.* Injection into the submucosa at the back of the anorectal ring. *B.* Injection directly into hemorrhoid. *C.* Care must be taken in both techniques to inject the sclerosant into the submucosa. Injection into the mucosa produces blanching and subsequent necrosis and ulceration. Record the site and amount of sclerosant injected.

given directly into or in the submucous tissue adjacent to the hemorrhoid (Fig. 21–9 *B* and *C*). A record should be made of the sites and amount of sclerosant injected. Great care must be taken not to inject the sclerosant into the mucosa or too deeply, i.e., outside the bowel wall. Injection into the mucosa produces an intense white area, and this should be a warning to stop. If injection is too deep, no distension occurs and there is also resistance to the injection.

Postoperative Management

The patient should be advised not to move his bowels until the day after injection, as this may precipitate bleeding. Otherwise, there are no special precautions, and the patient may return to work immediately.

The patient should be re-examined in six weeks, by which time all swelling and induration in the anal canal caused by the injections usually has resolved. Further injections may then be given if the symptoms still persist. Two series of injections are usually enough to control bleeding but may not be sufficient if prolapse is the prominent symptom. The limiting factor in this therapy is the submucosal fibrosis which is produced and prevents further injections. Injections can be given between the primary pile sites until these sites are also fibrosed.

When submucosal fibrosis prevents further injection in the pedicle of the hemorrhoid, injections may be given directly into the hemorrhoid. The 5 per cent aqueous solution of quinine urea hydrochloride is probably the best for this treatment, given 1 cc at a time. This technique may produce brisk bleeding, or, if too much solution is injected, prolapse and occasionally thrombosis of the hemorrhoid. It does, however, allow injection therapy to be prolonged. Care must be taken to keep injections above the dentate line in order to avoid pain and discomfort. If carefully used in properly selected patients, injection therapy can control the patient's symptoms for many years.

Complications

The following complications may occur. Serious complications are, however, rare.

FAINTNESS. Occasionally the patient may feel faint after the injections.

BLEEDING. An injection made straight into the hemorrhoid may puncture a hemorrhoidal artery radicle and produce brisk bleeding.

Treatment: This usually can be easily controlled by either injecting more sclerosant submucosally around the bleeding site, or by applying pressure with a pledget of cotton wool soaked in 1:10,000 epinephrine.

PROLAPSE. If a large second degree or third degree hemorrhoid has been injected, the swelling in the anal canal may give the patient the desire to defecate. In trying to do so, the hemorrhoid may prolapse, bleed and subsequently thrombose if not replaced.

Treatment: The hemorrhoid should be replaced if possible and the patient confined to bed for 24 to 48 hours until swelling has resolved.

INJECTION ULCER. This occurs at the site of injection by either injecting the sclerosant directly into the mucosa or occasionally putting too much sclerosant in one spot. Ulceration occurs after about a week. It is well-circumscribed, usually with surrounding induration, and may feel and look like a small carcinoma. It may be asymptomatic and found on follow-up or it may present with bleeding. Usually this is small in amount, but occasionally it may be massive enough to require transfusion. The hemorrhoids take a further three to six weeks to heal, and obviously no further injections should be given during this period.

Treatment: Pressure with a pledget of cotton wool soaked in 1:10,000 epinephrine is usually sufficient.

RARE COMPLICATIONS. (a) Submucosal abscess produced by injection at site of injection. This usually discharges spontaneously; and (b) hematuria and prostatic abscesses have been reported when injection has been made too deeply.

Ligation of Hemorrhoids

The technique of outpatient ligation of hemorrhoids was first described by Blaisdell[4] in 1958 and subsequently modified and developed by Barron (1964).[3] More recent studies have confirmed its value as a simple, effective treatment.[1] The objective is to place a latex band around the mucosal part of the internal hemorrhoid so that it becomes ischemic, necroses and sloughs away, leaving a clean granulating wound. The ring must not include the lining of the anal canal below the dentate line, as this is somatically innervated and inclusion produces severe pain.

The advantage of this technique is that it is simple and almost painless. There are no medical contraindications, and no local or general anesthetic is required. There is also no need for hospitalization or time off work.

Indications

(1) Any patient with internal hemorrhoids may be treated by this method. The most suitable are those with secondary or small third degree hemorrhoids. Those patients with large third degree hemorrhoids and associated external hemorrhoids are less likely to have a successful result. However, Barron (1964)[3] and Rudd (1970)[36] have found that in the large majority of patients with combined internal and external hemorrhoids, the external hemorrhoid will shrink or disappear when

the internal hemorrhoid is removed. Any residual skin tags can be removed under local anesthetic or by cryosurgery if they cause symptoms when the hemorrhoids have been treated.

(2) Acute prolapsing hemorrhoids may be safely treated by this method.

(3) Small degrees of rectal mucosal prolapse may be effectively treated.

Contraindications

(1) Associated pathological conditions in the anal canal or rectum, e.g., anal fissure or fistula.

(2) Obese patients with large associated external hemorrhoids, as they frequently have a short anal canal and require repeated ligations.

Preoperative Preparation

The rectum should be empty, as it is important to have a clear view of the rectum and anal canal to permit accurate placement of the latex band. The patient should be placed in the left lateral position.

Technique (Fig. 21–10 *A-F*)

The latex rings are first loaded onto the ligator. Two rings should be used for each hemorrhoid. The proctoscope is then inserted into the anal canal to the level of the dentate line and positioned so that the hemorrhoid protrudes into it. The ligator is inserted so that the drum surrounds the hemorrhoid, which is then grasped and drawn into it by a pair of grasping forceps. The inferior edge of the drum should be at least 1/4 inch above the dentate line to avoid including the skin of the lower end of the anal canal in the ligature. The two rubber bands are then pushed off by closing the handles of the ligator. This produces a cherrylike internal hemorrhoid which rapidly becomes cyanotic. A little local anesthetic solution can be injected

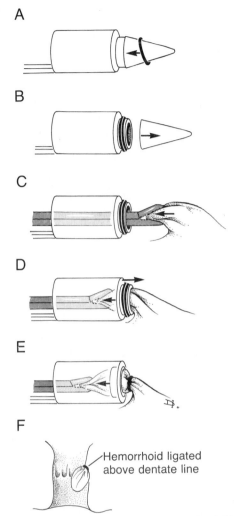

A

B

C

D

E

F

Hemorrhoid ligated
above dentate line

Figure 21–10 Technique of hemorrhoidal ligation. *A* and *B*. Method of rolling the rubber rings onto the drum of the ligator. *C*. The ligator is inserted through a proctoscope and the mucosal part of the hemorrhoid is drawn into it with the forceps. The inferior margin of the ligator drum must be at least ½″ above the dentate line. *D* and *E*. The rings are pushed off the drum onto the hemorrhoid by closing the handles of the ligator. *F*. Rings in place around base of the hemorrhoid.

into the cherry. This causes quicker separation, and diffusion may reduce late pain. The ligated hemorrhoid sloughs in three to six days. Two hemorrhoids may be ligated at a time, provided that the bands are applied at opposite sides of the anal canal.

Postoperative Management

The patient should be advised to avoid defecation, if possible, until the following day. A bulk laxative should be prescribed..

The procedure may be repeated after a few weeks. There is no limit to the number of ligations, but they should only be continued as long as the symptoms persist. Williams and Crapp[1] in a survey of 200 patients found that 46 per cent throughout had satisfactory results after one application of bands, 36 per cent required two applications, 10 per cent required three and 7 per cent required four or more.

Complications

These are unusual if the correct technique has been used.

PAIN. At the time of application of the band, the patient may feel some discomfort, but this should last only a few minutes. A few patients have more persistent, dull, aching pain in the rectum which lasts for about 48 hours and can be controlled with analgesics. If the anal canal below the dentate line is caught in the band the pain will be immediate, severe and persistent. The latex band must then be removed by cutting with scissors or a knife. Occasionally, when the band fails to separate, pain may occur about seven days postoperatively. The band may be removed if symptoms are severe.

BLEEDING. Bleeding may occur from tearing the hemorrhoid with the grasping forceps. This is controlled when the latex band is in place. Secondary hemorrhage occurs in about 2 per cent of cases 10 to 16 days postoperatively If the hemorrhage does not stop spontaneously or is severe, the patient should be admitted to the hospital. A simple quick way to stop the bleeding is to insert a well-lubricated 30 F Foley catheter into the rectum and inflate the bag with 20 to 30 cc of water (Fig. 21–11 *A*). Traction is then applied to the catheter, which compresses the internal hemorrhoidal vessels at the level of the anorectal ring. It should be kept in position by strapping to the thigh for 48 hours, then slowly removed. Alternatively, a thick rubber tube with paraffin gauze wrapped round it may be placed in the anal canal through a proctoscope, which is firmly gripped by the anal sphincter when the proctoscope is removed (Fig. 21–11 B). This also should be removed after 48 hours. The rubber tube is very uncomfortable and has no great advantage over the Foley catheter. Otherwise, the bleeding vessel must be ligated under a general anesthetic.

It is important to keep the bowel movements soft temporarily, as a constipated stool may cause a recurrence of the bleeding.

These techniques are also applicable to secondary hemorrhage following hemorrhoidectomy.

THROMBOSED EXTERNAL HEMORRHOIDS. This occurs in about 3 per cent of cases. Interestingly, it does not necessarily occur adjacent to the previously treated internal hemorrhoid and is probably related to altered hemodynamics in the area.[36] It may be precipitated by straining at stool.

Cryosurgery

Lewis[25] introduced this technique for the treatment of hemorrhoids. Its aim is to produce destruction of the hemorrhoidal tissue by rapid cooling to at least $-20°C$. A variety of probes may be used. The two main types cool by:

(1) the vaporization of liquid nitrogen, producing a probe temperature of $-180°C$.

(2) the sudden expansion of the gas nitrous oxide (Joule Thomson effect), producing a probe temperature of $-75°C$.

The lesion so produced is well circumscribed and painless.

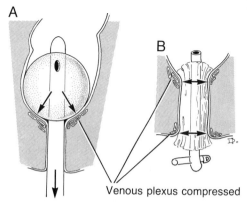

Venous plexus compressed

Figure 21–11 Methods of controlling secondary hemorrhage after hemorrhoidectomy. A. Traction on a large Foley catheter. B. Direct pressure on bleeding point by paraffin gauze surrounding a rubber tube.

Indications

This technique is suitable for second and third degree hemorrhoids and for treatment of associated skin tags.

Contraindications

Associated pathological conditions of the anal canal, for example, anal fissure or fistula.

Preoperative Preparation

No special preparation is required.

Technique

The procedure is carried out in the left lateral prone position. An open sided proctoscope is inserted and the hemorrhoid prolapses into it. The probe is applied at the base of the pile at the level of the anorectal ring. After a few seconds, the probe adheres to the mucosa, which becomes white and hard. Freezing should be carried out for no more than two minutes. If the hemorrhoid is too large to freeze with one application, the probe is switched off and then reapplied until all the hemorrhoid tissue becomes white and hard. It is important to make sure that only the hemorrhoidal tissue is frozen and not the underlying structures. The frozen hemorrhoid after treatment should be movable on the underlying muscle. The proctoscope is then rotated and the process repeated on the other hemorrhoids. Care is taken to leave muscosal bridges between each treated hemorrhoid.

Postoperative Management

The treated hemorrhoids become black and necrotic some 48 hours after treatment and slough at 10 to 14 days. There is usually a serous discharge, which may initially be profuse. The patient should be advised to wear a pad. Frequent sitz baths are advisable and a bulk laxative should be taken.

The anal mucosa heals with no obvious scar formation in three to four weeks. The patient should be seen for a check-up after six weeks.

Complications

1. PAIN. This may be experienced during freezing but is not usually a problem. Mild analgesics may be required.

2. SEROUS DISCHARGE. A watery discharge occurs in most cases which may be heavy for three to four days and persist for several weeks. Some patients, however, do not notice a discharge at all.

3. HEMORRHAGE. Serious hemorrhage is a rare complication. The serous discharge may sometimes be blood stained.

4. ANAL CANAL ULCERATION. Occasionally there is delayed healing at the site of treatment. The ulceration invariably heals without complication.

Manual Dilatation of Anus (MDA) (Fig. 21–12)

Lord[27] introduced this technique as a day case procedure for the treatment of hemorrhoids. It is based on the clinical findings that the majority of patients with symptomatic hemorrhoids have a constriction of the anal canal. The anal canal fails to dilate normally on defecation, producing a rise in intraluminal pressure in the rectum which causes congestion of the anal vascular cushions so producing hemorrhoids. Manual anal dilatation restores the normal functioning anal canal by breaking this constriction and so relieving the vascular congestion. It has been shown by Hancock and Smith[19] that the high pressure in the anal canal associated with hemorrhoids is returned to normal after this procedure. The principle advantage of this technique is that it cures the hemorrhoids without the tissue destruction of other techniques.

Indications

The majority of patients with symptomatic hemorrhoids may be treated by this technique. However, it is probably best carried out in cases of second and third degree hemorrhoids.

Age is no contraindication, but care should be exercised in elderly patients because of the possible risk of incontinence and also in those patients with colitis or conditions associated with loose stools.

Preoperative Preparation

No specific preparation is required. If the rectum is loaded, suppositories should be given. The patient should be anesthetised in the left lateral position — the position for the operation. Intravenous Pentothal should be used and may be supplemented by nitrous oxide, oxygen and halothane. Muscle relaxants should not be used.

Operative Technique

Instruments required are shown in Figure 21–12A. The patient should

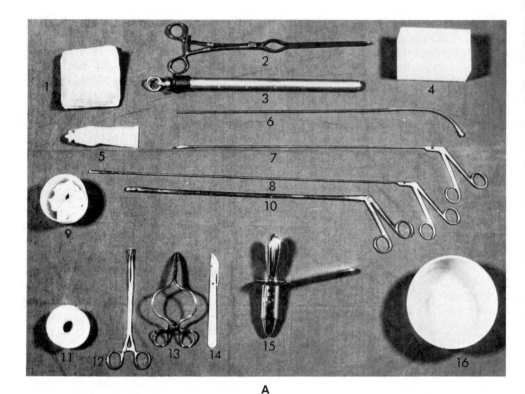

A

Figure 21–12   Manual and dilatation treatment for hemorrhoids.

A. Instruments and supplies used in anal dilatation. (1) Gauze swabs; (2) sponge insertion forceps; (3) sigmoidoscope; (4) sponge; (5) K-Y Jelly; (6) sucker; (7) biopsy forceps; (8) alligator forceps; (9) pledgets of cotton wool; (10) biopsy forceps–cup; (11) zinc oxide tape; (12) sponge skin holding forceps; (13) hemostatic clamp; (14) scalpel; (15) proctoscope; (16) bowl.

B. Digital dilatation begun. Two fingers have been inserted, and the right index finger is used to stretch constricting bands. *C.* Digital dilatation continued. Four fingers inserted. *D.* Digital dilatation nearly complete. Six fingers inserted. Eight fingers may eventually need to be inserted to stretch all bands. *E.* Lord sponge holder, loaded. *F.* Sponge holder in place, with sponge. The holder is then removed, one blade at a time. Sponge is left in place for one hour, then removed.

first have a rectal examination, to exclude any abnormality in the pelvis, followed by a sigmoidoscopy.

To assess the constriction bands in the anal canal, the surgeon stands at the patient's back and inserts two fingers, index and middle of the left hand, and pulls upwards. The index finger of the right hand is then inserted and pressed downwards (Fig. 21–12*B*). The types of constriction bands vary from a single tight band encircling the anal canal at about the level of the dentate line to several bands around the upper anal canal and lower rectum. The nature of these bands is not known, as they have not yet been demonstrated on histological examination. The principle of the dilatation is to stretch these bands and restore the normal anal diameter.

The procedure should be carried out gently, starting with the three fingers, then increasing the number of fingers up to eight as the bands are felt to give way. It is most important not to tear the anal mucosa, which is most likely to give way in the midline anteriorly and posteriorly where the sphincter is weakest. The force of dilatation should therefore be exerted on the lateral aspects of the sphincter by the most lateral of the inserted fingers (Fig. 21–12 *C, D*).

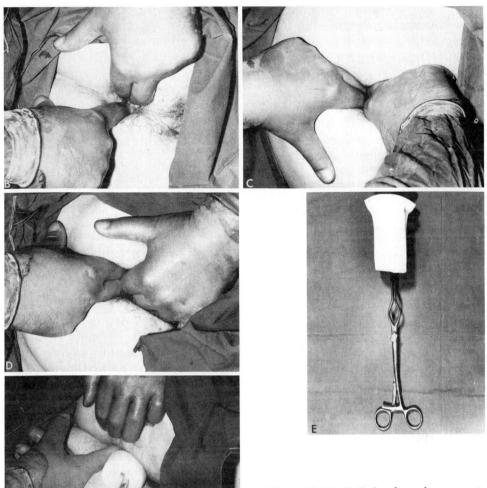

Figure 21–12   *B–F*. See legend on opposite page.

The dilatation is complete when all the constriction bands have given way. This may occur in some patients before eight fingers have been inserted.

Before the surgeon's fingers are removed, the nurse, using sponge holding forceps, inserts a sponge, soaked in 1:20,000 aqueous Hibitane, into the anal canal. The Lord pattern sponge holder has been designed to facilitate its easy removal following insertion. Care must be taken to see that the tip of the sponge holder does not protrude beyond the end of the sponge, other-wise the rectum may be damaged during the insertion (Fig. 21–12 *E, F*). The sponge exerts pressure on the walls of the lower rectum and anal canal, reducing the risk of hematoma formation.

The sponge is left in situ for at least one hour before being removed. It is advisable to give Demerol, 100 mg intramuscularly, prior to its removal as this may cause some pain to the patient.

Skin tags may be clamped across the base with a hemostatic clamp and excess skin excised with the scalpel. The Lord pattern clamp illustrated is then left in position for one hour postoperatively and removed at the same time as the sponge.

Postoperative Regimen

The patient may go home when he has fully recovered from the anesthetic. A bulk laxative is prescribed to produce a soft, well-formed stool so as to naturally dilate the anus. The addition of bran to the diet is also helpful. Lord advises the use of his specially designed dilator to prevent any narrowing of the anal canal. He recommends that this be inserted initially once a day after a hot bath. Then, as it passes more easily, the frequency of insertion can be reduced from once a day to twice a week over the next month.

The patient is seen two weeks after the procedure for check-up and at two months for a final check.

Complications

INCONTINENCE. True incontinence does not occur with this method provided the proper technique is used. However, most patients are usually incontinent for flatus for two or three days; in a few cases it may last for up to three weeks. During this period there may be some slight soiling of the underclothes. If the sphincter is torn during the procedure by poor technique, especially in the midline posteriorly, this may heal with a gutter formation allowing mucus and fecal leaking and thus anal soreness.

HEMATOMA FORMATION. Some degree of bruising occurs in all cases. Occasionally it is severe and painful, requiring analgesics for a few days.

MUCOSAL PROLAPSE. This may occur in a minor degree especially after dilatation of third degree hemorrhoids. It usually resolves spontaneously. If it is still troublesome at the two month check-up it may be dealt with by banding or cryosurgery.

The complications of urinary retention and fecal impaction associated with ligation and excision of hemorrhoids do not occur with this technique.

Treatment of Thrombosed Hemorrhoids

They may be managed conservatively or by immediate hemorrhoidectomy.

CONSERVATIVE TREATMENT. The patient should be put to bed with the foot elevated on 9 inch blocks. Dressings soaked in ice-cold saline should be applied to the prolapsed hemorrhoids every one to two hours. Analgesics, e.g., Demerol, should be given initially to control pain and also prior to the first defecation. Stool softeners should also be given. Systemic antibiotics should be administered if sloughing or sepsis occurs. On this regimen, the acute symptoms and perianal edema will usually settle in three to seven days. The patient will then be well enough to return to work in 14 to 21 days. If sloughing or sepis occurs, the convalescence will be longer.

The patient should be reviewed four to six weeks after the acute episode has subsided, and the residual hemorrhoids treated either by injection, ligation or hemorrhoidectomy.

MANUAL DILATATION (MDA). If the patient is seen within the first 48 hours of the prolapse and a gentle MDA is carried out, the results are often dramatic, with rapid relief of pain and shrinkage of the hemorrhoidal mass. If the hemorrhoids have been prolapsed for some time, an MDA may help their resolution but the external effects will not be so obvious. The procedure must not be attempted if the prolapsed piles are sloughing or infected.

HEMORRHOIDECTOMY. Immediate hemorrhoidectomy is widely practiced on the grounds that it rapidly relieves the symptoms. The convalescence is no longer than with the conservative method, and a second hospital admission is not required.

The operation is usually very straightforward, but great care must be taken in the presence of perianal edema not to excise too much skin and risk the subsequent development of a stricture. If there is extensive perianal edema, it is probably safer to treat the initial episode conservatively.

External Hemorrhoids

External hemorrhoids occur at the anal verge and in the perianal region. According to the symptoms and signs they produce, they are usually divided into two groups — chronic skin tags and thrombosed external hemorrhoids (anal hematomas).

Chronic Skin Tags

These may be classified into two groups according to their etiological factors:

(1) Primary or idiopathic. The majority of people examined have skin tags. In this group, there are no obvious etiological factors.

(2) Secondary. These occur in association with internal hemorrhoids, anal fissure or chronic pruritus ani or following the resolution of an anal hematoma.

EXAMINATION. A full local rectal examination must be carried out to exclude any associated pathology.

TREATMENT. Idiopathic skin tags which do not give trouble require no treatment. Frequently, however, they may cause discomfort and difficulty in cleansing the anal region after defecation. They may be removed under local anesthetic. Care must be taken not to excise too much skin and to make sure that the wound is pear-shaped, the narrow end toward the anus so that it will heal flat, from the anus out. If the tag is simply cut off without attention to the shape of the wound, it will result in the formation of more skin tags.

The treatment of secondary skin tags is primarily directed at the causal lesion. If they are still troublesome when this has been treated, then they may be removed as above.

Thrombosed External Hemorrhoids (Anal Hematoma)

In this condition, rupture occurs of one of the veins of the external hemorrhoidal plexus lying subcutaneously at the anal verge (Fig. 21–13 A). The blood clots and a tense, painful swelling is produced. It may be caused by straining at stool or prolonged sitting, squatting or other effort with legs apart. Frequently there is no obvious precipitating cause.

Figure 21–13 Excision of perianal hematoma. *A.* Technique of injecting local anesthetic. *B.* Excision of clot through an elliptical skin incision.

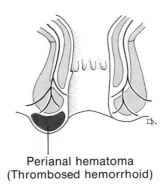

Perianal hematoma
(Thrombosed hemorrhoid)

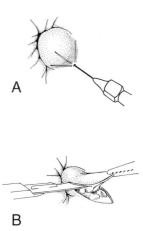

A

B

CLINICAL FEATURES. The condition usually presents with the sudden onset of an exquisitely painful swelling at the anal verge. Sometimes, however, there is no associated pain and it is not diagnosed until the patient notices the swelling. The hematoma may rupture spontaneously, producing bleeding and relief of pain. If untreated, the pain generally subsides after 48 hours. The untreated hematoma gradually resolves leaving a residual skin tag.

EXAMINATION. On examination there is a small, tense, bluish-tinged swelling at the anal verge. Occasionally there may be more than one hematoma (conglomerate hematomata).

TREATMENT. Treatment depends upon the degree of pain experienced by the patient.

(1) *Expectant.* If the patient presents after 48 hours with subsiding symptoms or a painless hematoma, it is best to use conservative treatment. The patient should be reassured that the swelling will resolve spontaneously and that no treatment is required. The treatment should also be conservative if the hematoma is in the midline either anteriorly or posteriorly, as these wounds take a long time to heal, and also if multiple hematomas are present.

(2) *Operative.* If the patient presents within 48 hours of the onset of the pain and swelling, then evacuation of the clot will produce instant relief of symptoms.

TECHNIQUE (FIGS. 21–13 A AND B). The skin and subcutaneous tissues around and beneath the hematoma are infiltrated with 1 per cent lidocaine containing epinephrine 1:100,000. A small radial elliptical incision is made over the swelling and the skin and clot are excised. The incision should not extend into the anal canal.

The patient should take daily sitz baths and stool softeners until the wound is healed. If internal hemorrhoids are present, they should be treated by sclerosant therapy if suitable. If

they are of third degree, elective hemorrhoidectomy should be carried out when the wound has healed.

ANAL FISSURE (FISSURE–IN–ANO)

An anal fissure is a crack in the skin lining of the lower part of the anal canal (Fig. 21–14A and B). It is a common and exquisitely painful condition. The majority occur in the midline posteriorly. Some 20 per cent occur anteriorly in females, but only 1 per cent in males.

Etiology

Fissures-in-ano are most probably produced by a combination of straining at stool and constipation. The passage of hard stool tears the squamous epithelium of the anal canal because it is firmly attached to the underlying internal sphincter by the mucosal suspensory ligament and therefore is relatively unelastic. It is believed that the tear occurs in the midline posteriorly because there is a deficiency of the subcutaneous external sphincter at this site.

Pathology

In the acute state the condition consists of a crack in the skin, the base being formed by the fibers of the longitudinal muscles. If it persists and fails to heal, the fissure deepens, exposing the white circular fibers of the lower quarter of the internal sphincter. This chronic fissure is usually associated with a tag of skin at its inferior end, the sentinel pile. The anal valve above this fissure may also become edematous and subsequently fibrose, producing a hypertrophied anal papilla. Persistent untreated fissure may produce fibrosis and stricture formation in the inferior part of the internal sphincter.

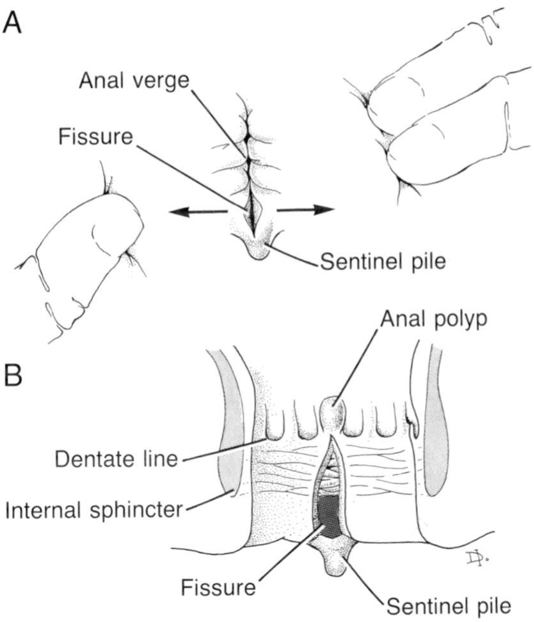

A

Anal verge

Fissure

Sentinel pile

Anal polyp

Dentate line

Internal sphincter

B

Fissure

Sentinel pile

Figure 21–14 Anal fissure. A. Demonstration of a chronic anal fissure on lateral separation of the anal verge. B. Anatomy of a chronic anal fissure.

Clinical Presentation

The classic symptom is severe pain during and after defecation. The pain, which produces sphincter spasm, may be such that the patient becomes afraid to defecate. Constipation develops and aggravates the condition. Often associated is bright red bleeding on defecation which streaks the outside of the stool and appears on the toilet tissue, and there may also be a mucous discharge.

Examination

This should be carried out with great gentleness. The fissure can usually be seen by lateral separation of the anal verge (Fig. 21–14A). However, this may be difficult owing to the associated spasm of the anal sphincter. The use of topical anesthetic jelly, e.g., 4 per cent Xylocaine, may make the examination easier. If there is much spasm, digital and proctoscopic examination should be avoided at the first visit. In these cases, it is often possible to pass, without causing too much discomfort, a well-lubricated, small-bore sigmoido-

scope in order to examine the rectum. A complete examination should be carried out on the second or third visit when the fissure is healing, or under general anesthetic during operative treatment.

Differential Diagnosis

The diagnosis is usually self-evident. It must be remembered, however, that fissures are commonly associated with ulcerative colitis and Crohn's disease. These are usually atypical, chronic and fail to heal. There may or may not be evidence of colonic disease. Fissures in these conditions should not be treated until the colonic lesions have been fully evaluated. Rarely, carcinoma of the anus may present as a fissure, but it is usually atypical and its edges are hard and raised.

The anus is not an uncommon site for the primary chancre of syphilis and acute inflammation due to gonorrhea. If there is any doubt about the nature of the anal fissure, a biopsy should always be made. If syphilis is suspected, a smear should be prepared for dark-field examination.

Treatment

Conservative

Conservative treatment should be tried first in cases of acute fissure. The most important factor is the avoidance of constipation, as the repeated trauma of hard feces on the anal canal will prevent the fissure from healing. The bowels should be regulated with a mild laxative, e.g., Milpar or Metamucil, to produce a soft, formed stool. Care must then be taken to make sure that a regular bowel habit is maintained.

The use of an anal dilator will also facilitate healing. It is used to overcome the anal spasm so that the fissure can heal with the sphincters relaxed. A fissure will not heal with the sphincters in spasm as each bowel action will re-open it.

The dilator, lubricated with 4 per cent Xylocaine ointment, should be inserted up to the flange and left in position for two minutes. It should be passed by the patient twice a day and also after defecation, and he should be thoroughly familiar with the technique before leaving the clinic. This method of treatment may be tried for two or three weeks, or longer if the fissure shows signs of healing. If, after this time, the patient is still experiencing pain and the fissure remains unhealed, operative treatment should be carried out.

Operative Treatment

ANAL SPHINCTER STRETCH. This is a simple, effective method. The technique is the same as that described for the treatment of hemorrhoids (see MDA, p. 1129).

The dilatation must be gentle, and care should be taken not to split the anal skin. The patient may go home after recovery from the anesthetic and should be re-examined in one month's time.

INTERNAL SPHINCTEROTOMY. The use of internal sphincterotomy for chronic fissure was first described by Eisenhammer. Under local anesthetic, he divided the lower part of the internal sphincter in the midline posteriorly, usually through the fissure. Although the recurrence rate was only 7 per cent, the wounds took a long time to heal and there was a high incidence of minor imperfections of anal continence. Eisenhammer[11] suggested that lateral sphincterotomy might have fewer complications. Hawley[20] reported no recurrence, fecal leak or soiling in 24 patients on whom this technique was used.

Operative Procedure. The simplest and most satisfactory outpatient technique is that of lateral subcutaneous internal sphincterotomy.[22] The operation is performed under general or local anesthetic. The patient is put in the lithotomy position and a bivalve speculum is inserted into the anal canal. Its handle is then rotated to the patient's right, so that the blades lie anteriorly and posteriorly (see Fig. 21–15A). The blades are then gently opened to approximately two finger breadths. This exposes the left lateral wall of the anal canal and makes the lower edge of the internal sphincter in that region taut and therefore easily palpable. The sphincterotomy is performed with a Von Graefe knife or a No. 10 blade on a long Bard-Parker handle. It is inserted through the perianal skin immediately lateral to the lower edge of the internal sphincter and passed vertically upwards in the intersphincteric plane until its point lies at, or just above, the dentate line (Fig. 21–15B). The lower half only of the internal sphincter is then divided by gentle cutting strokes made toward the anal canal.

Care must be taken not to penetrate the lining of the anal canal. Hoffmann and Goligher suggest that this may be avoided by leaving a few of the innermost fibers undivided; these may then be ruptured by lateral pressure of the finger in the anal canal after the knife has been removed. Firm pressure is then maintained over the myotomy site to achieve hemostatis. Sentinel tags

A

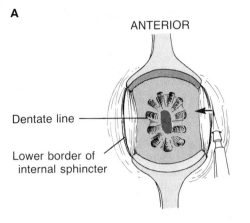

ANTERIOR

Dentate line ——

Lower border of
internal sphincter

B

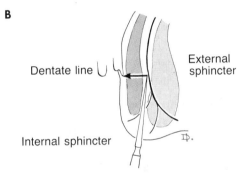

Dentate line

External
sphincter

Internal sphincter

Figure 21–15 Lateral subcutaneous internal sphincterotomy *A.* Bivalve speculum in position, displaying the left lateral wall of the anal canal. *B.* Knife inserted lateral to lower edge of internal sphincter which is divided up to the level of the dentate line.

and hypertrophied anal papillae should then be removed if large and troublesome. A cotton wool pad and T-binder are then employed.

Postoperative Management. The patients may go home after they have fully recovered from the anesthetic. They are given Demerol to control pain for 48 hours, and they should be advised to take a mild aperient such as mineral oil to soften the stool. They should have frequent sitz baths, preferably after defecation, and should apply a dry gauze or cotton dressing if there is any discharge. The use of toilet paper should be avoided until the wound has healed. Patients should be encouraged to return to work in about four to seven days.

Complications. These are minimal. Reactionary hemorrhage may occur rarely and this can easily be controlled by pressure. Alterations in anal sphincter function, such as flatus control, occur temporarily in 5 per cent of cases.

This technique gives complete and permanent relief of pain in the majority of cases, and the fissure usually heals within a month. Hoffmann and Goligher[22] had a 3 per cent failure rate in 99 cases that were followed for an average of 11 months.

ANORECTAL ABSCESS

This is a common painful condition in which suppuration occurs in the tissue around the anus and rectum. Anorectal abscesses are classified according to their site (Fig. 21–16): (1) perianal; (2) ischiorectal; (3) intersphincteric; (4) high intermuscular; and (5) pelvirectal.

Perianal and ischiorectal abscesses are the commonest and occur more frequently in men than in women. The common infecting organisms are *E. coli* and *Staph. aureus.*[16]

Etiology

In the majority of cases, no obvious cause can be found. However, perianal

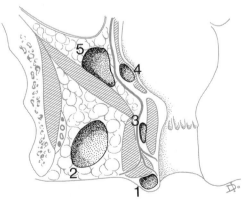

Figure 21–16 Classification of anorectal abscesses. (1) Perianal. (2) Ischiorectal. (3) Intersphincteric. (4) High intramuscular. (5) Pelvirectal.

infections are a common complication of ulcerative colitis and Crohn's disease. Other systemic disease, such as diabetes or leukemia, may also predispose to these infections. Therefore, before treatment, conditions such as these should be excluded. The most accepted theory is that the infection starts in the anal glands.[12, 34] Suppuration in these glands produces an intersphincteric abscess lying between the internal and external sphincter muscles. From this site, it may then extend through the external sphincter to the ischiorectal space, inferiorly to the perinal space and superiorly, giving a high intermuscular abscess. However, this theory is disputed by Goligher, Ellis and Pissidis[15] who carefully examined 29 cases of anorectal abscess for evidence of an internal opening at the level of the anal valves. They could find only five cases with an internal opening, and these were associated with perianal abscess; none were demonstrated with ischiorectal abscess.

Clinical Features

PERIANAL. This abscess presents as an exquisitely tender swelling immediately adjacent to the anus. It is red, well localized and may or may not be fluctuant. There is usually no constitutional upset. Rectal examination reveals no induration or tenderness deep in the ischiorectal fossa.

ISCHIORECTAL. These abscesses also present with perianal pain. In the early stages, there may be few clinical signs apart from tenderness in the perianal region, localized to the ischiorectal fossa on rectal examination. If untreated, a diffuse tender indurated area develops in the perianal skin with similar findings on rectal examination. Fluctuation occurs late. There is frequently an associated pyrexia. In patients who have received antibiotics, the abscess may become cold and nontender, and may not be diagnosed until fluctuation occurs.

INTERSPHINCTERIC. An intersphincteric abscess presents with acute pain in the anal region. There is no obvious swelling in the perianal or ischiorectal spaces. However, it can be diagnosed by finding an exquisitely tender spot on palpating the lower border of the internal sphincter, usually within the anal canal at the level of the dentate line.

INTERMUSCULAR. This kind of abscess is usually called a submucous abscess but is in fact a rectal wall abscess. It usually presents with rectal pain and may be difficult to diagnose. There are no signs in the perianal region, but rectal examination may reveal a smooth, tender indurated swelling in the rectal wall. Occasionally these abscesses have ruptured by the time of presentation. They are rare.

PELVIRECTAL. Pelvirectal abscesses are very rare. Their presentation is usually insidious with a pyrexia but no anal or rectal symptoms. There may be a recent history of pelvic infection. Rectal examination reveals a tender mass high in the pelvis.

Treatment

The treatment is surgical. Antibiotics may theoretically abort the early infection process, but usually by the time patients present at the clinic, pus is present and must be drained. A full rectal and sigmoidoscopic examination must be carried out. This preferably should be done while the abscess is being drained, or shortly after, since anesthesia is usually required for the examination.

PERIANAL. This may be drained under local anesthetic. If, however, there is any doubt as to the site of the abscess, then the procedure should be carried out under general anesthetic.

A very small radial or cruciate incision over the abscess (Fig. 21–17A and B) is all that is necessary. A Eusol dressing is then applied. Daily sitz baths should be taken until the wound is healed.

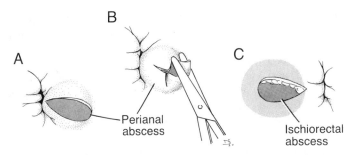

Figure 21-17   Methods of drainage of perianal and ischiorectal abscesses.

ISCHIORECTAL. This should be drained through a small pear-shaped or cruciate incision (Fig. 21-17C), and the minimum of skin should be removed. A finger may be inserted into the ischiorectal fossa to break down adhesions. Under no circumstance should the cavity be probed with a clamp or a pair of sinus forceps, for if undue force is used, a fistulous opening may be made into the rectum or into the supralevator space. It is important to remember that the abscess may extend above the urogenital diaphragm. Rarely, the abscess may extend posteriorly to the other ischiorectal fossa. In this case, a more extensive incision should be made passing posterior to the anus in order to drain both sides, or a separate drainage incision may be made on the opposite side.

The wound should be covered with a gauze dressing soaked in Eusol backed with a cotton wool pad and held in postition with a T-binder. It is not necessary to pack the ischiorectal cavity with gauze, as there is natural dependent drainage and it is also very uncomfortable for the patient. Antibiotics may be given if there is an associated constitutional upset, but usually such symptoms are relieved by drainage. The patient should take daily baths, after which the wound should be redressed. Stool softeners are helpful in the first postoperative week. The wound should be inspected twice a week to make sure that the wound edges do not heal prematurely. They usually take four to six weeks to heal completely. Ideally, the patient should be hospitalized for the first three to six postoperative days.

INTERSPHINCTERIC. The site of maximum tenderness should be marked before the anesthetic is given. With the patient in the lithotomy position, a small incision is made over this site and a pair of sinus forceps is pushed up in the intersphincteric plane until the abscess is entered (Fig. 21-18). A small rubber drain may be left in the cavity for 48 hours and then removed. Daily sitz baths should be taken until the wound is healed. The patient should be hospitalized for 24 to 48 hours.

HIGH INTERMUSCULAR AND PELVIRECTAL. The patient must be admitted to hospital for the treatment of these abscesses and their underlying causes.

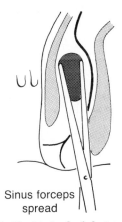

Sinus forceps
spread

Figure 21-18   Method of drainage of an intersphincteric abscess.

Associated Fistula-in-Ano

In the majority of cases of perianal and ischiorectal abscess, no fistula can be demonstrated at the time of abscess drainage. It is commonly taught that these patients should be reexamined after a week to see if a fistula is present, and if so, laid open. I do not think that this is necessary, as the majority of these abscess cavities heal uneventfully. In a small percentage, the abscess may recur, and in these patients a fistula should be sought.

Immediate Fistulotomy

If there is an obvious low level fistula present, i.e., with an opening at or below the anal valves, the fistula can be laid open when the abscess is drained.[38] The procedure, however, is only for the experienced surgeon; a careless division of the internal sphincter may lead to incontinence.

Immediate fistulotomy is contraindicated:

(1) In the presence of a high level fistula with opening above anal valves.

(2) When the fistula is associated with ulcerative colitis, Crohn's disease or anorectal tuberculosis, the latter condition now being rare.

(3) When there is doubt as to the level of the fistula.

(4) If the abscess is large and there is gross perianal induration and edema.

TECHNIQUE. A general anesthetic should be given and the patient placed in the lithotomy position. A bivalve speculum is then placed in the anal canal and an attempt is made to identify the internal opening before the abscess is drained. In a posterior abscess, the internal opening of a fistula is almost always in the midline. An anterior abscess usually has the opening within a crypt directly adjacent to the point of maximum swelling (Goodsall's rule). If an internal opening is present, pus may frequently be seen oozing from it, especially if pressure is applied to the abscess. A probe may then be gently inserted into the tract — no force should be used. The abscess is then drained as above. If the probe is visible in the abscess cavity, the fistulotomy is carried out by first dividing the skin, subcutaneous tissue and the sphincter muscle down to the probe. The probe should be positioned so that the sphincter muscle is cut in a radial rather than an oblique plane. This causes minimal damage to the sphincter and facilitates healing.

If no internal opening can be found, the abscess cavity is first drained. A probe is then passed gently from the abscess cavity toward the suspected crypt in an attempt to identify the fistulous tract. If a tract is found, fistulotomy is carried out as above (Fig. 21–19A, B and C). Great care, however, must be taken not to create a false tract with forceful use of the probe.

Postoperative Management

The wound is covered but not packed with a gauze dressing soaked in Eusol. This should be removed after 24 hours and daily sitz baths taken. Stool softeners should be given. The patient is kept in the hospital for at least 48 hours. The wound should be examined initially twice a week to make sure that it is healing from its base and to prevent premature closure of the wound edges.

FISTULA–IN–ANO

A fistula-in-ano is an abnormal tract between the anal, rarely rectal, mucosa and the perianal skin. It has a fibrous wall and is lined with granulation tissue.

Etiology

It probably arises in the majority of cases as a sequel to anal gland infec-

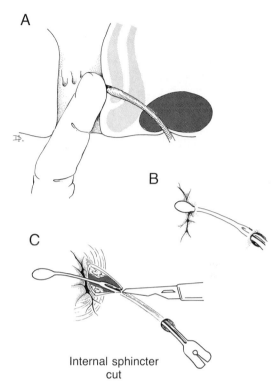

Figure 21-19 Method of immediate fistulotomy for low level anal fistula associated with ischiorectal abscess. *A.* Grooved probe is passed through fistula into the anal canal. Great care must be taken not to create a false tract. *B.* Probe in position. *C.* Fistula laid open by cutting onto probe.

Internal sphincter cut

tion, as was discussed in the etiology of anorectal abscess.[34] Some 10 to 20 per cent occur secondary to lesions of the bowel such as ulcerative colitis, Crohn's disease or tuberculosis.

Classification

They may be classified as follows:

Anal	Subcutaneous
	Submucosal
	High and low anal
Anorectal	

The fistulous tracts may be single or multiple, and the posterior ones commonly have a horseshoe configuration.

The important distinction between the two groups is the relationship of the internal opening to the anorectal ring. In the anal group, the internal opening is below the ring, usually at the level of the dentate line. The anorectal group, in which the opening is above the an-

orectal ring, is fortunately rare. These are much more difficult to treat because if the anorectal ring is divided, incontinence will result (Fig. 21-20 *A*).

The horizontal disposition of the fistulae follow, in the majority of cases, Goodsall's rule.[17] He said that if a transverse line is drawn across the midpoint of the anus, fistulae with their external openings anterior to this line usually run directly to the anal canal, while those with openings behind the line tend to take a curved course to an opening in the midline of the posterior wall of the anal canal (Fig. 21-20 *B*). The tracts of posterior and horseshoe fistulae lie at the level of the anorectal ring, to which they are closely applied. However, their internal openings are usually at the level of the dentate line.

Clinical Features

The patient presents with a chronic purulent anal discharge. In patients

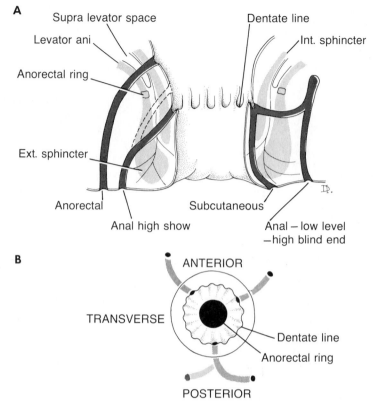

A

Supra levator space

Levator ani

Anorectal ring

Dentate line

Int. sphincter

Ext. sphincter

Anorectal

Anal high show

Subcutaneous

Anal – low level
—high blind end

B

ANTERIOR

TRANSVERSE

Dentate line

Anorectal ring

POSTERIOR

Figure 21–20 *A.* Classification of fistula-in-ano. *B.* Diagram illustrating Goodsall's rule.

with anal fistulae the onset of symptoms may or may not be related to a perianal abscess. Patients with anorectal fistulae, however, usually give a history of abscess drainage, followed by recurrent abscess or intermittent discharge. The discharge is irritating and is therefore often associated with pruritus ani. If the fistulae are secondary to ulcerative colitis or Crohn's disease, for example, there may be associated symptoms of these diseases.

Examination

A full examination should be made to exclude any cause for the fistula. Inspection of the perianal skin will show one or more fistulous openings. These are usually marked by a little spout of granulation tissue and pressure will produce a discharge from the opening. A note should be made of any scars from previous operations.

The perianal tissues and anal glands should then be palpated to determine the direction of the tract. In the low anal fistula, it can be felt as a hard subcutaneous cord.

Proctoscopy is important to determine the level of the internal opening, whether it is above or below the anorectal ring. The internal opening may be revealed by pressure on the tract expressing from it a bead of pus. A fine rectal probe may be used to define the tract. Great care and gentleness must be used to avoid creating a false passage. The probe may be passed from either the internal or external opening. If there is any difficulty, the probing must be stopped until the patient can be fully examined under anesthetic.

Sigmoidoscopy and barium enema are used to exclude a lesion of the bowel.

Differential Diagnosis

Chronic suppurative hidradenitis may produce a picture resembling anal fistula. However, there is no internal opening to the sinuses and no associated induration in the anal canal.

Treatment

Associated bowel lesions must first be treated, or there may be difficulty in healing of the anal wound, especially in ulcerative colitis and Crohn's disease. The ancient treatment of laying open a fistula (Fig. 21–19 *A, B* and *C*) and allowing the wound to granulate is still the treatment of choice. This should not be undertaken in outpatients, except perhaps in the anal fistulae of the subcutaneous type.

POLYPS OF COLON AND RECTUM

A polyp is a tumor which projects from the surface of the intestinal mucosa. It may be either sessile or pedunculated, multiple or single.

Pathology

Polyps may be classified into four main groups:[28] neoplastic, hamartomatous, inflammatory and unclassified (metaplastic).

Neoplastic Polyps

SOLITARY. Although these tumors have a varying gross appearance, microscopically they all present the same features in that they are all part of the spectrum of intestinal mucosal neoplasia. There is considerable evidence that these lesions are premalignant,[13] but the incidence of malignant change is difficult to estimate. However, the size of the polyp is a useful guide to its malignant potential. Grinnell and Lane[18] found that the benign adenomatous polyps were usually 1 to 2 cm in size and the average diameter of polyps with carcinoma was 2.1 cm. Although invasive carcinoma can develop in small polyps, a useful rule to follow is that polyps less than 1 cm in size rarely become malignant, polyps 1 to 2 cm in diameter should be carefully watched, and polyps over 2 cm should be excised. All polyps within reach of the sigmoidoscope should be excised regardless of their size.

A high percentage of villous adenomas will develop an area of invasive carcinoma, particularly if the lesion is over 6 cm in diameter.

Clinical Features. Adenomatous polyps may present with bleeding. In the majority of cases they are, however, asymptomatic. Villous adenomas usually present with a mucous discharge. If the lesion is large, this discharge may be so profuse as to produce a spurious diarrhea and occasionally weakness and lassitude due to electrolyte depletion, especially of postassium.

Examination. On rectal examination, adenomatous polyps are smooth,

Type	Solitary	Multiple
Neoplastic	Adenoma	Familial adenomatous polyposis
	Papillary adenoma	
	Villous adenoma	
Hamartomatous	Juvenile	Juvenile polyposis
	Peutz-Jeghers syndrome	Peutz-Jeghers syndrome
Inflammatory	Benign lymphoid polyp	Benign lymphoid polyposis
		Inflammatory polyposis
Unclassified	Metaplastic polyp	Multiple metaplastic polyps

lobulated and firm to palpation. However, they may be difficult to feel, particularly if they are small or have a long stalk. A villous adenoma feels soft, and because of this it may be difficult to detect, or to define its extent. It is important to remember that the presence of palpable induration in the polyp or its base may be the first sign of malignancy. The presence of a nodule or induration at the site of a previously excised polyp should also be regarded with suspicion.

Sigmoidoscopy is mandatory, as the majority of these lesions occur in the rectum and lower sigmoid, and excisional biopsy will give a tissue diagnosis. It is usually possible to distinguish grossly between adenomatous and villous polyps, although this may be difficult if bleeding occurs. A villous adenoma is generally larger and is characterized by a purple, pink color and a shaggy surface.

Investigations. (1) A biopsy should be first made of all sessile polyps, but pedunculated polyps must be removed together with their stalks (Fig. 21–21). A villous adenoma biopsy may initially be undertaken to confirm the diagnosis, but it must subsequently be removed completely to exclude malignant change.

(2) An air contrast barium enema should be carried out to determine whether other polyps are present in the colon.

Treatment. Diathermy excision or coagulation is the treatment of choice for those adenomatous polyps within reach of the sigmoidoscope (Fig. 21–21). This technique may be used on small villous lesions, but preferably these should be excised completely through the anus, if small, or by either the Kraske approach, the transphincteric approach or abdominoperineal excision if large.

FAMILIAL ADENOMATOUS POLYPOSIS (POLYPOSIS COLI). This condition is transmitted by a dominant gene and therefore affects both sexes.[10] The polypoid changes first appear in the colon

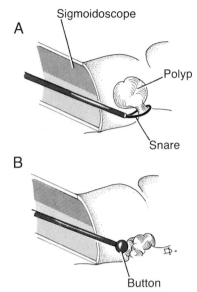

Figure 21–21 Methods of removing rectal polyps. *A.* Diathermy snare. *B.* Diathermy button.

and rectum around the age of puberty and, if left untreated, will usually undergo malignant change by the age of 35 years.

A full family history must be obtained and all potentially involved members examined.

Clinical Features. Symptoms such as mild diarrhea first occur between the ages of 15 and 20. Later, mucous discharge and bleeding occur and are frequently a sign of malignant change.

Diagnosis. On sigmoidoscopy, multiple small sessile and pedunculated polyps are present in the rectum and lower sigmoid. A barium enema should be carried out to ascertain their extent in the colon and a biopsy should be done to confirm the diagnosis.

Treatment. If no carcinoma is present in the rectum, then a colectomy and ileorectal anastomosis should be performed, ideally between the ages of 15 and 20 years. The polyps in the rectum are treated by fulguration. The patient must then be reexamined indefinitely at six-month to yearly intervals so that any new polyps can be fulgurated as they appear, or if malignant change occurs, the rectum can be removed at an early stage.

Hamartomatous Polyps

A hamartoma is a tumor composed of an abnormal mixture of normal tissues. There is no evidence that they are premalignant.

JUVENILE POLYP. The juvenile adenoma is commonly found in children, but occasionally in adults. It is a smooth round bright scarlet polyp with characteristic histological features.[24]

Treatment. A biopsy should be performed to confirm the diagnosis and the polyp should be removed if causing symptoms.

JUVENILE POLYPOSIS. This condition presents before the age of 10 years in contradistinction to familial adenomatosis. It is a pathologically distinct entity often associated with congenital abnormalities.[37]

Treatment. Polyps should be removed if they cause symptoms.

PEUTZ-JEGHERS SYNDROME. This syndrome is inherited as an autosomal dominant trait. It is characterized by melanin spots on the buccal mucosa and lips, and multiple polypoid lesions in the small intestine. In 50 per cent of cases, the large bowel is also involved. The polyps occasionally become malignant.

The syndrome usually presents with intermittent abdominal pain, episodes of bleeding and small bowel intussusception.

Treatment. The polyps are usually left alone until symptoms occur, at which time the polyps should be excised through multiple enterotomies.

Inflammatory Polyps

BENIGN LYMPHOID POLYP. This polyp is commonly found in the rectum and terminal ileum and is pale or yellowish in color. Occasionally it can be multiple. It is composed of normal lymphoid tissue.[9]

Treatment. Perform biopsy to make the diagnosis.

INFLAMMATORY OR PSEUDOPOLYPS. Occurring principally in chronic ulcerative colitis, these polyps are islands of inflamed mucosa produced by extensive mucosal ulceration. They occur in the lower sigmoid, but may extend into the rectal ampulla.

Treatment. Directed at primary pathology.

Metaplastic Polyps

These are the very small, often multiple, mucosal-colored polyps which are frequently seen in the rectum or during an otherwise normal sigmoidoscopy. Histologically, they have a distinct structure and are benign.[2]

Treatment. None is necessary except a biopsy if the diagnosis is in doubt.

Rectal Polypectomy

Pedunculated Polyp

Adenomatous pedunculated polyps should be treated in the first instance by local excision, subsequent treatment being based on the histological report. The whole polyp and stalk must be removed together. Biopsy should be avoided unless the size precludes primary local excision. The reason is that a biopsy will remove only a superficial part of the polyp, and this may not be representative of the whole lesion. In addition, by removal of the whole polyp, the pathologist can ascertain the completeness of excision if an invasive carcinoma is found.

In all cases where a polyp is found, the whole colon must be examined by double contrast enema for other polyps and any associated neoplasms.

Instruments. A wide bore operating sigmoidoscope, approximately 1 inch in diameter, should be used so that a good view can be obtained. A wire diathermy loop, as illustrated, should be used for removing the polyp. Ideally, a nonconductive sigmoidoscope of bakelite or plastic should be used. The same effect may be achieved when using a metal sigmoidoscope if the sheath of the diathermy loop is insulated with plastic or rubber tubing, and care is taken to avoid grounding the metal tip on the sigmoidoscope.

Preoperative Preparation. The rectum should be cleared, if necessary, by a disposable enema, e.g., Fleet's enema given one to two hours prior to operation. A general anesthetic is preferable for the procedure. The patient may be placed in either the Sims' or the lithotomy position.

Technique. The sigmoidoscope is introduced. The wire snare is then passed over the polyp and tightened round the stalk (Fig. 21–21 A). The polyp is then gently pulled away from the wall, at the same time a low cutting diathermy current is applied intermittently until the stalk is divided. After the removal of the polyp, the site should be checked for bleeding. If there is a brisk oozing, this may be controlled by pressure with a pledget of cotton wool soaked in epinephrine 1:1000.

Postoperative Management. It is advisable to admit the patient overnight. If the lesion, however, is below 7 cm, i.e., below the peritoneal reflection, he may be allowed to go home.

Sessile Polyp

It is not safe to use a diathermy snare on these polyps, as perforation is a very real risk, especially above the peritoneal reflection.

Technique. The procedure is the same as for the pedunculated polyp, only a diathermy button electrode is used and the polyp is fulgurated (Fig. 21–21 B). The polyp should be touched at several points on its surface and short bursts of a low coagulating current applied. It is important not to overfulgurate the lesion, as subsequent tissue

destruction is always greater than appears at time of treatment.

Postoperative Management. Patients with lesions treated above the peritoneal reflection should be admitted overnight. Another sigmoidoscopy should be done in three weeks and any residual tumor cauterized again with diathermy.

Villous Adenoma

These lesions are rarely suitable for primary outpatient treatment. If, however, they are small or have occurred after previous treatment, then they may be fulgurated, provided biopsy shows no evidence of malignant change.

Complications

SECONDARY HEMORRHAGE. This may occur from the sixth to the tenth day and may be minor or profuse. If profuse, it is advisable to give a short general anesthetic, so that the rectum can easily be cleared of blood clots and the bleeding point identified. The bleeding may then be stopped by pressure with an epinephrine-soaked swab, or by diathermy or suture-ligation to the bleeding point. The patient should be admitted until the bleeding has completely stopped for 48 hours.

PERFORATION OF THE BOWEL. Great care should be taken with all polyps above 7 cm, i.e., above the peritoneal reflection, as excessive traction on the polyp and too high a current when dividing the stalk of a pedunculated polyp or fulgurating a sessile polyp may easily perforate the bowel. If perforation is recognized immediately, laparotomy should be carried out and the perforation sutured. It is not always necessary to carry out a proximal colostomy in these cases. However, if the perforation is missed and peritonitis develops subsequently, a laparotomy, drainage and proximal colostomy must be carried out.

RECTAL PROLAPSE

Prolapse of the rectum is defined as a protrusion of the rectum through the anus. If only mucosa prolapses, it is called mucosal or incomplete prolapse (Fig. 21–22 A). If all layers of the rectum prolapse, then it is a complete prolapse (Fig. 21–22 B).

Incidence

Prolapse commonly occurs at the extremes of life. In children, the highest incidence occurs in the first two years of life and is rare after the sixth year.[8] The majority of these prolapses are of the mucosal type.

In adults, however, the majority of prolapses are complete. Eighty per cent occur in women, with increasing incidence after the fifth decade. In men the maximum incidence is before the age of 40.[23]

Etiology

The etiological factors are not fully understood. In children, it is probably

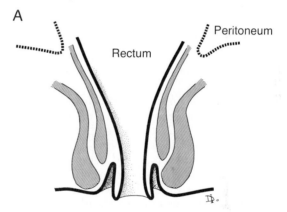

Mucosal (incomplete) prolapse

Figure 21–22   Coronal section of rectum and anal canal showing A, mucosal (incomplete) prolapse, and B, complete prolapse.

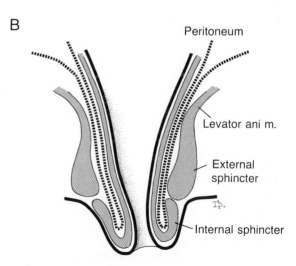

Complete prolapse

produced by constipation or persistent coughing. Obsessive toilet-training may be a factor. In adults there is no obvious cause in the majority of cases. In a small percentage, there may be a neurological cause, e.g., a cauda equina lesion. The principal etiological factors in adults are thought to be a weakness of the muscles of the pelvic diaphragm and straining due to constipation. Constant straining at stool causes the weak pelvic muscles to stretch and the rectum to descend. In support of this concept, Parks, Porter and Hardcastle (1966)[35] have shown that there is a tendency of the muscles of the pelvic floor to respond to straining by a sustained decrease in tone.

Clinical Features

On physical examination, it is important to establish three facts: (1) the degree of prolapse; (2) the state of continence; and (3) the exclusion of any pathology in the rectum and colon.

The degree of prolapse may be determined by asking the patient to strain down. (A receptacle should be placed at the anus!) In complete prolapse, the rectum protrudes to a length of 4 inches. The mucosa is usually inflamed and edematous and is thrown into concentric circular folds. If a finger is inserted into the lumen of the prolapsed bowel, the double layer of rectal wall can be palpated. This characteristic feature is missing in the cases of mucosal prolapse. However, a large mucosal prolapse may sometimes be difficult to distinguish from an early complete prolapse. A patulous anus, which may easily admit three or four fingers, is commonly found in complete prolapse.

It is important to establish whether the patient has had any history of incontinence. A history of previous anorectal surgery may be important in this context. If the patient has true fecal incontinence, he is very unlikely to benefit from any surgical treatment.

Patients frequently have a profuse mucus discharge, which may be stained by feces or blood produced by the prolapse. The prolapse may also make control of defecation difficult, especially if the patient is constipated. However, these patients are usually aware of any fecal soiling, whereas those with true incontinence are not. All patients must have a full proctoscopic and sigmoidoscopic examination to exclude any pathological factors in the rectum and lower colon. If surgical treatment is contemplated, a barium examination of the colon must also be carried out.

Differential Diagnosis

In children, the apex of an intussusception may rarely present at the anus. This is usually easily distinguished from a prolapse by the history and the fact that the examining finger will pass into the rectum lateral to the intussusception but will not in a prolapse. In adults, large third degree piles or a prolapsing rectal polyp may simulate a prolapse.

Treatment

Outpatient treatment is limited to small mucosal prolapses and to the occasional early complete prolapse in the elderly. Before any treatment is undertaken, it is important to correct constipation to prevent the patient from straining at stool.

Mucosal Prolapse

CHILDREN. Correction of constipation and bowel training is of paramount importance along with psychiatric consultation in selected cases. On this regimen the condition will resolve spontaneously in the majority.

OPERATIVE TREATMENT. Submucosal injection of 5 per cent phenol in almond oil given at the level of the anorectal ring as for hemorrhoids, is the simplest and most effective treatment. The submucosal fibrosis produces retraction of the mucosa.

The injection should be given under a short general anesthetic with the patient either in the lithotomy or left lateral position. About 3 ml of sclerosant should be given submucosally in four quadrants at the level of the anorectal ring. The patient should be reassessed in six weeks and further injection given as necessary.

ADULTS. Submucosal sclerosant therapy is also the most simple and effective treatment for small degrees of mucosal prolapse. The technique employed is the same as for children, but it may be carried out without anesthetic. Patients with greater degrees of mucosal prolapse or those who have failed to respond to sclerosant therapy should be treated by hemorrhoidectomy.

Complete Prolapse

For those patients with a complete prolapse, abdominal repair should be carried out. However, in a small percentage of patients, who are usually aged and unfit for operation, the Thiersch operation may be tried. It may also be used to correct a patulous anus after an abdominal repair.

THIERSCH OPERATION (Fig. 21–23 A to C). This may be carried out under local anesthetic by infiltration of the perianal tissues with 1 per cent lidocaine containing epinephrine 1: 100,000.

The patient should be placed in the lithotomy position and the perianal tissues cleansed. Two small incisions are made in the midline 1 inch in front and behind the anal verge. A half circle needle is passed from the posterior to the anterior wound in the subcutaneous plane. One end of either a 20 S.W.G. silver wire or a monofilament No. 1 nylon is passed through the eye of the needle which is then withdrawn through the posterior wound. The needle is then reinserted on the opposite side of the anus and the other end of the wire or nylon is also withdrawn through the posterior wound. It is advisable to use three strands of the monofilament nylon. An 18 Hegar dilator or an assistant's index finger is inserted into the anus. The wire or nylon is then pulled up around the dilator or finger, making sure it is not kinked, and tied. The proximal interphalangeal joint of the index finger should be able to pass comfortably through the anus.

The knot should be buried and the skin incision closed with a silk stitch or Michel's clips.

POSTOPERATIVE MANAGEMENT. Fecal impaction is the major problem. Therefore, mild aperients, e.g., Senna, milk of magnesia and suppositories if necessary should be given from the first postoperative day. A rectal examination should be carried out at least at

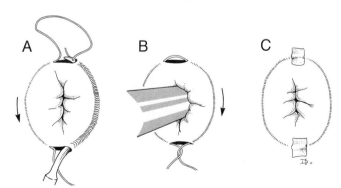

Figure 21–23 The Thiersch operation. A. Insertion of wire around the anus. B. Dilator or finger inserted into anus to adjust tension of wire before tying. C. Skin incisions closed.

weekly intervals initially to ensure that the rectum is being emptied and the patient's bowel movements are regular. The skin sutures may be removed after seven days. The patient should have regular follow-up to ensure that the wire remains intact, that the prolapse is controlled and that fecal impaction does not occur. The wire may be replaced on several occasions if necessary.

PILONIDAL SINUS DISEASE

A pilonidal or postanal sinus is a tract lined by squamous epithelium which occurs in the natal cleft overlying the sacrococcygeal region (Fig. 21–24 A). There may be one or several openings to the tract. Frequently in this condition there are several shallow midline pits in the natal cleft, which may or may not communicate with the sinus. The sinus characteristically contains loose hairs and debris (Fig. 21–24 B). Occasionally there may be only a cyst at this site containing fluid and epithelial debris.

Etiology and Incidence

Hodges[21] suggested that the primary postanal sinus may be the result of a congenital predisposition due to hirsutism, or a deep sacrococcygeal pit or a combination of these factors. Although some sinuses may be congenital in origin, it is now believed that the majority are acquired.[6] Buttock movements drill loose local hair into the skin of the natal cleft. Squamous epithelium proliferates into this puncture wound to form the primary pit in which hairs and debris accumulate. Pilonidal sinuses occur most frequently in males between the ages of 18 and 30. The majority are dark and hirsute, although the lesion is rare in blacks.

Pathology

Once the sinus is formed, the majority sooner or later become secondarily infected, and the subcutaneous cavity then becomes lined by granulation tissue. The natural history is then one of intermittent suppuration and discharge, with incomplete healing. This in turn causes a gradual extension of the sinus in a cephalad direction, and — if left untreated long enough — laterally out into the buttocks.

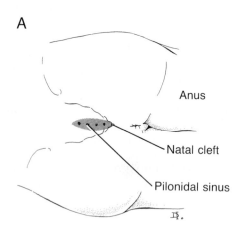

A

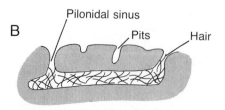

B

Figure 21–24 Pilonidal sinus. *A.* Sinuses occur in midline some two inches above the anus in the natal cleft. *B.* Longitudinal section showing sinuses and pits.

Clinical Presentation

The patients usually present with either an intermittent or chronic purulent discharge or an acute abscess in the natal cleft. The diagnosis is made on the site, the presence of hair and the direction of the sinus away from the anus. Rectal examination is generally normal.

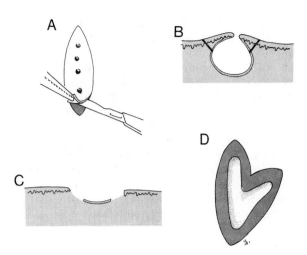

Figure 21–25 Excision of pilonidal sinus. *A–D*. The sinus openings and pits should be excised down to the underlying cavity. Any lateral extensions of the cavity should also be laid open.

Treatment

A pilonidal sinus is a foreign body sinus and the principle of treatment, therefore, is to remove all the hair and facilitate free drainage by laying it open. The techniques described below are, in my experience, the simplest and most effective, and are suitable for use in outpatients.

Uncomplicated Pilonidal Sinus

Ideally, the sinus should be treated in the early stage of its development before extensive tracts have formed.

OPERATIVE PROCEDURE (Fig. 21–25 *A–D*). The patient may be given a short general anesthetic, although local infiltration with 1 per cent lidocaine containing 1:10,000 epinephrine is very effective. The patient is placed on the table in either the left lateral position with an assistant retracting the right buttocks, or prone. The area should be thoroughly shaved and cleansed.

The sinus opening and midline pits are excised with an elliptical incision down the underlying cavity approximately 0.5 cm to each side of the midline removing a minimum of skin. All hair and debris are removed by curettage. Any lateral tracts should be laid open in a similar way. The wound should then be packed with a Eusol dressing and the patient sent home when he has recovered from the anesthetic. The pack should remain in position for 24 to 36 hours, after which time it may be removed and frequent sitz baths taken. The patient should be seen once a week until the wound has healed, usually in four to six weeks. Care must be taken to see that the wound heals from the bottom. Any regrowth of surrounding hair should be shaved until the wound is healed. The patient may, however, return to work in two to three days.

COMPLICATIONS. The only major complication likely to be encountered after this procedure is hemorrhage, and this can easily be controlled by pressure dressings. The patient should therefore be instructed that if this occurs at home, he should apply more gauze to the wound and sit on it! In a series of 33 patients treated by this technique and followed up for six months to two years, there was apparent cure in 32.[26]

Acute Pilonidal Abscess

Simple incision results in a high recurrence rate. Simple incision plus excision of the midline pit and sinus openings does not predispose to recurrence.[29]

OPERATIVE PROCEDURE. A general anesthetic is preferable, but local anesthetic can be used if there is not extensive surrounding inflammation. The position of the patient and the technique of excision of the sinus openings and pits are the same as those described for uncomplicated pilondal sinus. All pus and debris are removed from the cavity, and the region is thoroughly shaved. It is not necessary to remove the granulation tissue from the wall of the sinus. The wound is packed with Eusol dressing for 24 to 36 hours, then removed and daily sitz baths taken.

There is no need subsequently to pack the wound provided the skin edges remain apart, but it should be covered with a dry gauze dressing. It should be inspected at weekly intervals to make sure that it is healing from the bottom of the cavity and to break down any fibrinous bridges which may prematurely close the wound. If these precautions are not taken, there is a high incidence of recurrence. The patient can usually return to work in two to three days.

If extensive infection of the tracts and local cellulitis occur, it is advisable to admit the patient to the hospital.

Recurrent Pilonidal Sinus

The late recurrence rate appears to be equal despite the method of treatment used. Recurrences are principally caused by failures of technique and adequate follow-up, although some late recurrences may be new sinuses.[32] If the recurrent sinus is small, it may be treated on an outpatient basis, as described earlier. If, however, the sinus is multiloculated and infected, or if there have been multiple unsuccessful operations, the patient should be admitted for treatment.

Alternative Techniques

MARSUPIALIZATION. This is a popular modification of the basic operation described above for the uncomplicated case. The skin edges are sewn to the floor of the sinus with silk or nylon for eight days.[7] This technique usually necessitates the removal of more skin than is necessary and may be difficult to achieve in the obese person. I do not think that it makes the basic operation any more effective.

EXCISION AND PRIMARY SUTURE. In this technique the sinus cavity and tracts are widely excised and the defect closed with deep tension sutures. This method is not suitable for outpatient treatment.

PROCTITIS

Proctitis is a nonspecific term used to describe inflammation of the rectal mucosa. It may be limited to the rectum or it may be part of a more extensive colitis (proctocolitis).

Etiology

The condition may be primary, or idiopathic, or secondary.
  1. Primary
      a. Idiopathic proctitis
      b. Ulcerative colitis
      c. Crohn's disease
  2. Secondary
      a. Infection:
          (1) Bacillary — Shigella, dysentery, gonorrhea
          (2) Viral — lymphogranuloma venereum
          (3) Protozoal — amebiasis, balantidiasis
          (4) Helminthic — schistosomiasis
      b. Radiation
      c. Carcinoma

Clinical Features

Symptomatology depends on the causative condition. A mild proctitis is essentially asymptomatic except for a slightly increased frequency of bowel movements, whereas in severe cases frequent small, loose motions with tenesmus, hemorrhage and mucus are the main symptoms.

Investigations

(1) Full medical history
(2) General examination
(3) Rectal examination

INSPECTION. The presence of perianal infection, fistula or fissures in association with proctitis is suggestive of Crohn's disease or ulcerative colitis.

RECTAL EXAMINATION. This is usually normal in mild cases, but if acute, the mucosa may be tender and feel swollen. In Crohn's disease, the lower rectal mucosa may feel thick and nodular. The mucosa may also feel nodular in lymphogranuloma venereum and there may be evidence of a tubular stenosis in the late stage of the disease.

SIGMOIDOSCOPY. Proctoscopy is of little diagnostic help, but sigmoidoscopy is most important to determine the nature and extent of the mucosal inflammation.

In idiopathic proctitis and ulcerative colitis, mucosal changes may range from mild inflammation with mucosal vessels visible, to red and granular with loss of mucosal vessels, and finally to friable edematous mucosa with contact bleeding and purulent discharge. In idiopathic proctitis these changes are confined to the rectum and do not generally extend more than 8 to 10 cm from the anus.

In Crohn's disease, the main feature is edema with scattered areas of ulceration in normal-looking mucosa. In severe cases, however, it may be difficult to distinguish Crohn's disease from ulcerative colitis. Bacillary dysentery produces mucosal edema and, if severe, superficial ulceration which may become confluent with an associated fibropurulent exudate.

Acute gonococcal proctitis is rarely seen. It produces a very irritating yellow frothy discharge. The chronic form is difficult to diagnose, as the mucosa is only mildly red with streaks of pus. It should be suspected in all male homosexuals.

The acute stages of lymphogranuloma venereum produce a hyperemic, swollen mucosa covered with nodules and variably sized shallow ulcers.

Ulcers of *Entamoeba histolytica* or *Balantidium coli* occur early in the disease and are found predominantly in the sigmoid and upper rectum. They are multiple and small, with undermined hyperemic edges and a yellow necrotic floor which discharges pus. However, the changes may be nonspecific and diagnosed on biopsy. An ameboma of the rectum appears as a soft dark red mass with a friable ulcerated surface. Balantidiasis should be diagnosed and treated as early as possible, for perforation is the ultimate result of an untreated infection.

Rectal Biopsy

Mucosal biopsy should be carried out in all cases, especially of ulcerated regions, if present. Multiple small snips of mucosa should be taken if schistosomiasis is suspected.

Examination of Stools

For cysts and ova of *Entamoeba histolytica*, *Balantidium coli* or schistosoma.

Stool Culture

For bacillary dysentery and gonorrhea. If gonorrhea is suspected, a smear of pus should be examined directly for gram-negative intracellular diplococci, in addition to the cultures.

Barium Enema

This should be carried out in all cases to ascertain the extent of the mucosal changes and to exclude any other pathology in the colon.[40]

Blood Tests

Hemoglobin, white count and sedimentation rate.

Specific serological tests may include complement fixation tests for lymphogranuloma venereum, schistosomiasis, gonorrhea and serological tests for syphilis.

Skin Test

The Frei test is an intradermal antigen-antibody reaction specific for lymphogranuloma venereum. A specific skin test can also be used in schistosomiasis.

TREATMENT. The treatment of proctitis is directed at the primary cause. Idiopathic proctitis may be controlled by prednisolone or acetarsal (triple arsenical) suppositories. Salazopyrine, 2 to 4 grams per day in divided doses, and prednisolone retention enemas may be given if suppositories are not effective. Systemic steroids may be needed if symptoms are not controlled. The benign but recurrent nature of the condition should be explained to the patient.

Crohn's disease and ulcerative colitis, once diagnosed, should be referred to the Gastroenterology Department.

Bacillary dysentery may be treated with either streptomycin 1 gram intramuscularly every six hours or chloramphenicol 250 mg four times a day — both for five days.

Gonorrhea usually responds to penicillin, but antibiotic treatment and its duration should be determined by the sensitivity of the organism.

Lymphogranuloma venereum may be effectively treated by chloramphenicol or erythromycin given in the acute stage.

Amebiasis should be treated with emetine hydrochloride injections 60 mg per day for an adult for three days,

then oral emetine bismuth iodide 180 mg daily for ten days. It should be remembered that emetine, besides having a tendency to make the patient vomit, has a toxic effect on the myocardium. Metronidazole has recently been used with satisfactory results and less toxicity.

Balantidiasis requires immediate hospitalization and treatment outlined by a specialist in tropical diseases. Schistosomiasis is treated with either trivalent organic antimony compounds or new oral agents such as Neridazole.

Radiation proctitis has no specific treatment. Symptomatic treatment with stool softeners and prednisolone enemas may be helpful.

Carcinomas should be treated by radical surgical excision on an inpatient basis.

PRURITUS ANI

Pruritus ani is the condition of itching of the anal and perianal skin. It is a troublesome condition which may occur at any age in either sex, and is frequently difficult to treat.

Etiology

It occurs in association with many conditions, which may be classified as follows:

(1) *Anorectal conditions,* for example: skin tags, and fissures and fistulae, hemorrhoids and prolapse.

(2) *Dermatological lesions,* which may be either localized to region or manifestations of a generalized condition.

Examples are intertrigo, seborrheic dermatitis, psoriasis, contact dermatitis, leukoplakia and the rare lesions, Bowen's disease and extramammary Paget's disease, both of which are "premalignant."

(3) *Infections,* which may be of several types:

Bacterial: usually mixed. Erythrasma[5]

Specific: primary chancre of syphilis

Yeast: *Candida albicans*

Fungi: not common, often associated with tinea pedis

Parasites: pediculosis, scabies, pinworm *(Oxyuris vermicularis)*

Viral: condylomata acuminata

It is important to exclude a vaginal discharge as the source of the perianal infection.

(4) *General diseases,* for example, uncontrolled diabetes, Hodgkin's disease, jaundice, uremia, and gout.

(5) *Idiopathic.* A significant group exists in which no associated organic lesion can be found. Some of these cases are undoubtedly psychological in origin, but great care must be taken not to assign a patient to this group without an exhaustive search for a primary cause.

Clinical Features

Itching is the main complaint. It may be transient or persistent. In severe cases there may be associated soreness, bleeding and a weeping discharge.

Investigations

All patients with persistent symptoms must have:

(1) Full medical history

(2) General, vaginal and rectal examination

(3) Skin scrapings for candida and fungi

(4) Bacteriological swab

(5) Ultraviolet light examination for erythrasma

(6) Scotch tape test for pinworms

(7) Urinalysis for glucose

(8) Further tests dependent on above findings

Treatment

SPECIFIC TREATMENT. If there is a demonstrable cause for the pruritus, it should be treated. A biopsy should be made if there is any doubt about the nature of the lesion. Anorectal conditions should be treated surgically. Contact dermatitis is commonly caused by prolonged use of local anesthetic, antiseptic and antibiotic creams. If their use is stopped, the condition usually resolves rapidly, but improvement may be accelerated by a short course of 1 per cent hydrocortisone or 0.1 per cent betamethasone cream.

Erythrasma, caused by *Corynebacterium minutissimum,* responds to oral erythromycin 250 mg four times per day for 14 days. Candidiasis may be treated by local nystatin, and other fungi by systemic griseofulvin or topical Whitfield's ointment. Scabies may be treated with benzyl benzoate. Pediculosis should be treated with baths and DDT powder. Pinworms respond to piperazine, but may require several doses at two-week intervals. If pinworm infestation is present, all members of the family should be treated and careful hygiene observed.

Condylomata should be treated by podophyllin or excision.

The idiopathic group is the most difficult to treat. If there are obvious psychological problems, psychotherapy should be given. Symptoms can usually be controlled by hygiene, sitz baths, judicious use of cortisone creams and topical anesthetic (e.g., Nupercaine) and sympathetic handling. The operations of tattooing, undercutting and subcutaneous injection of ethyl alcohol have all been recommended for intractable pruritus ani. Their value, however, is doubtful, and most cases can be controlled as described above. The diagnosis must be kept constantly under review in these cases, and it is advisable to seek a dermatological opinion.

GENERAL TREATMENT. The patient should first be instructed on the importance of anal hygiene and given a simple regimen to follow. He should be advised to avoid those factors which aggravate the condition, e.g., scratching, heat, tight underclothes, prolonged sitting, excessive use of topical preparations and scented or harsh soaps to wash the anal region. If the symptoms disturb his sleep or work, a hypnotic and a tranquilizer may be prescribed.

Diet plays an important but variable role in pruritus ani. In general, patients should reduce or eliminate spicy foods, coffee and tea from their diets. Some patients have allergies to specific foods, which should be removed from the diet, especially if they cause diarrhea. Tomatoes, garlic, gin, fresh fruits and shellfish are common offenders. Sweets, particularly chocolate, and tobacco may provoke pruritus ani in some patients.

CONDYLOMATA ACUMINATA (ANAL WARTS)

These arise in the skin of the anal canal and perianal region, are multiple and occur more commonly in men. Anal warts are very common in homosexuals. They are viral in origin.

The diagnosis is usually obvious. Rarely, however, they may be confused with the condylomata lata of secondary syphilis. If these are suspected, serology and dark ground illumination of a smear should confirm the diagnosis.

Treatment

CONSERVATIVE. The application of a 25 to 40 per cent solution of podophyllin in tinct. Benzoin compound on the surface of the wart is the simplest and most effective treatment. The solution should be carefully painted on each wart with a cotton-tipped swab.

Care should be taken not to get it on the perianal skin, as it is highly irritating. The podophyllin should dry before the patient is allowed to dress. A pledget of cotton wool should then be placed at the anus to prevent the podophyllin on the warts coming into contact with the skin. The patient should be told to have a bath four hours after the application. He should be examined at weekly intervals, and further applications made if necessary. The warts have a strong tendency to recur, but they can be effectively treated by the meticulous use of this method.

OPERATIVE. Under local anesthetic, the warts may be cut off with a pair of scissors and the base is excised by diathermy. Care should be taken to remove any warts in the anal canal, for if these are not removed, a general recurrence will take place. *Postoperative Care:* Daily baths should be taken and a dry dressing applied. The patient should be reexamined after two weeks and any remaining warts removed.

REFERENCES

1. Alexander-Williams, J. and Crapp, A. R.: Conservative management of hemorrhoids. Clin. Gastroenterol., 4(3):595–618, 1975.
2. Arthur, J. F.: Structure and significance of metaplastic nodules in the rectal mucosa. J. Clin. Pathol., 21:735–743, 1968.
3. Barron, J.: Office ligation of internal hemorrhoids. Am. J. Surg., 105:563–570, 1963.
4. Blaisdell, P. C.: Prevention of massive hemorrhage secondary to hemorrhoidectomy. Surg. Gynecol. Obstet., 106:485–488, 1958.
5. Bowyer, A. and McColl, I.: The role of erythrasma in pruritus ani. Lancet, 2:572–573, 1966.
6. Brearley, R.: Pilonidal sinus. A new theory of origin. Br. J. Surg., 43:62–68, 1955.
7. Buie, L. A.: Practical Proctology. Springfield, Ill., Charles C Thomas, 1960.
8. Carrasco, A. B.: Contribution à l'Étude du Prolapsus du Rectum. Paris, Masson, 1935.
9. Cornes, J. S., Wallace, M. H. and Morson, B. C.: Benign lymphomas of the rectum and anal canal. A study of 100 cases. J. Pathol. Bacteriol., 82:371–382, 1961.
10. Dukes, C. E.: Familial intestinal polyposis.

Ann. Roy. Coll. Surg. Engl., *10*:293–304, 1952.

11. Eisenhammer, S.: The evaluation of internal anal sphincterotomy operation with special reference to anal fissure. Surg. Gynecol. Obstet., *109*:583–590, 1959.

12. Eisenhammer, S.: The anorectal and anovulval fistulous abscess. Surg. Gynecol. Obstet., *113*:519–520, 1961.

13. Enterline, H. T., Evans, G. W., Mercado-Lugo, R., Miller, L. and Fitts, W. T.: Malignant potential of adenomas of colon and rectum. J.A.M.A., *179*:322–330, 1962.

14. Goligher, J. C., Leacock, A. G. and Brossy, J. J.: The surgical anatomy of the anal canal. Br. J. Surg., *43*:51–61, 1955.

15. Goligher, J. C., Ellis, M. and Pissidis, A. G.: Critique of anal glandular infection in the aetiology and treatment of idiopathic anorectal abscesses and fistulas. Br. J. Surg., *54*:977–983, 1967.

16. Goligher, J. C.: Surgery of the Anus, Rectum and Colon, 3rd ed. Boston, London, Bailliere, Tindall and Cassell, 1975.

17. Goodsall, D. H. and Miles, W. E.: Diseases of Anus and Rectum. Part 1. London, Longmans, 1900.

18. Grinnel, R. S. and Lane, N.: Benign and malignant adenomatous polyps and papillary adenomas of the colon and rectum: An analysis of 1,856 tumors in 1,335 patients. Int. Abstr. Surg., *106*:519–538, 1958.

19. Hancock, B. J. and Smith, K.: The internal sphincter and Lord's procedure for haemorrhoids. Br. J. Surg., *62*:833–836, 1975.

20. Hawley, P. R.: The treatment of chronic fisure-in-ano. A trial of methods. Br. J. Surg., *56*:915–918, 1969.

21. Hodges, R. M.: Pilo-nidal sinus. Boston Med. Surg. J., *103*:485–486, 1880.

22. Hoffmann, D. C. and Goligher, J. C.: Lateral subcutaneous internal sphincterotomy in the treatment of anal fissure. Br. Med. J., *3*:673–675, 1970.

23. Hughes, E. S. R.: Discussion on prolapse of the rectum. Proc. R. Soc. Med., *42*:1007–1011, 1949.

24. Knox, W. G., Miller, R. E., Begg, C. F. and Zintel, H. A.: Juvenile polyps of the colon: A clinicopathological analysis of 75 polyps in 43 patients. Surgery, *48*:201–210, 1960.

25. Lewis, M. I., de la Cruz, T. and Gazzaniga, D. A.: Cryosurgical haemorrhoidectomy. Dis. Colon Rectum, *12*:371–374, 1969.

26. Lord, P. H. and Millar, D. M.: Pilonidal sinus: A simple treatment. Br. J. Surg., *52*:298–300, 1965.

27. Lord, P. H.: A day case procedure for the cure of third degree haemorrhoids. Br. J. Surg., *56*:747–749, 1969.

28. McColl, L., Bussey, H. R. J. and Morson, B. C.: Polyps and polyposis. *In* Morson, B. C. (Ed.): Diseases of Colon, Rectum and Anus. New York, Appleton-Century-Crofts, 1969.

29. Millar, D. M. and Lord, P. H.: The treatment of acute postanal pilonidal abscess. Br. J. Surg., *54*:598–599, 1967.

30. Morson, B. C. and Pang, L. S.: Rectal biopsy as an aid to cancer control in ulcerative colitis. Gut, *8*:423–434, 1967.

31. Nesselrod, J. P.: Clinical Proctology. Philadelphia, W. B. Saunders Co., 1964.

32. Notaras, M. J.: A review of three popular methods of treatment of postanal (pilonidal) sinus disease. Br. J. Surg., *57*:886–890, 1970.

33. Parks, A. G.: The surgical treatment of haemorrhoids. Br. J. Surg., *43*:337–351, 1956. (Anatomy)

34. Parks, A. G.: Pathogenesis and treatment of fistula-in-ano. Br. Med. J., *1*:463–469, 1961.

35. Parks, A. G., Porter, N. H. and Hardcastle, J. D.: The syndrome of the descending perineum. Proc. R. Soc. Med., *59*:477–482, 1966.

36. Rudd, W. W. H.: Hemorrhoidectomy in the office: Method and precautions. Dis. Colon Rectum, *13*:438–440, 1970.

37. Veale, A. M. O., McColl, I., Bussey, H. R. J. and Morson, B. C.: Juvenile polyposis coli. J. Med. Genet., *3*:5–16, 1966.

38. Waggener, H. U.: Immediate fistulotomy in the treatment of perianal abscess. Surg. Clin. North Am., *49(6)*:1227–1233, 1969.

39. Young, A. C.: The "instant" barium enema in proctocolitis. Proc. R. Soc. Med., *56*:491–494, 1963.

The Foot 22

DAVID S. WOLF, D.P.M.,
and WILLIAM R. ROSS, D.P.M.

INTRODUCTION

Podiatric medicine is that profession of the health sciences which deals with the examination, diagnosis, treatment and prevention of diseases, conditions and malfunctions of the foot by medical, surgical or other means.

This chapter is designed to be used by physicians in their offices, in Outpatient Clinics and Emergency Rooms, in which ambulatory procedures may be performed with ease by the busy practitioner. The ambulatory patient is able to return to work or home on the day of surgery, which is more advantageous and cost-effective than hospitalization. It is not our purpose to give a thorough review of all foot disorders, but to demonstrate practical applications of minor surgery of the foot on an outpatient basis.

It was noted by Ferguson[2] that ambulatory patients develop fewer complications than hospitalized patients. He concluded that end results are equally satisfying with outpatient procedures as with those performed in the hospital.

It has been our experience that patients have less postoperative pain in an outpatient setting owing to familiarity with their surroundings. In most cases, the home atmosphere provides less chance of contracting secondary infections than an inpatient hospital setting. Nevertheless, ambulatory surgery requires the same techniques, skill, time and postoperative care as that given to the hospitalized patient, to ensure its effectiveness and success.

INTEGUMENT

Disorders of the Nails

Diseases of the nails are more frequent than are diseases of any other part of the foot. Krauss[7] tabulated the nail disorders in 9,500 patients who had skin problems of the foot; 5,890 of the patients, or 62 per cent, had nail disorders. In a later study, 61 per cent of his patients with nail disorders suffered from club nail or hypertrophic nail and 75 per cent reported with onychocryptosis (ingrown toenails).

The function of the nail plate is to protect the distal ends of the toe and its ungual phalanx. Poor hygiene and improper trimming are major causes of nail pathology.

Incurvation is the most frequent affliction of the nail plates and occurs at any age. The medial side of the hallux is generally first involved. Anterior elongation of the first metatarsal and valgus rotation of the hallux increase the trauma on the nail plate. At first the patient complains of tenderness in the nail groove. As time advances, the nail plate commences to incurvate, and the removal of a small edge of the nail plate is necessary. If temporary removal of the nail spicule is the only method employed to relieve the symptoms, incurvation is destined to become chronic and increasingly severe.

Ingrown Toenail (Onychocryptosis)

A confusing variety of procedures have been advocated for this condition in the podiatric surgical and orthopedic literature.

The pathology of ingrown toenail is shown in Figure 22–1. The nail is formed on the dorsal aspect of the distal phalanx in a manner that corresponds with the hair root. The margins of the nail do not ordinarily connect with the adjacent soft tissue.

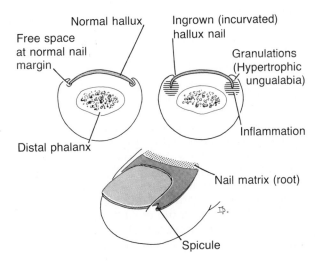

Figure 22–1 Pathology of ingrown toenail. The normal free space at nail margin is obliterated by inflammation and granulation tissue, which is caused by improper nail trimming, trauma to the matrix and faulty foot gear.

Normal hallux

Ingrown (incurvated) hallux nail

Free space at normal nail margin

Granulations (Hypertrophic ungualabia)

Inflammation

Distal phalanx

Nail matrix (root)

Spicule

Ingrown toenails are largely caused and made symptomatic by shoes that wedge the forefoot into the compressing toe of the shoe. High heels compound the problem by directing the weight onto the fore part of the foot. Pronation of the foot produces increased pressure on the forefoot.

An ingrown toenail is often complicated by improper treatment. Improper trimming destroys the nail groove, which then becomes hypertrophied and may overgrow the nail margin. Infection of the soft tissue complicates the clinical picture.

There are three major types of ingrown toenail.

SUBCUTANEOUS NAIL. As a result of improper trimming of the nail, a prominence may grow distally beneath the soft tissue surrounding the nail. The nail is normal, but it produces irritation by growing into the soft tissue.

INWARD DISTORTION OF NAIL PLATE. The lateral margins of the nail plate may be pressed inward by the surrounding soft tissues. The interfaces between the soft tissue and the nail plate become inflamed. A dorsal extension of the nail plate usually forms a subungual exostosis. The displaced nail hypertrophies.

HYPERTROPHY OF THE LATERAL LIPS OF NAIL. The nail may be normal, but the lips of the nail overgrow it. Inflammation occurs beneath the hypertrophied soft tissue.

SURGICAL TREATMENT. *Anesthesia*: After preparation, the toe is anesthetized with approximately 1.5 to 3 ml of lidocaine or Carbocaine (Fig. 22–2). Anesthesia is produced by injecting the great toe at its fibular side, toward its plantar aspect. The needle is then retracted slightly and redirected horizontally, dorsiflexing the toe so that the needle will pass under the extensor hallucis longus tendon. The dorsum of the toe is infiltrated toward its tibial side. The needle is next inserted on the plantar side of the great toe at its fibular side and directed diagonally upward, until an anesthetic wheal has

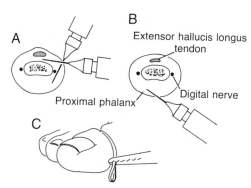

Figure 22–2 Anesthesia for surgery on ingrown toenail. Disposable 25 gauge ⅞ inch needle used to inject 1 per cent lidocaine and to block lateral, dorsal and plantar aspects, as shown. Maximum volume of lidocaine is 1.5 to 3.0 ml. Tourniquet is then applied and removed when operative procedure is completed.

been created around the base of the toe.

Procedure: The offending nail margin is split from its distal end back almost to its base with an English nail splitting forceps, taking care not to incise the epidermal tissue (Fig. 22–3). The remainder of the nail is split with a T-shaped nail chisel. A small elevator similar to a dental spatula is inserted under the offending section of nail, which is lifted from its bed. The exposed nail bed is then rubbed with 88 per cent carbolic acid (phenol) applied with a cotton-tipped applicator for two minutes. The applicator must be vigorously applied to the nail bed without spilling excess phenol on the adjacent normal tissues. If this happens, wipe off spillage with an alcohol-soaked sponge. Chemical cautery produces a mild sloughing of the nail bed and matrix, inhibiting recurrence of the nail margin. The patient will rarely complain of postoperative pain after adequate phenol cautery, since it destroys the superficial digital nerve endings.

After two minutes the area is sponged dry with another cotton-tipped applicator and the wound is dressed with Cortisporin* ointment

---

*Polymyxin B–neomycin-gramicidin-hydrocortisone (Burroughs Wellcome)

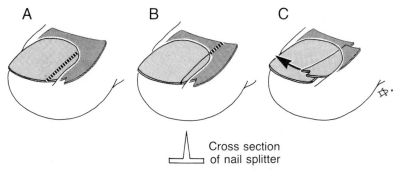

Cross section
of nail splitter

Figure 22–3 Surgery for ingrown toenail. Nail is split with nail forceps or sharp, heavy scissors. T-shaped chisel or nail splitter completes division of nail deep to eponychium following nail striations, and loose nail segment is then removed. Exposed nailbed is cauterized with 88 per cent phenol (carbolic acid).

and a compression bandage for 24 hours. The patient then returns to the office for redressing, which usually consists of a Band-aid and more Cortisporin ointment. In several days a straw-colored exudate will appear. Slight drainage may be experienced for several weeks. Showers and baths are permitted.

The same technique can be used for matrix destruction of the entire toenail. We have found no complications with balance or function after this procedure, for the purpose of the toenail is simply to protect the distal end of the toe.

Fungal Infection (Onychomycosis)

This is the most common disease entity of the nail plate. A mycotic toenail is an abnormal nail that exhibits growth deformity, causing the nail to be incurvated and hypertrophic with possible underlying subungual exostosis on the distal phalanx. The most common types of fungi that affect the nail plate are *Trichophyton rubrum, T. mentagrophytes* and *Candida albicans.*

DIAGNOSIS. Onychomycosis simulates a number of other nail conditions and must be differentiated from the following: psoriasis, atopic dermatitis, eczema and lichen planus. Many patients will present with a history of trauma followed by distortion and incurvation of the nail plate, which may become infected with fungus.

Fungus involvement of the nail causes elevation of the nail plate from the nail bed, makes the nail plate thickened, yellow and brittle, and may predispose to nail incurvation (onychocryptosis) and secondary cellulitis.

Fungus first appears at the distal tip of the nail plate as a scaly striation with radiating strains along the nail plate. This progresses until the nail plate is brittle and hypertrophic and has a powdery consistency involving all the nail components, including the nail matrix.

Before therapy is begun, fungal infection must be differentiated from trauma and other pathological conditions, such as subungual melanoma, through culture and microscopic examination of the nail tissues. Some offices employ Sabouraud's agar or Mycokit culture tubes to obtain a faster growth.

TREATMENT. As recently as 1956, onychomycosis of the toenails was thought to be incurable,[12] but the value of griseofulvin was described two years later. It was first administered in tablets of 250 mg, four times daily for 16 to 18 months. We have found that griseofulvin (Fulvicin-U/F — Ultra Fine) administered in 500 mg tablets, twice daily, results in resolution of the nail mycosis in approximately 9 to 12 months. If Fulvicin causes undue gastric upset, headaches or nausea, it should be discontinued or reduced. Over the last few years, it has been our experience that long-term use of oral antifungal agents is undesirable owing to cost and excessive long-term systemic effects. Onycho-Phytex (Unimed) has been used widely for the topical treatment of nail fungus. This preparation is composed of a borotannic complex derived from boric and tannic acids and salicyclic acids dissolved in ethyl alcohol. Mycotic nails can be treated atraumatically by avulsing the nails and then applying Onycho-Phytex twice a day for at least four weeks.[5] Treatment with Onycho-Phytex is not ordinarily effective without avulsion of the nail. If the fungus radiates to the eponychium and nail matrix, topical application will be ineffective.

Other modes of therapy include disinfection of the shoes with formalin, routine débridement of the nail plate with Betadine (povidone-iodine) scrubs, complete avulsion of the nail plate and subungual application of tolnaftate (Tinactin) drops.

For hypertrophic onychomycotic nails associated with brittle yellow discoloration involving all the nail components, the most effective treatment is atraumatic avulsion of the nail plate and phenolization of the matrix (Fig. 22–3).

Neoplasms

Neoplasms in or around the nail plate may affect its blood or nerve supply. Neoplasms thus produce disturbances of the nail matrix (root cells), causing abnormal color or growth patterns. Many benign neoplasms and even some malignant tumors have been misdiagnosed as calloused nail grooves. The following neoplasms should be considered before any treatment is instituted.

CHONDROMA. Chondroma is a new growth consisting of cartilage cells. It usually develops directly under the nail plate and causes elevation or deformation of the nail. It is not as dense as subungual exostosis, which is a true bony proliferation. Pain may be severe when pressure is applied to the nail. Treatment consists of surgical excision of the tumor. It is often seen in patients with chronic recurrent ingrown toenails when there is an irritation of the underlying dermal structures.

GRANULOMA PYOGENICUM. This is a pedunculated red fungating benign tumor in which the granulation tissue contains masses of staphylococci. It is most frequently seen in the nail groove and may range in size from that of a pinhead to that of a coffee bean. The granuloma occasionally covers the entire nail surface. It bleeds easily but is ordinarily not too painful. This condition is one of the complications of the ingrown toenail. Antibiotics will not cure granuloma pyogenicum. Resection of the offending portion of the nail plate is the treatment of choice, followed by electrodesiccation of the granuloma.

MELANOMA. Melanomas are highly malignant tumors of pigmented melanocytes. They usually develop in the matrix or in the nail fold. When found under the nail, the bluish color of the lesion will usually show through the nail plate. The lesion causes elevation of the nail from the bed and produces distortion of the nail. Most melanomas are black, bluish black or dark brown, but occasionally one will be found with no distinguishing color (amelanotic). Melanomas metastasize early. Amputation of the involved digit is the recommended treatment. A general surgical consultation should be obtained so that further evaluation and therapy may be performed as indicated.

VERRUCAE. Verrucae are benign tumors caused by a filterable virus. When they appear around the nail, they usually elevate the structure. They are fairly common and resemble

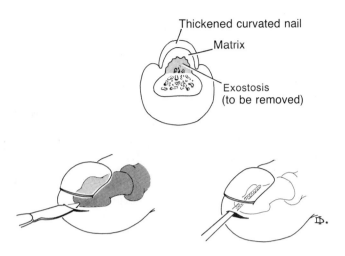

Figure 22–4 Subungual exostosis. Nail is thickened and encurvated, overlapping the rough exostosis (shaded area). This is removed by rasping with a No. 8 Bell dental file, which is inserted through a small transverse incision at the distal aspect of the toe. The incision should be just ventral to the plane of the terminal phalanx.

other types of verrucae, bleeding profusely upon superficial débridement. Because of the potential danger to the nail bed, we suggest chemotherapy utilizing mono- or trichloroacetic acid as the destructive agent. We have been pleased with the results obtained using Cantharone, which is well tolerated even by children.

SUBUNGUAL EXOSTOSIS (Fig. 22–4).

Diagnosis: A subungual exostosis is an osteogenic growth usually found on the dorsum of the distal phalanx of the great toe. Lateral radiographic projections readily identify it as a dome-shaped elevation creating pressure under the nail plate. Exostoses frequently occur distal to the nail plate. Upon pressure, pain is felt equally at the site of the exostosis and on the nail plate. Both areas are subject to weight-bearing and shoe pressure, which accentuate the discomfort. Subungual exostoses are benign and are often associated with a prior history of trauma.

The overlying nail plate is frequently involved and is often elevated and tender upon pressure. This condition is often misdiagnosed as an ingrowing nail, but efforts to produce relief by resecting the nail margins will be unsuccessful.

Surgical Procedure: Bone Planing. A 1 cm incision is made at the distal end of the hallux, just below the level of the ventral plane of the distal phalanx. With a No. 15 blade the opening is extended to the distal tip of the phalanx, and soft tissue is separated at the periosteal level. Care must be exercised to minimize soft tissue damage.

A small curved tenotomy forceps is then inserted into the wound to further detach soft tissue proximal to the exostosis. The reason for starting below the distal phalangeal level is to prevent embarrassment of the nail blood supply. A Bell dental file is inserted into the wound and the exostosis is rasped smooth.

Benign Soft Tissue Tumors of the Foot

Lipoma

Lipoma is an abnormal deposit of fatty tissue that may be found in the foot and ankle. It usually occurs as a circumscribed lobulated mass but may arise where fat does not normally occur. It may appear beneath fascia and periosteum as well as in muscles and joints. A lipoma may also be found in the subcutaneous tissue as a soft, movable mass. Lipomas may be single or multiple. Treatment consists of surgical excision with linear closure.

Ganglion

Ganglionic cysts apparently arise from degeneration in the connective tissue outside of the joints. These lesions are benign. A ganglion presents as a lobular mass over a joint capsule or tendon sheath, often over a bony prominence, and it contains colorless or straw-colored gelatinous material.

Conservative treatment by aspiration of the cavity usually results in refilling within a few days. Surgical treatment is therefore the preferred therapy. Complete excision of the mass should be performed.

Morton's Metatarsal Neuroma (Plantar Interdigital Neurofibroma, Perineurofibroma, Morton's Metatarsalgia)

Morton's neuroma is an entrapment of an interdigital nerve. It is found most commonly where the interdigital nerve branches into the contiguous compartments of the digits, most often the third interspace (between the third and fourth toes).

Lasker[8] observed that the condition was most common in middle-aged women. Neuritic pain radiates from the area of the metatarsal heads into the toes. Pain initially occurs only on weight-bearing but later occurs even at rest. A desire to remove the shoe and massage the foot suggests the diagnosis of neuroma. The major differential diagnosis is metatarsalgia, which causes pain at the plantar aspect of the metatarsal heads. If a neuroma is present, it can be compressed against the adjacent metatarsals by pressing against the web space with a pen, thus eliciting pain. Neuroma may also produce numbness or cramping of the contiguous toes.

TREATMENT. Conservative treatment consists of injections of steroid, 1 cc Xylocaine (lidocaine) and 1 cc Decadron (dexamethasone) for temporary relief of symptoms and metatarsal

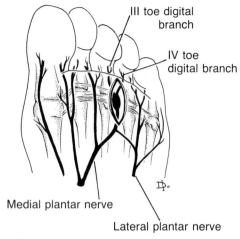

III toe digital
branch

IV toe
digital branch

Medial plantar nerve

Lateral plantar nerve

Figure 22–5 Morton's metatarsal neuroma. The tender neuroma between metatarsal rays III and IV is excised through a 4 cm incision on the dorsal or plantar aspect of the foot.

pads to redistribute weight to nonpainful areas.

Surgical treatment is the preferred method (Fig. 22–5). A 4 cm linear incision is made on the dorsal or plantar aspect of the foot between the metatarsal rays of the third and fourth metatarsals, extending distally between the metatarsal heads. Sharp and blunt dissection is carried down between the metatarsal heads, at which time the tumor becomes visible, bulging into the wound. The neuroma is then grasped with a tenaculum and excised. The proximal nerve trunk is cauterized with 88 per cent phenol. The wound is closed in layers and covered with a nonpressure sterile dressing. Ambulation is begun in a Reese postoperative shoe immediately.

Hyperkeratosis

The term *keratosis* includes conditions sometimes referred to as hyperkeratosis, hematoma and callous thickening of the outer layer of the epidermis. Hyperkeratosis may be a solitary or diffuse collection of plantar thickening. Calluses represent a mild inflammatory response of the body to long-standing intermittent pressure or function that is confined to certain areas of the skin. It is in these areas that the skin undergoes shearing or frictional forces to induce callus formation. If a metatarsal head becomes hypertrophied or an abnormal parabola of the metatarsals exists, intractable plantar keratoma might occur. Other biomechanical abnormalities, such as hammertoes and hallux valgus, cause callus formation owing to structural change that creates additional pressure and friction.

Plantar Warts (Verrucae Plantaris) (Fig. 22–6)

Verrucae plantaris are benign lesions of the papillary layer of the skin caused by a filterable virus that is autoinoculable and quite contagious. In-

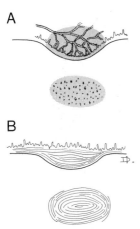

Figure 22–6 Plantar wart (verruca). Plantar wart (A) has a thin layer of callus, underneath which is a rich blood supply identified by multiple tiny blood vessel endings which can be seen when callus is removed. A keratoma or plantar callus (B) differs from a verruca in having a thick layer of keratin and no abnormal vascularity.

Treatment of a plantar wart is enucleation of the diseased tissue (shaded area) by blunt dissection under local anesthesia. The base and sides of the residual cavity are hyfercated to coagulate the blood vessels.

fection of several members of a family is not uncommon.

Verrucae vary widely in their clinical course. A single lesion may appear and persist relatively unchanged for many years. However, a single lesion may also be followed by the development of satellite verrucae. The mode of spreading may be minor injuries or breaks in the skin of the sole of the foot.

DIAGNOSIS. Verrucae located on the dorsum of the foot present a spongy consistency, while those on the plantar aspect have a thin layer of callous tissue covering them. They are not necessarily found on weight-bearing areas and they occur in both children and adults. The verrucae are exquisitely tender on compression and they bleed profusely when debrided. Verrucae have an affinity for the foot, since it is usually enclosed in a dark, damp shoe. This alkaline, moist environment seems most conducive to growth.

TREATMENT. There are approximately 20 different treatments for warts, and none are entirely satisfactory. Therapeutic modalities vary from suggestion therapy to surgical excision. Verrucae may respond well to escharotics; e.g., salicylic acid, 88 per cent phenol, sulfuric or nitric acid, or repeated applications of silver nitrate. Dry ice "snow" (CO_2) and liquid nitrogen have been employed with moderate to good results.

Curettage Method. Curettage has been used as a means of eliminating verrucae. The curettage method involves circumscribing the wart shallowly with a knife and then, using a combination of prying and scraping motions, scooping out the verrucae with a Spratt bone curette, down to the basal fascial layer only.

Enucleation Technique. The enucleation technique is preferred by many, being relatively atraumatic and usually successful. The foot is soaked in warm soapy water for one-half hour to soften the overlying callus, following which the area is dried carefully, prepared aseptically and draped. Local anesthetic is injected near the margins of the plantar wart and deep to it and is gently massaged into the tissues until anesthesia is complete. Careful blunt dissection is begun with a curved "mosquito" (Halsted) clamp in the plane between the central core and the adjacent normal tissue. If a heavy callus is present on the surface, it may be carefully shaved with a razor blade until the plane between the central core (wart) and the surrounding tissue is apparent. The blunt dissection continues around and deep to the wart until the base is fully exposed. The wart can then be lifted out. The base usually has several small but briskly bleeding vessels, which respond nicely to hyfercation (unipolar electrocoagulation) or silver nitrate stick cautery. A small gauze sponge is cut and shaped to fill the defect that is present. This sponge is pressed into the defect for five minutes and then removed to permit inspection of the base of the defect. If bleeding is then absent or minimal, a fresh, shaped gauze sponge is placed in the defect and secured with Elastoplast adhesive. The patient may walk on the foot immediately, although it should be kept elevated for a few days when the patient is not ambulating. The dressing is changed completely in the office after two or three days and redressed thereafter by the patient until healing is complete. Postoperative discomfort is usually minimal.

MUSCULOSKELETAL DEVELOPMENTAL DISEASES

Corns (Dorsal Helomas) (Fig. 22-7)

A corn is a localized overgrowth of skin with or without a central core. It is a circumscribed, cone-shaped impaction of the horny layer of the epider-

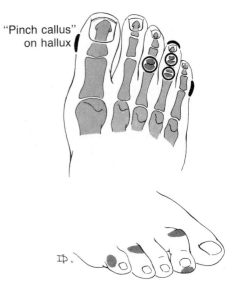

Figure 22-7 Corn (heloma) locations. Common locations are on great toe (medial), fifth toe (lateral) and middle toes (dorsal or at distal aspect).

mis. When external pressure impinges on the sensitive papillae, pain is produced.

Corns occur because of the continuous or intermittent pressure produced by shoes. In many instances, the style, design or dimension of the shoe causes pressure on the foot, contributing to corn formation. However, corns are not due solely to poorly fitting shoes. Very often elongation, pronation or supination of the foot inside the shoe will also produce pressure and hence a corn. The most common locations of corns are on the sites on the foot where the greatest localized pressures are exerted, such as the lateral side of the fifth toe, the dorsum of the middle toes or the medial side of the hallux. In a contracted toe (hammertoe), the location of the painful heloma is frequently at the distal end of the toe, just inferior to the distal margin of the toenail or at the highest part of the toe.

Conservative Treatment

The corn is softened with a wet pledget immersed in warm tincture of green soap solution. The wet pledget will soften or macerate the hardened underlying callus, thus facilitating débridement. Then, using a Bard-Parker No. 10 blade, the surface of the corn is debrided carefully without penetrating vital underlying tissue and creating capillary hemorrhage or pain for the patient. When the superficial layers of the impacted epithelial tissue or corn have been removed, the deeper segment of the corn may be enucleated using a smaller No. 15 blade. The work should be done carefully and deftly to avoid pressing on the inflamed subcutaneous tissue. When most of the corn has been removed, the toe is dried and prepared to accept an aperture pad. The skin around the corn is painted with either tincture of benzoin or rubber cement, which acts as an adherent. The skin is permitted to dry and a corn pad is applied. These pads may be purchased ready-cut or may be fashioned from adhesive felt of varying thicknesses. Adhesive felt or moleskin 1/16 inch thick is preferred. An anesthetic ointment such as Americaine, benzocaine, Nupercaine or Diothane can be placed on the irritated lesion within the aperture. A thick piece of adhesive tape is then placed over the aperture to retain the ointment and the padding in place. Next, the corn pad itself is wrapped to the toe using lamb's wool or self-adhering gauze, i.e., gauze tape or Gauztex. If a lamb's wool wrapping is used, it can be made to adhere more firmly by brushing the surface lightly with flexible collodion. This creates a water-resistant dressing. It is bulky but very soft and conforms to the interior of the shoe.

Operative Treatment

Before attempting any surgical procedures for corns, x-ray studies should be made during weight-bearing. In order to delineate the position of the corn in relation to the underlying os-

seous tissues, each corn is encircled with a piece of soft copper wire held in place with Scotch tape. On the film, a white identifying ring that encircles each lesion may be seen, specifically locating the corn and the underlying osseous tissue or the condyle that is the etiological factor.

There are various surgical techniques used to eradicate chronic corns (helomata). Those that we perform on an outpatient basis are:

1. SOFT TISSUE PROCEDURE (PHALANGEAL SET) (Fig. 22–8). *Phalangeal set* is a term used to indicate a manipulative surgical procedure for the treatment of lesser toe deformities. Phalangeal set and soft tissue procedures offer an alternative simplified technique, in contrast with complex arthroplastic procedures used for the treatment of hammertoes, mallet toes, underlapping (varus) toes, overlapping toes and other toe deformities. This method is indicated for flexible (nonrigid) digital deformities. In most instances with this soft tissue procedure it is possible to release toe contractures and superimposition of the phalanges, increase joint space and correct malalignment.

The procedure is performed under digital block anesthesia. A small plantar longitudinal incision is made (preferably under tourniquet control) beginning at the distal interphalangeal

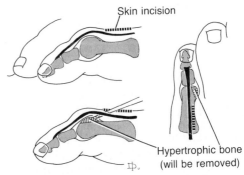

Figure 22–8 Subdermal rasping technique. Dorsal skin incision parallel to extensor tendon preserves tendon from injury. Hypertrophic bone (shown cross-hatched) is removed with No. 8 Bell dental file.

joint crease and extending proximally beyond the proximal crease. The flexor tendons are pulled out through the incision with a small blunt hook and the tendon sheaths are opened (tenotomy). The skin is then coapted with two or three sutures, and a sterile dressing is applied. Ambulation is initiated on the following day. Corrective splinting is accomplished with tape that is incorporated in the bandage, and the sutures are removed on the eighth postoperative day.

Phalangeal set surgery limits the grasping action of the toes but allows for more important pressing action, enabling the straightened toes to stabilize against the metatarsal heads in a foot in which the hypermobility and biomechanical factors have been controlled.

2. DIGITAL ARTHROPLASTY (Fig. 22–9). The toe is anesthetized at its base with 2 cc of 1 per cent Xylocaine. After the digital block is accomplished, hemostasis is achieved with a pneumatic cuff applied to the ankle at approximately 50 to 75 mm Hg above the patient's systolic blood pressure. After anesthesia has been induced and the foot and toes are carefully shaved, scrubbed, prepared and draped, the tourniquet is removed. Hemostasis is continued with a Martin (Esmarch) bandage or a pneumatic cuff applied just proximal to the malleoli and inflated to 50 mm Hg above the patient's systolic blood pressure. The corn is encircled with two semi-elliptical incisions that pass transversely through the skin, made by a No. 10 blade. The outlined corn is then grasped with a small Allis clamp and resected, using a deep No. 15 blade. The skin margins are next underscored and the toe is then plantar-flexed, exposing the involved interphalangeal joint directly below the resected corn. The joint space is located and opened, simultaneously severing the extensor tendons. A small-sized dental collar and crown scissors are then inserted into the joint to free the collateral ligaments. Next, a

closed Backhaus towel clamp is looped around and under the head of the proximal phalanx. The head of the phalanx is then elevated from the wound to enable a bone rongeur to sever it at its surgical neck. The phalangeal head is removed and the shaft is smoothed with a rasp. Three deep vertical mattress sutures are used to close the wound. The sutures are inserted so that the base of each stitch includes capsule and tendon, while the superficial part of the suture includes only the skin. A helpful hint in placing mattress sutures is to leave 1 cm of suture material exposed at its distal loop where it appears outside the skin. This serves to prevent strangulation of the tissue and allows ready access to the sutures when the time comes to remove them. The wound is dressed with sterile 2 inch square cotton gauze and 1 inch Kling dressing. Sutures are removed in 10 to 14 days.

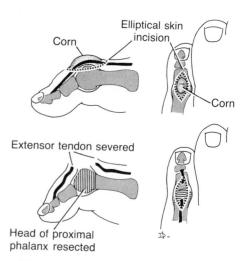

Figure 22–9 Digital arthroplasty. Elliptical incisions are made around dorsal corn. The extensor tendon is severed. The proximal phalangeal head is grasped with a towel clamp and resected at surgical neck with large double-action rongeur. Bone edges are smoothed with rasp. Capsule, tendon and skin are coapted with three deep mattress sutures.

Soft Corns (Heloma Molles)

Soft corns may occur between any of the toes. The causes of soft corns are: (1) apposition of adjacent skin surfaces, (2) excess heat or friction, (3) excess production of moisture, either by perspiration or retention of bath water, that cannot evaporate and (4) bony prominences or exostoses on the phalanges that impinge on the skin.

The lesion can be one of the most painful and insidious conditions of the foot. The most common site is the fourth digital space where moisture accumulates (Fig. 22–10).

Chronic irritation and pressure from narrow footgear cause condyles on adjacent bone surfaces to enlarge and lie in close apposition, thereby precipitating this interdigital lesion. Frequently, sinus formation in the interdigital web may lead to an acute infection. Subsequently, cellulitis develops that forces the patient to seek treatment.

Lesions that are left untreated often develop an underlying bursa or cyst. Roentgenograms of the area are necessary and will reveal underlying osseous hypertrophy.

Fungal infection is the main problem in differential diagnosis.

Conservative Treatment

The use of wider shoes and properly applied pads to separate the toes will encourage resolution of these lesions. The most common conservative thera-py is surgical débridement of the soft corn and the application of accommodative padding. Prior to employing any treatment, the patient's pedal circulation as well as his peripheral neurological status must be thoroughly evaluated.

Surgical Treatment

It is our experience that when the soft corn is of a chronic nature, i.e., when the condyles are enlarged and the digits are in close apposition, the following surgical procedure is recommended for the best results.

Under local anesthesia obtained by means of a digital block, a linear incision is made over the dorsomedial aspect of the digit. The incision commences at the base of the distal phalanx and terminates at the base of the proximal phalanx. The collateral ligament and capsular tissue of the involved articulation are dissected free. The underlying osteophytic hypertrophy is then completely resected. It is usually necessary to resect the contiguous condyles of the involved articulation of each phalanx so that the remaining surface presents a smooth, flat plane. This can be accomplished with bone rongeurs or with bone forceps to reduce the condylar enlargement. Preoperative radiographic studies and digital palpation during surgery reveal the necessity of the latter phase of the procedure.

Plantar Callus (Keratosis, Keratoma, Intractable Plantar Keratoma)

Diagnosis

Calluses are differentiated from corns by their anatomical location on the foot. Routinely, the corn (heloma) is found on the dorsum of the digits. The callus or plantar keratosis is found on the plantar aspect of the foot, usually under weight-bearing areas.

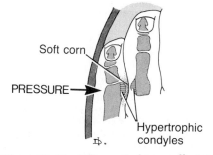

Figure 22–10 Soft corn (heloma molles). Lateral pressure on fourth interdigital space causes soft corn to form as shown. Adjacent bone surfaces (cross-hatched) become hypertrophic.

On microscopic examination, the plantar callus presents the following findings: the epithelium on the central portion of the lesion is indented and there is striking hyperkeratosis of the center in comparison with the marginal portions. There is localized elongation of the rete pegs which extend into the corium. Many small, shrunken nuclei can be seen throughout the thickened stratum corium. The corium does not show any abnormality.

On an outpatient basis, this lesion is often misdiagnosed as a plantar wart (verruca). (See previous discussion of verrucae plantaris.)

The verruca plantaris is caused by a filterable virus, whereas the plantar callus is produced by pressure. Microscopically these lesions appear similar, and for this reason they are often misdiagnosed and subsequently treated incorrectly.

On clinical examination the plantar callus is found on weight-bearing areas, whereas the plantar verrucae usually are not. The plantar callus is found primarily in female adults, since high-heeled shoes transfer weight-bearing to the metatarsal heads. The plantar keratosis is heavily cornified. When debrided, it presents a small, pearl-gray avascular center. The verruca plantaris has multiple papillae that are discernible upon superficial débridement. Verrucae are also distinguished by a many-dotted appearance caused by numerous coagulated capillary endings, plus an encircled connective tissue capsule. Verrucae are more sensitive to pressure than are plantar calluses.

Conservative Treatment

Conservative therapy should invariably be tried for relief of symptoms. Conservative measures are identical to those used for corns. A plaster impression can be taken of the foot and a molded inlay fabricated from it to redistribute pressure away from the met-

atarsal heads. The pad may also be placed proximal to the metatarsal head to alleviate forefoot imbalance.

Surgical Treatment

PLANTAR CONDYLECTOMY (Fig. 22–11). This procedure is indicated when the metatarsal head is enlarged or rotated in its axis, or both, and causes an intractable plantar keratoma.

The operative technique is adapted from Duvries.[1] An ellipitical incision large enough to include the entire

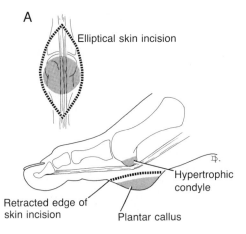

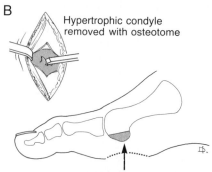

Figure 22–11 *A.* Plantar condylectomy for plantar callus. Procedure is indicated for intractable callus on metatarsal heads 2, 3, 4 or 5. Elliptical incision is made around the keratoma (callus), which is then removed. Flexor tendons are retracted laterally. *B.* Hypertrophic condyle on metatarsal head is removed with osteotome. Bone is smoothed and skin closed. Another technique (osteoclasis) is described in text.

keratoma is made on the plantar aspect of the foot. Sharp dissection is carried down into the fatty tissue, freeing the lesion so that it pops up and out into the wound space. The keratoma is then grasped with a tenaculum and dissected in one piece. Through this opening the dissection is extended to the flexor tendons, which are retracted laterally to expose the joint capsule. The capsule is then incised, and with the aid of a bone elevator, the metatarsal head is brought into view. Then using an osteotome, rasp and chisel, the plantar condyle is removed and the bone surface rasped smooth. The metatarsal is repositioned and the joint capsule is closed. The wound is closed in layers. The superficial gap caused by removal of the keratoma is filled with chromic sutures prior to coapting the skin edges. The area is then covered with a sterile nonpressure dressing. Ambulation may be permitted 48 hours postoperatively in a cut-out shoe.

2. FLOATING HEAD OSTEOTOMY (OSTEOCLASIS). This is a relatively new procedure for plantar keratosis in which the metatarsal head just proximal to the surgical neck is fractured without stabilization. The rationale for metatarsal osteotomy without stabilization is based on our experience that patients with plantar keratomas experienced resolution of their lesions when fractures of the metatarsals occurred after physical injury, e.g., march fractures.

The metatarsal head should be pushed back or up into its proper position by natural pressure forces. The exact degree and amount will be determined by postoperative ambulation (upward pressure from the ground). After osteotomy, a hard bony callus is formed around the fracture site. This has the advantage of maintaining the integrity of the metatarsophalangeal joint that has caused the subluxated toes, the shortened toes, and toes that do not function fully. The patient may walk from the office in a postoperative shoe.

COMPLICATION. Keratotic lesions may be transferred to other metatarsal heads and subluxated or shortened toes. This condition can be obviated with careful preoperative evaluation as well as weight-bearing x-ray evaluation of the metatarsal length pattern. We have found excellent results with proper postoperative follow-up, balancing the patient's foot with orthoses or molded inlays.

Hallux Valgus

Definition: Hallux Valgus and Bunion (Fig. 22–12)

Hallux valgus is one of the most common chronic disorders seen in our podiatric practices. Hallux valgus is an angulation of the great toe away from the midline of the body or toward the other toes, with a valgus or tibial rotation of the great toe.

A *bunion* is an inflammation of the great toe joint. It is not an exostosis of the medial condylar process of the metatarsal head. Therefore, "exostectomy" is incorrect and "condylectomy" is correct. "Bunionectomy" is also a misnomer. There is, at best, no more than 1/8 inch cortical hypertrophy over the medial condyle. The condition is therefore one primarily of partial dislocation.

Etiology

PREDISPOSING FACTORS. There is an hereditary tendency to flaccid ligamentous structures as well as long narrow feet. Also inherited may be variations in the morphology of the articular surface of the first metatarsophalangeal joint (an increased obliquity). An increase in the angle of the first metatarsocuneiform articulation is also a contributing factor. The more oblique the angle, the more the individual is predisposed to the hallux valgus formation.

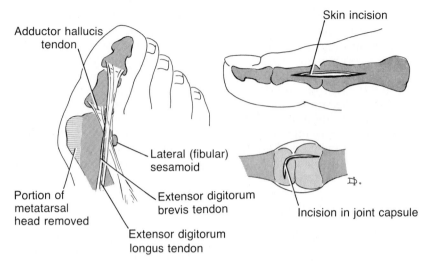

Figure 22–12 Hallux valgus. Hallux is angled toward the other toes, with valgus (tibial) rotation of great toe and partial dislocation of M-P joint. When joint is inflamed, the lesion is termed a "bunion." Surgery is usually necessary for correction.

McBride procedure (illustrated here) uses longitudinal skin incision, inverted "L" capsulotomy, and resection of shaded area of metatarsal head with rongeur. The lateral (fibular) sesamoid is then removed completely and the dorsal tendons inserting at the base of the proximal phalanx are severed. The tendons to be severed are the adductor hallucis and extensor digitorum brevis, which lie deep to the extensor digitorum longus. Tendons and sesamoid are exposed by retracting skin incision dorsally and laterally.

DIRECT FACTORS. (1) *Short shoes* are the most important direct factor. (2) The abducted gait, pronation, flatfoot and the patient's occupation may predispose to the development of hallux valgus. (3) Fatigue factors may cause elongation and pronation of the foot, with resultant progression of the forefoot in the narrow confines of the toe box of the shoe.

Pathological Anatomy

The proximal and distal phalanges of the great toe are directed toward the fibula and occasionally rotated toward the tibia, i.e., overlapping the second toes or underlying first toes. The first metatarsal is directed medially (tibially) and exhibits slight tibial rotation. The tibial capsule of the first metatarsophalangeal joint is stretched and the fibular aspect of the base of the proximal phalanx of the hallux is shortened. The abductor hallucis tendon, which inserts into the medial aspect of the base of the proximal phalanx of the hallux, is stretched and the extensor hallucis longus and extensor hallucis brevis are sometimes shortened.

Treatment

PALLIATIVE. One or more of the following may be rendered to accomodate the condition but will not correct the hallux valgus deformity.

1. *Physical therapy:* (a) hydrotherapy, i.e., whirlpool baths, hydrocollation to increase hyperemia and reduce congestion, stress and inflammation; (b) paraffin baths and (c) diathermy and ultrasound.

2. *Injection* of steroid hormones in combination with local anesthetic agents to break up the pain cycle and institute an anti-inflammatory effect.

3. Applying an *accommodative shield* utilizing soft felt or sponge to prevent further irritation.

4. *Shoe therapy* is necessary. Consult a reliable shoe fitter for proper footgear. In the fitting of shoes it must be noted that the size of the shoe is measured from the ball (the metatarsophalangeal joint) to the posterior aspect of the heel. Therefore, the ball of the foot must be contiguous with the break of the shoe (a diagonal transverse line drawn across the sole from the first metatarsophalangeal joint to the fifth metatarsophalangeal joint). Flexion of the fore part of the foot (metatarsophalangeal joints one through five) with the break of the shoe will cause binding and secondary restrictions of movement, with blistering and subsequent calluses along the dorsum of the foot. If the metatarsals flex at the break of the shoe, there must be a finger's breadth of room distal to the toes upon weight-bearing. This defines the long vamp shoe. The higher the heel, the greater the propulsive driving force influences the force of the foot in the toe box, so low-heeled shoes should be worn. When all these conditions are met, the patient's foot is comfortable and symptoms are alleviated. If none of these procedures is effective, the practitioner should resort to surgical treatment.

PHILOSOPHY OF BUNION SURGERY. Before listing the different surgical approaches that we have found effective in permanent treatment of this disorder, we would like to outline our philosophy of bunion surgery. In our hands, unilateral uncomplicated hallux surgery on an outpatient basis has been more successful than prolonged hospitalization with subsequent circulatory complications, e.g., phlebitis, osteoporotic demineralization and other changes associated with disuse atrophy. The patient may ambulate immediately with a postsurgical shoe (Reese or Ortho mold) that promotes blood flow and ventilation but without loss of muscle tone due to immobilization of the affected part. With the following unilateral surgical approaches, the patient may use the other foot without suffering excessive emotional or physical disability.

The surgical correction of any foot deformity should be performed with caution, since the foot is the most distant organ in the vascular tree. Diminution of circulation and weight-bearing are factors that interfere with wound healing.

Surgical Reduction

SILVER PROCEDURE (JONES OPERATION). This procedure is indicated only when there is a mere prominence of bone at the metatarsophalangeal joint without any partial dislocation of the joint. If the patient is elderly or debilitated, surgical relief is indicated, but functional realignment is not necessary. This procedure is the least traumatic and will remove the original symptoms.

The technique commences with a curvilinear incision medial to the extensor digitorum longus tendon. The medial capsule is incised and shortened by making a reverse L-shaped incision which is followed by a medial osteotomy. This is varied by severing the adductor hallucis through a stab wound to help take the hallux out of the valgus position.

Postoperative care consists of splinting the toe for approximately six weeks to maintain proper alignment. Osteotomy and capsule shortening alone will not straighten the toe. In a very short time, the position of the bones will revert to their preoperative state.

MODIFIED McBRIDE PROCEDURE (Fig. 22–12). The rationale behind a McBride bunionectomy is the removal of the lateral sesamoid. Its resection actually removes part of the internal cubic content of the fibular aspect of the first metatarsophalangeal joint. Upon resection of the lateral sesamoid, the joint capsule is released on its fibular aspect, permitting the first metatarsal to move back into proper approximation to the second metatarsal. The primus varus angle is thereby reduced.

A dorsal longitudinal midline incision is made in the skin over the first metatarsophalangeal joint, extending from midshaft of the first metatarsal distally to midshaft of the proximal phalanx. The incision is deepened through the fascial plane and is undermined to the medial and lateral aspects of the joint. The extensor hallucis brevis tendon is next located deep to the longus tendon. The brevis tendon is elevated and a section of it is excised. An inverted L capsulotomy is performed along the dorsal and tibial aspects of the joint. The flap thus created is freed and retracted. The metatarsal head is also freed from the capsule along the dorsum. The head is then elevated out of its capsule with a periosteal elevator. The redundant bone is resected with a bone rongeur from the dorsal and tibial aspects of the head. The remaining surface is smoothed. Care is taken to smooth the tibioplantar aspect of the head without sacrificing the condyle at that point. The presence of the condyle is helpful in protecting against overcorrection of the position of the tibial sesamoid, which could result in a hallux varus.

The incision is then retracted to the fibular side of the joint and a self-retaining retractor is inserted in the first metatarsal interspace. Dissection is carried down to the floor of the interspace. An incision is then made parallel to and just dorsal to the fibular sesamoid. This incision in the capsule is approximately parallel to the long axis of the first ray. It extends distally to a point just dorsal to the insertion of the adductor hallucis tendon. The scalpel is re-introduced in the same incision and is backed up in the incision until the cutting edge of the blade is just proximal to the sesamoid. The flat edge of the blade is pressed against the plantar surface of the tendon. A short-

stroke sawing action is begun distally with the instrument. The edge of the sesamoid is encountered as the blade begins to cut between the sesamoid and the tendon fibers. As cutting progresses distally, the blunt edge of the blade is gradually raised so that the cutting edge of the instrument contacts the sesamoid at approximately a 35 to 45 degree angle. In this way, the flat edge of the blade retracts the tendon while the cutting edge separates the tendon from the sesamoid. This permits freeing of all the attachments of the sesamoid with the exception of the intrasesamoidal ligament.

The hallux should be flexed sharply and the metatarsal head elevated. The blade can then be placed plantarly and parallel to the sesamoid bone with the blade's cutting edge directed against the ligament from beneath. The sesamoid can then be grasped and removed. The adductor hallucis tendon is then grasped with a clamp and is sharply cut from its attachment to the phalanx. The tendon is freed adequately to permit its attachment under physiological tension into the bone at the neck of the first metatarsal. The hallux is manipulated into overcorrection to ensure that no deforming influence remains and to be certain that the first metatarsal moves into position beside the second metatarsal.

Returning to the tibial side of the joint, the hallux is placed in correct alignment and held while the capsule is closed. The longitudinal portion of the L-shaped capsular incision is closed first along the dorsum of the metatarsal head. With the hallux in correct alignment, the excess joint capsule is then removed with a vertical capsulectomy. The vertical portion of the joint incision can now be closed. In instances where rotation of the hallux may have been present along with valgus angulation, the sutures are placed obliquely in closing the vertical portion of the capsular incision. Oblique placement of sutures will retain correction of the derotation which has been accomplished by this surgery.

When the extensor hallucis longus tendon is excessively short, it is lengthened by Z-plasty. More often, it is simply positioned in its best alignment and sutured to the joint capsule at the metatarsal neck with a double-turn 000 plain or chromic catgut suture. This retains the position of the tendon in relation to the joint during the initial weeks of healing and prevents malposition of the hallux postoperatively as a result of extensor muscle spasm. The fascial plane is next replaced and sutured carefully and completely with multiple 000 plain catgut sutures. The skin is closed with nonabsorbable sutures.

Sterile gauze bandaging is applied over suitable sterile padding. The bandaging is applied in such a way that it assures retention of the correct alignment. A fresh dressing is usually applied after three or four days and a similar bandage is reapplied. One-half of the sutures are removed at five to seven days and the remainder of the sutures at the next redressing, usually at 10 to 14 days after surgery. Once sterile bandaging is unnecessary, the foot is painted with skin adherent and a cohesive gauze supportive bandage is applied so that it will retain the correction. In instances where drifting of the toe may seem evident, the cohesive gauze is reinforced with multiple corrective layers of adhesive tape. Such a bandage can remain in place for up to two full weeks. It may be replaced in problem cases. More often, we apply molded polyurethane retainers three weeks postoperatively and return the patient to a closed, newly fitted round-toe oxford. We require the wearing of such a shoe for approximately two full months from fitting. Orthotic needs are met as required by the patient.[11]

HISS BUNIONECTOMY. The Hiss bunionectomy is a tendon balance procedure designed to transplant the abductor hallucis tendon into the dorsal aspect of the proximal phalanx. The hallux is thereby brought into normal alignment, while at the same time the sesamoids are brought back to their original articulating facets.

Procedure. A linear incision is made 0.5 cm on the fibular side of the tuberosity of the base of the first proximal phalanx. A short Sistrunk dissecting scissors is inserted into the incision, and the adductor hallucis tendon is severed at its attachments by following the contour of the bone. The scissors points are now utilized to sever the fibular portion of the joint capsule. A medial longitudinal incision approximately 5 cm long is made just above the heavy skin of the sole of the foot and below the calloused area of the metatarsal head. Retraction is accomplished to expose the abductor hallucis tendon while it is dissected free. Note the location of the medial branch of the medial plantar nerve which runs along the lower border of the adductor tendon. The abductor hallucis is reflected back at its insertion into the inferior aspect of the proximal phalanx. The joint capsule is opened with a longitudinal incision. The edges of the joint capsule are then detached and an exostectomy is performed at the enlarged head of the first metatarsal. The sesamoid bones are brought back to their normal alignment by replacing the abductor tendon into the base of the proximal phalangeal base, thereby taking the hallux out of the valgus position.

KELLER BUNIONECTOMY. Three procedures have been recommended for correction of hallux limitus or rigidus with or without hallux valgus: the Mayo, Keller and Stone procedures. The Mayo procedure has generally been discredited because of the infliction of trauma to the first metatarsophalangeal joint. The Keller procedure is most widely used. It is indicated in patients over 50 years of age in whom the metatarsal joint is destroyed or the normal joint space is lost. The Stone procedure is little known, but we have found it generally preferable to the Keller procedure because of the loss of function that follows the latter.

Technique. A medial osteotomy of the first metatarsal is performed in the Keller procedure, along with amputation of the proximal one-third to one-half of the base of the proximal phalanx. A curvilinear incision is made over the first metatarsophalangeal joint, followed by a U-shaped incision through the capsule with the apex distally. A medial osteotomy is accomplished, followed by resection of the base of the proximal phalanx. The toe is then sutured into proper alignment.

Complications. (1) All four insertions (flexor hallucis brevis, extensor hallucis brevis, adductor hallucis, abductor hallucis tendons) to the base of the proximal phalanx are destroyed. (2) The great toe has little residual function and is frequently dorsiflexed. (3) Calluses develop presently under second, third and fourth metatarsal heads with possible marked proximal shifting of second, third and fourth digits. (4) Marked proximal shifting of the sesamoids occurs along the metatarsal shaft.

STONE PROCEDURE. The Stone procedure is a modification of a procedure first described by Fessler in 1926. Fessler removed the prominence of the medial aspect and lateral corner of the first metatarsal head but left the plantar weight-bearing area intact.

The main advantage of the Stone procedure over the Keller procedure is functional. Shortening of the hallux is minimal and metatarsus primus varus is overcome when a hallux valgus deformity is present. Full function of the first metatarsophalangeal joint is maintained because the intrinsic structures are left intact.[10]

Technique. Make a longitudinal incision approximately 6 cm long medial to the extensor hallucis longus. The incision extends from midshaft of the hallux's proximal phalanx to just behind the head of the first metatarsal. The incision is carried deep through the fascial layers to the capsule both medial and lateral to these fascial structures.

The capsule is opened with a longitudinal incision extending from the metatarsophalangeal joint to just behind the head of the metatarsal. The head of the metatarsal is freed with care from the surrounding capsular structures completely enough so that the head can be retracted free from the wound.

The medial prominence of the head is excised with a mallet and osteotome if a hallux valgus deformity is present. A dorsal cut is made on the bone with a mallet and osteotome extending dorsally downward at approximately a 45 degree angle. The dorsal cut extends to the articular margin of cartilage on the plantar surface of the metatarsal head. Nearly 1 cm of space should be left between the cut metatarsal head and the articular surface of the base of the proximal phalanx.

The exposed area of bone left after excision is denuded of any sharp edges and rasped smooth. Care should be taken to leave the articular surface of the base of the phalanx alone. Any lipping on the dorsum or sides of the base of the phalanx may be removed.

At this time, the hallux should be dorsiflexed 90 degrees. Any limitations of movement should be evaluated and corrected at this time. If a hallux valgus angulation is present, it may be necessary to do a Z-plasty on the extensor hallucis longus to prevent the proximal phalanx from drifting into a valgus position again.

The joint capsule is then closed with 3–0 chromic catgut sutures. Subcutaneous tissue is closed with 4–0 plain catgut. The skin is closed with nonabsorbable sutures and a sterile compression dressing is applied, with the toe maintained in a corrected position.

Postoperative Care. Postoperative

care consists of letting the patient ambulate with a Reese shoe within 36 hours. Sutures should be left in approximately ten days to two weeks. Physical therapy must be given soon after suture removal to retain motion of the first metatarsophalangeal joint. Patients may return to normal foot gear two days following suture removal with appropriate splinting. The patient may return to work in four to six weeks.

Heel Pain

Heel Spur (Inferior Calcaneal Spur; Calcaneal Exostosis)

DESCRIPTION. A heel spur is an osteophytic outgrowth just anterior to the tubercle of the calcaneus. The mass extends over the entire width of the tuberosity. It is approximately 2 cm wide with its apex in the plantar fascia.

ETIOLOGY. The exact cause is unknown, but heel spur is probably due to mechanical trauma and stress. The condition often is associated with a weak foot or strained foot. Patients standing or working on concrete floors often develop this condition.

OCCURRENCE. Heel spur is found most commonly in middle age (40 to 60 years). It is more prevalent in females (often concomitant with menopause), but it is also seen in males. It is seen most frequently in obese persons, and it is often unilateral.

ANATOMY. The plantar fascia arises from the plantar surface of the calcaneus and the area immediately above it. The area of attachment, over the medial and lateral tubercles, is about 2 cm wide and ½ cm thick. From its origin, the plantar fascia fans out over the entire plantar surface of the foot and inserts into or blends with the soft tissues of the five metatarsal heads. The plantar fascia acts as a bowstring to the longitudinal arch. Therefore, excessive strain will be absorbed by the origin of the fascia. This strain will gradually tend to induce osteophytic proliferation, ultimately producing a characteristic spur. The plantar fascia resembles a trapezoid; the spur resembles a wedge.

PATHOLOGY. The earliest change is mild chronic inflammation, with or without pain. As the condition advances, osteophytic changes take place in the sulcus anterior to the tuberosity. The accumulation of bone is self-limiting and the final spur may vary greatly in size and shape, the most common shape being a triangular block.

TYPES: (1) Those that are *massive* in size but *asymptomatic* because the angle of growth is on a plane with the plantar fascia; these often are discovered inadvertently. (2) Those that are *massive* in size and *symptomatic*; they are painful because the angle of gravity crosses the plane of the plantar fascia. (3) Those causing *acute pain* but with *no visible spur* ascertainable in a radiograph.

SYMPTOMS AND SIGNS. Patients state that they have excruciating pain when they get up in the morning and again late in the afternoon. The onset is usually insidious, and if untreated the heel may be painful for years. Patients usually exhibit: (1) pinpoint *pain* and tenderness under the heel at the area of the *medial tubercle*, (2) mild *discomfort* and tenderness in the *arch* and (3) mild *discomfort* and tenderness in the medial side of the heel *up to the ankle*. When the condition is treated, the heel gets better at first, but there still will be mild pain in the arch and ankle for some time. Infrequently, bursitis develops deep to the plantar fascia, simulating heel spur symptoms.

PALLIATIVE TREATMENT. 1. *Removal of stress* or weight on the heel. Fitting proper shoes, e.g., laced oxfords with wide Thomas heels.

2. *Elevation of heels* adds to relief pattern: (a) insertion of felt or sponge *heel lifts* in shoes, (b) wearing of shoe

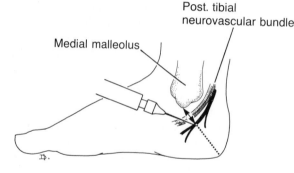

Medial malleolus

Post. tibial
neurovascular bundle

Figure 22–13 Posterior tibial nerve block. Injection site is identified 4 cm posteroinferior to medial malleolus, on the line between medial malleolus and posterior projection of heel. Usual volume required is 5–10 ml 1 per cent lidocaine. Hyperemia of the sole is present when anesthesia is obtained.

types that have *raised* heels, e.g., cowboy boots or lumberjack boots.

3. Injection techniques. (a) *Posterior tibial block* (Fig. 22–13) breaks the pain cycle and permits painless injection of steroids. (b) *Steroids* can be injected directly into central pain area.

4. Physical therapy: (a) whirlpool baths, (b) diathermy, (c) ultrasound radiation, (d) paraffin baths.

SURGERY. Many authorities believe that there is no need for corrective surgery since results may be obtained palliatively. If symptoms persist following conservative management, excision of the spur and plantar fasciotomy are indicated.

Haglund's Disease (Albert's Disease, "Pump Bump")

DESCRIPTION AND DISCUSSION. Haglund's disease is a protuberance of the posterior-superior surface (usually the fibular aspect) of the calcaneus. It usually occurs in young girls (ages 14 to 21) when they start to wear high heels (Fig. 22–14).

SYMPTOMS AND SIGNS. (1) *Callus* at the posterior-lateral aspect of calcaneous. (2) *Pain* over heel cord. (3) Occasional *sinus tract*. (4) Retrocalcaneal *bursitis*.

CONSERVATIVE TREATMENT. (a) *Pad* the foot and later pad the counter of the shoe. (b) Employ a heel lift. (c) Use *physiotherapy*. (d) *Steroid* injections.

SURGICAL TREATMENT. With the patient prone, the bursa and the protruding bone are removed carefully, so as not to sever the sural nerve. A posterior splint is applied with the foot in plantar flexion.

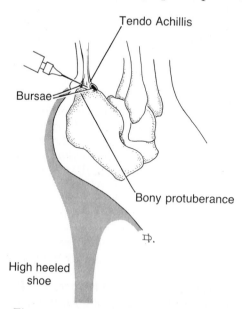

Tendo Achillis

Bursae

Bony protuberance

High heeled shoe

Figure 22–14 Haglund's disease ("pump bump"). Bony protuberance develops on posterosuperior aspect of calcaneus in young women wearing high-heeled shoes. Treatment is by injection therapy (as shown) or resection of bursae and the protuberance (see text).

CONGENITAL CONDITIONS

Hammertoe

Definition

Hammertoe is a contraction type of toe deformity in which one or more

bones of a toe are subluxated or ankylosed, resulting in limited motion.

Etiology

STATIC DEFORMITIES. Hammer-
toes often were originally long flaccid
toes confined in short-fitting shoes.
This condition may also be caused by
an imbalance in the intrinsic musculature of the foot.

SYSTEMIC DISEASES. Other forms
of muscular imbalance may result from
high fever, such as in scarlet fever or
measles.

CONGENITAL TYPES. These are
usually multiple and are associated
with different types of talipes equinus
or pes cavus deformities.

POST-POLIOMYELITIS. This type
usually involves paralysis following
poliomyelitis. The digital deformities
usually are multiple and there is a
pathological contracture.

GREAT TOE. When the great toe is
involved, it is usually the result of
muscular imbalance or high fever.

Anatomy

GREAT TOE. The head of the proximal phalanx is displaced dorsally and
the inferior surface lies immediately
above the head of the metatarsal. The
dorsal capsule of the interphalangeal
joint is stretched and the plantar capsule is contracted. The extensor hallucis longus is also contracted (Fig. 22–
15).

THREE LESSER TOES (MID-
DLE). There are three types of hammertoe affecting the lesser toes:

1. The *proximal phalanx is dorsiflexed* with the head dislocated dorsally in 90 per cent of the lesser toe
hammertoes. The middle phalanx
plantar-flexes and the distal phalanx
extends.

2. *Double contraction* occurs in 5
per cent of lesser hammertoe conditions, with dorsal dislocation of the

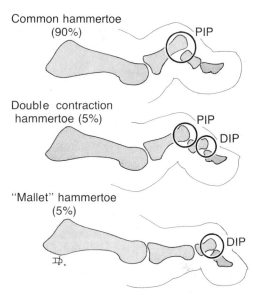

Figure 22–15 Hammertoe pathology. The
three types of hammertoes are shown. The most
common type, dislocation of proximal interphalangeal joint, occurs in 90 per cent of patients.
The double contraction and mallet toe deformities each occur in 5 per cent of patients.

head of the proximal phalanx and a
dorsal dislocation of the head of the
middle phalanx.

3. *Mallet toe* occurs in 5 per cent of
the lesser toe deformities. In this condition, the proximal interphalangeal
joint is not misaligned, but the distal
interphalangeal joint has a dorsal dislocation on the head of the middle phalanx.

Treatment

Digital arthroplasty is the procedure
of choice (see Fig. 22–9). Whenever a
joint has had both articulating surfaces
removed and the raw surfaces come in
contact, they eventually will fuse if
motion is eliminated. If motion is not
eliminated, pain and fibrosis will result. Therefore, at least one surface
must be capped or replaced with an
artificial surface of the same type of
soft tissue in the interspace to maintain
the integrity of a functional joint. It is

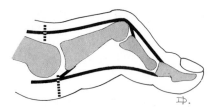

Figure 22–16 Hammertoe correction by tenotomy. Digital arthroplasty is the preferred technique (see Fig. 22–9), but an alternate technique for congenital hammertoes is tenotomy, shown here. Extensor and flexor tendons are divided at the locations illustrated. The toe is manipulated dorsally into normal alignment and splinted to the adjacent digit with tape.

better to preserve at least one surface, leaving the articular surface intact. One preserved surface will permit function of that joint. Nearly all lesser hammertoe surgery can be done effectively by this method.

An alternative method in congenital hammertoe deformity with good functional joints is the tenotomy procedure shown in Figure 22–16.

Overlapping Toes

This is a condition in which one toe lies on the dorsum of an adjacent toe, most commonly, the fifth toe over the fourth. The second most common type involves the second toe overlapping the first.

Fifth Overlapping Toe

This is usually due to a congenital deformity or a flaccid type of foot, in which there is a short extensor tendon, skin shortening and a contracted dorsal capsule.

TREATMENT. Conservative treatment consists of teaching the parent or child to tape the toe down or attaching an elastic sling from the toe to the heel. This therapy usually must be started immediately after birth in order to be effective. Surgical treatment (Fig. 22–17) utilizes a Z-lengthening of the skin, in which the interphalangeal web

is incised, followed by a tenotomy and capsulotomy. Suturing is performed with the toe in a plantar-flexed position.

Second Overlapping Toe

The second toe usually overlaps the first toe as the direct result of hallux valgus deformity. Sometimes the condition may be due to a long second toe. Often there is a partial or complete dislocation at the metatarsophalangeal joint. Short shoes are a contributing factor. Of all the joints in the foot, the second metatarsophalangeal joint exhibits the greatest frequency of dislocation, occurring most commonly with a second hammertoe.

TREATMENT. When associated with hallux valgus, the hallux valgus angulation must be reduced at the same time. When overlapping is not associated with hallux valgus, a simple tenotomy and capsulotomy will resolve the condition. The procedure should be followed by eight weeks of

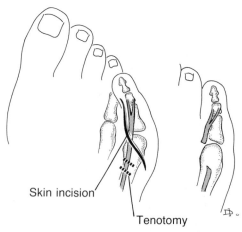

Figure 22–17 Overlapping toes. Fifth overlapping toe is treated as shown here. A dorsal Z-incision is made. The interphalangeal web is then incised. The extensor tendon is divided and the joint capsule relaxed by a dorsal incision. The toe is sutured in a plantar-flexed position. The operation for uncomplicated second overlapping toe requires only tenotomy and capsulotomy.

splinting the toe in a plantar-flexed position with a rubber digital prosthesis.

Webbed Toes

This is a congenital deformity in which the toes are joined together at the web space of the digit. Webbed toes are rarely symptomatic and surgical treatment is performed only for cosmetic reasons.

METABOLIC DISEASES

Diabetes

Location of Problems Encountered

The major diabetic problems encountered by the podiatrist are usually readily discerned. These problems vary from a simple tyloma to gangrene and bone destruction. Points of pressure and trauma are the areas most likely to undergo pathological changes. Areas likely to be affected by pressure are the plantar aspects of the metatarsal heads, the lateral sides of the first and fifth metatarsal heads, the dorsal aspects of the middle and distal phalangeal articulations, the opposing articulations of the digits, the distal aspects of all phalanges, the lateral nail grooves, the lateral aspect of the base of the fifth metatarsal and the inferior lateral aspect of the heel.

Problems primarily or secondarily caused by various types of foot imbalance are often seen in the diabetic. Whether the conditions are congenital or are caused or aggravated by improper foot gear, obesity or misuse (which present additional problems to the diabetic patient), they all produce undue pressure or trauma.[9]

Treatment

PROPHYLACTIC THERAPY. As this is an outpatient surgical text, it will be noted that foot surgery must be approached with extreme caution. Prophylactic treatment is the procedure of choice and must be utilized before surgical treatment is considered.

Routine débridement is utilized with extra caution, as described in the section on conservative therapy for corns. It should be noted that the patient must be instructed and educated in the proper care of the foot and must avoid "bathroom surgery" or the utilization of "store-bought" cures. Surface padding should be kept to a minimum and should be nonocclusive if possible. Dressings should be worn for only a short period of time, as they tend to cause maceration and lead to bacterial or fungal infections.

Nail Care

Careful débridement of the toenails is of the greatest importance because nail clipping can be potentially hazardous. Diabetic patients with normal nails should be trained to trim their toenails, teaching them to bear in mind never to progress beyond the junction of the lateral nail edge and lateral nail fold. The corners should not be cut out of sight. The idea that cutting a "V" in the center of the nail will "train the corners out" is a misconception. Patients with mycotic, thickened, incurvated nails should be referred to a podiatrist for partial nail avulsion, and if the diabetic patient is under the control of an internist or family practitioner, a more permanent surgical procedure may be attempted. (Please refer to the section on surgical treatment of disorders of the nails.)

The following instructions may be given to a diabetic patient with foot problems:

CORNS AND CALLUSES. Both corns and calluses are caused by the building up of hard skin at points where shoes cause pressure. In general, they should be treated gently with a fine emery board or pumice stone. Consult your physician or podiatrist.

BATHING.   Bathe your feet daily in luke-warm (not hot) water, using a mild soap. After thorough rinsing, dry them gently; use a soft towel and a "blotting" technique. Pay special attention to the skin between the toes. If your feet are rough or dry, rub them gently with a moisture-restoring cream or lotion. If your feet sweat exces-sively, rub them gently with alcohol and dust them with foot powder.

SOCKS.   Heavy cotton or wool socks (or stockings) are recommended. They should be of the correct size and need to be free of seams and darns. To ensure cleanliness, it is important to change your socks every day. Loose woolen socks may be worn at night to keep your feet warm.

EXERCISE.   Walking is the best exercise for your feet. Your doctor may advise spe-cial exercise.

SHOES.   Soft leather oxford shoes are recommended for daily wear. Shoes should have a leather sole and a flat low heel and should conform to the shape of your foot. New shoes should be worn only for short periods during the first week of wear (for example, two hours daily). Casual shoes should be worn for short periods. All shoe corrections should be done on the advice of your physician or your podiatrist.

TOENAILS.   Trim or file your toenails straight across so that they are even with the skin on the ends of your toes. A coarse metal file with a blunt tip is a satisfactory instrument to use. (A nail clipper may be used.)

INSPECTION.   Inspect your feet every day. If you notice any redness, swelling, cracks in the skin or sores, consult your physician or your podiatrist.*

Ulcers of the Foot in Diabetics

One of the more common findings in diabetics is the formation of ulcers of the foot. The most frequent site is the plantar surface, usually under a meta-tarsal head. The ulcer is usually of long standing and if gently pressed will

---

*Reprinted from: U.S. Department of Health, Education and Welfare, Public Health Service, Division of Chronic Diseases, Diabetes and Ar-thritis Program, Washington, D.C. 20201

demonstrate a purulent discharge. The ulcer is always surrounded by a heavy, tough callus.

Pressure is believed to be an impor-tant factor in diabetic ulcers of the feet. The failure to heal properly is proba-bly due to a vascular defect rather than to abnormal sugar metabolism.

TREATMENT.   Débridement of ne-crotic tissue is carried out after aseptic preparation. More complete drainage is established, followed by accommo-dative padding and topical proteolytic enzyme therapy. A felt pressure pad aperture dressing is used to accommo-date the lesion (Fig. 22–18).

Gout

The usual presentation of gouty ar-thritis is a painful, tender, reddened great toe. There is usually no history of direct trauma and infection is not pres-ent. The pain is severe in the morning as well as in the afternoon, in contrast with osteoarthritis, in which pain is worsened by the activities of the day. Diagnosis is made by the finding of elevation in serum uric acid levels. The disease is differentiated from dia-betes and rheumatoid arthritis by blood tests. Blood sugar and serology for rheumatoid factor should therefore also be obtained when patients pre-sent with a painful erythematous toe.

We believe that the systemic treat-ment of gout, diabetes and rheumatoid arthritis is best performed by an in-ternist, and we limit our treatment for these conditions to management of the local problems in the foot.

Treatment of the painful toe consists of relieving pressure on the first meta-tarsal head by fabrication of an accom-modative orthotic inlay, which the pa-tient may transfer from shoe to shoe. Wedging of the shoe can be performed if necessary, in cases in which the pa-tient is not improved sufficiently by the accommodative inlay. Wedging is considerably more expensive, since

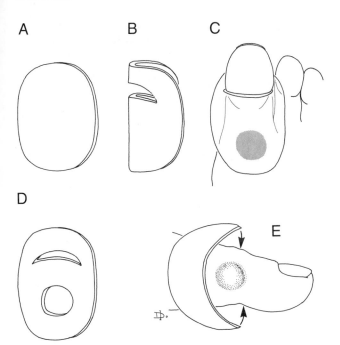

Figure 22–18 Diabetic foot ulcer dressing. A pressure aperture dressing is constructed from felt (*A*) as shown. A slit is made (*B*), through which the toe is inserted (*C*). The area of the ulcer, which is usually on the ventral aspect of the metatarsal head, is marked on the pad. The pad is removed and an aperture is cut out (*D*). The pad is then placed again on the toe.

For lateral ulcers, the same technique is used, except that the pad is rotated 90 degrees and the toe slit is proximal rather than distal (*E*).

each pair of shoes must be wedged to be effective.

BIOMECHANICS OF THE FOOT

Biomechanics is the term used to designate functional orthopedics. To a large extent it also encompasses the medical and surgical management of orthopedic problems along with functional or mechanical control. By mechanical control, we do not imply support or accommodation but rather the establishment of motions and positions that will allow optimum function in the feet and entire skeletal complex so that mechanical symptoms such as corns, calluses, cramps, fatigue, strain and so on can be alleviated by attacking the underlying pathology.[14]

Simply speaking, biomechanics is the study of foot motion and function. Many variables affect the motion of the foot, including foot type, neuromuscular status, leg influence (length, presence of knock knees), body weight and flexibility of joints. These influences can cause the foot to compensate by excessive motion, which in turn produces fatigue, arch strain, corns, calluses, heel spurs, muscle atrophy, joint deviations and subluxations (hammertoe and hallux valgus deformities). Excessive motion of the foot is referred to as *terminal pronation*, meaning an outward rolling of the heel and flattening of the arch.

REFERENCES

1. Duvries, H. L. (ed.): Disorders of synovia and fascia. *In* Surgery of the Foot. St. Louis, C. V. Mosby Co., 1959, pp. 231–232.
2. Ferguson, L. K.: Surgery of the Ambulatory Patient, 4th ed., Philadelphia, J. B. Lippincott Co., 1966.
3. Frost, L.: Atraumatic nail avulsion with a novel ungual elevator. J. Am. Podiatry Assoc., 48:51, 1958.
4. Frost, L.: A treatment for paronychia with concomitant onychocryptosis. J. Am. Podiatry Assoc., 49:197–201, 1959.
5. Frost, L.: Onychomycosis — treatment by avulsion and onychophytax. J. Am. Podiatry Assoc., 50:283–287, 1960.
6. Frost, L.: Root resection for incurvated nail. J. Natl. Assoc. Chiropody, 40:19, 1950.

7. Krauss, C. E.: Surgery of nail disorders. J. Am. Podiatry Assoc., *40*:11, 1966.

8. Lasker, A. S.: Intermetatarsal neuroma. Curr. Podiatry, *19*:March, 1970.

9. Levin, M. E., and O'Neal, L. W. (eds.): The Diabetic Foot. St. Louis, C. V. Mosby, 1973.

10. Macdonald, R. G.: The Stone Procedure. Hopedale Medical Complex Podiatry Staff, 4th Annual Surgical Seminar Manual — A Case Report. Hopedale, Ill., 1971.

11. McGlamry, E. D., and Feldman, M. H.: A treatise on the McBride procedure. J. Am. Podiatry Assoc., *61*:170–171, 1971.

12. Pillsbury, D. M., Shelley, W. B., and Kligman, A. M.: Dermatology. Philadelphia, W. B. Saunders Co., 1956. pp. 631–635.

13. Taub, J., and Steinberg, M.: *Porokeratosis Plantaris Discreta*, a previously unrecognized dermatological entity. Int. J. Dermatol., *9*:83, 1972.

14. Wernick, et al.: A Practical Manual For a Basic Approach to Biomechanics, Vol. II. Deer Park, N.Y., Langer Acrylic Lab, Inc., 1972.

23 Pediatric Surgery

JOHN D. BURRINGTON, M.D.

GENERAL APPROACH

The initial contact between physician and child often determines the magnitude of a surgical procedure that the patient will tolerate as an outpatient.[8, 9] If the child is frightened and hurt during the initial examination, much time will be lost in evaluating his problem, and the valuable initial rapport may not be achieved. One effective method of contacting the child is through the parent or adult accompanying him to the Emergency Room. A few words to the parents establishes the exact time and nature of the injury as well as the duration of symptoms and the status of the child's immunizations. Most important, it indicates to the child that you are a friend who is accepted by the parent. The child follows the questions carefully, and once he senses that you are a friend interested in his injury, he will let you examine him. The physician who bursts into the examining room and attempts to overwhelm the child with attention may be greeted by shrieks and complete withdrawal.

Detailed sensory examinations are difficult in an injured child under four or five years of age. However, the observant physician will note the position of the child's hand or finger as an indication of tendon injury and the temperature and texture of the ex-

1185

tremities as indications of possible nerve injury. Also, a very adequate motor examination can be obtained utilizing the child's natural tendency to reach for shiny or desirable objects and his willingness to play simple games, such as holding a file card between various fingers or wiggling his digits on command. Try it with the normal hand first, and then switch to the injured side.

Immunization

Most children over one year of age brought to an Outpatient Department have had their basic immunization

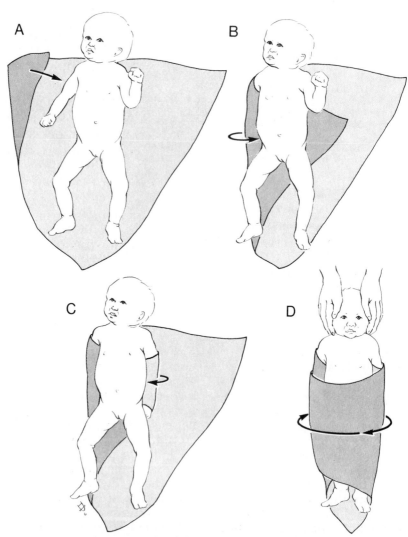

Figure 23–1   Restraint with a folded sheet. *A.* In wrapping the child for restraint it is important to have the sheet or towel large enough to restrain the infant from feet to shoulders. A bed sheet folded as illustrated is preferable. *B.* The first fold goes over the arm, under the body and then, *C,* over the opposite arm and back under the body. *D.* The opposite flap then completely encircles the child and is wrapped snugly to keep him from kicking his feet or legs. A single piece of tape may be necessary to keep the wrapping intact during a prolonged procedure. When working on the face, it is helpful to have an assistant hold the child's head gently as illustrated.

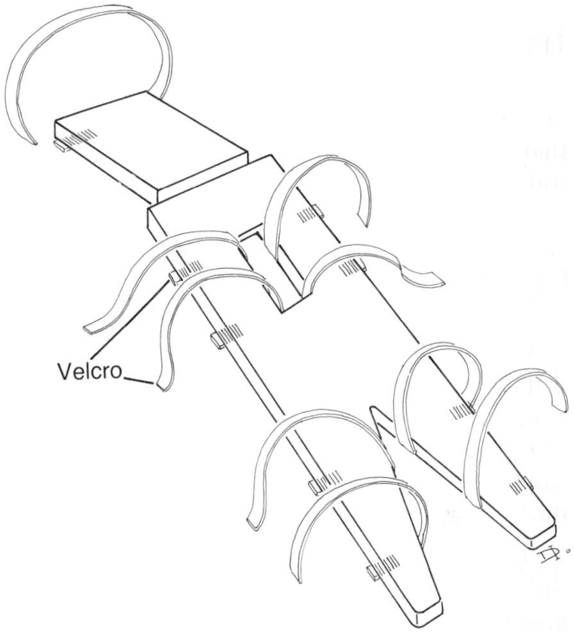

Figure 23–2 Restraint board. This is one of many types of board suitable for restraint. They are excellent for circumcisions or suturing lacerations on the trunk or thighs. However, they are not suitable for treatment of lacerations on the hands, feet or face.

Velcro

against tetanus. If they have had one or more of their D.P.T. immunizations, a single booster of 0.5 ml of tetanus toxoid should establish adequate immunization.[4] It is superfluous to given an additional injection to a child who has completed his basic immunization and has had a booster shot within three years. If an unimmunized child suffers a burn or a penetrating or crushing injury or is injured in an area frequented by farm animals, he should receive 1 cc of human hyperimmune globulin. After the lesion has healed, the child must then receive full, active immunization with three doses of tetanus toxoid. In all cases in which an injection is required, it should be administered after débridement, repair and bandaging are complete. By then the child realizes that you are helping him and often accepts the injection stoically. Giving the much-feared "needle" before the injury has been treated will destroy any early rapport the physician may have established.

Restraint

Whenever possible, the nurse who will assist in the outpatient procedure should be introduced to the child and his parents simultaneously. An understanding nurse experienced in working with injured children can be of immeasurable help in getting the child to cooperate. However, virtually all children under eighteen months of age and many children under three years of age require some form of restraint during a surgical procedure or an uncomfortable examination. Wrapping the child with a folded sheet (Fig. 23–1) or a standard padded restraint apparatus (Fig. 23–2) will immobilize the child without undue discomfort. While we all abhor physical restraint of a child, I believe it is often misplaced kindness to leave the child unrestrained. His wiggling may prevent complete débridement and cleansing of the wound and may compromise the meticulous closure necessary for a good cosmetic result.

For facial lacerations, I prefer to have the extremities immobilized in a folded sheet and then to have a nurse complete the immobilization by holding the sides of the child's head gently but firmly. The emotional problems caused by such restraint are far less than those created by an unsightly scar or a mismatched vermillion border that can result from inadequate restraint.

Local Anesthesia

A few drops of local anesthetic dripped directly into an open wound anesthetizes the margins sufficiently so that the remainder of the infiltration can be carried out through the edges of the wound. While it is theoretically undesirable to inject clean tissue through a contaminated area, the degree to which the surrounding skin can be cleansed in the presence of an unanesthetized wound probably renders it not much cleaner than the wound itself. When injecting local anesthetic, it is most important to inject slowly through a 25 gauge needle, since rapid injection distends the tissue and causes local pain. In most cases local anesthetic with dilute epinephrine can be used safely in children to aid hemostatis, although it is rarely necessary except in procedures about the face and mouth.

Topical sprays of local anesthetics or ethyl chloride to "freeze" an injury have little or no place in surgery. Local anesthetics are not well absorbed through intact skin, and ethyl chloride may cause an unpleasant burning sensation when the area rewarms. Ethyl chloride may actually damage wound edges and interfere with normal wound healing.

LACERATIONS

Lacerations occur predominantly about the toddler's head and face. Because of his large head and unsteady gait, the head absorbs an enormous amount of trauma from the age of about 12 to 36 months. The forehead and lips seem particularly prone to such injuries and are, of course, most likely to develop unsightly scars. Virtually all of these can be handled in the Outpatient Department with the toddler wrapped in a sheet and his head gently restrained by an assistant. Since these lacerations are often irregular and have sustained some crushing, the edges must be carefully debrided with iris scissors or a small scalpel blade and closed accurately with 5–0 or 6–0 silk. Rarely is sedation with barbiturates or opiates of much value in treating such lacerations, since doses sufficiently large to render the child somnolent during the procedure induce sedation to such an extent that observation for three or four hours before discharge is usually required. If the facilities are available, general anesthesia with Fluothane is just as quick and often safer than make-shift sedation. Ketalar, given intramuscularly, is also an excellent drug when working around a child's face.

Preparation and draping of a child for suture of a facial laceration must be planned so that he does not feel suffocated by the drapes and, when possible, he should be allowed to look around and see the face of the physician or assistant. Constant verbal reassurance is also very important.

A child's face heals very rapidly if the wounds are properly cleansed and debrided. Early removal of sutures prevents the "cross-hatching" of scars that may ruin an otherwise perfect result.[5] In most instances, one half of the sutures can be removed on the second or third day and the remainder on the fourth or fifth day. If the wound does not appear sufficiently healed to go unsupported, the edges can be reinforced in stages with Steritapes as the sutures are removed. Steritapes may be unsatisfactory for preliminary closure of facial lacerations, especially when the child is crying and hot and his skin is moist. In no case is Steritape or any other nonsuture technique a short cut to wound closure. Débridement, cleansing and meticulous approximation of wound edges are essential regardless of how the skin is to be approximated. When Steritapes are used, the skin adjacent to the larceration should be painted with tincture of benzoin without allowing any of it to touch the open wound. When the benzoin is "tacky" skin tapes will hold, even when the child's skin is moist from crying.

In an older child lacerations tend to occur on the extremities and knees. Whenever possible, the hand or extremity should be examined in the exact position it was in at the time of the injury. This often exposes damaged structures and hidden foreign material not apparent during the initial inspection and cleansing. If there is any question of the laceration involving a tendon, nerve or joint space, the entire repair should be performed in an operating room with the child under general anesthesia or a local block so that the wound can be explored and repaired under optimal conditions. It is often possible to send the child home within several hours after completion of nerve or tendon repair, but a busy Outpatient Department is not the place to attempt such delicate procedure with a wiggling or screaming child.

Many of the childhood injuries involve large areas of abrasions in which gravel or clothing may be deeply imbedded. These wounds can be completely cleansed with sponges moistened with saline or dilute benzalkonium chloride solution. If there still is residual dirt within the wound and the area is not amenable to complete infiltration or to a nerve block, it may be necessary to anesthetize the child for complete débridement. Any dirt not removed at this time will become imbedded in the tissues and result in permanant tattooing. Once the débridement is complete, large or deep abrasions should be treated as a second degree burn of equal magnitude.

Intraoral lacerations or lacerations involving the lip and mouth are very common in childhood. The typical intraoral laceration is sustained when the child falls with a ruler, popsicle stick or pencil in his mouth. These lacerations bleed very briskly when they first occur, although most have stopped by the time they are seen by a physician. Such intraoral lesions usually do not require any suturing and, as with most penetrating injuries, tight closure is contraindicated. The exception is the instance when a triangular flap has been raised from the buccal mucosa, tonsillar pillar or mucoperiostium of the palate. These flaps heal as polypoid protrusions of the mucous membrane which are then constantly traumatized by food and chewing. It is usually advisable to tack such a flap down with two or three sutures of chromic catgut. These lacerations should not be closed tightly, and rarely is there any indication to use nonabsorbable suture material. Lacerations that penetrate the soft palate and leave a hole should also be closed, since any perforation of the palate is likely to interfere with speech and will also permit liquid and food to enter the nasopharnyx during swallowing.

Tongue lacerations usually result from a fall with the tongue protruding, so that the teeth are driven forcibly into it when the mandible strikes the ground. Again, most of these lesions do not require suturing and heal very rapidly on their own. Any flap raised on the top or lateral aspect of the tongue requires closure with buried cutgut stures or complete excision of the flap. When such intraoral lesions are repaired under local anesthesia, the infiltration can be rendered virtually painless by applying a cocaine- or Xylocaine-soaked sponge directly to the surrounding mucosa. The physician who sutures such a laceration without placing a mouth gag or a piece of thick-walled plastic tubing between the molars to prevent the child from biting does so at his or her own risk. In general, a child under five years of age should have general anesthesia for intraoral surgery.

FOREIGN BODIES

Undoubtedly far more foreign bodies are ingested than ever come to the attention of the parents or physician. Coins are most generally ingested and rarely, if ever, require any therapy. As a general rule, any coin smaller than a quarter will pass unimpeded through the gastrointestinal tract of any child old enough to put the object in his mouth. Quarters usually pass without delay in a child two years or over; consequently, I rarely obtain x-rays of such foreign bodies. If the child is eating well, does not have excess salivation indicating esophageal obstruction, and has no evidence of bowel obstruction, the only therapy is to reassure the parents and warn them of the specific symptoms of obstruction.

Sharp objects, including screws, hatpins, bobby pins and so on, also pass in an astounding number of children without causing any symptoms whatsoever. If there is a fairly clear-cut history of ingestion of a sharp object, I usually obtain a single chest and abdominal x-ray at the time of the first visit. If the foreign body can be seen within the digestive tract, the parents are warned to return immediately should the child develop anorexia, abdominal pain, tenderness or an unexplained fever. The child is then re-examined every three to four days, and if at the end of a week the object has not passed, I repeat the abdominal x-ray to be sure that the foreign body has moved. Any sharp foreign body remaining in the same position for more than 48 hours usually has impaled the bowel wall and will not progress further. Failure of the pointed foreign object to move, any vomiting, signs of peritonitis and local irritation are the only indications for surgical removal of a foreign body from a child's digestive tract. This, however, is quite uncommon, and only rarely does a child require surgery for removal of a foreign body (Figs. 23–3 and 23–4).

Flexible fiberoptic endoscopes are now available with a diameter of 5.5 mm and a channel for foreign body forceps. Extraction of a foreign body from a child's stomach with this instrument requires general anesthesia and therefore should be undertaken only if the foreign body has been in the stomach for one or more weeks and is causing symptoms. The surgeon should be prepared to remove the foreign body by gastrotomy if endoscopy fails.

Coins and marbles frequently become lodged in the esophagus, most commonly at the thoracic inlet, above the aortic arch or at the cardioesophageal junction. In children with strictures resulting from previous esophageal surgery, peptic esophagitis or lye ingestion, the foreign body lodges at the level of the stricture.

Marbles are extremely difficult to

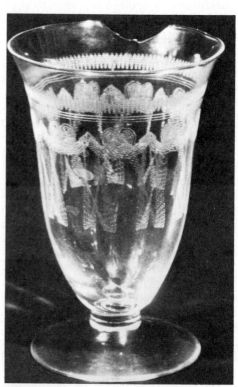

Figure 23–3 Goblet bitten by child. A two year old child bit a large piece of glass from this goblet. He then swallowed the glass fragment intact.

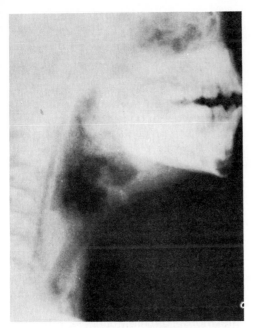

Figure 23–4 Cervical esophagus laceration by goblet fragment. This is a lateral x-ray of the child four hours later. There is considerable free air in the neck and a column of air between the posterior wall of his esophagus and the anterior margin of the spine. He has clinically obvious crepitus in his neck and has sustained a laceration of the cervical esophagus. The glass, however, passed completely unimpeded through the rest of his GI tract.

grasp, but frequently they can be removed with a Fogarty embolectomy catheter. The catheter is passed well beyond the foreign body, the balloon inflated and the catheter withdrawn slowly, bringing the marble up into the pharynx where it can be spit out.

Coins also can usually be removed by passing a Fogarty or Foley catheter and then inflating the balloon. Under fluoroscopic control the catheter is passed through the child's nose, and the balloon then inflated with dilute contrast material. The patient is then placed prone or on his side, with the head of the fluoroscopic unit lower than the foot. The catheter is slowly withdrawn under fluoroscopic control and the foreign body is drawn up into the pharynx, where it can be spit out or removed with a forceps. The catheter

balloon is then deflated and the catheter is removed.

This technique is not safe for removal of irregularly shaped objects, sharp objects or those not visible on x-ray because of the possibility of esophageal perforation. All such foreign bodies should be removed from the esophagus under general anesthesia, using a rigid esophagoscope.

Foreign bodies in the tracheobronchial tree are extremely common, and again, they may not come to medical attention until days or weeks after aspiration. The vast majority of nonpointed objects can be recovered by a program of postural drainage and vigorous pulmonary physiotherapy.

No foreign body, no matter how benign its appearance, should be left in the tracheobronchial tree for longer than a few days at most, since sepsis distal to the object invariably develops and destroys the pulmonary parenchyma distal to the obstruction.

Aspirated aspirin tablets initiate an especially intense tissue reaction in the tracheobronchial tree. They inevitably fragment as soon as they come in contact with the wet bronchial mucosa, so they can rarely be removed intact. All possible fragments should be removed as quickly as possible, and the area should then be washed with copious amounts of sterile 0.9 molar sodium bicarbonate solution. A child often becomes febrile after aspiration and bronchial lavage and may develop bronchial obstruction secondary to local edema. If this occurs, he should be admitted until all atelectasis has resolved. Decadron administered at the time the child is first seen may reduce endobronchial reaction after aspirin aspiration, but this has not been proven.

Around Halloween one is likely to see an epidemic of aspirated beans and split peas coincident with the use of peashooters. Once the dried pea or bean lodges in a bronchus, the bronchial mucosa becomes edematous and entraps the object. It has been stated that dried beans and peas swell in the bronchus, although I have never been impressed by any significant change in the size and texture of such aspirated beans.

Peanuts and popcorn initiate intense bronchial reaction, probably in response to salt and vegetable oils covering them, and a child may develop total bronchial obstruction even after the peanut or popcorn has been removed.

If there is an unequivocal history of aspiration and the child is old enough to cooperate, he can usually point to the place where the foreign body is lodged. This is of inestimable help in planning the physiotherapy, since it gives a clue as to which bronchus contains the foreign body. Position the child on pillows so that the suspected bronchus is dependent, have him inhale some isoproterenol (a "Medihaler" is very convenient for this), and then have him cough vigorously while his chest wall is percussed rapidly with cupped hands. The isoproterenol reduces the profound bronchoconstriction created by the foreign body in the tracheobronchial tree and aids in clearing the bronchus.

The history of foreign body aspiration can be difficult to document. The child using a peashooter against his parents' advice or pilfering peanuts from the cupboard may not volunteer this information. In fact, he may not be brought to a physician until he is coughing, wheezing or feverish. Preliminary chest examination may reveal local or generalized wheezing, atelectasis, pneumonia or a combination of all three. Only detailed history and a practice of bronchoscoping all children with localized unresolved pneumonia can lead to a proper diagnosis.

If the child is seen soon after aspiration of a radiolucent foreign object and is too frightened or young to indicate its location, inspiratory and expiratory chest x-rays usually aid in locating it. The lung tissue supplied by a partially obstructed bronchus fills more slowly on inspiration and empties more slowly on expiration. On x-ray then, the obstructed area appears underinflated on inspiration and overinflated on expiration. The mediastinum may shift toward the lesion on inspiration and away from it on expiration.

If the foreign body has not been dislodged by physiotherapy or if it is pointed or sharp, the child should have it removed under direct vision, using either a flexible or a rigid bronchoscope.

Beans, dried peas and buttons seem to be favored objects for children to insert in their noses and ears. Most foreign objects in the ear can be washed out using a syringe and warm water. Foreign bodies in the nose are best removed under direct vision using topical Xylocaine or cocaine to anesthetize the nasal mucosa, although this procedure may require the use of Ketalar or a brief general anesthetic.

I am always amazed at the number of children who step on pins or needles and have the ends break off within the foot. If they have been disobeying their parents by going barefoot, they may not reveal the incident until they have a noticeable bump. Removal of such a foreign body is never an emergency and rarely should be attempted under local anesthesia. When a parent or physician calls me about such a child, I arrange to see the child the following morning after he has been fasting for at least five hours. If x-rays confirm the presence of a foreign body, I explore the foot under general anesthesia with x-ray or fluoroscopy available.

The incision should be placed when possible so that the scar will not be on a weight-bearing surface. In the forefoot, the incision is best placed between the metatarsal heads and approximately parallel to the metatarsals.

If I do not find the pin or needle within ten minutes, I insert three No. 25 needles in a circle, all aimed at where I think the object is. AP and lateral x-rays will then show the relative position of the foreign body to the three needle tips and facilitate removal. If fluoroscopy is available, this type of "triangulation" is not necessary.

I do not hesitate to close these wounds with 4–0 silk, but I do drain them with a sterile elastic band if there has been inflammation or sepsis along the needle tract. I check the wound in 48 hours and remove the drain at that time. If there is cellulitis, I remove at least one suture and begin the child on frequent soaks, elevation and reduced activity. Immunization should be the same as for any puncture wound or contaminated laceration.

Any chronic draining sinus on the foot of a child should be suspected to be the result of a foreign body. Splinters of wood, glass and plastic are not radiopaque and will not be detected on routine x-ray. Xerography, when available, will often outline such objects. If xerography is not available, or if no foreign object is detected, the sinus should be explored carefully.

BURNS

The vast majority of thermal burns in children can be treated in the Outpatient Department.[7] Any burn is a very painful and frightening episode for a child, and if he can be spared the additional experience of a hospital admission, so much the better. Also, the problems with cross-infection that are inevitable in any hospital ward are much less likely to occur at home. I have found that most mothers are capable of doing excellent dressing changes and even local débridement if they are properly instructed and encouraged.

Hot water burns or scalds are the most common burns sustained from infancy through age four or five. Typically, these accidents involve a cup of coffee or soup being spilled down the child's face, shoulder and arm. The burn produced is a superficial partial

thickness burn (second degree) and heals very nicely without scarring if kept clean. Initial treatment should consist of a gentle cleansing with a dilute solution of pHisoHex or Betadine to insure that all food particles, grease and foreign matter are gently removed.

Superficial partial thickness burns heal rapidly with little scarring as long as they are kept clean and free of infection. While dressings of Vaseline gauze, Xeroform, Furacin and scarlet red have all proved satisfactory, I currently favor the use of pigskin xenografts, available commercially from the Burn Treatment Skin Bank, Phoenix, Arizona. The skin can be used fresh or frozen. It is applied directly to the burned surface after careful cleansing and débridement, just as when placing an autograft (Figs. 23–5 through 23–7). The skin is held in place with bulky dry dressings. There is almost immediate relief of pain, so the child is much more comfortable and can move without discomfort.

The dressings are checked in 24

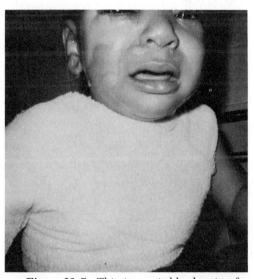

Figure 23–5 This is a suitable dressing for the usual scald burn involving the face and chest. This child had all loose skin debrided, and the burn was washed with Betadine. After drying thoroughly, commercially available pigskin was applied directly to the burn.

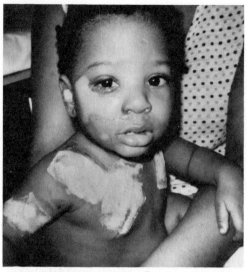

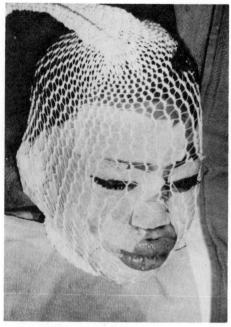

Figure 23–6 Two days later the dressings were removed. The pigskin was adherent to the burned area, and there was no pus beneath it. The pigskin is then left in place until it falls off spontaneously. There is no vascularization of the graft and no rejection.

Figure 23–7 This is a suitable dressing for second degree burns that occur mainly about the face. This scald burn was debrided, cleansed and covered with pigskin. A Flexi-Net head dressing was then prepared. This material conforms very well to any irregular surface and will hold dressings or pigskin in place.

hours, and the graft should be adherent without pus underneath. If this is so, the skin is left alone, since it will peel off when healing is complete.

Vaseline gauze should be prepared with a small amount of Vaseline in a coarse-meshed gauze. The interstices of the gauze between the fibers must not be occluded with Vaseline, so that if blisters drain, the fluid can seep into the dressing applied over the Vaseline gauze. These dressings must be sufficiently bulky and absorbent to accommodate all serum draining from the burn, since an occlusive dressing or a nonabsorbent dressing allows the moist serum to stay in contact with the burn and provides an ideal culture medium for all bacteria, especially *Pseudomonas*.

Deeper partial thickness burns with a white, waxy layer of denatured collagen on the surface are not suitable for pigskin dressings, since the collagen readily becomes infected. These burns are more safely treated with topical Silvadene (silver sulfadiazine), which is a potent bactericidal preparation in a bland base. The burned area must be cleansed thoroughly every eight hours and fresh Silvadene applied to it. For ambulatory patients the Silvadene should be covered with bulky dry dressings to keep the ointment in contact with the burned area.

For the first 24 hours the diet should be restricted to fluids and bland foods, since the fear, pain and crying accompanying the burn lead to aerophagia and resultant anorexia or vomiting.

The initial dressing should be performed by a physician with the parents watching so that they can do subsequent dressing changes at home. The child can then be seen at two to three day intervals until epithelium has completely regenerated. Then only a bulky dry dressing need be applied to protect the healing area from further trauma.

Children from ages four to six or

seven are particularly susceptible to flame burns when their pajamas or light clothing ignite. Often these burns are limited to one flank, the axilla and shoulder. If the areas are quite clearly third degree and constitute less than ten per cent of the surface area, the child is an excellent candidate for admission and for early excision and grafting. If only portions of the burned area appear to be third degree, these can be managed in the Outpatient Department until the granulating bed is ready for skin grafting. The hard eschars of the third degree burn can be debrided at home in the bathtub in a solution of two cups table salt in a full tub of warm water. Silver sulfadiazine is applied after each débridement. When the granulating bed is suitably clean, the child can be admitted to the hospital for a short time until grafting is complete.

All burns that are freshly healed and all recent skin grafts should have lanolin or cocoa butter applied liberally to keep the new skin soft, supple and free of small cracks. This will reduce the itching and hyperpigmentation that are often troublesome.

Electrical burns in childhood are almost exclusively limited to the mouth (Fig. 23–8). Curious toddlers bite into electrical cords, or careless parents leave the charged end of an extension cord within the child's reach.[1] Although electrical burns can cause devastating cosmetic problems, they rarely pose any immediate threat to the child's life. The electrical circuit is completed locally in the tissues surrounding the mouth so that the child does not suffer systemic effects from the current. Initial estimation of the tissue destruction can be extremely misleading. Within the first few minutes or hours after the burn is sustained, the child may have only edema and a tiny area of white coagulum on the mucous membranes. Over the next 48 hours the true extent of the tissue destruction becomes apparent, although the devitalized tissue usually

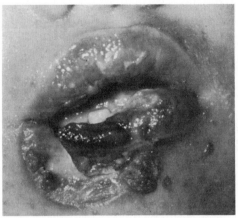

Figure 23–8 Electrical burn of the mouth. This is the appearance of a 13 month old boy who bit into an electrical cord. The current coagulated a large portion of his lower lip and alveolar ridge. The child when first seen may have only a small blister on the lip and a peculiar pallor on the adjacent skin. Electrical burns are always much more extensive than they first appear. Initially, the child may have difficulty with alimentation and drooling from the corner of the mouth. At about 8 to 10 days when the coagulum sloughs, the child may bleed from the limbal artery of the lip. All such lesions should be allowed to heal spontaneously and then revised one to two years later if the scar interferes with alimentation.

does not separate completely until the seventh to tenth day. When this coagulum separates, there may be alarming bleeding from the limbal vessels. A child is often difficult to feed at this stage because the mouth lesion is painful, and the slough from the lower lip may be so great that food and saliva constantly trickle out his mouth. If the parents are reliable and live reasonably close to the hospital, I believe that most of these children can be treated as outpatients for the first five or six days after the burn. However, they must be admitted when the coagulum is about to slough so that bleeding from the raw edges can be controlled by pressure on the limbal vessels or by topical epinephrine solution. During the entire interval between the burn and cicatrization, the child should be kept in a jacket with stiffened sleeves so that he cannot bend his elbow to put the hands or foreign objects into his mouth.

Acid and lye burns are distressingly common, although fortunately most of them do not have serious sequelae. The burns sustained from powdered lye consist of small punctate lesions about the hands and mouth. Flushing with large quantities of water or cold milk is the best treatment. The standard recommendation to give vinegar or lemon juice for the treatment of lye burns has always seemed to be nonsense. Have any of these authorities ever tried to get a toddler to drink vinegar? Cold water and milk are readily available and are much more acceptable to the child. They are also more effective in limiting the local tissue injury.

Ingestion of powdered lye is not nearly as likely to damage the esophagus as is ingestion of a lye solution. Even the most inquisitive toddler will not put sufficient powdered lye in his mouth to do more than raise some vesicles or areas of white coagulum on the tongue and soft palate. When there is no evidence of injury to the mucous membranes of the pharynx, the child can be sent home as soon as the local hand and oral lesions have been treated. However, if there is reddening or apparent burning of the pharyngeal wall or uvula or if the child was seen to play in a lye solution, he should be admitted immediately and, if possible, induced to swallow a string as a guide for dilators in case later dilations are necessary. If he seems to have excess salivation or appears to be unable or unwilling to swallow, it must be assumed that he has sustained a significant lye burn, and he should be admitted.

Passing a string into the stomach is usually easier than it sounds. Older children can be induced to swallow a string with one or two pieces of lead shot attached to the end. Younger children can have the string attached to the end of a nasogastric tube with half a gelatin capsule. After the tip of the tube has been in the stomach for 15 to 20 minutes, the capsule dissolves and the tube can be withdrawn, leaving the weighted string in the stomach.

The role of esophagoscopy in the evaluation of esophageal lye burns is still much debated. Direct visualization of burned esophageal mucosa will prevent prolonged therapy in children who do not have a significant injury. The procedure is not without risk, however, and under no circumstances should the esophagoscope be passed through a burned area because of the great risk of perforation.

I personally have never seen a significant burn sustained by ingesting ammonia or any of the standard sodium hypochlorite bleach solutions, and these ingestions require only induced emesis.

RECTAL BLEEDING

A child is frequently brought to the Outpatient Department after he has passed some blood mixed with stool or has had blood spotting on his diapers or underclothing. A detailed history and physical examination usually lead to the proper diagnosis, although in some instances the source of bleeding is never discovered.[6]

Anal fissures are quite common in children in the diaper age. The etiology is not clear, but once the fissure has become painful the child develops anal spasm and has difficulty with defecation. He then may get into the vicious circle of spasm, constipation, more pain, and then more spasm. Infants with an acute or chronic fissure usually cry and have obvious discomfort associated with defecation. A tiny amount of blood-streaking appears on the outside of the stool, and a small amount of red blood may stain the diaper after defecation. With the child in the frogleg position, the fissure is readily apparent when the physician firmly separates the buttocks (Fig. 23–9). If the buttocks are held apart for

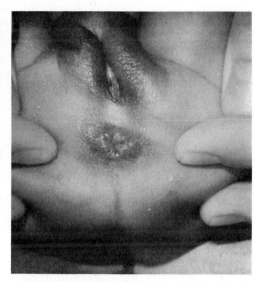

Figure 23–9 This three day old infant had blood-streaked stools. Gentle sustained pressure on the buttocks was adequate to evert the entire mucocutaneous junction, which shows marked fissures at 2, 5, 7 and 10 o'clock.

several seconds, the anal sphincter begins to relax, and in most cases the entire anal verge can be viewed directly. Anoscopy, utilizing a tapered centrifuge tube, has been widely described, although I find it of little value. When there is an apparent fissure I apply a small amount of Xylocaine ointment to the painful region and then perform a fairly vigorous anal dilatation. This should be accomplished by slow, gentle pressure in all four directions, and in most cases the sphincter can be felt to relax considerably. Once the dilatation is complete, it is important to insure that the child has soft stools during the time the fissure is healing. If there is a history of constipation, the addition of Metamucil and extra sugar to the formula or extra fruit juice to the diet is usually adequate to keep the stools soft. Local hygiene is also most important. The child's anus should be carefully washed after each defecation, and the perianal area dried carefully with a soft, absorbent towel. The area should then be dusted with cornstarch or talcum powder applied with a cotton fluff

or powder puff. If too much starch or talcum powder is applied, it tends to cake and the area remains moist. Only rarely do anal fissures require excision in infancy, and then only when they become chronic or neglected and persist after two weeks of conservative therapy.

Painful or extensive fissures occurring in older children may be due to Crohn's disease. If the fissures do not heal after two to four weeks of conservative therapy, the child should undergo sigmoidoscopy and biopsy of the fissures under general anesthesia.

A fistula-in-ano may present with bleeding on the diaper, although more often it presents as a perirectal abscess. Fistulas must be treated vigorously, and the principles are exactly the same as for an adult. The tract is identified at anoscopy and laid open. Most of these fistulas are superficial to the sphincter and heal without significant scarring or debility.

Dilated hemorrhoidal veins often appear on routine anoscopy or sigmoidoscopy, but they rarely bleed or thrombose in otherwise normal children. A child with prominent hemorrhoids and bleeding usually has some other underlying pathology, especially portal hypertension. Investigation, management and treatment of the hemorrhoids is again the same as for adults.

Large bowel polyps in children present as bright red rectal bleeding associated with defecation.[2] There may be an occasional blood clot passed with little or no stool present. The amount of blood lost can be significant, and the children often have a mild to moderate iron deficiency anemia associated with chronic occult bleeding. The blood loss is painless and rarely associated with blood spotting of the underclothes. Since about 90 per cent of these polyps occur within the sigmoid colon or below, many of them can be removed through a sigmoidoscope (Fig. 23–10). In children older than about six years, this can be done

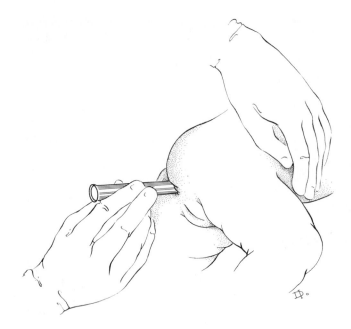

Figure 23–10 Sigmoidoscopy. Sigmoidoscopy in the small child is best performed in the lateral position. With one hand on the abdomen, the tip of the sigmoidoscope can be palpated and loops of colon manipulated onto the end of the sigmoidoscope. This greatly facilitates examination of the sigmoid colon.

under sedation with Demerol, 2 mg per kg, given subcutaneously one half hour before the examination to minimize the cramping pain that often accompanies sigmoidoscopy. Smaller children should be anesthetized or sedated with the mixture of Thorazine, Phenergan and Demerol used in preparing children for cardiac catheterization (Table 23–1). Ketalar is unsatisfactory anesthesia for sigmoidoscopy or anal procedures because of poor relaxation and frequent laryngeal spasm produced by the anal stretching. Virtually all colon polyps in children are juvenile polyps, which are morphologically quite different from the adenomatous polyp of the adult. The juvenile polyp has no potential for malignant degeneration, and in most

TABLE 23–1 Sedative Mixture for Outpatient Procedures in Children

Each ml of sedative mixture contains:
Demerol	25 mg
Thorazine	6.5 mg
Phenergan	6.5 mg

Dosage:
1.0 ml per 10 kg
Maximum dose 1.5 ml

cases it will pass spontaneously. The only indication for admitting such children for open colotomy is the presence of multiple polyps, a family history of multiple polyposis, or persistent bleeding sufficiently severe to cause symptomatic anemia. In most cases, a barium enema followed by an upper GI series and small bowel follow-through should be performed before sigmoidoscopy.

A Meckel's diverticulum may cause passage of a large quantity of bright red clotted blood through the rectum. There may or may not be pain associated with the bleeding. Contrast studies rarely outline a Meckel's diverticulum, although a ^{99m}Tc pertechnetate scan will diagnose about 80 per cent of diverticula that contain sufficient gastric mucosa to produce bleeding.

Intussusception typically occurs in children between the ages of six and eighteen months. About half the children will be seen because of hematochezia, and probably all of the children with intussusception will develop bleeding if diagnosis is delayed. The blood passed is partially clotted and dark in color and has been likened to currant jelly in appearance.

In about 40 per cent of the children a sausage-shaped mass will be palpable in the epigastrium. If the diagnosis of intussusception is seriously considered, a barium enema should be given immediately, since it will prove the diagnosis and may be therapeutic.

If no source of bleeding is demonstrated, the child should be followed at regular intervals and checked for occult blood and anemia. If he develops episodes of abdominal pain, he should be examined with the presumptive diagnosis of a bleeding Meckel's diverticulum. However, a large number of children never have the bleeding site identified, and it often ceases spontaneously. Some believe that this type of bleeding is from hemangiomas of the bowel, similar to those frequently seen on an infant's skin. These slowly thrombose and probably bleed intermittently during the process.

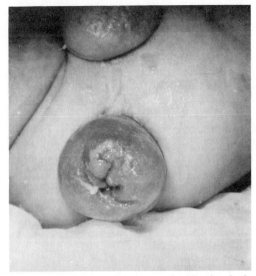

Figure 23–11 This 13 month old infant had a marked rectal prolapse that had been out for at least a day. Note the breakdown and ulceration within the mucosa. Once reduced, the buttocks must be taped tightly together to prevent recurrence of the prolapse, since the local edema and swelling causes tenesmus.

RECTAL PROLAPSE (Fig. 23–11)

Idiopathic rectal prolapse is most common in children aged one to three years and coincides with toilet training. Typically the mother has several other small children, and so puts the patient on the potty and leaves him there until he produces. Occasionally there is a history of constipation or difficulty with defecation, although this occurs in surprisingly few patients. Initially, I recommend that the parents abandon toilet training for several months, explaining to them the hazard of leaving the child on the toilet for long periods of time.

On initial examination it is important to notice if the prolapse is concentric. When the lumen of the prolapsed bowel either is not visible or is markedly displaced posteriorly, there may be an associated enterocele. Also on initial examination it is most important to be sure that prolapse reduces completely, since occasionally an ileocolic intussusception will present with the intussusceptum prolapsed through the anus.

The parents must be taught how to reduce the prolapse promptly whenever it recurs. Once the prolapse has been out several hours, it may become so edematous that replacement is very difficult. Once the rectum becomes edematous, the infant feels a constant urge to defecate and continues to grunt until frequently he produces a prolapse again. When this happens, wide vertical strips of adhesive tape should be applied to both buttocks. A wad of Vaseline gauze is then placed over the anus and a bulky dry dressing is placed between the buttocks. This is taped securely in place with transverse strips, thus keeping the rectum from prolapsing. The dressing must be replaced immediately after each defecation, but the deep vertical layer of tape on the buttocks is left in place. This prevents excoriation from the frequent dressing changes.

Occasionally a child with cystic fibrosis presents with frequent or persistent rectal prolapse, so a careful family history as well as a history of bowel habits must be obtained. If these are suggestive of cystic fibrosis, the child should have his sweat chlorides measured.

Complicated abdominoperineal prolapse repairs are rarely justified in children. In cases of persistent prolapse or in families in which the parents cannot cope, I occasionally use the Lockhart-Mummery procedure, in which the retrorectal space is opened just behind the anus and packed with iodoform gauze. This causes dense fibrosis between all layers of the rectum and presacral fascia. This can be done on an outpatient basis, and recurrences are infrequent. Only rarely is it necessary to amputate the prolapse from below, although this procedure is usually curative.

Children with severe myelomeningoceles or other causes of paraplegia may be plagued by rectal prolapse. Such children can usually be helped by placing two concentric purse string sutures of monofilament nylon subcutaneously about the anus. Placed much like a Thiersch wire, the sutures are tied just tight enough to make the anus snug about the surgeon's little finger. This can, of course, be done without anesthesia since children with this type of prolapse invariably have an anesthetic perianal region. All the sutures eventually cut out and may have to be replaced. Often, however, there is no recurrence of symptoms after placement of the first pair of sutures. With sutures in place, the child may require intermittent laxatives or enemas to prevent fecal impaction.

CHRONIC ABDOMINAL PAIN

The typical child with chronic abdominal pain is a girl between the ages of eight and ten years. She is a perfectly stable and well-adjusted child who does not appear to use her complaint as a means of getting attention. When having pain, she becomes pale and lethargic, and often her parents can tell at a glance that she is having an "attack." Physical examination at this time shows only a pale, asthenic girl complaining of moderately severe pain throughout her lower abdomen. All physical and laboratory parameters are entirely normal. How much of a work-up is indicated? After the initial physical evaluation I usually examine a clean-catch urine, check the stool for occult blood, ova and parasites, examine a peripheral blood smear and check the sedimentation rate and sickle cell prep if indicated. If all these are normal, I reassure the child and her parents and encourage them to note the patterns of her pain to see if it can be associated with eating, ingestion of large quantities of fluid, or any particular activities. An intravenous pyelogram or a barium enema may be indicated if there is any suggestion from either the history or from the laboratory that the bowel or urinary tract is involved. Should the family become unduly concerned about these episodes of pain, it may be necessary to perform these x-ray examinations so that the family can be reassured that body systems are radiographically normal. The condition is usually self-limited, although a few children do come to laparotomy and incidental appendectomy. The large percentage of cures resulting from this surgical therapy must be explained on the basis of the art rather than the science, since rarely is any significant pathology discovered. Jackson's membrane kinking the appendix or small ovarian cysts may be noted in these children, but the incidence appears to be the same as in the general population.

When the sedimentation rate is elevated or if there is occult blood in the stool, the clinician must consider the possibility of colitis, enteritis or parasite infestation and proceed with further diagnosis and therapy as indicated.

HERNIAS

Children are often brought to the Outpatient Department because of a lump in the groin. The diagnostic possibilities include a hernia, a hydrocele of the cord or inguinal lymph nodes. The nodes, of course, are usually distal to the groin crease and can be readily differentiated from hernias, especially if one looks for a contributory lesion somewhere on the extremity. Ulceration of the urethral meatus can cause adenopathy above the inguinal ligament, so the clinician must examine the genitalia carefully. Femoral hernias do occur in children, although they are extremely rare under the age of ten. In older children, when the lump cannot be palpated, the examining physician can often produce the hernia by having the child cough, perform the Valsalva maneuver or jump rope.

One can often elicit the "silk glove sign" when the hernia sac is long. To do this properly, the physician examines the supine child and places gentle traction on the ipsilateral testis. This stretches out the cord structures so that they can be readily palpated just lateral to the pubic tubercle. If there is a significant sac at this level, the cord structures can be felt to slide as the two edges of the sac are rubbed together.

Incarcerated hernias are moderately common in infancy, and statistically the vast majority occur in children under one year of age. Typically, the hernia has not been noticed previously by either the parent or the physician and is first noticed at the time of incarceration. The very large infant hernias containing several loops of bowel almost never incarcerate and even less commonly strangulate. They can, however, cause testicular infarction because of the constant pressure of the viscera on the venous and lymphatic drainage from the testis.

In the infant with a tender, hard bulge at his external ring, the differential diagnosis between an acute hydrocele of the cord and an incarcerated hernia can be more difficult. In children under one year of age the examinating physician can usually palpate the internal inguinal ring with an examining finger in the rectum and the other hand over the region of the cord. If the mass is due to an incarcerated hernia, bowel can be felt entering and exiting through the internal ring. Unfortunately, even if the mass is an acute hydrocele, the testis can infarct if the mass is tense and contained within the rigid walls of the inguinal canal.

While most incarcerated inguinal hernias can be reduced by deep sedation with Nembutal and Demerol, I do not recommend this if facilities and personnel are available for safe emergency surgery, since the level of sedation that must be achieved to reduce the hernia usually borders on general anesthesia. The children are often so depressed that they must be watched for one to four hours before they can be discharged safely. I personally prefer to repair the hernia at the time of incarceration and to discharge the child four to six hours later (Fig. 23–12.) Not only have I seen testicles infarcted by prolonged delay in reducing the hernia, but I have seen several testicles ruptured by overzealous attempts to reduce a hernia associated with an ectopic or undescended testis. If suitable surgical facilities are not available, most hernias can be reduced by sedating the child and elevating the foot of the bed about 20 degrees.

If for some reason facilities are not available for a safe emergency herniorrhaphy or if the child has some additional medical contraindication to surgery, I believe that once the hernia is reduced the child should be discharged and scheduled for elective herniorrhaphy at least one week later. Rarely do hernias become reincarcerated within this length of time, and the one to two week interval allows all local edema and swelling to subside.

Elective hernia repair can be done

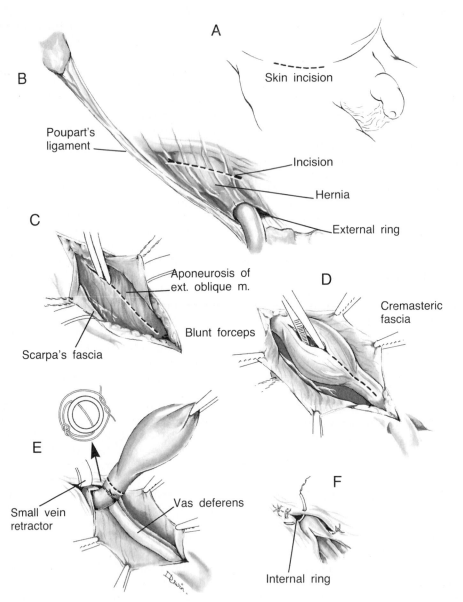

Figure 23–12 Inguinal herniorrhaphy. Infant hernias can be repaired on an outpatient basis. *A.* The skin incision is made in the lowermost abdominal skin crease starting above and slightly lateral to the pubic tubercle. *B.* The external oblique fascia is then exposed down to Poupart's ligament. This reflection is followed inferiorly until the external ring is completely cleared. *C.* The external oblique fascia is then opened in the plane of its fibers down to the external ring. *D.* The cremasteric fascia of the cord is then split in the plane of its fibers and the sac grasped with blunt forceps. *E.* The cord structures are dissected free from the sac, and with a retractor in the internal ring the sac is suture-ligated as high as possible. The excess sac is then trimmed off. *F.* In some cases it is necessary to repair the floor of the canal and internal ring with interrupted sutures. However, in most infants this type of repair is not necessary and only the external oblique fascia need be repaired. The skin is closed with subcuticular catgut in children wearing diapers so that there is little chance of forming stitch abscesses. The child can be discharged from the hospital approximately four hours after completion of surgery.

on an outpatient basis in most children. I check the urine and hemoglobin at the initial office visit and instruct the parents to bring the child to the hospital on the day of surgery with nothing to eat or drink during the previous four hours. On admission, the child is checked for rashes, upper respiratory illness and cleared for general anesthesia. Two to four hours after surgery, the child is discharged if he is afebrile and taking fluids well.

In general, I explore both groins in female infants, since I have found bilateral hernia sacs in about 70 per cent of the girls explored. In males whom I have operated upon, about 40 per cent of those with a clinical hernia on the left also have a sac or patent processus vaginalis on the right. When the hernia has been on the right, only about 10 per cent of the boys have a sac or patent processus vaginalis on the left. Therefore, in males I explore the clinically normal side only if the hernia is on the left side. Statistics on the advisability of exploring both sides vary widely and each surgeon must make up his or her own mind on the subject.

An acute hydrocele of the cord should be treated as an incarcerated hernia unless the physician can be certain of the diagnosis. Acute hydroceles within the scrotum rarely become as hard or as painful as those within the canal, and in most cases they can be dealt with electively.

When there is any tenderness within the testicle associated with the hydrocele, one must be certain that there is no underlying torsion of the testis or of the appendix testis. With torsion of the testis, the cord is usually thickened and foreshortened on the side of the torsion. The testis or cord is also exquisitely tender, and the child usually has anorexia or vomiting and a low-grade fever. The torsion of the appendix testis may be quite subtle at its onset and detectable only as a tender pea-sized nodule immediately adjacent to the testis. The scrotum may become erythematous or edematous soon after a torsion of either the testis or the appendix testis. Transillumination will help differentiate an acute hydrocele from a torsion of the testis. A torted testis seen soon after the onset can occasionally be reduced by the examining surgeon, but in most cases the swelling in the cord makes it difficult to tell which way the testis should be twisted, and the extreme discomfort experienced by the child makes this maneuver impossible.

A history of trauma to the scrotum often precedes torsion of the testis, but in any instance when the testis remains firm and tender after trauma it must be explored. Every time I have broken this rule I have regretted it.

Umbilical hernias and epigastric hernias rarely incarcerate bowel. They do, however, frequently cause acute pain when a nubbin of properitoneal fat or omentum becomes incarcerated within the sac. If possible these should be reduced, but complete reduction may be possible only at operation.

Most umbilical hernias regress spontaneously as the child grows older, although occasionally a small child has a hernia projecting two to three inches and resembling a ram's horn in shape. These have attenuated skin, and I personally have never seen such a hernia resolve spontaneously. Taping umbilical hernias serves only to cause excoriation and rarely, if ever, is it beneficial.

INFECTIONS

Although children have excellent circulation, and lacerations and abrasions normally heal promptly, their injuries are often heavily contaminated with dirt and debris. All foreign material must be carefully removed from the depths of the wound and all devitalized tissue debrided. Even when these precautions are taken, a small number become infected. However, if the parents are forewarned of the significance of erythema, drainage or increasing pain, they will bring the child back promptly and the infection can be treated simply by removing the sutures and instituting a program of soaks and immobilization. Lacerations about the face and especially the eyebrows seen to be prone to infection in spite of the excellent circulation. This area has the added risk of cavernous sinus thrombosis and, in general, any infection involving the portion of the face draining into the cavernous sinus should be treated by parenteral antibiotics with the child in the hospital. Other infections can usually be treated quite satisfactorily on an outpatient basis, although occasionally the child may have to be seen once or twice daily for antibiotic injections.

The prepatellar bursa and the olecranon bursa also frequently become infected after a trivial laceration, a deep abrasion or a small puncture wound in the area, even if the bursa was not entered during the initial injury. If the child develops erythema or edema over the region of the bursa, there is probably frank pus within the bursa itself. The child also will have rather marked limitation of motion in the involved joint, but no evidence of septic arthritis. With prepatellar bursitis the child limps with the knee slightly flexed. There is no tenderness over the posterior or lateral aspect of the joint, and the child does not keep it flexed as acutely as he would if the joint space were involved. If the erythema does not respond promptly to warm soaks, complete immobilization and parenteral antibiotics, the bursa should be drained.

Joint space infections result primarily from puncture wounds or lacerations that actually enter the joint. At times it may be difficult to differentiate between septic arthritis, hemorrhage into an injured joint and sympathetic effusion following a direct blow to the joint. If the physician is in doubt, the joint should be aspirated through sterile, undamaged skin and appro-

priate therapy initiated. All three conditions are symptomatically improved if as much fluid as possible is aspirated from the joint space.

Children between the ages of about six months and three years frequently present with cervical lymphadenopathy secondary to bacterial tonsillitis. The most common organisms are staphylococci or beta hemolytic streptococci, and if seen early the infection does respond to penicillin. After throat and nasopharyngeal cultures are taken, the child should be started on oral penicillin V, 250 mg four times a day. The parents should be instructed in the technique of warm soaks, which are best applied in this area using a small Turkish towel wrung out in warm water. The towel must be rewarmed frequently and applied for at least ten minutes four times a day. On this regimen many of the cervical lymph nodes regress and require no further therapy.

If the cervical lymph nodes have not shown marked regression after a week to ten days of therapy, I stop all antibiotics and continue only the soaks. Prolonged antibiotic coverage apparently delays markedly the normal process of suppuration, fluctuance and drainage, all of which are inevitable if the adenopathy has not responded to the initial regimen of heat and antibiotics. In no case should cervical lymph nodes be drained until they are unmistakably fluctuant. Premature incision of a hyperplastic lymph node leads to prolonged lymph drainage, and it may take months to heal. If the node is truly fluctuant it can be drained through a very small incision carefully placed in a skin crease. The cavity should be loosely packed for 48 to 72 hours, and then the pack can be removed. The drainage site usually heals completely within one week, and I have the parents continue daily soaks during the healing phase. The soaks, if kept warm, stimulate circulation in the skin edges and keep them apart so that the cavity can evacuate completely. The local cleansing keeps the edges free of crusts and debris that harbor bacteria. If the soaks are allowed to cool, they cause vasoconstriction in the skin, thereby defeating the major purpose of the treatment.

Inguinal abscesses can be seen in any age group, although they are most common among children in diapers. Older children may develop inguinal adenopathy in response to infections on the leg or foot, but only a very tiny percentage of these nodes suppurate. The small child who presents with irritability, fever and a palpable mass in the groin may cause difficulty for the physician in differentiating an inguinal abscess from an incarcerated hernia or an acute hydrocele of the cord. The abscesses are, of course, usually below the inguinal ligament and are associated with considerable edema and erythema. To minimize tension in the area of the abscess, the child frequently keeps the hip flexed when in the supine position. In contradistinction to the cervical nodes where the temptation is to drain them too early, the groin abscesses usually do not become fluctuant until there is a very large amount of pus present. If the skin over the node is erythematous and has pitting edema, there is usually a significant quantity of pus in or around the lymph node. Children rarely become toxic with inguinal abscess, and most do not require hospitalization.

Small pustular lesions on the hands and feet that do not heal promptly with adequate drainage and soaking usually have a foreign body within the depths. Routine x-rays of such draining areas show a surprising number of fairly large metal objects even though there is no clear-cut history of impalement by a foreign body. Even when x-rays are normal, exploration of any chronic draining sinus in the hand or foot usually produces a splinter or piece of glass.

Ingrown toenails are common in adolescents and usually involve the great toe. By the time these children see a surgeon, there is usually a three or four month history of cellulitis, suppuration and pain. In such cases there is no place for temporizing measures such as wedging pledgets of cotton under the toenail, since the area is so exquisitely tender that the child cannot tolerate a piece of cotton large enough to elevate the nail significantly. If there is surrounding cellulitis, it may be necessary for the child to soak the foot several times a day in warm water for three or four days. He or she should be instructed to keep off the foot and to keep it elevated. Once the acute cellulitis has regressed, the offending one third of the toenail must be removed completely under a local digital block or a more proximal nerve block. The operation must include complete destruction of the dorsal and ventral components of the nail-forming organ, or else the deformed nail will regrow and the child will have a recurrence of his symptoms within a year or two. If an elastic band is used as a tourniquet about the base of the toe, the incision remains sufficiently dry so that one can inspect the depths and identify the nail-forming organ. This can be removed with a No. 15 scalpel blade or with a small, sharp curette. Any large area of hypertrophic granulation tissue along with the lateral edge of the nailbed must also be curetted down to healthy tissue. After the entire area is clean and dry, firm digital pressure should be applied as the tourniquet is released, maintaining pressure for a full five minutes with the foot elevated.

Once the bleeding has stopped, a bulky dressing should be applied to absorb the inevitable drainage and also to protect this very tender toe from further trauma. A small gauze strip liberally covered with Neosporin ointment and placed in the raw area keeps the dressing from becoming foul and also minimizes pain and bleeding at the first dressing change. I have found that most children want to stay off the foot and keep it elevated for 24 hours after the excision, and I normally instruct the parents to soak the dressing off in a pan of warm water about 48 hours after excision. After the initial dressing has been removed, I encourage the parents to soak the foot three times a day and to keep the open area covered with a Band-Aid. In most cases healing is complete in seven to ten days.

Plantar warts are quite common on the weight-bearing surfaces of the feet (Fig. 23–13). Of the numerous treatments available, I find that those using salicylic acid are most likely to succeed, and there is minimal risk of further damage or painful scarring. The commercially available preparation called Compound W is very effective when used according to directions and is much cheaper than prescription medication.

Common warts on the hand respond just as quickly, and in children I prefer salicylic acid or Compound W to electrodesiccation or more caustic chemicals.

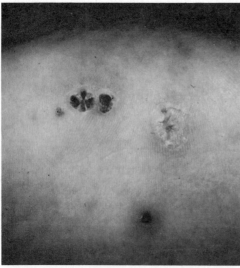

Figure 23–13   These are typical plantar warts on the sole of the foot. They characteristically are deeply pigmented in the center, and occasionally this hard pigmented material sloughs, leaving a pink or reddened base.

ANIMAL BITES

Children are frequently bitten by small household pets such as guinea pigs, hamsters, gerbils and other more exotic animals. The bites inflicted by small rodents are rarely very deep, and their jaws are not sufficiently powerful to cause any significant crushing or deep tissue necrosis. If the animal has been raised within the household, there is virtually no possibility that it is rabid, so that cleansing and soaking the extremity in warm water two to three times a day is usually adequate. Such bites become infected less often than human bites, and in general there is no need for local or systemic antibiotics.

The typical dog bite consists mainly of a crushing type of injury to the calf or buttock, with resulting hematoma and superficial skin abrasion. When the clothing has not been torn, the injury requires only adequate local cleansing and soaking. The edges must be debrided and the wound left open if there appears to be a significant component of puncture or laceration.

Dog bites sustained on or near the face are much more likely to be penetrating, and they often produce a jagged flap of skin and raised soft tissue (Fig. 23–14). Such wounds should be carefully debrided, cleansed with a dilute Betadine solution and closed loosely with a 5-0 or 6-0 silk. I have found that only about 3 per cent of the wounds do become infected, and the cosmetic result in the other 97 per cent is far superior if the wounds are closed surgically. It is imperative that the child be followed daily for five days so that sutures can be removed if there is any evidence of cellulitis or sepsis. Every effort should be made to salvage any piece of nose or ear tissue removed and to reapproximate it as a free composite graft. If it is properly cleansed and promptly sutured in place, a surprising number of these grafts will take in small children and

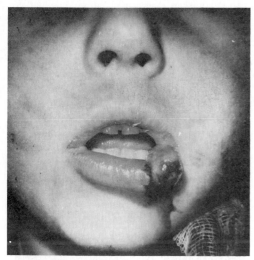

Figure 23–14 This five year old boy was bitten in the face by his pet dog. A dog bite about the face can be closed as safely as any other laceration of equal magnitude if it is carefully debrided and irrigated. If antibiotics are required, penicillin is usually adequate.

save them from a severe cosmetic defect.

Cats and dogs often harbor *Pasteurella multocida* in their mouths and, consequently, animal bites may become infected with it. While it is related to the organism that causes plague, this species behaves clinically like β-streptococcus and is sensitive to penicillin. Therefore, I treat all penetrating dog and cat bites with penicillin for ten days.

Any strange dog or wild animal that bites should be captured if possible and watched for at least three weeks to see if it develops rabies. In areas where rabies is endemic, any child bitten by a wild skunk, fox, bat, squirrel or mink should be given full active rabies immunization (see Table 4–1).

The physician working in an Outpatient Department should also familiarize himself with the state laws governing animal bites. In some states they must be reported, while in others antiquated laws require that they be treated with fuming nitric acid and other medieval remedies.

BREAST MASSES

Infants a week or so old are often brought to the Outpatient Department because of an apparent breast mass. This is, of course, the normal button of breast tissue that has hypertrophied under the effects of the maternal hormones. When the mother begins to bathe the infant at home, she notices these for the first time and may become alarmed. This tissue involutes rapidly and is normally gone within ten days. Staphylococcal abscesses can occur in an infant's breast at this stage and should be considered if there is asymmetry, local erythema or apparent tenderness. These abscesses should be incised and drained through a small circumareolar incision, and soaks should be applied often enough to keep the edges apart while the abscess drains. Such infants should have their daily bath and shampoo with hexachlorophene in an effort to prevent skin colonization with pathogenic staphylococci that were probably picked up in the hospital.

Many adolescent males are troubled with transient breast hypertrophy that may be unilateral or bilateral and that persists for a year or two. The patient most likely seeks medical help because he is extremely sensitive about his feminine bustline and because he suffers as the butt of jokes by his contemporaries. In all cases the breast enlargement consists of a firm disc of hypertrophied ducts and connective tissue just beneath the areola. The nipple is also usually somewhat conical in shape just as in the normal preadolescent girl. This condition of male gynecomastia is entirely self-limited, although occasionally the emotional and social problems become sufficiently serious to warrant excision. A simple mastectomy through a circumareolar incision can usually be accomplished as an outpatient procedure under general anesthesia.

When a preadolescent girl develops one breast before the other, she may complain of a tender lump in one breast. This appears as a plaque of firm breast tissue placed concentrically beneath a developing nipple, and there is no need for further evaluation. Both the patient and her parents are usually satisfied with an explanation and reassurance.

Obese girls may develop a moderate degree of breast tenderness in association with the onset of their menses. Typically their periods are quite irregular and unpredictable, and the breast tissue has a finely nodular feeling similar to that in an older woman with a mild degree of cystic mastitis. Referred to as adolescent mastitis, this condition is entirely self-limited and usually regresses at about the time that menses become regular. If the discomfort is sufficiently debilitating, it is promptly relieved by a three month course of any one of the combination birth control pills. There is, of course, the slight but significant risk of clotting problems associated with these pills, and the girls may develop ravenous appetites, become even more obese and thus more miserable than they were with the mastitis.

Solitary nodules in the breast of older girls are usually fibroadenomas. These are particularly common in black girls and others with dark skin. Such nodules can be excised completely under local anesthesia in the Outpatient Department. The incidence of carcinoma of the breast in children is so extremely low that there is no indication for an initial surgical procedure more extensive than excisional biopsy.

ABNORMALITIES OF THE NAVEL

Many newborns are left with a small granulating area at the base of the navel when the cord separates. This area should be completely epithelialized by the fourteenth day, although a small polypoid area of chronic granulation tissue may develop deep within

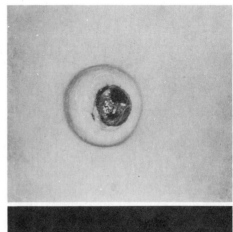

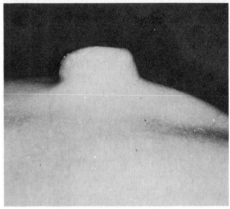

Figure 23–15 Patent omphalovitelline duct. This is the appearance of the navel of a one month old child who had intermittent greenish-brown staining from his navel. In appearance the navel was somewhat more raised than usual, and there was a small area of mucosa in the base. A small catheter threaded into the depths of the mucosa passed into the abdominal cavity. Injection of dye outlined terminal ileum and the diagnosis of a patent omphalovitelline duct was confirmed. The child was then hospitalized for surgery.

the depths of the navel. There is usually little or no drainage, and the child is brought in simply because of the navel's appearance. These polyps regress entirely with several applications of silver nitrate, or they can be removed initially with electrocoagulation. If there is a history suggestive of either bowel contents or urine draining through the navel, the area should be probed with a small blunt probe or sterile catheter. If there appears to be a communication through an omphalovitelline duct or a urachus, the child should be admitted for appropriate surgical correction (Fig. 23–15). X-ray studies may be of help, although the diagnosis can usually be confirmed on the basis of history or by passage of a catheter into the tract.

INTRAORAL LESIONS

Babies are frequently referred for release of tongue-tie because the frenulum appears short and tight owing to feeding problems, or because the parents have noticed the band. At ages three to five the children usually are brought to the physician because of speech impediments. Rarely, if ever, is the degree of tongue-tie sufficient to interfere with normal speech or normal eating. A child who has been swallowing normally must *a priori* have reasonable motion in the tongue, since the swallowing process is initiated by pressing the tip of the tongue against the roof of the mouth. Occasionally a small infant has a frenulum so tight that the tip of the tongue is actually notched and held tightly to the floor of the mouth. It is probably reasonable to release these surgically, but the vast majority of such bands cause no symptoms and require no therapy.

Release of a significant tongue-tie can be done in a minute or two. A Xylocaine- or cocaine-soaked pledget of cotton is applied to the mucosa over the frenulum, and the tongue is then elevated with the heart-shaped end of a grooved director (Fig. 23–16). This instrument has a small cleft in the middle which fits perfectly over the frenulum. When the tongue is elevated, the frenulum is put on the stretch and can be incised with a small pair of iris scissors. One must be careful to avoid injury to the lingual vessels. which are large and quite readily visualized. Any bleeding can be stopped with a few drops of 1:100,000 solution of epinephrine applied with the corner of a sponge.

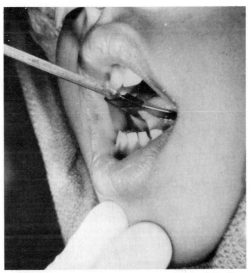

Figure 23–16 This nine year old girl had a tight tongue-tie that prevented her from extending the tip of her tongue beyond her lower teeth. Tongue-tie release is rarely indicated, but when necessary it can be performed easily on an outpatient basis using the spatulated end of a grooved director.

Inclusion cysts often appear about the lips and intraoral mucosa. These are typically thin-walled and contain thick mucus. While some of these cysts are congenital, some are formed in response to a viral infection. I find that they are most reliably removed by excising the outer portion of the cyst and coagulating the base after the mucous membranes have been suitably anesthetized with topical Xylocaine or cocaine. The coagulum separates in three to five days, leaving a clean new base of mucosa. When the cyst is excised surgically and the incision sutured, there is a reasonably high incidence of recurrence.

Ranulas occur in children of any age, although they appear most often in infants as a rather large inclusion cyst under the base of the tongue. They are soft and cystic and contain thick mucus. Again, I prefer to treat these by excising the transparent anterior wall with electrocautery. I make no effort to remove the deep portion of the cyst, and so far I have seen no recurrences.

INJURIES TO THE EXTERNAL GENITALIA

The commonest injuries to the female external genitalia are labial hematomas and lacerations in the region of the urethra resulting from falls, especially while riding bicycles or tricycles. The major problem is one of urinary retention caused by surrounding edema that is partially blocking the urethra. More often, the child withholds urine because it stings the recently traumatized genitalia. The vast majority of such children can be induced to void if they are allowed to sit in a bathtub filled with warm water and encouraged to void. When left alone for a few minutes and allowed to relax, they are usually able to urinate. Catheterization is necessary only when the bladder is palpable and all other conservative measures have failed. Few of these lacerations require suturing, although when the extent of the laceration is not clear or when the blood appears to be coming from within the introitus, the child must have a complete vaginal examination performed under general anesthesia. If there is a history of any sort of penetrating injury to the vagina or if the injury was inflicted during a sexual attack, the entire vagina must be inspected with the child anesthetized. Upright x-rays of the abdomen should be obtained prior to the anesthesia examination to determine the presence of free air or a foreign body in the abdomen. Either of these findings or a high, deep vaginal laceration necessitates a laparotomy.

Injuries to the male genitalia most often involve direct trauma to the testicles of sufficient magnitude to cause a hematoma within the tunica albuginea or in the spermatic cord (Fig. 23–17). In either case the child should be admitted to the hospital to have the

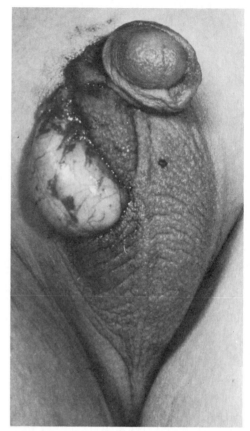

Figure 23–17 Scrotal laceration. This three year old boy lacerated his scrotum on a fence. The testicle was completely exposed at the time of admission. Under general anesthesia the scrotum was debrided and all blood clot and nonviable tissue removed from the testis. It was replaced in the scrotum, which was then closed loosely, and a small drain was led out through the base of the scrotum. The entire injury healed spontaneously and the testis remains normal.

hematoma evacuated surgically; in a surprising number of cases there will be an acute torsion of the testis.

Ruptures of the membranous urethra occur in children much less often than in adults, and I have seen this injury only in association with extensive pelvic fractures.

Paraphimosis results when the foreskin has been retracted for examination or cleaning of the glans and then has not been properly repositioned. This may follow a routine well-baby exam or may result from young parents who have not been sufficiently instructed in cleansing their infant's genitalia. Once the paraphimosis is recognized, it can usually be reduced easily in the Emergency Room, and nothing further is required at that time. If there is sufficient edema or cellulitis to prevent manual reduction, the child must have a dorsal slit of the foreskin. Circumcision should be deferred until all swelling, edema and cellulitis have subsided.

CIRCUMCISION

Since most circumcisions are performed in the newborn nursery for social or religious reasons, the older child presented for circumcision often has a definite indication for operation. Phimosis leading to urinary dribbling or balanitis is the usual presenting symptom. Occasionally a child presents for revision of an inadequate or asymmetrical circumcision performed in infancy.

I personally prefer to do all circumcisions "free hand" under general anesthesia (Fig. 23–18). Starting with dorsal and ventral slits carried down to the reflection of the mucosa and the glans, I then connect the two incisions. All bleeding points are carefully ligated with 5-0 chromic catgut and then the skin and mucosa are approximated with interrupted 4-0 catgut sutures. I dress the glans with Vaseline and several layers of gauze.

At the time of discharge from the recovery room I instruct the mother to apply Vaseline or Obtundia ointment to the glans at each diaper change to prevent irritation and superficial ulcers that will develop if the glans rubs on dry diapers.

The Gomco clamp is widely used, but great care must be taken to excise the foreskin symmetrically and to remove excess skin. The clamp must be left engaged at least five minutes, or bleeding will begin when the foreskin is excised.

The "Plastibell" (Fig. 23–19) seems to work well, although I have treated numerous children with balanitis resulting from this type of circumcision. If the ligature is not tied tightly enough, the foreskin swells and becomes edematous but will not separate.

In my hands, the free-hand circumcision is easier, less likely to bleed or become infected, and gives the best cosmetic result.

THE BATTERED CHILD

The physician should suspect child abuse whenever he or she sees a child with an unusual combination of injuries or when there are multiple injuries of different ages and the history does not seem compatible with these injuries. Lacerations or bruises involving both sides of the head, bruises over the head, shoulders or buttocks, or long, linear bruises indicate that the child has been beaten. Hot water burns in a glove or stocking distribution on an extremity or any deep burn in an unusual place may also indicate maltreatment. Evidence of healing skull fractures, multiple long bone fractures of different ages, and rib fractures are all radiological signs of the battered child syndrome or "trauma X." Rib fractures especially are rare in children under the age of three and should arouse the physician's suspicion that the child has been beaten.

Burns as a result of child abuse are distressingly common. The child may have the palms of both hands held against a hot stove or radiator, may be placed in a tub of boiling or very hot water or may be burned with cigarettes. Hot water burns involving the plantar surface of both feet usually indicate that the child was placed in hot water, since the area of contact with the floor is invariably spared when hot liquid is spilled on a standing child.

In most states the physician is obligated to report any suspected battered

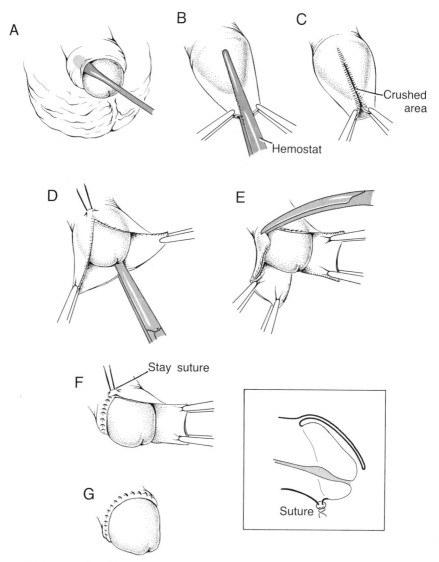

Figure 23–18 "Free hand" circumcision. Circumcision is frequently performed on an outpatient basis. I prefer to use the "free hand" technique of circumcision, which is fully described in the text. *A.* The most important preliminary step is to be sure that the foreskin is completely free of the glans. In the newborn there may be some synechiae between the two structures that must be completely broken down. The foreskin can then be retracted completely to allow adequate cleansing and to be sure that the level of circumcision is correct. *B.* The dorsal portion of the foreskin is crushed with a clamp to minimize subsequent bleeding. *C.* An incision is made along the crushed line. In *D,* the dorsal slit has been completed and mosquito clamps are placed on the corners of the incised foreskin. The ventral portion is then crushed in a clamp. *E.* The ventral cut is made well up along the frenulum. There is often a blood vessel in this area that must be suture-ligated. *F.* The dorsal and ventral incisions are then connected by an incision that removes the redundant foreskin and mucosa. Interrupted 5-0 chromic catgut sutures are then used to approximate the skin and mucosa and to suture-ligate any bleeding points. *G.* The finished circumcision. I instruct the mother to apply Vaseline or Obtundia ointment to the entire glans and sutured area at each diaper change. This minimizes the chance of a meatal ulcer caused by irritation of the diaper on the freshly exposed mucous membrane. Within about ten days the glans becomes sufficiently toughened to withstand the constant irritation of diapers.

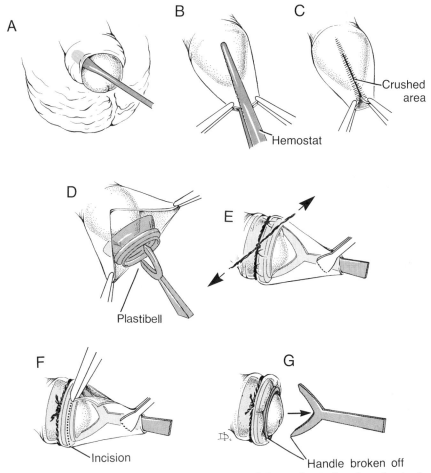

Figure 23–19 "Plastibell" circumcision. Steps *A*, *B* and *C* are identical to those for the free hand circumcision. *D*. The Plastibell is then inserted over the glans and *E*, the suture is tied tightly around the foreskin, holding it against the plastic ring. *F*. The excess foreskin is then removed about 4 or 5 mm beyond the ligature. *G*. The plastic handle is then broken off, leaving the small plastic ring and suture in place. Five to seven days later the foreskin sloughs through the portion crushed by the suture and the entire plastic ring and distal foreskin separate.

children to the police, sheriff or state welfare agency. Separate conversations between the physician and each parent, rather than with both parents together, often reveal the parent's relationships with his or her child and spouse. It is then usually possible to tell which parent is doing the battering, although it can be both parents or occasionally a babysitter, an older sibling, or another adult who is to blame. In addition to reporting the incident to the appropriate social and law enforcement agencies, the physician should be sure that the family obtains appropriate professional counseling.

ALLEGED SEXUAL ASSAULT (Rape and Molestation)

Any physician who sees a large number of children in an Outpatient Department should be thoroughly familiar with the local laws governing his or her responsibilities in examining children who have allegedly been sexually molested. In most states the physician is obligated to report all such cases, and in a few states it is a misdemeanor for him or her to examine the child before the child has been examined by a physician from the office of the Coroner or State Attorney. In recording the history, it is most important to make it quite clear which statements are attributable to the patient, parents or witnesses. After determining the circumstances of the alleged assault, the child should be examined for any signs of physical mistreatment. All clothing, especially underclothing, should be examined for blood or stains that might be attributable to seminal fluid. The garments must be retained and turned over to local authorities for further laboratory examination.

The child should be examined for evidence of any trauma about the introitus, rectum and perineum. The status of the hymen must be carefully noted and recorded. When there is evidence of such trauma, the vagina should be examined using an appropriately sized nasal or vaginal speculum.

Any fluid in the vagina should be examined microscopically for the presence of sperm, with a small aliquot sent to the laboratory for acid phosphatase determination. The presence of either sperm or acid phosphatase presents incontrovertible evidence of recent sexual contact. Rarely are the local injuries sufficiently serious to require hospitalization, although occasionally it is necessary to admit the child temporarily to remove her from the surrounding in which the attack occurred. When the offender is not immediately apprehended for examination, the child should have a two week course of penicillin therapy followed in four to six weeks by a VDRL determination. If there is extensive tearing of the introitus or if there appears to be any blood in the posterior fornices, the child should be observed closely for 24 hours to rule out the possibility that the peritoneal cavity has been entered.

BLEEDING DISORDERS

In any large pediatric population some children with known bleeding disorders will be encountered. For the surgeon the most significant of these are classic hemophilia and Christmas disease. The severity of the defect varies widely, so it is difficult to formulate general rules for the care of these children. However, in most cases a fracture, laceration or sprain sufficiently severe to bring the child to a physician requires treatment with blood products.

Lacerations large enough to require sutures or those that have not stopped bleeding within 30 minutes require specific replacement with blood products as part of their therapy. In children having documented factor VIII or IX deficiency, treatment of major lacerations without specific clotting factor replacement results in catastrophe. They will continue to bleed into the depths of the wound and will return with the wound bulging. Such hematomas inevitably become infected, so the wound must be opened and allowed to granulate. This process may take as long as a month, and the child must be given infusions of specific blood factors daily or every other day until the wound is completely epithelialized.

Whenever I see a child with known hemophilia or Christmas disease who has sustained a laceration, I administer sufficient plasma or cryoprecipitate to raise the blood level to about 40 per cent of normal. Then the wound responds as it would in a normal child. The child should return to the Outpatient Department daily or every other day for infusions until all sutures are out and the laceration is completely healed.

A hemophiliac with a significant sprain or with evidence of bleeding into a joint must be hospitalized and given specific replacement therapy; the extremity should be immobilized and as much blood as possible should be aspirated from the joint. Once the bleeding has stopped, the patient may begin active and passive exercises and may soon resume normal activity, although he must receive factor VIII or factor IX replacement for a minimum of two weeks after such an injury. Occasionally it is possible to keep circulating blood levels of these specific factors in a safe range by administering infusions on alternate days. This must be individualized, however, and carefully documented by determining circulating blood levels.

Hemophiliacs who sustain fractures should be started immediately on specific replacement therapy prior to reduction. In general, they must receive daily infusions until the fragments are stable and callus has begun to form. Premature cessation of replacement therapy may result in late bleeding into the fracture site and in markedly delayed union.

WRINGER INJURIES

In spite of the trend toward automatic washing machines, there are still many homes with only the roller type of clothes wringer. The temptation of such a wringer seems irresistible to a small child, who either puts his fingers directly into the moving rollers or forgets to let go of a piece of clothing he introduced. The result is that the arm is drawn in between the rollers up to the wrist, elbow or axilla (Fig. 23–20). Here the rollers continue to turn, creating a tremendous amount of friction with the skin. The result is a combination of crushing injury to the entire extremity as well as a significant thermal burn to the area stuck between the rollers. On initial inspection there may be little to see other than some erythema caused by the turning rollers. Over the next several hours, however, there may be considerable swelling as well as skin necrosis in association with the thermal injury. The

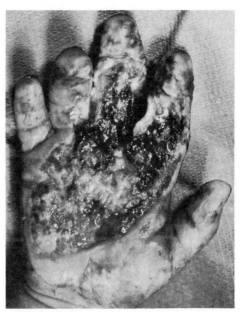

Figure 23–20 Wringer injury. This two year old child put his right hand in a wringer. The hand went in only as far as the palm and the constant rotary motion of the rollers caused extensive tissue destruction. The damage is often more extensive than is initially estimated because of thermal injury caused by the friction of the rubber rollers on the skin. Such injuries should be debrided carefully and dressed daily for several days until the extent of the injury is clear. The child should then have early grafting to preserve as much function as possible in the hand.

acute injuries are rarely associated with fractures and at worst include only an area of third-degree burn. However, because of the crushing nature of the injury, there may be great swelling in the muscle compartments of the forearm that can lead to Volkmann's contracture. Many such tragic late complications have developed when the extent of injury was not initially appreciated.

In the past many hospitals have made it a policy to admit all children with wringer injuries and to treat them with tight wrapping and elevation. This was designed to minimize the chance of late ischemia problems. In recent years I have tended to treat most of these children on an outpatient basis. After initial evaluation to see the extent of the crushing and thermal injuries, I treat the abraded or blistered area just as a second-degree burn and immobilize the arm in a sling. If the injury is acute, I believe that wrapping the extremity in a Turkish towel and then in ice for 20 minutes of each hour for four hours does reduce the edema considerably. If the injury is more than four hours old, the ice seems to have little or no effect. I then arrange to see the child or have the child seen by a responsible physician at 12 hour intervals for at least the first 48 hours. Usually by that time the swelling has subsided remarkably, with the area of tissue necrosis clearly outlined. During the examination in the first two days, I note carefully the capillary filling in the nail beds, the ability to move all fingers, the nature of the radial and ulnar pulses, and the amount of pain in the forearm.

After the initial threat of vascular compromise passes, the area of thermal injury must be treated like a burn of similar severity. In most wringers only the lower of the two rollers has direct power, and conseqently the burned areas are usually on the volar aspect of the wrist, on the medial aspect of the arm, or within the axilla. About one child in ten has sufficient tissue destruction to require eventual skin grafting.

BICYCLE INJURIES

Children frequently injure their feet by catching them in a bicycle wheel. If the child is sitting astride the luggage carrier on the rear fender or on the crossbar, the dorsum of the foot is forced against the metal frame of the bicycle. The result is a triangular laceration based distally and associated with considerable crushing. Even with meticulous care, many of these flaps slough and require eventual grafting. Bicycle spokes may slice off a circle or ellipse of skin from the heel or ankle that is very slow to heal. Many of these injuries require extensive bedrest and eventual skin grafting.

GILL ARCH ANOMALIES

Anomalies involving the development of the first and second gill arches as well as their pouches produce cosmetic problems in childhood. Most common is the first gill cleft remnant which presents as a preauricular sinus. The actual skin dimple may be anywhere in the area anterior to the exterior auditory canal, but it invariably communicates with a sinus or cyst connected to the cartilaginous portion of the external auditory canal. The sinuses and cysts have a strong familial tendency and often three or more generations are involved. Typically, the deeper portions of the sinus become infected, and the child presents with purulent drainage from the skin dimple or a small abscess just anterior to the tragus. When there is infection, every effort should be made to treat the infection and cellulitis conservatively and then to arrange for elective excision of the sinus at a later date. Such excision should always be performed under general anesthesia and in a fully equipped operating room. The dissection is often tedious and involves removing the entire sinus and often some anomalous pieces of cartilage just anterior to the exterior auditory canal. Some of the sinuses come into close approximation to the facial nerve, and local anesthesia is rarely satisfactory, since few children are capable of lying still in awkward positions for the required length of time.

First arch remnants appear as small bits of redundant skin or cartilage along a line from the external auditory canal to the angle of the mouth (Fig. 23–21). These may be unilateral or bilateral and often are multiple. These are all very amenable to excision under local anesthesia and rarely have any deep connections.

Branchial cleft sinuses and cysts are

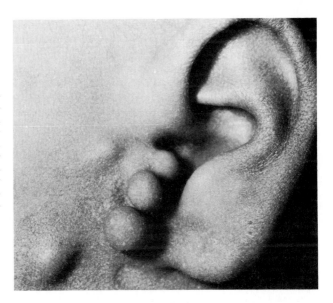

Figure 23–21 Gill arch remnants. This child had a rather unusual accumulation of first gill arch remnants. There may or may not be associated sinuses from the first gill cleft that extend down into the middle ear. All such anomalies should be removed under general anesthesia, since the cartilaginous portion is often much more extensive than is apparent.

remnants of the second gill cleft and appear anywhere along the anterior border, of the sternocleidomastoid muscle. Most are associated with a skin dimple, and they usually present as asymptomatic swellings slightly above the area of the dimple. Occasionally the sinus drains a few drops of mucousy material, and of course it may become secondarily infected. These sinuses always connect with the pharynx in the region of the anterior tonsillar pillar and usually pass through the bifurcation of the carotid artery. Because of the extent of this dissection, it must always be done under general anesthesia. Abscesses and infected cysts must be drained and all cellulitis cleared before the definitive operation is undertaken.

TORTICOLLIS

This relatively common childhood condition is frequently misdiagnosed and often mistreated.[3] Like many chronic diseases of unknown etiology causing no serious debility, it is quite tempting to temporize and defer definitive treatment. In spite of the many theories about the cause of torticollis,

none explains the clinical course and microscopic findings.

Typically the child is normal at birth, and a firm nodule is noted with the sternocleidomastoid muscle sometime during the first month of life. Since babies at this age have short necks and are often quite chubby, it may not be apparent initially that the nodule arises within the muscle. Many children are treated for cervical adenopathy, and I have seen drainage attempted in several cases. There is never any associated skin discoloration and never any microscopic evidence of extravasated blood, so it is doubtful if the nodule results from a hematoma in the stenocleidomastoid muscle.

Whatever the cause infants at this stage can be treated conservatively. Because of the anatomical arrangement of the sternocleidomastoid muscle, it is stretched to its longest length when the head is turned towards the side of the nodule. I instruct the parents in turning the head through a full range of motion. This consists of holding the child's shoulders firmly against the surface of the changing table and rotating the child's head to both sides so that the chin nearly touches the point of the shoulder. This should be done five times to each side at each diaper change. I then have the parents position the child's bed so that the window or doorway with the most light is on the side of the nodule when the child is prone. This encourages him to keep the head turned in the proper direction. Some believe that direct massage in the region of the nodule is beneficial, though I have found it of little value. I continue conservative therapy until the child begins to show evidence of facial asymmetry, which begins with a flattening of the malar region and is usually associated with a prominence in the occipital region on the other side. If this deformity develops while the child is undergoing conservative therapy, I then excise the involved area of the sternocleidomastoid muscle as well as a broad sheet of fascia on either side of the nodule. This excision can be performed under general anesthesia on an outpatient basis, and I normally reinstitute active and passive therapy about one week after surgery. Surgery without adequate postoperative manipulation is doomed to failure. The excision must be extensive, but care should be taken to preserve the spinal accessory nerve (XI).

In preoperative evaluation it is essential to differentiate between true torticollis with fibrosis of a portion of the sternocleidomastoid and a tight muscle caused by cerebral palsy or some other form of spasticity.

THYROGLOSSAL CYSTS AND SINUSES

As the thyroid descends from the base of the tongue to its normal position in the neck, there may be remnants of thyroid tissue and occasionally cysts and sinuses left along its track. These are characteristically midline masses just below the hyoid bone. The cyst may become infected and present as an abscess in the anterior portion of the neck. When these ab-

scesses are drained, a chronic fistula may form with intermittent discharge of muscus or pus. When all cellulitis has subsided, the sinus should be excised. Since this always involves a rather extensive dissection with resection of the middle third of the hyoid and removal of the sinus on the base of the tongue, I believe that the procedure should always be done under general anesthesia with the patient hospitalized for at least 48 hours after surgery.

Occasionally a midline neck nodule represents ectopic thyroid and is the only functioning thyroid the child has. This has led some centers to obtain thyroid scans on all children before surgery on thyroglossal duct cysts or sinuses. I rarely obtain a scan, although I do warn the parents preoperatively that the nodule may be the only thyroid tissue present. At operation I explore the region of the normal thyroid digitally. If there is no normal thyroid, I divide the nodule in half, leaving the upper pole vessels intact, and transplant the two portions deep to the sternocleidomastoid muscles. This preserves the child's functioning thyroid tissue and eliminates the rather unsightly bulge in the neck. An alternate treatment involves administering two grains of thyroid a day in an effort to shrink the ectopic thyroid tissue as much as possible.

Acute bacterial thyroiditis is relatively rare, although one still sees an occasional staphylococcal or streptococcal thyroid infection following severe upper respiratory tract infection. The gland will be diffusely tender, and the child will appear quite ill. If the infection does not respond to penicillin therapy, an abscess will form that can be drained like any other abscess. During the phase of acute bacterial infection there may be marked abnormalities in the thyroid function tests, and the uptake will be virtually zero. Yet once infection subsides, function returns to normal.

Thyroid nodules are extremely common in children, especially in adolescent females. Typically the gland is enlarged with one or more firm nodules, and laboratory tests show an increase in thyroglobulin, a decrease in triiodothyromine, and an elevated thyroglobulin antibody. This picture is virtually diagnostic of Hashimoto's thyroiditis, and no biopsy is necessary. If the laboratory findings are not conclusive or if the diagnosis is questioned on clinical ground, I prefer an open biopsy of a palpable nodule, although a needle biopsy will often suffice. Open biopsy can be performed on an outpatient basis and causes little more morbidity than a needle biopsy. The incision need be only two centimeters long and so positioned that it can be extended into a classic thyroid incision if indicated.

I personally believe that all thyroid nodules in children should be treated for at least three months with suppressive doses of thyroid before any thought is given to biopsy. Since the activity of thyroid extract tends to be variable, I prefer the more easily standardized synthetic medication.

There are only about 50 cases of thyroid cancer reported annually in the United States among children 14 years or younger. Of these, about 75 per cent present as palpable nodules outside the thyroid and represent node metastases. Thus, a nodule in a child's thyroid has only a very tiny chance of being malignant when compared with the numbers of children who have Hashimoto's thyroiditis or nodular goiter.

DERMOIDS

Dermal inclusion cysts appear very frequently along the lateral aspect of the eyebrow. Initially, they are usually noticed in the first year of life, and they grow slowly as firm, round, movable nodules. There may be an indentation in the skull at the site of the cysts. They may occur at almost any area around the skull, although the vast majority are in the eyebrow region.

Classically, skull x-rays should be obtained before excising any of these cysts so that any underlying cranial defects that might indicate a dumbell-shaped cyst with an intracranial extension will be detected. While this complication does occur, it is extremely uncommon, and in the last seventy patients I have not obtained x-rays. One child had a small tract from the base of the cyst through the calvarium, which I tied off. A few months later the child had a very limited craniectomy with the removal of the intracranial portion. I believe this is a perfectly suitable way of managing the rare case with intracranial extension.

For cosmetic reasons I prefer an incision within the upper margin of the eyebrow. The cysts are quite circumscribed and shell out without difficulty. After closing the incision with a subcuticular suture, I apply a pressure dressing to prevent blood from extravasating beneath the skin into the eyelids. This prevents the massive "black eye" that can result from cyst excision. All these cysts can be excised on an outpatient basis.

A much rarer position for dermoids is in the midline between the nasal bones. These are much more formidable lesions and usually communicate with the vomer and occasionally with the meninges at the base of the skull. All these must be performed with the patient in the hospital since they require an extensive dissection with splitting of the nasal bones and tracing of the cyst to its origin. Dissection in this location must never be attempted on an outpatient basis.

BIOPSIES

Lymph node biopsies are commonly required in children and can usually be performed on an outpatient basis. Prior to any biopsy of a lymph node draining an extremity, the area should be examined carefully for any site of infection. If the node is discrete and not attached to the skin or to deep tissues, it should be watched for two to four weeks, since most such nodes result from local infection and are self-limited.

Cervical and jugular nodes are also most likely a result of local pharyngeal, ear or scalp infection if they are discrete and tender. Nodes involved with bovine tuberculosis or atypical myobacteria are usually matted, multiple and nontender. The child will also have a positive skin test with intermediate strength PPD.

Nodes involved with Hodgkin's disease occur more commonly in older children than does cervical adenitis from pharyngitis. The Hodgkin's nodes are usually nontender and tend to be matted or adherent to deeper structures. Chest x-rays may show mediastinal widening.

All biopsies should be planned so as to remove the entire node, since cutting across a hyperplastic node or one involved with TB may result in a chronic draining sinus. Skin incisions should be placed in natural skin folds and closed carefully.

Muscle biopsies are required in children to confirm the diagnosis of muscular dystrophy or in the differential diagnosis of locomotor difficulties. The muscle selected for biopsy is often dictated by the clinical findings, and when only one muscle or muscle group is involved, this is, of course, the one on which biopsy should be performed. For a generalized disease, however, biopsies around the shoulders and chest should be avoided because of the tendency to develop hypertrophied scars in these areas. A biopsy of the gastrocnemius muscle or of the quadriceps femoris is easier to perform and will give suitable results for any disseminated disease. Local field block is usually adequate for anesthesia, and the muscle itself is relatively anesthetic. It is important to avoid any injections of local anesthetic into the tissue being removed for biopsy. In general, I prefer a transverse incision over either the body of the quadriceps femoris or the gastrocnemius muscle.

Once the fascia has been divided, a suitable muscle bundle can be isolated by placing suture ligatures of 3–0 or 4–0 silk above and below the muscle to be removed. The muscle bundles are then divided beyond the ligatures so that they can be used to deliver the specimen. This prevents distortion of the muscle from the pressure of forceps or other instruments. The specimen can then be tied to a tongue blade to keep the muscle fibers properly oriented and to prevent them from shrinking during fixation. The fascia should be closed carefully to prevent herniation of the muscle through the defect.

Nerve biopsies may also be required to diagnose various dystrophic diseases. The sural nerve is accessible and the biopsy, if properly done, does not leave a significant motor or sensory defect. When the sural nerve is isolated over the midportion of the gastrocnemius muscle, it is usually in the midline and superficial to the investing fascia of the leg. When biopsy is performed on the sural nerve at this level, there is usually no permanent anesthesia over the lateral part of the foot, since there are many interconnections with other sensory nerves in the area. Sural nerve biopsies taken at the level of the lateral malleolus often result in an annoying area of anesthesia over the lateral portion of the foot.

The rectal biopsy in a child with frequent constipation or diarrhea, performed to rule out the possibility of Hirschsprung's disease, can be done quite suitably in the Outpatient Department. The pathologist likes to have a full-thickness rectum, but from the surgeon's viewpoint this causes undesirable fibrosis that interferes with the definitive operation. Most pathologists are willing to make the diagnosis of Hirschsprung's disease if ganglion cells are absent in the submucosal Meissner's plexus, especially if there are hypertrophied nerve fibers in that area.

A suitable biopsy can be performed without anesthesia in small infants. A long nasal speculum is passed into the anus with the infant held in the lithotomy position. The biopsy specimen should be taken from the posterior wall more than 1 centimeter above the pectinate line with a sharp biopsy forceps. If a larger piece is required, a single suture of 3–0 catgut can be placed at the apex of the biopsy site and a long ellipse of tissue can be removed with scissors. The mucosa and submucosa can then be closed by running the catgut suture along the biopsy site. It is most important to immobilize the biopsy specimen before fixation by trying it to a piece of tongue depressor and noting which end is distal and which is proximal. Then if ganglion cells are absent in one portion, you will know where the area of transition occurs.

URINARY RETENTION IN CHILDREN

While urinary retention is uncommon in children, the distended bladder is easily palpable and the child will complain of lower abdominal pain. He may have vomiting and fever, and it is often difficult to determine when he last voided. The physical exam is more rewarding than the history. The usual causes are:

1. Fecal impaction
2. Bladder tumors, usually rhabdomyosarcoma
3. Spinal cord compression, usually from tumor or leukemia
4. Hydrometrocolpos
5. Prolapsed ureterocele

Rectal examination is usually completely diagnostic, since fecal impaction will be quite obvious, and any significant neurological lesion will render the anal sphincter loose or even patulous. Tumors of sufficient size to cause urinary retention are quite readily palpable as mass lesions indenting the anterior rectal wall or causing extension in the region of the trigone.

If the urinary retention results from simple fecal impaction, the bladder should be decompressed with a small straight catheter, and then the catheter should be removed. Fecal impaction can be relieved by digital disimpaction followed by oil retention and soapsuds enemas. The mechanism for this form of urinary retention appears to be upward displacement of the bladder neck by the bolus of feces in the pelvis. Since micturition is initiated by descent of the bladder neck, voiding is impossible if the bladder neck is held by an extrinsic mass. Once the impaction is removed, bladder function returns immediately.

If a neurological lesion or tumor is encountered, a small Foley catheter should be inserted to provide continuous drainage. When a tumor is suspected, a cystogram performed through the Foley catheter will usually outline the tumor in the region of the bladder neck or trigone. Obviously, bladder tumors or spinal cord compression require urgent inpatient evaluation and therapy.

Careful examination of the perineum in a child with urinary retention may show a cystic or polypoid mass protruding from the urethra. Seen almost exclusively in females, this finding represents prolapse of a ureterocele. As the ureterocele grows in size, it soon extends to the region of the bladder neck. It then can prolapse when the child voids and will function like a stopper in a bottle. On a cystogram the ureterocele will show as a smooth, round filling defect in the region of the ureteral orifice. Pyelography will frequently show duplication of the ureter on the side of the ureterocele. Correction requires endoscopic resection of the ureterocele followed in some cases by reimplantation of the involved ureter.

HYDROCOLPOS AND HYDROMETROCOLPOS

While these two conditions are often grouped together, they occur at different ages and have quite different natural histories. Hydrocolpos is usually encountered within the first three months of life and may cause symptoms soon after birth. Either the vagina is atretic or the hymen has failed to open normally. The result is a buildup of mucus and fluid that causes marked distention of the vagina. The mass may be grapefruit-sized and clearly visible as a lower abdominal mass, or it may cause urinary retention by anterior displacement of the bladder and bladder neck. The mass may be misinterpreted as a distended bladder, but of course this can be ruled out by simple bladder catheterization. Rectal examination reveals a fairly large pelvic mass anterior to the rectum. These are best treated in the hospital unless the bulging membrane of the intact hymen can be easily visualized. It is always safest to aspirate with a needle before incising the membrane.

In older girls, hydrometrocolpos almost invariably results from an imperforate hymen. The child has well-developed secondary sexual characteristics but has had no menses. Examination of the perineum shows a bulging purplish hymen that when incised drains copious amounts of old blood. Once drainage has been established the vagina will return rapidly to its normal size and configuration. Hymenotomy can easily be performed in the office or Outpatient Department by applying topical Xylocaine in the form of viscous jelly or Xylocaine-soaked sponges to the hymen itself. After several minutes the line of incision can be injected directly if the hymen is thicker than just the membrane. Addition of a small amount of epinephrine to the Xylocaine will minimize local bleeding from the incised edges.

REFERENCES

1. Gross, R. E.: An Atlas of Children's Surgery. Philadelphia, W. B. Saunders Co., 1970.
2. Jones, P. G.: Clinical Pediatric Surgery. Philadelphia, F. A. Davis Co., 1970.
3. Jones, P. G.: Torticollis in Infancy and Childhood. Springfield, Ill., Charles C Thomas, 1968.
4. Kempe, C. H., Silver H. K., and O'Brien, D.: Current Pediatric Diagnosis and Treatment, 5th ed. Los Altos, Cal., Lange Medical Publications, 1978.
5. McGregor, I. A.: Fundamental Techniques of Plastic Surgery, 6th ed. New York, Longman, 1975.
6. Mustard, W. T., et al., (ed.): Pediatric Surgery, 3rd ed. Chicago, Year Book Medical Publishers, 1979.
7. Polk, H. C., and Stone, H. H. (eds.): Contemporary Burn Management. Boston, Little, Brown and Co., 1971.
8. Potts, W. J.: The Surgeon and the Child. Philadelphia, W. B. Saunders Co., 1959.
9. Redo, S. F.: Surgery of the Ambulatory Child. New York, Appleton-Century-Crofts, 1961.
10. Rickham, P. P., Soper, R. T., and Stauffer, U. G.: Synopsis of Pediatric Surgery. Chicago, Year Book Medical Publishers, 1976.
11. Tarnay, T. J.: Surgery in the Hemophiliac. Springfield, Ill., Charles C Thomas, 1968.

24 Transplantation

ISRAEL PENN, M.D.

This work was supported by research grants from the Veterans Administration MRS 6–9850–1, by grants RR-00051 and RR-00069 from the general clinical research centers program of the Division of Research Resources, National Institutes of Health and grants AM-17260, AM-07772 of the United States Public Health Service.

1223

INTRODUCTION

Many readers have expressed surprise that a chapter on transplantation should be included in a book dealing with outpatient surgery. However, there are currently several thousand organ transplant recipients who are living at home and are being followed periodically in the Outpatient Clinic. The number of such patients is steadily increasing.

In this chapter we shall discuss the indications for transplantation of various tissues and organs, the preoperative and postoperative outpatient care, and complications that may be encountered.

Up to the present time a wide variety of tissues and organs have been transplanted as autografts, homografts or even heterografts. Many transplants have involved relatively simple tissues, including blood cells, bone, cartilage, tendons, blood vessels, skin, heart valves, hair, middle ear ossicles and corneas. Transfers of these tissues generally do not require immunosuppressive therapy and will not be discussed further in this chapter, nor will reimplantations of severed digits or limbs. In recent years much experience has been gained with transplantation of complex internal organs and tissues, including the kidney, liver, heart, lung, pancreas, bone marrow, spleen, thymus, larynx and small bowel. As most experience has been gained with transplantation of the kidney, the outpatient management of patients undergoing this procedure will be described in detail. Treatment of recipients of other organs or tissues will be discussed briefly.

HISTORICAL BACKGROUND

The possibility of transplantation of parts of the body from one individual to another or between members of different species has stirred man's imagination since antiquity. Figures in Greek mythology such as Pegasus and the satyrs are such examples, as are the Sphinx and Thoth of ancient Egypt. The legend of Daedalus and Icarus concerns an attempt to escape imprisonment on an island with the use of heterologous wings. Unfortunately, the beeswax used to attach the wings to the body of Icarus melted in the sun and the escape failed.

Among the earliest known transplants in man was a method of nasal reconstruction using a skin flap that was performed by the Hindu surgeon Sushruta in the sixth century B.C. In the fourth century A.D., Saints Cosmos and Damian were credited with having transplanted a leg from a cadaver to a faithful churchgoer suffering from gangrene. Apparently no problems with rejection were encountered and the transplant was a success! Today Cosmos and Damian are regarded as the patron saints of transplantation.

In 1597, an Italian surgeon, Gaspar Tagliacozzi, performed elaborate rhinoplasties to reconstruct noses destroyed by syphilis or dueling injuries. In 1804 Baronio first demonstrated the survival of free skin autografts. Crude attempts were made by eighteenth and nineteenth century surgeons to perform transplants of various organs and tissues. John Hunter, the founder of scientific surgery, was among the early workers in this field and was one of the first to use the term "transplanting."

The modern era of transplantation commenced early in the present century when Alexis Carrel and Charles Guthrie perfected techniques of vascular anastomosis and showed in experimental animals that it was technically possible to transplant kidneys, hearts, lungs, thyroids, ovaries, limbs and heads.

Sporadic attempts to transplant various organs subsequently were made in man but were doomed to failure because of a lack of understanding of the immunological problems involved. During the second World War a major breakthrough came with the work of

Medawar and his colleagues, who produced convincing evidence that graft failure was immunologically mediated. Their work opened up avenues for the treatment of rejection and set the stage for successful transplantation of major organs in man.

The work of Willem Kolff from the 1940s onward established hemodialysis as a method of keeping uremic patients alive. In the early experience, the cannulated peripheral vessels were sacrificed after each dialysis, thus seriously limiting the number of treatments that each patient could receive. Long-term patency of the cannulated vessels was assured by the introduction in 1960 of external arteriovenous shunts by Quinton and his colleagues.[87] The ability to maintain patients on hemodialysis for prolonged periods was enhanced by the development in 1966 of subcutaneous arteriovenous fistulas by Brescia and associates.[13] These advances, together with improvements in dialysis equipment and technique, made it possible to keep patients with chronic renal failure in good condition preparatory to renal transplantation.

Although kidney transplantation in man was attempted as early as 1902, the significant developments in this field came in the early 1950s in Chicago, Paris, Boston and Toronto. No immunosuppression was used in these early cases, and no long-term function was accomplished except in transplants between monozygotic twins.

Immunosuppression with total body irradiation was introduced in 1958 to prevent rejection in transplants between individuals other than identical twins. The following year this therapy was superseded by the use of 6-mercaptopurine and in 1961 by the closely related compound, azathioprine (Imuran). In 1963 the use of a combination of azathioprine and prednisone was reported. Histocompatibility testing was introduced in 1964, and two years later antilymphocyte globulin (ALG) was used to augment immunosuppression with azathioprine and prednisone. In its evolution kidney transplantation has served as the prototype for the transfer of other major organs. Today it can no longer be looked upon as an experimental procedure but as an accepted method of treatment.

The first liver transplant in man was performed by Thomas Starzl in Denver in 1963, while in the same year the first human lung graft was accomplished by James Hardy in Jackson, Mississippi. In the following year Dr. Hardy transplanted a chimpanzee heart into a patient. The first transplantation of a human heart was performed by Christiaan Barnard in Cape Town, South Africa, toward the end of 1967. Transplantation of the pancreas was performed by Drs. W. Kelly and Richard Lillehei in 1966 in Minneapolis. The latter surgeon performed the first graft of the small bowel in the following year.

KIDNEY TRANSPLANTATION

Much of the management of renal recipients and their living donors can be handled on an outpatient basis.

Selection of Kidney Recipients

Renal transplantation is performed for uremia caused by glomerulonephritis or pyelonephritis in 67 per cent of patients.[2] Less common indications include diabetes mellitus, amyloidosis, polycystic kidney disease, familial nephritis, Goodpasture's syndrome, medullary cystic disease, cystinosis, Alport's syndrome, amyloidosis, Fabry's disease, gout, obstructive uropathy, hemolytic uremic syndrome, analgesic nephropathy, lupus nephritis, oxalosis, ethylene glycol nephropathy and renal malignancy.

In the early experience with renal transplantation the operation was restricted to a select group of relatively young patients who had no other serious illnesses apart from chronic renal failure. The indications for the procedure have been liberalized very considerably during recent years.[72, 74, 102] The following factors should be taken into consideration:

1. AGE. Most pediatric patients do well after renal transplantation.[59] Our youngest recipient was about eight weeks old. At the opposite extreme of life the physiological age of the recipient is more important than the chronological age when kidneys from related donors are used, and patients can be treated up to about 60 to 65 years of age. Those over the age of 45 years who receive kidneys from cadaver donors have a substantially increased risk of mortality and morbidity. In fact, some workers[72] advise chronic dialysis for patients over 45 years of age who do not have living related donors.

2. GENERAL PHYSICAL CONDITION. Renal homograft recipients often have anemia, hypertension and even heart failure, so a history of previous myocardial infarcts is not a contraindication to transplantation. In fact, the patient with severe cardiac disease will probably do better with a kidney graft than with dialysis therapy,[72] since cardiovascular complications are the leading cause of death in dialysis patients.

Infectious complications are the major cause of death following transplantation. Therefore, patients with chronic infections such as diverticulitis, bronchiectasis or active pulmonary tuberculosis should not undergo transplantation until these disorders have been eradicated.

Hepatitis B antigenemia is common in dialysis patients, many of whom are persistent asymptomatic carriers. It also occurs in 19 to 51 per cent of renal homograft recipients.[31, 114] Some authors[19, 31, 92] believe that it has no effect on patient survival or homograft function, while others describe a fivefold increase in deaths from liver disease,[84] or an increased incidence of graft rejection in recipients with antibodies to hepatitis B surface antigen.[61] In the present state of our knowledge patients should not be denied transplantation because they are hepatitis B antigen carriers.[109] However, extra precautions are necessary in their management, as they constitute a reservoir of infection and thus pose a significant hazard to the individuals responsible for their care.[114]

As there is an increased incidence of malignancy after transplantation,[80, 82, 83] caution is necessary in the management of patients with pre-existing cancers. Our current policy is to keep potential recipients, with the exception of those with low-grade skin cancers, on dialysis for at least one year following treatment of the neoplasms. Then if there is no evidence of recurrence or metastasis, transplantation may be undertaken. Occasionally this waiting period may have to be shortened, as in the case of very young children suffering from Wilms' tumors, who may be difficult to maintain on dialysis for prolonged periods.[83]

3. MENTAL STATUS. Uremia is sometimes complicated by a toxic psychosis. Furthermore, the stress of a serious and potentially fatal illness is often responsible for mental symptoms. These are not contraindications to operation, as they will often clear up following successful transplantation. However, the existence of a long-standing functional psychosis or severe behavior disorder is a deterrent to operation, because patients with these problems are very difficult to manage postoperatively.

4. PRIMARY RENAL DISEASE. Insulin-dependent juvenile onset diabetic patients do very poorly on dialysis therapy. While the risks of transplantation are substantially greater than in nondiabetic individuals, they are less than those encountered with dialysis. The University of Minnesota group has accumulated great experience in the management of these patients.[74]

Some renal diseases are associated with a moderate to high risk of recurrence in the homograft. An example of moderate risk is glomerulonephritis[98] and of high risk, oxalosis.[72] Many years of good homograft function have been obtained in patients in the moderate risk category, but in the high risk category transplantation would appear to be unwise.

5. STATUS OF THE LOWER URINARY TRACT. Obstruction of the bladder neck or urethra is a contraindication to transplantation unless the underlying lesion is treated. This may be done before transplantation[33] or, in the case of posterior urethral valves, a few days after homograft insertion, when a good urinary stream will help to maintain an adequate urethral lumen and prevent scarring and stricture formation.[16] Even bladders that have been nonfunctional for years may function satisfactorily.[16, 33] If the lower urinary tract cannot be satisfactorily reconstructed, ileal segment urinary diversion may be performed several weeks before transplantation is undertaken.[66]

6. IMMUNOLOGICAL FACTORS. ABO blood group compatibility between donor and recipient is necessary to prevent hyperacute homograft rejection. The place of human leucocyte antigen (HLA) typing in transplantation is unclear. While good results can be expected in transplants between HLA-identical siblings, opposing conclusions have been published about the value of HLA typing in transplantation from cadaver donors.

Of great importance is the cross-match between the recipient's serum and the donor's lymphocytes. The recipient may have pre-formed antibodies as a result of previous exposure to foreign antigens through blood transfusions, multiple pregnancies or previous transplants. In the presence of such antibodies the risk of hyperacute rejection of the homograft is a very serious one, and transplantation should not be performed. However, sensitization to B-cells only is not a contraindication to transplantation.

Preoperative Management

Preoperative Preparation of the Recipient

A full history and thorough mental and physical examination are essential. The following studies (Fig. 24–1) are performed: a chest radiograph, full blood count, fasting blood sugar, two hour postprandial blood sugar, electrocardiograph, urinalysis, culture of the urine, blood urea nitrogen, serum creatinine, creatinine clearance, and serum levels of sodium, potassium, chloride, calcium, phosphorus and magnesium.[95] In the course of his illness the patient may have received blood transfusions and been exposed to the risk of hepatitis. Evidence for this is sought by measuring the serum bilirubin, alkaline phosphatase, SGOT, serum proteins and prothrombin time and by testing for the hepatitis B antigen.[114] If active hepatitis is present then transplantation should be deferred for several months, owing to the risk of further liver injury by the immunosuppressive drugs.

Immediately before admission to the hospital, routine cultures of the throat, sputum, urine, feces and skin are taken.[95]

In cases when the status of the patient's lower urinary tract is doubtful, studies such as voiding cystourethrograms, cystoscopy, retrograde pyelography and cystometrograms may be necessary.

The patient's blood is typed for ABO, Rh and HLA antigens. A direct cross-match between the recipient's serum and the donor's lymphocytes is always performed. A wide variety of other immunological tests are being evaluated in an attempt to detect sensitization to the antigens of potential donors.[104] As yet, none has received widespread acceptance.

A few patients do not require management with dialysis prior to transplantation. However, the great majority need this treatment to correct fluid and electrolyte imbalance, acidosis,

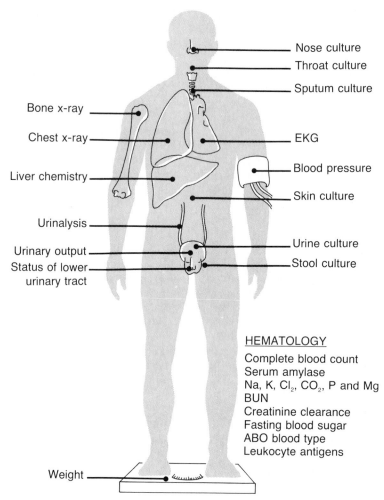

Figure 24–1   Investigations in a potential renal homograft recipient.

hypertension and pulmonary edema, if present (Fig. 24–2). In most cases dialysis is handled by the renal medicine department, and details will not be discussed here. Most nephrologists prefer hemodialysis to peritoneal dialysis (PD) because the latter is much less effective than the former and is associated with numerous complications. PD may be indicated in small children, in whom vascular access is difficult, and in patients who have lost all vascular access routes.[28]

Arteriovenous Shunts and Fistulas for Hemodialysis

Currently some 10,000 patients are being maintained on chronic intermittent hemodialysis throughout the United States.[43] Provision of vascular access for hemodialysis has therefore become an important surgical activity in many hospitals. Many ingenious techniques have been devised, and in this chapter we shall consider the more commonly used methods. Most can be performed on an outpatient basis under local anesthesia.

Vascular access is provided by construction of an external arteriovenous shunt or an internal arteriovenous fistula. When a short period of treatment is required, the use of an external shunt is adequate. This is usually constructed between a peripheral upper limb artery such as the radial or ulnar and an adjacent vein (Figs. 24–3 and

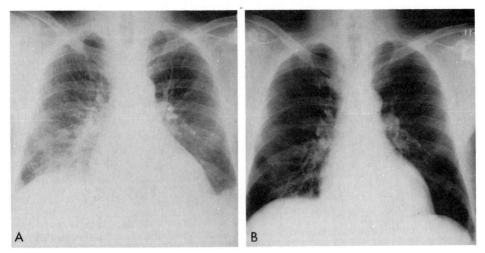

Figure 24–2 *A.* Chest radiograph of a 45 year old physician with chronic renal failure who came to the hospital in pulmonary edema. *B.* Repeat chest radiograph several hours after hemodialysis showing marked improvement in the radiographic appearance.

24–4). The shunt is usually placed on the nondominant extremity to restrict the patient's activities as little as possible. In instances in which the distal vessels have previously been used, the same artery is cannulated a centimeter or two more proximally. In those patients requiring repeated shunt revisions, even multiple ligations of one forearm artery have not produced distal vascular insufficiency. In these cases the final shunt in that forearm

may lie quite close to the elbow (Fig. 24–4).

The two types of shunts most commonly used are the standard shunt, with a U-shaped Silastic tube that has a step at the point of exit through the skin, and the straight tube, which has a wing just distal to the tip, with or without a step. The cannula tips are made of Teflon and are available in several sizes. A straight tube is easier to declot than a curved tube but has a minor

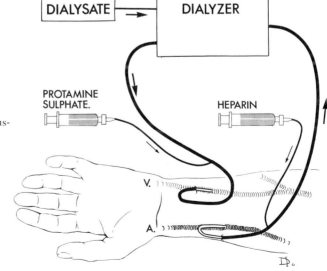

Figure 24–3 Hemodialysis using an arteriovenous shunt.

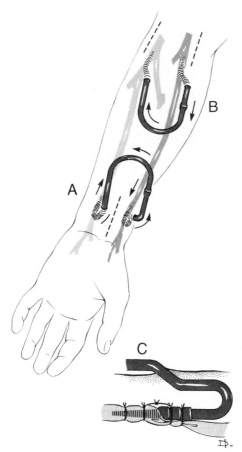

Figure 24–4 *A.* Standard arteriovenous shunt in lower part of forearm. *B.* Shunt near elbow. Direction of tubes is opposite to that in *A* to avoid crossing the antecubital fossa. Dotted lines in *A* and *B* represent incisions used, and arrows indicate direction of blood flow. *C.* Detail showing cannula firmly secured in blood vessel, and buried subcutaneous portion of Silastic tube emerging through the skin.

disadvantage in that the site of insertion must be higher in the limb than with conventional shunts because the connecting tube must lie distally rather than proximally. This results in a loss of arterial length and may be important in patients requiring long-term dialysis.

When vessels in the forearms are unsatisfactory because of thrombosis caused by multiple venipunctures and intravenous infusions or because of multiple previous shunts, lower extremity shunts may be necessary.[30] Satisfactory types are shown in Figure 24–5 between either the anterior or posterior tibial arteries and the long or short saphenous veins. Occasional patients are seen in whom the distal vessels in the upper and lower limbs have been previously used and have undergone thrombosis. In such instances one may anastomose a free graft of the saphenous vein to the superficial femoral artery to provide access to the arterial circulation and use the proximal divided end of the vein for the venous return (Fig. 24–6).

In children it is frequently possible to construct shunts in distal arm or leg vessels. However, if these vessels are too small, shunts between the brachial artery and cephalic vein or between the profunda (deep) or superficial femoral artery and the saphenous vein may be used.[14] Ischemic changes are minor, infrequent and transitory after the use of femoral arteries because of the abundant collateral circulation in children.

The survival rate for well-constructed external shunts varies considerably from one center to another, ranging from 2 to 24 months. In most series there have been an average of three shunt revisions per patient per year of dialysis.[43] The most common cause of failure is thrombosis.[44, 45] Declotting of a thrombosed shunt is often possible by means of syringe suction, an Intracath catheter, a Fogarty balloon catheter, irrigation with heparinized saline or instillation of fibrinolysin to dissolve clot that cannot be removed mechanically. Shunt angiography (Fig. 24–7) is often valuable to establish whether there is a mechanical cause, such as marked angulation of a cannula tip or a stricture in a vessel requiring revision of the affected limb. In the absence of a mechanical fault, repeated clotting may be an indication for systemic anticoagulant therapy.

Infection is another frequent complication, occurring in 17 to 50 per cent of patients.[43] The most common organ-

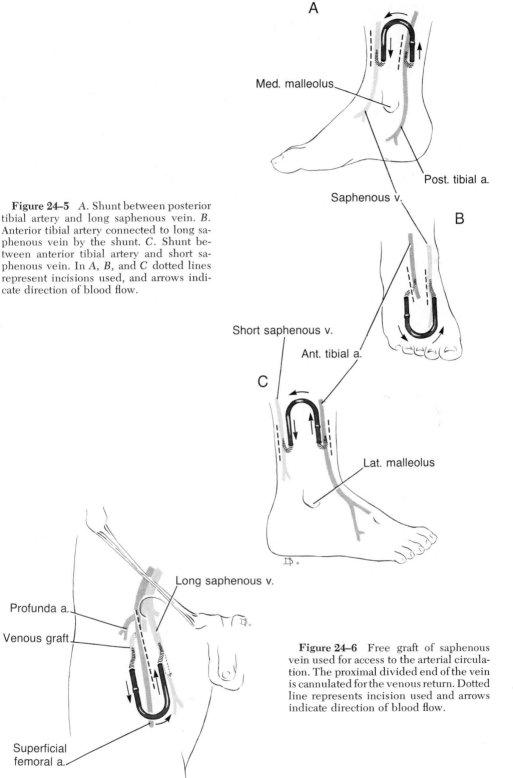

A

Med. malleolus

Post. tibial a.

Saphenous v.

B

Short saphenous v.

Ant. tibial a.

C

Lat. malleolus

Figure 24–5 *A.* Shunt between posterior tibial artery and long saphenous vein. *B.* Anterior tibial artery connected to long saphenous vein by the shunt. *C.* Shunt between anterior tibial artery and short saphenous vein. In *A*, *B*, and *C* dotted lines represent incisions used, and arrows indicate direction of blood flow.

Long saphenous v.

Profunda a.

Venous graft

Superficial femoral a.

Figure 24–6 Free graft of saphenous vein used for access to the arterial circulation. The proximal divided end of the vein is cannulated for the venous return. Dotted line represents incision used and arrows indicate direction of blood flow.

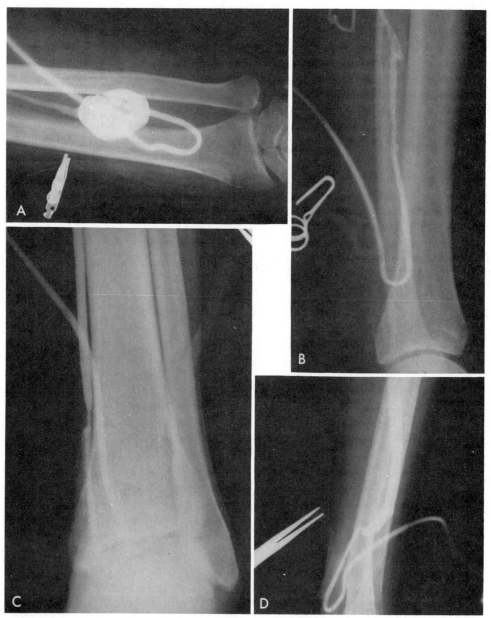

Figure 24–7 Shunt angiograms. *A.* Left forearm with arterial false aneurysm at site of cannula insertion. *B.* Right lower leg with irregular filling defects caused by thrombi in the long saphenous vein. *C.* Right lower leg with stricture of long saphenous vein just above cannula tip. *D.* Left forearm with marked angulation of cannula and stricture of vein.

isms are *Staphylococcus aureus* and the Pseudomonas group. Septic phlebitis, septic embolism, generalized septicemia, endocarditis and pulmonary abscesses may occur. Most infections can be treated successfully with

antibiotic therapy. Failure of such treatment or the development of systemic sepsis is an indication for removal of the shunt.

Other problems encountered with shunts are erosion of the skin overly-

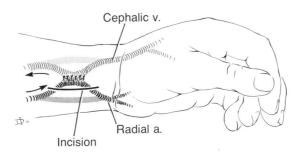

Figure 24–8 Side-to-side arteriovenous fistula. Solid line shows incision used and arrows indicate direction of blood flow.

ing the buried portion of the tube, hemorrhage around the cannula and false aneurysm formation at either the arterial or venous end (Fig. 24–7). The high incidence of complications and the necessity for repeated surgical revisions of the shunts contribute to the psychological fixations that some patients develop about dialysis.

Construction of an internal arteriovenous fistula is the procedure of choice for obtaining access to the patient's circulation for hemodialysis, particularly when a prolonged period of treatment is necessary.[45, 63] A few weeks after creation of such a bypass the veins become arterialized, remain

distended, and can be punctured easily.

Most fistulas are placed in the distal portion of an upper limb by performing a 5 to 8 mm side-to-side anastomosis between the radial or ulnar artery and an adjacent vein (Figs. 24–8 and 24–9). Alternatively, an end-to-end or end-of-vein-to-side-of-artery anastomosis can be constructed. An advantage of an end-to-side anastomosis is preservation of continuity of the artery should the vein or fistula become clotted. The artery usually remains patent and the second artery in the same extremity can be used with impunity, if it is needed.[45] Even when the radial arte-

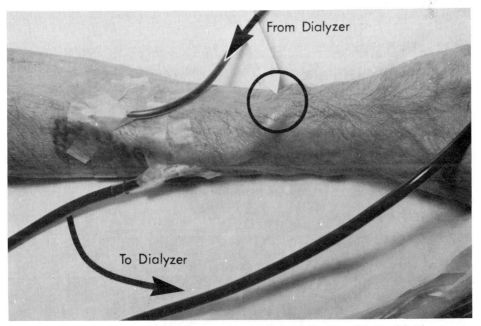

Figure 24–9 Radial artery cephalic vein arteriovenous fistula (indicated by circle). The prominent cephalic vein has been punctured and blood is being returned from the dialyzer through the tube (at the top of the photograph) which is connected to a needle in another forearm vein.

ry has been interrupted at several points between the elbow and the wrist, a radial pulse may be palpable distally, and when a fistula is created using this distal arterial stump, flow via palmar arch collaterals is adequate for dialysis.[70]

A useful procedure when there are no suitable veins in the distal forearm is to place a saphenous vein graft subcutaneously as a straight conduit between the radial or ulnar artery at the wrist and one of the antecubital veins.[45] Occasional patients have unsuitable distal forearm arteries, e.g., patients who are old or diabetic or who have other peripheral vascular diseases. In such individuals a fistula can be made between the lower part of the brachial artery and an adjacent vein or between the proximal radial artery and the cephalic vein or a large vena comitans, taking care to ligate the multiple deep venous channels that would direct the flow away from the cephalic system.[113] Alternatively, a segment of long saphenous vein can be placed as a gentle loop in the subcutaneous tissues of the forearm by end-to-side anastomosis with the distal brachial artery and a similar union with the cephalic vein just at or below the elbow.

After numerous previous procedures some patients have no usable veins in the forearm or antecubital area. Fistulas with long-term patency can be constructed in these individuals by inserting a graft in the upper arm between the distal brachial artery and the cephalic or basilic vein at the shoulder.[3] The graft lies subcutaneously in front of the biceps muscle. An alternative procedure is to mobilize the basilic vein from the axilla to the antecubital fossa, divide the lower end, relocate the vein in a subcutaneous tunnel along the anterior aspect of the arm, and then anastomose the lower end to the brachial artery in the antecubital fossa. This provides a straight, long, easily accessible fistula capable of maintaining high flow rates.[23]

When the upper limb vessels are unsuitable, a fistula may be constructed in a lower extremity[30] (Fig. 24–10). However, this is not as successful as one in the upper extremity because the venous pattern is not as well developed or as accessible.[55] The best exposure is obtained in thin people who have a tendency to varicose veins. Occasional patients are seen whose peripheral vessels in all extremities have become thrombosed after the repeated use of external shunts. In such cases division of the long saphenous vein in the midthigh and anastomosis of the proximal end to the superficial femoral

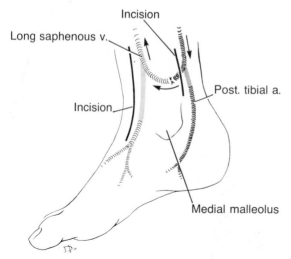

Figure 24–10 End-to-end arteriovenous fistula. Solid lines represent incisions used and arrows indicate direction of blood flow.

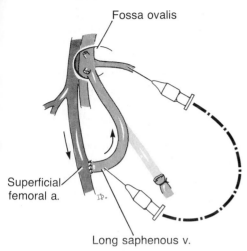

Figure 24-11   End-to-side arteriovenous fistula in the proximal thigh. Arrows indicate direction of blood flow. Syringes show sites of venipuncture for obtaining access to the circulation.

artery will provide a subcutaneous arteriovenous conduit that can be punctured readily whenever necessary (Fig. 24–11). An alternative procedure is division of the long saphenous vein at the knee, translocation of the vein into a subcutaneous tunnel, and then end-to-side anastomosis to the popliteal artery.[60]

Besides the use of segments of autogenous vein, vascular conduits have been constructed with venous or aterial homografts,[3] modified bovine heterografts,[119] Sparks mandril-grown grafts,[9] preserved fetal umbilical cord veins[69] and various prosthetic materials.[34, 49]

Very occasionally, arterial access alone may be used as a last resort to provide access for hemodialysis. An external shunt may be placed to bridge or bypass a segment of the superficial femoral artery.[55] Alternatively, a 6 to 7 inch segment of this vessel may be mobilized and placed in a subcutaneous position, where it can be punctured for hemodialysis whenever necessary.[55] Another method is to place a graft subcutaneously connecting an artery in the upper part of a limb with another

lower down in the same extremity.[15, 45]

Although the initial failure rate for A-V fistulas may be as high as 15 to 25 per cent, once they are established the incidence of late failures is small, being less than 5 per cent after six months on dialysis.[43] There are many patients who have been maintained on dialysis for more than five years using the same fistula.

Most patients prefer an internal fistula to the external shunt. Complications are less frequent and the patient is not restricted from using the affected extremity for work or recreation. When a shunt must be removed because of malfunction it is sometimes possible to construct a side-to-side fistula in the same artery and vein proximal to the site of shunt removal. In such cases the vein is already arterialized and the fistula can be used immediately.[93] Disadvantages of the internal fistula are the necessity for two venipunctures for each dialysis, lower blood flow rates than those obtained with shunts and less freedom for the patient to move about while being dialysed, for fear of dislodging the dialysis needles. Venous hypertension in the hand may occur because of retrograde venous arterialization.[44] It manifests itself with massive edema, pain or discomfort, skin induration, hyperpigmentation and eventual ulceration similar to that seen with chronic venous insufficiency in the lower extremities. In addition, there have been occasional reports of ischemic changes in the limb, with gangrene, thromboembolic complications, venous aneurysms, cardiac embarrassment, or infection leading to frank septicemia or bacterial endocarditis.[43-45, 56, 63, 108]

Ischemic and hemodynamic problems are more prone to occur with the more proximal fistulas. Some can be prevented by the avoidance of large-sized proximal anastomoses and by the use of end-of-vein-to-side-of-artery fistulas instead of the side-to-side variety with its associated "steal" phenomenon and retrograde venous hypertension. Occasionally it is necessary to close a fistula because of a serious complication.

The patient with a shunt or fistula may require dialysis two or three times a week for periods of 6 to 12 hours at a time, in preparation for transplantation.

In between dialyses he is maintained on a 2 gm sodium diet containing 30 to 50 gm of protein and 2000 to 3000 calories. In addition to the water content of the diet the patient is permitted a daily fluid intake of 600 ml plus an allowance equivalent to the previous day's urine output. Antihypertensive drug therapy may be necessary.

The recipient is managed on an outpatient basis until he is ready for transplantation, unless he requires admission for a preliminary operative procedure. Depending on circumstances he may require a gastric operation to control pre-existing peptic ulcer disease, a urological procedure to provide relief of lower urinary tract obstruction, parathyroidectomy for severe hyperparathyroidism, or bilateral nephrectomy. The last-named operation is performed if renal infection is present, as in pyelonephritis or congenital polycystic disease, for severe hypertension that cannot be controlled by dialysis and drugs, for progressive subacute glomerulonephritis, or for Goodpasture's syndrome. In these cases the nephrectomies may precede transplantation by several weeks or months. In the meantime the patient is maintained on regular hemodialysis as an outpatient.

Preoperative Preparation of the Living Donor

In our center approximately 60 per cent of renal transplants are obtained from related living donors. Whenever a patient becomes a candidate for transplantation, his family is contacted for possible volunteers, all of whom are fully informed about the procedure. Those wishing to proceed are screened by performing ABO blood grouping, HLA typing and the mixed lymphocyte culture (MLC) test. ABO incompatibility between the donor and the recipient automatically eliminates that volunteer.[95] The ideal donor-recipient combination is identical twins, but these are rarely available. The next best pairing involves siblings who have double haplotype identity on HLA typing. Favorable combinations can also be identified by the MLC test because grafts obtained from donors who are low stimulators have a good clinical course.[91] HLA typing is of limited predictive value in intrafamilial donor-recipient pairings other than those who show double haplotype identity. The decision about who is to be the donor under these circumstances is often made on social, vocational or general medical grounds. A substantial number of potential donors are rejected on the grounds of ABO histo-incompatibility, unsatisfactory general condition, psychological unsuitability, serious renal disorder or, in occasional instances, when the recipient's renal disease is of recognized familial type.

The selected individual is then thoroughly evaluated as to his general physical and mental condition and renal function.[78] After a full history and physical and mental evaluation, the volunteer undergoes the following tests: chest radiography, electrocardiography, full blood count, fasting blood sugar, two hour postprandial blood sugar, serum electrolytes, urinalysis, microscopic examinations of the urine, urine cultures, BUN, creatinine, creatinine clearance and intravenous pyelography.[78] Serum is also tested for the hepatitis B antigen to exclude a carrier state. Any positive reactors are excused as donors. Only if all the investigations are satisfactory is the patient subjected to the final test, abdominal aortography. This demonstrates whether single or multiple arteries supply the kidneys and whether there is any unsuspected disease involving these vessels. This examination permits the surgeon to choose a kidney that is supplied by a single artery or — if bilateral double renal arteries are present — the kidney with vessels that will be easiest to anastomose in the recipient. Slight abnormalities, such as atheromatous plaque at the origin of the renal artery, are not a contraindication to donation. The "abnormal" kidney is removed and transplanted to the recipient. Aortography provides protection to the donor, since serious but unsuspected disorders are sometimes present and contraindicate operation in that volunteer.[78] All studies on the donor can be performed on an outpatient basis. The donor is admitted to the hospital 24 to 48 hours prior to the transplant operation.

Postoperative Management

Postoperative Management of Living Donors

Most donors can be discharged from the hospital 7 to 10 days after the operation. They require little treatment at this stage and their convalescence is usually uneventful. Rarely, a patient may need outpatient care for a complication such as wound infection or persistent incisional pain. We have had no deaths among more than 450 living donors at our center. Very occasional fatalities (five in the author's knowledge) have occurred elsewhere.

Immediately following kidney donation renal function is halved. This situation improves rapidly, so that by the end of the first postoperative week the creatinine clearance reaches approximately 70 per cent of preoperative values. Thereafter there is little further change. None of our donors has developed postoperative renal insufficiency.[78]

Postoperative Management of Renal Homograft Recipients

Two aspects are important: (1) maintenance therapy with immunosuppressive drugs and other agents and (2) prevention and treatment of complications.

1. MAINTENANCE THERAPY. The average patient is discharged from the hospital three to five weeks after transplantation. Our immunosuppressive regimen consists of three agents: azathioprine (Imuran), prednisone and antilymphocyte globulin (ALG).[96] By the time the patient is discharged from the hospital he has completed a three to four week course of ALG therapy. We shall therefore not discuss the use of this agent in this chapter. At the time of discharge the dose of azathioprine is relatively stable but that of prednisone will require reduction in the ensuing weeks.

In our center azathioprine administration is commenced at 5 mg per kg and is then reduced to daily maintenance levels of 1.5 to 2.5 mg per kg. Dosage depends on the white blood cell count, which is initially made on a daily basis, but by the time the patient is discharged from the hospital it is performed once or twice a week and later, less frequently. We are guided more by sudden changes in the count than by the absolute number of cells. A sudden large drop is an indication for reduction in dosage or, if severe, for omission of the drug until the leukocytes have recovered. Daily counts are again performed until the downward trend has been reversed. If the level falls below 2000 cells per cu mm the patient should be admitted to the hospital and placed in reversed isolation because of the risk of serious infection.

During episodes of threatened rejection the dosage of azathioprine should not be increased, because the drug is partially excreted by the kidney and toxic levels may develop rapidly in the presence of impaired renal function.

We prefer instead to use larger doses of prednisone.

Another toxic effect of azathioprine is liver injury.[76, 95, 96, 114] Liver chemistry tests are therefore performed once a month for the first six months and, thereafter, every three months. Evidence of jaundice or serious alteration of liver function is an indication to hospitalize the patient for further investigation to exclude other possible causes, particularly hepatitis. If azathioprine is believed to be responsible, dosage is reduced or another immunosuppressive agent, such as cyclophosphamide, is substituted.[114]

Azathioprine may also have teratogenic effects. While animal studies have shown that it may cause fetal abnormalities,[35] the risk in man appears to be small. Thus far our male and female patients have been responsible for more than 59 live births, with congenital abnormalities in four of the offspring.[64] These abnormalities were relatively minor in two cases. In addition, there was a strong family history of spina bifida in one child who was born with a myelomeningocele.

Prednisone dosages vary from time to time. Currently we are using a schedule in which an adult patient initially receives 200 mg per day. The dosage is progressively reduced, so that by the time the patient is discharged from the hospital he receives 60 mg per day. About once a month thereafter the daily dose is reduced by 5 to 10 mg till a final maintenance level of 0.2 to 0.3 mg per kg per day or less is reached. Occasional patients have had their prednisone therapy discontinued permanently.

If threatened rejection occurs, it is managed by an increase in steroid dosage. We have used several different methods of treatment. One technique is to increase dosage to 100 or 200 mg per day and then to reduce the level progressively, provided of course that the rejection episode is satisfactorily aborted. An alternative method is to give 1 gm of methyl prednisolone intravenously as soon as rejection is suspected and to increase the daily maintenance dose of prednisone by 20 to 30 mg. If the rejection is severe the intravenous doses may be repeated daily, or every second or third day if necessary, until a total of three doses have been given. Thereafter, the daily prednisone dose is gradually reduced toward the original maintenance level. The large intravenous doses cause drastic reductions in the peripheral lymphocyte counts and are very useful in reversing severe rejection episodes.

The corticosteroids have many toxic side effects.[95, 96] In all transplant centers it has been noted that a large percentage of the morbidity following organ transplantation can be attributed to the use of these agents. Obesity is common, mainly because of the tremendously increased appetite engendered by the steroid therapy aided by relaxation of the dietary restrictions that the patient may have experienced for many months or years before the transplant operation. Moon face, acne, obesity and other manifestations of Cushing's syndrome are a source of considerable distress to some patients, particularly young females. Hypertension is another common problem that requires therapy and is discussed later in the chapter. Osteoporosis is a frequent complication of prolonged steroid administration and may cause pathological fractures. Avascular necrosis of bone (Figs. 24–12 and 24–13) occurs in 5 to 18 per cent of patients maintained on steroids for more than one year.[26] The joint most commonly involved is the hip, followed by the knee, ankle, shoulder, elbow and wrist. Once the disease process starts there is no evidence that reduction of steroid dosage, partial weight-bearing or other measures will retard or stop the pathological process. When pain or limitation of motion is severe, joint replacement is effective in restoring function and alleviating pain.

Steroid-induced diabetes mellitus is

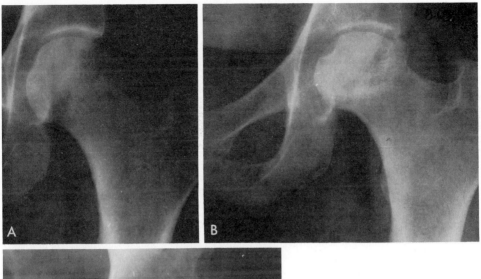

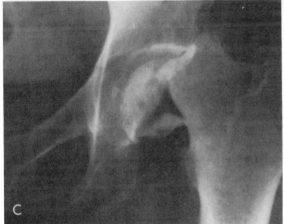

Figure 24–12 Pathologic fracture of head of femur. *A.* Normal appearance of left hip soon after transplantation. Radiograph taken during routine intravenous pyelography. *B.* Sixteen months post-transplantation. Aseptic necrosis of the head of the femur is present. *C.* Fifteen months later a pathologic fracture of the head of the femur is evident.

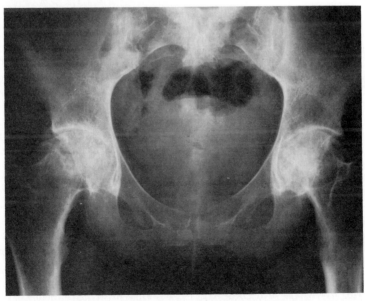

Figure 24–13 Bilateral aseptic necrosis of the femoral heads six years after renal transplantation. The condition had been present for several years at the time the radiographs were taken.

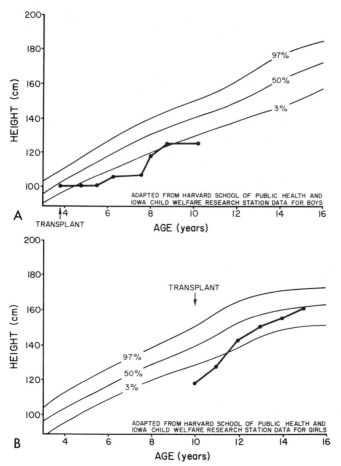

Figure 24–14 *A.* Height percentile growth curve of a three year old boy. At the time of renal transplantation he was in the 40th percentile. Although he grew 23 cm over the subsequent six and two-thirds years, growth rate was now subnormal and he is now below the third percentile. *B.* Height percentile growth curve in a ten year old girl who was far below the third percentile at the time of renal homotransplantation. She reached the 50th percentile five years after surgery. (By kind permission of the Editor, Pediatrics, 47, 548–557, 1971.)

looked for by periodic measurements of the fasting blood sugar and examination of the urine. Treatment includes reduction of prednisone dosage if possible, dietary restriction and administration of oral hypoglycemic agents or insulin if necessary. In many instances we have observed that when steroid therapy is reduced below a critical level the diabetes will resolve itself completely.

Large doses of prednisone in children may cause stunting of growth (Fig. 24–14). If steroid dosage is reduced below a critical level, normal growth is restored (Fig. 24–14).[59] Attempts have been made to reduce the incidence of this and other complications by the use of alternate-day steroid administration. Some workers

have reported satisfactory results, but many have encountered an increased incidence of rejection and have abandoned this approach.

The question as to whether or not steroids cause gastroduodenal ulceration is highly controversial.[21, 26] However, many surgeons are concerned about this risk. Our policy is to treat patients with known ulcers surgically before the transplant operation in order to avoid exacerbation of symptoms and complications such as perforation or gastrointestinal bleeding, which we encountered in 8 of 184 patients (4.3 per cent) who were studied.[75] After transplantation all patients are treated prophylactically with antacids. Initially these are administered every two hours, day and night. As the steroid dosage is reduced the frequency of antacid administration is decreased to every four to six hours during the day, with a double dose before retiring for the night.

The corticosteroids may also contribute to the high incidence of colonic complications observed in organ transplant recipients. Massive bleeding from ulceration may occur.[26] Perforation is seen in 2 to 4 per cent of patients[18] and may result from diverticular disease or occur spontaneously. Most perforations are in the left side of the colon. As with gastroduodenal perforation, the corticosteroids tend to mask the clinical features and cause delay in diagnosis. The mortality rate is high. Best results are obtained with resection or exteriorization of the perforated segment together with a proximal colostomy.[18]

Prednisone may also cause fatty infiltration of the liver. This may account for some of the abnormalities in hepatic function that occur postoperatively.[76, 114]

Psychiatric disorders, particularly depression and lethargy, may result from steroid therapy. In some cases a severe toxic psychosis may occur.[79] Symptoms improve with reduction in dosage.

Posterior subcapsular cataract formation is a common complication of steroid therapy and may be unilateral or bilateral. The incidence appears to be related to dosage and duration of administration. Treatment is symptomatic, but if visual acuity is severely impaired, cataract extraction may be necessary.

Pseudotumor cerebri, caused by brain edema and manifested by headache, nausea, vomiting, diplopia, drowsiness and stupor, occasionally occurs shortly after a change in steroid dosage.[26] Examination reveals bilateral papilledema, and the electroencephalogram is abnormal. The pressure of the cerebrospinal fluid is normal, as is the protein content, but computerized axial tomography may reveal an abnormal position of the ventricles. Treatment consists of an increase in the daily steroid dosage followed by a gradual reduction.

Other complications include pancreatitis,[81] an increased risk of pulmonary tuberculosis and a higher incidence of infection and disruption of operative incisions.[26]

Cyclophosphamide (Cytoxan) may be used instead of azathioprine as a part of the immunosuppressive regimen.[99, 100] It may be used on a long-term basis from the outset or as a short-term substitute for azathioprine in patients who have suffered toxic reactions, such as hepatic damage, from this agent. Cyclophosphamide is as potent and as safe as azathioprine when used in low doses in combination with prednisone and ALG. The incidence of side effects, including bone marrow depression, serious infection and gastrointestinal morbidity, is similar to that of azathioprine.

The dosage of cyclophosphamide in transplant patients is considerably less than that used in cancer chemotherapy, where it has a reputation of being very toxic. Complications such as anorexia, nausea, vomiting, diarrhea, alopecia and hemorrhagic cystitis either are uncommon or are not observed at all. The dosage of cyclophosphamide per body weight is about 40 per cent of that of azathioprine. When used from the outset, cyclophosphamide is given in a dose of 3 to 5 mg per kg, which is then reduced to a daily maintenance level of 1 mg per kg or less. Dosage depends on the white blood cell count, which is followed closely, as already described for azathioprine therapy. When cyclophosphamide is substituted for azathioprine at some stage in the patient's post-transplantation course, the initial dose is approximately two-thirds of the existing azathioprine level and is then adjusted according to the patient's white blood cell count.

Outpatient visits are initially made once or twice weekly following the patient's discharge from the hospital.

The intervals between clinic visits are then increased progressively so that patients may be seen once every 6 to 12 months. Recipients who are seen infrequently at our clinic have periodic checkups performed by their own physicians.

At each clinic visit the patient is questioned regarding any untoward symptoms. His weight, blood pressure, height (if a child) and temperature are recorded. The abdominal incisions and kidney homograft are examined and evidence of peripheral edema is sought. Further examinations are carried out as indicated by the patient's symptoms. A complete blood count is performed as a guide to therapy with azathioprine or cyclophosphamide. Adjustments in dosage of immunosuppressive agents and other drugs are made. Other studies include BUN, serum creatinine, creatinine clearance, urinalysis, microscopic examination of the urine, urine culture, and measurement of protein, urea, creatinine, sodium, potassium and chloride in a 24-hour specimen.[95] Liver function tests (bilirubin, SGOT, alkaline phosphatase, prothrombin time and serum protein electrophoresis) and tests for the hepatitis B antigen[76, 114] are performed every one to three months. An intravenous pyelogram is obtained once every 6 to 12 months or as indicated. Serum calcium, phosphorus, magnesium, amylase and fasting blood sugar measurements are obtained every one to three months or more frequently if necessary.

Chronic renal failure is almost always associated with parathyroid gland hyperactivity,[27] which may have important clinical sequelae in blood vessels and in bone. After uremia has been corrected by transplantation the hyperplastic parathyroid glands often will involute, although this may take a considerable time. Persistent hyperparathyroidism may contribute to the development of aseptic necrosis of the femoral head. A frequent cause of postoperative hypercalcemia is the use of phosphate-binding antacids. In many cases we have found that adjustment of the phosphate intake with the use of phosphate-containing compounds such as Phosphaljel (Wyeth) or K-Phos (Beach) will readily control the hypercalcemia.[4] In occasional patients with persistent hyperparathyroidism subtotal parathyroidectomy may be necessary.

2. PREVENTION AND TREATMENT OF COMPLICATIONS. The renal homograft recipient is liable to a great variety of complications. The most frequent problems are infection and rejection. The two conditions frequently occur together[98] and one may predispose to the other.

Acute Renal Homograft Rejection

This usually occurs within the first few weeks or months after transplantation. Rejection is usually recognized by evidence of deterioration of renal function or its effects[95] — albuminuria, reduced urinary output, elevated BUN, decreased creatinine clearance, sudden weight gain with peripheral edema, and hypertension. The patient complains of feeling out of sorts and may have fever and leukocytosis. The kidney is often enlarged and tender and there may be edema of the overlying skin. In severe cases the patient requires admission to the hospital for treatment, which can later be continued on an outpatient basis, while the less severe attacks can be treated wholly on an outpatient basis.

Chronic Rejection

Chronic rejection of a renal homograft manifests itself by a slow deterioration of renal function with elevation of the BUN and decline of the creatinine clearance. Albuminuria may become severe, with a loss of as much as 20 gm of albumin per day, and hypoproteinemia may ultimately develop. Marked hypertension is often present.

Attempts have been made to prevent this type of rejection using long-term anticoagulation and the administration of platelet deaggregators,[53] but the results have not been impressive. Furthermore, there is no effective treatment for the established condition. The patient should continue on immunosuppressive therapy as long as worthwhile renal function can be retained without serious hazard. As renal function fails, arrangements should be made for another renal homograft or for maintenance on permanent hemodialysis.

Infection

Infection is the most frequent complication of immunosuppression and is the most common cause of death in transplant recipients. Factors contributing to this problem include leukopenia (especially neutropenia), poor kidney function, hyperglycemia, high dose prednisone therapy and age over 40 years.[29] Immunosuppressive therapy reduces the patient's resistance to a wide variety of bacterial, fungal, viral and protozoal agents. The risk of infection is greatest when immunosuppression is at its height. This is usually at the time of threatened rejection of the organ. Any fever should be regarded with the greatest suspicion. A thorough physical examination should be performed and if no obvious cause is found, a chest radiograph, as well as cultures of throat, sputum, urine and blood, should be obtained. Mild to moderate fevers can be investigated on an outpatient basis, but if the patient obviously appears ill he should be hospitalized for investigation and treatment.

Common types of infection are herpes labialis and moniliasis involving the mouth and lips. These will usually respond to reduction in immunosuppressive dosage and to topical therapy with deoxyuridine or mycostatin, respectively. Occasionally, moni-

lial infection may spread to involve the pharynx, larynx or blood stream. Such cases will require admission for more intensive therapy.

Herpes zoster is another common infection. Most recipients with this disorder can be managed on an outpatient basis. However, if there is any suspicion that herpes is spreading, the patient should be hospitalized immediately for vigorous treatment, because disseminated herpes often has a fatal outcome.

Virus warts (verrucae vulgaris) occur in about 40 per cent of patients. Most involve the hands, but in several instances we have found extensive lesions on the scrotal skin. Large warts may require excision, not only for cosmetic reasons but also because they may be difficult to distinguish clinically from carcinoma, which has occurred in several of our patients (Fig. 24–15).

Bacteriuria has been reported in 40 to 80 per cent of recipients in several large series during the early post-transplantation period.[97] Most cases respond well to treatment with the appropriate antibacterial agent. Persistent urinary tract infections occur in 6 per cent of cases and may require prolonged therapy, particularly when caused by Proteus or Pseudomonas organisms. A possible mechanical cause for persistent infection should always be excluded.

Pneumonia is the most common of the more serious infections.[95, 98] A chest radiograph is therefore mandatory in any patient complaining of fever, breathlessness, cough or chest pain. Besides bacterial and viral pneumonias, fungal infections are by no means rare, as also is true of the pneumonia caused by the protozoon *Pneumocystis carinii*. The last-named condition frequently manifests itself by breathlessness. Physical examination of the chest is often normal but the diagnosis is suggested by cyanosis, a bilateral infiltrate in the lower lung fields (Fig. 24–16) and evidence of desaturation of the arterial

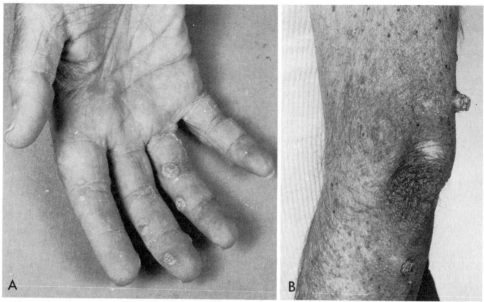

Figure 24-15 *A.* Multiple warts of right hand which appeared approximately one year after renal transplantation. Patient had numerous lesions on both upper extremities and face. *B.* Seventy-four months after transplantation the patient presented with the large lesions near the left elbow. The lower lesion was a squamous cell carcinoma while the upper was a wart. During the following year the patient had multiple lesions excised from the upper limbs and head. The majority were warts but in addition there were multiple squamous cell carcinomas.

blood. All patients with proven or suspected pneumonia should be hospitalized forthwith.

Infections of the central nervous system, causing meningitis or brain abscess, are not uncommon. Any patient who develops fever and neurological symptoms must be immediately admitted for investigation.

In our experience, wound infections are uncommon and most are superficial. Deep infections usually occur

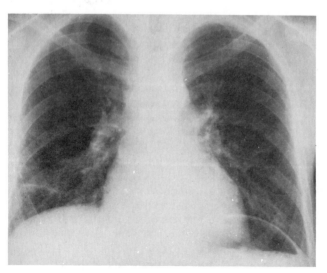

Figure 24-16 Chronic *Pneumocystis carinii* pneumonia in a 15 year old renal homograft recipient. The patient had breathlessness, cough and fever for many weeks. The linear density at the right base is the result of open pulmonary biopsy which was necessary to establish the diagnosis in this case.

while the patient is still hospitalized and may delay his dismissal considerably. After this occurs the wounds may still require repeated irrigation and dressing, and steroid dosage must be kept as low as possible to permit healing.

Performance of routine liver function tests has shown that 60 per cent of our patients have evidence of hepatic dysfunction at some stage of their postoperative course.[76, 96, 114] Most disturbances occur during the early months after transplantation and are usually mild and of short duration. Azathioprine, prednisone or other hepatotoxic drugs may be responsible for some of the changes, but at least half the cases are caused by virus hepatitis, including hepatitis A and B and cytomegalovirus. The infection is frequently low-grade but may be very persistent. The dangers of hepatitis are twofold. First, it may contribute to the patient's death. Second, it has the potential to spread to other patients and to the medical and nursing staff. Great care must be exercised when drawing blood samples or performing surgical procedures on individuals with hepatitis.

Cytomegalovirus infection is very frequent in transplant patients. In one series, evidence of clinical infection was found in 38 per cent of patients, manifesting as a prolonged fever, hepatitis, pneumonia or profound leukopenia.[89] Its effect on the white blood cells and the lung may predispose to fatal superinfections. In any unexplained febrile illness, evidence for this infection should be sought by viral isolation and demonstration of at least a fourfold rise in complement-fixing antibody.[89]

Fungal infections are also common in transplant patients.[8] These agents should always be sought for in the work-up of any patient suspected of having an infection. Besides Monilia, the more frequently encountered fungi are Aspergillus, Nocardia, Cryptococcus and Phycomycetes. While many patients with low-grade monilial or nocardial infections can be handled on an outpatient basis, all of the more severe infections require hospitalization.

Other Complications

A great variety of other complications are seen in renal transplant recipients. Only the more common ones will be mentioned here.

RENAL. In transplants between identical twins a high incidence of recurrence of the original disease has been described in patients who require transplantation for glomerulonephritis.[71] This has not been our experience in a small series of cases. Because preformed antiglomerular basement membrane antibodies and immune complexes have been implicated in the pathogenesis of the recurrent disease, prophylactic immunosuppressive therapy has been recommended in an attempt to prevent this complication.

In nontwin transplant recipients we have found a high incidence of glomerulonephritic changes.[98] Definite evidence of this disease was found in 47.6 per cent of 105 patients studied by conventional light microscopy, and another 21.9 per cent had more subtle findings detectable only by ultrastructural or immunofluorescent techniques. In approximately 22 per cent of the cases the pathological features were suggestive of recurrence of glomerulonephritis, but in the remainder they were probably manifestations of chronic rejection.[98]

UROLOGICAL. Urological complications have occurred in the transplanted kidney or ureter in approximately 10 per cent of our patients.[97] These include persistent urinary tract infections, ureteral stricture, ureteral calculus, hydronephrosis, compression of the ureter by a pelvic lymphocele (Fig. 24–17) and urinary fistulas. Apart from fistulas that occur early in the postoperative period while the patients are still hospitalized, the problems are usually recognized by studies performed at

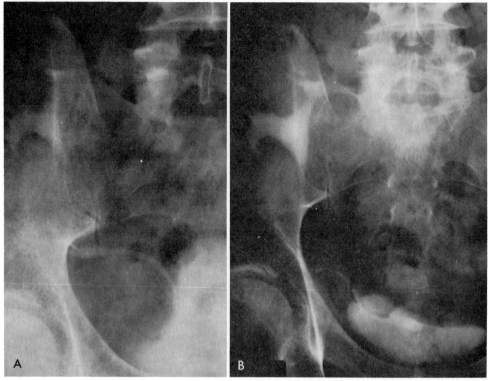

Figure 24–17 *A.* Marked upward and medial displacement of homograft ureter and compression of the bladder by a large lymphocele. This appeared within a few weeks of transplantation and persisted unchanged for many months without causing hydronephrosis. *B.* Intravenous pyelogram after surgical drainage of lymphocele two and a half years after transplantation showing marked improvement in the course of the ureter and absence of previous filling defect in the bladder outline.

routine outpatient follow-up visits. If the complications are mild, the patients are followed on an outpatient basis with urine cultures and serial intravenous pyelograms. Recipients with more severe lesions require admission to the hospital for corrective surgery.

Libido and potency are markedly decreased in male patients with end-stage renal failure. Following transplantation, the majority of recipients with satisfactorily functioning kidneys regain at least the pre-illness level of sexual function.[90] However, sexual impairment may persist in some, while in others it may develop for the first time after transplantation. We have occasionally seen patients who improved following reduction of steroid or hypertensive medication or following administration of testosterone. Whether these

therapeutic changes were responsible or whether psychological factors played a role is not known. In occasional patients it has been necessary to insert a penile prosthesis.

CARDIOVASCULAR. Hypertension is commonly seen in renal homograft recipients. We have observed this at some stage in at least 50 per cent of our patients. There are several possible causes for it, including acute rejection of the transplant, chronic rejection with thickening of the vascular endothelium and reduced blood flow, high dosage steroid therapy, stenosis at the arterial anastomosis or in the homograft artery, and persistent hypertension in patients whose own diseased kidneys have not been removed. The recipients are managed with a restricted sodium intake and the administration of one or more of the following antihypertensive drugs: hydrochlorothiazide, furosemide, propranolol hydrochloride, hydralazine, L-methyl dopa, and guanethidine. If the maximum therapeutic dose of one agent is unable to control the blood pressure, other drugs are added as necessary. Other aspects of treatment will vary with the cause of the hypertension. Acute rejection is usually reversed with increased immunosuppressive therapy. Blood pressure often decreases with reduced steroid dosage, but removal of the native kidneys occasionally may be necessary if severe hypertension persists despite drug therapy. Excision of a stenotic arterial segment is necessary in rare instances. Frequently it is possible to reduce or completely eliminate antihypertensive drug therapy as rejection episodes are reversed or steroid therapy is reduced. However, many patients must remain on antihypertensive drug therapy indefinitely.

There is an increased incidence of venous thromboembolism after transplantation. Possible causes include steroid therapy, an increased platelet count following splenectomy, thrombus formation at the renal vein anastomotic line, or stasis in the stumps of the host renal veins. Any complaint of calf pain or swelling, chest pain, breathlessness or fever requires thorough investigation. Except for patients with mild superficial thrombophlebitis, all suspected cases of thromboembolism should be admitted for treatment. Subsequent to discharge from the hospital, the patient is seen regularly as an outpatient to monitor long-term anticoagulant therapy and to prevent any sequelae of deep vein thrombosis of the legs.

Cardiovascular problems are more frequent in transplant patients than in people in the general population in the same age range. Atheroma is a striking feature of untreated uremia. Factors contributing to its are hypertension, hyperlipidemia, secondary hyperparathyroidism and possibly immunological processes.[32] The extent of arterial occlusive disease present before transplantation will determine the incidence of postoperative cardiovascular complications.[2] After transplantation, steroid-induced hyperlipidemia may compound the problem. Complications such as myocardial infarctions, strokes and peripheral vascular occlusions have been relatively uncommon in our experience but are frequently encountered in programs in which substantial numbers of diabetic patients undergo transplantation. In one series the incidence of myocardial infarction was 11 per cent in diabetic patients compared with 2 per cent in nondiabetic recipients.[74] Whereas no amputations were performed in a large number of nondiabetic patients, almost all of 132 diabetics had some peripheral vascular disease at the time of transplantation, and subsequent amputations of fingers, toes or legs were necessary in 32 recipients.[74]

MUSCULOSKELETAL. Most of the complications involving the musculoskeletal system are the result of steroid therapy. They include osteoporosis with vertebral collapse, pathological fractures and myopathy. Thirty-eight per cent of a group of our patients who were studied showed other evidence of connective tissue disorders, including avascular necrosis of bone, synovitis, arthralgia and diffuse musculoskeletal pain.[12] "Steroid pseudorheumatism" appears to be the underlying cause of many of these problems,[88, 94] but hyperparathyroidism may contribute to some of the osseous lesions. Bone and joint sepsis is rare, though hand infections are occasionally seen. Preexisting uremic neuropathy usually improves after successful transplantation, but recovery may be incomplete even after one year.[10]

GASTROINTESTINAL. Gastrointestinal complications are often the result of steroid therapy. As mentioned earlier, we try to prevent peptic ulceration with intensive antacid therapy. Despite this it is sometimes necessary to admit the patient to the hospital because of gastrointestinal bleeding or perforation of a peptic ulcer.[75]

Intestinal obstruction may be caused by adhesions resulting from previous intra-abdominal surgery and may require admission for treatment.[75]

Acute colitis occurs in from 0.9 to 3.8 per cent of transplant patients. It may result from acute ischemia or infection with staphylococcus, monilia or cytomegalovirus. Perforation of the colon and other colonic lesions are also observed following transplantation.[18, 77] These often require treatment on an inpatient basis.

Acute pancreatitis or pancreatic pseudocysts are occasionally encountered, usually early in the postoperative period. These lesions may be related to operative trauma during splenectomy and host nephrectomy, to high dosage steroid therapy, hyperparathyroidism, or azathioprine or chlorothiazide toxicity, may be associated with systemic infection, hepatitis or cytomegalovirus infection, or may be related to renal failure.[81]

Despite the young age of most of our patients we have seen less than half a dozen cases of acute appendicitis in more than 650 renal transplant recipients. For this reason we do not perform prophylactic appendectomy as has been advocated by some workers.[48]

OBSTETRICAL AND GYNECOLOGICAL. A gratifying feature of successful renal transplantation in most patients is the restoration of sexual function and the opportunity for parenthood, should this be desired. Females are advised against pregnancy during the first 18 to 24 months after operation to be certain that kidney function remains stable. Thus far, 25 of our patients have become pregnant on 35 occasions.[64] Twenty-two pregnancies resulted in live births, four are currently in progress, seven required abortions, one was an ectopic pregnancy and one terminated in a stillbirth. Frequent outpatient monitoring is necessary, because toxemia occurs in 32 per cent of the pa-

tients. In recipients with satisfactory pregestational renal function, we observed a few whose function deteriorated during pregnancy but returned to pre-existing levels in the postpartum period. Thus far, none of our patients has developed persistent renal functional impairment attributable to the pregnancy, although this has been described by other authors.[64]

There are also increased risks to the infant. Most of these occur early in the neonatal period, but occasional congenital defects may require outpatient management.

Dysplasia of the cervix uteri has been observed in female renal transplant recipients receiving immunosuppressive therapy.[42, 52] In addition, carcinoma of the cervix, usually *in situ*, has occurred in at least 32 patients, including three of our own recipients.[82] We therefore strongly believe that females should have a pelvic examination and vaginal smear before transplantation and at regular intervals thereafter. If a carcinoma of the cervix is detected, the patient should be admitted for definitive treatment.

The Problem of Malignancy

The use of immunosuppressive agents causes an increased risk of *de novo* malignancies and may enhance the growth of neoplasms inadvertently transplanted with kidneys taken from donors who have cancer.[80, 82] In our own series we have found an approximately 6 per cent risk of the development of *de novo* malignancies. We have collected data on 453 tumors that developed in 432 organ transplant recipients treated in centers all over the world.[82] The average period of time after transplantation for development of the lesions is 34 months. About 70 per cent are of epithelial origin (Fig. 24–15), most commonly carcinomas of the skin, lip or uterine cervix, but highly malignant carcinomas of the internal organs also occur. Solid lymphomas, mostly reticulum cell sarcomas, make up 23 per cent of the neoplasms, in contrast with a 3 per cent incidence in the general population. Whereas central nervous system involvement by lymphomas occurs in less than 2 per cent of patients in the general population, it occurs in 48 per cent of transplant recipients.

It is important to be aware of the danger of malignancy so that any unusual symptoms can be investigated promptly. Most of the patients will require admission to the hospital for appropriate therapy, but tumors of the skin or lip often can be treated on an outpatient basis with surgical excision, radiotherapy or topical chemotherapy. In addition, *in situ* carcinoma of the uterine cervix can sometimes be completely removed by performing a wide cone excision during a brief stay in the hospital.

Psychiatric Complications

The stress of a potentially fatal illness coupled with a major surgical procedure and prolonged postoperative care is associated with the development of psychiatric symptoms in 32 per cent of patients.[79] Episodes of anxiety and depression are common, particularly when complications mar the postoperative course. An organic psychosis may result from several causes, including large doses of steroids, infectious complications and poor renal function. The antihypertensive drugs may also cause psychological side effects. The patient often has adjustment difficulties, since a successful operation may convert him from a dependent status to one in which he must once again become independent and cope with life's problems. Occasional recipients who are unable to adjust may manifest suicidal tendencies. Those with the more severe psychiatric symptoms should be hospitalized for treatment. The other patients need assurance and guidance, and much can be accomplished in the Outpatient Clinic to help them deal with their problems and resume useful places in the community.

LIVER TRANSPLANTATION

Selection of Liver Recipients

Patients requiring liver transplantation are in the end stages of hepatic disease. Their life expectancy is a matter of days, weeks or perhaps a few months. The main indications[85, 86, 96, 101] for the operations are as follows: (1) congenital biliary atresia in cases in which no reconstructive surgery is possible, (2) chronic aggressive hepatitis, (3) alcoholic cirrhosis, (4) primary hepatic malignancies such as hepatoma, cholangiocarcinoma and hemangioendotheliosarcoma, which are too extensive to be treated by hepatic lobectomy, (5) liver-based metabolic disorders. Hepatic homografts retain their metabolic specificity after transfer to a new host.[96] Certain liver-based metabolic disorders might be treatable with hepatic replacement in patients who are severely incapacitated and cannot be treated adequately by more conservative measures. Thus far, patients with Wilson's disease, alpha$_1$-antitrypsin deficiency, tyrosinemia, and Niemann-Pick disease have been successfully treated. (6) Other benign hepatic diseases may be indications for transplantation. Prolonged survival has been achieved after liver replacement in patients with primary biliary cirrhosis and the Budd-Chiari syndrome. However, no long-term successes have yet been obtained in patients with acute liver failure from fulminant hepatitis or other toxic agents.

In the selection of patients for transplantation the criteria are similar to those used for renal recipients except, of course, that there is usually no concern about the status of the lower urinary tract. Candidacy for this formidable undertaking should be limited to those under 45 years of age. Investigations should be undertaken to exclude disorders involving other organs, particularly in children with biliary atresia, in whom other serious congenital anomalies may contraindicate transplantation. Efforts should be made to rule out metastases in patients with primary hepatic malignancies. Since no artificial support system comparable to hemodialysis is available to potential liver transplant recipients, their period of candidacy is necessarily much shorter than that of chronic renal failure patients. In consequence, a relaxation of criteria for donor-recipient selection is necessary if they are to be treated at all. If the patient's deteriorating condition warrants doing so, the standard immunological restrictions may be ignored, and an ABO-incompatible or cross-match positive organ may be inserted. Unlike renal transplantation, in which such action is likely to precipitate hyperacute rejection, the liver appears to be quite resistant to this immunological complication.[85, 86]

Preoperative Management

Many candidates for liver transplantation are so ill that they cannot be treated as outpatients. Those who can be managed on this basis require supportive therapy until a suitable donor can be found. Treatment includes dietetic control (protein and salt) to prevent hepatic coma and reduce ascites; the latter condition may also necessitate the administration of diuretics. If the patient is jaundiced and shows a tendency to hypoprothrombinemia, vitamin K is given parenterally. Severe itching may be ameliorated with cholestyramine. Gastrointestinal bleeding, hepatic pre-coma or serious infections will, of course, necessitate admission to the hospital. All infections, no matter how minor, must be eradicated as quickly as possible so that the patient is in the best possible condition to receive a transplant whenever a donor becomes available.

Postoperative Management

Maintenance Therapy

Because liver transplantation and the postoperative convalescence are much more complicated than renal transplantation, the patient is kept in the hospital for a longer time. After being discharged he is maintained on immunosuppression with azathioprine and prednisone, as described earlier in the chapter. Rejection is much less of a problem than after cadaveric renal transplantation so the daily doses of azathioprine are usually smaller (averaging 1.2 mg per kg).[17, 96] Antacids are also administered. Hypertension is rare after liver transplantation[96] but if present may require drug therapy. Usually there are no fluid or dietary restrictions.

The patient periodically attends the follow-up clinic where he is examined for signs of rejection or other complications. Liver function tests are performed, including serum bilirubin, alkaline phosphatase, SGOT, prothrombin time and serum protein electrophoresis. Hepatitis B antigen studies are done at regular intervals.[114] When indicated, liver scans are also made. The same hematological tests performed for renal homograft recipients are done, as well as urinalysis, BUN and creatinine clearance. Chest radiographs and cultures of the sputum, urine, throat, blood and stool are performed if there is any suspicion of infection.

Prevention and Treatment of Complications

Many of the complications described in renal recipients are seen also in hepatic homograft patients with the exception, of course, of most of the urinary tract complications and hypertension. The most frequent problems are infection, rejection, bile duct obstruction and recurrence of malignancy.

Infection

Hepatic homograft recipients are prone to any of the infections described under renal transplantation. Infection is a major cause of morbidity and mortality in these patients.

The homograft itself may be the site of infection. Viral hepatitis may occur, particularly if the indication for transplantation was hepatitis B antigen–positive liver disease.[86] Routine studies for this antigen are essential in establishing the diagnosis of recurrent hepatitis.[114] It is important to identify this disorder, because otherwise the associated clinical and biochemical changes may be misinterpreted as rejection, and immunosuppressive therapy may be intensified. Instead, the dosage level should be maintained or reduced to permit the host to control the infection. Satisfactory recovery of hepatic function may occur, although the patient may remain a chronic carrier of the antigen.

The liver is repeatedly exposed to enteric organisms, which reach it through the portal vein or the biliary passages. Infection is likely to occur during rejection episodes when the poorly functioning organ is unable to deal with portal bacteremia, and septicemia may occur. Ischemic areas in the liver may become colonized by gram-negative organisms with resultant abscess formation. A far more important cause of intrahepatic sepsis is infection superimposed on mechanical obstruction of the extrahepatic biliary system.[103] Twenty-four of 93 patients who underwent orthotopic liver transplantation developed this complication.[101] If this problem is suspected, the patient must be admitted to the hospital for transhepatic cholangiography and liver biopsy. Prompt surgical correction of the obstruction may be life-saving.

Rejection

Technical and mechanical problems, especially those of biliary duct reconstruction, and systemic infections are the major causes of death after liver transplantation.[17, 101] Surprisingly, rejection plays a relatively small role, accounting for less than 10 per cent of the deaths. Rejection is much less of a problem than after cadaveric renal transplantation.[17, 85, 86]

Acute rejection usually occurs in the early weeks after transplantation while the patient is still hospitalized, but occasional instances are seen in the Outpatient Clinic. The degree of rejection may vary from a mild anicteric episode to a severe rejection crisis. Mild rejection may be detectable only by elevation of the SGOT levels and by changes in the liver scan, but with severe rejection the patient may become seriously ill in a few hours.[96] Warning symptoms are anorexia, extreme fatigability, fever, pain in the back, nausea and vomiting. Fluid retention may be manifested by weight gain and periorbital and dependent edema. The liver is enlarged and tender and the patient may be frankly icteric. The serum bilirubin and alkaline phosphatase levels are increased and often there are elevations of the serum enzymes. Polymorphonuclear leukocytosis may be present. Radioisotope scans usually show enlargement of the homograft. Sometimes, however, the organ may be clinically enlarged but the scan shows a paradoxically small liver owing to reduced blood flow with consequent poor uptake of the isotope. Irregular filling defects may also be seen in areas of poor perfusion. All cases of suspected acute hepatic rejection should be admitted promptly to the hospital for treatment.

Chronic rejection occurs several months or years after transplantation. The clinical picture resembles obstructive jaundice, with elevation of serum bilirubin and alkaline phosphatase levels, dark urine and pale stools.[96] The condition results from gross narrowing of the arteries and arterioles within the liver, causing marked interference with blood flow, necrosis, collapse of lobules, cholestasis and, ultimately, fibrosis. Serial liver scans show a slow but steady shrinkage of the organ. Deterioration of liver function progresses relentlessly, and the eventual clinical picture is of chronic hepatic insufficiency with prominent abdominal wall collateral vessels, spider angiomata, peripheral edema and ascites.

In patients with severe, unrelenting rejection, whether acute or chronic, retransplantation is advisable rather than persisting with intensive immunosuppressive therapy in an attempt to prolong graft survival. Successful retransplantations have been performed on several occasions.[85, 86, 101]

The development of jaundice following successful transplantation does not necessarily indicate that rejection is responsible. Other important causes are biliary tract obstruction, viral hepatitis and liver cell damage from drugs, especially azathioprine.[85, 86, 101] Immediate diagnostic procedures are necessary, including serological testing for hepatitis B antigen, transhepatic cholangiography and liver biopsy. Unless the correct diagnosis is made the patient may be subjected to unnecessary increase in immunosuppressive therapy, which frequently is fatal. If the other causes are excluded and azathioprine hepatotoxicity is suspected, this agent should be discontinued and cyclophosphamide should be substituted.[101]

Recurrence of Malignancy

A disappointing feature of orthotopic liver transplantation performed for primary hepatic malignancies has been the high incidence of recurrent tumor. Of 38 patients followed for a minimum of two months and for periods of up to 88 months, 22 (58 per cent) died with recurrent or metastatic tumor.[83] The actual figure may prove to be higher, since several of the apparently tumor-free survivors have been followed only for a short time.

The most common sites of the lesions were the lungs and the homografts themselves, and they were recognized on serial chest radiographs and liver scans. In addition, serum α_1-fetoprotein levels remained persistently elevated in patients with hepatoma, suggesting the presence of residual tumor.

The high incidence of recurrent neoplasia has prompted some workers[85, 86, 101] to regard patients with large primary hepatic malignancies as highly questionable candidates for liver replacement. Exceptions are made if the tumor is an incidental finding in a liver afflicted with another disease and in young patients who have cholangiocarcinomas arising at the bifurcation of the hepatic ducts.[101]

HEART TRANSPLANTATION

Selection of Cardiac Recipients

In the selection of cardiac transplant recipients the cardinal rule is that the patient has terminal heart disease that is not amenable to any other surgical procedure or medical treatment. Since most heart disease is caused by coronary arteriosclerosis, this is the most common reason for cardiac transplantation.[22, 62] Cardiomyopathy is another indication[51] despite the theoretical danger that the immune factors responsible for the original disease could damage the homograft. Rheumatic multivalvular disease, although often correctable by valve replacement, may have caused such severe damage that cardiac transplantation is required. Severe congenital anomalies that are not amenable to surgical correction also warrant excision of the organ and its substitution by a healthy one.

Definite contraindications are infection, carcinoma and severe systemic disorders such as diabetes. Patients with multiple organ disease who are not expected to benefit from improved cardiac function should not undergo cardiac transplantation. Age over 50 to 55 years is a contraindication to transplantation, as is the presence of severe pulmonary hypertension.

Preoperative Management

Most potential recipients are so ill that they require hospitalization. A few can be managed as outpatients with supportive therapy, including digitalis, quinidine, diuretics and oxygen. All foci of infection should, of course, be eliminated as expeditiously as possible.

Postoperative Management

Maintenance Therapy

After discharge from the hospital the patient is initially seen twice a week and later at progressively increasing intervals. Immunosuppression is similar to that described for kidney transplantation, and the patients also receive antacid therapy. Besides the hematological, urinary and liver studies mentioned earlier, the cardiac status is evaluated by clinical and laboratory observations. Exercise tolerance is assessed from the history and by tests such as the Master two-step test and, if desired, by measurement of the cardiac output before and after exercise.[22] Serial electrocardiographs are a valuable guide to the diagnosis of acute rejection.[39, 62, 105] Ultrasound cardiography permits estimation of total heart size and chamber dimensions, as well as left ventricular wall thickness.[105] Other tests for rejection are serial measurements of the enzymes LDH, CPK and SGOT.

Acute rejection injury appears to be most intense in the subendocardium, particularly of the right ventricle. This can be diagnosed readily by endomyocardial biopsy[39] obtained by percutaneous introduction of a biopsy forceps through the right internal jugular vein into the apex of the right ventricle, from which several samples are removed. The procedure is performed under local anesthesia and can be repeated as often as is required. It is a relatively safe procedure.

Prevention and Treatment of Complications

As with transplantation of other organs the major problems are rejection and infection.[22, 62, 105]

ACUTE REJECTION. Decrease in exercise tolerance is a warning sign of impending rejection. Clinical findings in the early stages are the appearance or accentuation of a previously present pericardial friction rub and the development of abnormal diastolic heart sounds, usually an early diastolic gallop, although a presystolic gallop has also been noted.

The electrocardiogram serves as the primary index of acute rejection. Characteristic and reversible changes include decreased electrocardiographic voltage, atrial arrhythmias, rightward deviation of the mean electrical axis and ischemic type ST segment changes.[105] Ultrasound cardiography shows increased total heart and right ventricular chamber size, thickening of the left ventricular wall and variable decreases in the transverse diameter of the left ventricular cavity.[105] Changes in the levels of the enzymes LDH, CPK and SGOT unfortunately reflect the severity of the rejection process rather than provide an early warning system.[62] The introduction of endomyocardial biopsy has proved to be a major improvement in the management of acute rejection.[39]

Because there is danger of development of a sudden arrhythmia with potentially lethal consequences, all patients with suspected acute rejection should be hospitalized for treatment immediately.

CHRONIC REJECTION. This results from intimal thickening in the coronary arteries and their branches and has been responsible for many of the late deaths following transplantation.[22] It is postulated that the initiating event is immune injury to the intima, causing deposition of fibrin and platelets, followed by a process of proliferative repair. Infiltration of plasma lipids into the damaged area occurs, accentuating the inflammatory process and provoking additional intimal proliferation and formation of atheromatous plaques. Based on this hypothesis, some workers[39] advocate the chronic administration of the anticoagulant warfarin and the platelet deaggregator dipyridamole together with attempts to control the plasma lipids with a diet low in cholesterol and saturated fat and calorie restriction designed to maintain normal body weight. Annual coronary arteriography may be performed in all patients to assess the development of graft atherosclerosis. This program has proved remarkably successful in reducing the problem of coronary arteriosclerosis in the homograft.

Chronic rejection manifests itself by a progressive reduction in exercise tolerance and the development of cardiac failure, which requires the appropriate medications to keep it under control.

Cardiac retransplantation can be carried out successfully in the early postoperative period for severe acute rejection and also can be done later if the development of coronary atherosclerosis becomes life-threatening.[39]

LUNG TRANSPLANTATION

Selection of Pulmonary Recipients

The prime candidates for this procedure are patients who are gravely ill with primary pulmonary hypertension or restrictive lung disease.[25, 118] Unilateral transplantation in patients with chronic obstructive pulmonary disease has failed, largely owing to a serious ventilation-perfusion imbalance between the homograft and the host's residual lung. Attempts have been made to overcome this problem with bilateral lung replacement. Occasional transplants have also been performed for acute respiratory insufficiency caused by toxic pneumonitis or trauma.[118]

Preoperative Management

Most candidates are so ill that they are already in the hospital. Those few who are outpatients will require workup to exclude other serious nonpulmonary problems. Supportive pulmonary therapy is essential, and foci of sepsis must be eradicated, particularly in the lungs, or else there is a grave danger of cross-infection involving the transplanted organ.

Postoperative Management

Little can be said of postoperative care because thus far very few patients have survived long enough to be treated on an outpatient basis. Besides immunosuppressive therapy the patient needs careful clinical and radiological follow-up; with periodic studies of arterial blood gases and pulmonary function.

Acute rejection is heralded by general malaise, cough, dyspnea, fever, leukocytosis, the rapid appearance of an infiltrate on a chest roentgenogram, a decrease in arterial oxygen tension and, importantly, no change in the sputum bacteriology as determined by serial Gram stains.[116] Unfortunately, pneumonia has many of the same features, and it may be very difficult to distinguish between the two disorders.

PANCREATIC TRANSPLANTS

Selection of Pancreatic Recipients

Transplantation is indicated in patients with severe juvenile onset diabetes complicated by marked retinopathy and nephropathy.[57, 58] In many cases the kidney damage is so marked as to necessitate renal replacement at the same time as the pancreatic transplantation. However, the combined procedure greatly increases the risks in this particularly ill group of patients, and it has largely been abandoned in favor of staged procedures or even of pancreatic transplantation before renal failure has occured.[50] The transplants have consisted of the pancreas and duodenum (providing drainage of pancreatic exocrine secretions) or of the body and tail (either with ligation of the pancreatic duct or with anastomosis to the recipient ureter) or, more recently, of islet cell tissue isolated by enzymatic digestion of human cadaveric pancreases.[36, 37, 50, 73]

Preoperative Management

Preoperative care is the same as that already described for renal transplantation, with the additional problem of control of severe diabetes. There are difficulties in treating these patients with dialysis, which has a high morbidity and mortality.[57, 72] The extent of the vascular damage caused by the diabetes needs to be assessed carefully. Particular emphasis is placed on the elimination of septic foci.

Postoperative Management

Maintenance Therapy

After discharge from the hospital the patient's care is much the same as that already described for renal transplantation. If the pancreatic homograft is functioning satisfactorily the patient does not require insulin, and the fasting blood sugar and glucose tolerance tests are normal.

Additional follow-up studies include periodic measurements of the fasting blood sugar, glucose tolerance, blood insulin, amylase and lipase levels, and the effects of tolbutamide stimulation.[57, 110]

Prevention and Treatment of Complications

When the duodenum and kidney are transplanted along with the pancreas, more difficulties seem to arise from the other organs than from the pancreatic homograft itself. Whether this is due to technical factors or to a greater susceptibility of the duodenum and kidney to rejection is unknown.[36] Pancreatic rejection is infrequent but should be suspected by recurrence of diabetes or elevation of the serum amylase or lipase level.[57, 110] Threatened rejection of any of the transplanted organs is best handled on an inpatient basis. Other major problems are repeated infections and failure of the graft to reverse such complications as advanced retinopathy, peripheral neuropathy or atherosclerosis.[37] Patients are prone to vascular complications, including stroke and gangrene of the extremities necessitating amputation.

BONE MARROW TRANSPLANTATION

Selection of Bone Marrow Recipients

Bone marrow transplants are usually performed in patients who are seriously ill with one of the following disorders[115] that has failed to respond to other forms of treatment: (1) severe combined immune deficiency (SCID), (2) severe aplastic anemia and (3) chemotherapy-resistant acute leukemia. The aim of bone marrow replacement in SCID is to reconstitute the immune system and in aplastic anemia to repopulate all hemopoietic tissues. In leukemia the object is not only to restore depleted blood elements but to provide immunocompetent cells that, it is hoped, will destroy residual malignant cells that have persisted after other forms of therapy.

Preoperative Management

Preoperative donor work-up should exclude the possibility of transmittable infections or malignant disease. For successful bone marrow transplantation the ideal donor is an identical twin, as there is no need for immunosuppressive therapy in this case. Otherwise, a relative who is carefully matched for the ABO, Rh and HLA antigens should be used. The "one-way mixed lymphocyte culture test"[7] seems to be particularly useful in selecting well-matched combinations. In the absence of a familial volunteer, an unrelated donor — either living or cadaveric — may be used. However, at the present time almost all worthwhile long-term results have been obtained in transplants between ABO- and HLA-identical siblings.

Care of the recipient before admission to the hospital for the transplantation is purely supportive and depends on the condition being treated. It may include blood transfusions and antibiotic treatment of infections, which are common in these patients. Many recipients are so ill with severe anemia, granulocytopenia, thrombocytopenia or pancytopenia and associated complications that they must be hospitalized.

In marrow transplantation we try to obtain persistent immunological tolerance between donor and host cells. The immunosuppressive regimen is different from that used in transplantation of the other organs described previously. Before transplantation, patients with aplastic anemia are conditioned with large doses of cyclophosphamide or a combination of procarbazine, antithymocyte globulin (ATG) and cyclophosphamide or by total body irradiation.[107] Leukemia patients are conditioned with large doses of cyclophosphamide followed by total body

irradiation, or a combination chemotherapy-radiation regimen called SCARI (six-thioguanine, cyclophosphamide, arabinosyl cytosine, Rubidomycin and irradiation).[111, 112] SCID is unique in that there are virtually no immunological barriers, and therefore conditioning of the patient is not required.[115]

Postoperative Management

The donor needs no special treatment after discharge from the hospital.

Maintenance Therapy

A major problem after transplantation is the development of graft versus host disease (GVHD), a disorder in which immunologically competent donor cells become established and react to the host's tissues as if they were foreign. In order to prevent this complication, the immunosuppressive regimen after transplantation consists of methotrexate given on days 1, 3, 6 and 11 and weekly thereafter for 100 days.[107, 111] Thereafter all immunosuppressive therapy is discontinued.

Frequent outpatient hematological studies are necessary to establish that the grafted bone marrow is functioning and that a state of partial or complete chimerism has been established. The proliferation of the transfused cells is determined by means of erythrocyte or leukocyte antigenic markers, or both. Depending on the patient's condition, transfusion of whole blood or blood constituents such as platelets or granulocytes may still be necessary.

Prevention and Treatment of Complications

The most frequent problems are recurrence of leukemia, infection, failure of engraftment, and GVHD. Recurrence of leukemia occurs in 31 per cent of patients.[112] Attempts are being made to reduce this high incidence by more intensive antileukemic therapy before transplantation or by doing the graft at an earlier time when the leukemia cells are not resistant to therapeutic modalities, when the body burden of leukemia cells is minimal, and when the patient is in relatively good clinical condition.[111]

There is a high risk of fatal infectious complications because many patients already have impaired immune responses that may be further reduced by the immunosuppressive agents. These complications frequently are indications for hospitalization of the recipients.

Failure of engraftment is uncommon in SCID[115] and acute leukemia[112] but may occur in up to one-third of patients with aplastic anemia.[115] It is heralded by a disappearance of the initial symptomatic and hematological improvement. The patient may require admission because of hemorrhage or infection, and further transplantation attempts may be made.

GVHD is difficult to prevent and even more difficult to treat. It is clinically recognizable in approximately two-thirds of patients and is life-threatening in one-fifth.[111] The main organs affected are the intestines, the liver and the skin. GVHD causes an illness characterized by malaise, anorexia, diarrhea, malabsorption, weight loss, exfoliative dermatitis, jaundice and fever. It is usually associated with a severe immunological deficiency. Consequently, the usual terminal event is an infection by bacterial, viral or fungal opportunistic organisms.[111] The disorder may occur despite HLA identity,[38, 68] suggesting that antigenic differences must reside at as yet undetected non-HLA sites. GVHD occurs in two forms: an acute type that begins within a few days of transplantation and terminates either in early death of the host or in attenuation of reactivity and recovery within four to six weeks, and a chronic syndrome that occurs more than 30 days after transfusion.

Attempts have been made to prevent or minimize GVHD by using grafts of hemopoietic stem cells with as few lymphoid cells as possible.[5] Pretreatment of the recipient with ALG or preincubation of the bone marrow with ALG has also been attempted.[67, 115] Of greater importance is the finding that X and Y chromosome–associated transplantation antigen systems play an important role in GVHD, and therefore a donor of the same sex should be chosen whenever possible.[111, 112]

Treatment of GVHD is with ATG, high dose steroids or other immunosuppressive agents.

LONG-TERM RESULTS OF TRANSPLANTATION

In the early 1960's the world experience of human organ transplantation consisted of a small number of renal homograft recipients. Apart from transplantation between identical twins, the outlook was dismal and survival was for short periods only. During the intervening years the picture has changed dramatically, and long-term function has been achieved with kidney, liver, heart, pancreas, lung and bone marrow transplants. In consequence, an increasing number of organ recipients are being treated on an outpatient basis.

In interpreting the results of transplantation we must constantly bear in mind the fact that the patients are in the end stages of their various diseases. They are seriously or even gravely ill. Without transplantation their life expectancy is very brief.

Throughout the world more than 25,000 kidney transplants have been performed.[1] Based on a sample size of 19,631 patients with follow-up information, 68 per cent are currently alive and 45 per cent have functioning grafts. With identical twin transplants survival for as long as 21 years has been accomplished, with fraternal twins 18 years, with related donors more than 14½ years, and with nonrelated donors more than 13 years. Patient and graft survival are far superior when organs from related donors are used, as compared with those obtained from cadavers. In our series 52 per cent of the first group of patients are alive after 10 years, compared with 11 per cent in the latter category.[102] In our center over 800 kidney transplants have been performed. Approximately 65 per cent of the recipients are currently alive, with postoperative intervals ranging from several weeks to 14½ years; 60 of these patients have survived 10 years or more.

The world experience with liver transplantation is much less extensive. Approximately 275 transplants have been performed. The Denver series constitutes about 40 per cent of this total experience.[85] Thirty patients (29 per cent) have survived at least one year, with the more recent figures ranging up to 45 per cent. Half of all one-year survivors are still alive. Fifteen patients have reached the two-year mark, eight have reached three years, and four are five-year survivors. The longest survivor in our series (and in the world) is almost 9 years post-transplantation and has normal liver function. Long-term survival, including one patient who lived over five years, has also been obtained in the Cambridge University–King's College Hospital series.[17]

Heart transplants have been performed in 354 patients throughout the world.[1] Results have shown that the procedure can rehabilitate very ill patients with secondary effects on the lungs, liver and kidneys, restoring them to satisfactory health for months or years. Seventy grafts are currently functioning, and the longest survivor is more than 9 years post-transplantation.[1] The largest experience has been of the Stanford group, who performed 130 transplant procedures in 124 patients, of whom 48 are currently alive.[106] Survival rates for the entire series are 53 per cent at one year and 25 per cent at five years. The results have been steadily improving, and currently one-year survival is 66 per cent and the three-year figure is 58 per cent. Ninety per cent of patients surviving one year or more have been rehabilitated to functional Class I status.

Lung transplants involving the whole lung, one lobe, or both lungs and the heart have been performed in 37 patients.[1] There have been only two long-term survivors; they lived for 6 months and 10 months, respectively.

Fifty-one attempts at transplanting the whole gland or the distal segment of the pancreas have been reported.[50] Despite numerous technical problems, four patients have lived at least six months with functioning grafts. The longest survivor died recently almost 4½ years after transplantation.[37] At least 10 islet cell transplantation procedures have been attempted, but satisfactory long-term function has not been achieved thus far.[73]

Bone marrow transplants have been performed in at least 600 patients.[115] The Seattle group, with a very extensive experience, have 31 of 73 HLA-matched patients with aplastic anemia alive from eight months to five years after grafting.[111] Of their 100 HLA-matched patients with acute leukemia, 18 are currently alive. The longest disease-free survivor is now 6½ years post-transplantation. There are 15 leukemia-free patients in the United States who are more than two years post-transplantation and who have not been on any form of maintenance chemotherapy following transplantation. Of 69 patients with SCID 29 per cent are currently alive with a functioning graft 6 to 92 months after transplantation.[11] Many patients with SCID do not have HLA-matched donors to permit bone marrow transplantation. Transplants of fetal liver, fetal thymus or cultured thymic epithelium have been used in such recipients with partial or complete correction of the immunological deficiency.[47, 115] Successes with thymic grafts have also been achieved in other states of immune deficiency, including the DiGeorge syndrome (congenital thymic aplasia) and Swiss type agammaglobulinemia.[6, 20, 24]

At least eight patients have received splenic homografts for the treatment of terminal carcinoma,[65] Gaucher's disease,[40] agammaglobulinemia[65] and hemophilia.[46] The results thus far have been disappointing, with no evidence of survival of the transplant for more than a few weeks.

Apart from the pancreas, transplants of endocrine tissue are rarely indicated, since satisfactory replacement therapy is readily available. Occasionally, however, parathyroid homotransplantation has been performed in renal homograft recipients who underwent total or near-total parathyroidectomy prior to receipt of their kidneys and who developed severe hypoparathyroidism after good renal function was restored. The patients were already receiving immuno-suppressive therapy, rejection did not occur, and the grafts functioned satisfactorily for prolonged periods.[41, 117]

Transplantation of the larynx has been performed in one patient who had a total laryngectomy for carcinoma. He died of recurrent cancer 10 months later.[54]

Small bowel replacements have been performed in less than a dozen cases. The longest survival was two and a half months.

Transplants of other organs such as the ovary, testis and uterus are not being done, because the risks of current immunosuppressive therapy are not justified in the replacement of non-life-sustaining organs.

The field of organ transplantation is rapidly expanding. In the coming years we can anticipate greater numbers of long-term survivors who will require treatment on an outpatient basis. It is therefore important for the surgeon to be familiar with the handling of these patients.

REFERENCES

1. ACS-NIH Organ Transplant Registry Newsletter, January 1977.
2. Advisory Committee to the Renal Transplant Registry. The 13th report of the human renal transplant registry. Transplant. Proc., 9:9–26, 1977.
3. Ahmed, N., Di Scala, V., Nielsen, E., et al.: Brachial artery to brachial vein preserved vein allograft fistulas for hemodialysis. J. Cardiovasc. Surg., 17:483–488, 1976.
4. Alfrey, A., et al.: Resolution of hyperparathyroidism, renal osteodystrophy and metastatic calcification after renal homotransplantation. N. Engl. J. Med., 279:1349–1356, 1968.
5. Amato, D., et al.: Review of bone marrow transplants at the Ontario Cancer Institute. Transplant. Proc., 3:397–399, 1971.
6. August, C. S., Levey, R. H., Berkel, A. I., et al.: Establishment of immunological competence in a child with congenital thymic aplasia by a graft of fetal thymus. Lancet, 1:1080–1083, 1970.
7. Bach, F. H., and Voynow, N. K.: One way stimulation in mixed leukocyte cultures. Science, 153:545–547, 1966.
8. Bach, M. C., Sayhoun, A., Adler, J. L., et al.: High incidence of fungus infections in renal transplantation patients treated with antilymphocyte and conventional immunosuppression. Transplant. Proc., 5:549–553, 1973.
9. Beemer, R. K., and Hayes, J. F.: Hemodialysis using a mandril-grown graft. Trans. Am. Soc. Artif. Intern. Organs., 19:43, 1973.
10. Bolton, C. F., Baltzan, M. A., and Baltzan, R. B.: Effects of renal transplantation on uremic neuropathy. A clinical and electrophysiologic study. N. Engl. J. Med., 284:1170–1175, 1971.
11. Bortin, M. M., and Rimm, A. A.: Severe combined immunodeficiency disease: characterization of the disease and results of transplantation. Transplant. Proc., 9:169–170, 1977.
12. Bravo, J. F., Herman, J. H., and Smyth, C. J.: Musculoskeletal disorders after renal homotransplantation. A clinical and laboratory analysis of 60 cases. Ann. Intern. Med., 66:87–104, 1967.
13. Brescia, M. J., Cimino, J. E., Appel, K., et al.: Chronic hemodialysis using venipuncture and a surgically created arteriovenous fistula. N. Engl. J. Med., 275:1089–1092, 1966.
14. Buselmeier, T. J., Santiago, E. A., Simmons, R. L., et al.: Arteriovenous shunts for pediatric hemodialysis. Surgery, 70:638–646, 1971.

15. Butt, K. M. H., and Kountz, S. L.: A new vascular access for hemodialysis: the arterial jump graft. Surgery, 79:476–479, 1976.

16. Butt, K. M. H., Meyer, A., Kountz, S. L., et al.: Renal transplantation in patients with posterior urethral valves. J. Urol., 116:708–709, 1976.

17. Calne, R. Y.: The present status of liver transplantation. Transplant. Proc., 9:209–216, 1977.

18. Carson, S. D., Krom, R. A. F., Uchida, K., et al.: Proceedings of the Third Annual Meeting of the American Society of Transplant Surgeons, Chicago, Illinois, June 3–4, 1977.

19. Chatterjee, S. N., Payne, J. E., Bischell, M. D., et al.: Successful renal transplantation in patients positive for hepatitis B antigen. N. Engl. J. Med., 291:62–65, 1974.

20. Cleveland, W. W., Fogel, B. J., Brown, W. T., et al.: Foetal thymic transplant in a case of DiGeorge's syndrome. Lancet, 2:1211–1214, 1968.

21. Conn, H. O., and Blitzer, B. L.: Nonassociation of adrenocorticosteroid therapy and peptic ulcer. N. Engl. J. Med., 294:473–479, 1976.

22. Cooley, D. A., et al.: Cardiac replacement: current status of cardiac transplants and prostheses. Ann. Int. Med., 73:677–681, 1970.

23. Dagher, F., Gelber, R., Ramos, E., et al.: The use of basilic vein and brachial artery as an A-V fistula for long term dialysis. J. Surg. Res., 20:373–376, 1976.

24. Dekoning, J., et al.: Transplantation of bone marrow cells and fetal thymus in an infant with lymphopenic immunological deficiency. Lancet, 1:1223–1227, 1969.

25. Derom, F.: Current state of lung transplantation. Transplant. Proc., 3:313–317, 1971.

26. Diethelm, A. G.: Surgical management of complications of steroid therapy. Ann. Surg., 185:251–263, 1977.

27. Editorial: Hyperparathyroidism after renal transplantation. Lancet, 1:343–344, 1977.

28. Editorial: Long-term peritoneal dialysis. Lancet, 1:18–19, 1974.

29. Eickhoff, T. C., Olin, D. B., Anderson, R. J., et al.: Current problems and approaches to diagnosis of infection in renal transplant recipients. Transplant. Proc., 4:693–697, 1972.

30. Faris, T. D., Alfrey, A. C., Schorr, W. J., et al.: Lower extremity shunts for hemodialysis. J.A.M.A., 203:344–346, 1968.

31. Fine, R. N., Malekzadeh, M. H., Pennisi, A. J., et al.: HBs antigenemia in renal allograft recipients. Ann. Surg., 185:411–416, 1977.

32. Finn, R., Nichol, F. E., and Coates, P.: Im-

munological factors in accelerated atheroma associated with renal disease (letter to the editor). Lancet, 2:1141–1142, 1976.

33. Firlit, C. F.: Use of defunctionalized bladders in pediatric renal transplantation. J. Urol., 116:634–637, 1976.

34. Flores, L., Dunn, I., Frumkin, E., et al.: Dacron arteriovenous shunts for vascular access in hemodialysis. Trans. Am. Soc. Artif. Intern. Organs, 19:33, 1973.

35. Githens, J. H., Rosenkrantz, J. G., and Tunnock, S. M.: Teratogenic effects of azathioprine (Imuran). J. Pediatr., 66:959–961, 1965.

36. Gliedman, M. L., Tellis, V. A., Soberman, R., et al.: Long-term effects of pancreatic transplant function in patients with advanced juvenile onset diabetes. Proceedings of the Third Annual Meeting of the American Society of Transplant Surgeons, Chicago, Illinois, June 3–4, 1977.

37. Gliedman, M. L., Tellis, V., Soberman, R., et al.: Pancreatic transplantation. Transplant. Proc., 7:729–733, 1975.

38. Graw, R. G., Jr., et al.: Graft-versus-host reaction complicating HL-A matched bone marrow transplantation. Lancet, 2:1053, 1970.

39. Griepp, R. B., Stinson, E. B., Bieber, C. P., et al.: Increasing patient survival following heart transplantation. Transplant. Proc., 9:197–201, 1977.

40. Groth, C. G., et al.: Splenic transplantation in a case of Gaucher's disease. Lancet, 1:1260–1264, 1971.

51. Groth, C. G., Hammond, W. S., Iwatsuki, S., et al.: Survival of a homologous parathyroid implant in an immunosuppressed patient. Lancet, 1:1082–1085, 1973.

42. Gupta, P. K., Pinn, V. M., and Taft, P. D.: Cervical dysplasia associated with azathioprine (Imuran) therapy. Acta Cytol., 13:373–376, 1969.

43. Haimov, M.: Vascular access for hemodialysis. Surg. Gynecol. Obstet., 141:619–625, 1975.

44. Haimov, M., Baez, A., Neff, M., et al.: Complications of arteriovenous fistulas for hemodialysis. Arch. Surg., 110:708–712, 1975.

45. Haimov, M., Singer, A., and Schupak, E.: Access to blood vessels for hemodialysis: experience with 87 patients on chronic hemodialysis. Surgery, 69:884–889, 1971.

46. Hathaway, W. E., et al.: Attempted spleen transplant in classical hemophilia. Transplantation, 7:73–75, 1969.

47. Hong, R., Santosham, M., Schulte-Wissermann, H., et al.: Reconstitution of B and T lymphocyte function in severe combined immunodeficiency disease after transplantation with thymic epithelium. Lancet, 2:1270–1272, 1976.

48. Hume, D. M.: Progress in clinical renal

homotransplantation. *In* Welch, C. E., (ed.): Advances in Surgery, Vol. 2. Chicago, Year Book Medical Publishers, pp. 419–498, 1966.

49. Jenkins, A. M.: Gore-Tex: A new prosthesis for vascular access. Br. Med. J., 2:280, 1976.

50. Jonasson, O., Reynolds, W. A., Synder, G., et al.: Experimental and clinical therapy of diabetes by transplantation. Transplant. Proc., 9:223–232, 1977.

51. Kahn, D. R.: Human heart transplantation for cardiomyopathy. Surgery, 67:122–128, 1970.

52. Kay, S., Frable, W. J., and Hume, D. M.: Cervical dysplasia and cancer developing in women on immunosuppressive therapy for renal homotransplantation. Cancer, 26:1048–1052, 1970.

53. Kincaid-Smith, P.: Modification of the vascular lesion of rejection in cadaveric renal allografts by dipyridamole and anticoagulants. Lancet, 2:920–922, 1969.

54. Kluyskens, P., and Ringoir, S.: Follow-up of a human larynx transplantation. Laryngoscope, 80:1244–1250, 1970.

55. Lawton, R. L., and Sharzer, L. S.: Vascular access for patients on maintenance hemodialysis. Surg. Gynecol. Obstet., 135:279–283, 1972.

56. Levi, J., Robson, M., and Rosenfeld, J. B.: Septicemia and pulmonary embolism complicating use of arteriovenous fistula in maintenance hemodialysis. Lancet, 2:288–290, 1970.

57. Lillehei, R. C., et al.: Pancreatico-duodenal allotransplantation: experimental and clinical evidence. Ann. Surg., 172:405–436, 1970.

58. Lillehei, R. C., et al.: Current state of pancreatic allotransplantation. Transplant. Proc., 3:318–324, 1971.

59. Lilly, J. R., et al.: Renal transplantation in pediatric patients. Pediatrics, 47:548, 1971.

60. Lindsey, E. S., McDonald, J. C., Olivio, B., et al.: Popliteal-saphenous fistula for dialysis (abstract). Proc. Am. Soc. Artif. Intern. Organs. Boston, Mass., April 8–9, 1973.

61. London, W. T., Drew, J. S., Blumberg, B. S., et al.: Association of graft survival with host response to hepatitis B infection in patients with kidney transplants. N. Engl. J. Med., 296:241–244, 1977.

62. Lower, R. R., et al.: Current state of clinical heart transplantation. Transplant. Proc., 3:333–336, 1971.

63. Lytton, B., Goffinet, J. A., May, C. J., et al.: Experience with arteriovenous fistula in chronic hemodialysis. J. Urol., 104:512–517, 1970.

64. Makowski, E. L., and Penn, I.: Parenthood following renal transplantation. *In* De Al-varez, R. R. (ed.): The Kidney in Pregnancy. New York, John Wiley and Sons, 1976, pp. 215–227.

65. Marchioro, T. L., et al.: Splenic homotransplantation. Ann. N. Y. Acad. Sci., 120:626–651, 1964.

66. Markland, C., Kelly, W. D., Buselmeier, T., et al.: Renal transplantation into ileac urinary conduits. Transplant. Proc., 4:629–631, 1972.

67. Mathé, G., et al.: Bone marrow graft in man after conditioning by antilymphocytic serum. Transplant. Proc., 3:325–332, 1971.

68. Meuwissen, H. J., et al.: Graft-versus-host reactions in bone marrow transplantation. Transplant. Proc., 3:414–417, 1971.

69. Mindich, B., Silverman, M., Elguezabal, A., et al.: Umbilical vein fistula for vascular access in hemodialysis. Trans. Am. Soc. Artif. Intern. Organs, 21:273–279, 1975.

70. Morgan, A. P., and Bailey, G. L.: The transpalmar fistula for hemodialysis. Arch. Surg., 104:353–354, 1972.

71. Murray, J. E., and Harrison, J. H.: Surgical management of 50 patients with kidney transplants including 18 pairs of twins. Am. J. Surg., 105:205–218, 1963.

72. Najarian, J. S., Kjellstrand, C. M., and Simmons, R. L.: High-risk patients in renal transplantation. Transplant. Proc., 9:107–111, 1977.

73. Najarian, J. S., Sutherland, D. E. R., Matas, A. J., et al.: Human islet transplantation: a preliminary report. Transplant. Proc., 9:233–236, 1977.

74. Najarian, J. S., Sutherland, D. E. R., Simmons, R. L., et al.: Kidney transplantation for the uremic diabetic patient. Surg. Gynecol. Obstet., 144:682–690, 1977.

75. Penn, I., et al.: Surgically correctable intra-abdominal complications before and after renal homotransplantation. Ann. Surg., 168:865–870, 1968.

76. Penn, I., et al.: Hepatic disorders in renal homograft recipients. *In* Zuidema, G. D., and Skinner, D. B. (eds.): Current Topics in Surgical Research, Vol. 1. New York, Academic Press, 1969, pp. 67–76.

77. Penn, I., et al.: Major colonic problems in human homotransplant recipients. Arch. Surg., 100:61–66, 1970.

78. Penn, I., Halgrimson, C. G., Ogden, D., et al.: Use of living donors in kidney transplantation in man. Arch. Surg., 101:226–231, 1970.

79. Penn, I., Bunch, D., Olenik, D., et al.: Psychiatric experience with patients receiving renal and hepatic transplants. Semin. Psychiatry, 3:133–144, 1971.

80. Penn, I.: Malignant Tumors in Organ Transplant Recipients. New York, Springer-Verlag, 1970.

81. Penn, I., Durst, A. L., Machado, M., et al.:

Acute pancreatitis and hyperamylasemia in renal homograft recipients. Arch. Surg., 105:167–172, 1972.

82. Penn, I.: Development of cancer as a complication of clinical transplantation. Transplant. Proc., 9:1121–1127, 1977.

83. Penn, I.: Transplantation in patients with primary renal malignancies. Transplantation, 24:424–434, 1978.

84. Pirson, Y., Alexandre, G. P. J., and Van Ypersele de Strihou, C.: Long term effect of HBs antigenemia on patient survival after renal transplantation. N. Engl. J. Med., 296:194–196, 1977.

85. Putnam, C. W., Halgrimson, C. G., Koep, L., et al.: Progress in liver transplantation. World J. Surg., 1:165–175, 1977.

86. Putnam, C. W., and Starzl, T. E.: Transplantation of the liver. Surg. Clin. North Am., 57:361–373, 1977.

87. Quinton, W., Dillard, D., and Scribner, B. H.: Cannulation of blood vessels for prolonged hemodialysis. Trans. Am. Soc. Artif. Intern. Organs, 6:104, 1960.

88. Rotstein, J., and Good, R. A.: Steroid pseudorheumatism. Arch. Intern. Med., 99:545, 1957.

89. Rubin, R. H., Cosimi, A. B., Tolkoff-Rubin, N. E., et al.: Infectious disease syndromes due to cytomegalovirus (CMV) and their significance among renal transplant recipients. Proceedings of the Third Annual Meeting American Society of Transplant Surgeons. Chicago, Illinois, June 3–4, 1977.

90. Salvatierra, O., Jr., Fortmann, J. L., and Belzer, F. O.: Sexual function in males before and after renal transplantation. Urology, 5:64–66, 1975.

91. Segall, M., Bach, F. H., Bach, M. L., et al.: Correlation of MLC stimulation and clinical course in kidney transplants. Transplant. Proc., 7:41–43, 1975.

92. Shons, A. R., Simmons, R. L., Kjellstrand, C. M., et al.: Renal transplantation in patients with Australia antigenemia. Am. J. Surg., 128:699–701, 1974.

93. Simonian, S. J., Stuart, F. B., Hill, J. L., et al.: Conversion of a Scribner shunt to an arteriovenous fistula for chronic hemodialysis. Surgery, 82:448–451, 1977.

94. Slocumb, C. H.: Symposium on certain problems arising from clinical use of cortisone; rheumatic complaints during chronic hypercortisonism and syndromes during withdrawal of cortisone in rheumatic patients. Mayo Clin. Proc., 28:655, 1953.

95. Starzl, T. E.: Experience in Renal Transplantation. Philadelphia, W. B. Saunders Co., 1964.

96. Starzl, T. E.: Experience in Hepatic Transplantation. Philadelphia, W. B. Saunders Co., 1969.

97. Starzl, T. E., et al.: Urologic complications in 216 human recipients of renal transplants. Ann. Surg., 172:1–22, 1970.

98. Starzl, T. E., et al.: Long-term survival after renal transplantation in humans (with special reference to histocompatibility matching, thymectomy, homograft glomerulonephritis, heterologous ALG, and recipient malignancy). Ann. Surg., 172:437–472, 1970.

99. Starzl, T. E., et al.: Cyclophosphamide and human organ transplantation. Lancet, 1:70–74, 1971.

100. Starzl, T. E., et al.: Cyclophosphamide and whole organ transplantation in human beings. Surg. Gynecol. Obstet., 133:981–991, 1971.

101. Starzl, T. E., Porter, K. A., Putnam, C. W., et al.: Orthotopic liver transplantation in 93 patients. Surg. Gynecol. Obstet., 142:487–505, 1976.

102. Starzl, T. E., Weil, R., and Putnam, C. W.: Modern trends in kidney transplantation. Transplant. Proc., 9:1–8, 1977.

103. Starzl, T. E., Putnam, C. W., Hansbrough, J. F., et al.: Biliary complications after liver transplantation: with special reference to the biliary cast syndrome and techniques of secondary duct repair. Surgery, 81:212–221, 1977.

104. Stiller, C. R., Dossetor, J. B., Carpenter, C. B., et al.: Immunologic monitoring of the transplant recipient. Transplant. Proc., 9:1245–1254, 1977.

105. Stinson, E. B., Griepp, R. B., Dong, E., Jr., et al.: Results of human heart transplantation at Stanford University. Transplant. Proc., 3:337–342, 1971.

106. Stinson, E. B.: Personal communication, 1977.

107. Storb, R., Weiden, P. L., Prentice, R., et al.: Aplastic anemia (AA) treated by allogeneic marrow transplantation: the Seattle experience. Transplant. Proc., 9:181–185, 1977.

108. Storey, B. G., et al.: Embolic and ischemic complications after anastomosis of radial artery to cephalic vein. Surgery, 66:325–327, 1969.

109. Strom, T. B., and Merrill, J. P.: Hepatitis B, transfusions and renal transplantation (editorial). N. Engl. J. Med., 296:225–226, 1977.

110. Teixeira, E. D., and Bergan, J. J.: Auxiliary pancreas allografting. Arch. Surg., 95:65, 1967.

111. Thomas, E. D., Fefer, A., Buckner, C. D., et al.: Current status of bone marrow transplantation for aplastic anemia and acute leukemia. Blood, 49:671–681, 1977.

112. Thomas, E. D., Buckner, C. D., Banaji, M., et al.: One hundred patients with acute leukemia treated by chemotherapy, total body irradiation, and allogeneic marrow

transplantation. Blood, *49*:511–533, 1977.

113. Toledo-Pereyra, L. H., Kyriakides, G. K., Ma, K., et al.: Proximal radial artery–cephalic vein fistula hemodialysis. Arch. Surg., *112*:226–227, 1977.

114. Torisu, M., et al.: Immunosuppression, liver injury and hepatitis in renal, hepatic, and cardiac homograft recipients: with particular reference to the Australia antigen. Ann. Surg. *174*:620–639, 1971.

115. Van Bekkum, D. W.: Bone marrow transplantation. Transplant. Proc., 9:147–154, 1977.

116. Veith, F. J.: Lung transplantation. Transplant. Proc., 9:203–208, 1977.

117. Wells, S. A., Jr., Gunnells, J. C., Leslie, J. B., et al.: Transplantation of the parathyroid glands in man. Transplant. Proc., 9:241–243, 1977.

118. Wildevuur, C. R. H., and Benfield, J. R.: A review of 23 human lung transplantations by 20 surgeons. Ann. Thorac. Surg., 9:489–515, 1970.

119. Zincke, H., Hirche, B., Amanoo, D., et al.: The use of bovine carotid grafts for hemodialysis and hyperalimentation. Surg. Gynecol. Obstet., *139*:350–352, 1974.

Cancer Chemotherapy 25

NANCY S. SCHER, M.D.,
and GEORGE J. HILL, II, M.D.

INTRODUCTION

Cancer chemotherapy is, by the strictest definition, the treatment of cancer with drugs and hormones. However, the use of chemotherapy should not be separated from the total care of the cancer patient.[35] Chemotherapy should not be used as the primary modality of therapy if either surgery or radiation is more likely to be curative. Patients receiving chemotherapy should be considered for reoperation or radiation therapy if previously unfavorable tumors become correctible by local eradication.

The cancer chemotherapist must be an oncologist — a student of the biology of neoplasms. The oncologist understands the statistical likelihood of survival as related to type and stage of tumor and knows the relative efficacy of available therapeutic modalities. He or she is familiar with the common patterns of tumor growth and metastasis, but is always alert for unusual manifestations of malignant disease. The oncologist is a clinical pharmacologist, willing to test the effects of some of the most dangerous drugs used in medicine. He or she observes closely for objective and subjective effects of therapy on the patient and the tumor,[36] measures dose-related consequences of therapy, and watches for the unexpected, unfavorable idiosyncratic effects of chemotherapy. The oncologist is skilled in the age-old techniques of physic: offering comfort, relief of pain, control of anxiety, and — when appropriate — sensible prognostication.[2]

GOALS

The major goals of cancer chemotherapy are (1) cure, (2) palliation and (3) research. These goals are interrelated.

Cure

Recent advances in chemotherapy have resulted in long-term remissions and apparent cures in a significant percentage of patients with acute lymphocytic leukemia of childhood, Wilms' tumor, choriocarcinoma, Hodgkin's and non-Hodgkin's lymphomas and metastatic carcinoma of the testis. However, the common malignancies of adults, such as carcinoma of the lung, gastrointestinal tract and breast, are not sufficiently responsive to chemotherapy available at this time to be cured by this modality of therapy alone.

Palliation

A major effort of cancer chemotherapy is the palliation of patients who have incurable cancer. We define palliation as the prolongation of useful life. Successful palliation is not achieved if the life prolonged is spent solely in the hospital or if the patient is made sicker by chronic administration of chemotherapy than he would have been if left untreated. Thus, toxic symptoms should be avoided when possible, although in the palliation of malignancy the promise of significant long-term gains may warrant moderate short-term toxicity. When protocols of demonstrated significant benefit are available they should be followed closely, because courses of therapy with inadequate drug dosages may provide no palliation at all.

In addition to using antineoplastic drugs, the chemotherapist must be liberal in the administration of sedatives, tranquilizers and narcotics. When required, reassurance should be combined with honesty in answering patients' questions, and the therapist must give sound advice to patients regarding finances and the use of accumulated time for vacations and sick leave. Other aspects of palliation include dietary instructions, brief hospitalizations for administration of intravenous fluids, laxatives and enemas. Since much of the success in palliation is undoubtedly due to nonspecific aspects of patient care, restoration or preservation of useful life cannot always be related to objective effects of chemotherapy.

Although the initial course of chemotherapy may be administered to the patient in the hospital, most commonly employed chemotherapy regimens lend themselves to outpatient administration. If the patient's clinical condition permits, he should be treated as an outpatient so as to minimize the disruption of useful life and time away from his family. Hospitalization should be reserved for brief courses of intensive chemotherapy, diagnostic evaluation, treatment of intercurrent complications of disease and therapy, and for terminal care.

Prolongation of life per se is not regarded as palliation, and heroic efforts to add days or weeks of life are usually not indicated. On the other hand, if a life-endangering complication results from chemotherapy, aggressive management is usually indicated; this may include hospitalization, antibiotics, intravenous fluids and transfusions. Likewise, aggressive management may be indicated for patients who exhibit sudden, unexpected deterioration. Examples include perforated viscus, tension pneumothorax, hematuria, cardiac tamponade[37] or paraplegia. Hospitalization and surgery should be strongly considered in such cases. However, the approach may be mitigated by the prognosis and reasonable expectation that chemotherapy will provide significant palliation if the patient survives the acute problem. Prolongation of life per se may be indicated when the patient needs to attend to specific personal problems, such as religious, family or legal matters. In these cases the physician should consult closely with his or her colleagues in the legal, ministerial and social professions. The presence of nurses and students who are unfamiliar with the entire problem places a special burden on the physician, who must take time to explain the rationale of management to them.

Research

Each patient should be observed closely for indication of subjective or — preferably — objective signs of improvement. In the absence of objective improvement, the benefit from chemotherapy may be difficult to distinguish from the results of supportive or psychological therapy or from other forms of palliation such as surgery or radiation therapy. The individual patient is, in this sense, his own control; most patients accept this notion readily and participate willingly in the measurements, blood tests and x-rays that are required for evaluation.

Research begins with establishment of protocols and records. The use of a standard form (Fig. 25–1), commonly called a "flow sheet," for the summarization of data is valuable both for management of an individual patient and for study of groups of patients. The record is updated on each visit. Sketches and measurements of lesions on the patient and on the x-ray are recorded promptly, before they are lost or hidden in files. Graphs and tables of data are prepared frequently as a continuing guide to therapy and for demonstration purposes.

Inevitably, patients read or hear of "new" methods of therapy. The chemotherapist must be conversant with current developments in order to provide answers to questions from patients, relatives and other doctors. Whether or not he or she is a participant in formal research projects, the cancer chemotherapist will frequently be challenged to attempt unfamiliar or recently developed methods. He or she must approach this work with caution and objectivity, keeping careful records, consulting with colleagues and obtaining written, informed consent from patients. The chemotherapist must maintain a candid relationship with the patient and his family and utilize the scientific method in his or her clinical research.

SEG CHEMOTHERAPY FLOW SHEET FOR SOLID TUMORS

PATIENT'S NAME_____ PROTOCOL NO. _____

        LAST   FIRST   M.I.

ON STUDY DATE_____ DIAGNOSIS_____ M^2 _____

Instructions on Back

		DATE								If drug(s) not given or dosage changed, give reason		REMARKS
		Rx DAY OR WEEK								Rx Day/Wk Reason		
ANTI TUMOR DRUGS & DOSE		1.										
		2.										
		3.										
		4.										
		5.										
Tumor Location and size		6.										
		7.								Abnormality Due to:		
		8.								Toxicity / Disease / Unknown / Other		
		9. TRANSFUSION										
		10. WEIGHT (lbs. or kg)										
		11. TEMPERATURE (°F or °C)										
SPECIFY		12. LIVER	cm.									
		13. FLUID RETENTION*	0-4									
		14. FOOD INTAKE*	0-4									
		15. PERFORMANCE (Karnofsky)	%									
		16. PAIN*	0-4									
		17. NAUSEA & VOMITING*	0-4									
		18. DIARRHEA*	0-4									
		19. STOMATITIS*	0-4									
		20. INFECTION*	0-4									
SYMPTOMS:		21. BLEEDING*	0-4									
		22. SKIN*	0-4									
		23. HAIR*	0-4									
		24. NERVOUS SYSTEM*	0-4									
		25. RESPIRATORY*	0-4									
		26. RENAL*	0-4									
		27. CARDIAC*	0-3									
		28. HGB or HCT										
		29. WBC	x1000									
		30. GRANULOCYTES	x1000									
		31. LYMPHOCYTES	x1000									
		32. PLATELETS	x1000									
		33. SERUM ALBUMIN	gm/dl									
		34. GLOBULIN/TOTAL PRO	gm/dl									
		35. BUN/CREATININE	mg/dl									
		36. BILIRUBIN TOTAL OR D/I	mg/dl									
		37. SERUM CALCIUM	mg/dl									
LABORATORY		38. ALKALINE PHOS	IU/L									
		39. SGOT or SGPT (Circle One)	IU/L									
		40. CPK	IU/L									
		41. LDH	IU/L									
		42. URIC ACID	mg/dl									
		43. URINE PROTEIN										
		44. EKG										
		45. CHEST X-RAY										
		46. CREATINE CLEARANCE										
		47. OTHER										

PS-1540

Figure 25-1 Therapy record used by Southeastern Cancer Study Group (SEG). At each visit, blood counts, drug dosage and clinical findings are recorded.

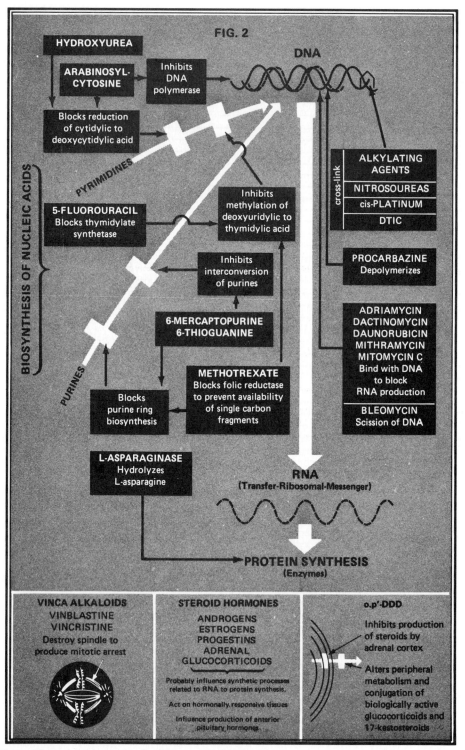

Figure 25–2 Inhibition of cellular growth by biochemical action of anticancer drugs. (From Krakoff, I. H.: Cancer chemotherapy agents. CA, 23:208–219, 1973.)

TABLE 25-1 Antimetabolites

CHEMICAL OR GENERIC NAME	COMMERCIAL OR OTHER NAME	ABBREVIATION	MECHANISM OF ACTION AND COMMENTS	FORMULATION	DOSE WHEN USED ALONE (APPROXIMATE)
5-Fluorouracil	Fluorouracil	5FU	Pyrimidine analogue. Inhibits thymidylate synthetase	500 mg vials	12–15 mg/kg IV per week or 12 mg/kg IV daily × 5 q. 5 weeks
6-Mercaptopurine	Purinethanol	6MP	Purine analogue. Competes with hypoxanthine and inosinic acid in DNA formation	50 mg tablets	50–150 mg PO daily
Methotrexate	Amethopterin. 4-amino-n[10] methyl pteroylglutamic acid	MTX	Folic acid analogue. Prevents methylation by inhibition of tetrahydrofolate reductase	2.5 mg tablets $\overline{5}$ and 50 mg vials	2.5 mg PO daily $\overline{25}$–50 mg/m^2 IV weekly
Cytosine arabinoside	Cytarabine, Cytosar	AraC	Ribose analogue. Blocks incorporation of normal purines and pyrimidines into DNA	100 mg and 500 mg vials	100 mg/m^2 IV continuous infusion daily × 5–7

THEORY

Several types of therapeutic agents are available that affect cells in different aspects of metabolism and replication[18, 19, 22, 41] (Fig. 25–2).

Antimetabolites

Antimetabolites are analogues of normal biochemical molecules that interfere with cellular metabolism and synthesis by competitive inhibition. The most commonly used antimetabolites are analogues of pyrimidines, purines and folic acid. Pyrimidines and purines are the nitrogenous bases from which the molecules of DNA and RNA are formed. Folic acid is a necessary coenzyme in reactions that incorporate carbon into DNA and amino acids. Examples of antimetabolites in common use are shown in Table 25–1.

Antimetabolites are, in general, "cycle-active" drugs and are potentially effective upon all cells that are in the S phase (DNA synthesis) of the cell cycle (Fig. 25–3). Cells in other phases of cell life are relatively protected from the effects of antimetabolites. Cells in the resting phase (G_0) or the postmitotic and premitotic phases (G_1 and G_2) are relatively insensitive to antimetabolites unless a residual concentration of the drug is present when the cell again enters the S phase. Since antimetabolites may also interfere with RNA synthesis, which occurs in the G phases, antineoplastic effect and drug toxicity are produced by the presence of residual concentrations of drugs. The emergence of drug-resistant cell populations occurs during prolonged therapy, a phenomenon that is shown in the clinical course of the patient in Figure 25–4.

In order to avoid the emergence of drug-resistant tumor cell populations, cycle-active drugs such as ara-C (cytosine arabinoside) have sometimes been utilized in brief, continuous

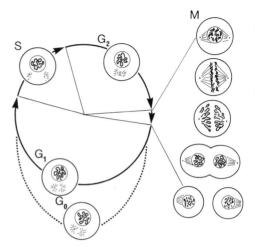

Figure 25–3   Cell cycle. Theoretical diagram of the cell cycle.*

Phase	Usual Duration
G_1–Postmitotic phase (Minimum resting phase) RNA and protein synthesis at normal rate DNA synthesis for repair only Rapid increase in RNA synthesis immediately prior to S phase	hours to days (usually constant for one cell line)
S – DNA synthetic period RNA and protein synthesis at normal rate DNA synthesis for replication	8–30 hours
G_2 – Premitotic phase RNA and protein synthesis at normal rate DNA synthesis stops	30–90 hours
M – Mitotic phase RNA and protein synthesis diminish abruptly Segregation of DNA into daughter cells	30–90 minutes
G_0 – Nondividing cells Cells which are in resting phase longer than the obligatory minimum period.	indefinite

*Adapted from De Vita, Vincent T. Cell kinetics and the chemotherapy of cancer. Cancer Chemotherapy Reports. Part 3, Vol. 2, No. 1:23–33, 1971.

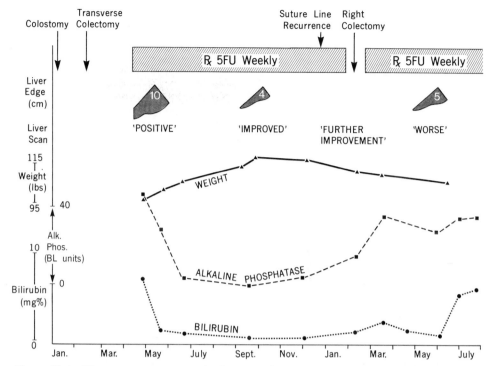

Figure 25–4 Therapeutic response and subsequent drug resistance. Treatment with antimetabolite 5FU produced initial improvement, followed by local tumor recurrence and subsequent deterioration in liver function. Resumption of chemotherapy again produced benefit, but only temporarily.

courses. Other efforts to avoid drug resistance in tumors have utilized drug combinations to reduce the populations of drug-resistant cells by simultaneous exposure to drugs with different mechanisms of action.

In practice, the use of antimetabolites is more often governed by empirical decisions than by theoretical considerations. Our basic knowledge of the rate of cell turnover, the percentage of resting cells, the percentage of drug-resistant cells, and optimum drug combinations is based mainly on work with transplantable mouse tumors and cultured cell lines. However, human tumors appear to be distressingly variable *in vivo*, and drug toxicity is a greater problem in humans than in mice. Strenuous efforts in the 1950s and 1960s using toxic courses of antimetabolites in solid tumors in humans resulted in a high mortality rate from toxicity and few cures — except in choriocarcinoma. In contrast, a surprisingly high percentage of responses and excellent palliation have been achieved by the use of antimetabolites in long-term, nontoxic therapy on a daily or weekly basis. A high percentage of cells in human tumors may be in the resting phase *in vivo*. If this is the case, long-term, low-dosage administration of antimetabolites would provide the best accessibility of the drug when DNA synthesis is begun by the resting tumor cells.

Alkylating Agents

Alkylating agents are drugs that add alkyl groups to molecules within the body. In the simplest sense, alkyl groups are methyl groups and straight-chain hydrocarbons. Many alkylating agents are complex chemicals that also contain aromatic rings and other atoms in addition to carbon and hydrogen. The most commonly used alkylating agents are shown in Table 25–2. The

TABLE 25-2 Alkylating Agents

Chemical or Generic Name	Commercial or Other Name	Abbreviation	Mechanism of Action and Comments	Formulation	Dose When Used Alone (Approximate)
Mustards					
Nitrogen mustard	Mechlorethamine Mustargen	HN2	Intense local irritant	10 mg vials	0.4 mg/kg in single or divided doses q. 3–4 weeks
Cyclophosphamide	Cytoxan		Phosphoric acid amide mustard. Inactive until enzymatic activation takes place	50 mg tablets 100, 200 and 500 mg vials	50–150 mg/day PO 10–15 mg/kg/wk IV 25–50 mg/kg IV q. 3–4 weeks
Chlorambucil	Leukeran		Aminophenylbutyric acid mustard	2 mg tablets	2–6 mg/day PO
Melphalan	Alkeran	L-PAM	L-phenylalanine mustard	2 mg tablets	2–4 mg/day PO 0.2 mg/kg/day × 5 q. 4–6 weeks
Nonmustards					
Triethylenethio-phosphoramide	ThioTEPA	TSPA	Relatively free of local irritating effects; nausea minimal compared with other alkylating agents	15 mg vials	Initial dose: 30 mg IV or 60 mg intracavitary. Subsequent doses individualized weekly.

BCNU; carmustine	BiCNU		Bone marrow suppression occurs at 4–6 weeks after administration of nitrosoureas.	100 mg vials	200 mg/m² IV q. 4–6 weeks
CCNU; lomustine	CeeNU		Cumulative marrow toxicity occurs with multiple courses of therapy with nitrosoureas	100 mg, 40 mg and 10 mg capsules	130 mg/m² PO q. 4–6 weeks
Methyl CCNU[a]				Capsules	200 mg/m² PO q. 4–6 weeks
Dimethyltriazeno-imidazole carbox-amide	Dacarbazine	DTIC, DIC	Alkylating and antimetabolite properties	200 mg vials	250 mg/m² IV daily × 5 q. 3 weeks
Cis-diamine-dichloroplatinum	Cis-platinum Cis-DDP		Renal toxicity is dose limiting. Severe nausea and vomiting. Ototoxicity and myelotoxicity.	10 mg vials	20 mg/m² IV daily × 5 q. 3 weeks or 50 mg/m² IV × 1 q. 3 weeks with appropriate diuresis

[a]Available for investigational use only.

alkylating agents first used were derivatives of mustard gas (sulfur mustard), a poison manufactured for military purposes. Nitrogen mustard (HN_2), a soluble mustard, was first used for cancer chemotherapy in 1946.[31] The symbol used for nitrogen mustard is apparent from its formula:

$$\downarrow \quad \quad \downarrow \quad \quad \quad \quad \quad \downarrow$$
$$H_3C—N—(CH_2—CH_2—Cl)_2$$

Nonmustard alkylating agents now in use include a phosphoramide (thio-TEPA) and busulfan (an ester of sulfonic acid). The drugs DTIC, *cis*-platinum, and the nitrosoureas are believed to function at least in part as alkylating agents. Alkylating agents are said to be "radiomimetic" because they induce cellular damage similar to that produced by ionizing radiation. The critical mechanism of action of these drugs is believed to be the cross-linking of DNA strands by an alkyl bridge between adjacent nitrogenous bases, leading to fracture or failure of separation of the strands during transcription.

Alkylating agents exhibit a phenomenon known as "log kill," which refers to the observation in animal tumors that a specific percentage of cells is killed by a given dose of drug, and the same percentage is killed each time the dose is repeated. This phenomenon may produce a cure if successive doses are administered until virtually no living cells are left, unless drug-resistant cells are present or toxicity precludes administration of the drug at sufficiently frequent intervals.

Inhibition of RNA Synthesis

The later phases of cell life may be summarized as transcription (formation of RNA), translation (protein synthesis) and cell division. RNA is a single-stranded molecule of nucleic acid formed along a pattern (template) of nuclear DNA. Three types of RNA are known: (1) messenger RNA (mRNA), along which the amino acids are assembled as the "message" of the genetic code is translated, (2) transfer RNA (tRNA), which is the intracellular carrier for individual amino acids, and (3) ribosomal RNA (rRNA), the function of which is still relatively obscure.

DNA-dependent RNA synthesis is blocked in sensitive cells by the antibiotics actinomycin D and mithramycin (Table 25–3), which are derivatives of Streptomyces species. Actinomycin D is highly toxic, even in small doses, but has a valuable therapeutic role in chemotherapy because it may eradicate all residual tumor in some instances — particularly in Wilms' tumor, choriocarcinoma, rhabdomyosarcoma and carcinoma of the testis. Kinetics analysis reveals a similarity to the "log kill" action of alkylating agents (Fig. 25–5).

Inhibition of Protein Formation

L-Asparaginase is an enzyme that hydrolyzes L-asparagine, an amino acid necessary for protein synthesis. Most normal cells are able to synthesize L-asparagine, whereas certain tumor cells are unable to do so and are sensitive to the drug. L-Asparaginase has been most effective in the therapy of childhood leukemia.

Mitotic Inhibitors

Cell division is arrested in metaphase by the plant alkaloids vinblastine and vincristine (Table 25–4). These complex molecules are derived from the periwinkle (*Vinca rosea* Linn.), a common garden plant used for ground cover. Like most other chemotherapeutic agents, the vinca alkaloids exhibit toxic effects on the marrow and gastrointestinal tract and also produce neurological toxicity that may be subtle in onset but of permanent consequence.

TABLE 25-3 Antitumor Antibiotics

Chemical or Generic Name	Commercial or Other Name	Mechanism of Action and Comments	Formulation	Dose When Used Alone (Approximate)
Adriamycin (doxorubicin)		Intercalating agent. High incidence of myocardiopathy above total dose of 550 mg/m²	10 mg vials	60 mg/m² IV q. 3-4 weeks
Bleomycin	Blenoxane	Causes scission of DNA. Total dose should not exceed 400 units because of incidence of pulmonary fibrosis	15 unit vial	15 units/m² IV or IM once or twice weekly
Mitomycin C	Mutamycin	Myelosuppression that may be cumulative	5 mg vials	20 mg/m² IV q. 6-8 weeks
Actinomycin D (dactinomycin)	Cosmegen	Blocks DNA-dependent RNA polymerase	0.5 mg vials	10-15 µg/kg/day IV × 5 q. month
Mithramycin (aureolic acid)	Mithricin	Inhibits RNA synthesis and causes hypocalcemia	2500 µg vials	50 µg/kg IV every other day for up to 8 doses 1 mg IV push once or twice weekly for treatment of hypercalcemia

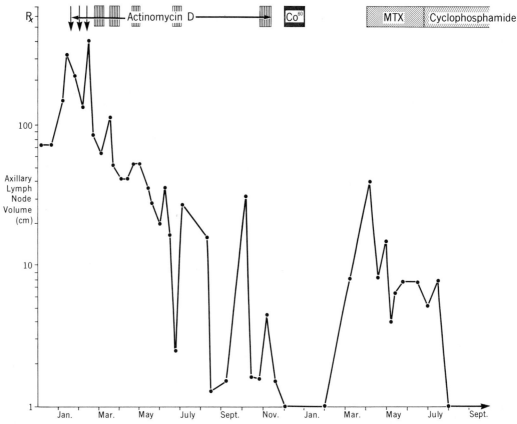

Figure 25–5 "Log kill" of tumor by chemotherapy. Logarithmic scale of tumor volume is used to illustrate percentage of cells killed by single doses and short courses of therapy. In this case, actinomycin D was used to treat metastatic rhabdomyosarcoma. Decrease in tumor volume from either 100 cc to 10 cc or 10 cc to 1 cc represents destruction of 90 per cent of tumor cells present.

Alteration of Hormonal Environment

Adrenal corticosteroids, natural or synthetic androgens, progestins, estrogens, and antiestrogens have an important role in cancer therapy (Table 25–4).

Many normal tissues and hormonally responsive tumor cells have cytoplasmic receptors for steroid hormones. The hormone forms a complex with the receptor. The complex is translocated to the cell nucleus, where RNA polymerase is induced, resulting in the formation of specific mRNAs that are translated into new proteins. These mediate specific hormonal effects by altering cellular metabolism.

The ability to measure estrogen receptor levels in tumor tissue has been a recent advance that makes possible a prediction of the likelihood of response of metastatic breast cancer to hormonal manipulation.[46] Up to 70 per cent of estrogen receptor-positive tumors will respond to endocrine therapy, whereas only 5 per cent of the receptor-negative tumors will respond. The importance of other steroid hormone receptors in predicting the therapy response of breast and other tumors is under investigation. Castration and androgens may be useful in premenopausal and perimenopausal women, while estrogens and synthetic antiestrogens may be of help in postmenopausal women with metastatic breast cancer. Progestational agents are used for carcinoma of the endometrium. Castration and estrogens are useful in metastatic prostatic carcinoma.

METHODS

Methods of Evaluation

Every possible effort should be made to obtain a record of the location and size of the tumor prior to starting chemotherapy, and observations should be made at regular intervals during therapy. A complete response is defined as the disappearance of any clinically detectable disease. A partial (objective) response is commonly defined as a 50 per cent or greater reduction in the product of the cross-sectional diameters of measurable lesions. Palpation, x-rays, photographs and radionuclide scans are the most common methods used for evaluation. A superficial lesion is more accurately measurable than a deep one. Lesions of 1.0 to 5.0 cm in size are particularly suitable for measurement. Chest x-ray usually provides more accurately measurable lesions than those seen on GI series, bone x-rays, IVPs or scans. However, any of these studies may be helpful in following specific lesions.

At the time of initial assessment and at regular intervals during therapy, the patient should also be evaluated as to his performance status. This is an index of the patient's overall level of function, a measure of the degree to which he is able to perform normal activities of life. Two classifications commonly used by oncologists to measure performance status are shown in Table 25–5.[1] Improvement of performance status in the symptomatic patient is an important goal of therapy. In addition, in many malignancies the performance status at the onset of treatment may be an important prognostic factor in terms of likelihood of response to chemotherapy.

One clinical classification system for the staging of cancer is the TNM classification developed by the American Joint Committee on Staging of Cancer.[1] It is hoped that this system will provide a uniform language to aid physicians to determine the most effective treatments and evaluate the results of management for given stages of disease. Tumors are described in terms of the size of the primary tumor (T) and the presence or absence of nodal (N) and distant metastases (M). Table 25–6 outlines the TNM system.

Chemistries should be done at regular intervals and may be helpful in monitoring the progression or regression of disease. Liver function tests are most commonly useful. Serum acid phosphatase level correlates with the response of prostatic cancer to therapy. Serum calcium value may be a guide to the healing of bone lesions or to the control of parathyroid carcinoma or medullary cancer of the thyroid; blood glucose level may be a guide in the management of retroperitoneal sarcoma or insulin-secreting tumors of the pancreas. Urinary excretion of hormones and their metabolites may be useful in following some tumors, such as trophoblastic tumors of men and women (chorionic gonadotrophin), metastatic carcinoid tumors (5-hydroxyindoleacetic acid), carcinoma of the adrenal gland (17-hydroxycorticosteroids and ketosteroids) and neuroblastoma (vanillylmandelic acid). Serum α-fetoprotein levels correlate with the mass of hepatoma present in some patients, and serum gastrin levels may be used to monitor the treatment of patients with metastatic Zollinger-Ellison tumors. Serum and urine levels of paraprotein may be followed in some patients with multiple myeloma. Urinary melanin excretion occasionally can be used to monitor the response to therapy in melanoma. Carcinoembryonic antigen (CEA) levels may be useful in following the response of colon carcinoma to therapy.

Toxicity

Rational management of the patient requires selection of an appropriate
Text continued on page 1283.

TABLE 25-4   Other Cancer Chemotherapeutic Agents

Chemical or Generic Name	Commercial or Other Name	Abbreviation	Mechanism of Action and Comments	Formulation	Dose When Used Alone (Approximate)
Vinca Alkaloids Vincristine	Oncovin	VCR	Mitotic inhibitor. Cell division blocked in metaphase. Neurotoxic	1 and 5 mg vials	1.4 mg/m²/week IV. Maximum single dose 2 mg.
Vinblastine	Velban	VLB	Same as above	10 mg vials	0.1–0.3 mg/kg/wk IV
Hormones and Hormonal Antagonists Cortisone acetate			Prolonged therapy with all corticosteroids will produce adrenal cortical atrophy. The use of ACTH should be considered when corticosteroid withdrawal is contemplated. Prolonged use at levels greater than physiologic equivalent doses will cause iatrogenic Cushing's syndrome and risk fatal reactions from peptic ulceration, pancreatitis, diabetes, hypertension, infections, fluid retention, hypokalemia and psychosis	5, 10 and 25 mg tablets 25 mg/cc, vials of 20 cc	25–37.5 mg/day for chronic replacement after adrenalectomy. 50–200 mg/day for leukemia therapy
Hydrocortisone sodium succinate	Solu-Cortef			100, 250, 500, and 1000 mg vials	300 mg IV/24 hr in continuous infusion for Addisonian crisis
Prednisone			Approximately 5 times as potent as cortisone	2.5 mg and 5 mg tablets	15–60 mg/day for responsive tumors, with dose reduced gradually as soon as possible
Prednisolone			Approximately 5 times as potent as cortisone	2.5 and 5 mg tablets	Same as prednisone
Methyl prednisolone	Medrol		Approximately 6 times as potent as cortisone	2.4 and 16 mg tablets	Same as prednisone

	Trade name		Description	Supplied	Dosage
Methyl prednisolone sodium succinate	Solu-Medrol		Approximately 6 times as potent as cortisone (for intravenous use)	40 mg in 1 cc vial; 125 mg in 2 cc vial	Same as prednisone
Methyl prednisolone acetate	Depo-Medrol		Approximately 6 times as potent as cortisone (for intramuscular or intra-articular injection)	40 mg/cc in 1 cc and 5 cc vials 20 mg/cc in 5 cc vials	Same as prednisone
Dexamethasone	Decadron		Approximately 33 times as potent as cortisone	0.25, 0.5, 0.75 and 1.5 mg tablets	0.75 to 16 mg PO/day to relieve signs and symptoms of cerebral tumors
Dexamethasone sodium phosphate	Decadron		Approximately 33 times as potent as cortisone (for intravenous use)	1 and 5 cc vials 4 mg/cc	3.0–6.0 mg IV for acute treatment of cerebral tumor signs
Fludrocortisone acetate	Florinef 9-α-fluorohydro-cortisone		Potent synthetic mineralocorticoid, used with cortisone in adrenal replacement therapy	0.1 mg tablets	0.1 mg every 1–2 days PO, with 25–37.5 mg cortisone daily, for adrenalectomized patients
Estrogens Diethylstilbestrol		DES	Synthetic estrogenic substance	0.1, 0.25, 0.5, 1.0 and 5 mg tablets	1 mg PO daily for prostate and 5–15 mg PO daily for breast cancer
Diethylstilbestrol phosphate	Stilphostrol		Synthetic injectable estrogenic substance. Used to test responsiveness of tumor to estrogen therapy	0.25 gm ampuls	0.5 gm in 300 ml N/S IV for 3 hrs; increase to 1 gm during next 4 days
Estradiol valerate	Delestrogen		Long-acting intramuscular preparation	10 mg/cc (1 and 5 cc vials) 20 mg/cc (1 and 5 cc syringes) 40 mg/cc (5 cc vials)	20–40 mg IM every 2–3 wks for elderly women with breast cancer
Chlorotrianisene	Tace		Long-acting oral estrogenic substance	12 and 25 mg tablets	12 or 25 mg per day for prostatic cancer

Table continued on following page.

TABLE 25–4 Other Cancer Chemotherapeutic Agents (*Continued*)

Chemical or Generic Name	Commercial or Other Name	Abbreviation	Mechanism of Action and Comments	Formulation	Dose When Used Alone (Approximate)
Estrogens, conjugated equine	Premarin		Injectable and oral preparations of natural equine estrogens	20 mg ampul and 1.25, 2.5, 0.625 and 0.3 mg tablets	Available for cautious trial in patients who do not tolerate synthetic estrogens
Androgens					
Testosterone ethanate	Delatestryl		Long-acting injectable androgen	200 mg/cc in 5 cc vials and 1 cc syringes	200 mg/2 weeks, IM for breast cancer in young women
Testosterone cyprionate	Depotestosterone		Long-acting injectable androgen	50 mg/cc (10 cc vials) 100 mg and 200 mg/cc (1 cc and 10 cc vials)	Same as above
Fluoxymesterone	Halotestin Ora-Testryl		Oral androgen, 5 times as potent as testosterone	2, 5 and 10 mg tablets	15–30 mg/day PO for breast cancer in young women
Progestins					
Hydroxy progesterone caproate	Delalutin		Synthetic injectable progestin	125 mg/cc (2 and 10 cc vials) 250 mg/cc (1 and 5 cc vials)	500–1000 mg IM twice a week for endometrial cancer or hypernephroma

Medroxyprogesterone acetate	Provera Depo-Provera	Synthetic progestin in oral and injectable forms	2.5 and 10 mg tablets 50 and 100 mg/cc in 1 cc and 5 cc vials	Doses are titrated by physician for endometrial cancer and hypernephroma. 500–1000 mg/wk is not unusual.
Megestrol acetate	Megace	Synthetic oral progestin	20 and 40 mg tablets	40–320 mg per day in divided dosage for breast and endometrial cancer
Antiestrogens Tamoxifen	Nolvadex	Nonsteroidal oral antiestrogen	10 mg tablets	10 mg b.i.d. for breast cancer
Miscellaneous Compounds *o,p'*-**DDD**	Mitotane, dichloro-dichloro-diphenyl-ethane, Lysodren	Destroys adrenal cortex	500 mg	2–10 gm/day
Procarbazine	Matulane	Alkylates and inhibits trans-methylation	50 mg tablets	100 mg/m² PO × 14 q. 4 weeks in MOPP regimen for Hodgkin's disease
Streptozotocin	Zanosar	Antibiotic with alkylating activity in the nitrosourea group	1 gm vials	500 mg/m² IV × 5 q. month for malignant pancreatic islet tumors
Hexamethylmelamine[a]		Active in ovarian, lung and breast cancers and lymphomas.	100 mg tablets	

[a] Available for investigational use only.

TABLE 25–5   Classifications of Performance Status*†

"PERFORMANCE STATUS" (KARNOFSKY SCALE)

Criteria of Performance Status (PS)

Able to carry on normal activity; no special care is needed	100	Normal; no complaints; no evidence of disease
	90	Able to carry on normal activity; minor signs or symptoms of disease
	80	Normal activity with effort; some signs or symptoms of disease
Unable to work; able to live at home and care for most personal needs; a varying amount of assistance is needed	70	Cares for self; unable to carry on normal activity or to do active work
	60	Requires occasional assistance but is able to care for most of his needs
	50	Requires considerable assistance and frequent medical care
Unable to care for self; requires equivalent of institutional or hospital care; disease may be progressing rapidly	40	Disabled; requires special care and assistance
	30	Severely disabled; hospitalization is indicated although death not imminent
	20	Very sick; hospitalization necessary; active supportive treatment is necessary
	10	Moribund, fatal processes progressing rapidly
	0	Dead

PERFORMANCE SCALE (PS) (ECOG)

Grade

0 – Fully active, able to carry on all predisease activities without restriction (Karnofsky 90–100)

1 – Restricted in physically strenuous activity but ambulatory and able to carry out work of a light or sedentary nature; for example, light housework, office work (Karnofsky 70–80)

2 – Ambulatory and capable of all self-care but unable to carry out any work activities. Up and about more than 50% of waking hours (Karnofsky 50–60)

3 – Capable of only limited self-care, confined to bed or chair more than 50% of waking hours (Karnofsky 30–40)

4 – Completely disabled. Can not carry on any self-care. Totally confined to bed or chair (Karnofsky 10–20)

*The ECOG/Zubrod scale and the Karnofsky scale are frequently used to record the physical state of the patients before treatment and at each subsequent examination.

†From: American Joint Committee for Cancer Staging and End-Results Reporting: Manual for Staging of Cancer 1977.

TABLE 25–6 The TNM Classification System for the Staging of Cancer*

Three capital letters are used to describe the extent of cancer

T	Primary tumor
N	Regional lymph nodes
M	Distant metastasis

Type of classification

c	Clinical-diagnostic
s	Surgical-evaluative
p	Postsurgical treatment-pathological
r	Retreatment
a	Autopsy

This classification is extended by the following designations:

TUMOR

TX	Tumor cannot be assessed
T0	No evidence of primary tumor
TIS	Carcinoma in situ
T1, T2, T3, T4	Progressive increase in tumor size and involvement

NODES

NX	Regional lymph nodes cannot be assessed clinically
N0	Regional lymph nodes not demonstrably abnormal
N1, N2, N3, N4	Increasing degrees of demonstrable abnormality of regional lymph nodes

METASTASIS

MX	Not assessed
M0	No (known) distant metastasis
M1	Distant metastasis present ____

*Developed by the American Joint Committee on Staging of Cancer.

drug and intelligent observation for both therapeutic benefit and toxicity. Most of the drugs used have toxic effects on both normal and neoplastic cells, so the clinician must be keenly aware of the toxic side effects of the drugs. In general, toxicity is greatest in cells of the hematopoietic system and the gastrointestinal tract, which are undergoing rapid turnover. Hepatic, renal, pulmonary and neurological complications are commonly observed from chemotherapeutic agents, and other organs occasionally show toxic manifestations during therapy. Toxicity may be difficult to distinguish from subtle or unusual aspects of progression of cancer, so it is occasionally necessary to discontinue chemotherapy to determine whether the patient is having a toxic reaction or whether the tumor is progressing. A common problem, for example, is nausea, which may be due to drug toxicity, cerebral metastases or progression of an intra-abdominal tumor.

Route of Administration

Cancer chemotherapeutic agents may be administered by a variety of routes. On an outpatient basis, the preferred methods are oral, intramuscular or intravenous "push." Less convenient (but often appropriate) methods are slow intravenous infusion, rapid injection into tubing of intravenous infusion, intracavitary injection (especially intrapleural and intraperitoneal) and chronic intra-arterial infusion. Direct injections into tumor nodules are occasionally performed.

Oral Therapy

This is clearly the most convenient mode of administration but obviously must be reserved for drugs that are satisfactorily absorbed via the gastrointestinal tract. Examples of drugs that may be given by the oral route include certain nitrosoureas, chlorambucil, procarbazine and cyclophosphamide.

Intramuscular

The intramuscular (IM) route is usually reserved for hormone injections or drugs such as bleomycin, methotrexate and thioTEPA, which are relatively free of reactions at the site of injection.

Intravenous

The intravenous (IV) "push" method refers to swift injection of the contents of a syringe. It is commonly used for drugs that have no serious immediate constitutional side effects when administered rapidly, and it is the most predictable mode of administration in terms of drug kinetics. Adriamycin, 5FU, methotrexate and the vinca alkaloids may be administered by the "push" method. A 23 gauge needle is suitable for most patients if the veins of the dorsum of the hand are used. Caution should be taken in intravenous "push" administration of adriamycin and the vinca alkaloids because extravasation will cause painful inflammation and tissue necrosis.

Slow intravenous infusion is recommended for large doses of cyclophosphamide (1000 mg or more). Patients who exhibit idiosyncratic syncope with "push" therapy often tolerate infusion therapy better.

Rapid injection into the side-arm of intravenous tubing of a well-running intravenous infusion is the recommended method of administering any cytotoxic drug that produces serious local reactions, such as HN_2 and actinomycin D.

Intracavitary

Intracavitary injections of thioTEPA and 5FU are easily performed in the Outpatient Clinic, and excellent palliation may be achieved with this method. The tolerable dosage of each drug is approximately doubled by using the intracavitary route, and the drug is thereby injected immediately adjacent to the tumor. However, the latter consideration may provide no definite advantage if the tumor is bulky.

Arterial Infusion

Infusions into the hepatic or external carotid artery have been used most commonly. Intra-arterial infusions are associated with a relatively high incidence of technical and toxic complica-

tions, so the method achieves greatest success when an experienced chemotherapist is managing the patient. Various devices may be used to maintain constant pressure. Our preference has been for the Fenwal system, utilizing a plastic bag filled with 1000 ml of glucose and water, plus desired amounts of heparin and the chemotherapeutic agent.[61] The bag containing the antineoplastic agent in solution is surrounded by an outer bag, in which pressure is regulated by a sphygmomanometer bulb and aneroid gauge. The rate of flow is maintained by a Hoffman screw clamp. An alternate method utilizes a constant infusion pump such as the USCI chroninfusor or the IVAC pump. Position of the catheter should be checked by injection of fluorescein or radiopaque dye at regular intervals, usually weekly. An alternative technique is "push" injection of drug once or twice a day, followed by injection of a concentrated solution of heparin (e.g., 10 ml physiological saline containing 5000 units of heparin).

DRUGS

Doses of drugs must be individualized carefully. Previous chemotherapy, especially with alkylating agents, or radiation therapy may limit tolerance to subsequent therapy. Doses should be based on ideal weight (Table 7–4) if ideal weight is less than actual weight. Blood counts should be checked frequently when therapy is initiated.

Antimetabolites

5-Fluorouracil (5FU, Fluorouracil)

5FU is a broad-spectrum pyrimidine analogue that is probably the antineoplastic agent most commonly used in treatment of solid tumors at the present time. It was synthesized in 1957[33] as an analogue of thymine. 5FU is activated *in vivo* to 5-fluorodeoxyuridine monophosphate, which inhibits thymidylate synthetase, a key enzyme in DNA synthesis. Another 5FU derivative, 5-fluorouridine monophosphate, may be incorporated into RNA, altering RNA synthesis and function, but this effect is of secondary importance to the inhibition of thymidylate synthetase.

5FU is useful in therapy of adenocarcinoma of the gastrointestinal tract, breast and ovary. It is occasionally helpful in the management of squamous carcinomas of the skin and oral cavity and carcinoma of the lung and prostate.

5FU is conjugated by the liver and excreted in part through the kidneys. However, it is remarkably well tolerated in the presence of deteriorating function in these organs and rarely is the cause of either renal or hepatic dysfunction. 5FU is primarily toxic to the hematopoietic system (predominantly polymorphonuclear leukocytes) and the gastrointestinal tract. It is rare to have a significant degree of thrombocytopenia occur in the absence of leukopenia. Serious gastrointestinal toxicity is usually preceded by nausea, vomiting, loose stools and stomatitis. Therefore, outpatient therapy can be regulated by observing the patient for mild GI toxicity and by maintaining a WBC of 3000 or more when the drug is given intravenously once a week.

5FU is relatively inexpensive in comparison with most other antineoplastic agents.

5FU is provided in ampules of 500 mg. The usual dose is approximately 12 to 15 mg per kg per week. The standard method of administration is "push" injection with a 23 gauge needle in a small vein of the hand or forearm. Therapy may be started with five daily doses of 500 mg each in patients with good general health, normal weight and normal bone marrow. Maintenance therapy is then given with 500 to 1000 mg per week. The drug is not absorbed reliably by the oral route, and this mode of administration is inferior to intravenous therapy.[12, 32, 60]

An alternative method for administration of 5FU is the use of monthly courses of therapy. Each course consists of 12 mg per kg per day IV for four to five days, at intervals of four to five weeks. Blood counts should be obtained mid-cycle for at least the initial course, and dosage should be adjusted downward when the WBC is less than 2000. The WBC should be normal before instituting the next course.

5FU topical formulations are available for treatment of multiple actinic keratoses. Efudex is prepared in 2 per cent and 5 per cent creams. Fluoroplex is supplied as a 1 per cent solution and a 1 per cent cream. 5FU solutions and creams are not recommended at present for chemotherapy of cancer, although their use in topical chemotherapy is now under investigation.

6-Mercaptopurine (6MP, Purinethol)

This drug is the most effective antineoplastic purine analogue, first used in 1952. Of the many sites of action of 6MP, the critical reaction is believed to be its competition with hypoxanthine and inosinic acid, which are converted to deoxyadenosine and deoxyguanosine diphosphates in the formation of DNA.

6MP and other purine analogues such as azathioprine (Imuran) and 6-thioguanine have potent immunosuppressive activity. For this reason caution is recommended when 6MP is used in chemotherapy, and the patient must be observed closely for acceleration in tumor growth. The most common use of 6MP at present is as one of a regimen of several drugs of maintenance of remission in childhood leukemia. Therapy is regulated by observation of white blood count, platelet count and symptomatic side effects, predominantly nausea.

Methotrexate (MTX, Amethopterin)

MTX is a broad-spectrum folic acid analogue closely related to the first antimetabolite (aminopterin) used in the chemotherapy of leukemia.

MTX is the only antifolate in common use at the present time. It is a potent inhibitor of dihydrofolate reductase, the enzyme that converts dihydrofolic acid to tetrahydrofolic acid. The latter is necessary for the synthesis of thymidylate, a precursor of DNA. Since the main action of MTX is to inhibit DNA synthesis, it affects only proliferative cells. For methotrexate to have a cytotoxic effect, it must reach an intracellular concentration greater than a certain threshold, which is variable for each tissue. The toxicity of the drug is a function of the duration of exposure to suprathreshold concentrations.[19]

A unique feature of MTX is the availability of an antidote, Leucovorin (5-formyl tetrahydrofolate), which can reverse the cytotoxicity of the drug if given promptly.

Methotrexate is useful in the treatment of choriocarcinoma,[34] head and neck cancer,[15] osteogenic sarcoma,[39] breast cancer[7] and other malignancies.

Methotrexate is excreted unchanged by the kidneys, and alteration in renal function causes profound alteration in MTX toxicity. It is generally advisable to require normal BUN and creatinine test results in patients before prescribing MTX, although very low doses may be used and increased cautiously in the presence of abnormal but stable renal function. The drug must not be continued in the presence of deteriorating renal function, whether due to intrinsic renal disease, obstruction or prerenal azotemia from dehydration (a common manifestation of drug toxicity). When conventional dosage schedules are employed, the usual toxic effects are myelosuppression, mucositis and gastrointestinal symptoms. MTX also produces chronic hepatic and pulmonary toxicity. Significant hepatic toxicity is usually associated with chronic oral administration[21] of the drug and may not be fully reversible. Pulmonary fibrosis from MTX is most commonly observed in children receiving long-term maintenance therapy for leukemia and has usually been reversible when detected in time. Since methotrexate has limited solubility in acid urine, high-dose regimens may be associated with precipitation of the drug in the renal tubules, resulting in acute renal toxicity, which in turn causes delayed drug excretion and may lead to fatal bone marrow toxicity.

Methotrexate is available in 50 mg and 5 mg vials and 2.5 mg tablets. Conventional dosage therapy is administered as a rapid IV "push" of 25 to 50 mg per m² once weekly. High-dose infusion regimens of 50 to 250 mg per kg over six hours followed by Leucovorin rescue, with concomitant diuresis and alkalinization of the patient's urine, should be used only by physicians experienced with this therapy. Methotrexate is also useful in the therapy of leukemic and carcinomatous meningitis when given intrathecally.

Cytosine Arabinoside (Ara-C, Cytarabine, Cytosar)[42]

Ara-C is an analogue of the normal cytidine nucleosides in which the five-carbon sugar arabinose is substituted for ribose. It is a cycle-active drug, blocking DNA formation through inhibition of DNA polymerase by the nucleotide derivative, arabinoside cytidine triphosphate. The drug is primarily useful in the treatment of acute leukemia. It is available in 100 mg and 500 mg vials. The usual mode of administration is continuous IV infusion of 100 mg per m² for five to seven days. Toxic effects include myelosuppression, nausea and vomiting, megaloblastosis and occasionally fever or hepatic toxicity.

Alkylating Agents

These drugs are radiomimetic and can cause cumulative bone marrow toxicity with loss of bone marrow reserve.

Mustards

NITROGEN MUSTARD (HN$_2$). Nitrogen mustard was the first synthetic drug used in cancer chemotherapy. It is employed in the chemotherapy of Hodgkin's disease in the MOPP regimen.[24] It is also useful in the management of malignant pleural effusion, where it exhibits specific antineoplastic cytotoxicity and acts as a sclerosing agent that obliterates the pleural space. HN$_2$ is highly irritating to tissues and should be used only after the manufacturer's brochure is studied thoroughly for guidelines regarding safety to patient and doctor. It is also unstable in solution and must be used as soon as possible after it has been dissolved.

The maximal dose of HN$_2$ is 0.4 mg per kg when given as a single intracavitary dose. However, the drug is absorbed systemically when given via this route, and caution must be exerted if other chemotherapy is to be given simultaneously.

CYCLOPHOSPHAMIDE (CYTOXAN).[30] Cyclophosphamide is one of many congeners (derivatives) of HN$_2$ that have been produced in the search for an improved therapeutic ratio. Cyclophosphamide is a cyclic phosphoric acid amide derivative of HN$_2$. It is hydrolyzed slowly in aqueous solution but is converted rapidly by liver enzymes to its active form. The drug is inactive until it has been metabolized, so both the acute toxicity and local side effects are much less than those of HN$_2$.

The usual toxic effects of cyclophosphamide include bone marrow depression, nausea and vomiting, and alopecia. Hemorrhagic cystitis is common owing to the excretion in the urine of cyclophosphamide metabolites, but it may be minimized by assuring adequate hydration. Sterility may occur with chronic therapy. Impairment of water excretion resembling the syndrome of inappropriate ADH secretion may occur occasionally. The massive doses used in conjunction with bone marrow transplantation rarely have been reported to cause fatal cardiac toxicity.

Cyclophosphamide is the most widely used of the alkylating agents at the present time. It is particularly effective in hematological malignancies and is frequently useful in the management of carcinoma of the ovary and breast and in neuroblastoma. It is of some use in palliation of carcinoma of the lung and sarcomas, particularly in combination with other drugs.

Cyclophosphamide may be given by mouth in tablet form (one to three tablets of 50 mg each per day) or intravenously in a higher intermittent dosage. The injectable form is provided in ampules of 100 mg, 200 mg and 500 mg. It must be dissolved in distilled water prior to use. Patience is required when it is used in a busy clinic, for it dissolves slowly, and a relatively large volume of water is required for making soluble the usual intravenous dose at the recommended concentration of 20 mg per ml.

CHLORAMBUCIL (LEUKERAN, AMINOPHENYLBUTYRIC ACID MUSTARD). The spectrum of action of this drug is similar to other alkylating agents, but it has the convenience of smaller doses required to produce similar responses and toxicity. The usual dose is 2 to 6 mg per day, the tablets being 2 mg each. It is useful in treating chronic lymphocytic leukemia, lymphomas and ovarian carcinoma.

MELPHALAN (ALKERAN, L-PHENYL-ALANINE MUSTARD, L-PAM). This mustard was one of many that were prepared to determine if selective incorporation in tumor cells would occur when natural amino acids were linked to alkylating groups. It was developed as a specific agent for the treatment of melanoma, since phenylalanine is the amino acid precursor of melanin. However, the spectrum of its activity appears similar to that of chlorambucil. It is commonly used with prednisone in the treatment of multiple myeloma and is also used to treat breast and ovarian carcinoma. The parenteral form remains under investigational use, and only the oral form is available for regular use on an outpatient basis.

The dose of melphalan is 2 to 4 mg per day in 2 mg tablets. It may be given in a high-dose, intermittent regimen of 0.20 mg per kg per day for five days every four to six weeks. Patients receiving prolonged therapy with melphalan may acquire increased bone marrow sensitivity to the drug and require a decrease in the maintenance dosage.

Nonmustard Alkylating Agents

TRIETHYLENETHIOPHOSPHORAMIDE (THIOTEPA). ThioTEPA is highly soluble, stable in solution, and causes relatively little systemic toxicity except pancytopenia. The ethylenimines similar to that of the mustards. ThioTEPA is no longer commonly used for systemic therapy of malignancies. However, it is occasionally instilled into body cavities for palliation of malignant pleural effusion and malignant ascites. In these circumstances the usual initial dosage would be 30 mg IV or IM or 60 mg intracavitarily for an average-sized adult with normal blood counts. The drug is absorbed from body cavities. Toxic effects include bone marrow depression (particularly thrombocytopenia), nausea and alopecia.

NITROSOUREAS. The nitrosoureas (BCNU, CCNU, methyl CCNU) are a relatively new class of drugs with alkylating activity. The chloroethyl moiety of the molecule has alkylating capacity, while the isocyonate portion is capable of carbomoylation of proteins and inhibition of repair of DNA. These drugs are highly lipid-soluble and therefore, unlike many chemotherapeutic drugs, can cross the blood-brain barrier. They are active in the therapy of malignant lymphomas, multiple myeloma, gastrointestinal carcinomas, malignant brain tumors, carcinoma of the lung and malignant melanoma.

BCNU (1,3-Bis[2-chloroethyl]-1-nitrosourea; carmustine), CCNU (1-[2-chloroethyl]-3-cycloheryl-1-nitrosourea; lomustine), and methyl CCNU (1-[2-chloroethyl]-3-[4-methyl-cyclohexyl]-1-nitrosourea) have similar toxic effects. They cause gastrointestinal toxicity, characterized by nausea and vomiting, and myelosuppression that is uniquely delayed, occurring three to five weeks after administration. Repeated administration results in cumulative bone marrow suppression, usually requiring a decrease in dosage after several courses of therapy. Because of the delayed marrow toxicity, the drugs in this class are usually administered at intervals of four to eight weeks.

BCNU is available in 100 mg vials as a powder that must be dissolved in absolute alcohol. It is further diluted in D5W or saline and then infused slowly because of local pain associated with administration. CCNU and methyl CCNU are both well absorbed by the oral route. Methyl CCNU is still investigational and not available for routine use.

DTIC (DIMETHYLTRIAZENOIMIDAZOLE CARBOXAMIDE; DACARBAZINE). DTIC has alkylating properties and may also function in part as an antimetabolite, since it is an analogue of a purine precursor, 5-aminoimidazole-4-carboxamide.

DTIC is the most active drug available against metastatic malignant melanoma.[43] The drug is also used, in combination, for therapy of disseminated sarcomas and Hodgkin's lymphoma.

The usual toxic effects include moderate leukopenia and thrombocytopenia and moderately severe nausea and vomiting. When the drug is given in the conventional five-day course every five weeks (250 mg per m² IV daily), patients frequently note less severe gastrointestinal toxicity during a given course after the initial few days of therapy. Some patients experience a flu-like syndrome as a minor toxic reaction.

The drug is supplied as a powder in 200 mg vials. It is easily dissolved in water but it is unstable in solution and must be used promptly.

CIS-PLATINUM (CIS-DIAMMINE-DICHLOROPLATINUM, CIS-DDP).[53] *Cis*-platinum is a new drug that is believed to have a mechanism of action similar to that of the alkylating agents. It has been very promising against a broad variety of solid tumors when used in combination with other drugs. It is active against cancer of the testis, ovary, bladder, lung, and head and neck.

Administration of the drug is associated with severe nausea and vomiting. It causes only modest myelotoxicity. Sequential audiograms may be indicated to evaluate ototoxicity that may occur. There have been reports of acute anaphylactoid reactions and neurotoxicity with *cis*-platinum. However, the major, dose-limiting toxicity is renal. Renal toxicity is dose-related and cumulative. Even with optimal administration technique, it is common to see a worsening of the creatinine clearance with repeated courses of chemotherapy. A variety of regimens are being evaluated that include saline and mannitol diuresis to limit the degree of renal toxicity.

Antibiotics

Anthracyclines (Adriamycin and Daunomycin)

Adriamycin (doxorubicin) and daunomycin (daunorubicin) are glycoside antibiotics, which differ chemically only by the presence of an extra hydroxyl radical on the former molecule. The drugs are believed to inhibit both DNA and RNA synthesis by intercalating the coils of DNA, causing it to uncoil partially. The cytotoxic action of the anthracyclines is maximal during the S phase of the cell cycle, but they are active during all phases.

Daunomycin is investigational and has been employed mainly in the treatment of acute leukemia. Adriamycin[6] has a broad spectrum of effectiveness and is used for therapy of lymphomas, breast carcinoma, soft-tissue sarcomas, and lung and thyroid carcinoma.

Toxic effects of the drug include myelosuppression, nausea or vomiting or both, stomatitis and alopecia. Cardiac toxicity, manifested by refractory congestive heart failure, is usually associated with high cumulative doses. The incidence of cardiomyopathy rises sharply with doses above 550 mg per m² to a frequency of 30 per cent.[6] For this reason the drug is discontinued when this dose range is reached, even in the absence of cardiac findings. There have been reports of clinically significant cardiotoxicity occurring within several weeks after a first or second course of therapy with anthracyclines.[9]

Adriamycin is available in 10 mg vials of powder, which is diluted prior to intravenous administration. Extravasation of the drug causes severe local tissue necrosis and must be scrupulously avoided. The usual dose is a 60 to 75 mg per m² IV push every three weeks when used as single-agent therapy, or 30 to 45 mg per m² when used in combination with other myelotoxic drugs. Some oncologists prefer to use lower-dose weekly therapy with adriamycin to avoid the episodes of severe toxicity that sometimes occur when the drug is given at three-week intervals. The usual weekly dose is 20 to 40 mg IV. Adriamycin must be used with caution and the dose modified in patients with liver dysfunction. Caution must also be used when the drug is given to patients who have had previous radiation therapy because of the ability of the anthracyclines to cause "recall" flares at sites of prior radiation damage.

Bleomycin

Bleomycin[19] is a mixture of polypeptide antibiotics derived from Streptomyces species. It causes scission of double-stranded DNA and is most active against cells that are proliferating, resulting in delayed progression through the G_2 and M phases of the cell cycle. It is useful in the treatment of lymphomas, squamous carcinomas and testicular carcinoma.

Bleomycin has minimal effect on bone marrow. Anaphylactoid reactions and febrile reactions have been reported, particularly in patients being treated for lymphomas. Its major sites of toxicity are the lung and skin. Cutaneous toxicity is manifested by induration and erythema of the fingers and hands and in areas of previous radiation therapy, with possible progression to desquamation. The major toxic effect is diffuse interstitial pulmonary fibrosis, which may be fatal. The incidence of this complication is increased above total doses of 400 mg, but it has been reported after total doses as low as 50 mg.

Bleomycin may be given as an intramuscular or intravenous injection of 15 mg per m² once or twice weekly. The drug is supplied in vials containing 15 mg (or units) of powder, which may be dissolved in saline or dextrose solution and administered over 10 minutes when given intravenously. Bleomycin has also been given as a continuous 24-hour infusion. In view of the incidence of anaphylactoid reactions, it is prudent, especially in patients with lymphoma, to give a one-unit test dose initially and then to observe the patient for 24 hours before giving a second five-unit test dose. After additional observation the regular therapeutic dose can be given.

Mitomycin C (Mutamycin)

Mitomycin C is an antibiotic derived from *Streptomyces caespitosus*. It inhibits DNA synthesis and may have a mechanism of action similar to that of alkylating agents.

It has some activity in gastric carcinoma and other malignancies. The usual toxic reactions are nausea or vomiting, or both, and severe myelosuppression, which may be cumulative. Stomatitis and alopecia may occur. Skin necrosis will occur if the drug is extravasated.

Mitomycin C is supplied in 5 mg vials as a powder that is reconstituted with sterile water. It may be given as 20 mg per m² in a single dose every six to eight weeks.

Actinomycin D (Dactinomycin)

Actinomycin D is believed to act by intercalation of adjacent DNA strands, thereby interfering with DNA-dependent RNA polymerase. It has an important role in the management of many neoplasms, such as choriocarcinoma, testicular tumors, sarcomas and Wilms' tumor.

The major toxic effects are myelosuppression, nausea or vomiting, or both, stomatitis, alopecia and chemical phlebitis. It will potentiate irradiation effects and should be used cautiously when the patient is receiving radiotherapy. It will cause severe soft-tissue damage if extravasated

The drug is supplied in ampules containing 0.5 mg of lyophylized powder. It must be mixed with sterile distilled water rather than sterile water containing preservative, for it will not dissolve well in the presence of the preservative. In adults, the usual dose is 10 to 15 μg per kg daily for five days, repeated at four to six week intervals.

Mithramycin (Mithricin)

This drug binds to DNA and also to metallic cations, inhibiting RNA synthesis and lowering serum calcium levels in many patients. It has a narrow spectrum of activity in human tumors, for it is effective in metastatic tumors of the testis but has remarkably little other antitumor activity.[11] It has been used in the treatment of hypercalcemia due to benign or malignant disease; the doses in this case are lower than the anticancer doses. The therapy of hypercalcemia is now its most important use, and other, more active drugs in combination are preferred for therapy of testicular tumors.

Severe coagulopathy has been reported in conjunction with the use of mithramycin at the usual doses for treatment of testicular carcinoma.

The drug is supplied in vials of 2500 µg, which are prepared by the addition of 4.9 ml of sterile water. The usual course of treatment for testicular tumors is 25 µg per kg per day for 10 days. The usual course for hypercalcemia is 1 mg IV push up to several times per week to maintain the desired serum calcium level.

Vinca Alkaloids – Vincristine (Oncovin) and Vinblastine (Velban)

The vinca alkaloids bind to the microtubular protein that makes up the mitotic spindle. The drugs are cell cycle–specific, causing metaphase arrest. Large doses can also kill cells in the S and G_1 phases. These drugs are employed in the therapy of leukemias, lymphomas, and lung, breast and testicular carcinomas.

The major toxic effect of vincristine is neurotoxicity, most commonly manifested by paresthesias, loss of deep tendon reflexes and constipation. Paralytic ileus may occur as a severe manifestation of autonomic nervous dysfunction. Alopecia and very mild bone marrow depression may occur. The dosage should be modified for patients with liver dysfunction, since the drug is to a large degree excreted in the bile. It may be given in a dose of 1.4 mg per m² IV push weekly, and 2.0 mg is the usual maximum single dose. It has a sclerosing effect if extravasated.

Significant neurological toxicity is much less common with vinblastine. The major toxic effect of the drug is bone marrow depression occurring at four to seven days. Other toxic effects include nausea, alopecia and sclerosing of tissue if extravasated. It is administered in a dose of 0.1 to 0.15 mg per kg weekly to a maximum of 0.3 mg per kg per week.

Hormonal Therapy

Corticosteroids

Adrenal corticosteroids are commonly used in cancer chemotherapy because of their profound effects on lymphocytes (lympholytic effect) and some therapeutic benefit in cancer of the breast. Corticosteroids are also required for replacement therapy (in the form of cortisone and Florinef) following surgical adrenalectomy or hypophysectomy and for control of symptoms and signs of primary or metastatic brain tumors (to reduce cerebral edema). Corticosteroids are occasionally used in therapy for other types of cancer and may produce good results in unexpected situations. Corticosteroids are also used in the management of hypercalcemia, superior vena cava syndrome, lymphangitic tumor spread in the lungs, fever due to necrotic tumor, and Addison's disease due to metastases in the adrenal glands.[38] Considerable palliation is sometimes produced by the euphoric side effect of corticosteroids, though generally this is better sought through the use of tranquilizers and mood elevators.

Prednisone, prednisolone and methyl prednisolone are probably the most commonly used corticosteroids in cancer chemotherapy. They have an excellent spectrum of the desired antineoplastic effects while causing relatively less retention of salt and water than that produced by cortisone or hydrocortisone. Cortisone, hydrocortisone and methyl prednisolone may be given either by mouth or by parenteral injection. In cancer chemotherapy, these agents are usually used for adrenal replacement or suppression. Dexamethasone (Decadron) is used for reduction of cerebral edema, particularly in patients with known or suspected brain tumors. Fludrocortisone acetate (9α-fluorohydrocortisone; Florinef) is used as an adjunct to cortisone in the treatment of adrenal insufficiency because it produces retention of sodium and chloride.

The dose of an adrenal corticosteroid hormone should always be the minimum dose required to produce the desired effect. Frequently, the initial dose is larger than the maintenance dosage in order to determine if an effect will be achieved or because a therapeutic emergency exists. Since the side effects initially are subtle, the dosage may be maintained inadvertently at an excessively high level, but the chemotherapist must be aware of the devastating, life-endangering complications that result from high doses of corticosteroids. The most common dangerous complications include activation of peptic ulcer and massive GI bleeding, immunosuppression with septicemia — an especially common phenomenon in patients with lymphomas and lymphatic leukemia — and iatrogenic, drug-induced Addison's disease. Also observed are: diabetes, hypertension, activation of tuberculosis, osteoporosis and psychosis. The equivalent dosage of various corticosteroids may be estimated from the relationship described in the formula:

For the initial management of the addisonian patient, intravenous hydrocortisone is begun at a rate of 300 mg per day, or higher if septicemia is suspected. Cortisone maintenance therapy for the adrenalectomy patient is usually sufficient at 37.5 mg per day, but some patients will require 50 mg and some are managed well with 25 mg per day. Florinef is administered in doses of 0.1 mg every one to two days. Therapy with prednisone (and its 1–2 dehydroanalogues, prednisolone and methylprednisolone) is usually initiated with doses of 25 to 100 mg per day and then tapered as quickly as possible to a level that provides satisfactory maintenance therapy. We find that 45 mg per day for one week provides a convenient test of prednisone therapy in most patients (three tablets, three times per day). The dosage may be increased, but substantial benefit in cancer chemotherapy is usually not seen at higher doses if no benefit is seen at the 45 mg daily dose. A convenient tapering routine is 30 mg per day for two weeks followed by 15 mg per day for maintenance therapy. Dexamethasone at 16 mg per day in divided dosage is employed for short-term relief of symptoms and signs of increased intracerebral pressure due to tumor. This dose may be cautiously tapered and perhaps discontinued in the patient who is rendered asymptomatic after the completion of whole brain radiation therapy.

Estrogens

Estrogens are available in several forms. Tablets, injections and intravenous preparations each have specific indications, and individual patients may tolerate the side effects of one preparation better than another. Estrogens in

cortisone 25 mg	*hydrocortisone* 20 mg	*prednisone or prednisolone* 5 mg
methyl prednisolone 4 mg	*dexamethasone* 0.75 mg	

cancer therapy are used mainly in metastatic cancers of the prostate and carcinomas of the breast in elderly men and women. Nausea and vomiting are acute effects that appear in many patients. Edema and cardiac decompensation are particularly difficult to manage if the patients have serious underlying heart disease. Increased libido or vaginal bleeding may be embarrassing complications in elderly women. Long-term, chronic administration of estrogens has been associated with the development of hypertensive and arteriosclerotic cardiovascular disease.

Diethylstilbestrol diphosphate (Stilphostrol) is available as a rapid-acting intravenous estrogen preparation. It provides a quick means to determine the responsiveness of a tumor to estrogen therapy. It should be given as a dose of 0.5 mg in 300 ml of saline or glucose solution over a period of one hour on the first day, followed by 1.0 gm on four or more subsequent days. Although nausea may appear, this therapy can be given in the Outpatient Clinic. If the patient develops severe pain in metastases with each infusion, long-term estrogen therapy will probably not be beneficial.

Diethylstilbestrol is a potent oral synthetic estrogen that often provides benefit in responsive tumors. It is usually given in doses of 1 mg daily for cancer of the prostate and 15 mg daily (5 mg t.i.d.) for carcinoma of the breast. In the latter case, it is prudent to begin therapy with a few mg per day, gradually increasing the dose while watching for serious toxicity, particularly hypercalcemia.

Estradiol valerate (Delestrogen) is a long-acting intramuscular preparation that may be given every two to three weeks. Doses of 20 to 40 mg are usually administered every two to three weeks in metastatic carcinoma of the breast after careful observation for serious side effects. This preparation is particularly useful in patients with responsive tumors who are not reliable enough to take therapy daily.

Chlorotrianisene (Tace) is a long-acting synthetic oral estrogen. It is commonly used in therapy of prostatic cancer in doses of 12 to 25 mg per day.

Androgens

Androgens may be used as specific therapeutic agents in premenopausal and perimenopausal women with metastatic carcinoma of the breast. These hormones also have been reported to produce benefit in some patients with hypernephroma.[5] Protein anabolism is enhanced and red cell formation is stimulated by androgens. These effects may be undesirable in some patients but may be exceedingly useful in others. Other side effects commonly observed are nausea and vomiting, fluid retention and hirsutism. Acceleration of tumor growth rate may occur and should be watched for closely when therapy is initiated. Hypercalcemia and cholestatic jaundice are less common but very troublesome complications. Several preparations are available that give a wide range of options in route of administration, dosage and rapidity of effect. Androgens should not be administered to men with carcinoma of the breast.

Testosterone ethanate (Delatestryl) is a long-acting injectable androgen in sesame oil, available in doses of 200 mg per cc. The usual treatment is 200 mg IM every two weeks. Testosterone cypionate (depo-testosterone) is similar in its effects and is usually used in the same dosage as testosterone ethanate. It is available in dilutions of 50, 100 and 200 mg per cc, which provides greater accuracy when small doses are given to patients who do not require or tolerate large doses.

Fluoxymesterone (Halotestin, Ora-Testryl) is a potent oral androgen with a relatively rapid action that allows easy titration of dosage. Because of its short action it should be given in divided doses, and the usual treatment for carcinoma of the breast is 15 to 30 mg per day. Fluoxymesterone is a halogenated methyl testosterone derivative that is said to be five times as potent as the parent compound.

Progestins

Progesterone derivatives have been highly effective in some patients with metastatic carcinoma of the endometrium or breast. These drugs have also been useful in some patients with hypernephroma. Natural progesterone cannot be tolerated in doses sufficient to produce significant effects, but the synthetic derivatives cause relatively less edema, nausea and local inflammation at the sites of injection. Thrombophlebitis and pulmonary embolism have also been reported in association with progesterone therapy.

Hydroxyprogesterone caproate (Delalutin) is a long-acting injectable progestin, which is given in doses of 500 to 1000 mg IM twice a week. It is supplied in potencies of 125 and 250 mg per cc.

Medroxyprogesterone acetate is available in a long-acting intramuscular form (Depo-Provera) and an oral form (Provera). The injectable preparation is supplied in concentrations of 50 and 100 mg per cc, and tablets are available at 2.5 and 10 mg. The dosage of medroxyprogesterone must be titrated by the physician for antineoplastic effect. The usual oral dose is 100 to 200 mg per day.

Megestrol acetate (Megace) is available in tablet form and has virtually no side effects. The usual dose ranges from 40 to 320 mg per day in divided dosage.

Antiestrogens (Tamoxifen)[44]

Tamoxifen (Nolvadex) is a nonsteroidal oral antiestrogen that has recently been approved for palliation of metastatic breast cancer in postmenopausal women. It binds to estrogen-receptor proteins in the cytoplasm; the complex is translocated to the cell nucleus where it affects the synthesis of mRNA, which codes for specific cellular proteins. The drug is less toxic than most other hormonal agents, but side effects may include nausea, vaginal bleeding or hypercalcemia. The usual dosage is 10 mg twice daily.

Aminoglutethimide[58]

Aminoglutethimide blocks adrenal steroidogenesis and may be as effective as surgical adrenalectomy in producing responses in selected patients with metastatic breast cancer. The drug is given in a dose of 1 gram per day in four divided doses. Dexamethasone, 1.5 to 3 mg per day, is given as replacement therapy. Some patients require Florinef (0.1 mg twice weekly) to prevent symptoms of mineralocorticoid deficiency. Adverse effects include lethargy, ataxia, nystagmus and skin rash.

Miscellaneous

Procarbazine (Matulane)

Procarbazine is a derivative of methylhydrazine. Its mechanism of action is believed to be similar to that of the alkylating agents. It is most useful in combination chemotherapy in Hodgkin's disease and carcinoma of the lung. The drug crosses the blood-brain barrier. Toxic effects include myelosuppression, nausea, hyperpigmentation and dermatitis, and central nervous system effects. Since it is a mild monoamine oxidase inhibitor, it may exert an antabuse-like effect if taken with alcohol.

o, p'-DDD (Mitotane; 1,1-dichloro-2-[o-chlorophenyl]-2-[p-chlorophenyl] ethane; Lysodren)

This experimental drug has a unique role in the treatment of adrenal cortical carcinoma. It has relieved the cushing-oid side effects of some patients with functioning adrenal tumors and has been useful in some patients with non-functioning adrenal cortical carcinoma. Regressions have been reported in up to 50 per cent of patients, persisting for ten months. *o*, *p'*-DDD suppresses adrenal cortical activity and produces anorexia, vomiting and diarrhea, plus toxicity in the central nervous system and other organs in some patients. It is supplied in tablets of 500 mg. The usual dose is 9 to 10 gm per day initially, with subsequent therapy adjusted for the desired effect or for toxicity.

Streptozotocin

Streptozotocin is an antibiotic with alkylating activity in the nitrosourea class of drugs. It has a selective effect on pancreatic islet cells. It is an investigational drug that is active against hormone-secreting malignant pancreatic islet cell tumors.[53, 59] It is also being studied in the therapy of malignant carcinoid tumors. It causes severe nausea, vomiting and renal toxicity but no significant bone marrow suppression.

Hexamethylmelamine[45]

Hexamethylmelamine is an investigational drug that structurally resembles the alkylating agent triethylenemelamine (TEM). Its precise mechanism of action is uncertain. It is active in ovarian cancer, carcinoma of the lung and breast, and lymphomas. Toxic effects include myelosuppression, nausea and neurological symptoms including depression and peripheral neuritis.

COMBINATION CHEMOTHERAPY

Recent reviewers have outlined the rationale for the use of drugs in combination for the treatment of can-cer.[16, 23, 25] By and large, the most effective chemotherapeutic regimens employ multiple agents. In general, only drugs that have significant activity against a given tumor when employed singly should be used in combination. Theoretically, drugs that work by different biochemical mechanisms are more likely to achieve synergy and overcome the problem of drug resistance that develops with prolonged therapy. If drugs with different toxicities are chosen, they can be employed in full doses in combination. Scheduling considerations must be carefully evaluated. For example, one drug may be used to synchronize the tumor population to obtain maximal cell kill by a second, phase-specific drug, given sequentially. Most combination regimens employ high doses of drugs given intermittently, every 2 to 4 weeks. The advantage of this approach is that the intermittent scheduling enables bone marrow recovery and some immunological recovery between cycles of chemotherapy.

THERAPY OF ADVANCED MALIGNANCY

This section describes some of the most effective drug regimens for selected adult malignancies (Table 25–7). It is not an exhaustive attempt to detail all chemotherapy regimens for all diseases.

Hodgkin's Disease

The treatment of advanced Hodgkin's disease with combination chemotherapy is one of the major success stories in medicine of the past decade. When single agents were employed the remissions were of very short duration. The MOPP[24] protocol (mustargen, Oncovin, procarbazine, prednisone) results in up to 80 per cent complete remissions, with half of these patients having long-term survival. Long-term

TABLE 25–7   Drug Therapy in Selected Malignancies

DISEASE	ACTIVE AGENTS	DRUG COMBINATIONS
Hodgkin's disease	Mechlorethamine, cyclophosphamide, vincristine, vinblastine, adriamycin, DTIC, bleomycin, BCNU, procarbazine, prednisone	MOPP (Mechlorethamine, Oncovin, procarbazine, prednisone)
Non-Hodgkin's lymphoma	Cyclophosphamide, chlorambucil, vincristine, adriamycin, bleomycin, methotrexate, procarbazine, prednisone, Ara-C, nitrosoureas	CVP (Cyclophosphamide, vincristine, prednisone) CHOP (cyclophosphamide, adriamycin, Oncovin, prednisone) BACOP (bleomycin, adriamycin, cyclophosphamide, Oncovin, prednisone) COMLA (cyclophosphamide, Oncovin, methotrexate with leucovorin rescue, Ara-C)
Breast cancer	Hormones, alkylating agents, 5FU, methotrexate, adriamycin, hexamethylmelamine[a]	CMF(P) (Cyclophosphamide, methotrexate, 5FU, prednisone) CAF (Cyclophosphamide, adriamycin, 5FU)
Testicular cancer (nonseminomatous)	Vinblastine, bleomycin, *cis*-platinum, adriamycin, cyclophosphamide, actinomycin D, chlorambucil, mithramycin, methotrexate	Einhorn regimen — vinblastine, bleomycin, *cis*-platinum VAB III — vinblastine, bleomycin, *cis*-platinum, cyclophosphamide, actinomycin D
Small cell lung cancer	Cyclophosphamide, adriamycin, vincristine, methotrexate, procarbazine, CCNU	Cyclophosphamide, adriamycin, vincristine Cyclophosphamide, CCNU, methotrexate
Colon carcinoma	5 FU, methyl CCNU[a]	5 FU and methyl CCNU[a]
Gastric carcinoma	5 FU, adriamycin, mitomycin C, BCNU	FAM (5FU, adriamycin, mitomycin C) 5FU and BCNU or methyl CCNU[a]
Ovarian carcinoma	Melphalan, cyclophosphamide, chlorambucil, adriamycin, 5FU, methotrexate, *cis*-platinum, hexamethylmelamine[a]	Hexa-CAF (hexamethylmelamine,[a] cyclophosphamide, methotrexate, 5FU) Adriamycin and *cis*-platinum
Sarcoma	Adriamycin, methotrexate, DTIC, cyclophosphamide, actinomycin D, vincristine	CYVADIC (Cyclophosphamide, vincristine, adriamycin, DTIC) Adriamycin and DTIC
Melanoma	DTIC, methyl CCNU[a]	
Head and neck cancers	Methotrexate, bleomycin, cyclophosphamide, 5FU, *cis*-platinum	*Cis*-platinum and bleomycin
Prostate cancer	Estrogens, adriamycin, cyclophosphamide, 5FU, *cis*-platinum	*Cis*-platinum and adriamycin

[a]Available for investigational use only.

survival and perhaps cure may now be predicted for 40 to 50 per cent of patients with advanced Hodgkin's disease who are treated appropriately. An alternate regimen (ABVD),[8] employing adriamycin, bleomycin, vinblastine and DTIC, is equally promising.

Non-Hodgkin's Lymphoma

For lymphomas with a good prognosis (e.g., lymphocytic nodular lymphoma) intensive chemotherapy probably offers no survival advantage over the use of single-agent alkylators in advanced disease.[52] However, in advanced lymphomas of poor prognosis, especially diffuse histiocytic and diffuse poorly differentiated lymphocytic lymphomas, the use of intensive combination chemotherapy has made a significant impact on survival and may be curing a significant number of patients. The most successful regimens are CHOP[49] (Cytoxan, adriamycin, Oncovin, prednisone), BACOP[56] (bleomycin is added) and COMLA[3] (Cytoxan, Oncovin, methotrexate with leucovorin rescue, and Ara-C.

Breast Cancer

The most effective chemotherapy of advanced breast carcinoma employs high-dose, intermittent combinations of cyclophosphamide, methotrexate and 5FU (CMF) or cyclophosphamide, adriamycin, and 5FU (CAF).[10, 13, 14, 57, 63] The response rate is 50 to 65 per cent, and the median duration of response is 24 to 32 weeks. This is superior to single-agent therapy for metastatic breast cancer. Additional agents with some efficacy when used as single agents include melphalan (L-PAM), Oncovin, BCNU and the investigational drugs hexamethylmelamine and dibromodulcitol.

Protocols employing combination chemotherapy and hormonal therapy are currently under investigation.

Malignant Testicular Tumors

Significant advances have been made in the chemotherapy of malignant metastatic nonseminomatous testicular tumors. Using an intensive regimen of cis-platinum, vinblastine and bleomycin, Einhorn and Donohue[27] attained 74 per cent complete and 26 per cent partial remissions in patients with widespread disease. Many of these remissions are long-term and may represent cure. Similar success has been reported by Cvitkovic and associates[20] employing a five-drug regimen that also includes cis-platinum. Combination chemotherapy is distinctly superior to single-agent therapy in this disease. Other drugs with significant activity include adriamycin, actinomycin-D, chlorambucil, methotrexate, cyclophosphamide and mithramycin.

Lung Cancer

Small cell carcinoma of the lung accounts for 15 to 20 per cent of all cases of lung cancer. Early dissemination, even in patients who appear to have localized disease, distinguishes this variety of lung cancer and renders inoperable at the time of diagnosis virtually all patients with small cell carcinoma. Chemotherapy has been shown to have an important role in the treatment of both clinically limited and extensive disease, often in conjunction with radiation therapy.[47] A variety of drugs are active in this disease, including cyclophosphamide, adriamycin, methotrexate, vincristine, CCNU and the investigational drugs VP-16 and hexamethylmelamine. Combinations of these drugs have definitely prolonged survival in a significant number of patients. Successful combinations include cyclophosphamide and vincristine, plus either methotrexate[26] or adriamycin.[48]

Chemotherapy of carcinoma of the lung other than the small-cell type is unrewarding. Although there may be limited responses to a variety of chemo-therapeutic agents, these responses are transient and generally of little survival value.

Cancer of the Gastrointestinal Tract

A review by Moertel[50] summarizes the current status of chemotherapy of gastrointestinal cancer. 5-fluorouracil has been the standard of therapy for many years. The objective response rate averages 20 per cent, and most responses are partial and transient and do not make a definite contribution to survival. In colon carcinoma, the addition of a nitrosourea[28] may increase the response rate but probably offers no advantage in survival over therapy with 5FU alone. The results of chemotherapy of pancreatic carcinoma are even less optimistic. Studies are now being made to determine whether there may be survival value in combinations of 5FU with adriamycin and mitomycin when employed in advanced gastric carcinoma.

Cancer of the Ovary

The majority of women with ovarian cancer have advanced disease at the time of diagnosis. Alkylating agents have been used most extensively in the chemotherapy of this disease, with response rates of 35 to 65 per cent, including about 15 per cent complete remissions.[62] However, the median duration of survival has been only about 10 to 12 months. Other drugs with significant activity in ovarian carcinoma include 5FU, adriamycin, methotrexate, and the investigational drug hexamethylmelamine. One study compares the efficacy of a combination of hexamethylmelamine, cyclophosphamide, methotrexate and 5FU (Hexa-CAF) with the oral alkylating agent melphalan in patients with advanced disease.[64] It reports an improved response rate,

more complete remissions and longer median survival using this combination but also reports more severe toxicity than when melphalan is used alone.

Sarcoma

The most effective regimen for treatment of metastatic soft tissue sarcoma in adults is the combination of cyclophosphamide, vincristine, adriamycin and DTIC (CYVADIC).[51] The less toxic combination of adriamycin and DTIC is promising and may prove to be as effective.

Malignant Melanoma

DTIC is the most effective chemotherapeutic agent for therapy of metastatic melanoma. The response rate is on the order of 25 per cent,[43] and responses are usually partial and of short duration.

Head and Neck Cancers

The majority of these lesions are squamous cell carcinomas involving the oral cavity, pharynx, larynx and sinuses. The single most effective and most-studied agent for this class of tumors is methotrexate. A variety of methods and routes of administration have been used, but weekly, low-dose intravenous therapy is probably as efficacious as any other approach.[4, 17] The response rate is approximately 50 per cent but is usually of short duration. Other active agents include bleomycin, adriamycin, cyclophosphamide, 5FU and *cis*-platinum. Studies employing combination chemotherapy and combined modality approaches (radiation therapy and chemotherapy) are being made.

Cancer of the Prostate

Estrogen therapy may provide dramatic palliation of bone pain and other symptoms. Chemotherapy has a low degree of effectiveness and is reserved for patients who have failed to respond to orchiectomy or estrogen therapy, or both. A small number of patients may achieve palliation from 5FU, adriamycin or cyclophosphamide, but no survival benefit has been shown. Regimens employing *cis*-platinum are being studied.

ADJUVANT CHEMOTHERAPY

Much attention has been directed in recent years to the possibility of increasing the cure rate of malignancies by employing chemotherapy at a time when patients have a minimal tumor burden. When the tumor burden is small, the growth fraction is greatest and tumors should be most responsive to certain chemotherapeutic agents.[54] Drugs and drug combinations of proven efficacy in advanced metastatic disease are employed postoperatively in patients who have tumors of poor prognosis. A significant number of such patients are expected to have residual microscopic disease even if all gross tumor has been removed, and therefore they have a high risk of recurrence and death from cancer. This is the rationale for adjuvant chemotherapy.

The efficacy of this approach has been established in a variety of malignancies of childhood. However, the use of adjuvant chemotherapy in the common adult solid tumors is still disputed. Since cancer chemotherapeutic drugs are, by and large, also immunosuppressive and carcinogenic, the use of adjuvant chemotherapy involves the possibility of harm as well as potential benefit. Studies of the adjuvant effect of chemotherapy usually require large institutions or interinstitutional cooperative groups.

Preliminary reports of the efficacy of postoperative adjuvant chemotherapy in patients with breast cancer at high risk of recurrence were extremely optimistic.[7, 27] However, more recent additions to the data have been less impressive. When the National Surgical Adjuvant Breast Project compared L-PAM with placebo, the recurrence rate for the treated patients was superior to placebo at 24 months only in premenopausal patients with one to three positive nodes. Likewise, the data presented by Bonadonna at the 1978 American Society of Clinical Oncology Meetings, giving a four-year update on the efficacy of cyclophosphamide, methotrexate and 5-fluorouracil (CMF) as adjuvant chemotherapy, show no decrease in the eventual recurrence rate for postmenopausal women. Hence, adjuvant chemotherapy may delay the initial time of recurrence in these women but does not appear to increase the cure rate.

Studies employing intravenous 5-fluorouracil as postoperative adjuvant therapy for colorectal cancer have failed to show a statistically significant survival benefit in this approach.[50] The search for effective adjuvant therapy in this and other diseases continues.

CONCLUSIONS

Recent advances in cancer chemotherapy have been due to the development of new, effective drugs and to the use of these drugs in combination, applying knowledge of tumor cell biology and pharmacology to the treatment of patients with cancer.

The cancer chemotherapist must be alert to new developments. He or she must be optimistic but realistic, honest with himself and with patients and willing to measure and record observations as a guide to further therapy. The chemotherapist must integrate the use of surgery and radiation therapy, palliative drugs and specific chemicals and hormones. Consultation and informed consent are important ethical and legal requirements for this work. His or her goal must always be both the cure of cancer and the relief of suffering.

REFERENCES

1. American Joint Committee for Cancer Staging and End-Results Reporting: Manual for Staging of Cancer. Chicago, Am. Joint Committee, 55 E. Erie Street, 60611, 1977, pp. 4–5.

2. Bean, W., and Featherman, K.: A time for dying. Curr. Med. Digest, 37:1039–1042, 1970.

3. Berd, D., Cornog, J., DeConti, R. C., et al.: Long-term remission in diffuse histiocytic lymphoma treated combination sequential chemotherapy. Cancer, 35:1050–1054, 1975.

4. Bertino, J. R., Boston, B., and Capizzi, R. L.: The role of chemotherapy in the management of cancer of the head and neck. A review. Cancer, 36:752–758, 1975.

5. Bloom, H. J.: The basis for hormonal therapy. Cancer of the urogenital tract: kidney. J.A.M.A., 204:605–606, 1968.

6. Blum, R. H., and Carter, S. K.: Adriamycin: a new anti-cancer drug with significant clinical activity. Ann. Intern. Med., 80:249–259, 1974.

7. Bonadonna, G., Brusamolino, E., Valagussa, P., et al.: Combination chemotherapy as an adjuvant treatment in operable breast cancer. N. Engl. J. Med., 294:405–410, 1976.

8. Bonadonna, G., Zucali, R., and DeLena, M.: Combination chemotherapy (MOPP vs. ABVD) plus RT in advanced Hodgkin's disease (Abstr.). Proc. Am. Soc. Clin. Oncol., 94:260, 1976.

9. Bristow, M. R., Thompson, P. D., Martin, R. P., et al.: Early anthracycline toxicity. Am. J. Med., 65:823–832, 1978.

10. Broder, L. E., and Tormey, D. C.: Combination chemotherapy of carcinoma of the breast. Cancer Treat. Rev., 1:182–203, 1974.

11. Brown, J. H., and Kennedy, B. J.: Mithramycin in the treatment of disseminated testicular neoplasms. N. Engl. J. Med., 272:111–118, 1965.

12. Bruckner, H. W., and Creasy, W. A.: The administration of 5-fluorouracil by mouth. Cancer, 33:14–18, 1974.

13. Canellos, G. P., DeVita, V. T., Gold, G. L., et al.: Combination chemotherapy for advanced breast cancer: response and effect on survival. Ann. Intern. Med., 84:389–392, 1976.

14. Canellos, G. P., Pocock, S. J., Taylor, S. Z., et al.: Combination chemotherapy for metastatic breast carcinoma: prospective comparison of multiple drug therapy with L-phenylalanine mustard. Cancer, 38:1882–1886, 1976.

15. Capizzi, R. L., DeConti, R. C., Marsh, J. C., et al.: Methotrexate therapy of head and neck cancer: improvement in therapeutic index by the use of leucovorin "rescue." Cancer Res., 30:1782–1788, 1970.

16. Capizzi, R. L., Keiser, L. W., and Sartorelli, A. C.: Combination chemotherapy — theory and practice. Semin. Oncol., 4:227–253, 1977.

17. Carter, S. H.: The chemotherapy of head and neck cancer. Semin. Oncol., 4:413–424, 1977.

18. Chabner, B. A., Myers, C. E., Coleman, C. N.: et al.: The clinical pharmacology of antineoplastic agents. N. Engl. J. Med., 292:1107–1113 and 1159–1168, 1975.

19. Chabner, B. A., Myers, C. E., and Oliverio, V. T.: Clinical pharmacology of anticancer drugs. Semin. Oncol., 4:165–191, 1977.

20. Cvitkovic, E., Hayes, D., and Golbey, R.: Primary combination chemotherapy (VAB III) for metastatic or unresectable germ cell tumors. Proc. Am. Soc. Clin. Oncol., 17:296, 1976.

21. Dahl, M. G., Gregory, M. M., and Scheuer, P. J.: Liver damage due to methotrexate in patients with psoriasis. Br. Med. J., 1:625–630, 1971.

22. DeVita, V. T.: Cell kinetics and the chemotherapy of cancer. Cancer Chemother. Rep., 2(3):22–33, 1971.

23. DeVita, V. T., and Schein, P. S.: The use of drugs in combination for the treatment of cancer. N. Engl. J. Med., 288:998–1006, 1973.

24. DeVita, V. T., Serpick, A. A., and Carbone, P. P.: Combination chemotherapy in the treatment of advanced Hodgkin's disease. Ann. Intern. Med., 73:881–895, 1970.

25. DeVita, V. T., Young, R. C., and Canellos, G. P.: Combination versus single agent chemotherapy: a review of the basis for selection of drug treatment of cancer. Cancer, 35:98–110, 1975.

26. Eagan, R. T., Maurer, H. L., Forcier, R. J., et al.: Small cell carcinoma of the lung: staging, paraneoplastic syndromes, treatment and survival. Cancer, 33:527–532, 1974.

27. Einhorn, L. H., and Donohue, J.: Cis-diamminedichloroplatinum, vinblastine, and bleomycin combination chemotheray in disseminated testicular cancer. Ann. Intern. Med., 87:293–298, 1977.

28. Falkson, G., and Falkson, H. C.: Fluorouracil, methyl-CCNU and vincristine in cancer of the colon. Cancer, 38:1468–1470, 1976.

29. Fisher, B., Carbone, P., Economou, S. G., et al.: L-phenylalanine mustard (L-PAM) in the management of primary breast cancer. N. Engl. J. Med., 292:117–122, 1975.

30. Gershwin, M. E., Groetzl, E. J., and Steinberg, A. D.: Cyclophosphamine use in practice. Ann. Intern. Med., 80:531–540, 1974.

31. Gilman, A., and Philips, F. S.: The biological actions and therapeutic applications of the B-chloroethyl amines and sulfides. Science, 103:409–415, 1946.

32. Hahn, R. G., Moertel, C. G., Schutt, A. J., et al.: A controlled comparison of intensive course 5-fluorouracil by oral vs. IV route in colorectal carcinoma. Proc. Am. Assoc. Cancer Res., 15:191, 1974.

33. Heldelberger, C., et al.: Fluorinated pyrimidines, a new class of tumour-inhibitory compounds. Nature, *179*:663–666, 1957.

34. Hertz, R., Lewis, J., Jr., and Lipsett, M. B.: Five years' experience with the chemotherapy of metastatic choriocarcinoma and related trophoblastic tumors in women. Am. J. Obstet. Gynecol., *82*:631–640, 1961.

35. Hickey, R. C. (ed.): Palliative Care of the Cancer Patient. Boston, Little, Brown and Co., 1967.

36. Higgins, G. A., and White, G. E.: Cancer chemotherapy and surgery. Surg. Clin. N. Am., *48*:839–850, 1968.

37. Hill, G. J., II, and Cohen, B. I.: Pleural pericardial window for palliation of cardiac tamponade due to cancer. Cancer, *26*:81–93, 1970.

38. Hill, G. J., II, and Wheeler, H. B.: Adrenal insufficiency due to metastatic carcinoma of the lung: case report and review of Addison's disease caused by adrenal metastases. Cancer, *18*:1467–1473, 1965.

39. Jaffe, N., Frei, E., III, Traggis, D., et al.: Adjuvant methotrexate and citrovorum-factor treatment of osteogenic sarcoma. N. Engl. J. Med., *291*:994–997, 1974.

40. Krakoff, I. H.: Cancer chemotherapy agents. CA, *23*:208–219, 1973.

41. Krakoff, I. H.: Systemic cancer treatment: A. Cancer chemotherapy. *In* Horton, J., and Hill, G. J., II, (eds.): Clinical Oncology. Philadelphia, W.B. Saunders Co., 1977, pp. 157–181.

42. Kremer, W. B.: Cytarabine. Ann. Intern. Med., *82*:684–688, 1975.

43. Larsen, R. R., and Hill, G. J., II: Improved systemic chemotherapy for malignant melanoma. Am. J. Surg., *122*:36–41, 1971.

44. Legha, S. S., Davis, H. L., and Muggia, F. M.: Hormonal therapy of breast cancer: new approaches and concepts. Ann. Intern. Med., *88*:69–77, 1978.

45. Legha, S. S., Slavik, M., and Carter, S. K.: Hexamethylmelamine: An evaluation of its role in the therapy of cancer. Cancer, *38*:27–35, 1976.

46. Lippman, M. E., and Allegra, J. C.: Receptors in breast cancer. N. Engl. J. Med., *299*:930–933, 1978.

47. Livingston, R. B.: Treatment of small cell carcinoma: evolution and future directions. Semin. Oncol., *5*:299–308, 1978.

48. Livingston, R. B., Moore, I. N., Heilbrun, L., et al.: Small-cell carcinoma of the lungs: combined chemotherapy and radiation. A Southwest Oncology Group study. Ann. Intern. Med., *88*:194–199, 1978.

49. McKelvey, E. M., Gottlieb, J. A., Wilson, H. E., et al.: Hydroxyldaunomycin (adriamycin) combination chemotherapy in malignant lymphoma. Cancer, *38*:1484–1493, 1976.

50. Moertel, C. G.: Current concepts in cancer: chemotherapy of gastrointestinal cancer. N. Engl. J. Med., *299*:1049–1052, 1978.

51. Pinedo, H. M., and Kenis, Y.: Chemotherapy of advanced soft tissue sarcomas in adults. Cancer Treat. Rev., *4*:67–86, 1977.

52. Portlock, C. S., Rosenberg, S. A., Glatstein, E., et al.: Treatment of advanced non-Hodgkin's lymphoma with favorable histologies. Blood, *47*:747–756, 1976.

53. Rozencweig, M., Von Hoff, D. D., Slavik, M., et al.: *Cis*-diamine-dichloroplatinum (II), a new anticancer drug. Ann. Intern. Med., *86*:803–812, 1977.

54. Schabel, F. M.: Concepts for systemic treatment of micrometastases. Cancer, *35*:15–24, 1975.

55. Schein, P. S., DeLellis, R. A., Kahn, C. R., et al.: Islet cell tumors: current concepts and management. Ann. Intern. Med., *79*:239–257, 1973.

56. Schein, P. S., DeVita, V. T., Hubbard, W., et al.: Bleomycin, adriamycin cyclophosphamide, vincristine and prednisone (BACOP) combination chemotherapy in the treatment of advanced diffuse histiocytic lymphoma. Ann. Intern. Med., *85*:417–422, 1976.

57. Smalley, R. V., Carpenter, J., Bartolucci, A., et al.: A comparison of cyclophosphamide, adriamycin, 5-fluorouracil (CAF) and cyclophosphamide, methotrexate, 5-fluorouracil, vincristine, prednisone (CMFVP) in patients with metastatic breast cancer. Cancer, *40*:625–632, 1977.

58. Smith, I. E., Fitzharris, B. M., McKinna, J. A., et al. Aminoglutethimide in treatment of metastatic breast carcinoma. Lancet, *2*:646–649, 1978.

59. Stadil, R., Stage, G., Rehfeld, J. F., et al.: Treatment of Zollinger-Ellison syndrome with streptozotocin. N. Engl. J. Med., *294*:1440–1442, 1976.

60. Stolinsky, D. C., Pugh, R. P., and Bateman, J. R.: 5FU therapy for pancreatic carcinoma: comparison of oral and intravenous routes. Cancer Chemother. Rep., *59*:1031–1033, 1975.

61. Wirtanen, G. W., Bernhardt, L. C., Mackman, S., et al.: Hepatic artery and celiac axis infusion for the treatment of upper abdominal malignant lesions. Ann. Surg., *168*:137–141, 1968.

62. Young, R. C.: Chemotherapy of ovarian cancer: past and present. Semin. Oncol., *2*:267–276, 1975.

63. Young, R. C. (moderator): NIH conference. Perspectives in the treatment of breast cancer, 1976. Ann Intern. Med., *86*:784–798, 1977.

64. Young, R. C., Chabner, B. A., Hubbard, S. P., et al.: Advanced ovarian adenocarcinoma. A prospective clinical trial of melphalan (L-PAM) versus combination chemotherapy. N. Engl. J. Med., *299*:1261–1266. 1978.

The Unconscious Patient 26

DENNIS BARTON, M.D.

INTRODUCTION

A physician's approach to the unconscious patient must be simultaneously diagnostic and therapeutic. This chapter's organization follows this approach. When faced with a completely unknown comatose patient who is nearing respiratory and cardiovascular collapse, one must think clearly and proceed in an orderly fashion.

Life-supporting techniques are outlined in the first portion of the chapter. They are described in the same order as they are applied during resuscitation.

After a measure of respiratory and cardiovascular stability has been achieved, or if it is already present, the physician may proceed with a differential diagnosis that encompasses the common causes of coma. Having arrived at a presumptive diagnosis, he or she then applies the appropriate treatment. Only those therapeutic measures that have emergency application will be discussed. At this point it will be necessary to utilize laboratory examinations to make or support the diagnosis. A compilation of the more useful laboratory values and their interpretation is given at the end of this chapter (Tables 26–2 through 26–5).

Presuming that the patient is comatose from an obscure cause, a more complex differential diagnosis is required. References will be listed so that the physician can pursue the treatment of these disorders. An exhaustive discussion of the infrequent causes of coma would exceed the purpose of this chapter.

LIFE-SUPPORTING TECHNIQUES — RESPIRATORY SYSTEM

In managing the comatose patient, establishment of adequate ventilation must be the first concern. The physician must train himself to recognize partial and complete airway obstruction. Complete obstruction of the airway may be manifested by a complete lack of air movement or by struggling respirations with suprasternal and supraclavicular retraction. The physician will be unable to inflate the lungs in this situation. Partial obstruction is manifested by air movement with snoring or by air movement in the presence of excessive secretions, blood or vomitus. The patient may appear to be moving air without obstruction. However, the respiratory rate may be rapid, the volume moved may be insufficient, or the respirations may be arrhythmic: gasps followed by several seconds of apnea or Cheyne-Stokes respiration.

Arterial hypoxemia may result from lung disease or failing circulation, even if the rate and volume of respiration appear to be adequate and breath sounds are clear to auscultation. Cyanosis is a helpful indicator, if detectable. The absence of cyanosis does not guarantee adequate oxygenation. Cyanosis visible to the human eye usually means that at least 5 gm of desaturated hemoglobin per 100 ml blood exist in the arterial blood. Cyanosis can be difficult to detect in anemic or hypovolemic patients, as well as those with darker skin coloration. The physician

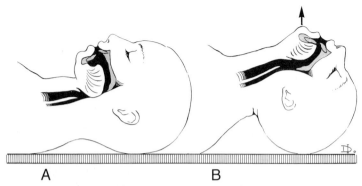

Figure 26–1   *A.* The tongue often falls onto the pharyngeal wall and occludes the airway. *B.* By extending the head and lifting the mandible upwards the tongue is pulled off the pharyngeal wall. By opening the mouth the soft palate can no longer act as a flap valve that blocks the nasal passages with expiration.

can be misled by peripheral vasoconstriction secondary to cold. Here peripheral cyanosis exists without arterial desaturation. Arterial hypoxemia can cause anxiety, disorientation, negativism, combativeness, tachycardia, sweating, and somnolence progressing to coma. Retained CO_2, another manifestation of hypoventilation, contributes to this symptom complex.

Forceful subdiaphragmatic compression is used to save the acutely asphyxiated victim by expelling a bolus of food or aspirated water.[39] This simple means of resuscitation is best used on the scene of the accident. In the Emergency Room the immediate goal of airway care in a comatose patient is to deliver 100 per cent O_2 to the alveoli. The percentage of oxygen delivered can be reduced after the patient is stabilized and his condition warrants the reduction. The airway must first be opened and cleared. As demonstrated in Figure 26–1*A* and *B*, the patient's neck must be extended and the head tilted backward, a maneuver that lifts the tongue off the posterior pharyngeal wall and opens the airway. One then displaces the mandible down and forward, which further lifts the tongue from the posterior pharyngeal wall and opens the mouth. An open mouth prevents the soft palate from flapping up and closing the nasal

passages with expiration. Excessive secretions, blood and vomitus are next suctioned or wiped from the mouth, and the patient is then ventilated. Either mouth-to-mouth resuscitation or bag and mask ventilation can be instituted. Mouth-to-mouth resuscitation is more effective for immediate delivery of air. Mask fit can sometimes be a real problem, especially in edentulous patients. However, a bag and mask system can quickly supply a high concentration of oxygen and should be utilized if possible. If the airway is still obstructed after these steps have been taken, an oropharyngeal or nasopharyngeal airway will be necessary. The insertion of an oropharyngeal airway is seen in Figure 26–2*A*. (The application of the breathing mask to the face is shown in Figure 26–2*B* and *C*.)

Intubation should be attempted only after the patient has been well oxygenated through a clear airway by a bag and mask system. Dr. Peter Safar has remarked, "Experienced personnel can perform endotracheal intubation more rapidly than tracheotomy. Prolonged attempts at intubation by inexperienced operators, however, have caused asphyxia and cardiac arrest. All hospitals treating seriously ill or injured patients should have personnel experienced in endotracheal intuba-

A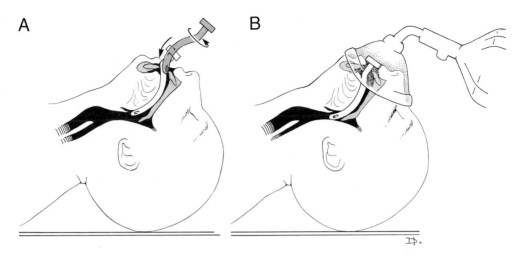

B

C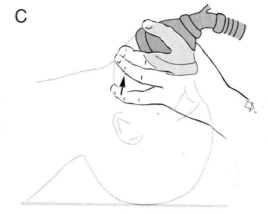

Figure 26–2 *A.* Insertion of the oropharyngeal airway is accomplished by placing the airway upside down against the hard palate. The airway is then rotated 180° and moved further down into the mouth. The final position of the airway is best seen in *B. B.* The oropharyngeal airway is now in position. It holds the tongue off the pharyngeal wall and permits an unobstructed airway. A mask has been applied to the face so that ventilation through both oral and nasal passages is permitted. *C.* The mask is being held here with the left hand. The thumb and forefinger press the mask down on the face. The remaining three fingers of the hand steady the mandible. The tips of the fingers rest on the ramus of the mandible so that pressure is not exerted on the soft tissue of the neck. The little finger hooks under the angle of the mandible and lifts the jaw forward. *D.* Intubation in a patient with a full stomach is hazardous because of the risk of aspiration. Compression of the cricoid cartilage against the bodies of the cervical vertebrae closes the esophagus during intubation. This is termed Sellick's maneuver. (From: Sellick, B. A.: Lancet, 2:404, 1961.)

D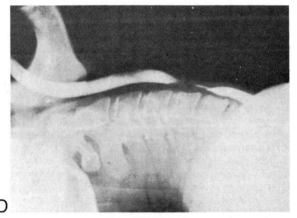

tion immediately available at all times."[74]

When considering intubation, the physician must choose between cuffed orotracheal or cuffed nasotracheal intubation. The nasotracheal tube can often be inserted by the experienced operator even in the presence of clenched teeth. Furthermore, the tube is more easily tolerated by the semicomatose patient, and with proper adjunctive care the tube can be kept in

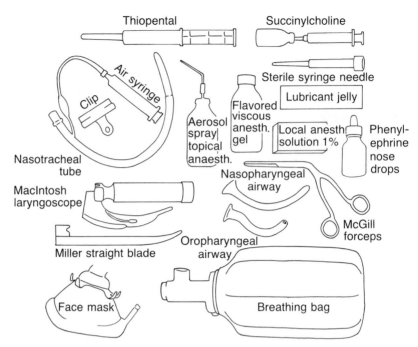

Figure 26–3   A selection of equipment for performing intubation. The components of the tray have been labeled. Airways and a bag and mask system are illustrated to remind the reader that no intubation should be attempted without adequate preoxygenation. Topical anesthesia in the form of viscous gel, liquid or aerosol spray can be used to anesthetize the upper airway if this is deemed necessary. Anesthesia and muscle relaxation can be provided by thiopental and succinylcholine, but great caution is urged when considering these drugs for use in the comatose patient. Phenylephrine nose drops are helpful in shrinking the nasal mucosa and thus facilitating the passage of a nasal tube. A broader description of the pharmacology of the drugs used with intubation is described in the chapter in this book on anesthesia. A cuffed endotracheal tube, two types of blades, and a Magill forceps are also shown. The operator will need a selection of various sizes of endotracheal tubes.

place for several days, thus avoiding a tracheostomy altogether. The orotracheal tube, however, is more swiftly inserted. A clenched jaw or inadequate visualization of the glottis can frequently be overcome by the injection of succinyldicholine. However, use of muscle relaxants will make aspiration of stomach contents more likely. Sellick's maneuver is helpful in emergency intubation of the patient suspected of having a full stomach. The cricoid cartilage is pressed inward to occlude the esophagus. The glottis remains visible during this maneuver (Fig. 26–2D).[76] Before attempting intubation, the operator must have a selection of equipment, best illustrated in Figure 26–3.

The accompanying drawings illus-

trate the basic differences in the two techniques. Orotracheal intubation is best accomplished with a MacIntosh laryngoscope and endotracheal tube with a well-lubricated stylet (Fig. 26–4). A straight (Miller) laryngoscope blade is sometimes useful if the patient's mouth can be only slightly opened (Fig. 26–5A and B). If the operator is relatively inexperienced, this blade may inadvertently injure the posterior pharyngeal wall. The patient's head is best supported by a small pillow (Fig. 26–4A). The MacIntosh laryngoscope is held in the operator's left hand and inserted into the right of the patient's mouth. The tongue is followed back (Fig. 26–4B), and pushed to the operator's left until the tip of the laryngoscope falls into the valleculum located at the base of the tongue and the epiglottis. The laryngoscope is then lifted, not levered (Fig. 26–4C). This motion moves the mandible, the tongue, and the epiglottis out of the operator's line of sight and exposes the glottis (Fig. 26–4D).

The tube is inserted through the glottis, and the operator is advised to keep it in sight as it passes through the glottis, lest he blindly drop it into the esophagus, which is posterior to the larynx. The tube must not be passed too far, or it will enter the right or occasionally the left main stem bronchus and deprive the contralateral lung of ventilation. Once the tube is placed, the chest must be inflated with positive pressure. Air will leak around the cuff of the tube. The cuff is then inflated with a volume of air sufficient to stop the leak, and no more. The operator must carefully auscultate the lateral aspects of both lung fields to assure that the breath sounds are equal and that a main stem bronchus has not

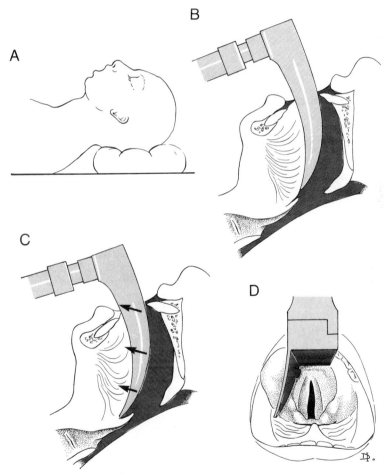

Figure 26–4 *A.* In performing intubation with the MacIntosh blade, the patient's head is placed, slightly flexed, on a small pillow. *B.* The laryngoscope blade follows the tongue back, pushing the tongue to the operator's left. The tip of the blade comes to rest in the valleculum between the epiglottis and the tongue. *C.* The blade is lifted (not levered) in the direction of the arrow. Under no circumstances should the teeth be used as a fulcrum for this maneuver. *D.* Glottic exposure accomplished with the MacIntosh blade. Note how the tongue has been moved to the left. For clarity the size of the tongue has been somewhat exaggerated.

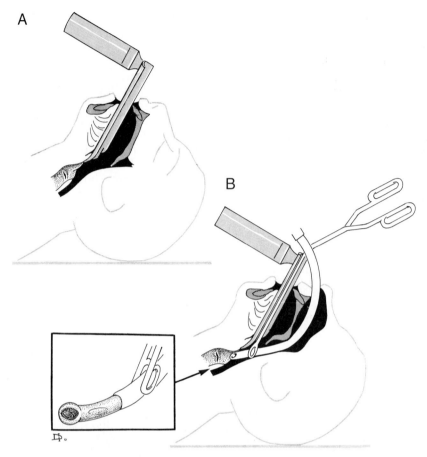

Figure 26–5 *A.* Here a Miller laryngoscope blade has been used. The blade presses the epiglottis against the tongue, thus permitting exposure of the glottis. Nasotracheal intubation is being accomplished in this drawing. *B.* The nasotracheal tube has been grasped with the McGill forceps and guided toward the glottis. This enlarged view shows the rounded Murphy tip of the nasotracheal tube. The authors have found this type of nasotracheal tube less traumatic to the nasopharyngeal mucosa.

been intubated. Secretions and aspirated material are cleared from the endotracheal tube. Only five seconds of suctioning is permitted between lung inflations with oxygen. This prevents hypoxemia caused by the suction catheter removing oxygen from the lungs. An oropharyngeal airway is inserted so that the patient will not occlude his airway by biting. The operator then cleans the skin of the patient's face, applies tincture of benzoin to the external portion of the endotracheal tube and the skin of the face, and firmly tapes the tube in place. Adhesive tapes are placed across the zygoma and circumferentially around the head. Ad-

equate ventilation may rouse a semicomatose patient enough so that he will pull out the endotracheal tube. Restraints are sometimes required to prevent this unfortunate event.

If nasotracheal intubation is the choice, the nasal passages are best suctioned clean, then sprayed with a vasoconstrictive agent such as ¼ per cent Neo-Synephrine. Insertion is also facilitated by anesthetizing the nasal and posterior pharyngeal mucosa with a topical anesthetic spray in order to avoid painful stimuli that will cause struggling in a semicomatose patient. Blind nasotracheal intubation depends on the operator's ability to hear breath sounds through the external portion of the nasotracheal tube. The operator begins by placing the patient's occiput on a small pillow and cautiously advances the nasotracheal tube. If the trachea is not entered on this attempt, the operator must *flex or extend* the neck of the patient in order to bring the cuffed end of the nasotracheal tube into alignment with the glottis, a matter of some trial and error. However, if a cervical fracture is known, or even suspected, the neck cannot be moved. Any history of head trauma, especially when force was applied to the vertex or anteroposterior aspect of the skull, should alert the physician to an associated cervical spine injury, commonly seen in the upper segments of the cervical spine.[83] If visualization of the glottis, or even of the posterior pharyngeal wall is possible with a laryngoscope, the operator can manipulate the cuffed end of the nasotracheal tube with a McGill forceps (see Fig. 26–5B) in order to bring the tube into proper alignment with the glottis. Once the tube is through into the trachea proper, cuff location and pressure must be maintained as with an orotracheal tube.

Skill in intubation cannot be gained simply by reading this description. The skill must be acquired in the morgue and in the operating room under instruction from someone skilled in intubation.

Percutaneous transtracheal ventilation has been recommended.[86] An intermittent jet of high-pressure oxygen is delivered through a needle placed in the trachea. The technique does not guard against the aspiration of vomitus.

LIFE-SUPPORTING TECHNIQUES — CARDIOVASCULAR SYSTEM

As soon as the airway is established, hopefully in a matter of seconds, the physician's attention is directed to the cardiovascular system. An absence of peripheral pulses and heart sounds immediately requires the institution of closed chest massage. Resuscitation should not be denied any patient until the full status of the patient is known. There are numerous instances of resuscitative efforts being denied to "hopeless" trauma patients, only to have these patients "revive" and live on, often with serious neurological deficits. Such patients, with proper resuscitation, could perhaps have resumed full and useful lives.

With the cessation of cardiac activity, physiological events occur that lead inexorably to death. Oxygen stores drop rapidly, leading first to CNS failure of function, which results in coma and apnea. Permanent CNS damage is the result of oxygen deprivation for three to five minutes. This time will be less if hypoxia preceded cardiac arrest. Brain survival in anoxia can continue only as long as energy stores (ATP) are present. The reduction in metabolic rate by anesthesia and hypothermia can prolong survival time.[58] As O_2 stores decrease, anaerobic metabolism increases with an increase in hydrogen ion and a fall in pH. Asphyxial death was studied in dogs,[44] where investigators found that PaO_2 of 5 to 10 torr* (control of 100 torr) or pH_a of 6.5 to 6.45 (control of pH_a 7.40) were both fatal. The effects of hypoxia and acidosis are additive, however, and death in dogs also occurs at a pH_a less than 6.8. Circulatory arrest was studied in monkeys.[54] In these animals untreated hypotension appears to account for the hemispheric brain injury occurring after short periods of circulatory arrest. Closed chest massage should continue to insure adequate cerebral blood flow (70 to 80 torr mean pressure), even with restored normal sinus rhythm. The rapid arrival of death following O_2 deprivation is illustrated in Figure 26–6A.

---

*One torr equals approximately 1 mm Hg.

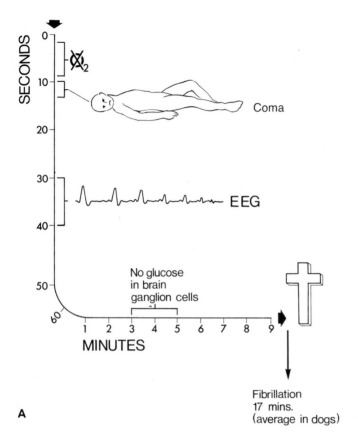

A

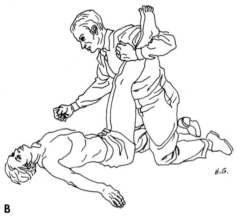

H.G.

B

Figure 26–6 Time is of the essence with cardiac arrest. The vulnerability of the brain is quickly demonstrated. Unconsciousness will ensue within seconds, and brain glucose disappears within minutes. A. The heart can survive longer than the brain. Ventilation with a hypoxic gas mixture will not produce cardiac fibrillation until 17 minutes have passed, but the brain has become functionless long before this.[44] B. The initiation of resuscitation is illustrated here. Raising the legs causes the return of venous blood to increase. A sharp blow to the sternum is about to be administered. This maneuver may start electrical activity in an asystolic heart.

Acidosis has negative inotropic effects on the myocardium and, if severe, can disrupt intracellular metabolism. An efflux of K^+ ions from the liver also occurs with severe hypoxemia. Excessive K^+ ions enter the right heart and increase the possibility of arrhythmia.[48] Disruption of intracellular metabolism eventually stops glycolysis, and blood glucose falls alarmingly. The brain is almost entirely dependent upon glucose for its metabolism[25] and will begin to die within minutes unless the glucose is replaced, even in the face of adequate oxygenation.

The physician begins resuscitation

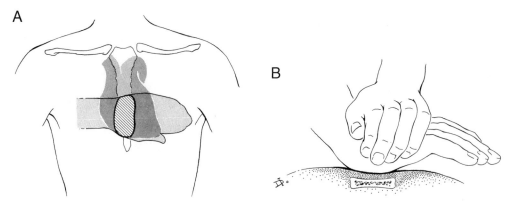

Figure 26–7 *A.* The hands are placed on the lower third of the sternum. *B.* If pressure is exerted only on the lower third of the sternum and not on the ribs, the incidence of rib fracture will be decreased.

by lifting the patient's legs high in the air and delivering a sharp blow to the lower sternum (Fig. 26–6*B*).[90] This maneuver will occasionally start an asystolic heart or ventricle. Some success in cardiac arrest has been achieved by continuous chest pounding. Each sternal blow initiates a myocardial contraction, making closed chest massage unnecessary.[98] Chest thumping has been noted to convert ventricular tachycardia to normal sinus rhythm[63] and to reverse ventricular fibrillation of recent onset. If effective cardiac action does not commence, closed chest massage is then begun with direct downward compression of the lower one-third of the sternum with the heel of the hand (Fig. 26–7*A*). A minimum distance of 1½ to 2 inches is advised. One hand is placed on the other, so that the strength of both arms can be used (Fig. 26–7*B*). The patient must be lying on a firm surface. Never push down on the xiphoid process. This can cause liver laceration. Closed chest massage pushes the sternum against the heart and in turn pushes the heart against the vertebral bodies. The increase in intrathoracic pressure forces blood into the systemic and pulmonary circulation (Fig. 26–8).

Resuscitation should be instituted immediately even if only one individual is present. Help is soon required. At least three operators are necessary for efficiency. One should handle the airway and ventilation, another should continue the massage, and the third should connect the monitoring device and administer the proper drugs.

Massage should continue at the rate of 60 times per minute in adults — half a second for the down stroke and half a second for the up stroke. After every five beats there should be a pause for a deep inflation of the lungs with 100 per cent O_2. If only one rescuer is pres-

Figure 26–8 Closed chest cardiac massage will move blood only if the heart is compressed down onto the vertebral bones by pushing down on the sternum. Adequate time (0.5 sec) is necessary to both empty and then fill the heart. (See text.)

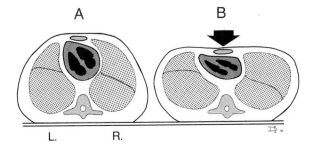

ent the formula is 15 beats of massage followed by two quick chest inflations. A single rescuer must therefore compress the chest 80 times per minute. Oxygen is most efficiently given through an endotracheal tube, but a bag and mask system may be satisfactory.

An intravenous catheter should be inserted and a slow infusion of 5 per cent D/W started as a route for administration of drugs. A greater saphenous vein cutdown at the medial malleolus or a subclavian vein catheterization has been the most useful IV route in our hospitals. (See Figs. 4–1 and 4–2.) Transcutaneous cardiac puncture for drug administration saves time but often results in unnecessary morbidity (pneumothorax, hemopericardium) and this approach should be used only if an intravenous line is unobtainable.

An electrocardiograph with either an oscilloscope or direct writer printout is mandatory if resuscitation is unsuccessful in the first minute. A defibrillator should be brought to the scene and used either if the diagnosis of defibrillation is established from an ECG tracing, or if the diagnosis is suspected in the absence of a proper ECG trace. Only one unmonitored defibrillatory shock is recommended, and this only in adult patients. Electrode paddle placement follows the precept that the shock is best delivered over the long axis of the heart (Fig. 26–9). One elec-

trode is placed in the region of the right first and second costal cartilages while the other is placed just lateral to the left anterior axillary line in the fifth intercostal space (Fig. 26–9). Direct current defibrillators are preferred. The defibrillator output is usually set at 300 watt-seconds (joules), but lesser output is frequently adequate.

The effectiveness of massage can be judged from the patient's color and pupil diameter. Fixed dilated pupils are indicative of ineffective circulation, while contracted pupils that constrict to light are a good prognostic sign. Brain stem activity in the form of swallowing, reaction to the endotracheal tube or unconscious movements may become evident with improved cerebral circulation. The patient may attempt purposeful movement and become fully aware of what is occurring. Palpation of pressure waves at various "pulse points" in the body does not indicate blood movement and tissue perfusion but merely pressure change in a column of liquid.[38] The effectiveness of the massage cannot be judged from the palpation of the pulse.

As might be expected, there are many differences between the normal heart and the arrested heart with assisted circulation.[32, 38] With circulatory arrest, venous pressure increases to 20 to 25 cm H_2O, with resultant cardiac distention. The distention increases the difficulty of defibrillation. Mitral and tricuspid valves become incompetent. This contributes to the observation that closed chest massage produces a cardiac output that is only 30 to 50 per cent of normal. Oxygenation of blood, even with an inspiratory oxygen concentration of 100 per cent, falls precipitously because of poor pulmonary perfusion. PaO_2 has been measured at less than 100 torr even with PIO_2 of 600 torr. This severe disturbance of the ventilation-perfusion relationship declines gradually after successful resuscitation. Adequate mean pressure (70 to 80 torr) to insure cerebral blood flow must be maintained after cardiac rhythm is restored. It may be necessa-

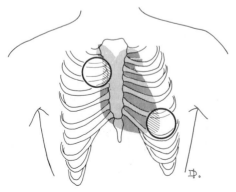

Figure 26–9 This shows the correct paddle placement for defibrillator paddles.

ry to continue closed chest massage despite restoration of normal sinus rhythm.

Adjunctive Drugs in Cardiac Arrest

The drugs that may be required in cardiac arrest are summarized in Table 26–1.

SODIUM BICARBONATE. The rapidly developing acidosis of circulatory collapse cannot be controlled by hyperventilation alone. Furthermore, acidosis reduces the effectiveness of many of the other drugs used in resuscitation. Sodium bicarbonate is used as a buffer. The initial dose is 1 mEq per kg of body weight. One-half this dose is repeated every 10 minutes. In infants or in patients with congestive heart failure, the continued use of this drug will result in a massive sodium load, which will increase the resuscitation problem. Excess bicarbonate administration during resuscitation may result in a marked dissociation between arterial and cerebrospinal fluid pH. This is a consequence of rapid CO_2 diffusion across the blood-brain barrier, which may result in postresuscitation CNS depression.[9]

EPINEPHRINE. This drug usually causes peripheral vasoconstriction by alpha-receptor stimulation. Its usefulness in cardiac resuscitation is probably due to increased myocardial perfusion and improved venous return following its administration.[85] Slow, low-voltage fibrillation is often converted to more rapid, higher voltage fibrillation with epinephrine, the latter electrical pattern being more susceptible to defibrillation. The drug is also useful with complete isoelectric cardiac activity. Epinephrine is a double-edged sword: overly enthusiastic use of the drug can lead to arrhythmia, myocardial ischemia and infarction in some patients.

CALCIUM CHLORIDE. Calcium increases contractility[32] by its action directly on the myocardial muscle cell membrane. Calcium chloride is used in states of decreased myocardial contractility when defibrillation has been achieved but tissue perfusion remains poor. It is especially useful in counteracting the myocardial depressant effects of hyperkalemia. Injudicious use of this drug will be followed by arrhythmia and even ventricular fibrillation, especially in fully digitalized patients. Direct injection of calcium chloride into the myocardium may cause an irreversibly sustained contraction termed "stone heart." Calcium gluconate is less irritating to veins and carries less risk of overdosage because of a smaller concentration of Ca^{++} ions. $CaCl_2$ may be preferred in emergency situations, however.

PROPRANOLOL (INDERAL). This drug blocks beta-adrenergic receptors. Propranolol also possesses antiarrhythmic properties unrelated to beta blockade, often referred to as "quinidine-like" activity.[101] It is useful in suppressing arrhythmias secondary to exogenous catecholamines or enhanced endogenous sympathetic nervous system stimulation. Cardiac arrhythmias that respond to this drug include atrial and ventricular tachycardias, as well as premature ventricular contractions. The drug is not a useful agent for arrhythmias associated with myocardial infarction. Rapid administration of propranolol may precipitate hypotension, and its use may exacerbate congestive heart failure. Its beta-blocking properties *contraindicate its use in asthmatics* and in those patients on insulin or other hypoglycemic drugs.

LIDOCAINE (XYLOCAINE). This drug increases the electric stimulation threshold of the ventricle during diastole. It is useful in ventricular tachyarrhythmias and premature ventricular contractions.[16] It is not useful in atrial or A-V junctional rhythms. Lidocaine produces no detectable circulatory depression in the doses recommended. Because it tends to maintain circulatory stability, the drug is an excellent

TABLE 26–1 Resuscitative Drugs for the Comatose Patient

DRUG (TRADE NAME)	SUPPLIED	DOSAGE ROUTE OF ADMINISTRATION	USES
NaHCO₃	Amps 44.6 mEq/amp	See text p. 1313.	Correction of metabolic acidosis, including the acidosis of cardiac arrest. Correction of respiratory acidosis if ventilation is adequate.
Epinephrine (Adrenalin)	Amps 1:1000 concentration	1 amp IV or rarely intracardiac	Cardiac arrest — see text.
CaCl₂	Amps 100 mg/cc. 1 gm	3–5 cc. IV slowly	Cardiac arrest — see text. Counteracts hyperkalemia.
Ca Gluconate	*Same*	*Same*	
Isoproterenol (Isuprel, Isoprenaline)	Amps of 1 mg/5 cc. 0.2 mg/cc	IV drip: 1–4 µg/min or rarely 0.02–0.04 mg intracardiac	Bradycardia secondary to heart block. Powerful myocardial stimulant (see text) with peripheral vasodilating properties.
Propranolol (Inderal)	Amps 1 mg/cc 1 cc/amp	1–3 mg — no faster than 1 mg/min. Total dose limit: 0.1 mg/kg body weight	Arrhythmias of sympathetic stimulation.

Phenytoin; Diphenylhydantoin (Dilantin)	Amps 250 mg crystals with diluent	100 mg q 5 min. Total dose limit: 1000 mg in adult	Arrhythmias of digitalis overdose (see text).
Lidocaine (Xylocaine, Lignocaine)	Vials 1.0-2% (without preservative)	1-2 mg/kg. then IV drip 20-50 μg/min	Ventricular arrhythmias, especially those of myocardial infarction (see text).
Atropine	Vials, various concentrations	0.3-0.4 mg increments IV	Sinus bradycardia, A-V dissociation (see text).
Digitalis Preparations:			
Ouabain	Amps 0.25 or 0.5 mg/ml	0.25-0.5 mg IV	3-10 minute onset of action; regresses after 8-12 hours.
Deslanoside (Cedilanid-D)	Amps 2-4 ml of 0.2 mg/ml	1.2-1.6 mg IV	10-30 minute onset of action; regresses after 16-36 hours.
Digoxin	Amps 0.25 mg/cc	0.5-1.0 mg IV	5-30 minute onset of action; regresses after 8-10 hours.

antiarrhythmic drug in myocardial infarction.

Lidocaine is best begun as a single intravenous bolus dose of 1 to 2 mg per kg. Blood levels of the drug are then maintained by an intravenous drip of 20 to 50 μg per kg per min, which is approximately 1.5 to 3.5 mg per min in a 70 kg man. This dosage avoids convulsions, which may occur if an excessive dose of the drug is given.[34] The metabolism of lidocaine may be grossly abnormal in patients with cardiac failure, cardiogenic shock or severe liver disease. The dosage should be watched closely in these patients to avoid lidocaine overdose.[69]

ATROPINE.   The emergency use of atropine should be given immediate consideration in a patient who is found to have a symptomatic bradycardia of unknown origin. Atropine blocks parasympathetic stimulation of the heart. It is useful in counteracting sinus bradycardia, A-V dissociation, A-V junctional rhythm or S-A block. Its effect is variable; in complete A-V block, there may be no response to atropine. It has been found most useful in the profound bradycardia of myocardial infarction. Large doses (1 mg) given intravenously may produce premature ventricular contractions, ventricular tachycardia or ventricular fibrillation.[52] Incremental doses of 0.3 to 0.4 mg are recommended. A heart rate around 60 is desirable. Higher rates may increase myocardial oxygen consumption and enlarge the myocardial infarct.

ISOPROTERENOL   (ISUPREL).   Isoproterenol is a strong beta receptor stimulator. Isoproterenol has therefore been recommended in various clinical situations. Both rate and force of myocardial contraction are increased. Additionally, peripheral vasodilation can increase peripheral perfusion by vasodilation and thus decrease the work of the heart. Isoproterenol has been suggested for use in such clinical emergencies as cardiogenic shock and A-V block. Nevertheless, Smith and

Corbascio state: "The implications that the seemingly beneficial hemodynamic actions of isoproterenol effectively reverse clinical shock and improve survival is as yet unproven."[85] The authors go on to point out that the inotropic effects of the drug increase oxygen consumption to the heart without increasing coronary blood flow, and the peripheral vasodilation occurs mainly in muscle, where increased flow is not necessary. Furthermore, the drug may produce myocardial lesions similar to those seen with hypoxia. The drug is also arrhythmiagenic. Great care should be exercised in its use.

DOPAMINE (INTROPIN).   This catecholamine exerts beta-stimulation on the heart and produces peripheral vasoconstriction. It does not constrict renal, mesenteric, pulmonary, coronary or intracerebral vascular beds.[31] One to 10 μg per kg per minute increases cardiac output and renal blood flow in most patients. Its cardiac effects are not blocked by propranolol or atropine, suggesting that a specific dopamine receptor exists. Dopamine has been suggested as therapy in shock states that are unresponsive to other forms of therapy.

CARDIAC GLYCOSIDES.   Rapid-acting preparations of digitalis are invaluable in many resuscitation attempts. There are several preparations that can be given intravenously for rapid effect: ouabain, deslanoside and digoxin. I am more familiar with digoxin, although ouabain has a slightly faster onset of action. The doses of these drugs are listed in Table 26–1. Digitalis' primary effect is a positive inotropic effect — the improvement in cardiac output often results in a slower pulse rate. The digitalis effect on electrical properties of cardiac muscle is much more complicated.[43] The end product of digitalis' electrical effect is to increase atrial-ventricular conduction time and decrease ventricular rate in atrial dysrhythmias. Other electrical effects, along with changes in autonomic tone, may revert supraventricular dysrhythmias to normal sinus rhythm.

Digitalis may be a hazard in cardiac resuscitation, for the stricken patient may already be taking the drug and indeed may be in a state of digitalis intoxication. Digitalis intoxication will result in many types of arrhythmias. Ventricular extra-systoles culminating in ventricular tachycardia or ventricular fibrillation are some of the more common arrhythmias seen with digitalis overdose. Digitalis toxicity is frequently encountered in hypokalemic patients on digitalis. For this reason serum K^+ is always measured. Slow intravenous K^+ administration in these patients will often result in abolition of the arrhythmia. Dilantin has been proposed as the most useful drug in combatting digitalis arrhythmia not due to hypokalemia.[102]

VASODILATORS. The judicious use of vasodilators in resuscitation has become widespread. Cardiac output can be increased and elevated pulmonary capillary pressure can be decreased by their use.[30] The greatest hazard in vasodilator therapy is the drastic lowering of the systolic pressure. These drugs are then lethal. Vasodilator drugs are best used during monitoring of both arterial pressure and pulmonary wedge pressure with the Swan-Ganz catheter. Pulmonary artery catheter pressure should not be allowed to fall below 15 to 18 torr. It is suggested that without this monitoring, hypertensive patients should not be allowed to have a reduction in peak systolic pressure of more than 20 torr, and hypotensive patients should not have a reduction in peak systolic pressure exceeding 5 torr.

Various vasodilators are available. Nitroprusside administered in an IV drip has achieved popularity. Metabolism of nitroprusside can result in cyanide poisoning[49] if high doses are used. A dose of 15 μg per min IV with increments of 5 to 10 μg per min, but totaling no more than 200 μg per min, has been recommended. Other vaso-

dilators include chlorpromazine (Thorazine), which has alpha-blocking properties, phentolamine (Regitine), another alpha blocker, and sublingual isosorbide (Isordil).

Chlorpromazine is given in 2.5 mg increments. The drug has a long duration of action, and small doses usually achieve therapeutic results. Phentolamine, 50 mg in 50 ml of IV solution, can be given at the rate of 0.5 to 1.0 mg per min. This drug has a rapid onset but short duration of action. Some clinicians have claimed good results with a combination of phentolamine with either levarterenol (Levophed) or metaraminol (Aramine). Here the clinician takes advantage of the beta-stimulating properties of levarterenol and metaraminol but blocks their adverse peripheral vasoconstricting properties. The use of the combination must be considered of unproven value.

The outlook for survival after cardiac resuscitation varies with the patient population. Those patients who are closely monitored in hospital intensive care wards or operating rooms have a better prognosis than those who are stricken at home. Improved survival rates for patients stricken in their homes have been seen by rushing trained teams in an ambulance equipped with monitors to meet cardiac emergencies. It would appear that many of the "at home" cardiac arrests are due to the sudden onset of ventricular fibrillation, often not associated with myocardial infarction.[7] The immediate availability of sophisticated technical equipment such as transvenous pacemakers or various mechanical circulatory assistance devices[99] may also improve prognosis. Occasionally successful electrical complexes are restored on the ECG, but there is no perceptible blood pressure. This is called the state of electromechanical dissociation and carries a very poor prognosis. Fixed dilated pupils for 15 to 30 minutes are clear criteria for abandoning resuscitation.

COMMON CAUSES OF COMA — CARDIOVASCULAR DISORDERS

Cardiogenic Shock

Coma can be caused by poor cerebral perfusion related to failure of the heart to function as a pump. The normal value for cerebral blood flow is around 44 ml/min/100 gm[46] or 750 ml/min for a 70 kg man. Cerebral blood flow is maintained constant when systolic arterial blood pressure is between 60 and 150 torr by the phenomenom of autoregulation.[45] When the blood pressure falls below 60 torr, cerebral blood flow decreases and cerebral venous PO_2 is lowered. Unconsciousness is produced[47] by a reduction of flow to roughly one-third of normal (15 ml/min/100 gm brain tissue) or cerebral venous O_2 saturation reduction to 24 per cent. These critical levels are rapidly approached — with cardiogenic shock — in the hypertensive patient or in the patient with arteriosclerotic cerebral vascular disease.

Patients with cardiogenic shock are most often the victims of severe myocardial infarction, although myocarditis, cardiac tamponade or massive pulmonary emboli may also present in this fashion. As the cardiac output begins to fall in these patients, adrenergic impulses cause increased peripheral vasoconstriction, which will maintain flow to critical parts of the body. As the cardiac output continues to fall, the patient is left hypotensive, with cold, wet, cyanotic extremities. The patient will then lapse into coma and cardiorespiratory collapse.

Treatment of coma due to cardiac failure is frustrating. The patient's arterial pressure, CVP, urine output and blood gases must be closely monitored. Application of balloon flotation catheter systems has allowed routine measurement of the filling pressure of the right and left ventricles and cardiac output.[93] It is recommended that pulmonary wedge pressure be kept at 20 torr or

at an optimal level determined by serial cardiac output studies. Peripheral arterial pressure is difficult to determine because of the intense vasoconstriction. Noninvasive monitoring, utilizing a blood pressure cuff and a Doppler blood flow detection device, avoids trauma to the artery. Controlled ventilation and administration of oxygen is usually mandatory. The real difficulties come when one attempts to support the cardiovascular system.[97] Digitalis is of little use. Methylprednisolone, 5 mg per kg, or 1 mg per kg dexamethasone has been advocated, especially in the presence of cerebral edema. Norepinephrine, metaraminol, or dopamine may be helpful. The drugs can be administered as a slow intravenous infusion with continuous monitoring.

Intra-aortic balloon counterpulsation can be instituted if available. This method is used to treat cardiogenic shock and medically refractory left ventricular failure. Most patients have such extensive disease that balloon placement is difficult. Furthermore, most can neither be weaned from balloon support nor undergo a successful infarctectomy or myocardial revascularization.[99] The mortality rate in cardiogenic shock remains distressingly high.

Malignant Hypertension

Hypertension can lead to cerebral events that are the cause of coma. It is sometimes difficult to determine if the coma is due to a cerebral hypertensive event or due to uremia related to a kidney disorder. If the coma is due to a cerebral hypertensive event, the bulk of these will be focal in nature: focal brain ischemia, cerebral or subarachnoid hemorrhages. Some patients may be comatose from these causes alone. Other patients may have convulsions related to these cerebral events. The syndrome of hypertensive encephalopathy is rare. It is a complication of acute glomerulonephritis, toxemia of pregnancy, or severe hypertension.[15, 27] Hypertensive encephalopathy is an acute *generalized* cerebral episode manifested by increasing blood pressure, headache, drowsiness, vomiting, visual impairment, convulsions and focal neurological signs without focal brain lesions.

The patient with malignant hypertension may present with a variety of neurological findings, including coma. Unfortunately, intracranial mass lesions with increased intracranial pressure can also present in this fashion. If the patient has an intracranial mass and secondary hypertension, lowering the blood pressure will reduce cerebral blood flow, often to fatal levels. The physician should support the airway and ventilation and, if the neurological lesion is due to malignant hypertension, should attempt to lower the blood pressure.

The objective of this therapy is to lower the diastolic pressure to 100 mm Hg without excessive risk from cerebrovascular ischemia, myocardial ischemia or renal shutdown. Trimethaphan camphorsulfonate (Arfonad) used as a drip has an immediate hypotensive action and has the advantage that its action is rapidly terminated when the drip is stopped. Tachyphylaxis to Arfonad can develop in some patients, however. The drug is made up as 1 mg/cc solution in D5W and the flow rate is adjusted so that the desired blood pressure is obtained. Nitroprusside, described in the section on vasodilators, has also been recommended.

Hypovolemic Shock

As with cardiogenic shock, coma is produced because cerebral blood flow falls below critical levels. Replacement of lost fluids is the goal of resuscitation. The mental status of the patient gives a clue to the volume of blood lost. An acute decrease of 20 to 25 per cent of the circulating blood volume produces anxiety, 30 to 35 per cent volume loss produces restlessness, and 35 to 40 per cent volume loss produces obtundation.[100] Loss of half the circulating volume will produce coma in patients with hypertension, cardiac impairment or cerebrovascular disease. Other symptoms of shock are pallor, intense peripheral vasoconstriction and sweating. Severe hemorrhagic shock also produces subendocardial hemorrhage, myocardial necrosis and alterations in myocardial muscle histology.[36] All these findings are related to the sympathetic discharge that is the body's defense in hypovolemic shock.

The diagnosis of massive blood loss is easy if there is obvious external trauma. Shock can also occur from blood loss associated with internal bleeding from a fractured femur, from occult gastrointestinal hemorrhage, and from blunt trauma to the chest or abdomen. Such patients can present in coma with few clues to the diagnosis.

There is no ideal substitute for human blood. Treatment of massive blood loss must inevitably utilize blood replacement. Unfortunately, patients may present with severe hypovolemia due not only to blood loss but also to loss or sequestration of plasma or electrolytes. Severe burns, prolonged vomiting or diarrhea may play a variable part in bringing these patients to collapse. The physician must judge what combination of fluids he or she will infuse. The judgment is based on the diagnosis. The physician's judgment is subject to revision during continuous monitoring of arterial and venous blood pressure, heart rate, EKG, urinary output, ventilation and pulmonary compliance. The last-named value is important in the early detection of pulmonary edema caused by fluid overload. Balloon flotation catheter systems[93] have greatly aided the treatment of shock. Controlled ventilation in the comatose or anesthetized shock patient allows the physician to gauge when increasing pressure is required to maintain a constant minute volume. (The decreased compliance evidenced here may be due not only to fluid overload but also to tension pneumothorax or an obstruction in the endotracheal tube.) CVP monitoring is a helpful guide during fluid replacement, although this measurement can be misleading. Volume-depleted patients may exhibit an abnormally high CVP during infusion of blood. This phenomenon is transitory, and the intense peripheral resistance recedes as volume is restored. If a high CVP (over 15 cm saline) persists, one should look for the cause: misplaced or blocked CVP line, occult tension pneumothorax, overtransfusion, congestive heart failure and so on. In the rush to restore blood volume, it is far too easy to resort to the infusion of balanced salt solutions such as Ringer's lactate. Such action is pardonable only when blood or plasma cannot be obtained.

The transfusion of blood can be hazardous to the patient if several rudimentary precautions are not taken. Blood that has been crossmatched with that of the patient is, of course, preferable. However, type specific, or even O^- or O^+ blood may be necessary for the rapidly dying patient. Administration of incompatible blood is disastrous but can easily occur in mass casualty situations where comatose patients are known only by numbers or fictitious names. Blood should be warmed. A thermostatically controlled water bath or a thermostatically controlled infrared oven are both quite suitable, but even a pan of warm water with extra coils of tubing on the blood line will do well in an emergency. If the blood is not warmed, the transfused patient may inadvertently be rendered hypothermic to the point of ventricular fibrillation.

Banked blood is acidic. Massive transfusion usually requires buffering with $NaHCO_3$. I give 1 ampule (50 mEq) $NaHCO_3$ with every three to five units of blood on an empirical basis. If blood gas analysis is available, frequent checks of the patient's pH and acid-base balance are advisable. Banked

blood is hyperkalemic, the potassium content rising with the age of the blood. Electrocardiographic monitoring may allow the early detection of hyperkalemia: increasing height of the T-waves leading to standstill and ventricular fibrillation.

Banked blood is buffered with citrate. Replacement with several units of transfused blood does not appear to significantly lower serum calcium. However, the massively transfused patient may exhibit a widened P-R interval on the electrocardioscope or may exhibit Chvostek's sign. (The latter is sometimes encountered after hyperventilation also.) In these instances the slow infusion of 100 to 500 mg IV $CaCl_2$ is advisable.

Banked blood has an altered oxyhemoglobin dissociation curve. The curve is shifted to the left with hypothermia. Furthermore, the hemoglobin of stored red cells shows an increased O_2 affinity secondary to reduced 2,3 DPG levels.[12] Both these effects prevent oxygen from reaching body tissue. The effects can be diminished by infusing warmed blood that is as fresh as possible.

Banked blood may have micro-aggregates, clumps of leukocytic debris and platelets. Massive transfusion may load the pulmonary vasculature with this material. Dacron-wool blood filters are the best means of preventing these micro-aggregates from reaching the circulation and lodging in the pulmonary vascular bed.[17]

Massive use of ACD blood will often result in a bleeding diathesis. The causes of this diathesis, arranged in order from the common to the rare, are as follows: (1) Dilutional thrombocytopenia. This is corrected by platelet transfusion or by the use of fresh whole blood. (2) Disseminated intravascular coagulation. This is marked by a decrease in platelets, labile clotting factors and fibrinogen. Heparin therapy may rapidly restore the platelet count and fibrinogen, thus attenuating the bleeding. Heparin therapy is reserved for severe cases. (3) Lack of the labile clotting factors V and VII. This is corrected by administration of fresh frozen plasma. (4) Primary fibrinolysis. This is corrected by the use of epsilon-aminocaproic acid (Amicar). Consultation with a pathologist knowledgeable in transfusion problems is helpful for diagnosis and treatment.[55]

Ventilation must be supported in the patient who is comatose from hemorrhagic shock. Pulmonary blood flow decreases, and the resultant poor perfusion of alveoli will drop the PaO_2. Intubation and ventilation with 100 per cent O_2 will be required to overcome this problem.

Severe Pulmonary Disease

Coma can result from severe cerebral hypoxia, severe hypercarbia or combinations of these two. All these states can be the result of severe pulmonary disease. Hypoxia is far more dangerous than hypercarbia, although hypercarbia and attendant acidosis certainly potentiate the deleterious effects of hypoxia. Neurological signs that may precede coma include a symptom complex of headache, papilledema, drowsiness, confusion, tremor and arrhythmic twitching reminiscent of hepatic coma.[6] Coma occurs from hypoxia when the normal O_2 consumption of the brain of 3.3 ml O_2/100 gm tissue/min falls to 2.0 ml O_2/100 gm tissue/min.[67] Cerebral autoregulation is lost within minutes. Hypercarbia, if severe, can cause convulsions and deep anesthesia, but the changes are reversible.[26] Hypoxia can result from exposure to high altitudes, impairment of O_2 diffusing capacity, and hypoventilation based on central or peripheral neurological problems, diaphragmatic impairment or obesity. However, most patients with coma induced by respiratory failure are the victims of intrinsic lung disease. Asthmatic or emphysematous patients will become comatose when their disease is exacerbated by pulmonary infection or severe bronchospasm. We have encountered ambulatory patients of PaO_2 levels of less than 50 torr. How thin a margin of pulmonary reserve these patients have! It is easy to see that a minor exacerbation of the patient's pulmonary disease can become a fatal illness. Small doses of sedative drugs to control "restlessness" from hypoxia can prove calamitous.

Diagnosis of coma caused by respiratory failure can be difficult, as outlined in the resuscitation portion of this chapter. Arterial blood gas analysis is essential in diagnosing and following the course of illness, and the reader is referred to the bibliography for more detail.[8, 66] The basis of treatment is the institution of artificial ventilation through a cuffed endotracheal tube. Immediate tracheostomy is not advisable as the goal of therapy in *short term* ventilatory support, since it carries an unnecessary morbidity and mortality for such short term support.

Two important warnings should be recalled when ventilation of these patients is undertaken: severely hypercarbic patients may be dependent on hypoxic drive to maintain ventilation. Exposing such patients to an oxygen-enriched atmosphere may result in hypoventilation. Such patients must have ventilatory support. On the other hand, abrupt change in pH by assisted ventilation (or intravenous buffering) may cause cardiac arrhythmia. This phenomenon can be explained by alkalosis in the presence of hypoxia, activation of catecholamines or hypokalemia. Rapid reversal of respiratory acidosis can also cause cerebral problems, manifested by convulsions, coma and sometimes death. The etiology of this complication appears to be in part related to changes of cerebral spinal fluid pH that accompanies sudden alkalosis.[19] Diamox (carbonic anhydrase inhibitor) has been used experimentally to combat central depression during correction of severe respiratory acidosis.

Once the cuffed endotracheal tube is

in place, ventilation is instituted with one of a variety of breathing bags. The use of these bags should be considered an intermediate step to the use of a mechanical ventilator.

Frequent checking of blood gases, minute volume, inspired O_2 concentration and so on are necessary when these machines are used. The reader is again referred to the bibliography for a further understanding of respiratory intensive care.[8, 66]

ENDOCRINE DISORDERS — GLUCOSE METABOLISM

Hypoglycemia is a common cause of coma. The brain is almost solely dependent on glucose for metabolism and will not survive long without an adequate blood glucose level. Patients can adapt to relatively low levels of blood glucose, so that the rate of the fall of blood glucose is also important.[25] It is thus difficult to cite a blood glucose level at which a particular patient will become comatose.

The most common cause of hypoglycemic coma is insulin overdose in diabetics. The patient may have taken too much insulin, may not have eaten his meals, or may have engaged in excessive physical exercise. Oral hypoglycemic agents are capable of precipitating comas that can be prolonged and difficult to treat.[21, 77] Alcoholism can precipitate hypoglycemia. Alcohol can act independently of insulin and inhibit hepatic gluconeogenesis.[3] Severe liver disease will also cause hypoglycemia by the same mechanism.

Hypoglycemia precipitated by an overnight fast is often caused by pancreatic islet beta cell tumors. Extrapancreatic tumors that produce hypoglycemic coma are infrequently encountered.[40]

The neurological manifestations of hypoglycemia include: (1) a spectrum of delirium from confusion to mania, (2) epileptic seizures with postictal

coma, (3) coma associated with hypothermia and hypotension with pupils which react to light and (4) a strokelike illness.[65] Severe diabetics are prone to brain stem encephalomalacia. As will be seen later in this chapter, lesions of the brain stem are frequent causes of coma.[4]

The diagnosis is easily made with Dextrostix analysis of the patient's blood. This procedure takes about one minute and should be done in any coma of unknown etiology. Treatment is equally simple. After a blood sugar sample is taken, the patient is given 25 gm of glucose intravenously. This is useful even in nonhypoglycemic coma because, as has been mentioned before, the brain utilizes glucose for all its metabolic needs. IV glucose is contraindicated in bacterial meningitis.

Hyperglycemia, with its associated metabolic disorders, can also be the cause of coma. Diabetic ketoacidosis frequently causes coma and demands prompt recognition and treatment. Diabetic ketoacidosis is found in untreated diabetics, in diabetics who do not take their insulin or who overeat, in diabetics who have severe infections, and in diabetics with alcohol overdose. The hyperglycemia results in osmotic diuresis leading to dehydration and electrolyte depletion. Lack of insulin also results in increased lipolysis with increased ketogenesis. The acidosis of this disorder results from both HCO_3^- ion loss in the osmotic diuresis and an increase in the H^+ ion from the ketogenesis. The exact cause of the coma is still not clear. Cerebral edema is seen in diabetic ketoacidosis.[35] Intravascular coagulation within cerebral vessels may contribute to death in diabetic coma. This coagulation phenomenom may be related to the cerebral edema.[94]

The patient presents with dehydration and often is febrile. There may be a detectable odor of acetone on the breath. Excess acetone is produced as the result of increased ketogenesis. The patient may initially hyperventilate as a result of acidosis, but if the coma has deepened, respirations may be depressed. A history of thirst and copious urinary output, as well as abdominal pain, may be obtained. Diagnosis is quickly made from blood glucose Dextrostix determinations, as well as urinary and serum acetone tests. Treatment of this disorder must begin with determining baseline measurements of the deranged aspects of the body's metabolism. Insulin therapy and correction of electrolyte imbalance follows. Basic laboratory determinations are blood glucose, electrolytes (Na^+, K^+, Cl^-, and HCO_3^-), blood gases (especially pH and base deficit determinations), and serum acetone. As there is often renal, pancreatic and cardiac disease associated with this disorder, BUN and amylase determinations as well as an EKG should be obtained. Urine output, urine glucose and urine acetone should be followed. The patient may require urethral catheterization. If the patient is comatose, aspiration of vomitus should be prevented with a cuffed endotracheal tube. Oxygen supplementation or even ventilatory assistance may be necessary, depending on the ventilatory status of the patient.

Insulin therapy for diabetic keto-acidosis is best given using small doses of insulin infused continuously into the vein. A loading dose of 2 to 12 units of soluble insulin is used, followed by a continuous infusion of 2 to 12 units per hour until ketosis is corrected. The insulin is placed in a small-volume syringe and delivered by a motor-driven pump. A small amount of human albumin may be added to the syringe to prevent adsorption of the insulin to the glass syringe.[78] It has been suggested that overvigorous insulin therapy in the treatment of diabetic coma may cause cerebral edema when glucose levels have been brought to values approaching normal.[35] Electrolyte imbalance is best corrected with saline and bicarbonate solutions. Bicarbonate correction increases sensitivity to insulin,[5]

and cautious use of bicarbonate is urged. Potassium supplementation is usually required as the acidosis is corrected. The reader is referred to an excellent source for further discussion of the treatment of diabetic ketoacidosis.[92]

Hyperglycemia without ketoacidosis is a feature of two other forms of coma in diabetics. Tissue hypoxia in the diabetic may result in coma with severe lactic acidosis. In other patients the blood sugar may rise to astronomical levels (1000 mg/100 ml or more). Seizures may result.[84] Treatment of this group of patients depends on rehydration as well as insulin therapy. The average water deficit may be 24 per cent of total body water. Cerebral edema may play a part in the production of this coma.[35]

HEPATIC COMA

There is still uncertainty as to why hepatic disease should cause coma. Ammonia, short-chain fatty acids, certain amino acids and false neurotransmitters have all been implicated as the cause of hepatic coma.[51] Three groups of patients may develop hepatic coma: those with chronic liver disease and progressive loss of hepatic function, those with acute liver failure secondary to infections, hepatotoxins or autoimmune reactions and, finally, those patients with hepatic encephalopathy due to shunting from portal circulation directly into the vena cava. Significant hepatic encephalopathy developed in 8 of 21 patients submitted to portacaval anastomosis procedures.[70]

The presentation of the patient has been epitomized as a "generalized disorder of movement coupled with a lack of external stimuli proceeding into coma."[1] Signs of severe liver disease may be quite evident in the patient: jaundice, ascites, spider angiomata, hepatomegaly and splenomegaly. However, all clinical signs of liver disease may be absent, and in this case, one must depend on laboratory diagnosis.

An elevated blood ammonia (normal 40 to 70 μg per 100 ml.) or BSP retention of greater than 5 per cent in one hour may be the only clues to the diagnosis of a deep coma.

A list of the less common causes of coma due to systemic disease is found at the end of this chapter.

DRUG OVERDOSE

This section will treat the common drug overdoses that cause coma. The complete list of drugs that cause coma is endless, and the reader is referred to the end of this chapter for the supplementary reading list.

Supportive care may be required. The patient who has attempted suicide may arrive in the Emergency Room appearing only sleepy but may deteriorate rapidly to a comatose, hypoventilating, hypotensive state. These patients may need intubation, ventilation, possibly cardiovascular support, and continuous monitoring by electrocardiogram.

Removing the offending drug from the gastrointestinal tract can be attempted in patients with recent ingestion of the drug. Gastric lavage can be done through an Ewald tube. Many drugs are adsorbed by activated charcoal. Activated charcoal can adsorb amphetamines, phenytoin (Dilantin), aspirin and dextropropoxyphene (Darvon). In general, charcoal should be administered within 30 minutes of the ingestion to prevent drug absorption from the gastrointestinal tract. Charcoal preparations include Norit A activated charcoal (Merck) and Nuchar C. The charcoal is mixed with tap water and administered as a slurry.[18]

Many central nervous system depressants can be antagonized. The narcotic antagonist naloxone (Narcan) will be discussed in the section on narcotic overdose. A central anticholinergic syndrome has been described in a wide variety of overdose problems. In this case physostigmine (Antilirium) may be of use. Symptoms of this syndrome are agitation, a toxic confusional psychosis, and peripheral signs of cholinergic blockade. These peripheral signs include dilated pupils, tachycardia, urinary retention and dry, hot skin. Drugs that may cause this syndrome include the phenothiazines, antihistamines, antispasmodics, anti-Parkinson drugs and over-the-counter sedatives that contain scopolamine.[33]

Physostigmine (Antilirium) is a cholinesterase inhibitor. Unlike other drugs in this category, physostigmine can pass the blood-brain barrier to exert central as well as peripheral cholinomimetic actions.[33] Physostigmine can be used to alleviate both the central and peripheral effects of cholinergic blockade. Tricyclic antidepressants (Elavil, Tofranil and Aventyl), described later, can also cause the central anticholinergic syndrome. Success has been achieved by using physostigmine in tricyclic antidepressant poisoning,[13] but caution is urged. Physostigmine may cause seizures or bradycardia in patients with tricyclic antidepressant poisoning.[57]

Barbiturates

Barbiturate coma may be preceded by nystagmus, ataxia and dysarthria. When coma appears, pupillary light reflexes are preserved and neurological signs are symmetrical, providing some clue in the differential diagnosis. The coma is accompanied by respiratory depression and later by circulatory depression. Death will occur unless respiration and circulation are supported.

Treatment begins with airway care, and the steps leading to intubation are performed as outlined earlier in this chapter. Cardiovascular instability must be treated with vasopressors. Gastric lavage is performed only in the presence of an endotracheal tube. An attempt should be made to identify the poison by the presence of empty pill boxes or by a history from friends and relatives. Laboratory analysis of blood or gastric juice should be done to identify the type of depressant drug.

Supportive hospital treatment with close monitoring of physiological functions produces an excellent survival rate.[89] Cerebral stimulant drugs are no longer recommended. There is controversy as to the effectiveness of diuresis or peritoneal dialysis as an adjunct in therapy. Osmotic diuresis may be effective in phenobarbital coma. Dialysis is reserved for the desperately ill.

Doriden (Glutethimide)

Doriden (glutethimide) produces an appearance of dilated or midposition pupils that may be unequal or fixed to light.[65, 103] The patient can sometimes be roused to movement by vigorous stimulation, only to lapse into immobility with cessation of stimulation. Hypotension, unresponsive to volume expansion, is seen. Supportive treatment is complicated by the fact that glutethimide coma exhibits a prolonged and unpredictable course. The cyclic nature of glutethimide coma has been attributed to enterohepatic circulation of the drug but may be due to accumulation of an active metabolite of the drug.[37]

Tricyclic Antidepressants (Elavil, Tofranil, Aventyl)

The fatal dose in this group of drugs is variable at 10 to 30 times the daily dose. These patients are notoriously difficult to manage.[79] Coma is accompanied by cardiovascular depression, cardiac arrhythmias, hypoventilation and disturbances of temperature regulation. Antiarrhythmic therapy and massive glucocorticoid dosage has been recommended. The picture may resemble the central cholinergic syndrome described previously. Success has been achieved using physostig-

mine, but this drug may exacerbate the cardiac arrhythmias.[57]

Alcohol (Ethanol)

Coma produced by ethanol ingestion alone is uncommon except among those who vaingloriously swallow an entire fifth at once. Ethanol in combination with other drugs or disease states figures prominently in any tabulation of comatose patients brought to the Emergency Room. Levels of ethanol above 110 mg per 100 ml blood produce staggering, mental confusion and perhaps euphoria. At 310 mg per 100 ml blood the patient is comatose or arousable only with vigorous stimulation. Assessment of coma due to ethanol is difficult, since ethanol is an analgesic. Ethanol also acts as a peripheral vasodilator, and the resultant heat loss may result in hypothermia. As blood ethanol rises, the patient becomes more liable to death by respiratory obstruction, vomiting with aspiration, and eventually respiratory arrest. Supportive airway care is mandatory. Alcohol disappears at the rate of 50 to 200 mg per kg per hr. If the drunken patient cannot be aroused within a few hours after cessation of drinking, other causes for his coma should be sought.

Alcoholism can be complicated by the simultaneous ingestion of other drugs. Barbiturates and other hypnotics are additive in their depressant effect. Phenothiazines, reserpine, meprobamate, amitryptylene, morphine and heroin are hyperadditive.[29] Alcohol derelicts have been known to ingest methyl alcohol,[42] isopropyl alcohol (rubbing alcohol)[41] and ethylene glycol (antifreeze) as substitutes for alcohol.[53, 62] Methyl alcohol metabolism produces formaldehyde, which is toxic to retinal cells. Methyl alcohol overdose can cause blindness, and inhibition of methyl alcohol metabolism is in order. This can be done by infusing ethanol to raise the blood alcohol level to 100 mg per 100 ml blood.

Chronic alcoholism can lead to a number of disease states that can, in turn, lead to coma.[14] Liver disease, either acute (as in acute fatty degeneration of the liver) or chronic (as in cirrhosis), can result. This in turn leads to coagulopathies. Thrombocytopenia, independent of portal cirrhosis and hypersplenism, can also occur. The coagulopathies make the patient quite susceptible to intracranial bleeding, for the alcoholic frequently falls and injures his head. Portal cirrhosis also leads to varices, which in turn lead to massive hemorrhage, shock and coma. Alcohol ingestion also can result in hypoglycemia, and this state can be complicated by liver disease.

Rarely one encounters alcoholics who are comatose from vitamin deficient states or thiamine deficient (Wernicke's) encephalopathy or in cardiogenic shock from alcoholic cardiomyopathy. This last-named state is unresponsive to thiamine in the majority of cases and appears different from beriberi heart disease.[61] Alcohol withdrawal is also associated with coma. The patient may be comatose from a postictal state following withdrawal seizures, or further on in the course of withdrawal he may be moribund from delirium tremens.

NARCOTIC OVERDOSE

Coma can be caused by opium, heroin, morphine, meperidine, paregoric and even methadone, a drug used in the treatment of heroin addiction.[88]

One type of coma encountered in narcotic overdose can be expected from the pharmacology of narcotics. The patient has slow, deep respiration and pinpoint pupils. The coma can be reversed with naloxone (Narcan). The naloxone dose will usually be between 0.2 and 0.8 mg IV, and the drug is best given in 0.2 mg increments. Naloxone has a short duration of action, and narcotic overdose symptoms are likely to

reappear. Further doses of naloxone may be necessary. The injection of naloxone may lead to an acute narcotic withdrawal syndrome characterized by hallucinations, fever, pain, perspiration and combative behavior. It is for this reason that the drug is given in small increments.

A second type of narcotic-induced coma is associated with pulmonary congestion and pneumonitis. The coma does not respond to narcotic antagonists but may be associated with increased intracranial pressure. Acute delirium and convulsions may also be seen.[72]

Propoxyphene (Darvon) poisoning is characterized by coma, severe respiratory depression, convulsions and pulmonary edema. Naloxone is a specific antidote for the respiratory depression.

SALICYLISM

Aspirin overdose is extremely common in children. Adults with aspirin overdose are less frequently encountered, but all age groups can present real problems in management. The comatose patient presents with hyperventilation and flushed, often cyanotic skin. The picture is reminiscent of diabetic ketoacidosis. High concentrations of salicylate stimulate respiration centrally and result in an initial respiratory alkalosis. This phase is followed by a metabolic acidosis due to an accumulation of keto and hydroxy acids. Under these conditions, mechanical hyperventilation to lower $PaCO_2$ would be beneficial. Late manifestations of salicylate overdose are hyperthermia — from salicylate-induced uncoupling of oxidative phosphorylation — and gastrointestinal hemorrhage. The presence of salicylate will cause development of a purple color when 5 ml of urine is tested with 1 ml of 10 per cent $FeCl_3$ solution. Serum salicylate levels above 30 mg per 100 ml blood confirm the diagnosis. However, there is a poor correlation of salicylate level in serum with clinical signs.[22]

Most patients will respond to intubation, gastric lavage (although the salicylates are rapidly absorbed) and osmotic diuresis (although kidney function must be intact). It is imperative to keep checking the progress of therapy with frequent analyses of the blood for acid-base status and salicylate levels. Prognosis for adult patients with salicylate levels of 70 mg per 100 ml is not good, and these patients may be candidates for hemodialysis.[10]

INTRACRANIAL PATHOLOGY

This section will discuss one of the major causes of coma, intracranial pathology. As the reader is aware, computerized axial tomography has changed the diagnostic approach to many intracranial problems. This section will emphasize the pathological mechanism and treatment of the common causes of coma caused by intracranial lesions. Brain edema occurs with all these lesions, and a brief review of this entity follows.

Brain edema can be divided into three types: (1) vasogenic edema, (2) cytotoxic edema and (3) interstitial edema. The first category, vasogenic brain edema, is the result of increased capillary permeability causing the accumulation of plasma filtrate, especially in the white matter of the brain. It is commonly caused by brain tumors, abscesses, trauma, brain infarction, severe hypertension and lead encephalopathy. Steroids are of benefit in the edema seen with brain tumor and abscess. Intravenous osmotic agents (mannitol, urea) caused only a temporary alleviation of vasogenic edema.

Cytotoxic brain edema is caused by brain cell swelling. The most common cause is hypoxia, although water intoxication can produce the same effect. Steroid therapy is not effective, and

only osmotic agents can be recommended for water intoxication.

Interstitial brain edema most frequently presents as a mixture of cytotoxic and vasogenic edema.[28] Steroids are thus given empirically in this instance.

As a general rule, supratentorial mass lesions alone rarely cause coma unless these lesions are both quite large and destructive. The most common types of intracranial disease that cause coma remain infratentorial lesions or herniating supratentorial lesions that compress the brain stem from above. Steroids may be effective if the lesion is producing vasogenic edema. Dexamethasone (Decadron) 10 mg IV, then 4 mg q.i.d., is recommended. Osmotic therapy is only temporarily effective.

Diagnosis

The progression of brain herniation with a supratentorial lesion can be quite orderly and can often be followed by successive physical signs. Every physician who handles comatose patients must recognize these signs and act upon his or her knowledge of them. Of prime importance to the physician are those lesions in which immediate operative intervention can be life-saving.

Every comatose patient must be evaluated for the presence of a head injury. Examination of the head may reveal obvious lacerations, hematomas, or blood in the external auditory canal — a sign of a basilar skull fracture. Less obvious signs are blood behind the tympanic membrane, a bruise or hematoma over the mastoid area, spinal fluid rhinorrhea, or even minor lacerations that the unwary physician may tend to dismiss as insignificant. Papilledema indicative of intracranial hypertension may be seen on fundoscopy.

Eye signs are of great importance. They often indicate increasing intra-

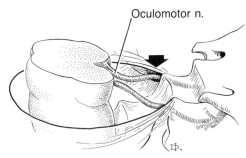

Figure 26–10 Downward pressure on the tentorium causes pressure on the oculomotor nerve. Damage to this nerve produces the dilated pupil of increased intracranial pressure.

cranial pressure and resultant temporal lobe herniation with compression of the vulnerable ipsilateral oculomotor nerve (Fig. 26–10). Oculomotor nerve injury may demonstrate the following sequence as the compression of the nerve progresses (Fig. 26–11 *A* to *D*): (1) Pupillary miosis appears secondary to parasympathetic stimulation. This sign may be absent or fleeting in its appearance. (2) Further compression which results in isolated sympathetic activity (Fig. 26–11*B*). This leads to the ominous dilated pupil of head injury. Consensual response to light in the contralateral pupil is not lost, since the dilated pupil is the result of oculomotor injury. Ophthalmic nerve damage will also cause a dilated pupil, but there will be no consensual light reflex. With complete pupillary dilation (Fig. 26–11*C*), oculomotor ophthalmoplegia occurs, and the eye assumes the characteristic outward and downward gaze of third nerve palsy.

The lesion may be difficult to localize by physical examination. For example, the dilated pupil is not always on the same side as the lesion. The dilated pupil may be contralateral to the actual mass lesion that is causing the temporal lobe herniation, especially if the patient has suffered a chronic increase in intracranial pressure. In addition, there may be bilateral mass lesions that complicate the diagnosis. Anisocoria, unrelated to head injury,

may have been present in the patient before the onset of his coma.

Bilateral dilated pupils (Fig. 26–11 *D*) are a grave sign and quite frequently indicate cerebral death or severe cerebral hypoxia. Rarely the cardiovascular system may appear to be intact and the bilateral pupillary dilation will be the result of bilateral optic nerve lesions accompanying frontal lobe trauma. We have seen this sign only with obvious external signs of trauma.

The presence of an oculocephalic response ("doll's eyes") is helpful in assessing head injury in coma. After ascertaining that there is no cervical spine injury, the physician turns the head to the left or right. The eyes nor-

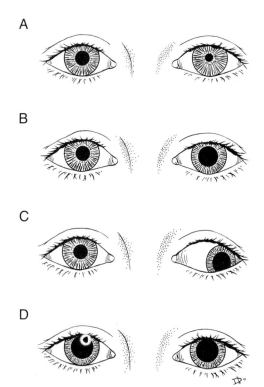

Figure 26–11 Progressive pupillary changes as might be seen with a progressive increase of intracranial pressure: *A.* Pupillary constriction secondary to irritation of the nerve is a transient sign and is often absent. *B.* Isolated sympathetic stimulation of the pupil leads to dilation. *C.* Motor paralysis results in an outward, downward gaze to the affected eye. *D.* Bilateral dilated pupils, frequently, but not always, connoting death.

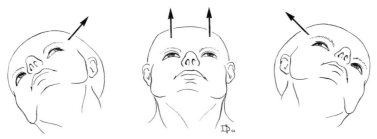

Figure 26–12 The oculocephalic response ("doll's eyes"). The eyes stare straight up, despite the head being turned. The presence of the reflex indicates that at least some brain stem activity has been preserved.

mally move so that they stare in the same direction despite the head being turned (Fig. 26–12). If the eyes remain centered, midbrain function is lost. Deep comas of systemic disease, poisoning or massive brain stem injury do not exhibit this response. Light systemic coma and supratentorial mass lesions that have not sufficiently damaged the brain stem will exhibit this response. Presence of the oculocephalic response in coma is thus a more favorable sign than its absence. Likewise the disappearance of the response with the course of time indicates deepening coma or further brain stem injury. If oculomotor ophthalmoplegia is present (see the preceding paragraphs), the oculocephalic response will be lost in the affected eye. If brain herniation has proceeded so far as to produce ophthalmoplegia, the brain stem may be so compromised that the oculocephalic response disappears altogether.

Brain stem function can also be assessed by caloric response. The placement of 5 to 20 ml of iced water in the ear will normally cause the eyes to deviate slowly toward the ear stimulated and to remain there for several minutes. This sign may be present even if the oculocephalic response is absent. Its absence or disappearance is a grave sign.[64, 68]

A wide variety of neurological signs indicative of upper motor neuron damage can sometimes be found. Vigorous stimulation may cause the comatose patient to move one side and demonstrate an occult hemiplegia. The patient may look toward the side with a cerebral hemispheric lesion or away from the side with a brain stem lesion. Abnormal respiratory patterns may be seen, indicating brain lesions. Central neurogenic hyperventilation, apneustic breathing that exhibits prolonged inspiration and a slow rate, and gasping respirations are often encountered. They may indicate brain stem lesions or pressure on the brain stem from above. Unfortunately, these signs do not satisfactorily localize all mass lesions, and emergency diagnostic procedures should be undertaken if the physician feels that the patient is stable enough to permit them. Echoencephalography is useful in detecting shifts of the brain midline that are indicative of a supratentorial mass lesion.[73] Skull x-rays are mandatory, and even films taken with difficulty from a struggling, semicomatose patient are of more use than no films at all. The physician must check for shifting of a calcified pineal gland (again indicative of a midline shift) and for fractures. The Waters' view is necessary for visualization of many basilar fractures, but the hyperextension required for x-ray should be avoided until the patient has been evaluated for the presence of cervical fractures or dislocation. Even a trained radiologist finds fractures difficult to locate at times. Computerized axial tomography, if available, is extremely informative in evaluating intracranial and intraventricular hemorrhage. This technique replaces invasive angiography and pneumoencephalography in many instances.[75]

In a patient who is rapidly deteriorating, neurosurgery is often begun on the basis of conclusions drawn only from the neurological examination and perhaps from skull films. It is therefore important that the physician constantly observe and record neurological signs at frequent intervals when treating a comatose patient suspected of head injury. Deterioration may be sudden and unexpected. Operative intervention is then forced to proceed with few, if any specific guidelines.

Treatment

Intracranial pressure monitoring has been used to elucidate many of the factors that increase intracranial pressure.[80] Consider the patient with increased intracranial pressure. In this patient small changes in intracranial blood volume, blood flow or brain size become increasingly critical. Between mean arterial pressures of 35 to 140 torr cerebral blood flow remains constant. This is the phenomenon of autoregulation. When arterial pressure falls below the autoregulatory range, cerebral ischemia may result. Above the autoregulatory range, increases in intracranial pressure may be dramatic, especially if increased intracranial pressure already exists.

It has been demonstrated that the hypertension that accompanies laryngoscopy and intubation will often result in a deleterious increase in intracranial pressure in a patient who has intracranial hypertension. Emergency intubation in the patient with increased intracranial pressure should be done with this phenomenon in mind.

On the other hand, most comatose patients with intracranial hypertension need intubation and many additionally require hyperventilation. These patients may be hypertensive and exhibit

bradycardia caused either by reflex or by direct cephalic hypoxia and vagotonia. These patients may exhibit cardiac arrythmias and even pulmonary edema,[96] although the latter is rare. These signs underscore the need for continuous monitoring.

Even before surgery begins, intracranial pressure should be decreased. Reduction of CO_2 by hyperventilation reduces cerebral blood flow and the size of the intracranial vascular compartment. A $PaCO_2$ of 25 torr is felt to be a safe level for this purpose[2] and represents a reduction of approximately 25 per cent in cerebral blood flow. Authorities all agree that hyperventilation does reduce intracranial pressure over the short term, but the usefulness of this technique for several days is still unknown. Other means of reducing intracranial pressure are often employed to gain time before surgical treatment. Hypertonic mannitol or urea infusion, hypothermia, and dexamethasone (dose: 10 mg IV) can be employed for this purpose.[104] The use of intravenous barbiturates to control intracranial hypertension is under study.[81] Hypothermia may not be effective. Cooling brain patients is merely prophylactic against the hyperthermia that may accompany brain injury.[82]

Major Causes

There is a wide variety of intracranial mass lesions that cause coma. Only the major varieties will be considered here.

EPIDURAL HEMATOMA. The most common cause of this lesion is laceration of the middle meningeal artery or its branches. The lesion is frequently associated with skull fracture. The enlarging mass of extravasated blood produces a rapidly progressive syndrome of increased intracranial pressure, temporal lobe herniation, brain stem compression, and death. Early homolateral pupillary dilation can be seen, and as herniation progresses, the contralateral eye also becomes affected.[91] Bilateral fixed and dilated pupils are a poor prognostic sign. Immediate operative intervention is mandatory (see Chapter 8).

SUBDURAL HEMATOMA. Acute and subacute hematomas are often found in conjunction with brain damage. The brain damage contributes to the high mortality of the disease.[71] Skull fracture is less common here than with epidural hematoma and may be opposite to the hematoma. Rapid enlargement of the hematoma makes the lesions clinically indistinguishable from acute epidural hematoma. Craniotomy, rather than burr hole placement alone, increases survival.

Chronic subdural hematoma can be notoriously difficult to diagnose correctly. The clinical picture may make the physician suspect brain tumor, various forms of cerebral vascular disease, senile dementia, encephalitis or psychosis. Computerized axial tomography will greatly facilitate the diagnostic evaluation.

The chronic subdural hematoma evolves with a definite lining or membrane. The interior is filled with decomposing blood and protein-rich fluid. Fresh blood can leak from the vessels in the containing membrane, and the hematoma enlarges further. As the hematoma enlarges, headache, progressive neurological signs and obtundation ensue. The symptoms may fluctuate, and the patient may appear to move in and out of a syndrome of brain stem compression.[65] As with other mass lesions, unconsciousness will result from central or temporal lobe herniation. Coma is a late and grave sign of subdural hematoma. Pupillary signs are often homolateral with respect to the lesions, but the physician cannot depend on it.

When the diagnosis of chronic subdural hematoma is suspected in a comatose patient, immediate steps must be taken to save the patient's life. Hyperventilation with oxygen through a cuffed endotracheal tube is instituted to reduce the brain size and to increase oxygen to the brain. Other methods to reduce intracranial pressure must also be undertaken. Surgical intervention must occur soon after the diagnosis, perhaps even before computerized axial tomography or cerebral angiography can be done.

Chronic and some acute subdural hematomas can be successfully aspirated with a syringe and needle in infants. Emergency drainage through the lateral aspect of the open fontanelle is indicated when the lesion is suspected. Forceful aspiration is not advised.[50]

OTHER SUPRATENTORIAL VASCULAR LESIONS. Coma associated with supratentorial hemorrhage is due to brain stem compression, the irritative effects of blood in the subarachnoid space, or severe intraventricular hemorrhage. The last-named catastrophe appears to affect the brain stem via pressure changes in the ventricular system.[65] Coma with supratentorial hemorrhage is usually due to (1) rupture of an intracerebral blood vessel, sometimes associated with subarachnoid hemorrhage (2) leakage or rupture of an arterial aneurysm at the base of the brain, with resultant hemorrhage, or (3) leakage or rupture of vascular malformations. Blood in the subarachnoid space appears to produce vascular spasm of blood vessels at the base of the brain with diffuse cerebral ischemia.[24] Chemical meningitis may also occur from blood. Blood in the subarachnoid space can thus cause diffuse neurological symptoms and even coma without brain stem herniation.

Patients with supratentorial vascular lesions are often hypertensive. If coma occurs, the onset is usually rapid, although preceded by headache and localizing signs. If there is no history of symptoms preceding the coma, the patient has suffered either infratentorial hemorrhage with direct damage to the brain stem or intraventricular hemorrhage. If coma ensues with supratentorial vascular hemorrhage, the prognosis is poor. Surgical intervention for bleeding aneurysm can be successful. Intervention is most frequently done to prevent rebleeding of the aneurysm after the patient's condition stabilizes. The surest way to complicate an already desperate situation is to fail to support ventilation with endotracheal intubation. Hyperventilation and other adjunctive measures to decrease intracranial pressure should be considered. There is some evidence that hyperven-

tilation will also reduce the area of cerebral infarction following vascular occlusion or hemorrhage,[87] but this approach must be considered not fully established.

SUBTENTORIAL VASCULAR LESIONS. Sudden coma is seen in the case of a brain stem hemorrhage, whereas coma preceded by occipital headache, nausea, dizziness and inability to stand is strongly suggestive of cerebellar hemorrhage. If the patient survives, the coma presents with varying discrete and localizing neurologi-

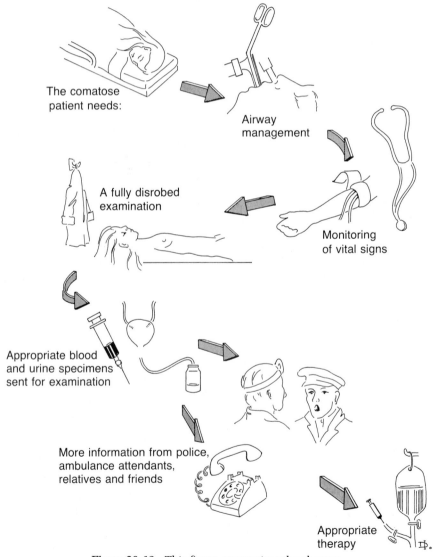

The comatose patient needs:

Airway management

A fully disrobed examination

Monitoring of vital signs

Appropriate blood and urine specimens sent for examination

More information from police, ambulance attendants, relatives and friends

Appropriate therapy

Figure 26–13   This figure summarizes the chapter.

TABLE 26-2 Electrolyte Determinations (Normal Values)

Ca — 9.0–10.6 mg/100 ml	Very high or very low values result in coma.
Mg — 1.8–3.0 mg/100 ml	Very high levels may result in cardiac arrest. Very low levels are associated with nutritional deficiency.
P — 3.0–4.5 mg/100 ml	
Na — 136–142 mEq/L	Extremely high or low values can accompany coma.
Cl — 95–103 mEq/L	If the value is abnormally low, excessive HCO_3 may be the cause. Excessive high values usually reflect Na overload. It is usually not necessary to measure Cl on an emergency basis.
K — 3.5–4.5 mEq/L	Extremely high or low values can be lethal.

cal signs. Coma associated with systemic disease or intoxication will produce no such discrete and localizing signs but rather overall dysfunction of the brain stem. It is difficult to separate cerebral herniation–brain stem compression comas from comas caused by direct brain stem injury. As a rule, brain stem compression proceeds as an orderly erasure of brain stem function, while direct brain stem injury has a spotty and variable presentation of loss of neurological function.[65] Brain stem vascular lesions are the result of occlusions of the basilar artery or its branches, pontine hemorrhage, or rupture of a vertebrobasilar artery aneurysm. Coma or death from acute head trauma, often attributed to cerebral contusion, is in fact frequently due to the brain stem lesions of ischemic necrosis, microhemorrhage, and foci of axonal degeneration.[20] Cerebellar hemorrhage is also a subtentorial event, and here coma is caused by compression or involvement of the brain stem. Aggressive neurosurgical intervention may salvage some

patients if this entity is recognized quickly.[59] Likewise basilar artery aneurysm has become more amenable to surgical correction.[23] Prognosis is poor for most patients with coma due to subtentorial hemorrhage.

Seizures

The physician will frequently encounter seizures in known epileptics, in alcoholics in the early stages of alcohol withdrawal, in patients with craniocerebral trauma, in patients with brain damage secondary to cardiac arrest or brain hemorrhage, and in patients with brain tumors or abscesses. Fortunately for the puzzled diagnostician, the ensuing postictal coma rarely lasts for more than an hour. Often the patient is a known epileptic, or there have been witnesses to the seizures. Tongue-biting occurs during a seizure, and may be a clue to the diagnosis. The airway should be secured in the postictal patient.

The physician is sometimes confronted with a patient having uncon-

TABLE 26-3 Acid-Base Values 37° C

	ARTERIAL	VENOUS
pH	7.37–7.44	7.35–7.45
Pco_2	34–45 torr	36–50 torr
Base	−2.4–+2.3 mEq/L	0–+5.0 mEq/L
Oxygen		
Sea Level	80–95 torr	
	96–97 per cent sat.	
Denver	67–76 torr	25–40 torr
	92–94 per cent sat.	40–70 per cent sat.

TABLE 26-4 Other Important Values (Endogenous)

AMMONIA	Collect with heparin, analyze immediately — 40–70 μg/100 ml
ACETONE	Serum — normal negative on qualitative exam with Acetest tablet
GLUCOSE	Collect with heparin-flouride — 65–100 mg/100 ml
LACTIC ACID	Draw without stasis — 5–20 mg/100 ml normal
UREA NITROGEN	8–20 mg/100 ml — abnormally high values are often associated with coma

TABLE 26–5   Exogenous Toxic Substances

ALCOHOL   Collect without cleansing the skin with alcohol.
  10–50 mg/100 ml: no influence
  50–250 mg/100 ml: increasing drunkenness
  250–300 mg/100 ml: "falling down" drunkenness
  300 mg/100 ml and up: coma

METHYL ALCOHOL   Fatal ingestion with 30–100 gm.

AMPHETAMINES   Amounts greater than 20 μg/ml in the urine are
  indicative of abuse

BARBITURATES   Can be detected in blood or stomach contents.
  3–9 mg/100 ml blood is observed in coma.

BROMIDE   100–200 mg/100 ml serum — toxic manifestations.

DILANTIN   2 mg/100 ml plasma — toxicity manifest.

DORIDEN (GLUTETHIMIDE)   3.0 mg/100 ml plasma produces coma.

LITHIUM   2–3 mEq/L plasma.

LSD   Detectable by thin layer chromatography.

MEPROBAMATE   12 mg/100 ml produces deep coma.

METALS
  Lead (Pb)
    Urine: 0.01–0.15 mg/day — normal
    Blood: 0.01–0.08 mg/100 ml — normal
  Arsenic (As) — Urine: 0.1 mg/24 hr indicative of arsenic poisoning.
  Mercury (Hg) — Urine: 30–100 μg/24 hr indicative of toxic symptoms.
  Iron (Fe) Avoid hemolysis when collecting blood. Toxicity at 50–150
    μg/100 ml serum.

OPIATES   These are better detected in the urine.
  Morphine: 0.01–0.2 mg/100 ml blood may be fatal.
  Methadone: Fatalities reported at levels similar to morphine.

SALICYLATE   30 mg/100 ml — toxicity.

trollable seizures. The airway should be secured and the patient given oxygen to increase the supply of oxygen to the brain. The patient can be given medication to control the seizure. Dilantin 500 mg IV,[95] Valium 5 to 10 mg IV, or phenobarbital in 100 to 200 mg IV doses have proven effective in the adult. Small intermittent doses of Valium or methohexital (Brevital) are often effective in children.[60] Seizures can sometimes injure a patient. The onset can be sudden, resulting in a fall with fractures and head trauma, or the muscular activity can become so violent as to result in dislocation, ligamentous strains or fractures. A trained anesthesiologist can administer a short-acting muscle relaxant such as succinylcholine in order to control muscular activity. Endotracheal intubation and a means of positive pressure ventilation with oxygen are re-

quired. This therapy is limited to seizures that cannot be easily controlled with sedation or in those instances when the seizures are the result of overdose with local anesthetic drugs.[56] In the latter case the seizures are limited in time, and oxygen and prophylactic muscle relaxants are all that are required. Surprisingly, however, IV lidocaine is effective in controlling status epilepticus.[11]

SUMMARY AND LABORATORY VALUES

The preceding sections survey the common causes of coma as they present in the Emergency Room. Various emergency diagnostic and therapeutic measures to identify and alleviate the coma are reviewed. They are summarized in Figure 26–13. The tables that follow (Tables 26–2 through 26–5) list laboratory blood examinations that are helpful in differentiating the causes of coma. The section (following the cited references (Supplementary Reading) will present references to causes of coma not covered by this chapter.

The author gratefully acknowledges the assistance of Dr. Steven Wyte, Dr. Homer McClintock and Dr. Ralph Lehman in preparation of this chapter.

REFERENCES

1. Adams, R. D., and Foley, J. M.: The neurological disorders associated with liver disease. Assoc. Res. Nerv. Ment. Dis. Proc., 32:198–237, 1953.
2. Alexander, S. C., and Lassen, N. A.: Cerebral circulatory response to acute brain disease: Implications for anesthetic practice. Anesthesiology, 32:60–68, 1970.
3. Arky, R. A.: States of unconsciousness associated with alcohol. Surg. Clin. North Am., 48:403–413, 1968.
4. Aronson, S.: Intracranial vascular lesions in patients with diabetes mellitus. J. Neuropathol. Exp. Neurol., 32:183–196, 1973.
5. Assal, J-P., Aoki, T. T., Manzano, F. M., et al.: Metabolic effects of sodium bicarbonate in the management of diabetic ketoacidosis. Diabetes, 23:405–411, 1975.
6. Austen, F. K., Carmichael, M. W., and Adams, R. D.: Neurologic manifestations of chronic pulmonary insufficiency. N. Engl. J. Med., 257:579–590, 1957.
7. Baum, R. S., Alvarez, H., and Cobb, L. A.: Survival after resuscitation from out-of-hospital ventricular fibrillation. Circulation, 50:1231–1235, 1974.
8. Bendixen, H. H., Egbert, L. D., Hedley-Whyte, J., et al.: Respiratory Care. St. Louis, C. V. Mosby, 1965.
9. Berenyi, K. J., Wolk, M., and Killip, T.: Cerebrospinal fluid acidosis complicating therapy of experimental cardiac arrest. Circulation, 52:319–324, 1975.
10. Beveridge, G. W., Forshall, W., Munro, J. F., et al.: Acute salicylate poisoning in adults. Lancet, 1:1406–1409, 1964.
11. Bohm, E.: Treatment of status epilepticus with intravenous lignocaine. *In* Illustrated Handbook in Local Anesthesia. Copenhagen, Munksgaard, 1969.
12. Bunn, H. F., and Jandl, J. H.: Control of hemoglobin function within the red cell. N. Engl. J. Med., 282:1414–1421, 1970.
13. Burks, J. S., Walker, J. E., Rumack, B. H., et al.: Tricyclic antidepressant poisoning: reversal of coma, choreoathetosis and myoclonus by physostigmine. J.A.M.A., 230:1405–1407, 1974.
14. Carson, D. J. L.: Pathologic findings following alcohol. Anesth. Analg., 48:670–675, 1969.
15. Clarke, F., and Murphy, E. A.: Neurological manifestations of malignant hypertension. Br. Med. J., 2:1319–1326, 1956.
16. Collinsworth, K. A., Kalman, S. M., and Harrison, D. C.: The clinical pharmacology of lidocaine as an antiarrhythmic drug. Circulation, 50:1217–1230, 1974.
17. Connell, R. S., and Webb, M. C.: Filtration characteristics of three new in-line blood transfusion filters. Ann. Surg., 181:273–278, 1975.
18. Corby, D. G., and Decker, W. J.: Management of acute poisoning with activated charcoal. Pediatrics, 54:324–328, 1974.
19. Cotev, S., and Severinghaus, J. W.: Role of cerebrospinal fluid pH in management of respiratory problems. Anesth. Analg., 48:42–47, 1969.
20. Crompton, M. R.: Brain stem lesions due to closed head injury. Lancet, 1:669–673, 1971.
21. Cushman, P., Jr., Dubois, J. J., Dwyer, F., et al.: Protracted tolbutamide hypoglycemia. Am. J. Med., 35:196–204, 1963.
22. Done, A. K.: Salicylate intoxication. Significance of measurements of salicylate in blood in cases of acute ingestion. Pediatrics, 26:800–807, 1960.
23. Drake, C. G.: Ligation of the vertebral (unilateral or bilateral) or basilar artery in treatment of large intracranial aneurysms. J. Neurosurg., 43:255–274, 1975.
24. Echlin, F.: Experimental vasospasm, acute and chronic, due to blood in the subarachnoid space. J. Neurosurg., 35:646–656, 1971.
25. Etheridge, J. E.: Hypoglycemia and the central nervous system. Pediatr. Clin. North Am., 14:865–880, 1967,
26. Ferguson, A., and Gaensler, E. A.: Respiratory failure and unconsciousness. Surg. Clin. North Am., 48:293–310, 1968.
27. Finnerty, F. A.: Hypertensive encephalopathy. Am. J. Med., 52:672–678, 1972.
28. Fishman, R. A.: Brain edema. N. Engl. J. Med., 293:706–711, 1975.
29. Forney, R. B., and Harger, R. N.: Toxicology of ethanol. Ann. Rev. Pharmacol, 9:379–392, 1969.
30. Forrester, J. S., daLuz, P. L., and Chatterjee, K.: Peripheral vasodilators in low cardiac output states. Surg. Clin. North Am., 55:531–544, 1975.
31. Goldberg, L. J.: Dopamine — clinical uses of an endogenous catecholamine. N. Engl. J. Med., 291:707–710, 1974.
32. Goldberger, E.: Treatment of Cardiac

Emergencies. St. Louis, C. V. Mosby, 1974.

33. Granacher, R. P., and Baldessarini, R. J.: Physostigmine: its use in acute anticholinergic syndrome with antidepressant and anti-Parkinson drugs. Arch. Gen. Psychiatry, 32:375–380, 1975.

34. Granelly, R., von der Groeben, J. O., Spivack, A. P., et al.: Effect of lidocaine on ventricular arrhythmias in patients with coronary heart disease. N. Engl. J. Med., 277:1215–1219, 1967.

35. Guisada, R., and Arieff, A. I.: Neurologic manifestations of diabetic comas: correlation with biochemical alterations in the brain. Metabolism, 24:665–679, 1975.

36. Hackel, D. B., Ratliff, N. B., and Mikat, E.: The heart in shock. Circ. Res., 35:805–811, 1974.

37. Hansen, A. R., Kennedy, K. A., Ambre, J. J., et al.: Glutethimide poisoning. A metabolite contributes to morbidity and mortality. N. Engl. J. Med., 292:250–252, 1975.

38. Harley, H. R. S.: Reflections on cardiopulmonary resuscitation. Lancet, 2:1–4, 1966.

39. Heimlich, H. J., Hoffman, K. A., and Canestri, F. R.: Food choking and drowning deaths prevented by external diaphragmatic compression. Ann. Thorac. Surg., 20:188–195, 1975.

40. Hurwitz, D.: Hypoglycemic and hyperglycemic coma. Surg. Clin. North Am., 48:361–370, 1968.

41. Juncos, L., and Taguchi, J. T.: Isopropyl alcohol intoxication. J.A.M.A., 204:732–734, 1968.

42. Keyvan Larijarni, H., and Tannenberg, M.: Methanol intoxication. Arch. Intern. Med., 134:293–296, 1974.

43. Koch-Weser, J.: Current concepts: mechanism of digitalis action on the heart. N. Engl. J. Med., 277:417–419, 469–471, 1967.

44. Kristofferson, M. B., Rattenborg, C. C., and Holaday, D. H.: Asphyxial death: the roles of acute anoxia, hypercarbia, and acidosis. Anesthesiology, 28:488–497, 1967.

45. Lassen, N. A.: Autoregulation of cerebral blood flow. Circ. Res., 15(Suppl. 1):201–204, 1964.

46. Lassen, N. A., and Lane, M. H.: Validity of internal jugular blood flow for study of cerebral blood flow and metabolism. J. Appl. Physiol., 16:313–320, 1961.

47. Lennox, W. G., Gibbs, F. A., and Gibbs, E. L.: Relationship of unconsciousness to cerebral blood flow and to anoxemia. Arch. Neurol. Psychiat., 34:1001–1013, 1935.

48. Lund, I., and Lind, B. (ed.): Aspects of resuscitation. Proceedings of the Second International Symposium on Emergency

Resuscitation. Acta Anesthesiol. Scand., suppl. 29, 1968.

49. McDowall, D. G., Kenaey, N. P., and Turner, J. M.: The toxicity of sodium nitroprusside. Br. J. Anaesth., 46:327–332, 1974.

50. McLaurin, R. L., Isaacs, E., and Lewis, H. P.: Results of nonoperative treatment in 15 cases of infantile subdural hematoma. J. Neurosurg., 34:753–759, 1971.

51. Maddrey, W. C., and Weber, F. C.: Chronic hepatic encephalopathy. Med. Clin. North Am., 59:937–944, 1975.

52. Massumi, R. A., Mason, D. T., Amsterdam, E. A., et al.: Ventricular fibrillation and tachycardia after intravenous atropine for treatment of bradycardia. N. Engl. J. Med., 287:336–338, 1972.

53. Michelis, M. F., Mitchell, B., and Davis, B. B.: Bicarbonate resistant metabolic acidosis in association with ethylene glycol intoxication. Clin. Toxicol., 9:53–60, 1976.

54. Miller, J. R., and Myers, R. E.: Neuropathology of systemic circulatory arrest in adult monkeys. Neurology, 22:888–904, 1972.

55. Miller, R. D.: Complications of massive blood transfusion. Anesthesiology, 39:82–93, 1973.

56. Moore, D. C., and Bridenbaugh, L. D.: Oxygen: the antidote for systemic toxic reactions from local anesthetic drugs. J.A.M.A., 174:842–847, 1960.

57. Newton, R. W.: Physostigmine salicylate in the treatment of tricyclic antidepressant overdose. J.A.M.A., 231:941–943, 1975.

58. Nilsson, B., Norberg, K., and Siesjo, B. K.: Biochemical events in cerebral ischemia. Br. J. Anaesth., 47:751–760, 1975.

59. Ott, K. H., Kase, C. S., Ojeman, R. G., et al.: Cerebellar hemorrhage: diagnosis and treatment. Review of 56 cases. Arch. Neurol., 31:160–167, 1974.

60. Pampiglione, G., and DaCosta, A. A.: Intravenous therapy and EEG monitoring in prolonged seizures. J. Neurol. Neurosurg. Psychiatry, 38:371–377, 1975.

61. Parker, D. M.: The effects of ethyl alcohol on the heart. J.A.M.A., 228:741–742, 1974.

62. Parry, M. F., and Wallach, R.: Ethylene glycol poisoning. Am. J. Med., 57:143–150, 1974.

63. Pennington, J. E., Taylor, J., and Lown, B.: Chest thump for reverting ventricular tachycardia. N. Engl. J. Med., 283:1192–1195, 1970.

64. Plum, F., and Caronna, J. J.: Can one predict the outcome of medical coma? In Outcome of Severe Damage to the Central Nervous System. Ciba Foundation Symposium. Amsterdam, Excerpta Medica, 1975.

65. Plum, F., and Posner, J. B.: The Diagnosis

of Stupor and Coma. Philadelphia, F. A. Davis, 1966.

66. Pontoppidan, H., Geffin, B., and Lowenstein, E.: Acute respiratory failure in the adult. N. Engl. J. Med., 287:690–698, 743–752, 799–806, 1972.

67. Posner, J. B., and Plum, F.: Toxic effects of carbon dioxide and acetazolamide in hepatic encephalopathy. J. Clin. Invest., 39:1246–1258, 1960.

68. Poulsen, J., and Zilstorff, K.: Prognostic value of caloric vestibular test in the unconscious patient with cranial trauma. Acta Neurol. Scand., 48:282–292, 1972.

69. Prescott, L. F., Adjepon Yamoah, K. K., and Talbot, R. G.: Impaired lignocaine metabolism in patients with myocardial infarction and cardiac failure. Br. Med. J., 1:939–941, 1976.

70. Read, A. E., Laidlaw, J., and Sherlock, S.: Neuropsychiatric complications of portacaval anastomosis. Lancet, 1:961–963, 1961.

71. Richards, T., and Hoff, J.: Factors affecting survival from acute subdural hematoma. Surgery, 75:253–258, 1974.

72. Richter, R. W., Pearson, J., Bruun, B., et al.: Neurologic complications of addiction to heroin. Bull. N.Y. Acad. Med., 49:3–21, 1973.

73. Rothman, J., and Gershowitz, M.: Ultrasonic diagnosis of subdural hematomas, epidural hematomas, brain edema, and brain atrophy. Am. J. Roentgenol. Rad. Ther. Nucl. Med., 122:531–537, 1974.

74. Safar, P.: Recognition and management of airway obstruction. J.A.M.A., 208:1008–1011, 1969.

75. Scott, W. R., New, P. F., Davis, K. R., et al.: Computerized axial tomography of intracranial and intraventricular hemorrhage. Radiology, 112:73–80, 1974.

76. Sellick, B. A.: Cricoid pressure to control regurgitation of stomach contents during induction of anaesthesia. Lancet, 2:404–406, 1961.

77. Seltzer, H. S.: Drug induced hypoglycemia. Diabetes, 21:955–966, 1972.

78. Semple, P. F., White, C., and Manderson, W. G.: Continuous intravenous infusion of small doses of insulin in treatment of diabetic ketoacidosis. Br. Med. J., 2:694–698, 1974.

79. Serafimovski, N., Thorball, N., Asmussen, I., et al.: Tricyclic antidepressant poisoning with special reference to cardiac complications. Acta Anesthesiol. Scand., 19(suppl. 57):55–63, 1975.

80. Shapiro, H. M., and Aidinis, S. J.: Neurosurgical anesthesia. Surg. Clin. North Am., 55:913–928, 1975.

81. Shapiro, H., Lafferty, J., Keykhah, M. M., et al.: Barbiturates and intracranial hypertension. *In* McLaurin, R. L. (ed.): Head Injuries. New York, Grune and Stratton, 1976.

82. Shenkin, H. A., and Bouzarth, W. F.: Clinical methods of reducing intracranial pressure. N. Engl. J. Med., 282:1465–1471, 1970.

83. Shrago, G. C.: Cervical spine injuries: association with head trauma. Review of 50 patients. Am. J. Roentgenol. Rad. Ther. Nucl. Med., 118:670–3, 1973.

84. Singh, B. M., Gupta, D. R., and Strobos, R. J.: Nonketotic hyperglycemia and epilepsia partialias continua. Arch. Neurol., 29:187–190, 1973.

85. Smith, N. T., and Corbascio, A. N.: The use and misuse of pressor agents. Anesthesiology, 33:58–101, 1970.

86. Smith, R. B., Schaer, W. B., and Pfaeffle, H.: Percutaneous transtracheal ventilation for anesthesia and resuscitation. Can. Anaesth. Soc. J., 22:607–612, 1975.

87. Soloway, M., Nadel, W., Albin, M. S., et al.: The effect of hyperventilation on subsequent cerebral infarction. Anesthesiology, 29:975–980, 1968.

88. Sopira, J. D., and McDonald, R. H., Jr.: Drug abuse — 1970. Disease-a-Month, November 1970.

89. Spear, P. W., and Protass, L. M.: Barbiturate poisoning, an endemic disease. Med. Clin. North Am., 57:1471–1479, 1973.

90. Standards for cardiopulmonary resuscitation (CPR) and emergency cardiac care. J.A.M.A., 222(Supplement), February 1974.

91. Sunderland, S., and Bradley, K. C.: Disturbances of oculomotor function accompanying extradural hemorrhage. J. Neurol. Neurosurg. Psychiatry, 16:35–46, 1953.

92. Sussman, K. E., and Metz, R. J. S. (eds.): Diabetes Mellitus. New York, Am. Diabetes Assoc., 1975.

93. Swan, H. J. C., and Ganz, W.: Use of balloon flotation catheters in critically ill patients. Surg. Clin. North Am., 55:501–520, 1975.

94. Timperly, W. R., Preston, F. E., and Ward, J. D.: Cerebral intravascular coagulation in diabetic ketoacidosis. Lancet, 1:952–956, 1974.

95. Wallis, W., Kutt, H., and McDowell, F.: Intravenous diphenylhydantoin in treatment of acute repetitive seizures. Neurology, 18:513–525, 1968.

96. Webb, W. R.: Pulmonary complications of nonthoracic trauma: summary of the National Research Council Conference. J. Trauma, 9:700–711, 1969.

97. Weisberger, C. L., Ruggiero, N., and Chung, E. K.: Treatment of cardiogenic shock. *In* Controversy in Cardiology. New York, Springer-Verlag, 1976.

98. Wild, J. B., and Grover, J. D.: The fist as a cardiac pacemaker. Lancet, 2:436–437, 1970.

99. Willerson, J. T., Curry, G. C., Watson, J. T., et al.: Intra-aortic balloon counterpulsation in patients in cardiogenic shock, left ventricular failure and/or recurrent ventricular tachycardia. Am. J. Med., 58:183–191, 1975.

100. Williams, L. F.: Hemorrhagic shock as a source of unconsciousness. Surg. Clin. North Am., 48:263–272, 1968.

101. Wit, A. L., Hoffman, B. F., and Rosen, M. R.: Electrophysiology and pharmacology of cardiac arrhythmias. IX. Cardiac electrophysiologic effects of beta-adrenergic receptor stimulation and blockade. Am. Heart J., 90:521–533, 665–675, 795–803, 1975.

102. Wit, A. L., Rosen, M. R., and Hoffman, B. R.: Electrophysiology and pharmacology of cardiac arrhythmias. VIII. Cardiac effects of diphenylhydantoin. Am. Heart J., 90:265–272, 397–404, 1975.

103. Wright, N., and Roscoe, P.: Acute glutethemide poisoning: conservative management of 31 patients. J.A.M.A., 214:1704–1706, 1970.

104. Zervas, N. T., and Hedley-Whyte, J.: Successful treatment of cerebral herniation in five patients. N. Engl. J. Med., 286:1075–1077, 1972.

SUPPLEMENTARY READING LIST

Coma

This list is arbitrarily divided by organ systems. Systemic diseases, such as myasthenia gravis, will be found under the organ primarily affected, e.g., the lung.

Adrenal

Egdahl, R. H.: Shock and the adrenal. Surg. Clin. North Am., 48:287–291, 1968.

Blood

Marsden, P. D., and Bruce-Chwatt, L. J.: Cerebral malaria. Contemp. Neurol. Ser., 12:29–44, 1975.

Portnoy, B. A., and Herion, J. C.: Neurologic manifestations in sickle-cell disease. Ann. Intern. Med., 76:643–652, 1972.

Smith, R. P., and Olson, M. V.: Drug induced methemoglobinemia. Semin. Hematol., 10:253–268, 1973.

Brain

Moreau, J. P.: Fat embolism. Can. J. Surg., 17:196–199, 1974.

Hasselmeyer, E. G., and Hunter, J. C.: Sudden infant death syndrome. Obstet. Gynecol. Annu., 4:213–36, 1975.

DeVivo, D. C., Keating, J. P., and Haymond, M. W.: Reye's syndrome: results of intensive supportive care. J. Pediatr., 87:875–880, 1975.

Malatinsky, J., Prochazka, M., and Samel, M.: Respiratory failure as a seizure phenomenon. Br. J. Anaesth., 47:1019–1022, 1975.

Krieger, A. J., and Rosomoff, H.: Sleep induced apnea. J. Neurosurg., 39:168–180, 181–185, 1974.

Nordgren, R. E., Marksbery, W. R., Fukuda, K., et al.: Seven cases of cerebromedullospinal disconnection: "locked-in" syndrome. Neurology, 21:1140–1148, 1971.

Johnson, R. T.: Slow viral infections and chronic neurologic disease. In Frontiers in Neurology and Neuroscience Research. Toronto, Canada, Neuroscience Institute, 1974.

Frank, G., Pazzaglia, P., Frank, F., et al.: Clinical course of post-traumatic coma. J. Neurosurg. Sci., 18:120–123, 1974.

Resnick, M. E., and Patterson, C.: Coma and convulsions due to compulsive water drinking. Neurology, 19:1125–1126, 1969.

Miller, R. B.: Central nervous system manifestations of fluid and electrolyte disturbances. Surg. Clin. North Am., 48:381–393, 1968.

Gitelman, H. J., and Welt, L. G.: Magnesium deficiency. Annu. Rev. Med., 20:233–242, 1969.

Plum, F., and Posner, J. B. (eds.): Vitamin deficiency: cofactor deficiency. In The Diagnosis of Stupor and Coma. Philadelphia, F. A. Davis Co., 1966.

Oxbury, J. M., and Whitty, C. W. M.: Causes and consequences of status epilepticus in adults. Brain, 94:733–744, 1971.

Ingvor, D. H., and Sourander, P.: Destruction of the reticular core of the brain stem. Arch. Neurol., 23:1–8, 1970.

Heart and Cardiovascular System

Kovach, A. G. B., and Sandor, P.: Cerebral blood flow and brain function during hypotension and shock. Annu. Rev. Physiol., 38:571–596, 1976.

Stephenson, H. E.: Cardiac Arrest and Resuscitation, 4th ed. St. Louis, C. V. Mosby, 1974.

Schumer, W., and Nyhus, L. M. (eds.): Treatment of Shock: Principles and Practice. Philadelphia, Lea & Febiger, 1974.

Hershey, S. G., Del Guercio, L. R. M., and
McConn, R. (eds.): Septic Shock in Man. Boston, Little, Brown & Co., 1971.

Glenn, T. M. (ed.): Steroids and Shock. Baltimore, University Park Press, 1974.

Hutchinson, E. C., and Stock, J. P. P.: The
carotid-sinus syndrome. Lancet, 2:445–449,
1960.

Kidney

Raskin, N.H., and Fishman, R. A.: Neurologic
disorders in renal failure. N. Engl. J. Med.,
294:143–148, 204–210, 1976.

Burks, J. S., Alfrey, A. C., Huddlestone, J., et al.:
A fatal encephalopathy in chronic haemodialy-
sis patients. Lancet, *1*:764–768, 1976.

Liver

De Matteis, F.: Disturbances of liver porphyrin
metabolism caused by drugs. Pharmacol. Rev.,
19:523–557, 1967.

Eales, L.: The porphyrins and the porphyrias.
Annu. Rev. Med., *12*:251–270, 1961.

Ware, A. J., D'Agostino, N., and Combes, B.:
Cerebral edema: major complication of massive hepatic necrosis. Gastroenterology,
61:877–884, 1971.

Lung

Bredenberg, C. E.: Acute respiratory distress.
Surg. Clin. North Am., *54*:1043–66, 1974.

Grant, J. L., and Arnold, W.: Idiopathic hyperventilation. J.A.M.A., *194*:119–122, 1965.

Thomas, A. N., and Stephens, B. G.: Air embolism, a cause of morbidity and death after
penetrating chest trauma. J. Trauma, *14*:633–
638, 1976.

Pruitt, B. A., Erickson, D. R., and Morris, A.:
Progressive pulmonary insufficiency and
other pulmonary complications of thermal injury. J. Trauma, *15*:369–379, 1975.

Engel, W. K., Festoff, B. W., Patten, B. M., et al.:
Myasthenia gravis. Ann. Intern. Med., *81*:225–
246, 1974.

Rochester, D. F.: Current concepts in the pathogenesis of the obesity-hyperventilation syndrome. Am. J. Med., *57*:402–420, 1974.

Jenkins, M. T., and Luhn, N. R.: Active management of tetanus. Anesthesiology, *23*:690–
709, 1962.

Heurich, A. E., Brust, J. C. M., and Richter, R.
W.: Management of urban tetanus. Med. Clin.
North Am., *57*:1373–1381, 1973.

Sankaran, S., and Wilson, R. F.: Factors affecting
prognosis in patients with flail chest. J.
Thorac. Cardiovasc. Surg., *60*:402–409, 1970.

Pancreas

Toffler, A. H., and Spiro, H. M.: Shock or coma
as the predominant manifestation of painless
acute pancreatitis. Ann. Intern. Med., *57*:655–
659, 1962.

Parathyroid

Kreisler, B., Dinbar, A., and Tulcinsky, D. B.:
Postoperative atetanic hypocalcemic coma; report of a case. Surgery, *65*:916–918, 1969.

Wilson, R. E., Bernhard, W. F., Polet, H., et al.:
Hyperparathyroidism: the problem of acute
parathyroid intoxication. Ann. Surg., *159*:79–
93, 1964.

Pituitary

Blau, J. N., and Hinton, J. M.: Hypopituitary
coma and psychosis. Lancet, *1*:408–409,
1960.

Thyroid

Newmark, S. R., Himathongkam, T., and Shane,
R.: Myxedema coma. J.A.M.A., *230*:884–85,
1974.

Mackin, J. F.: Thyroid storm and its management. N. Engl. J. Med., *291*:1396–8, 1974.

Coma: Secondary Exogenous Factors

This list is divided into several arbir-
trary headings.

Poisons — General

Arena, J.: Poisoning: Toxicology, Symptoms,
Treatment, 3rd ed. Springfield, Ill., Charles C
Thomas, 1974.

Gosselin, R. E., et al.: Clinical Toxicology of
Commercial Products. Baltimore, Williams &
Wilkins Co.,1976.

Mofenson, H. C., and Greensher, J.: The unknown poison. Pediatrics, *54*:336–342, 1974.

Schreiner, G. E., and Teehan, B. P.: Dialysis of
poisons and drugs: annual review. Trans. Am.
Soc. Artif. Intern. Organs, *18*:563–599, 1972.

Holland, J., Massie, M. J., Grant, C., et al.: Drugs
ingested in suicide attempts and fatal outcome. N.Y. State J. Med., *75*:2343–2349,
1975.

Dreisbach, R. H.: Handbook of Poisoning: Diagnosis and Treatment, 8th ed. Lange Medical
Publications, Los Altos, Calif. 1974.

Poisons — Food

Lamanna, C., and Carr, C. J.: The botulinal, tetanal and enterostaphylococcal toxins: a review. Clin. Pharmacol. Ther., 8:286–332, 1967.

Brady, L. R.: Toxins of higher fungi. Lloydia, 38:36–56, 1975.

Cherrington, M.: Botulism: ten year experience. Arch. Neurol., 30:432–437, 1974.

Coma Secondary to Prescription Drugs

Westlin, W. F.: Desferal (deferoxamine) in the treatment of acute iron intoxication. Clin. Pediat., 5:531–535, 1966.

Adams, P., and Waite, C.: Isoniazid induced encephalopathy. Lancet, 1:680–682, 1970.

McBay, A. J., and Algeri, E. J.: Ataraxics and nonbarbiturate sedatives. Prog. Chem. Toxicol. 157–190, 1963.

Xanthaky, G., Freireich, A. W., Matusiak, W., et al.: Hemodialysis in methyprylon poisoning, J.A.M.A., 198:1212–1213, 1966.

Teehan, B. P., Maher, J. F., Carey, J. J. H., et al.: Acute ethchlorvynol (Placidyl) intoxication. Ann. Intern. Med., 72:875–882, 1970.

Finkelstein, R., and Jacobi, M.: Fatal iodine poisoning: a cliniopathologic and experimental study. Ann. Intern. Med., 10:1283–1296, 1937.

Wooster, A. G., Dunlop, M., and Joske, R. A.: Use of oral diuretic (Doburil) in treatment of bromide intoxication. Am. J. Med. Sci., 253:23–26, 1967.

Kerr, F., Kenoyer, G., and Bilitch, M.: Quinidine overdosage. Br. Heart J., 33:629–631, 1971.

Diamond, M. J., Brownstone, Y. S., Erceg, G., et al.: The reduction of coma time in lipophilic overdose using castor oil. Can. Anaesth. Soc. J., 23:170–175, 1976.

Holt, D. W., Traill, T. A., and Brown, C. B.: The treatment of digoxin overdose. Clin. Nephrol., 3:119–122, 1975.

Cohen, W. J., and Cohen, N. H.: Lithium carbonate, haloperidol and irreversible brain damage. J.A.M.A., 230:1283–1287, 1974.

Davis, J. M., Bartlett, E., and Termini, B. A.: Overdosage of psychotropic drugs: a review. Part I: Major and minor tranquilizers. Part II: Antidepressants and other psychotropic agents. Dis. Nerv. Syst., 29:157–164, 246–256, 1968.

Coma Secondary to Illicit Drugs and Psychotropic Agents

Swissman, N., and Jacoby, J.: Strychnine poisoning and its treatment. Clin. Pharmacol. Ther., 5:136–140, 1964.

Hart, J. B., and Wallace, J.: The adverse effects of amphetamines. Clin. Toxicol., 8:179–190, 1975.

Price, K. R.: Fatal Cocaine Poisoning. J. Forensic Sci. Soc., 14:329–333, 1974.

Linden, C. B., Lovejoy, F. H., and Costello, C. E.: Phencyclidine: nine cases of poisoning. J.A.M.A., 234:513–516, 1975.

Gilroy, J., Andaya, L., and Thomas, V. J.: Intracranial mycotic aneurysms and subacute bacterial endocarditis in heroin addiction. Neurology, 23:1193–1198, 1973.

McGlothlin, W. H.: Drug use and abuse. Annu. Rev. Psychol., 26:45–64, 1975.

Caldwell, J., and Sever, P. S.: The biochemical pharmacology of abused drugs. Clin. Pharmacol. Ther., 16:625–638, 737–749, 989–1013, 1974.

Poklis, A.: Aerosol propellant abuse and toxicity. J. Can. Soc. Forensic Sci., 8:87–95, 1975.

Freedman, D. X.: The psychopharmacology of hallucinogenic agents. Annu. Rev. Med., 20:409–418, 1969.

Poisoning Secondary to Industrial Products and By-products

Jenkins, R. B.: Inorganic arsenic and the nervous system. Brain, 89:479–498, 1966.

Fowler, B. A., and Weissberg, J. B.: Arsine poisoning. N. Engl. J. Med., 291:1171–1174, 1974.

Magos, L.: Mercury and mercurials. Br. Med. Bull., 31:241–245, 1975.

Whitfield, C. L., Ch'ien, L. T., and Whitehead, J. D.: Lead encephalopathy in adults. Am. J. Med., 52:289–298, 1972.

Chisholm, J. J., and Kaplan, E.: Lead poisoning in childhood: comprehensive management and prevention. J. Pediatr., 73:942–950, 1968.

Bank, W. J., Pleasure, D. E., Suzuki, K., et al.: Thallium poisoning. Arch. Neurol., 26:456–64, 1972.

Larkin, J. M., Brahos, G. J., Moylan, J. A.: Treatment of carbon monoxide poisoning: prognostic factors. J. Trauma, 16:111–114, 1976.

Stolman, A.: The absorption, distribution, and excretion of drugs and poisons and their metabolites. Prog. Chem. Toxicol., 5:1–99, 1974.

Heyndrickx, A.: Toxicology of insecticides, rodenticides, herbicides, and phytopharmaceutical compounds. Prog. Chem. Toxicol., 4:179–256, 1969.

Hayes, W. J.: Mortality in 1969 from pesticides, including aerosols. Arch. Environ. Health, 31:61–72, 1976.

DePalma, A. E., Kwalick, D. S., and Zuckerberg, N.: Pesticide poisoning in children. J.A.M.A., 211:1979–1981, 1970.

Coma from Hostile Environmental Factors

Ward, M.: Mountain Medicine — A Clinical Study of Cold and High Altitude. London, Crosby-Lockwood-Staples, 1974.

Andrews, I. C., and Orkin, L. R.: Environmental cold and man. Anesthesiology, *25*:549–559, 1964.

Lapp, N. L., and Jurgens, J. L.: Frostbite. Mayo Clin. Proc., *40*:932–948, 1965.

Wakim, K. G.: Bodily reactions to high temperature. Anesthesiology, *25*:532–548, 1964.

Levine, J. A.: Heatstroke in the aged. Am. J. Med., *47*:25–258, 1969.

Martin, D. W., Watts, H. D., and Smith, L. H.: Heatstroke. West. J. Med., *121*:305–312, 1975.

Perchick, J. S., Winklestein, A., and Shadduck, R. K.: Disseminated intravascular coagulation in heat stroke. J.A.M.A., *223*:637–640, 1975.

Rivers, J. F., and Golden, F.St. C.: The immersion incident. Anesthesia, *30*:364–373, 1975.

Elliott, D. H., and Hanson, R. D.: Treatment of the diving casualty. Anaesthesia, *31*:81–89, 1976.

Strauss, R. H., and Prockop, L. D.: Decompression sickness among scuba divers. J.A.M.A., *223*:637–640, 1973.

Lee, W. R.: The nature and management of electric shock. Br. J. Anaesth., *36*:572–580, 1964.

Apfelberg, D. B., Masters, F. W., and Robinson, D. W.: Pathophysiology and treatment of lightning injuries. J. Trauma, *14*:453–460, 1974.

Frazier, C. A.: Insect Allergy. St. Louis, W. H. Green, 1969.

Brown, J. H.: Toxicology and Pharmacology of Venoms from Poisonous Snakes. Springfield, Ill., Charles C Thomas, 1973.

Outpatient and Short Stay Fiberoptic Endoscopy 27

ROBERT W. BEART, JR., M.D.,
and JOHN A. HIGGINS, M.D.

INTRODUCTION

The technical advances in fiberoptic equipment since the late 1960s have revolutionized diagnostic and therapeutic endoscopy of the gastrointestinal and bronchial tracts. The capabilities currently available allow the use of a flexible endoscope as a primary diagnostic and therapeutic instrument, as well as enhancing its value for confirming and augmenting diagnostic impressions gained from other procedures. The value of these instruments in the investigation of a wide variety of conditions involving the gastrointestinal and respiratory systems and the safety of their use has now firmly established their role in medical and surgical practice. For these reasons, the inclusion of a discussion of the techniques and indications for fiberoptic

gastrointestinal and bronchial endoscopy seems appropriate for this volume.

Since the introduction of clinical fiberoptic endoscopy by Hirschowitz and associates[2] in 1958, there has been a steady progression of technical improvements in flexibility, optical quality, illumination, biopsy potential and, more recently, therapeutic capability. Although the instruments vary with respect to manufacturer's design and the organ for which use is primarily intended, all flexible endoscopes have fundamental features in common. A fiberoptic bundle transmits a high-intensity light from an external source to the surface being examined, and a similar channel transmits the image to the eye of the examiner. Smaller channels allow for the insufflation of air to distend the viscus and for the injection of liquid to cleanse the optical system. A final open channel allows the introduction of biopsy forceps, cytological brushes or the various devices used in the newer therapeutic instruments. The directions and degree of flexion of the distal tip of the instrument can be controlled by the endoscopist with variously designed external handles or knobs. Depending on the particular requirement of the examination, a model may be chosen that provides end-on, oblique or lateral direction of view. The capability of the flexible instrument to be adapted to the particular requirements of the individual examination have now essentially excluded the use of rigid endoscopes in diagnostic endoscopy of the upper gastrointestinal tract. A similar trend is developing in the field of bronchoscopy; however, fiberoptic instruments seem less likely to provide significant advantages over the rigid proctosigmoidoscope.

The flexibility and maneuverability of fiberoptic instruments should increase the safety of their use in all routine diagnostic procedures. The fact that this is not strikingly borne out in published experience[3, 5] may reflect a degree of casualness on the part of endoscopists resulting from the apparent simplicity of examinations with these remarkable instruments. Fiberoptic endoscopy is indeed a safe procedure but, as is the case in many fields of medical practice, improved instrumentation cannot replace the trained and careful sensitivity of the examining physician. This sensitivity will be enhanced if the endoscopist has been involved in some way in the evaluation of the clinical problem and the role of the proposed endoscopic examination in its resolution. To the degree that the endoscopist provides only a technical service, his or her evaluation may suffer in safety, accuracy and completeness. Adequate training under careful and expert supervision is an essential prerequisite for the performance of a competent endoscopic examination.

Although in most instances the technique can be learned relatively quickly, the interpretation of the visualized variation in structure develops only through repeated experience. The technique itself does not require previous specialized training but, as emphasized earlier, the value of the examination is influenced significantly by an understanding of the various anticipated diseases and a degree of involvement in the particular problem under evaluation.

It is essential in the performance of any diagnostic or therapeutic procedure to give careful consideration to its role in the management of a patient's illness. Procedures that will not influence management decisions, regardless of outcome, should not be performed. If adequate, accurate diagnostic information on which to base a sound therapeutic decision is available, further studies should be avoided. Endoscopic procedures are most likely to be helpful when they are used to complement diagnostic possibilities raised by a careful medical history, physical examination and other forms of testing. Therefore, the decision to proceed with an endoscopic examination should be made deliberately, with full knowledge of the patient's particular problem and the results of prior investigations and treatment, and in conjunction with the recommendations of others involved in his care.

ENDOSCOPY OF UPPER GASTROINTESTINAL TRACT

Indications

The most commonly performed fiberoptic endoscopic procedure is that of examination of the upper gastrointestinal tract from the cervical portion of the esophagus through the second part of the duodenum. With appropriate technique, virtually all of the mucosal surfaces of these segments can be clearly visualized. This being

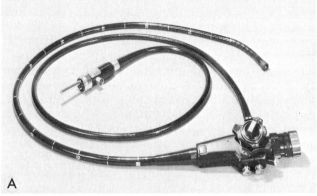

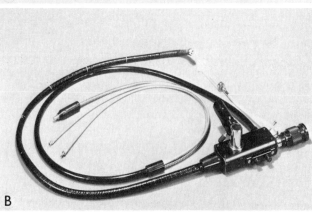

Figure 27–1 *A.* Olympus GIF-D3 end-viewing duodeno-scope (111-cm effective working length). *B.* ACMI Model F-8 end-viewing duodenoscope (105-cm effective working length).

A

B

the case, the flexible endoscope (Fig. 27–1 *A* and *B*) is the most accurate instrument for determining the presence or absence of mucosal lesions and for their evaluation — provided the examination is performed by a careful, experienced endoscopist. Thus, any circumstance in which a mucosal abnormality is a reasonable possibility can be considered as an indication for such an examination.

Gastric Ulcer

The most common indication for the examination is to provide further assessment of an ulcerating gastric lesion that has been identified previously by roentgenological study. The added capability for obtaining mucosal specimens for biopsy and brush cytology has significantly enhanced the accuracy of distinguishing benign and malig-

nant lesions, thus making possible more appropriate decisions of management. If radiological studies clearly indicate the probability of a malignant gastric lesion and if surgical treatment is required, endoscopic evaluation becomes unnecessary. Occasionally, in circumstances in which surgery would be associated with an unusually high risk, endoscopy with biopsy might be justified in the hope of finding a radio-sensitive tumor.

Duodenal Ulcer Symptoms With Normal X-ray

Radiologically demonstrated duodenal ulcer disease is a less compelling indication for endoscopic examination. Such lesions are uniformly benign, and management decisions are less likely to be influenced by further visualization of the ulcer. Nevertheless, duodenal deformity often produces a difficult roentgenographic interpretation; it is frequently associated with atypical symptoms, and the clear visualization of an active ulcer crater may significantly influence treatment options. Conversely, the endoscopic confirmation of duodenal deformity without active inflammation might be a critical factor in deciding against surgical treatment of an ulcer in a patient with atypical complaints. Experience at the Mayo Clinic[1] suggests that endoscopic evaluation is unlikely to be of additional help in patients with nonspecific dyspepsia whose x-ray studies have not shown any abnormality in the upper gastrointestinal tract; however, 20 per cent of patients with ulcerlike symptoms and normal roentgenograms were found to have significant erosive or ulcerative lesions.

Filling Defects

Filling defects of various configuration, noted on radiological examinations and possibly unassociated with the symptoms being evaluated, are usually considered to be appropriate indications for endoscopic study. The characteristic appearance of heterotopic pancreatic tissue, leiomyomas and other benign submucosal tumors usually suffices for diagnostic purposes, but the occasional demonstration of associated mucosal ulceration may influence the decision for surgical intervention. Newer capabilities for snaring pedunculated gastric polyps have added a further dimension to the endoscopic study of polypoid lesions in the stomach, and the availability of an entire lesion for histological study will provide a broader and firmer foundation for the evaluation of the malignant potential of such lesions than has previously been available. The question as to whether endoscopic removal of single or multiple gastric polyps will significantly influence the ultimate course of patients with these condi-

tions remains largely unresolved at this time.

The assessment of gastric distensibility and the evaluation of contour changes due to extrinsic conditions is generally more difficult for the endoscopist than for the radiologist, and the subtle changes associated with early scirrhous cancer of the stomach provide diagnostic difficulties for both.

Esophageal Disease: Dysphagia, Strictures and Reflux

Variations in esophageal contour are generally subtle, and the further evaluation of patients with dysphagia is a widely accepted indication for endoscopy. Biopsy of suspected carcinomas can be accomplished and the extent of the lesion can be more definitely documented. The benign nature of inflammatory strictures can be confirmed, the relationship to gastroesophageal reflux can be evaluated, and therapeutic dilatation can be performed by one of a variety of techniques. The diagnosis of achalasia usually will not be enhanced significantly by endoscopic study, although the occasional association of esophageal carcinomas or the clinical similarity of achalasia with some fundic neoplasms may provide adequate indications for endoscopic study in some patients with an apparent primary motility problem.

Postgastrectomy Symptoms

In patients with symptoms after gastrectomy, the gastroscopic examination is usually of more diagnostic value than the x-ray studies. Direct visualization of the area of a gastrojejunal or gastroduodenal stoma is the most reliable method of assessing the presence or absence of marginal ulceration or alkaline reflux gastritis or the patency of the anastomosis.

Bleeding

Upper gastrointestinal hemorrhage, manifested as hematemesis or melena, constitutes a compelling indication for endoscopic study. If bleeding is active, the endoscopic examination should be performed as soon as the patient's condition has become reasonably stabilized. In less urgent circumstances, the order of diagnostic procedures becomes less important, although barium studies may well preclude satisfactory endoscopic visualization of mucosal surfaces for a significant time. Esophageal varices and benign or malignant ulcers of the esophagus, stomach or duodenum usually can be demonstrated by either technique, whereas the bleeding associated with reflux esophagitis, hemorrhagic gastritis, stress ulcers or drug-induced erosions may only be detected endocopically. In addition, fiberoptic visualization has a significant advantage in identifying which of several potentially bleeding lesions may be the actual site of current hemorrhage. Techniques for electrocoagulation of bleeding sites are being evaluated currently but should undergo further refinement and testing before they are made widely available.

Foreign Bodies

The development of new instrumentation has made the extraction of foreign bodies from the esophagus and stomach possible by means of fiberoptic endoscopes. Grasping forceps of various designs allow the retrieval of most commonly swallowed objects. The use of a plastic sleeve that extends from the endoscope, into which sharp objects may be maneuvered for their retrieval, has also improved the effectiveness and safety of the nonoperative removal of these types of foreign bodies.

Contraindications

Contraindications to endoscopy of the upper gastrointestinal tract are few and, for the most part, relative. A totally uncooperative patient should not be examined, although this situation usually can be moderated with reassurance and the use of larger amounts of sedative drugs. This latter adaptation will increase the possibility of respiratory depression, and resuscitation equipment should be immediately at hand.

Recent acute myocardial infarction usually is considered a strong contraindication to endoscopic procedures. In most instances, the cardiac status will influence management decisions more definitively than the endoscopic findings. Other acute illnesses also may be influential in the decision for examination in a similar manner.

Conditions that affect the patency of the respiratory airway also may influence the approach to endoscopy of the upper gastrointestinal tract. Patients with vocal cord paralysis or other conditions producing stenosis of the upper respiratory tract probably are examined more safely with an endotracheal tube in place to prevent further limitation of the airway, should a degree of laryngospasm develop as a result of the endoscopic intubation.

It is worth reemphasizing in the context of contraindications for the examination that endoscopy probably should not be performed in a circumstance in which the outcome of the evaluation will not alter the diagnosis or management decision.

Technique

Endoscopy of the upper gastrointestinal tract is a safe, essentially painless procedure requiring only minimal preparation by the patient and the limited use of sedative drugs; it is rarely followed by sequelae requiring prolonged observation. As such, it is readily adaptable as an outpatient procedure.

A reliable and satisfactory examination requires that the stomach be free of retained food and secretions. Ordinarily this is accomplished adequately by an overnight fast. Patients with symptomatic obstruction of the gastric outlet or with postoperative gastric retention may require lavage with a large-bore tube before examination.

A safe and satisfactory endoscopic examination also requires a reasonably high degree of cooperation from the patient. This is best achieved by providing an opportunity for the endoscopist to discuss the procedure with the patient, outlining in adequate detail the rationale, expectations and risks of the study. In most instances, the apprehension generated in anticipation of the examination far exceeds that of the actual experience. There is no substitute for the establishment of a confident rapport between the endoscopist and the patient.

Premedication is not essential to a successful examination, although pharyngeal anesthesia and mild sedation do add to the patient's comfort and, therefore, contribute to his cooperation. If attention is paid to possible allergic history and to doses administered, these drugs are safe and effective. After the patient is gowned and dentures have been removed, the oral pharynx and base of the tongue are anesthetized with topical agents available as sprays (Cetacaine), gargles, or lozenges. Most endoscopists will then follow with a supplemental sedative, usually monitored amounts of diazepam (Valium) administered intravenously. In the normal 70 kg man, 5 to 10 mg of intravenous Valium at the time of the examination is usually adequate. Injection is made slowly and

carefully to minimize irritation, and the effects are evaluated by the patient's response to questioning. If the injection is stopped at the first indication of slurred speech or mental slowing, then significant respiratory depression can be avoided and adequate sedation usually will result. In any event, more than 10 mg of diazepam is rarely necessary for a satisfactory effect. Some endoscopists favor the concomitant use of an anticholinergic drug to control secretions and to inhibit motility. Atropine (0.1 mg) can be given intravenously during the course of the examination and is effective immediately. EKG monitoring is usually not necessary for healthy patients, although pulse and blood pressure monitoring are advisable. (See Table 27–1.)

Most endoscopists prefer to place the patient in a left lateral position while introducing the endoscope. In this position, the patient is solidly supported by the examining table, the head is comfortably rested in midposition, and the examiner can begin the intubation either while sitting or standing. The patient is instructed to breathe regularly and quietly and to avoid holding the breath. The endoscope is advanced to the base of the tongue, the tip being guided by the index finger of the free hand to keep the instrument in the midline. In small, careful increments the tip is advanced further until resistance of the cricopharyngeal ring, the upper esophageal sphincter, is encountered — usually slightly less than 20 cm from the incisor teeth. At this point, the pa-

TABLE 27-1 Upper GI Endoscopy Medication*

DRUG	DOSAGE	ROUTE
Atropine	0.1–0.2 mg	IV — Slowly
Valium	5–10 mg	IV — Slowly
Glucagon	1 mg	IV — Slowly
Cetacaine Spray	—	Spray retropharynx

*Suggested doses for healthy 70 kg male.

tient is instructed to swallow and, as the sphincter area relaxes, the endoscope is carefully advanced into the upper part of the esophagus. Advancement should never be forced against significant resistance and generally is accomplished with less reaction from the patient if it is attempted in several short steps. Unusual coughing usually indicates that the tip has been misdirected into the laryngeal area. It is usually difficult to visualize the pharynx adequately with the flexible instrument during intubation.

The examination begins with the upper portion of the esophagus and extends through the remainder of the esophagus, the region of the esophagogastric junction, the body of the stomach, the antrum, the pylorus, the duodenal bulb and the postbulbar duodenum to the extent of the instrument or until the diagnostic questions serving as the indication for the study have been satisfactorily answered. The gastroscope rarely should be advanced blindly and most certainly not against significant resistance. Remaneuvering and repositioning the tip almost always will result in an adequate forward view. The examination while withdrawing the endoscope is as important as that while introducing it; often it allows the visualization of areas inadequately seen earlier or improved views of questionable abnormalities. The exact sequence of the examination is at the discretion of the endoscopist; generally, if lesions have been identified earlier for further evaluation, it is wise to complete that assessment before turning to the remaining areas. A complete examination of all mucosal surfaces, however, is a requisite to satisfactory endoscopic study. Visualization of the gastric fundus and the region of the cardia, performed with the endoscope in the retroflexed position, can be done either early in the study or as the tube is being withdrawn.

An endoscopic examination of the upper gastrointestinal tract can be performed better with an endoscopic assistant. The additional reassurances provided to the patient by a calm and competent assistant often make a difficult examination much easier and safer. The need for suctioning secretions, for observing the patient's condition, for efficiently handling biopsy devices, cytology brushes and tissue specimens make assistance nearly mandatory for the satisfactory completion of most examinations.

When the study has been completed, the patient is carefully monitored in the recovery area for at least 1½ to 2 hours until all evidences of lingering sedative effects have cleared and the stability of the recovery indicates that significant bleeding from biopsy sites has not developed. Even so, the patient must be accompanied by a relative or friend and must not drive a car for several hours after the examination.

As of this writing, the value of flexible fiberoptic endoscopy of the upper gastrointestinal tract is overwhelmingly diagnostic. Therapeutic endoscopy is in its infancy, but there is every indication of a bright future in electrosurgery of focal lesions, coagulation of bleeding sites, injection of pharmacological agents or other maneuvers. Advances in technique and instrumentation will be so rapid as to make any description of these procedures obsolete well in advance of publication.

Complications

The use of flexible endoscopic instruments has resulted in various complications. Perforation can and does occur.[3, 5] Improved equipment and technique should continue to reduce the incidence of injury as the result of diagnostic procedures. Significant bleeding after mucosal biopsy is unusual, but the possibility does require attention to coagulation factors in appropriate clinical situations. Experience with therapeutic endoscopic techniques does not yet allow an adequate assessment of the risk and benefit factors. Although early experience seems promising, outcome data are insufficient for a satisfactory evaluation of the increased risk of complications that will accompany electrosurgical maneuvers.

COLONOSCOPY

Colonoscopy has become a procedure that can be safely performed on an outpatient basis without general or local anesthesia. Sedation, however, is usually necessary. Colonoscopes are available in two lengths — 105 to 110 cm and 160 to 186 cm (Fig. 27–2). The shorter model is useful for examination of the left colon and sigmoid, whereas the longer instrument is necessary to

inspect the right colon and cecum. This increased length makes the handling of these instruments more difficult; however, most colonoscopists accept this disadvantage in return for the opportunity to visualize the entire colonic mucosa with a single intubation.

Colonoscopy is a useful adjunct to traditional radiological examination of the colon. It has been estimated that an additional 20 to 50 per cent of colonic pathology can be identified by using both of these procedures.[4] The extent of disease, particularly inflammatory bowel disease, can be evaluated more fully with the colonoscope, although disagreement between colonoscopic and radiological findings is not great. It should be noted that the incidence of additional unsuspected pathological findings is probably great enough to

Figure 27–2 *A.* Olympus Model TCF-2L two-channel operating colonoscope (173-cm effective working length). *B.* Olympus Model BF5-B2 fiberoptic bronchoscope.

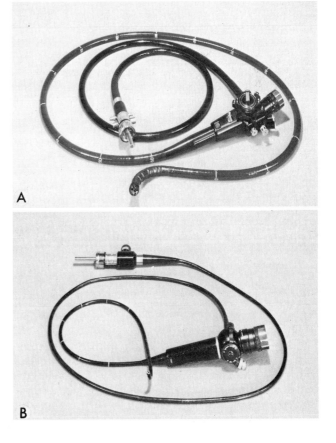

A

B

warrant a thorough colonoscopic examination when evaluating polyps or carcinoma.

Indications

The need for colonoscopy must be as clear and concise as possible if maximal diagnostic and therapeutic advantages are to be gained and morbidity and mortality reduced.

Diagnosis

Although some authors[9] express the opinion that colonoscopy is indicated regardless of the results of x-ray studies, it is most often used for further amplification of findings on a roentgenological examination. Less commonly, colonoscopy is performed when x-ray studies appear entirely normal but suspicious colonic symptomatology is present. Colonoscopy may be useful in the bleeding patient, although in patients who are bleeding actively the mucosa can be obscured and adequate preparation may be difficult. In patients with minimal or occult bleeding, colonoscopy may provide necessary verification of x-ray findings or may reveal mucosal lesions not visualized with standard radiological techniques. In patients who previously have had a polyp removed or a portion of colon resected, the postoperative changes are often confusing on x-ray examination. For this reason, colonoscopy is of great value in examining the mucosa for recurrence or additional disease.

Treatment

Therapeutic colonoscopy is more advanced than therapeutic endoscopic examination of the upper gastrointestinal tract. The colonoscope has proved to be a valuable aid in the diagnosis and management of colonic polyps. When complete removal of the polyps is not possible, a negative biopsy of the polyps may be reassuring. Whenever a malignant polyp is removed and cancer is demonstrated to invade deeper than the lamina propria, surgical excision of that portion of the colon is required.

Contraindications

Colonoscopic examination is sometimes contraindicated. Whenever the colon is poorly prepared, the incidence of perforation and inadequate examination increases. The presence of an acute inflammatory process greatly increases the risk of bleeding and perforation. Inflammatory bowel disease is particularly susceptible to this complication, although acute stages of diverticulitis, ischemic colitis and radiation colitis are also high-risk situations for colonoscopy. After pelvic surgery or irradiation, the bowel can become fixed and angulated, making colonoscopy more difficult and dangerous. Finally, recent operation often results in suture lines that are easily disrupted either by the instrument itself or by gas insufflation.

Pre-endoscopic Preparation

Most endoscopists are of the opinion that general anesthesia for colonoscopy should be avoided; the conscious patient can warn of unanticipated symptoms and thereby help avoid a complication. The use of sedation is similar to that for endoscopy of the upper gastrointestinal tract. Diazepam (Valium) (5 to 10 mg) and meperidine hydrochloride (Demerol) (50 to 75 mg) may be given before the procedure. Such doses generally produce safe, appropriate sedation without seriously interfering with the patient's ability to recognize significant pain.

Various regimens are available for preparation of the colon. Adequate cleansing almost always results with a regimen of (1) clear liquid diet for 24 hours before examination, (2) oral cathartic (castor oil [15 to 30 cc] or Phospho-Soda [15 to 30 cc]) 12 hours before examination and (3) cleansing tap water enemas two hours before the procedure. A "saline flush" preparation in which 3 to 6 liters of saline solution are given orally over two to four hours the night before endoscopy has been another effective mode of preparation. These regimens are well tolerated by healthy individuals. The importance of a clean bowel in terms of avoiding complications and detecting pathological lesions cannot be overemphasized. If the preparation is inadequate, the examination must be postponed.

Examination

The technique of colonoscopy is somewhat more difficult than upper gastrointestinal endoscopy or bronchoscopy. Before inserting the instrument it is important to check each of its functions to make sure it is in proper working condition. The examination usually begins with the patient in the left lateral decubitus position. After the patient is suitably sedated, the knees are flexed and the well-lubricated tip of the instrument is inserted into the anus and, with a combination of manual and visual guidance, is passed into the sigmoid. From this point on, the instrument is advanced only under direct vision. Air is insufflated as necessary to identify the lumen. Passage continues under direct vision until the mucosa blanches or the patient complains of pain. The most difficult portion to negotiate is the loop at the junction of the sigmoid and descending colon. This may require a so-called alpha maneuver in which the instrument is inserted to the midsigmoid, rotated 180 degrees counterclockwise, and then advanced into the descending colon. At the splenic flexure, the alpha loop is straightened by a 180 degree clockwise rotation and slight withdrawal of the colonoscope. This straightens out the loops of the bowel that are now telescoped over the end of the colonoscope. It is important to remember that throughout endoscopy, the tip should be advancing as fast as the colonoscope is fed into the anus. If this is not happening, then a loop is forming at some point along the path of the instrument and excessive pressures may result.

Landmarks are available as the procedure progresses. While traversing the sigmoid colon, it is rarely possible to see ahead for more than a few centimeters and the tortuosity of the sigmoid is obvious. Once into the descending colon, the first straight portion of colon is noticeable. The transverse colon has a triangular shape and has internal haustrations much like the descending colon. At the hepatic flexure, the liver may be seen as a bluish stain on the mucosa of the inflated bowel.

If fluoroscopy is utilized to determine the location of the instrument, the patient should be rolled into the prone position. Whenever possible, the examination should proceed to the full length of the colon. Once the endoscope is fully inserted, it is slowly and carefully withdrawn. As with endoscopy of the upper gastrointestinal tract, frequently the best view of the intestine is gained on withdrawal of the instrument; the endoscopist should use the left hand to control the distal tip and air-water controls while the right hand is used to withdraw, advance and rotate the instrument. Circular inspection of the lumen is used to identify pathological lesions. Occasionally such lesions may "hide" behind a fold or angulation, so compulsive care is necessary to assure complete evaluation. Telescoped bowel may move quickly past the end of the instrument; when this occurs, the endoscope must be reinserted and this portion of bowel must be visualized. The colonoscope is carefully withdrawn and reinserted until the entire bowel is inspected.

Because of the associated incidence of synchronous cancers and benign tumors, whenever possible the full length of the colon should be scrutinized. Fluoroscopy may be helpful when unusual length or angulation of the colon is encountered; it may also aid in confirming the location of the tip of the instrument in an area of previously identified pathological development. The use of fluoroscopy also should be minimized, since x-ray exposure accelerates the deterioration of fiberoptic bundles and results in a yellow image.

Further descriptions of the technical aspects of this procedure are available elsewhere.[7, 8]

Therapeutics

Therapeutic colonoscopy has been confined largely to the snaring and removal of pedunculated polyps and to biopsy of mucosal lesions, both of which are easily and safely performed. So far, there has been no extensive experience reported with the coagulation of bleeding sites. As mentioned previously, if cancer is found in an excised polyp, the excision may be adequate therapy if the entire polyp has been removed and the tumor is found to be confined to the portion of the polyp superficial to the lamina propria. If, however, the tumor penetrates below the lamina propria, surgical excision of that portion of the colon is required, as lymphatic metastasis may have already occurred.

Complications

As experience with colonoscopy is gained, the incidence of complications is minimized. The literature does not address itself carefully to the morbidity and mortality of this procedure, but several authors have attempted to survey the experiences of several colonoscopists. It is important to realize that these figures probably represent a minimal estimate. In 7,959 colonoscopies (6,290 diagnostic procedures and 1,669 polypectomies), the incidence of complications was 0.7 per cent; 0.1 per cent of these occurred with diagnostic procedures and 0.6 per cent occurred with therapeutic procedures.[6] These complication rates appear to be relatively low, particularly when compared with the morbidity and mortality of surgical exploration, and they support the diagnostic and therapeutic use of colonoscopy whenever possible.

BRONCHOSCOPY

Bronchoscopy with the flexible fiberoptic bronchoscope (Fig. 27–2 *B*) can be a safe and simple procedure for an outpatient.

Indications

Indications are essentially the same as those for rigid bronchoscopy and include the evaluation of (1) bronchial lesions, (2) pulmonary lesions, including brush and direct biopsies as well as cytological studies, and (3) an atelectatic lung. As a rule, the rigid bronchoscope is more valuable for the retrieval of foreign bodies.

Technique

Preparation of the patient is similar to that used for endoscopy of the upper gastrointestinal tract. Anesthesia, however, is somewhat more extensive. Atropine (0.4 mg subcutaneously) is used to decrease secretions from the bronchial tree. The instrument frequently is passed through the nares and, for this reason, it is necessary to anesthetize the nasal passages with 5 to 10 ml of lidocaine (Xylocaine) jelly. Sedation can be used but is frequently not necessary. Retropharyngeal anesthesia with topical application of one of the local anesthetics (as used in endoscopy of the upper gastrointestinal tract) is also necessary. As the instrument is passed through the pharynx and into the main stem bronchus, injection of 2 to 4 ml of 4 per cent lidocaine facilitates the passage of the endoscope and the comfort of the patient. This anesthetizes the endobronchial lining. The injection usually can be introduced directly through the instrument. The procedure can be done with the patient in the sitting, recumbent or decubitus position, and the landmarks are much the same as noted with the rigid bronchoscope. After the instrument is passed through the nares, the epiglottis is visualized and the instrument is passed into the main stem bronchus. The small flexible bronchoscope can be passed into the third and fourth generations of the bronchial tree. The extent of visualization is thus greatly improved over that obtained with the traditional rigid scope. Once the bronchoscope has entered the terminal portions of the bronchia, it is possible to aspirate fluid after injection of 3 to 4 ml of saline solution. This is a useful technique for obtaining specimens for cytology and cultures. Specimens for brush and punch biopsies can be taken through the flexible instrument. Transbronchial needle biopsies of lesions under fluoroscopic control are done routinely. These, however, are usually done on inpatients because of the risk of bleeding and pneumothorax. Biopsy, even of peripheral lesions, is possible with transbronchial techniques, but lesions of the mid to central lung fields are the ones that are most commonly approached. With the flexible fiberscope, an accurate view of the nasopharynx and hypopharynx as well as of the cords and pyriform sinuses is easily obtainable. The extreme flexibility of the instrument allows good visualization of the upper lobe, which is virtually impossible with the rigid bronchoscope.

Operative Bronchoscopy —The Rigid Bronchoscope

The flexible fiberoptic scope is a less adequate instrument for operative bronchoscopy and insufflation of large volumes of air. Retrieval of foreign bodies is difficult with the instrument. This is due to the lack of an adequate channel through which to pass a surgical instrument. Therefore, the rigid bronchoscope continues to be valuable for the retrieval of foreign bodies and the manipulation of large masses within the bronchus The biopsy forceps in the flexible instrument are small, and frequently the larger biopsy forceps that can be passed through a straight, rigid scope are necessary to obtain adequate specimens. It is clear that in bronchoscopic examinations, as opposed to upper gastrointestinal examinations, the straight and rigid scopes are mutually complementary, and skills with both are necessary if one is to be a good bronchoscopist.

SUMMARY

Endoscopy is a rapidly developing and changing field. The techniques necessary to become competent in the upper gastrointestinal, lower gastrointestinal and bronchoscopic evaluations are all different and all require appropriate training and experience. In this chapter we have attempted to describe some of the basic techniques, but we have also emphasized the importance of knowledge of the appropriate indications for the use of the procedures. All endoscopic examinations are potentially lethal and can be associated with serious complications. These complications can be reduced if the endoscopist is well trained, experienced, and attentive.

REFERENCES

1. Cameron, A. J., and Ott, B. J.: The value of gastroscopy in clinical diagnosis: a

computer-assisted study (abstract). Gastrointest. Endosc., 23:224, 1977.

2. Hirschowitz, B. I., Curtiss, L. E., Peters, C. W., et al.: Demonstration of a new gastroscope, the "fiberscope." Gastroenterology, 35:50, 1958.

3. Katz, D.: Morbidity and mortality in standard and flexible gastrointestinal endoscopy. Gastrointest. Endosc., 15:134–141, 1969.

4. Kirsner, J. B., Rider, J. A., Moeller, H. C., et al.: Polyps of the colon and rectum: statistical analysis of a long term follow-up study. Gastroenterology, 39:178–182, 1960.

5. Mandelstam, P., Sugawa, C. , Silvis, S. E., et al.: Complications associated with esophagogastroduodenoscopy and with esophageal dilation. Gastrointest. Endosc., 23:16–19, 1976.

6. Overholt, B. F.: Colonoscopy: a review. Gastroenterology, 68:1308–1320, 1975.

7. Smith, L. E, and Nivatvongs, S.: Complications of colonoscopy. Dis. Colon Rectum, 18:214–220, 1975.

8. Williams, C., and Teague, R.: Colonoscopy. Gut, 14:990–1003, 1973.

9. Wolff, W. I., and Shinya, H.: Modern endoscopy of the alimentary tract. Curr. Probl. Surg., January 1974, pp. 1–62.

28 Outpatient Surgery in Developing Countries

ROBERT R. LARSEN, M.D.

INTRODUCTION

The opportunities for the Western-trained surgeon to serve in a developing country are constantly expanding. Traditionally these opportunities were limited to only a few career medical missionaries, but today a large number of surgeons are finding challenge in short-term service through the American Peace Corps, A.I.D., Ford Foundation, HOPE Foundation and the British Ministry of Overseas Development. At the same time, many group medical practices and medical schools allow members of their staff to take extended "vacations" or sabbatical years for such service. Such an experience is indeed a challenge, but the satisfactions so far outweigh the frustrations that the opportunity should not be bypassed.

Frustrations result when the surgeon does not understand his or her role in the developing country. A visiting surgeon is not merely an exporter of Western medicine and techniques. He or she will seldom have any administrative authority but must be willing to work under a local doctor, who is likely to view the visitor's ideas with distrust and skepticism. In general, the role of the visiting surgeon will be that of teacher, organizer, supervisor and consultant. He or she must be pre-

pared to adapt personal methods of medical care to meet the financial as well as physical limitations of the patients within the framework of available medicines, materials and trained supportive personnel. I strongly recommend that any physician who is to practice medicine in a developing country should first read *Medical Care in Developing Countries*, edited by Maurice King.[15] Additional material of value to the surgeon who is planning to work in a developing country can be found in the texts of Bowesman,[1] Chatterji,[2] Davey,[7] Hunter,[12] Kerr,[14] and McNair.[18]

In these circumstances the adaptable surgeon will find it necessary to extend his or her indications for outpatient surgery.[25] There are three reasons for this:

1. Financial. Costs must be kept to an absolute minimum.

2. Patient. Many patients will refuse surgery because of fear or the inconvenience of staying in a hospital.

3. Beds. Inpatient beds are always in short supply.

Therefore, the list of surgical procedures that can be done satisfactorily in the outpatient operating room will include many operations usually considered to be inpatient procedures only. A partial listing includes:

breast biopsy

skin or lymph node biopsy
scar revisions
skin grafts (small)
pedicle graft advancement
abscess drainage
cleft lip repair
carpal tunnel release
endoscopy
vasectomy
tubectomy
D and C
hemorrhoids, fissures, fistulas
circumcision
hernia repair
hydrocelectomy
digit amputations
mallet finger repair

Certain precautions are necessary to assure successful surgery in these circumstances.[16]

1. The patient should be free of additional anesthetic risk, such as anemia or old age.

2. A friend or relative must be available to attend the patient at home until his first return visit to the hospital.

3. The patient must agree to prompt follow-up return. (Using nonabsorbable sutures helps to assure the patient's return.)

The advantages to the patient and to the hospital outweigh the risks of complications if these guidelines are followed.

ANESTHESIA

In developing countries there are two factors that restrict anesthesia: the lack of trained personnel and the limited availability of equipment and materials. In most hospitals anesthesia is the responsibility of the operating surgeon. The surgeon must, therefore, promptly become familiar with the use and limitations of a few simple, safe, inexpensive agents and techniques. A book such as *Regional Block* by D. C. Moore[19] will be of more value than an expensive gas anesthesia machine.

For setting fractures or for procedures of less than half an hour's time on the extremities, intravenous local anesthesia (the Bier block) is safe and simple. This procedure and several other commonly used regional blocks are adequately described in Chapter 3. Because the Bier block with intravenous local anesthesia utilizes a blood pressure cuff tourniquet, this technique should not be used in areas of the world where sickle cell disease is prevalent (see following discussion).

Regional block is ideal for outpatient operative procedures, but unfortunately few American-trained surgeons have sufficient experience with the technique to obtain good results. Familiarity with axillary, digital, pudendal, pericervical, ulnar, radial, median and sciatic nerve blocks is extremely valuable (see Chapter 3). Do not expect success right away, but persist in your efforts to master one technique for each block. Use 0.05 per cent solutions for infiltration of peripheral nerve blocks so that larger volumes will be possible without the risk of reaction. It is seldom necessary to use solutions with epinephrine, and the complications produced by improper use of epinephrine are serious. It is advisable to keep anesthetic solutions containing epinephrine well apart from the usual anesthetic solutions.

Systemic toxic reactions to anesthetic solutions must be treated immediately and properly to avoid death. If the reaction appears to be an allergic response manifested by angioneurotic edema, asthma or other histamine-type symptoms, give 50 mg of diphenhydramine (Benedryl) intravenously (IV) and 0.3 cc of epinephrine 1:1000 intramuscularly (IM). If, however, an anaphylactic allergic reaction or a reaction from high blood levels of the agent occur, much more aggressive therapy is indicated.

1. Maintain ventilation by giving oxygen through an endotracheal tube.

2. Start an IV.

3. Maintain the blood pressure with IV vasopressors.

4. Monitor the cardiac action by EKG.

5. Stop convulsions with frequent 50 mg doses of thiopental in or with 40

mg of succinylcholine, and assist ventilation.

Single dose spinal (subarachnoid) anesthesia is suitable for outpatient use under some circumstances. It is convenient for hernia repairs, lower extremity operations and perianal or genital procedures. These operations are seldom considered to be outpatient procedures in the United States but are commonly done on an outpatient basis in countries with limited inpatient beds, so the technique will be reviewed here.

1. Start an IV.

2. Have an assistant hold the patient on his side with the knees drawn up to his face or sitting upright with the back arched towards the anesthetist and the head held down on the assistant's chest.

3. Aseptically prepare the skin of the entire back with an iodine solution.

4. Locate the L3-L4 interspace just cephalad to an imaginary line connecting the two iliac crests.

5. Make a wheal in the skin overlying the interspace and infiltrate the underlying interspinous ligament with 1 per cent procaine solution.

6. A 24 or 25 gauge spinal needle is then inserted through the interspace into the subarachnoid space by aiming at the umbilicus. It will pass through the interspinous ligament and ligamentum flavum with moderate resistance, then less resistance will be felt when it reaches the epidural space, and finally the "pop" will be felt as it pierces the dura.

7. At this point the stylet is withdrawn and the needle is checked for spinal fluid return, with frequent rotations of the needle. If fluid does not return, slowly advance the needle another 5 mm and check again.

8. A syringe containing 0.2 cc epinephrine 1:1000 solution plus 1.0 cc (10 mg) of tetracaine (Pontocaine) plus 1.2 cc of 10 per cent dextrose solution is attached to the spinal needle. Spinal fluid is aspirated until the syringe con-

tains a total of 3.0 cc, and then it is slowly reinjected over a period of three minutes. Before removing the needle a small amount of spinal fluid is again aspirated and reinjected, to be sure that the anesthetic solution was injected in the subarachnoid space.

9. The patient is put in the supine position with the head and shoulders on a pillow, adjusting the table to achieve the proper level of anesthesia. (The anesthetic solution is hyperbaric and will therefore flow downhill.) *Do not* put the patient in Trendelenberg position.

10. Every 30 seconds for 15 minutes, monitor the patient's blood pressure and test the level of anesthesia with a pinprick. After 15 minutes the solution is "fixed."

11. Once the level is fixed a nurse can safely be trusted to monitor the patient's vital signs and responses every 15 minutes during the operative procedure.

The spinal anesthetic agents that are least expensive and most readily available are tetracaine and procaine. One hundred mg of procaine crystals dissolved in 2.0 cc of distilled water or normal saline solution produce a hyperbaric solution with a shorter duration of anesthesia. When using prepared solutions be sure to check whether they are hyperbaric or hypobaric before starting the procedure. Hypotensive complications are more common with the longer-acting agents and in patients with a low circulating blood volume because of the vasodilatory effect of this form of anesthesia. This hypotension will nearly always respond rapidly to Methedrine, Neo-Synephrine or other mild vasopressors.

General anesthetics have very limited usefulness in outpatient surgery, but a few words of advice are in order. In developing countries personnel who are capable of handling general anesthetic agents and equipment are rarely available. It is therefore essential that very simple techniques be

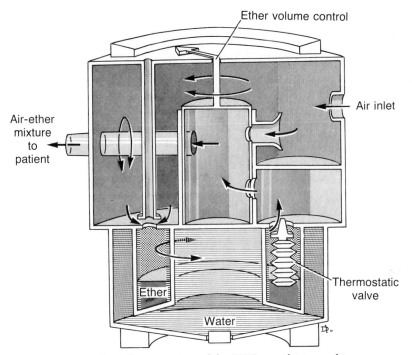

Ether volume control

Air inlet

Air-ether
mixture
to
patient

Thermostatic
valve

Ether

Water

Figure 28–1 Cutaway view of the EMO anesthésia machine.

used and that the operating surgeon constantly be aware of the patient's level of anesthesia. He or she must observe respiratory motions and ask the nurse-anesthetist frequently about the patient's status. The narrow margin of safety of the intravenous barbiturates limits their use as a sole agent to those surgeons who are very experienced with this technique. In many countries chloroform is still used but, again, its margin of safety is much less than that of ether. Chloroform provides more rapid induction and avoids the hyperexcitability that ether produces during induction. Ether evaporates readily in the tropics. Its use can be taught quickly to a nurse-anesthetist, but the surgeon must still be constantly aware of the patient's level of anesthesia. The open drop technique seems somewhat crude to the sophisticated surgeon and is difficult to use for induction, but it is safe in inexperienced hands with a little guidance.

Many hospitals in developing coun-

tries use the EMO (Epstein, Macintosh, Oxford) inhaler with the Oxford inflating bellows (Fig. 28–1). This machine is very simple, quite safe and has the convenience of use with either a mask or endotracheal tube (Fig. 28–2). The volume of ether vapor is controllable and of a concentration independent of the air temperature. The surgeon must be thoroughly familiar with the machine, for death can occur with its use in endotracheal anesthesia by not allowing for blow-off of CO_2 during expiration. The Oxford inflating bellows are particularly useful, for they afford the surgeon a constant visual indicator of the patient's respiratory volumes.

Before leaving the subject of anesthesia, a few comments concerning sickle cell disease are in order. Although this is primarily a disease of patients of African descent, it is wise for the surgeon to keep it constantly in mind. Hemoglobin S is an inherited defect in the globin portion of the hemoglobin molecule, where one gluta-

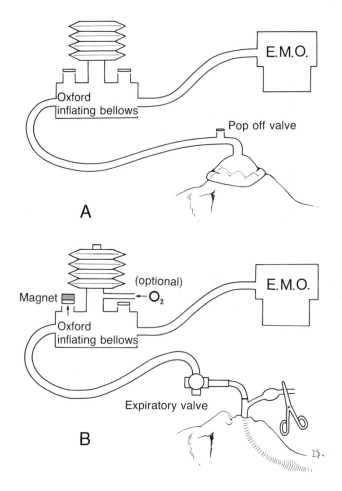

A

B

Figure 28-2 The EMO machine with the Oxford inflating bellows. *A.* With expiratory valve and mask; *B.* with an endotracheal tube.

mic acid group is replaced by a valine group. In the heterozygous patient with sickle cell trait, up to 40 per cent of the hemoglobin will be hemoglobin S, but this is insufficient to produce clinical symptoms. Whenever the capillary Po_2 of the patient with sickle cell disease falls below 45, the erythrocytes become distorted to the sickle shape. These cells then tend to tangle and clump and, along with fibrin formation, block the capillaries, resulting in tissue infarction. The following anesthetic conditions may lead to a local or general fall in tissue Po_2 and are therefore potentially lethal to the patient with sickle cell disease or trait: (1) hypoxia, (2) acidosis, (3) hypothermia, (4) hypotension and (5) use of tourniquets. Even minor surgery

should not be done on a patient of African descent until the hematocrit has been checked. If the hematocrit is less than 30 ml per 100 ml, sickle cell disease must be ruled out prior to surgery. To prepare for emergency surgery in patients with sickle cell disease, exchange about 70 per cent of the patient's blood with nonsickling blood; in addition, use sodium bicarbonate to prevent acidosis and avoid the just-named conditions during the procedure.

KELOIDS, SCARS AND SKIN GRAFTING

When working with dark-skinned patients, the surgeon must constantly keep in mind the principles of wound healing and scar formation. Unsightly hypertrophic scars and keloids can develop even after minor procedures or result from minor infections such as acne. To prevent both keloids and hypertrophic scars a few facts must be remembered.

1. The presternal and upper back skin is particularly susceptible to keloid formation.

2. The incision must extend to the fatty subcutaneous layer in order for a keloid to form. Keloids do not form in the scrotum or penis, where the skin contains no fat.

3. Always make the skin incision parallel to the lines of skin tension. To demonstrate these lines, pinch the skin in two perpendicular directions and observe the natural crease.

4. The wound must be absolutely free of tension when closed.

5. Avoid "cross-hatching" marker scratches, and when possible avoid skin sutures by careful closure of the subcutaneous layer. When possible use tapes for sutureless skin closures.

6. Trauma to the skin edges, wound hematoma and infection must be avoided.

Because of the difference in treatment and result, the differentiation between a keloid and a hypertrophic scar is essential. Histologically the two are indistinguishable. In time (up to three years) a hypertrophic scar will gradually shrink to a normal-appearing scar. Both may be associated with itching and redness. The keloid, however, behaves like a nonmalignant neoplasm. Following are some characteristics of a hypertrophic scar:

1. Confined to the area of the original scar.

2. Appears early (within weeks of the injury).

3. Frequently is associated with burn scars.

4. More common than keloids.

5. Usually has associated signs and symptoms of irritation.

Treatment of hypertrophic scar is primarily that of reassurance and patience. Local injection with hydrocortisone is helpful but also painful unless mixed with equal parts of 1 per cent lidocaine solution. This needs to be repeated monthly for several injections to get good results. A simple method of injecting hydrocortisone into the upper 4 to 5 mm of skin is using the Dermajet injector. A local anesthetic need not be added when this device is used. If the hypertrophic scar is particularly distressing to the patient, local excision and simple closure with a subcuticular pull-out nylon suture will usually produce a normal scar.

The treatment of keloids is much less satisfactory. Often they can be anticipated, for the patient will already have evidence of keloids from previous wounds, ear piercings or infections. In the known keloid former, meticulous atraumatic technique should be used for any surgical wound. As soon as sutures are out, treat the wound with low dosage radiotherapy or hydrocortisone therapy, either local or systemic. Neither radiotherapy nor steroids are adequate treatment for a mature keloid. Total surgical excision is possible but the recurrence rate is high, since the new wound must be larger than the initial wound. This requires undermining the skin edges to relieve all tension on the new wound, minimizing trauma to the skin edges, avoiding sutures on bleeders (better to twist-control the blood vessels) and closing with a subcuticular pull-out suture of monofilament nylon, followed by steroid therapy locally or systemically. Better results are reported by partial excision and grafting. With this technique, most of the keloid is excised but the subcutaneous fatty layer is not entered. The defect in the dermis is closed with a split-thickness skin graft from the keloid itself or from the anterior thigh. No sutures are used to hold this graft in place. A very thin split-thickness graft should be used, or else a single keloid may be converted

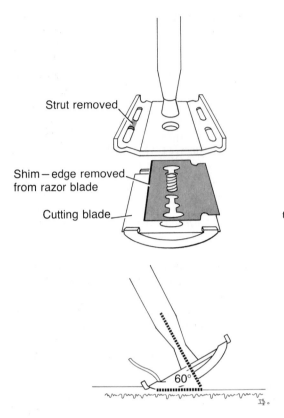

Strut removed

Shim — edge removed
from razor blade

Cutting blade

Figure 28–3 The safety razor dermatome.

60°

into two keloids — one at the donor site also. Do not be trapped into treating presternal keloids, for in this location all forms of treatment result in a larger keloid than before.

Skin grafting, especially in the tropics, is the most controversial outpatient procedure discussed. Except for very small grafts, it should be done as an inpatient procedure because of the high incidence of infection. Small grafts can be taken free-hand by the skilled surgeon, but a useful tool is the safety razor dermatome (Fig. 28–3).[23] The central strut supporting the skin guard must be filed off on one side of an ordinary household safety razor. Shims are made from old blades by placing the blade in a vise with only the beveled cutting edge exposed and then tapping off this edge with a screwdriver and hammer. The thickness of the graft to be taken can be varied by adding shims below the cut-

ting blade. One shim under the blade will cut the skin 0.010 inch thick, and each additional shim will increase the thickness by 0.004 inch. The split-thickness skin is removed by keeping the donor site under tension and holding the razor dematome at a 60 degree angle to the skin. Then, pressing gently, rapid side-to-side oscillations of about one-half inch are made. This process can be made even easier by utilizing the vibrating safety razor, but this is a much more expensive tool.

ABSCESSES AND INFECTIONS

In tropical countries the maxim of early incision and drainage (I and D) of subcutaneous abscesses does not always apply. For example, I and D is not the treatment of choice in parasitic abscesses caused by Onchocerca, Dracunculus, or *Diphyllobothrium latum*. These infections are not only confused with bacterial abscesses but are often mistaken for inguinal or femoral hernias.

Tropical Pyomyositis

Tropical pyomyositis due to *Staphylococcus aureus* is one of the most common infections seen in the tropics. These abscesses occur deep in large muscle masses and usually do not involve subcutaneous and cutaneous tissue until late. As a result, pain, erythema and local heat are often absent, making them confusing to the Western surgeon. A hard, woody swelling is usually preceded by fever, but even fever may be absent when the patient presents at the Outpatient Department. Often the abscesses are multiple. They affect all races in the tropics and do not seem to be related to the nutritional status of the patient. They are often associated with parasitic infection. These abscesses may be confused with abscesses of perforated appendicitis or diverticulitis but lack the signs and symptoms of peritonitis. Frequently they contain a large volume of pus (up to several liters) that provides a pure culture of *Staphylococcus aureus*. Surgical drainage is the primary treatment. If a concomitant antibiotic is to be used, a beta-lactamase–resistant penicillin is recommended.

Onchocerciasis

Onchocerca volvulus (Africa, Central and South America) is a filarial nematode whose larvae migrate from the site of the host black fly's bite to bony prominences around the iliac spines, greater trochanter or the sacrococcygeal area. Here the adults and their microfilaria soon produce a 2 to 3 cm irregular nodule or adenolymphocele. Needle aspiration and smear with a drop of saline will reveal the microfilaria. These nodules are best treated by excision, not incision. As many nodules as possible should be excised. Surgical treatment should be combined with diethylcarbamazine (Hetrazan).

Dracunculosis (Guinea Worm Abscesses)

Dracunculus medinensis or guinea worm (Africa, South America, India) is a nematode that gains entrance to the systemic circulation following ingestion and then spends the next few months burrowing subcutaneously. Some adult worms eventually die and disintegrate, but most come to the skin surface. Here the female worm produces local cellulitis and emerges, or forms a 2 to 10 cm cyst or abscess. The emerging worm should be "helped out" by winding it on a matchstick or by careful surgical removal. The worm should be killed previously by systemic treatment with diethylcarbamazine, metronidazole or thiabendazole. Persistent cysts or abscesses take 4 to 6 weeks to heal and may require excision.

Diphyllobothrium Abscesses (Sparganosis)

Similar to the guinea worm abscess in the tropics is the abscess of *Diphyllobothrium latum* (sparganosis) of colder climes (East Asia, Europe, Middle East, USA, Africa). The ingested tapeworm larvae invade the subcutaneous tissue, where they form localized abscesses. Frequently the patient describes the feeling of something moving in the lump, and the surgeon may be greeted by the moving tapeworm. Preferred treatment is incision and removal of the worm or excision of the nodule along with systemic nicosamide or paromomycin.

Leishmaniasis

Cutaneous leishmaniasis or oriental sore (Africa, India, Near East) is transmitted by the sandfly and produces a suppurating granuloma or exudating ulcer on the face or exposed surfaces. These should not be excised or incised but will usually heal within a year if left alone. Intramuscular trivalent antimonials such as ethylstibamine are helpful. A more destructive form of this infection called espundia is found in Central and South America. This requires local and systemic antibiotics along with the trivalent antimonials.

Amebiasis

When evaluating cutaneous ulcers keep in mind that amebiasis, which is almost universal in developing countries, may cause skin ulcers or skin amebomas. These should be treated in the same way as other extraintestinal amebiasis with metronidazole followed by diiodohydroxyquin.

Groin Infections

Infections and ulcerations of the groin, perineal and genital areas are particularly common in tropical areas. Diagnosis can be difficult, but specific treatment requires accurate diagnosis.

Syphilis

Syphilis is a major public health problem throughout the world and should always be considered first when there is a painless superficial ulcer with firm indurated margins on or near the genitalia and regional lymphadenopathy. Dark field examination of the exudate from the ulcer or the aspirate from the lymph nodes is too difficult to be reliable. The simplest diagnostic test is the VDRL, but it is important to remember that patients with leprosy will give false-positive

reactions. Often the FTA test is available through the regional WHO office, and this test does not give false-positive reactions in leprosy patients. The treatment of choice is 1.2 million units of benzathine penicillin in each buttock for a total dose of 2.4 million units.

Lymphogranuloma Venereum

Lymphogranuloma venereum can be very difficult to distinguish from syphilis. To complicate matters, it may produce a low titer false-positive VDRL reaction. This contagious, viral venereal disease is characterized by genital ulceration and suppurative inguinal bubos. In contrast with syphilis, these lymph nodes are usually soft and fluctuant with pus and tend to develop draining sinuses and fistulas. Rectal and vaginal involvement can become so severe that a diverting colostomy is necessary for management and control. The intradermal Frei test may or may not be helpful for diagnosis. The preferred treatment is systemic tetracycline and aspiration (not I and D) of the bubos.

Granuloma Inguinale

Granuloma inguinale is a chronic genital or perineal ulcerative infection caused by a relative of Klebsiella. The shallow ulcer may closely resemble a chancre but has a base of granulation tissue, and bubos are less prominent. A VDRL test should always be given to rule out syphilis. Tissue scrapings or secretions show characteristic Donovan bodies when stained with Wright's stain. Treatment consists of local cleansing, débridement and systemic tetracycline.

Tropical Ulcer

Ulceration of the skin and soft tissues in the region of the ankle, calf or foot are so common in the tropics that this condition is often considered a separate disease called "tropical ulcer." Factors contributing to these ulcers are malnutrition and vitamin deficiency, lack of shoes, lack of pure water for cleansing minor wounds, and contamination of wounds with fusiform bacilli. Before the diagnosis of "tropical ulcer" is made other causes, such as foreign bodies, leprosy, guinea worm, schistosomiasis, rhinoscleroma, tuberculosis, amebae, syphilis or other treponemal diseases, leishmaniasis, spider or other insect bites and carcinoma, must be ruled out. "Tropical ulcers" may simply be due to staphylococcus, streptococcus or diphtheria organisms, but commonly they contain a mixture of fusiform bacilli and Vincent's spirochetes. They may penetrate deeply to involve underlying bone. Most respond dramatically to penicillin and cleansing débridement. Large chronic ulcers may require excision and grafting, but this should be an impatient procedure.

Cancrum Oris

Cancrum oris is a similar infective process that occurs in the mouth. Again, it is a mixed infection of fusiform bacilli, spirochetes and secondary bacteria that proceeds uncontrolled in a debilitated patient. Deep invasion of periodontal tissue, gingiva, lips, cheek and even nose proceeds to necrosis and sloughing, resulting in grotesque scarring and disfigurement. Even trismus may become a late manifestation of the intense scar formation. In the early phase débridement, antibiotics and restoration of the patient's nutritional state will arrest the infection, but unfortunately patients seldom consult the physician early. Even in a late phase the infection can be controlled, but the disfigurement necessitates extensive and complicated plastic reconstruction procedures to produce a new face.

Tuberculous Cervical Lymphadenitis

Tuberculous cervical lymphadenitis (Fig. 28–4) is still commonly seen in developing countries, especially in children. Tuberculosis must be kept in mind whenever the surgeon is about to perform I and D on a fluctuant neck mass. Since it is common to find associated tuberculous lesions elsewhere in the body, antibiotics are the treatment of choice. In some cases radical excision of involved lymph nodes may shorten the length of treatment. An acid-fast stain of any cervical ulcer or draining sinus should always be done before planning surgical treatment.

Burkitt's Lymphoma

Burkitt's lymphoma (Fig. 28–5) is a virus-induced neoplastic condition and is the most common tumor in the jaws of children in tropical Africa. The maxilla is more often involved than the mandible, and the child frequently

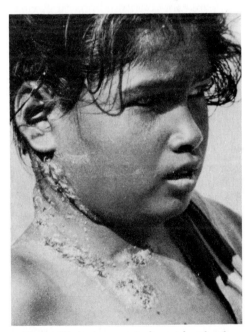

Figure 28–4 A young Indian girl with tuberculous cervical lymphadenitis.

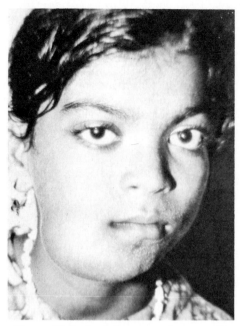

Figure 28–5 Lymphoma in the jaw of a young girl—probably Burkitt's lymphoma.

presents with a complaint of loose molars or premolars. The orbit is involved early in the course of the disease, making Burkitt's lymphoma the commonest cause of exophthalmos in African children. The tumors are often bilateral and usually multiple. Associated features may be abdominal tumors and CNS involvement with paraplegia. Outside Africa this disease is usually manifested by abdominal tumors, and only one of ten cases has facial bone involvement. The treatment of choice is cyclophosphamide (Cytoxan), which produces a 60 per cent remission rate. Do not expect remission, however, if the bone marrow or CNS is involved. Sometimes cyclophosphamide produces rapid, massive tumor regression with a resulting severe fall in the serum potassium level. Being alert to this possibility may prevent disaster.

Foot Infections

Mycetoma Pedis

Since footwear is seldom used in developing countries, a high incidence of foot infections is not surprising. Mycetoma pedis (Madura foot) is the result of inoculation with a variety of fungi or the bacteria actinomycetes when the patient, usually a male, steps on either a piece of thorn bamboo or acacia shrub. Swelling of the foot, multiple draining sinuses and a discharge containing black, yellow or red granules (Fig. 28–6) slowly develop. The process may extend over a period of several years. Gradually it progresses to involve bones and joints. Pain is seldom a prominent feature. Roentgenograms show cystic cavitation, osteoporosis and bone erosion. Any new bone formation is totally disorganized, usually at right angles to the cortex.[9] Medical treatment is generally discouraging. *Nocardia brasiliensis,* one of the yellow granule producers, is susceptible to prolonged streptomycin or sulfone treatment, and actinomycosis is best treated with penicillin. Other organisms have shown no consistent *in vivo*

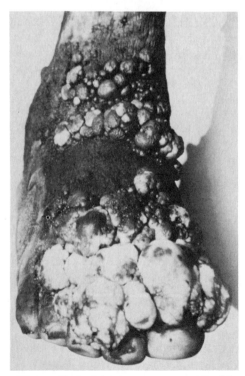

Figure 28–6 Severe mycetoma pedis (Madura foot).

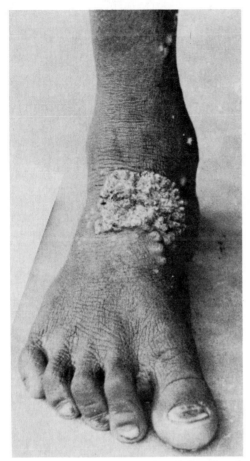

Figure 28–7 Chronic combined fungal and bacterial infection of the foot. This type of infection is commonly seen during the monsoon season and is not to be confused with early mycetoma.

susceptibility to agents currently available. Prior to amputation, a course of treatment with one of the systemic antifungal agents such as amphotericin B is advisable. Surgical excision is satisfactory for the early lesion that is confined to soft tissues, but the lesion is seldom seen early.

Superficial Infections

The newcomer may confuse the early stages of mycetoma with the superficial fungal and bacterial infections of the skin so commonly seen during the monsoon season (Fig. 28–

7). This more superficial infection will respond to systemic and local treatment with combined antibacterial and antifungal agents.

Ainhum

Ainhum is another foot problem seen throughout both Africa and Asia. Although fungus infection is often blamed for the disease, there is no good evidence to support this theory. All cases that I have seen occurred in barefoot patients, and many of them remembered relatives who had experienced the same disease. Just distal to the plantar digital fold, a groove forms and spreads towards the dorsum of the toe (Fig. 28–8). Slowly the groove widens and deepens, and later it may ulcerate. By this time it has the appearance of an encircling constriction of the soft tissue around the toe. Most commonly the fourth or fifth toe is involved, but it has been reported on the fingers as well. Eventually, bone becomes involved in the groove, resulting in slow autoamputation. In the late stages, pain may be a prominent feature, and often the patients come at this stage requesting the surgeon to complete the amputation for pain relief. It is possible simply to complete the amputation at the level of the groove, but the preferred treatment is amputation at the metatarsophalangeal joint under local anesthesia. In addition to attention to aseptic technique, a course of tetanus toxoid before surgery is advisable. If the disease is seen before ulceration or bone involvement has occurred, the toe can be saved by performing two or three Z-plasties on the constricting groove.

Cosmetic Wounds

It is customary in most tropical countries for people to create various holes, scars or wounds for cosmetic or therapeutic purposes. Ear piercing is widespread, and the jewelry may consist of

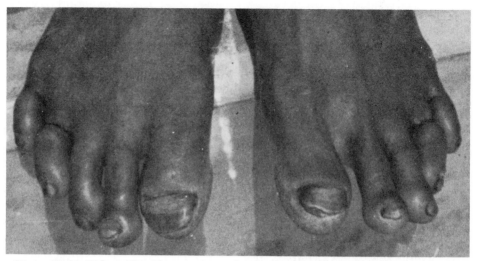

Figure 28-8 Ainhum. Note the constricting bands of ainhum on the fourth and fifth digits.

large pieces of bamboo or ivory that necessitate very large holes. Tattoos are often used for permanent cosmetics. Incisions made in intricate designs on the face or abdomen are used for tribal markings in Africa. Indian women often perforate the nasal alae for jewelry. Lip perforations for the insertion of ivory pegs are seen in both Africa and Asia. Constricting bands are applied as bracelets or necklaces in Indochina. In most developing countries the common methods of treatment for pain used by the local medicine men are burn escharification, moxibustion and hot cupping. It is frequently possible to make a diagnosis simply by observing the locations of these scars. It is amazing how rarely these various wounds become infected, in spite of the septic conditions under which most of them are produced. Tetanus, however, can be a complication of these wounds, and they should not be considered totally harmless. Occasionally with educational achievement people find these tribal marks or facial cosmetics distasteful and come to the surgeon to request their removal.

LEPROSY

Leprosy is a worldwide disease not limited to developing countries, but it does have a high incidence in Africa and Asia. Most people have the ability to resist infection, destroying the *Mycobacterium leprae* bacilli following exposure. Those few who lack this resistance, because of malnutrition or for some unknown reason will eventually begin to show manifestations of this disease. Often they will not appear until years after exposure.

Clinical Aspects

The early manifestation of this disease is a hypopigmented macule with or without associated sensory loss, called indeterminate leprosy. If untreated, this stage may heal by itself or may progress to the tuberculoid or the lepromatous form of the disease or, as usually happens, to a mixture of these two forms. The tuberculoid form is a result of a relative degree of patient resistance that is characterized by a vigorous defense reaction against the bacilli, manifested by a tuberculoid follicle consisting of giant cells surrounded by epithelioid cells. This reaction affects skin appendages and melanocytes, resulting in patches of skin devoid of hair, sweat and pigment. The lepromatous type (Fig. 28-9) has minimal host reaction and is

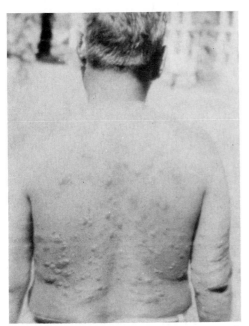

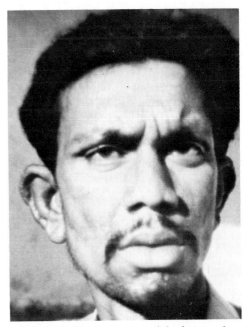

Figure 28–9 Lepromatous leprosy. Each nodule is teeming with *Mycobacterium leprae.*

Figure 28–10 Beginning of the leonine face of leprosy—frontal bossing, loss of eyebrows, nodules on the ear lobes.

characterized by nodules of granulation tissue and bacilli often located in the peripheral nerves.

Laboratory Studies

The diagnosis is usually made by the clinical picture, but to confirm this suspicion and follow the response to therapy the laboratory is essential (Fig. 28–10). Smears of the serum from the papillary dermis bordering an active lesion or from the mucosa of the nasal septum are used for this test.[13] A positive test may be difficult to obtain in the tuberculoid form. In those cases the lepromin test or surgical biopsy of a lesion may be helpful. The latter is easiest if a 4 mm punch biopsy tool is used to obtain a specimen from the margin of a lesion. In general, the lepromin test is much less reliable and should not be considered diagnostic.

To make a smear, prepare the skin with alcohol and then squeeze a skin fold between the left thumb and index finger to eliminate as much blood as possible from the area so that primarily serum will be obtained. Then make a 5 mm incision into, but not through, the papillary dermis. Scrape the sides of the incision with the blade to obtain the clear juice and pulp, smear this onto a glass slide, and stain it with Ziehl-Neelsen* stain. Since the nasal mucosa is the last area to become negative on therapy, a smear from this area is best for following the response to therapy. After removing any nasal mucus, scrape the hyperemic mucosa or a nodule with a blunt scraper. (A

---

*Technique of the Ziehl-Neelsen stain:
1. Fix the film on the glass slide by passing it once or twice through a flame.
2. Cover the slide with strong carbol fuchsin and heat gently for five minutes, letting the stain steam but not boil.
3. Wash in running water and drain.
4. Cover slide with 0.5 per cent acid alcohol for three to five minutes. (Use 3 per cent acid alcohol for TB preparations.)
5. Wash rapidly and drain.
6. Counterstain momentarily with malachite green or 2 per cent picric acid.
7. Wash and rapidly dry.

portion of a bicycle spoke hammered to a fusiform flat end makes a good nasal scraper.) Then smear it on the slide and stain as above. If blood is obtained, repeat the procedure, for blood will make it difficult to interpret the smear. One last word of precaution — remember that the leprosy patient often produces a false-positive VDRL reaction.

Treatment

The primary treatment of leprosy is medical, namely, diaminodiphenylsulphone (DDS, dapsone). Patients are started on a low dosage such as 25 mg twice weekly and then, over a period of three months, this is gradually increased to as much as 50 mg daily. Two new drugs that may ultimately replace DDS are clofazimine and rifampin, but they are still experimental. For the Western surgeon entering an endemic area, the question of prophylaxis may arise. BCG has long been considered of prophylactic value, but a recent Word Health Organization study indicates that this has little value. Low dose DDS orally, or the long-acting injectible DADDS are probably the only recommendable methods of prophylaxis. Generally, prophylaxis is not recommended at all.

In order to avoid the mistakes commonly made, the surgeon should be thoroughly familiar with this disease and its management when he or she is asked to enter into the patient's care. Many talented young surgeons have seen their technically beautiful surgical procedures totally wasted because the extremity was treated instead of the patient. Before the surgeon operates, he or she must consider certain principles:

1. Be sure everything possible is being done to prevent deformity. Time spent in prevention of deformity will reap more benefit than time spent in correction of deformity.

2. Freedom from ulceration is more important to a patient than fine dexterity.

3. Physical and occupational therapy programs must be planned and started long before and continued long after any surgical procedures are performed.

4. In many cultures the stigmata of leprosy prevent a patient from returning to his or her village even after arrest of the disease. Amputation of a deformed foot may therefore do more for a patient than an intricate tendon transfer.

5. Lost sensation is never restored by surgery.

6. The patient's motivation is more important than the surgeon's motivation.

When there is definite indication for surgical intervention in leprosy, many of the procedures can be done in the outpatient operating room with little or no anesthesia. The complications of leprosy most frequently requiring surgical treatment are ulcers, cosmetic repair of deformities, acute neuritis, acute reaction in the eye or hand and paralytic conditions of the hand or foot.

Prevention and Treatment of Ulcers

The primary treatment of ulcers is prevention. Constant education will make the patient aware of the three principles of preventing ulcers:

1. Care to avoid trauma

2. Inspection of hands and feet daily

3. Protective footwear

Chronic ulcers are best treated conservatively with frequent cleansing, dressings and antibiotics. As a last resort, conservative amputation may be necessary for severe multiple nonhealing ulcers. Both skin and serum zinc concentrations have been found to be low in all leprosy patients, but it has not yet been demonstrated that preparations with zinc are particularly helpful in the management of trophic skin ulcers.

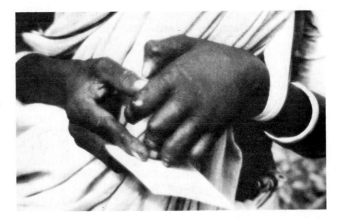

Figure 28-11 The paralyzed arm and claw-hand contracture of late lepromatous neuritis.

Cosmetic Repair

Cosmetic repair need not be elaborate but is based upon correcting those factors considered to be stigmata of the disease by the community. Simple procedures such as a full-thickness graft of hair-bearing skin to replace lost eyebrows or correction of gynecomastia may be all that is needed. Madarosis (loss of eyebrows) is a particular problem in lepromatous leprosy and socially is as damaging as a brand across the forehead.

Neuritis

Neuritis, with its crippling pain, can be a severely limiting problem (Fig. 28-11). Most commonly involved are the facial, ulnar, median and common peroneal nerves. Invasion into the nerve by *Mycobacterium leprae* causes inflammation and edema, which in turn cause a partial ischemia that can eventually produce paralysis. Conservative measures include plaster casts to put the extremity at rest, systemic steroids and injection of the involved nerve with anesthetic agents with hydrocortisone. Neurolysis to relieve the inflammatory swelling can provide tremendous relief from the pain. It may be necessary to incise along the entire length of a swollen nerve sheath to accomplish this. At the same time, abscesslike cavities may be noted and should be evacuated. Do not confuse these with bacterial abscesses, for these pockets are sterile. The wounds can be closed primarily. The ulnar nerve is particularly prone to neuritic involvement and is quite accessible for surgical procedures. Besides neurolysis and longitudinal incision in the nerve sheath, it may be helpful to transpose the nerve anteriorly by detaching the flexor muscles from the medial condyle and epicondyle.[20] If paralysis is complete, these procedures will probably bring little if any motor recovery, but they are worth doing for the pain relief alone.

Other Problems

Acute iridocyclitis should be recognized and treated early to prevent blindness. Treatment consists of bed rest, eye patches, twice daily instillation of atropine, systemic steroids and daily injection of 0.1 or 0.2 mg of cortisone subconjuctivally.

Most paretic and paralytic conditions will respond to conservative nonoperative care, including splints, massage, wax baths and faradic stimulation of weak muscles. Interphalangeal arthrodesis can be done with a very small incision and no anesthesia, holding the bone surfaces together by means of Kirschner wires. This will not only remove some of the dreaded stigmata but will provide useful grasping and pinching ability. Tendon transfers, such as the sublimis tendon transfer to provide opposition and abduction actions of the thumb, are reserved for highly motivated patients or those with skilled jobs requiring these functions.

Whenever the decision is made to admit a patient into a general hospital, the question of isolation will arise. Patients diagnosed in the hospital or those who have had less than two weeks of treatment should be admitted to a private room, but isolation precautions are not necessary. Patients who have been receiving regular treatment require no isolation but, unfortunately, other patients' attitudes may make isolation unavoidable. It takes a great deal of preparation and education of other patients and their families before the patient with obvious stigmata of leprosy can be placed in a ward with noninfected patients.

BITES AND STINGS[4]

Snakebite

Of the 3500 species of snakes in the world, about 200 are poisonous. These are generally classified by physical characteristics (Table 28–1). Subclassification by type of venom action is difficult, for no venom has a single mode of action. It is nevertheless possible to classify venoms by their primary mode of action. Most local residents classify snakes as either "highly toxic" or "not so toxic," and this may actually be the best classification.

Cobra venom is responsible for more deaths than any other venom. It is reported to be 10,000 times more toxic than botulinum toxin A. The primary action of cobra, krait and mamba venom is neurotoxic. Russell's viper, phoorsa and adder venom is cytotoxic or hematoxic. Pit viper venom may be neurotoxic or cytotoxic or mixed, in which case no action may be called primary. All poisonous snakes have proteolytic toxins that produce local destruction and swelling of tissues, but the viperine group produce the most intense local reaction. The wise physician will become acquainted early with the appearance and venom of the poisonous snakes in his or her area.

An unusual variety of cobra is the spitting cobra found in Africa and Southeast Asia. It attacks by projecting venom, which often reaches the eyes of its victim. Injury ranges from simple conjunctivitis to permanent blindness.[24] Treatment consists of immediate irrigation of the eyes with water. Then, using fluoroscein stain, careful examination should be done. If any ulceration is evident antibiotics and atropine should be applied. Do not use steroids, for they may be harmful.

Not all bites from poisonous species of snakes are dangerous. Generally, bites in children are more dangerous than in adults because of the greater relative concentration of toxin. A snake that bites after a recent kill may have little or no stored venom. Other factors that determine the toxic effect include depth of the bite, weather conditions, site of the bite and even the mood of the snake. As with rabies, head and trunk bites are more serious.

Treatment

Because of rapid-acting toxins, the treatment of cobra, krait, Russell's viper, mamba and pit viper bites must be prompt and vigorous. Immediate application of a tourniquet above the bite is helpful, with suction applied to remove as much of the uncirculated venom as possible. With these species, death may come in minutes to hours, with an average of eight hours from bite to death. Polyvalent antivenom vaccine is always indicated but does not insure saving the patient's life. Large doses (30 to 200 ml) should be given intravenously as soon as possible. Children require more than adults because they receive a relatively higher dose of venom per kilogram of

TABLE 28-1 A Simple Classification of Common Poisonous Snakes

GROUP NAME	IDENTIFICATION	PRIMARY TOXIC EFFECT	COMMON EXAMPLES		
			Asia	*Africa*	*Americas*
Colubrine	Back fang	Hematoxic		Boomslang	
Elapine	Fixed front fang	Neurotoxic	Cobra Krait	Mamba Cobra	Coral snake
Viperine	Hinged front fang	Hematoxic Marked local reaction	Russell's viper Phoorsa	Puff adder	
Crotaline (pit viper)	A pit between the eye and nostril	Mixed hema-toxic or neurotoxic	Malay pit viper Habu		Bushmaster Rattlesnake

body weight. Anaphylactic reactions to horse serum are a danger but can usually be controlled with epinephrine and hydrocortisone. Skin testing of the patient prior to administration should be done, but even with a negative skin test serum sickness is likely to occur. Unfortunately, the conventional preparations of antivenom have a short half-life of potency and must be discarded about six months after preparation. Many countries now have available a freeze-dried preparation that has a two- to three-year duration of potency. If respiratory paralysis occurs in spite of these measures, respiratory assistance is indicated, for the heartbeat will persist long after respiratory arrest has occurred.

As soon as the IV is established and antivenom given (if available), ice bags are applied to the bite site, and fluids are given in amounts sufficient to maintain adequate blood pressure. The patient is then prepared for surgery. Since the bite often produces immediate anesthesia, only supplemental local anesthesia is necessary. The bite site is opened longitudinally. Ecchymotic skin and subcutaneous tissue is excised. Then the underlying fascia is opened. If muscle is bulging out, the fascia incision is extended proximally as far as necessary until no more bulging occurs. All necrotic muscle must be debrided.[8] Blood vessels are ligated or cauterized, and the wound is irrigated thoroughly. Incisions are generally not closed but dressed open for later closure or, more likely, for later skin grafting.

Other snakebites have a slower response and a longer time available for therapy. Morbidity or mortality is the result of bleeding, fluid loss from swelling, and necrosis of local tissues. Although hemolysis frequently occurs, hemorrhage is a more common problem. The venom initiates abnormal coagulation which exhausts fibrin and fibrinogen, leading to a bleeding diathesis. Alertness to this problem will prompt early study and correction of the coagulation factors with fresh blood. It appears that heparin or epsilon-aminocaproic acid (Amicar) may reverse this coagulopathy. Following viper and adder bites, swelling of an extremity can be considerable. In the early phase the patient may become oligemic from the loss of serum and blood into the extremity. This must be corrected with intravenous colloid solutions or plasma expanders to prevent shock. At the same time, frequent evaluation of the perfusion of the swollen extremity must be done, and fasciotomy should be performed whenever there is evidence that the swelling is obstructing arterial flow.

Recent work with rattlesnake bites in the United States indicates that one gram of hydrocortisone IV every six hours for 72 hours, combined with immediate fasciotomy from the joint above to the joint below the bite, prevented tissue loss from necrosis and made antivenom unnecessary. This should be kept in mind in handling other pit viper bites. (See also Chapter 4.)

Gila Monster Bite

There is a great deal of similarity between Gila monster (*Heloderma suspectum*) bites and snakebites. Local reaction produces edema and arteriospasm in the involved extremity, and fasciotomy should be considered if there is any question of peripheral circulation.[21] Supportive therapy for systemic symptoms is usually sufficient. EKG changes suggestive of myocardial infarction have been reported but are only transient. The venom is usually classified as primarily hemotoxic. Fatalities are rare except in very young children.

Insect Bites

With the exception of certain spiders, insect venoms are more a problem of hypersensitivity than of serious envenomization. Insect venoms are composed of histamine, phospholipases, serotonin and acetylcholine, and most contain hyaluronidase for rapid dissemination. Pain, vasodilatation and hypotension are common symptoms. General treatment consists of removal of the stinger, injection of local anesthetics for pain, ice packs to slow the release of histamine and the use of systemic antihistamines. More often the major problem is hypersensitivity reactions. The prompt use of epinephrine, IV hydrocortisone, bronchodilators and vasopressors may be life-saving in these circumstances.

Black Widow Spider Bite

The hemolytic and neurotoxic effects of the black widow spider (*Latrodectus mactans*) bite are much more serious. The female of this species, recognizable by the red or yellow "hourglass" on her belly, is often found in crawl spaces or around outhouses. A short stinging bite is soon followed by generalized or abdominal muscular pains and spasms, convulsions, nausea, vomiting, variable CNS symptoms and shock. Often these symptoms are confused with those of acute abdominal surgical crises. In the United States there is a commercial antivenom available for treating these bites but it is seldom available in developing countries. In addition to the antivenom, pain relief, IV calcium gluconate and muscle relaxants are indicated.

Brown Recluse Spider Bite

The brown recluse spider (*Loxosceles reclusa*) is found almost worldwide in similar hiding places to those of the black widow. This centimeter-long brown spider is identified by a dark "violin" on its back. Often the bite goes undetected, with no initial symptoms, but pain ensues within a few hours. Hemolysis and necrosis are the trade-marks of this spider's venom. Initially only erythema and bleb formation are noted at the bite site, but in two to four days necrosis results in the formation of a large ulcer, several centimeters in diameter. Even underlying joints may be destroyed. Fever, malaise, nausea, vomiting, convulsions, muscle spasms and arthralgia may accompany these local effects. The hemotoxin may produce hemolytic anemia, thrombocytopenia, jaundice and even death. Local treatment consists of cold compresses and extremity immobilization, and early excision of the bite site should be considered. Systemic treatment depends upon the severity of symptoms. If severe systemic reaction has occurred, antihistamines, steroids and antibiotics are indicated. Ulcers tend to be chronic and very slow to heal. Débridement and skin grafting are helpful once the extent of tissue necrosis is well demarcated.[10] It may be possible to undermine the edges of and close up the defect of a small ulcer when the base is clean. Generally, periosteum, nerves and major blood vessels are spared the necrotic effects. (See also Chapter 4.)

Scorpion Stings

Unlike the insects, the scorpion has four rather than three pairs of legs and an anterior claw-pincer for grasping its prey. They are usually found in moist, cool places, such as under rocks or logs. Venom varies between species, but in general it is composed of phospholipase, neurotoxin and proteinase.[11] In the U.S.A. most scorpion stings are innocuous, producing only local pain and swelling, but more serious varieties are found in the American Southwest and much of the tropical world. These produce significant systemic effects and even death. Systemic reactions may include salivation, mydriasis, hypertension, gastric distention, convulsions, respiratory arrest, pulmonary edema and the EKG changes of an acute myocardial infarction. Treatment of the local site of the sting includes the injection of local anesthetics, the application of ammonia and the local injection of 65 mg of emetine hydrocholoride. The treatment of the severe systemic reactions is more difficult. Morphine and meperidine (Demerol) accentuate the effect of the venom and are definitely contraindicated. Barbiturates, calcium gluconate and atropine will provide some control of symptoms, and the aim of systemic therapy is to control the severe symptoms until the effect of the venom subsides. Antivenom is available from the Arizona State University.

Venomous Marine Life

When a jellyfish is disturbed it fires nematocysts from its tentacles. These nematocysts in turn release a polypeptide toxin that causes an intense stinging sensation. Attempting to wash off the nematocysts with fresh water causes increased release of toxin. Instead it is recommended that they first be fixed with alcohol or vinegar and then scraped off with sand or a scraper. There is controversy about the effectiveness of papain in detoxifying the effect of the polypeptide toxin. Nevertheless, it has been reported that the cut surface of papaya is helpful in relieving the stinging sensation of the toxin.

Stingrays are usually found in shallow water, partially buried in the sand. When they are surprised they attack by lashing out against the foe with their powerful tail, which contains a stinger. Inside the integumentary sheath of this stinger is the venom, which is released at once. The resulting local pain is excruciating. Systemic effects include nausea, vomiting, respiratory distress, hypotension and shock. If the sting lodges in a vital area such as the chest, it may be fatal. Since the toxin is acid-sensitive and also thermolabile, treatment with vinegar and hot compresses is effective. Local injection with anes-

thetic agents and systemic IV pentazocine (Talwin) also help to relieve the pain. At this point, surgically remove any of the stinger remaining and debride the wound. To prevent anaphylactic reactions to this venom, steroids are also indicated.

Like the stingray, the scorpion fish also has a thermolabile venom, so that immediate application of hot compresses to the site of the wound or immersion of the wound in water of 110 to 115° F. for 30 minutes will considerably minimize the toxic effects. Local anesthetic infiltration, IV pentazocine, and steroids and vasopressors for shock are also indicated.[17]

The Portuguese man-of-war and the sea anemone (sea nettle) have similarities in the action of their venom, which is injected through tentacles that attach to their victims. Symptoms produced include severe pain, local swelling and anaphylactic shock. Pre-existing heart disease in elderly persons may be aggravated and may even produce death. Treatment consists of first removing any adherent tentacles (while wearing protective gloves), washing the area with water and dilute ammonia, treating shock, administering antihistamines or steroids for anaphylaxis and giving IV calcium gluconate.

Probably the most lethal fish is the stonefish. Venom from sacs located under the skin is released along grooves in 13 short, sharp spines. This venom has powerful effects on the circulatory and CNS systems, and death can result within an hour after encounter. The pain is unbearable. Antivenom for some varieties is available in the United States.

One of the most fascinating fish (both marine and freshwater) is the catfish. Some species migrate from one body of water to another across land. One variety in India crawls onto the trunks of trees to lay its eggs in the bark so that they will hatch with the next monsoon season. Another variety has the ability to "talk" and chatters constantly while trying to sting the unwary fisherman as he removes the fish from the hook. A tiny Amazonian variety delights in entering the urethra of the human swimmer, where it lodges with its barbed head and produces an intense inflammatory reaction. The marine catfish (*Plastos pineatus*) possesses very dangerous neurotoxin and hemotoxin that may cause death.[22] Ordinary freshwater catfish have stingers in the dorsal and pectoral fin spines. The venom of these generally causes a local stinging sensation that lasts a few hours and requires only symptomatic treatment. Whenever fishing for catfish, the wearing of heavy canvas gloves is advisable.

Large Animal Bites and Wounds

Wounds produced by wild animals are best treated in the same way as open human bites, with special emphasis on prevention of sepsis, especially gas gangrene and other anaerobic infections. Generally speaking, delayed closure of these wounds following extensive débridement is advisable. Crocodiles seize their victims by an extremity and try to pull them into the water. The result is either a stripping injury or avulsive amputation or disarticulation. It is amazing how well most of these injuries heal, but they should be left open. Elephants and water buffalo produce crushing and goring wounds. Damage to thoracic or abdominal viscera frequently requires exploration. Since hippopotami are herbivorous, delayed primary closure is satisfactory for their enormous bites.

Other Bites

Human, cat and monkey bites are always heavily contaminated and are notoriously prone to infection. They should be debrided thoroughly and left open. One possible exception is bites on the face, in which accepting the risk of infection may be preferable to disfiguring scar formation, so that closure may be considered following débridement and copious irrigation. Monkey bites may transmit viral encephalomyelitis with symptoms ensuing several days after the bite. All of these bites should be treated with systemic penicillin or cloxacillin.

In contrast, dog bites are relatively clean and have an infection risk of only 10 to 15 per cent. Following careful débridement and irrigation cleansing, most of these can be closed primarily. Antibiotic coverage with penicillin will further reduce the risk of infection.

Rabies

Rabies is the dreaded outcome of bites by jackals, monkeys, bats and especially of stray dogs. Unprovoked attack by any of these animals should alert the physician to the possibility of the animal being rabid. Symptoms of rabies infection in an animal include snapping, drooling, vocal cord paralysis and unusual purposeless movements. Seldom is a biting animal impounded in developing countries, so the physician must make a decision based upon the patient's impressions and descriptions. In most developing countries rabies is endemic, and rabies vaccine is used more liberally than in the United States. Nevertheless, remember that both the sheep brain vaccine and the duck embryo vaccine may produce lethal anaphylactic reactions, and this risk must be weighed before committing the patient to treatment. The management recommended by the World Health Organization for treatment of exposure to rabies is outlined in Table 28–2. Do not overlook the local treatment. Antirabies serum is not available in all countries but is indicated in cases of severe exposure.

Once symptoms of rabies occur in the patient, only supportive measures are indicated. The risk of infection must be understood by all who treat patients who have clinical rabies. The mortality rate is essentially 100 per cent, al-

TABLE 28–2 WHO Guide for Treatment of Exposure to Rabies[26]

A. Local Treatment of Wounds Involving Possible Exposure to Rabies

(1) Recommended in all exposures

(a) *First-aid treatment*

Immediate washing and flushing with soap and water, detergent or water alone (recommended procedure in all bite wounds including those unrelated to possible exposure to rabies).

(b) *Treatment by or under direction of a physician*
  (i) Adequate cleansing of the wound.
  (ii) Thorough treatment with 20% soap solution and/or the application of a quaternary ammonium compound or other substance of proven lethal effect on the rabies virus.[1]
  (iii) Topical application of antirabies or its liquid or powdered globulin preparation (optional).
  (iv) Administration, where indicated, of antitetanus procedures and of antibiotics and drugs to control infections other than rabies.
  (v) Suturing of wound not advised.

(2) Additional local treatment for severe exposures only.
(*a*) Topical application of antirabies serum or its liquid or powdered globulin preparation.
(*b*) Infiltration of antirabies serum around the wound.

---

[1]Where soap has been used to clean wounds, all traces of it should be removed before the application of quaternary ammonium compounds because soap neutralizes the activity of such compounds.

B. Specific Systemic Treatment

Nature of Exposure	Status of Biting Animal (Irrespective of Whether Vaccinated or Not)		Recommended Treatment
	At Time of Exposure	*During Observation Period of Ten Days*	
I. No lesions; indirect contact	Rabid	—	None
II. Licks:			
(1) unabraded skin	Rabid	—	None
(2) abraded skin, scratches and unabraded or abraded mucosa	(*a*) healthy	Clinical signs of rabies or proven rabid (laboratory)	Start vaccine[1] at first signs of rabies in the biting animal
	(*b*) signs suggestive of rabies	Healthy	Start vaccine[1] immediately; stop treatment if animal is normal on fifth day after exposure
	(*c*) rabid, escaped, killed or unknown	—	Start vaccine[1] immediately
III. Bites:			
(1) mild exposure	(*a*) healthy	Clinical signs of rabies or proven rabid (laboratory)	Start vaccine[1,2] at first signs of rabies in the biting animal
	(*b*) signs suggestive of rabies	Healthy	Start vaccine[1] immediately; stop treatment if animal is normal on fifth day after exposure
	(*c*) rabid, escaped, killed or unknown	—	Start vaccine[1,2] immediately
	(*d*) wild (wolf, jackal, fox, bat, etc.)	—	Serum[2] immediately, followed by a course of vaccine[1]
(2) severe exposure (multiple, or face, head, finger or neck bites)	(*a*) healthy	Clinical signs of rabies or proven rabid (laboratory)	Serum[2] immediately; start vaccine[1] at first sign of rabies in the biting animal

TABLE 28–2 WHO Guide for Treatment of Exposure to Rabies (*Continued*)

B. Specific Systemic Treatment

| Nature of Exposure | Status of Biting Animal (Irrespective of Whether Vaccinated or Not) | | Recommended Treatment |
	At Time of Exposure	During Observation Period of Ten Days	
(2) severe exposure (multiple, or face, head, finger or neck bites)	(b) signs suggestive of rabies	Healthy	Serum[2] immediately, followed by vaccine; vaccine may be stopped if animal is normal on fifth day after exposure
	(c) rabid, escaped, killed or unknown		
	(d) wild (wolf, jackal, pariah dog, fox, bat, etc.)	–	Serum[2] immediately, followed by vaccine[1]

[1] Practice varies concerning the volume of vaccine per dose and the number of doses recommended in a given situation. In general, the equivalent of at least 2 ml of a 5% tissue emulsion should be given subcutaneously daily for 14 consecutive days. Many laboratories use 20 to 30 doses in severe exposures. To ensure the production and maintenance of high levels of serum-neutralizing antibodies, booster doses should be given at 10 days and at 20 or more days following the last daily dose of vaccine in *all* cases. This is especially important if antirabies serum has been used, in order to overcome the interference effect.

[2] In all severe exposures and in all cases of unprovoked wild animal bites, antirabies serum or its globulin fractions together with vaccine should be employed. This is considered by the Committee as the *best* specific treatment available for the post-exposure prophylaxis of rabies in man. Although experience indicates that vaccine alone is sufficient for mild exposures, there is no doubt that here also the combined serum-vaccine treatment will give the best protection. However, both the serum and the vaccine can cause deleterious reactions. Moreover, the combined therapy is more expensive; its use in mild exposures is therefore considered optional. As with vaccine alone, it is important to start combined serum and vaccine treatment as early as possible after exposure, but serum should still be used no matter what the time interval. Serum should be given in a single dose (40 IU per kg of body weight) and the first dose of vaccine inoculated at the same time. Sensitivity to the serum must be determined before its administration.

though one recovery has been reported following the onset of symptoms.

UNUSUAL WOUNDS, FOREIGN BODIES AND TETANUS

The variety of wounds and foreign bodies seen by the surgeon in developing countries is unlimited.

The wounds of bamboo, particularly of thorn bamboo, have already been discussed in relation to the feet. Thorn bamboo is commonly used for fencing material and is therefore a common cause of hand wounds as well. Thorn bamboo wounds are slow to heal and tend to form chronic draining sinuses. Such drainage usually indicates that a piece of the bamboo is still buried and will have to be removed before healing can occur. Frequently these thorns can be visualized by radiograph using a soft tissue technique.

Fishhooks imbedded in the finger or foot are a common problem everywhere in the world. The classic method of removal is to rotate the hook, advancing the point until it emerges from the skin, and then to cut the shaft of the hook and pull the hook out by the point (see Fig. 4–5). This technique requires local anesthesia (usually digital block) and increases the trauma to the digit. An alternative method first reported by Dr. Theo Cooke[6] is painless and requires no anesthesia but does require courage to attempt it the first time (Fig. 28–12). The technique described by Dr. Cooke is as follows: "The person who is to remove the hook makes a loop of ordinary string and winds the end securely around his right index finger. The loop, about 18 inches long, is slipped over the shank of the hook. The finger (or foot) which the hook has entered is placed on a firm surface with the eye of the hook pointing to the left of the manipulator, who then takes the

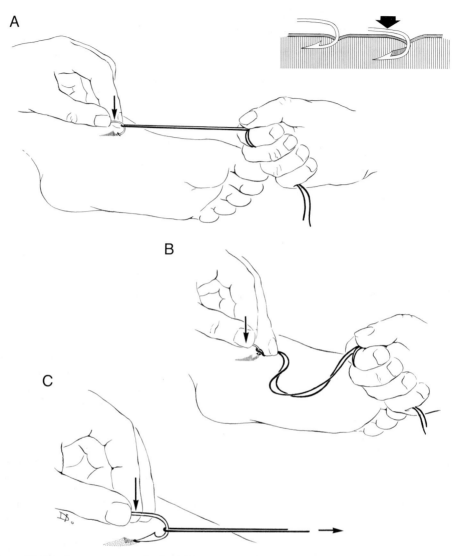

Figure 28–12   Stepwise removal of a fishhook. *A.* A doubled length of string is wound around the finger of the person who is removing the fishhook and looped over the shank of the hook. *B.* The shank is depressed with the thumb of the left hand, disengaging the hook from the tissues (see inset). The middle finger of the left hand is used to secure the loop of string in the middle of the curve of the hook, at the point of entry into the skin. *C.* After a slow test maneuver to insure that unobstructed motion of the right hand is possible, the hook is removed by a sudden jerk on the string, with a full follow-through of the right hand.

eye and shank between the thumb and index finger of his left hand. Holding the shank rigidly, he depresses it, painlessly disengaging the barb unless the hook is moved sideways. He slowly straightens the loop of the string horizontally in the plane of the long axis of the shank. This is a test maneuver to make sure the loop will not become tangled on coat buttons and to bring the center of the loop gently against the curve of the hook. The tip of the operator's left third finger then holds the center of the loop against the finger (or foot) at the point where the hook enters. The operator brings his right hand back to the hook and suddenly jerks it away in the same direction as in the test maneuver, with full follow-through. The hook is spun back out of the finger without enlarging the track or the hole of entry."

In parts of Egypt, the Sudan and Nigeria, unusual wounds include ritual circumcision of the female. This disappearing tribal ritual varies from trimming the labia minor and the tip of the clitoris to radical procedures that may damage the urethra and that include infibulation (an attempt to produce vulvar stenosis by encouraging the raw edges of the labia to adhere across the midline). In many parts of the world, caustics are commonly inserted into the vagina to treat gonorrhea. The management of most of these wounds is not an outpatient procedure and must be done meticulously to avoid damage to the urethra.

Tetanus

As long as it is common practice in some areas to treat wounds with mud, cow dung, or other excrement, tetanus will be a problem. Compounding these habits is the lack of pediatric immunization. The sanitary disposal of human excrement is unusual in these areas, so all soil should be considered contaminated with *Clostridium tetani* organisms. Puncture wounds into bare feet are a daily occurrence. In fact, the high incidence of tetanus is not surprising; indeed, it is surprising that there are not more cases.

After an average incubation period of six to ten days, the prodromal symptoms begin: stiffness in the jaw, restlessness, yawning and headache. These symptoms last for about 24 hours. If there is no treatment, the neurotoxin causes progressive trismus, tonic contracture of skeletal muscles, abdominal pain, convulsions and finally death. The exact cause of death is not known, but certainly hypoxia from the sustained convulsions is a major factor.

Seldom do patients come to the hospital with puncture wounds. But there are other wounds containing dead or dying tissue and a low local tissue PO_2 that are prone to tetanus. These include burn wounds, gunshot wounds, open fractures, gorings, wounds from arrows or spears, and neglected lacerations. For the prophylactic management of these patients, see the American College of Surgeons' guidelines (Table 28–3). Human tetanus immunoglobulin is

TABLE 28–3 Recommendations for Prophylactic Treatment of Rabies Based on Guidelines of American College of Surgeons*

| Type of Wound | Patient not Immunized or Incompletely Immunized | Patient Immunized Time Since Last Booster Dose | | |
		1–5 Years	5–10 Years	Over 10 Years
Clean, minor	Begin or complete immunization per schedule Tetanus toxoid 0.5 cc	None	Toxoid 0.5 cc	Toxoid 0.5 cc
Clean, major or tetanus-prone	Toxoid 0.5 cc and complete series Human tetanus immunoglobulin 250 mg	Toxoid 0.5 cc	Toxoid 0.5 cc	Toxoid 0.5 cc Human tetanus immunoglobulin 250 mg
Tetanus-prone with delayed or incomplete débridement	Repeat above and add penicillin or tetracycline	Toxoid 0.5 cc	Toxoid 0.5 cc and antibiotics	Repeat above and add antibiotics

*Bull. Am. Coll. Surg., 57:32–33 (Dec.), 1972.

unavailable in many countries. The only choice in this situation is horse serum antitoxin. This should not be given without first testing the patient for horse serum sensitivity. Use 0.1 to 0.2 cc of the antitoxin intradermally. If there is no sensitivity reaction, give at least 3000 units. If a sensitivity reaction occurs, begin immunization with toxoid and use antibiotics, but do not give the antitoxin.

Emergency Treatment of Tetanus

The management of the patient with prodromal or active symptoms is not an outpatient procedure, but since the program of treatment is usually started or outlined in the Emergency Room, the measures are included here:[3, 5]

1. *Maintenance of an adequate airway.* This means early tracheostomy in all except the very mild forms that present with a long incubation period prior to the onset of symptoms.

2. *Wound care.* Thorough débridement without closure of the primary wound.

3. *Neutralization of the toxin.* If human tetanus immune globulin is available, give 1000 to 1500 units in multiple IM injections, particularly in the suspected area of the infection. If this is unavailable, give 50,000 to 100,000 units of equine tetanus antitoxin IV and inject an additional 50,000 units into and around the wound following débridement. Since recent evidence questions the value of this measure, it is not advisable to give any equine antitoxin if the patient is sensitive to horse serum.

4. *Control of tetanospasms.* Paraldehyde, up to 12 cc IM every four hours, or diazepam (Valium) 5 to 20 mg and chlorpromazine 25 to 50 mg IM every four hours, combined with meperidine (Demerol) and barbiturates as necessary.

5. *Antibiotics.* These have no effect on the neurotoxin producing the symptoms, but it is advisable to give penicillin prophylactically, 10 million units per day IV, and kanamycin, 0.5 mg IM every eight hours.

6. *Maintenance of respiration.* In the severe fulminating form with a two or four day incubation period, it is usually necessary to perform a tracheostomy. The patient is then given curare and ventilatory assistance by means of a respirator. These patients develop rigidity of the face and neck muscles but have no convulsions. They can be managed adequately with ordinary nursing care and supportive measures as indicated.

Tetanus in Septic Abortion

It has been my experience that tetanus complicating attempted abortion is unusually severe and fulminant, with a high mortality rate. The plentiful culture medium and rich blood supply for rapid transport of the neurotoxin may be responsible for this. One or two hours after administration of the human tetanus immune gobulin or the antitoxin, the uterus should be removed, preferably by vaginal hysterectomy. This should be followed by the same measures outlined for severe tetanus.

Tetanus is a reversible disease. The patient will recover with no physiological or anatomical sequelae if careful attention is paid to the six measures of management outlined in the previous section.

Neonatal Tetanus

The same basic principles of treatment apply to neonatal tetanus. This disease usually begins between the fifth and tenth day of life. The mother first notices poor sucking, and within 36 hours the typical spasms are manifest. Again, paraldehyde is an excellent agent for sedation and control of the spasms (0.2 cc per kg every four to six hours IM). Aspiration is more likely to occur in the infant. Since feeding via a nasogastric tube is unwise, nutrition must be maintained by using 10 per cent dextrose solutions or, preferably, a parenteral hyperalimentation formula. Neither adult nor neonatal tetanus should have a mortality of greater than 40 per cent in any hospital.

MISCELLANEOUS

Family Planning

No concerned surgeon can practice in a developing country without becoming involved in family planning programs. In countries where the literacy rate is low, the birth rate per thousand is two or three times greater than in countries with a high rate of literacy. All progress in developing countries is hindered by a high birth rate and exploding rate of population growth. Rare are the hospitals today that do not have Family Planning Clinics or mobile clinics or do not conduct family planning camps. Taking their example from Japan, many countries are liberalizing abortion laws in an attempt to lower the birth rate. Vasectomy, D and C and even tubectomy are being done as outpatient procedures. See Chapters 19 (Urology) and 20 (Gynecology) for procedures.

Postmortem Examinations

In many countries it is impossible to obtain permission for postmortem examination of a body. One solution to this problem is the percutaneous biopsy needle. With a little practice, tumor masses as well as all major organs of the body can be sampled postmortem by a percutaneous needle biopsy. Few hospitals in developing countries stock these needles and they are seldom purchasable. It is therefore advisable to become familiar with a nondisposable variety and to take one with you.

SUMMARY

Half of the world's population live in developing countries. Most of these people are hungry, undernourished and have little access to even basic medical care. The United States has one doctor for every 750 people, whereas India has only one doctor for every 5000 people and northern Nigeria has only one doctor for every 140,000 people. Complicating this picture, developing countries are burdened with high unemployment rates, high birth rates, low per capita income, a large rural population and little foreign exchange for importing medical supplies and equipment. Although this situation is changing rapidly, doctors from medically advanced countries will be needed for several generations to share their skills.

It has not been the purpose of this chapter to discuss all the potential surgical procedures to be done in the outpatient operating room of a hospital in a developing country. Most of the cases presenting to the surgeon in a developing country involve principles of therapy discussed in other chapters of this text. Instead, this has been an attempt to discuss those conditions peculiar to tropical or developing countries.

REFERENCES

1. Bowesman, C.: Surgery and Clinical Pathology in the Tropics. Baltimore, Williams & Wilkins, 1960.
2. Chatterji, K. K.: Tropical Surgery and Surgical Pathology. London, John Bale Sons and Danielson, Ltd., 1927.
3. Christensen, N. A., and Thurber, D. L.: Current treatment of clinical tetanus. Mod. Treat., 5:729–757, 1968.
4. Christy, N. P.: Poisoning by venomous animals. Am. J. Med., 42:107–128, 1967.
5. Cole, L., and Youngman, H.: Treatment of tetanus. Lancet, 1:1017–1019, 1969.
6. Cooke, T.: How to remove fish-hooks with a bit of string. Med. J. Aust., 1:815–816, 1961.
7. Davey, W. W.: Companion to Surgery in Africa. Baltimore, Williams & Wilkins, 1968.

8. Glass, T. G.: Early débridement in pit viper bites. J.A.M.A., *235*:2513–2516, 1976.

9. Green, W. O., and Adams, T. E.: Mycetoma in the United States. A review and report of seven additional cases. Am. J. Clin. Pathol., *42*:75–91, 1964.

10. Hershey, F. B., and Aulenbacher, C. E.: Surgical treatment of brown spider bites. Ann. Surg., *170*:300–308, 1969.

11. Horen, W. P.: Insect and scorpion sting. J.A.M.A., *221*:894–898, 1972.

12. Hunter, G. W., Schwartzwelder, J. C., and Clyde, D. F.: Tropical Medicine, 5th ed. Philadelphia, W. B. Saunders Co., 1976.

13. Jacobson, R. R., and Trautman, J. R.: The diagnosis and treatment of leprosy. South. Med. J., *69*:979–985, 1976.

14. Kerr, W. F.: Surgery. London, Oxford University Press, 1957.

15. King, M.: Medical Care in Developing Countries. London, Oxford University Press, 1966.

16. Lewis, A. A. M.: Outpatient surgery in developing countries. Lancet, *1*:910–912, 1975.

17. Linaweaver, P. G.: Toxic marine life. Milit. Med., *132*:437–442, 1967.

18. McNair, T. J. (ed.): Hamilton Bailey's Emergency Surgery. Baltimore, Williams & Wilkins Co., 1967.

19. Moore, D. C.: Regional Block: A Handbook for Use in the Clinical Practice of Medicine and Surgery, 4th ed. Springfield, Ill., Charles C Thomas, 1971.

20. Palande, D. D.: Review of 23 operations on the ulnar nerve in leprous neuritis. J. Bone Joint Surg. (Am), *55*:1457–1464, 1973.

21. Roller, J. A., and Davis, D. H.: Gila monster bite. J.A.M.A., *235*:249–250, 1976.

22. Sciggin, C. H.: Catfish stings. J.A.M.A., *231*:176–177, 1975.

23. Shoul, M. I.: Skin grafting under local anesthesia using a new safety razor dermatome. Am. J. Surg., *112*:959–963, 1966.

24. Warrell, D. A., and Olmerod, L. D.: Snake venom ophthalmia and blindness caused by the spitting cobxa in Nigeria. Am. J. Trop. Med. Hyg., *25*:525–529, 1976.

25. Williams, J. A.: Outpatient operations. I. The surgeon's view. Br. Med. J., *1*:174–175, 1969.

26. World Health Organization. Technical Report Series, no. 321. Expert Committee on Rabies, 5th report.

29 Surgery and Medicine in the Field

BRUCE C. PATON, M.R.C.P. (Ed.), F.R.C.S. (Ed.),
and BEN EISEMAN, M.D.

INTRODUCTION

The average physician is poorly prepared to play an effective role in assisting in the rescue of a patient hurt or seriously ill in a remote area. An increase in the number of people seeking solitude and recreation in remote areas provides a concomitant increase in the frequency with which a physician lacking any prior training may be asked to perform in this unaccustomed milieu.

It is not possible to estimate how many people in the United States walk, climb or camp in the mountains, but nearly three million visitors came to the Rocky Mountain National Park, Colorado, in 1978. A distressing majority is neither trained for preventing injury nor prepared for the unexpected event that so often precedes an accident. The American Alpine Club annually records and analyzes fatal accidents that occur in the mountains of the United States and

1385

TABLE 29–1   Search and Rescue in
Colorado, 1978

No. of rescuers	3,400
No. of missions	1,100
Man-hours	500.000
Value @ $7.00/hour	$3,500,000

Canada. The number of fatal climbing accidents in the U.S.A. has risen from an average of 14 per year between 1951 and 1966 to 24 in 1978. The number of serious (nonfatal) accidents increased from 75 in 1974 to 210 in 1976. About one-third of accidents involved inexperienced, untrained climbers.

The time and effort expended by volunteer groups on search and rescue operations is enormous and increasing. Estimated statistics for Colorado in 1976 are given in Table 29–1.

Although most people probably go to the mountains or the seashore, the deserts, canyonlands and rivers all attract large numbers of vacationers, and with their increasing accessibility, many thousands trek annually into remote mountain areas such as Nepal. The types of accidents and the possible complications depend upon all aspects of the environment, including terrain, temperature, season and remoteness from and availability of help.

CALL FOR HELP AND EARLY ORGANIZATION

Disaster may strike, but two principles minimize delay in rescue: (1) All parties should leave a detailed climbing or camping plan with a responsible agency (Forest Service) or friend; and (2) No one should make solitary expeditions or climb alone.

These principles, however, are often overlooked. Unnecessary delays occur because it is not recognized that a party is overdue, or the loca-

tion of a possible accident is only vaguely known.

Time is of the essence in evacuating a casualty. Exposure to wind, rain, cold and high altitude may complicate enormously even a relatively simple injury. Indeed, cold injury may be fatal to a poorly equipped person immobilized by a simple extremity injury. It must be remembered that cold injury is the product of temperature plus time plus the chill factor (Table 9–2) of wind and humidity. One cold, wet night in the wind at high altitudes may be uncomfortable to a casualty. A second may be lethal. If the accident occurs during winter, these factors are readily obvious to everyone. But even in the summer, temperatures at high altitudes may drop to dangerously low levels, especially when cold is combined with wind and rain.

The physician should seldom organize the search and rescue operation. This is a job for professionals, who should be called at once. The best trained, equipped and manned group in the United States is the Mountain Rescue Association, which has branches adjacent to most recreation areas. The Forest Service and police usually know how to reach these groups, who maintain a 24-hour, 365-day-a-year watch.

Successful location, care and retrieval of a casualty in a remote area is largely a matter of organization, logistics and discipline. By its demands, a search closely resembles a military operation. The Director of the search establishes a base of operations at which he or she gathers trained personnel and equipment and from which he or she has good communication both with the outside and with the searchers on the site of the accident.

Locating a missing person in a remote area is a fascinating science and art but is not germane to this discussion, since the physician will probably play no important role in its activation. Details of search and rescue vary with terrain, weather and available rescue equipment.

Once the injured party is located, a well-equipped and strongly manned contact party is sent to the scene. Unless the physician is very fit (and a strong climber), it is best not to try to keep up with this initial group, which is apt to keep a quick pace.

Although the main purpose of the initial contact group is to assess the injury and the locale of the accident, its members should have splints, bandages and other basic first aid equipment, as well as sleeping bags, food and warm clothing. Their primary aim is to report back by radio or messenger an accurate assessment of the situation. One or two of its members will then stay with the casualty.

The physician should be close to the Director at the base camp and should make certain that all equipment is in order and that all means have been prepared for casualty evacuation (by helicopter, sled, litter, horse and so on) and hospitalization.

As soon as the exact status and location of the casualty are known, the physician should set off, taking not only the necessary medical equipment, but also warm clothes, gloves, parka and sleeping bag, for he or she may have to spend at least one night with the casualty in an exposed area.

Although it is the Director's responsibility to see that sufficient manpower is sent with the physician to accomplish the task of evacuation, it is well for the physician to remember that 10 to 18 people may be required to evacuate each casualty.

HELICOPTER EVACUATION

In the absence of more highly trained personnel, the physician may have to select and prepare a helicopter casualty evacuation site. The following principles should be kept in mind:

1. Do not risk the life of helicopter personnel by choosing a risky site, if a safe site can be reached by carrying the casualty farther. Unwarranted alarm may overtake the uninitiated under the conditions of a rescue, and unnecessary risks are often urged. Speed of evacuation is not always essential once the condition of the patient is stable.

2. Ability of a helicopter to land and lift off may be limited at altitudes over 10,000 feet. Factors to be considered are power of the machine available, load and temperature. There is less lift in warm air than in cold.

3. Size of landing zone. Although a straight vertical ascent requires a clearing greater than 100 feet on a side, risks increase directly with the surrounding clearing. In general, no area cleared less than 100 yards square should be considered. Low trees or bushes can compromise this minimum, but each encroachment increases the risk, particularly in windy, exposed landing zones.

4. Ground cover. Stumps, boulders, brush and even high grass can interfere or exclude a landing zone. The pilot will usually weigh the factors previously mentioned, but the ground party must confirm the safety of the terrain for him or her.

5. Recovery while hovering is extremely difficult and should be avoided unless both pilot and rescuer have been specially trained in this useful but hazardous technique.

6. Marking the zone. In wooded terrain, it may be difficult for the pilot to locate the landing zone. Brightly colored parkas are adequate substitutes for the panels used in military medical evacuation operations. Radio communication between ground and air is ideal but not always available in civilian life.

PRINCIPLES OF FIRST AID

A general scheme for organizing a medical evacuation is given in Figure 29–1.

Forewarned is forearmed. Since re-

TRANSPORTATION   SITE   ACTION

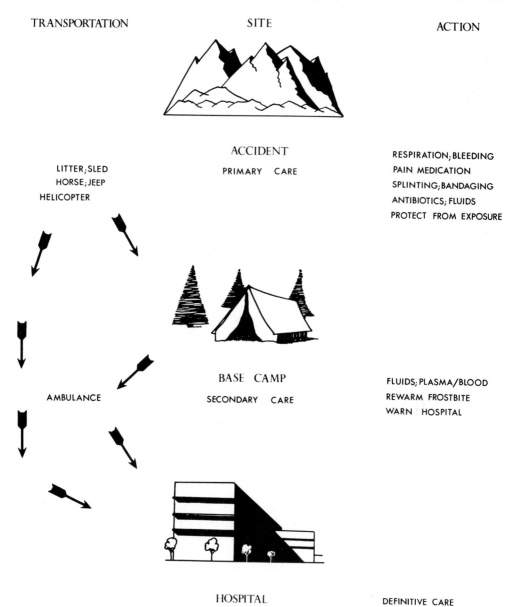

ACCIDENT
PRIMARY   CARE

LITTER;SLED
HORSE;JEEP
HELICOPTER

RESPIRATION;BLEEDING
PAIN MEDICATION
SPLINTING;BANDAGING
ANTIBIOTICS; FLUIDS
PROTECT FROM EXPOSURE

BASE CAMP
SECONDARY   CARE

AMBULANCE

FLUIDS; PLASMA/BLOOD
REWARM FROSTBITE
WARN   HOSPITAL

HOSPITAL   DEFINITIVE CARE

Figure 29–1 Scheme for action to be taken at various sites during evacuation of victim from mountain accident..

ports of accidents are often vague and even erroneous, as accurate a description of the emergency as possible should be obtained before the rescue party starts off from the base. Don't carry splints to a case of appendicitis. Make suitable arrangements for the treatment of the injured after they are brought off the mountain. The most

important principle in handling all problems, both medical and surgical, is: "Do the minimum necessary to make the patient safe and comfortable for transportation." If this principle is followed, unnecessary time will not be spent undertaking measures that are better done at a lower level or under more advantageous circumstances. Do not neglect to make as full an examination as time and circumstances permit. Do not neglect the first aid of a serious injury because of failure to make an examination. Vital signs should be recorded when the patient is first seen and regularly thereafter, depending upon the injury or illness. A label detailing all medications given and the time of administration should be attached to the patient, especially if the doctor cannot accompany the patient to the hospital.

ENVIRONMENTAL HAZARDS

Injuries and illness in the field usually are a combination of a disease or injury plus the complicating factor of exposure to the elements. The physician obviously must consider both but, for simplicity, hazards of the environment will be identified and means of treatment indicated.

High Altitude Sickness

Campers, climbers and hunters often become ill or injured in high mountains, a complication not often considered by the hospital-based surgeon.

Altitude is unlikely to be of serious consequence below 7000 feet, unless the patient has a pre-existing cardiac or pulmonary lesion. Partial pressure of oxygen in dry air at 5000 feet is about 130 mm Hg. Arterial oxygen tension at 5000 feet is 55 to 75 mm Hg. Only above 9000 feet is there a serious threat of hypoxia from altitude per se complicating the problems of the injured.

High altitude sickness is a syndrome that may variously occur at any height above 9000 feet.[1] Although the critical altitude varies in different parts of the world (U.S.A. above 8500 feet; Himalayas and Andes, 11,000 to 12,000 feet), the factors involved are altitude, exercise, conditioning and duration of exposure. During the Chinese invasion into India in 1966, more than 2000 cases occurred in unacclimatized Indian troops who rushed from lowlands to the Himalayas.

The manifestations of acute mountain sickness may be primarily respiratory and cardiovascular (dyspnea, cough, pulmonary edema), cerebral (headache, dizziness, unconsciousness), gastrointestinal (anorexia, nausea, vomiting, abdominal pain) or general tiredness and weakness. Insomnia, sometimes exacerbated by Cheyne-Stokes respiration, is very common. Individual patients may present primarily with one of these groups of symptoms or with a combination of types. Retinal hemorrhages may occur above 13,000 ft and may either cause obvious visual field defects or be undiscernible by the patient.

Nausea, anorexia, headache, insomnia and confusion have been recognized for many years by mountain climbers as part of the intrinsic hazards and discomforts of climbing at high altitudes. But it is only in recent years that pulmonary and cardiovascular problems — especially pulmonary edema — have been clearly defined as secondary effects of altitude hypoxia.

Pulmonary edema develops either in those who normally reside at high altitudes, go to lower levels for two or three weeks, then return to the original altitude; or in those who have never previously been at high altitudes and are rapidly transported to high country. In either case, pulmonary edema usually develops within about three days of exposure or re-exposure to altitude. The onset may be acute and explosive with the patient rapidly becoming moribund, or it may be insidious. The patient usually has associated symptoms of mountain sickness, with headache, anorexia, and sometimes oliguria. For two or three nights before the development of severe symptoms, he may experience shortness of breath and coughing and have to sit up in order to regain his breath.

The amount of exertion during the first few days at high altitude does not necessarily determine who will develop symptoms. Some people develop pulmonary edema although sedentary, while others are able to exert themselves without symptoms. Occasional individuals develop edema on repeated occasions.

Circulatory responses vary. Blood pressure may be higher or lower than normal. The pulse rate may be faster or slower than normal. Total blood volume does not change, but pulmonary blood volume increases as much as 80 per cent, and peripheral blood volume decreases. Pulmonary artery pressure is high, secondary to an increase in precapillary arteriolar resistance, but pulmonary wedge pressures and left atrial pressures are normal.

The treatment of high altitude sickness and high altitude pulmonary edema is based upon three principles: (1) Increase arterial P_{O_2}; (2) decrease pulmonary blood volume by giving diuretics; and (3) reduce overall activity by rest.

Arterial P_{O_2} can be increased either by administration of oxygen by face mask or by evacuation of the patient to an altitude lower than 9000 feet. Two to three liters of oxygen per minute may be sufficient to relieve symptoms.

Diuretics have been strongly advocated both for cure of established sickness and prophylactically during the first few days of exposure to high altitude. Furosemide, 40 to 120 mg twice daily for two to three days on arrival at high altitude, may reduce the incidence of severe symptoms. Furosemide may induce a rapid diuresis and relieve symptoms during acute pulmonary edema.

Morphine sulfate 5 mg given intravenously with a diuretic has been found to be very effective. Morphine and furosemide together may induce a greater diuresis than furosemide by itself. No danger of respiratory depression has been encountered by the use of IV morphine under these circumstances.

If cerebral symptoms are severe and cerebral edema is thought to be present, dexamethasone, 10 mg IV, should be given in conjunction with a diuretic. There is no evidence that pulmonary symptoms are helped by steroids. Patients with cerebral edema must be brought to a lower altitude as quickly as possible; awaiting evacuation may require too long a delay.

Activity should be reduced to a minimum. Reduction in bodily activity and evacuation to a lower altitude may, by themselves, result in marked improvement in many patients.

Effect of High Altitude on Fluid and Caloric Requirements

Climbing at high altitudes requires the expenditure of much energy and results in dehydration. Estimates of this dehydration should be taken into account when rehydration with intravenous fluids is attempted. Mountain explorers have found that a fluid intake of 3 to 4 liters per day is necessary to maintain a urine output of 1500 cc per day. At moderate altitudes of 10,000 to 15,000 feet, caloric requirements for an active climber may be as high as 4500 kcal per day. For the victim of an accident, however, the caloric requirements are of secondary importance compared with the maintenance of an adequate airway. Most victims of mountain accidents are healthy and young and, with appropriate indications, can be given 500 to 1000 cc lactated Ringer's solution intravenously in 60 minutes without fear of overloading the circulation. If the patient has pulmonary edema or a primary cardiac condition, this volume of fluid would be contraindicated.

Avalanche Victims

Occasionally a physician skier will be drafted to join an avalanche rescue team. Usually he or she is unfamiliar with the problems that must be faced. The following precepts are helpful:

Speed in reaching the victim is the essence of success because death is due to suffocation, freezing and blunt injuries. Of victims located within 15 minutes, 85 per cent survive; within 35 minutes, 75 per cent live; and within one hour 55 per cent are saved. This is the golden period, and all efforts and even reasonable risks should be taken to reach the victim within one hour. It is well to hurry to the scene but not to risk the lives of the rescuers two hours after an avalanche.

Density of new snow may be as little as 5 per cent that of water and is thus mostly air.[3] Avalanche snow is usually much more dense but is reasonably permeable to air. Depending on the type of snow in the slide, the victim may obtain some air for exchange if not too deeply buried.

While the search team looks and probes for the victim, the physician should set up an aid station near the base of the slide area. Once a slide has occurred, there is no immediate danger of another avalanche in the same slide path.

First aid supplies should include an endotracheal tube, an ambu bag or other means of ventilation, splints, warm clothes and intravenous resuscitative solutions. Once set up, the physician and the search Director should locate and prepare a helicopter evacuation area if such is appropriate.

Frostbite [5]

Immediate treatment is influenced by those factors that seriously influence ultimate injury and accentuate tissue damage. Remove wet cloth-ing and socks and replace them with dry clothes from the rescuers' packs. Shelter the victim because of the additional cooling factor of wind. The chilling effect of wind is related to several factors including the air temperature, wind velocity, the insulating properties of clothing, the activity of the victim and the amount of exposed skin. In order, therefore, to reduce the effects of wind, the patient should be sheltered, well-insulated and completely covered. Contact between the exposed part and wetness or metal greatly accelerates heat loss and increases the likelihood of loss of tissue.

Reflex vasodilatation induced by warming the rest of the body is a good method for restoring circulation in a frozen limb. While the victim is being removed from the scene of the accident, keep the rest of his body as warm as possible. Alcohol induces vasodilatation, but increases heat loss; avoid its use (until the end of the rescue mission)!

The best definitive treatment of frostbite is rapid rewarming in water no hotter than 42° C (107.6° F) after the patient has been brought to a care center or base camp beyond which good transportation is assured. Do not attempt rewarming of a frozen foot in exposed conditions when continued warmth of the part is not assured. Under extreme circumstances, it is possible to walk on a frozen foot. Walking on a thawed-out, painful foot, too swollen for a boot, is an impossibility.

After rewarming, the frostbitten part should be carefully protected with loose, preferably sterile padding during further transportation. In the hospital the part may be exposed on sterile sheets.

Generalized Body Hypothermia

In addition to frostbite, a localized condition, accident victims often develop generalized body hypothermia. General body hypothermia may be lethal. If body temperature falls below 27° C cardiac arrhythmias and, ultimately, ventricular fibrillation ensue. Atrial fibrillation is the commonest arrhythmia to develop first, followed by conduction disturbances, ventricular arrhythmias and ventricular fibrillation.

Cardiac arrhythmias usually disappear upon rewarming and do not require specific treatment. If atrial fibrillation should persist at a rapid rate, digitalis would be indicated.

The treatment of hypothermia is rewarming. Blankets, hot water bottles, heating pads or warm water tubs are all suitable agents. Cold tissues are, paradoxically, more easily burned than normothermic tissues. Therefore, great care should be taken to ensure that the temperature differential between the patient and the rewarming modality is not more than 10° C, and the maximum temperature for the rewarming medium should be 40° C (104° F). When cold tissues are rewarmed, a metabolic acidosis may develop as acidic metabolic end products re-enter the circulation. Obviously, acidosis cannot be detected in the field, although it may be suspected. In the hospital, appropriate measurements should be made of blood gases and other acid-base parameters, and the acidosis should be treated with sodium bicarbonate.

Lightning [4]

Approximately 300 people die each year in the United States after being struck by lightning. Most are either golfers or mountain climbers. The former usually either take refuge under a tree or are caught in the open after refusing to quit when a lightning storm approached. Mountaineers are usually caught on an exposed ridge where their bodies act as a lightning rod. Approaching lightning danger is often predicted by Saint Elmo's Fire — audible and visible discharge of electricity from hair or metal equipment. Given such warning, the mountaineer or sportsman must quickly minimize his or her exposure. Mountaineers must familiarize themselves with such techniques. Wherever the threat occurs, a group must disperse so one bolt cannot immobilize potential assistance.

Lightning kills immediately by cardiac arrest and injures by burning. It consists of an enormous electrical discharge (millions of volts and up to 20,000 amps) through the atmosphere into the victim's body. If the victim is standing near a tree that is struck, the electrical charge may jump from the tree to the victim. The repulsive charge thus built up may throw the victim many feet.

Immediate therapy consists of external cardiac massage and artificial ventilation. Cardiac rhythm should be determined electrocardiographically as soon as possible and the patient should be defibrillated if indicated. Because many victims are young and without underlying vascular disease, the possibilities of resuscitation are good, and attempts to restore a normal cardiac action should be continued for at least one hour.

Associated injuries include temporary deafness, often with a perforated ear drum, confusion or even coma, arterial spasm of major vessels in the legs where the discharge travelled up the legs, burns and late appearance of cataracts.

The arterial spasm will usually disappear spontaneously, but we have used both heparin and sympathetic blocks on occasion. Seldom is either necessary.

Lightning victims with cardiac arrhythmias should be hospitalized and monitored for several days, as would be routine after an acute myocardial infarction.

Heat Exhaustion and Hyperthermia

Physiology

Dissipation of heat is a constant physiological requirement. Of the 2000 calories used daily, only a fraction is used as work; the rest must be lost to the environment. Exercise in a hot environment obviously places stress on this thermoregulatory mechanism. Factors that increase such stress include high humidity, excessive clothing and obesity. The first two factors minimize heat loss by evaporation (64 calories per ml of water or sweat). Obesity decreases the surface-to-volume ratio and minimizes efficient heat loss. Clinically, hyperthermia is usually associated with dehydration and hyponatremia — the latter by way of sodium loss in sweat. One mechanism of heat adaptation is minimizing salt concentration in both sweat and urine.

Metabolic rate increases approximately 10 per cent for each degree centigrade of temperature. Unreplaced calories may result in depletion of liver glycogen stores and hypoglycemia.

When body temperature exceeds 106° F (47° C), normal physiological mechanisms become inoperative, and irreversible cerebral and renal damage occurs. Violent exercise, especially if associated with hyperthermia, may cause rhabdomyolysis, a release of myoglobin from damaged skeletal muscle that interferes with glomerular and tubular filtration. Rhabdomyolysis combined with dehydration and hyponatremia, acidosis and decreased renal perfusion pressure may result in fatal renal damage.

Epidemiology

Hyperthermia, or heat exhaustion, is most likely to occur in the obese, nonacclimatized, overdressed newcomer exercising excessively in a hot, humid, windless environment. The scenario can obviously be altered in a number of ways. Inexperienced hikers and climbers wear too much clothing and perspire as they exercise. The cognoscenti start walking cold and warm to their task. They also wear several layers of clothing that can be removed seriatim. Garments that button or zip up the front allow finer temperature readjustment for each layer, rather than the "all or nothing" effect of removal of a pullover sweater.

Symptoms

Serious hyperthermia and dehydration usually present with headache, fatigue and confusion. Symptoms of thirst so prominent in the early phases may be unmentioned by the confused or disoriented patient. Body temperature usually exceeds 40° C, and the skin is hot and flushed. The pulse is fast and full until shock intervenes. Urine is scanty and concentrated.

Prevention

Prevention consists of acclimatization to heat before exercise, adequate hydration, prophylactic salt tablet intake and proper clothing to minimize heat loss and exposure. Although the head and neck represent only 9 per cent of the body surface, they count for more than this share of surface blood flow, emphasizing the need for head covering to protect against the sun.

Treatment

Early stages of hyperthermia and heat exhaustion can be treated symptomatically with oral intake of water and salt. However, salt tablets taken on an empty stomach may cause vomiting by reason of local gastric mucosal irritation.

If body temperature is over 40° C homeostatic decompensation becomes a threat, and the patient should immediately be cooled by dousing with cool water, and maximum body surface should be exposed to circulating cool air. In the field all of these criteria usually cannot be met, and compromise obviously is necessary. The threat of hypoglycemia and brain and liver damage can be met by oral feeding of sugar or another carbohydrate.

Severe cases should be treated with immediate intravenous administration of 1000 to 2000 ml of 5 or 10 per cent glucose in saline solution in addition to the procedures just outlined. Urine should be alkalinized with intravenous $NaHCO_3$, if necessary, to minimize renal damage. Brain and renal damage occurs with even short periods of hyperthermia, so vigorous prompt cooling, rehydration and sodium restoration are mandatory.

Drowning

The problem of treating a person drowned in either fresh or salt water is one of clearing the airway and establishing artificial ventilation. As with suffocation beneath an avalanche, the duration of hypoxia must be minimized. Although victims of fresh water drowning absorb water from their alveoli and develop detectable hemolysis, anoxia — not hemolytic anemia — is the prime cause of death.

The physician should be ready to administer artificial respiration by mouth-to-mouth or mechanical means (ambu bag) using 100 per cent oxygen if available. Endotracheal intubation is ideal to allow better delivery of psoitive pressure ventilation, to avoid gastric distention from air forced into the mouth and to improve endotracheal suction. Ideally, some means of suction should be available to remove airway secretions.

A blanket or warm clothes should be available, since most victims of drowning feel very cold after resuscitation and may even be hypothermic.

Snakebite

Any camping group or expedition passing through snake-infested country should be familiar with the types of snakes likely to be encountered.

Space is insufficient to describe in detail all the many types of snake likely to be encountered throughout the world, or even in North America. Certain principles, however, can be stated briefly and should be kept in mind when treating snakebite.[2]

Specific antivenom should always be used whenever toxic symptoms are of sufficient severity to endanger life or limb. Because antivenom is derived from horse serum its use carries a risk of allergic reactions. If symptoms are not severe, judgment must be used in deciding whether the risks of using horse serum are justified. In severe cases of envenomation specific antivenom must be used, and other subsidiary forms of treatment such as tourniquets, incision and suction are inadequate substitutes.

The use of cold has been widely advocated as treatment for rattlesnake bite, but ill-advised and prolonged immersion of bitten limbs in ice water may result in greater tissue loss than from the snakebite alone. Ice packs, immersion in ice water or similar treatment should be used only as a temporary expedient until adequate treatment with antivenom is available. Incision, suction and tourniquets are of limited use and may be either inadequate or dangerous, depending upon the care, knowledge and energy with which they are applied.

Most venoms are absorbed via the lymphatics; lymphatic flow rates are increased by motion and therefore immobilization of the bitten limb reduces the rate of absorption of venom.

In the United States, polyvalent crotalid antivenom (Wyeth) is suitable for treating the bites of rattlesnakes, moccasins and copperheads. It will keep for many years at room temperature.

The dose of antivenom depends upon the severity of symptoms and the response to treatment. About three to five 20 cc vials are necessary for treating an average bite in an adult. Intramuscular administration is best, but the intravenous route may be used in severe emergency with the additional administration of hydrocortisone 100 mg to diminish chances of an allergic reaction. Fasciotomy to relieve tension within a muscular compartment may be limb-saving.

Immediate excision of a bite is an effective treatment if a doctor with appropriate instruments is available. Methyl prednisolone (30 mg per kg IV) may be used in addition to antivenom and is a good alternative treatment in patients allergic to horse serum. The combination of steroids and fasciotomy has been used with good results.

SURGICAL AND MEDICAL EMERGENCIES

Nontraumatic surgical emergencies, such as appendicitis and ruptured peptic ulcer, may occasionally occur in the field. Immediate evacuation to a hospital is mandatory. Nasogastric intubation and the administration of intravenous fluids are within the realm of first aid management, especially if the patient has been vomiting, is dehydrated, and faces a litter trip of several hours' duration.

First Aid Care of Injuries

Shock

The clinical manifestations of shock are the same, even at moderately high altitudes, as at sea level. Resting pulse rates are higher at high altitudes and the response of the pulse rate to work is greater at high altitude than at sea level. Therefore, in a resting man at a high altitude a rapid pulse may not have the same significance as in a patient seen in the Emergency Room. Low blood pressure, very rapid pulse, pallor. clammy sweating and vasoconstriction have, however, their usual significance.

Above 10,000 feet the resting respiratory rate may be increased by two to four breaths per minute. Hyperventilation and dyspnea should, therefore, be regarded as important signs of respiratory difficulty.

Soft Tissue Injuries

Do not attempt to debride or repair soft tissue injuries. Gross contamination by wood, grass or rock fragments can be dealt with immediately, provided that no more than a few minutes are taken for this task. Stop hemorrhage by pressure, or rarely, by the application of a hemostat and ligature. Leave ligature ends long for subsequent identification of the bleeding point. A dry, sterile dressing should be applied and copiously bandaged in position. If hemorrhage is likely during the evacuation, try to arrange the patient in such a way that bandages can be examined for blood with minimum disturbance.

Fractures

LIMBS. All limb fractures should be splinted using available materials, inflatable or cardboard splints. Do not set fractures except to obtain roughly correct alignment of the limb. Check circulation in the distal part of the limb before and after applying the splint. If compromise of the circulation is a possibility (e.g., with a supracondylar fracture of the humerus or injuries around the knee), keep the distal part of the limb available for frequent inspection. Overinflated inflatable splints may diminish circulation, especially if it is already decreased for other reasons. Fractures of the major bones, such as the femur, may be associated with blood loss of 2 to 3 liters into the soft tissues of the limb. Blood loss of this magnitude should be recognized in making calculations for fluid replacement and may be as great a cause for shock as exposure or exhaustion. If a patient has both a skull laceration and a fractured femur, do not forget that more blood may be lost into the thigh than through the more obvious scalp wound.

SKULL. A careful evaluation should be made of:

1. State of consciousness, including a history of lucid periods, deepening or lightening of coma.

2. Obvious neurological defects, such as hemiplegia, speech difficulties, gross sensory and motor loss.

3. Scalp and oropharyngeal lacerations. Do they communicate with intracranial contents? Is the airway compromised now or likely to be compromised by subsequent swelling?

4. Bleeding or escape of CSF from ears or nose.

Lacerations of the scalp may bleed profusely. Bleeding can be controlled by finger pressure around the bleeding area, compressing the scalp against the cranium.

Closed skull fractures require no special management and may not be amenable to superficial clinical diagnosis. Compound fractures should not be explored, but should be dressed copiously. The circular "doughnut" hematoma that sometimes develops after a blow on the head may be mis-taken for a depressed fracture. Resist the temptation to elevate the "depressed" fragment.

Mannitol or urea to diminish cerebral swelling is not indicated. Decadron (dexamethasone sodium phosphate) 4 to 10 mg IM or IV, may be valuable for the reduction of edema in severe cerebral injury.

Unconscious or semiconscious victims should be transported in the semiprone position, with constant attention to maintenance of the airway and with vigilance for the possibility of vomiting. During transportation the head should be kept uphill to reduce intracranial pressure and diminish bleeding from scalp lacerations.

SPINAL COLUMN. Notice areas of local pain and make a careful examination for motor and sensory deficits. Because of the obvious danger of neurological complications, actual or suspected victims of vertebral column injuries must be moved with maximum care. Keep the patient as straight as possible. No advantage is gained by adopting positions of flexion or extension. Movement must be avoided during transportation. A fixation collar is valuable in suspected cervical injuries. If the patient is already paraplegic and a prolonged evacuation of several hours is anticipated, a urethral catheter should be passed and attached to any convenient drainage system, or clamped and released every two hours. An inflatable splint makes a convenient urine container.

Chest Injuries

Simple chest injuries such as fractures of one or two ribs require only support of the patient in the litter and medication for pain.

Pneumothorax is treated by needle aspiration, which can be repeated as necessary. Open sucking wounds of the chest should be plugged by a large, bulky dressing made as airtight as possible.

In all cases of serious thoracic injury, additional oxygen may be not only valuable but life-saving, especially if ventilation is impaired and the accident has occurred at high altitude.

Abdominal Injuries

Little can be done for closed abdominal injuries. Fluids and volume expanders must be given intravenously if the patient is in shock because of a ruptured viscus or blood loss. Give only the minimal doses of narcotics needed to make transportation comfortable.

Penetrating abdominal injuries should be covered by a sterile dressing. Cover bowel that is visible in the wound with Vaseline gauze or a saline-soaked sponge. Intact, healthy, unperforated bowel should be washed with sterile saline and replaced in the abdominal cavity. The wound should be covered securely by a large dressing to prevent repeated evisceration. Bowel left protruding from a small wound can become strangulated by the abdominal wall. Give large doses of antibiotics. If the bowel is gangrenous or has ruptured, do not replace it within the peritoneum. Keep it exteriorized and covered adequately by dressings.

Vascular Injuries

Hemorrhage must be stopped by pressure. Clamping or ligation is advisable only if a large bleeder is clearly seen. Even large vessels, such as the brachial artery, may stop bleeding if completely torn across. It is, however, unsafe to transport someone with the proximal end of a large artery unsecured even if no bleeding is occurring from it. The vessel should be ligated and the ends of the ligature left long for future identification.

Speed is essential in the evacuation of patients with major vascular injuries. Much can be done surgically to restore blood flow, but time is important and the sooner definitive care is given the better are the chances of recovery.

Traveller's Diarrhea

Diarrhea is probably the commonest illness experienced by travellers. It may be annoying, frustrating, uncomfortable, embarrassing, debilitating and, rarely, dangerous. "Turista," an acute, self-limited syndrome, should be distinguished from other forms of diarrhea. The usual cause of turista is the ingestion of strains *E. coli* that are newcomers to the intestinal tract of the victim. Other diarrheas are caused by bacteria (Staphylococcus, *Vibrio cholerae*, Shigella, Salmonella), viruses and parasites (*Giardia lamblia, Entamoeba histolytica*).

Some forms of diarrhea may be prevented by avoidance of fresh foods and vegetables, sterilization of water and personal hygiene (especially in the cook!).

Prophylactic use of drugs does not eliminate the possibility of turista. The most rational therapy in the absence of specific bacteriological proof is replacement by mouth of fluids, electrolytes and sugar lost from the intestine. A simple formula containing 3.5 gm table salt, 2.5 gm baking soda, 1.5 gm potassium chloride, 20 gm sugar and 1000 ml water is effective for replacement therapy.

CARDIAC EMERGENCIES

Angina or frank myocardial infarct will frequently first occur in the middle-aged, overweight, unconditioned, enthusiastic, occasional outdoorsman when in a remote area. The relief of pain and hypoxia is a prime consideration. Oxygen should be administered, especially at altitudes above 5000 feet, and narcotics should be used to relieve pain. It is safer to use small frequent doses of narcotics rather than large doses, which may depress respiration.

Occasional patients develop cardiac arrhythmias in response to exertion and hypoxia. If atrial fibrillation develops with a rapid ventricular response the patient should be given digitalis and evacuated by means other than walking. If the patient has anginal pain and an arrhythmia suspected of being ventricular in origin, Xylocaine (lidocaine), 50 to 100 mg IV, followed by 0.5 to 1.0 mg per minute in an IV drip may be life-saving by averting ventricular tachycardia.

In all patients with cardiac symptoms exertion should be reduced to an essential minimum.

DRUGS AND SUPPLIES

The list of drugs in Table 29–2 is based upon the most likely requirements, both medical and surgical. Table 29–3 lists essential supplies. Because the doctor will almost certainly have to carry his or her own supplies, nothing is gained by too elaborate a kit. All drugs should be clearly labeled with name and dose so that a nonmedical rescue worker could administer them if necessary.

TABLE 29–2   Drugs and Medications

Morphine, Demerol	Digitalis, aminophylline
Chlorpromazine	Isuprel, nitroglycerine
Barbiturate,	Adrenaline,
chloral hydrate	antihistamine
Dilantin, dexameth-	Aspirin, Darvon
asone	50 per cent glucose
Penicillin, tetracycline	pHisoHex
Lactated Ringer's,	Diuretic, furosemide
dextran 70	Water purifying tablets
Lomotil	Furacin gauze
Xylocaine	Valium
Sunburn ointment	

TABLE 29–3   Basic Supplies

Bandages	Band Aids
Sterile dressings	Adhesive tape
Safety pins	Triangular bandages
Hemostats	Scissors
Note pad and pencil	Oral thermometer
Stethoscope	Clinical thermometer
Otoscope	Sphygmomanometer
Ophthalmoscope	Laryngoscope, endotra-
	cheal tubes

Razor blades or sterile scalpel blades
IV fluid administration sets
Disposable syringes, needles
Instant soups, bouillon
Small mountain stove, fuel, pan, matches, flashlight

Drugs

NARCOTICS. Morphine or Demerol. Morphine is the better analgesic but may induce vomiting, undesirable in a patient already nauseated from altitude. Small doses intravenously at frequent intervals are preferable to larger doses intramuscularly or subcutaneously, especially in cold, shocked patients. The recommended dose of morphine sulfate is 5 mg IV or 10 mg IM, and for Demerol, 80 to 100 mg IM. The doses for children are morphine sulfate 1 mg per 10 kg and Demerol 1 mg per kg, both IM.

ANTIBIOTICS. Wide-spectrum antibiotics capable of being given intramuscularly. Alternatives should be carried, because of frequent allergies to penicillin.

TRANQUILIZERS AND ANTIEMETICS. Nausea and vomiting are common at high altitudes and after injury. Chlorpromazine (25 to 50 mg IM) is effective in reducing nausea and as a general tranquilizer. Given intravenously, chlorpromazine induces vasodilatation and hypotension and should not be given to patients in shock unless adequate intravenous fluid replacement is available.

CARDIAC DRUGS. Digoxin acts within 30 to 45 minutes after intravenous administration. The total digitalizing dose for a previously undigitalized patient is 0.75 mg to 1.25 mg IV. An initial dose of 0.5 mg IV can safely be given to adults and repeated within four hours.

Diuretics may be of value in a patient with pulmonary edema, especially if several hours are likely to elapse before evacuation to a lower altitude. Furosemide (80 mg IV) has been shown to be of value.

Nitroglycerine is indicated for ischemic myocardial pain.

Xylocaine (lidocaine) may occasionally be of great value in treating ventricular arrhythmias (see Cardiac Emergencies).

ANTICONVULSANTS. Convulsions may occur after head injuries. The development of convulsions during a difficult evacuation might obviously be hazardous to patient and rescuer alike. Dilantin is the most effective anticonvulsant and does not depress respiration. The dose is 150 mg to 250 mg IV at a rate not greater than 50 mg per minute.

FLUIDS. Fluids are heavy to carry, but may be life-saving. The most useful fluid for intravenous use is lactated Ringer's solution. Its use presents neither problems of sensitivity nor bleeding complications. It is a safe temporary blood volume expander and simultaneously restores extravascular deficits in dehydrated patients.

Dextran 70 is a better plasma volume expander than Ringer's solution, but as an "all purpose" fluid, the latter is preferable. None of the physiological intravenous solutions is of high enough concentration to inhibit freezing at temperatures likely to be encountered during a winter rescue mission. If the fluid freezes, it can be thawed by putting it inside the clothing of a rescuer.

Basic Supplies

Bandages, dressings, tape, and other supplies that are considered necessary are listed in Table 29–3.

Numbers, quantities and doses are not given because these may vary with individual requirements. The list should serve as a checklist for anyone preparing a first aid supply kit.

MAJOR EXPEDITIONS

Medical logistic support for a major expedition requires the thought, planning and presence of an˙ expert climber and physician. Surprisingly little is written on the subject. Lessons learned in support of such expeditions involving dozens of people, isolated for many weeks, can be applied to planning for less ambitious outings. Medical needs of an expedition are analogous to those of astronauts embarking on space travel, both as to scope and weight restriction.

Individual packets should be bound in rugged plastic bags, small enough to fit into each person's pack.

TABLE 29–4 Items for Physician-Climber's Pack on Major Mountain Expedition

pHisoHex in small container
Dexedrine, 12 pills
Blistex, 1 tube
Nevafil ointment, 1 tube
Band Aids, 25
Dial soap, 1 bar
Moleskin for blisters, 12 × 12
Adhesive tape, one 2" roll
Darvon compound (65 mg), 15
Zinc oxide, 1 tube
Lasix (furosemide), 5 amps, 5 cc syringe and 20g needle
4 × 4 bandage, 2 packages of 2
Lomotil, 30
Neosporin ophthalmic ointment, 1 tube
Tetracaine ointment, 1 tube
Gelusil, 10 tablets
Vibramycin, 7 tablets
Pen V-K, 250 mg #30
Ornade, #20
Humatin (puromomycin), 16 tablets
Barbiturate (Seconal, gr 1½), 12
Chloral hydrate (500 mg), 12 (or other sleeping pill as per individual choice)

TABLE 29–5   Surgical Packs for a Major Expedition

Small Instruments × 3
Size 8 gloves, 3 pairs
Eye drape, 1
Small curved clamp, 2
Suture pack, 4/0 silk, 2
Suture pack, 2/0 chromic gut, 2
4/0 silk on curved cutting needle, 6
Suture scissors, 1
Adson pickups, 1
Pickups with teeth, 1
Knife handle, disposable, 3
Bard-Parker #15 blades, 3
Bard-Parker #11 blades, 3
Needle holder, 1

Chest Tube Tray
5 cc syringe, 1
Size 8 gloves, 2 pairs
Trocar, 1
Curved Kelly, 2
Small eye drape, 1
Chest tube with Heimlich valve
Suture scissors, 1
Needle holder, 1
4/0 silk on cutting needle, 1
Vaseline gauze, 2 strips
4 × 4 gauze, 4 packages
50 cc plastic syringe with threeway stopcock
Disposable scalpel handle with blades

Tracheostomy Set
Eye drape, 1
#34 Portex cuffed tube, 1
#36 Portex cuffed tube, 1
Bard-Parker #15 blade with appropriate handle,
  1
Curved mosquito clamp, 2
Curved Kelly clamp, 1
Trachea hook, 1 (or towel clip)
Army-Navy retractor, 2
Trachea spreader, 1
Allis forceps, 1
4/0 silk on a curved cutting needle, 2
4/0 silk suture pack, 1
#14 red French catheter, 1
4 × 4 flats, 8
5 cc syringe with #20 1½ inch needle, 1

Neurosurgical Pack
Plastic disposable razor with blade, 1
#10 Bard-Parker blade with appropriate handle, 1
Eye drape
Hemostats, small and curved, 2
Straights, 3/0 silk suture pack, 1
4/0 silk on a curved Kelly needle, 2
3/0 chromic on tapered needle
Duroclips, 2
Silver nitrate cautery sticks, 4
Trephine (not drill), hard type, 1

Emergency Laparotomy Set
Disposable paper drape set, 1
Vidrape, 1
Abdominal lap pads, 12
Brush, detergent-impregnated scrubbing, 1

Sponges, 4 × 4, 24
Knife handle, Bard-Parker #3, 2
Knife blades, Bard-Parker #10, 2
Knife blades, Bard-Parker #11, 2
Knife blades, Bard-Parker #15, 2
Clamps, towel clips, 4
Clamps, hemostat, Crile, 6
Clamps, curved Kelly, 4
Clamps, Mayo-Robson, GI, 10 inch, 2
Clamps, Babcock, 2
Needle holders, Mayo Hegar, 8 inches, 1
Needle holders, Crile-Wood, light, 6 inches, 1
Retractors, Deaver, medium, 2
Retractors, Harrington, 1
Pickup forceps, without teeth, medium, 1
Pickup forceps, without teeth, long, 1
Pickup forceps, two teeth, Adson, 1
Scissors, suture, 1
Scissors, tissue, 1
Scissors, Metzenbaum, 1
Sutures, silk, 3/0, precut, 6
Sutures, silk, 4/0, tapered needle, 3
Sutures, silk, 5/0, tapered needle, 3
Sutures, silk, 1/0, tapered needle, 3
Sutures, chromic gut, 2/0, dispensing reel, 3
Sutures, chromic gut, 3/0, dispensing reel, 3
Sutures, chromic gut, 2/0, tapered needle, 4
Needles, assorted pack, 1

Anesthesia Set
Syringes, 2 cc, 2
Syringes, 5 cc, 2
Syringes, 10 cc, 2
Spinal needles, 22 g, 2
Needles, 25 g, 2
10% dextrose, 30 cc
Pontocaine 1%
Xylocaine 1%
Procaine 1%
Epinephrine, 1:1000
Towels, 18″ × 27″, −4

Urinary Catheterization Tray
Foley catheters, three sizes, 5 cc bag
Lubricant
Towels, 18″ × 27″, 2
Syringe, 5 cc, 1
Clamp, catheter, 1

General Supplies
Syringes, disposable
Needles, re-usable, all metal
Towels, drapes
Gloves, sterile, 7½ and 8
Solution for skin preparation
Solution for cold sterilization of instruments
Pan for boiling instruments
Presterilized commercially available packed kits
  for urinary catheterization, spinal tap, etc.
  May be preferable to above listed items, but
  these cannot be resterilized.
Dental instruments — syringes, local anesthetic
  and extraction forceps, temporary fillings

Packaging should be color-coded, and each item should be available without destroying the packaging of the remaining items. Brief indications and dosage should be included with each drug. Resupply should be from the expedition's major medical source. All oral antibiotics can be kept in one bottle with color-coded directions on the outside.

The items suggested for the climber's pack are listed in Table 29–4. Much of this equipment is dispensed en route to porters and local population.

Table 29–5 lists the presterilized and double-packed surgical equipment packs necessary for a major expedition.

REFERENCES

1. Hackett, P. H., Rennie, D., Levine, H. D.: The incidence, importance and prophylaxis of acute mountain sickness. Lancet, 2:1149–57, 1976.
2. Paton, B. C.: Treatment of snake-bite. *In* Kyle, J. (ed.): Pye's Surgical Handicraft, Bristol, John Wright and Sons, 1969.
3. Snow Avalanches. Handbook of Forecasting and Control Measures. U.S. Department of Agriculture Handbook No. 194. Washington D.C., U. S. Government Printing Office 1968.
4. Taussig, H. B.: "Death" from lightning and the possibility of living again. Amer. Sci. 57:306–316, 1969.
5. Washburn, B.: Frostbite: What it is — How to prevent it — Emergency treatment. N. Eng. J. Med., 266:974–989, 1962.
6. Wilkerson J. A. (ed.): Medicine for Mountaineering. Seattle, Washington, The Mountaineers, 1967.

Index

Note: Page numbers in *italics* refer to illustrations; those followed by (t) refer to tables.